AF322992

IAES
Textbook of
Endocrine Surgery

IAES
Textbook of
Endocrine Surgery

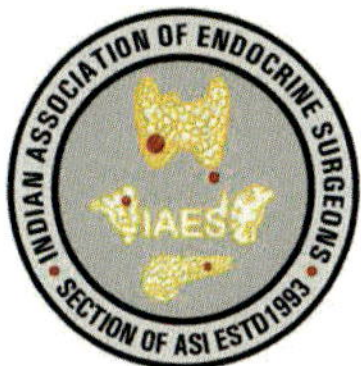

Indian Association of Endocrine Surgeons

Editor-in-Chief
Amit Agarwal
MS FRCS (Eng) FICS FAMS FCSSL (Sri Lanka)
Professor and Head
Department of Endocrine Surgery
Sanjay Gandhi Postgraduate Institute of Medical Sciences
Lucknow, Uttar Pradesh, India

Editors

Roma Pradhan
MS MCh (Endocrine Surgery)
Breast and Endocrine Surgeon
Associate Professor and Head
Department of Endocrine Surgery
Dr Ram Manohar Lohia Institute of Medical Sciences
Lucknow, Uttar Pradesh, India

Dhalapathy Sadacharan MCh
Professor and Head
Department of Endocrine Surgery
King George's Medical University
Lucknow, Uttar Pradesh, India

Anand Kumar Mishra
MS PDCC MCh FACS FICS
Professor and Head
Department of Endocrine Surgery
King George's Medical University
Lucknow, Uttar Pradesh, India

Deepak Abraham MS PhD
Professor
Department of Endocrine Surgery
Christian Medical College
Vellore, Tamil Nadu, India

Forewords
Gerard M Doherty
Sivapatham Vittal

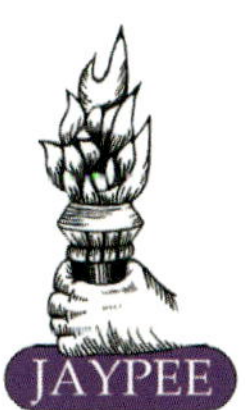

JAYPEE BROTHERS MEDICAL PUBLISHERS
The Health Sciences Publisher
New Delhi | London

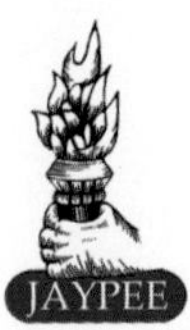 **Jaypee Brothers Medical Publishers (P) Ltd**

Headquarters

Jaypee Brothers Medical Publishers (P) Ltd
EMCA House, 23/23-B
Ansari Road, Daryaganj
New Delhi 110 002, India
Landline: +91-11-23272143, +91-11-23272703
+91-11-23282021, +91-11-23245672
Email: jaypee@jaypeebrothers.com

Corporate Office

Jaypee Brothers Medical Publishers (P) Ltd
4838/24, Ansari Road, Daryaganj
New Delhi 110 002, India
Phone: +91-11-43574357
Fax: +91-11-43574314
Email: jaypee@jaypeebrothers.com

Overseas Office

JP Medical Ltd
83 Victoria Street, London
SW1H 0HW (UK)
Phone: +44 20 3170 8910
Fax: +44 (0)20 3008 6180
Email: info@jpmedpub.com

Website: www.jaypeebrothers.com
Website: www.jaypeedigital.com

© 2023, Jaypee Brothers Medical Publishers

The views and opinions expressed in this book are solely those of the original contributor(s)/author(s) and do not necessarily represent those of editor(s) or publisher of the book.

All rights reserved. No part of this publication may be reproduced, stored or transmitted in any form or by any means, electronic, mechanical, photocopying, recording or otherwise, without the prior permission in writing of the publishers.

All brand names and product names used in this book are trade names, service marks, trademarks or registered trademarks of their respective owners. The publisher is not associated with any product or vendor mentioned in this book.

Medical knowledge and practice change constantly. This book is designed to provide accurate, authoritative information about the subject matter in question. However, readers are advised to check the most current information available on procedures included and check information from the manufacturer of each product to be administered, to verify the recommended dose, formula, method and duration of administration, adverse effects and contraindications. It is the responsibility of the practitioner to take all appropriate safety precautions. Neither the publisher nor the author(s)/editor(s) assume any liability for any injury and/or damage to persons or property arising from or related to use of material in this book.

This book is sold on the understanding that the publisher is not engaged in providing professional medical services. If such advice or services are required, the services of a competent medical professional should be sought.

Every effort has been made where necessary to contact holders of copyright to obtain permission to reproduce copyright material. If any have been inadvertently overlooked, the publisher will be pleased to make the necessary arrangements at the first opportunity. The **CD/DVD-ROM** (if any) provided in the sealed envelope with this book is complimentary and free of cost. **Not meant for sale**.

Inquiries for bulk sales may be solicited at: jaypee@jaypeebrothers.com

IAES Textbook of Endocrine Surgery

First Edition: **2023**

ISBN: 978-93-90595-05-1

Printed at Nutech Print Services - India

Dedications

I dedicate this book to all students of Endocrine Surgery!!
- *Those who have learnt from me and are now themselves accomplished Endocrine Surgeons;*
- *Those who are presently under training and are eager to practice Endocrine Surgery; and*
- *Those future trainees who desire to become Endocrine Surgeons*

–Amit Agarwal

Dedicated to my teachers and students of Endocrine Surgery

–Roma Pradhan

Dedicated to my late dad Thiru P Sadacharan
and,
To my respected teachers, dear students and esteemed patients

–Dhalapathy Sadacharan

Dedicated to my late mother Vimala Mishra, Papa Shri SP Mishra,
my wife Anjana
and
To all my patients

–Anand Kumar Mishra

I dedicate this book to all the students of Endocrine Surgery who have passed through the portals of the institution and have spurred me to make learning a joyful experience through problem-based learning.

–Deepak Abraham

Aarathi Vijayashanker MS DNB MRCS
Senior Clinical Fellow
Department of Liver Transplantation
Surgery
King's College Hospital and NHS
Foundation Trust
London, UK

Abhinav Arun Sonkar
MS FACS FUICC FRCS
Professor and Head
Department of Surgery
King George's Medical University
Lucknow, Uttar Pradesh, India

Akshay Anand MS (General Surgery)
Associate Professor
Department of General Surgery
King George's Medical University
Lucknow, Uttar Pradesh, India

Alok Thakar MS FRCSEd
Professor and Head
Otolaryngology and Head-Neck Surgery
All India Institute of Medical Sciences
New Delhi, India

Amit Agarwal MS FICS FCSL (Sri Lanka)
FACS FRCS (Eng)
Professor and Head
Department of Endocrine Surgery
Sanjay Gandhi Postgraduate Institute
of Medical Sciences
Lucknow, Uttar Pradesh, India

Anand Kumar Mishra
MS PDCC MCh FACS FICS
Professor and Head
Department of Endocrine Surgery
King George's Medical University
Lucknow, Uttar Pradesh, India

Anil D'Cruz MS DNB FRCS
Director–Oncology
Department of Surgery
Apollo Hospital
Mumbai, Maharashtra, India

Anish JC MCh (Endocrine Surgery)
Professor
Department of Endocrine Surgery
Christian Medical College
Vellore, Tamil Nadu, India

Anukriti Sood MS MCh
(Breast and Endocrine Surgery)
Consultant
CK Birla Hospital
Jaipur, Rajasthan, India

Aravindan Nair MS
Former Professor and Head
Department of Endocrine Surgery
Christian Medical College
Vellore, Tamil Nadu, India

Archana Gupta MD (Radiology)
Professor
Department of Radiodiagnosis
Sanjay Gandhi Postgraduate Institute
of Medical Sciences
Lucknow, Uttar Pradesh, India

Arjun Raja A MCh
Resident
Department of Endocrine Surgery
Sanjay Gandhi Postgraduate Institute
of Medical Sciences
Lucknow, Uttar Pradesh, India

Aromal Chekavar S MBBS MS MCh
Consultant Endocrine and Breast Surgeon
Travancore Medicity Medical College
Kollam, Kerala, India

Chakravarthy Marx Sadacharan PhD
Clinical Professor (Anatomy)
Department of Biological Sciences
Tilman J Fertitta Family College of Medicine
University of Houston
Houston, Texas, USA

Chanchal Rana MD
Associate Professor
Department of Pathology
King George's Medical University
Lucknow, Uttar Pradesh, India

Chitresh Kumar
MS (General Surgery) MCh (Endocrine Surgery)
Associate Professor
Department of Surgical Oncology
All India Institute of Medical Sciences
Bilaspur, Himachal Pradesh, India

CS Bal MD DNB DSc
Professor and Head
Department of Nuclear Medicine
All India Institute of Medical Sciences
New Delhi, India

Deepak Malviya MD (Anesthesia) FICA
Professor and Head
Department of Anesthesiology
and Critical Care Medicine
Dr Ram Manohar Lohia Institute
of Medical Sciences
Lucknow, Uttar Pradesh, India

Deepak Abraham MS PhD
Professor
Department of Endocrine Surgery
Christian Medical College
Vellore, Tamil Nadu, India

Deepak Paul MS
Assistant Professor
Department of General Surgery
Sree Gokulam Medical College
and Research Foundation
Trivandrum, Kerala, India

Deependra Narayan Singh
MS MCh (Endocrine surgery) FICS FAES
Consultant Endocrine and Breast Surgeon
Department of Diabetes and
Endocrine Science
CK Birla Hospital
Jaipur, Rajasthan, India

Dhalapathy Sadacharan MCh
Professor and Head
Department of Endocrine Surgery
King George's Medical University
Lucknow, Uttar Pradesh, India

Dileep Ramesh Hoysal MCh
Resident
Department of Endocrine Surgery
Sanjay Gandhi Postgraduate Institute
of Medical Sciences
Lucknow, Uttar Pradesh, India

Edwina C Moore
BMedSc MBBS (Hons) FRACS
Surgeon
Department of Endocrine Surgery
Peninsula Private Hospital
Melbourne, VIC, Australia

Elanthenral Sigamani MD (Pathology)
Associate Professor
Department of Pathology
Christian Medical College and Hospital
Vellore, Tamil Nadu, India

Farheen Khan MCh
Resident
Department of Endocrine Surgery
Sanjay Gandhi Postgraduate Institute
of Medical Sciences
Lucknow, Uttar Pradesh, India

Gouri Pantvaidya MS DNB MRCS
Professor and Surgeon
Department of Surgery
Tata Memorial Centre
Mumbai, Maharashtra, India

Gyan Chand MS FICS FMAS
Professor
Department of Breast and Endocrine
Surgery
Sanjay Gandhi Postgraduate Institute
of Medical Sciences
Lucknow, Uttar Pradesh, India

Han Boon Oh MBBS FRCS (Edin)
Consultant
Department of Endocrine Surgery
National University Health System
Singapore

Harsha Yadav CT MBBS MS (ENT)
Senior Resident
Otolaryngology and Head-Neck Surgery
All India Institute of Medical Sciences
New Delhi, India

Himagirish K Rao MS MCh
Associate Professor
Department of Surgery
St John's Medical College and Hospital
Bengaluru, Karnataka, India

Jiunn Wong MBBS MRCP MMed
Consultant
Department of Renal Medicine
Singapore General Hospital
Singapore

Jnaneshwari Jayaram
MS (General Surgery) MCh (Breast Endocrine
and General Surgery)
Assistant Professor
Department of Surgical Oncology
Father Muller Medical College
Mangaluru, Karnataka, India

Julie A Miller BA MD FRACS
Surgeon
Department of Endocrine Surgery
The Royal Melbourne Hospital
Melbourne, VIC, Australia

Kailash C Mohapatra
MS (General Surgery)
Professor
Department of Surgery
Link Polyclinic and Hospital
Cuttack, Odisha, India

Kamaludeen MS
Former Head
Department of Endocrine Surgery
Madras Medical College
Professor of Surgery
Madurai Medical College
Madurai, Tamil Nadu, India

Karthik Rao MS (ENT)
Senior Clinical Fellow
Department of Surgery
Tata Memorial Centre
Mumbai, Maharashtra, India

Kul Ranjan Singh
MS MCh FACS FICS
Associate Professor
Department of Endocrine Surgery
King George's Medical University
Lucknow, Uttar Pradesh, India

Kushagra Gaurav
MS (General Surgery) MCh (Endocrine Surgery)
Assistant Professor
Department of General Surgery
King George's Medical University
Lucknow, Uttar Pradesh, India

Loreno E Enny
MS (General Surgery) MCh (Endocrine Surgery)
Assistant Professor
Department of Endocrine Surgery
King George's Medical University
Lucknow, Uttar Pradesh, India

Madan Kapre FRCS DLO
Director
Department of ENT and Head
and Neck Surgery
Neeti Clinics
Nagpur, Maharashtra, India

Mallika Dhanda
MS (General Surgery) MCh (Endocrine Surgery)
Assistant Professor
Department of Endocrine Surgery
Dr Ram Manohar Lohia Institute
of Medical Sciences
Lucknow, Uttar Pradesh, India

Manish Gutch MD DM (Endocrinology)
Associate Professor
Department of Endocrinology
Dr Ram Manohar Lohia Institute
of Medical Sciences
Lucknow, Uttar Pradesh, India

Manju Chandran MD FACP FACE FAMS
Senior Consultant and Director
Osteoporosis and Bone Metabolism Unit
Department of Endocrinology
Singapore General Hospital
Singapore

Manohar H Martis
MS (General Surgery)
Fellowship in Endocrine Surgery
Assistant Professor
Department of General Surgery
Father Muller Medical College
Mangaluru, Karnataka, India

Maruthu Pandian MS
Former Head of Surgery and Dean
Madurai Medical College
Madurai, Tamil Nadu, India
Governing Council Member
National ASI and TN Medical Council

MJ Paul MS DNB FRCS
Professor and Head
Department of Endocrine Surgery
Christian Medical College and Hospital
Vellore, Tamil Nadu, India

Mohamed Salmon M MS
Assistant Surgeon
Department of General Surgery
Government Hospital
Sivakasi, Tamil Nadu, India

Mohanty Arun K MS (Surgery)
Associate Professor
Department of Endocrine Surgery
Srirama Chandra Bhanja Medical College
and Hospital
Cuttack, Odisha, India

Mohanty Biswa N MS (Surgery)
Chief Consultant and
Endocrine Surgeon
Department of Surgery
Link Polyclinic and Hospital
Cuttack, Odisha, India

Munita Menon Bal
MD (Pathology) DNB (Pathology)
Professor
Department of Pathology
Tata Memorial Centre
Mumbai, Maharashtra, India

Muthukumar S
MS MCh (Endocrine Surgery)
Assistant Professor
Department of Endocrine Surgery
Madurai Medical College
Madurai, Tamil Nadu, India

Nada Santrac MD
General Surgeon
Clinical Assistant in Surgery, ESSO Fellow
Surgical Oncology Clinic
Institute for Oncology and Radiology
of Serbia
Pasterova, Belgrade, Serbia

Narendra Krishnani MD DM
Assistant Professor
Department of Histopathology
Postgraduate Institute of Medical
Education and Research
Chandigarh, India

Natarajan Dorairajan
MS FRCS FICS FACS FICA
Professor Emeritus
The Tamil Nadu Dr MGR Medical
University
Chennai, Tamil Nadu, India

Neeti Kapre MS DNB (ENT) Fellowship Head
and Neck Oncology
Surgeon
Neeti Clinics
Nagpur, Maharashtra, India

Nelson George PhD
Post-Doctoral Visiting Fellow
Section of Cellular Differentiation
NICHD, NIH
Bethesda, Maryland, USA

Niraj Kumari MD DNB MNAMS
Professor
Department of Pathology and
Lab Medicine
All India Institute of Medical Sciences
Raebareli, Uttar Pradesh, India

Pankaj Sharma MBBS DMRD DNB PDCC
EBIR Fellowship (VIR)
Associate Professor
Department of Radiodiagnosis
All India Institute of Medical Sciences
Rishikesh, Uttarakhand, India

Pooja Ramakant
MS DNB MCh MNAMS FACS
Professor Jr Grade
Department of Endocrine Surgery
King George's Medical University
Lucknow, Uttar Pradesh, India

Poongkodi K MS MCh FAES
Senior Civil Surgeon and Assistant
Professor
Department of Endocrine Surgery
Government Mohan Kumaramangalam
Medical College
Chennai, Tamil Nadu, India

Pradeep PV MS DNB MRCS (Edin) FRCS
(Glasg) FACS MCh (Endocrine Surgery)
Senior Consultant
Department of Endocrine Surgery
Baby Memorial Hospital
Kozhikode, Kerala, India

Prateek Mehrotra DNB MCH
Consultant Endocrine Surgeon
Sahara Hospital
Lucknow, Uttar Pradesh, India

Punita Lal MD DNB
Professor
Department of Radiotherapy
Sanjay Gandhi Postgraduate Institute
of Medical Sciences
Lucknow, Uttar Pradesh, India

R Chandra Shekar Reddy
MBBS MS (ENT)
Senior Resident
Otolaryngology and Head-Neck Surgery
All India Institute of Medical Sciences
New Delhi, India

R Dayananda Babu MS MNAMS FRCS
Professor Emeritus
Department of General Surgery
Sree Gokulam Medical College and
Research Foundation
Trivandrum, Kerala, India

(Late) Radan Dzodic MD
General Surgeon–Oncologist
Professor of Surgery
Medical School
University of Belgrade
Dr Subotica 8, Belgrade, Serbia

Rajeev Parameswaran
BSc MBBS FRCSI MPhil FRCS UK FAMS
Senior Consultant and Head
Department of Endocrine Surgery
National University Health System
Singapore

Ranil Fernando
MS FRCS FCPS FAIS FCS PhD
Senior Professor of Surgery
University of Kelaniya, Colombo
Dean Faculty of Medicine
University of Moratuwa, Moratuwa
Universities of Kelaniya and Moratuwa
Sri Lanka

Ravikumar MS MCh (Endocrine Surgery)
Consultant Endocrine Surgeon
Department of Endocrine Surgery
Royal Care Hospital
Coimbatore, Tamil Nadu, India

Rekha Singh MD DM
Additional Professor and Head
Department of Endocrinology
and Metabolism
All India Institute of Medical Sciences
Bhopal, Madhya Pradesh, India

Roma Pradhan
MS MCh (Endocrine Surgery)
Breast and Endocrine Surgeon
Associate Professor and Head
Department of Endocrine Surgery
Dr Ram Manohar Lohia Institute
of Medical Sciences
Lucknow, Uttar Pradesh, India

S Babu MS
Former Head
Department of Surgery
Government Sivagangai Medical College
and Hospital
Sivagangai, Tamil Nadu, India

Sabaretnam M MS MCh
Additional Professor
Department of Endocrine Surgery
Sanjay Gandhi Institute of Postgraduate
in Medical Sciences
Lucknow, Uttar Pradesh, India

Sai Krishna Vittal
MS DNB FRCS FICS FAIS FAES FCSSL
Consultant
Department of Endocrine Surgery
Sree Sai Krishna Hospital, Vittal's Institute
of Endocrine Surgery and Apollo Hospitals
Chennai, Tamil Nadu, India

Sai Vishnupriya Vittal
MRCS DNB MCh (Endo) FRCS (Glasg)
FICS FAIS FAES
Assistant Professor
Department of Endocrine Surgery
Madras Medical College
Consultant
Sree Sai Krishna Hospital, Vittal's Institute
of Endocrine Surgery and Apollo Hospitals
Chennai, Tamil Nadu, India

Santosh Menon
MD (Pathology) DNB (Pathology)
Professor
Department of Pathology
Tata Memorial Centre
Mumbai, Maharashtra, India

Sapana Bothra Jain MBBS MS MCh
Consultant Endocrine and Breast Surgeon
Mahatma Gandhi Medical College
and Hospital
Jaipur, Rajasthan, India

Sarah Idrees MCh
Resident
Department of Endocrine Surgery
Sanjay Gandhi Postgraduate Institute
of Medical Sciences
Lucknow, Uttar Pradesh, India

Sasi Mouli MCh 3rd year
Senior Resident
Department of Endocrine Surgery
King George's Medical University
Lucknow, Uttar Pradesh, India

Saurabh Arora MD (Nucl Med)
DM (Therapeutic Nucl Med)
Senior Resident
Department of Nuclear Medicine
All India Institute of Medical Sciences
New Delhi, India

Sendhil Rajan MS MCH
Specialty Registrar
Department of General and
Endocrine Surgery
Aberdeen Royal Infirmary
Scotland, UK

Shagun Misra MD DNB
Additional Professor
Department of Radiotherapy
Sanjay Gandhi Postgraduate Institute
of Medical Sciences
Lucknow, Uttar Pradesh, India

Shaleen Kumar MD DNB
Additional Professor
Department of Radiotherapy
Sanjay Gandhi Postgraduate Institute
of Medical Sciences
Lucknow, Uttar Pradesh, India

Shilpi Misra MD (Anesthesia)
Associate Professor
Department of Anesthesiology
and Critical Care Medicine
Dr Ram Manohar Lohia Institute
of Medical Sciences
Lucknow, Uttar Pradesh, India

Shreyamsa M MCh 3rd year
Senior Resident
Department of Endocrine Surgery
King George's Medical University
Lucknow, Uttar Pradesh, India

Siddhartha Chakravarthy N MS MCh
Senior Consultant
Department of Endocrine Surgery
Apollo Hospitals
Hyderabad, Telangana, India

Sidharth Pant MD
Senior Resident
Department of Radiotherapy
Sanjay Gandhi Postgraduate Institute
of Medical Sciences
Lucknow, Uttar Pradesh, India

Sivapatham Vittal
MS FRCS FICS FAIS FAES FIMSA FTASc DSc (Hon)
Emeritus Professor and Senior Consultant
Department of Endocrine Surgery
Sree Sai Krishna Hospital, Vittal's Institute
of Endocrine Surgery and Apollo
Hospitals
Chennai, Tamil Nadu, India

Sudhi Agarwal MS MCh FMAS DMAS
Consultant and Head
Department of Breast and Endocrine
Surgery
Nutema Hospital
Meerut, Uttar Pradesh, India

Suneel Mattoo MS MCh
Consultant Endocrine and Breast Surgeon
JK Medicity
Jammu, Jammu & Kashmir, India

Supriya Sen MCh (Endocrine Surgery)
MS (Surgery) MRCS
Assistant Professor
Department of Endocrine Surgery
Christian Medical College
Vellore, Tamil Nadu, India

Surabhi Garg MS MCh (Endocrine Surgery)
Assistant Professor
Department of Endocrine Surgery
King George's Medical University
Lucknow, Uttar Pradesh, India

Surendra Kumar Agarwal
MS MCh FRCS
Professor
Department of Cardiothoracic
and Vascular Surgery
Sanjay Gandhi Postgraduate Institute
of Medical Sciences
Lucknow, Uttar Pradesh, India

Sushil Gupta MD DM DNB
Professor
Department of Endocrinology
Sanjay Gandhi Postgraduate Institute
of Medical Sciences
Lucknow, Uttar Pradesh, India

Sushobhan Pradhan
MCh (Endocrine Surgery)
Senior Resident
Department of Endocrine Surgery
Sanjay Gandhi Postgraduate Institute
of Medical Sciences
Lucknow, Uttar Pradesh, India

Suvradeep Mitra MD DM
Assistant Professor
Department of Histopathology
Postgraduate Institute of Medical
Education and Research
Chandigarh, India

Uma Devi MS MCh
Assistant Professor
Department of Endocrine Surgery
Madras Medical College
Chennai, Tamil Nadu, India

V Sucharitha MS FRCS(Ed) FICS FAIS FAES
Consultant
Department of Endocrine Surgery
Sree Sai Krishna Hospital and Vittal's
Institute of Endocrine Surgery
Chennai, Tamil Nadu, India

Yuvraj Devgan MCh
Resident
Department of Endocrine Surgery
Sanjay Gandhi Postgraduate Institute
of Medical Sciences
Lucknow, Uttar Pradesh, India

Foreword

Endocrine surgery includes the care of patients with diseases of the thyroid, parathyroid, adrenal and pancreas glands, as well as the neuroendocrine system distributed throughout the neck, chest and abdomen. There are special considerations that require management of both the functional aspects, and the oncologic aspects of the tumors that arise in these organs. In addition, there are several familial syndromes, some with known genetic origins that demand longitudinal management across the lifetime of the patient. The complexity of this field demands dedicated practitioners with specialized knowledge.

Professor (Dr) Amit Agarwal has been an international thought leader in endocrine surgery throughout his career. From my perspective as an endocrine surgeon, and Past President of both the International Association of Endocrine Surgeons, and the American Association of Endocrine Surgeons, he has been extraordinarily effective not only by advancing the field of endocrine surgery

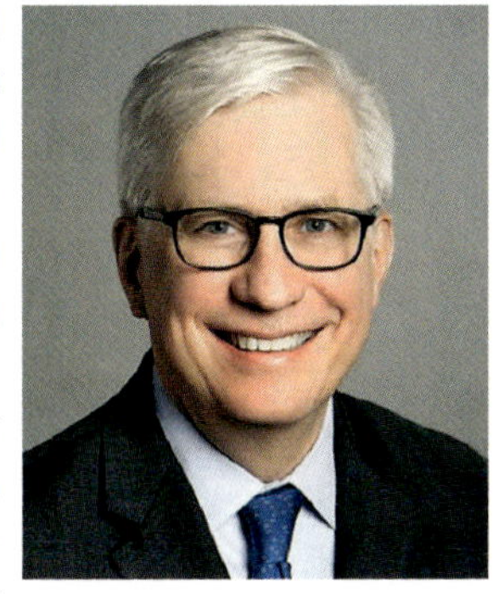

including our global understanding of the expressions of these diseases in the Indian subcontinent, but also by bringing this information to a wide audience. He has trained myriad surgeons and other specialists, delivered lectures, founded journals and edited books.

This latest textbook from Dr Amit Agarwal, along with several other members of the Indian Association of Endocrine Surgeons (IAES), adds to his record of stellar contributions. The coverage of the text is broad, and the execution of the individual chapters is expert. I know that this will be a valuable reference for both the initiate into endocrine surgery who needs broad coverage and clear explanations, as well as the expert surgeon seeking the most up-to-date information. I deeply appreciate the craftsmanship that is expressed here, and express my admiration for Dr Amit Agarwal, his co-editors and all of the authors. This book is a great addition to our libraries.

Gerard M Doherty MD
Moseley Professor of Surgery
Harvard Medical School
Surgeon-in-Chief and Crowley Family
Distinguished Chair of Surgery
Brigham and Women's Hospital
Surgeon-in-Chief
Dana-Farber Cancer Institute
Boston, Massachusetts, USA

Foreword

I deem it a privilege and honor to write a foreword for this book authored by Dr Amit Agarwal and his editorial colleagues which include Dr Deepak Abraham, Dr Anand Kumar Mishra, Dr Dhalapathy Sadacharan and Dr Roma Pradhan. I am delighted that Dr Amit Agarwal has taken the initiative to conceive a *Textbook of Endocrine Surgery* on behalf of Indian Association of Endocrine Surgeons (IAES), first of its kind by any Endocrine Surgical Association in the world.

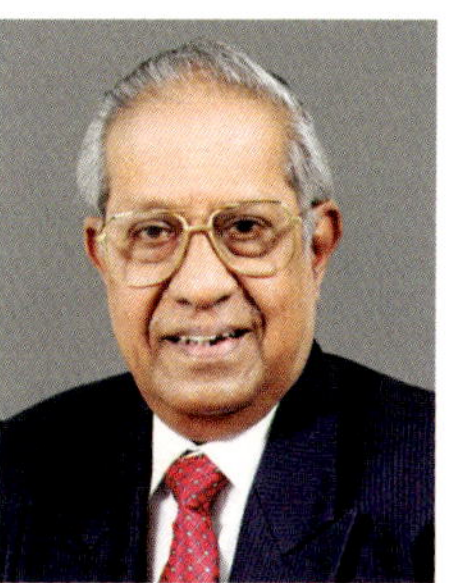

The chapters in this textbook cover the length and breadth of Endocrine Surgery. The editors have taken upon themselves to choose all the authors from the membership of Indian Association of Endocrine Surgeons, an outstanding feat indeed. This would reflect the disease pattern, presentation and management of endocrine surgical disorders especially with regard to India. This book would be of immense help to all endocrine surgeons, general surgeons with interest in endocrine surgery as well as trainees in endocrine surgery.

To go back memory lane, the Indian Association of Endocrine Surgeons was formed in 1993 as a section of Association of Surgeons of India with the aim to disseminate the principles and practice of endocrine surgery. To watch the Indian Association of Endocrine Surgeons, metamorphose into a vibrant organization involved in a lot of academic deliberations is indeed very heartwarming to me.

I would once again like to congratulate Dr Amit Agarwal and the entire team for their far-sighted venture and hard work for bringing out this book and I strongly recommend this book to all aspiring as well as established endocrine surgeons.

Professor Sivapatham Vittal
MS FRCS FICS FAIS FAES FIMSA FTASc DSc (Hon)
Emeritus Professor and Senior Consultant
Department of Endocrine Surgery
Sree Sai Krishna Hospital, Vittal's Institute of
Endocrine Surgery and Apollo Hospitals
Chennai, Tamil Nadu, India
Padma Shri Awardee, Dr BC Roy Awardee
Founder President
Indian Association of Endocrine Surgeons (IAES)
Past President, Association of Surgeons of India
Past President and Past Trustee
International College of Surgeons, Indian Section

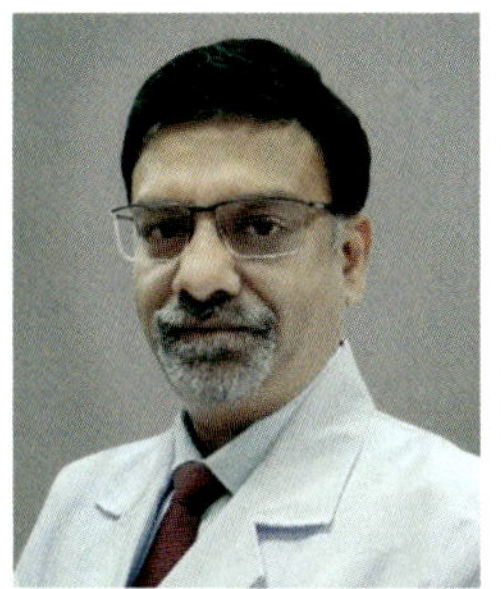 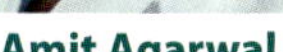 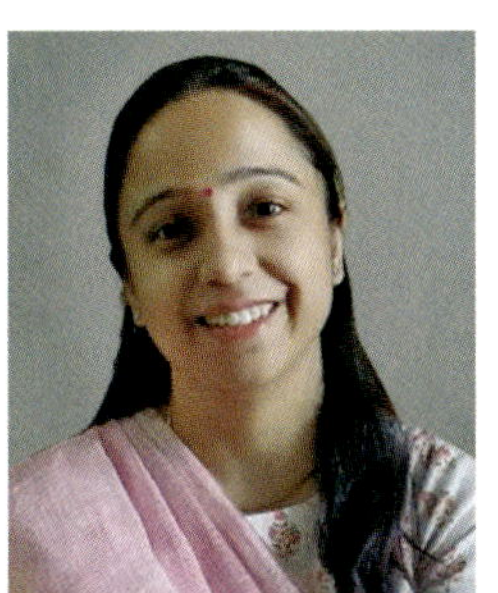 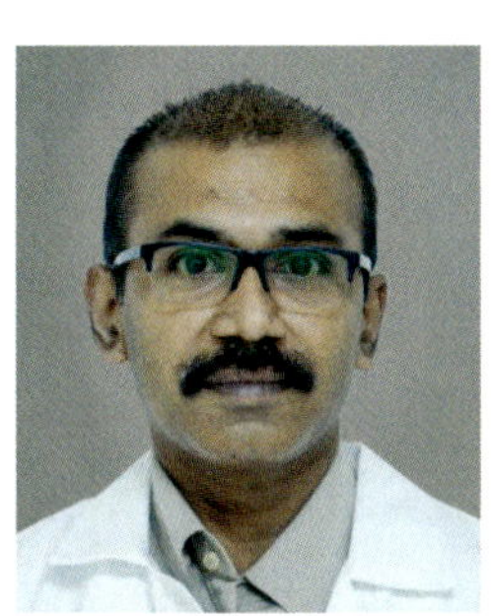 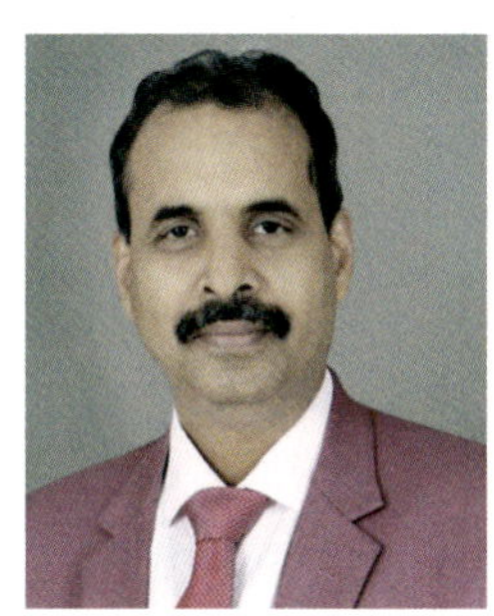 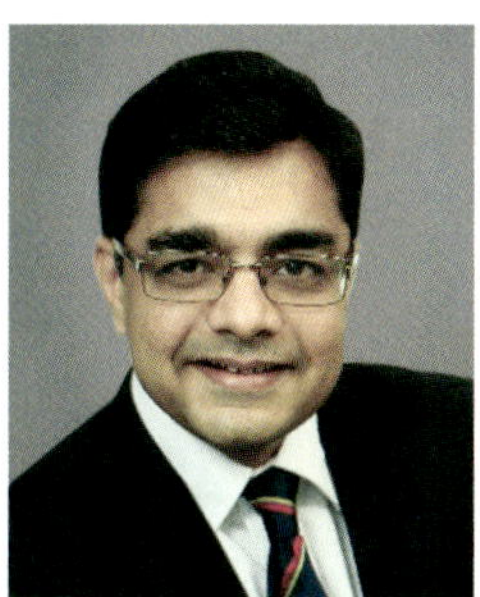

Amit Agarwal **Roma Pradhan** **Dhalapathy Sadacharan** **Anand Kumar Mishra** **Deepak Abraham**

After a struggle of more than 35 years, the super-specialty of Endocrine Surgery has come of age in India, with more than 70 formally trained endocrine surgeons in different parts of India and 6 academic centers offering 3-year MCh courses in Endocrine Surgery. Being one of the early students of endocrine surgery, we all know the trials and tribulations of having chosen this specialty against all odds. However, over 3 decades we have come a long way: from not having any dedicated section in the library to now a well-stocked section with many books of endocrine surgery; from skeptical super-specialists to appreciative colleagues, from few parathyroids/adrenals in a year to daily parathyroid/adrenal operations; from having no dedicated endocrine pathologists and radiologists to surgeon performed ultrasound and cytology; from being considered soft specialty to a specialty offering opportunity to perform aggressive and thrilling surgeries such as mediastinal clearance of LN in a case of MTC or extensive organ resection for an adrenal cancer with atrial thrombus, invading IVC, liver, kidney, pancreas; from the perception of a technology bereft specialty to a heavily equipped endocrine operation theater with neuromonitoring, ICG dye infusion equipment, endoscope and robot; from a small group of self-proclaimed but highly committed general surgeons/endocrine surgeons to a large, vibrant and leading association with more than 500 members. Endocrine operations are the epitome of a surgeon's skill, be it the meticulous dissection during thyroidectomy or the art of finding and dissecting the tiny parathyroid tumors. We felt the need of a book which would teach the students such nuances of endocrine surgery and prepare them to handle the endocrine surgical diseases. The association tasked one academic endocrine surgeon from each of the 5 Endocrine Academic Institutes of the country to take up this challenge. Almost all of the Members of the Indian Association of Endocrine Surgeons (IAES) were invited to contribute to this herculean task and we are happy that almost all of them responded and contributed actively to the book chapters. We are sure that the *IAES Textbook of Endocrine Surgery* will serve as a handbook for ready referral for practicing endocrine surgeons both in India and overseas. The topics covered and the style of presentation with emphasis on clinical pearls as a take home message in each chapter will help in simplifying complex problems in the clinic as well as improve patient-related outcomes. We are grateful to all the members of the IAES and other eminent contributors to have done justice to this objective. We are also grateful to Professor Gerard M Doherty and Professor Sivapatham Vittal for agreeing to write foreword for this book and we are indebted to their inspiring words. We also acknowledge our publishers for the beautiful processing of the book.

Contents

CHAPTER 1

Applied Embryology and Surgical Anatomy of the Endocrine Glands

Chakravarthy Marx Sadacharan

An understanding of the applied embryology and thorough knowledge of the gross anatomy of the endocrine glands are of paramount importance to the endocrine surgeons for the successful surgery.

THYROID GLAND

◇ EMBRYOLOGY OF THYROID GLAND AND DEVELOPMENTAL ANOMALIES

The first gland of endocrine origin during the embryonic development is the thyroid, under the influence of fibroblast growth factor (FGF) signaling pathways, approximately 24 days postfertilization. Development of the thyroid is from the floor of the primordial pharynx and the neural crest. In the floor of the pharynx, the epithelial cells of the endoderm proliferate, and soon form a small outpouching, the thyroid primordium that will form the follicular elements of the thyroid tissue **(Figs. 1A and B)**. The mode of descent of thyroid primordium starts in front of the pharyngeal gut in the midline of the neck, hyoid bone, and the laryngeal cartilages and reaches the front of the trachea finally. The thyroid primordium soon becomes a solid mass of cells and divides into right and left lobes that are connected by the isthmus of the thyroid, which lies anterior to growing second and third tracheal rings. Thyroglossal duct remains as a connecting narrow canal between the thyroid and the pharyngeal floor during this migration. This duct later disappears. The thyroid begins to function approximately during the 11th week of embryo. The follicular cells produce thyroxine and triiodothyronine. The neural crest of the ultimobranchial bodies from the fourth and fifth branchial pouches migrates to the lateral lobes of the developing thyroid to become parafollicular cells or C cells that serve as a source of calcitonin. Dorsal endoderm gives rise to the parathyroids from the third branchial pouch (PIII; parathyroid gland III) and fourth branchial pouch (PIV; parathyroid gland IV) and joins the thyroid lobes at the posterior border. The cardiac neural crest mesenchyme gives rise to the connective tissue capsule, which carries neurovascular and lymphatic supply to the thyroid.[1-4]

Anomalies of embryonic development of the lateral lobes result in a large variety of shapes and sizes. The absence of the thyroid gland or one of its lobes is a rare anomaly (<0.1%).

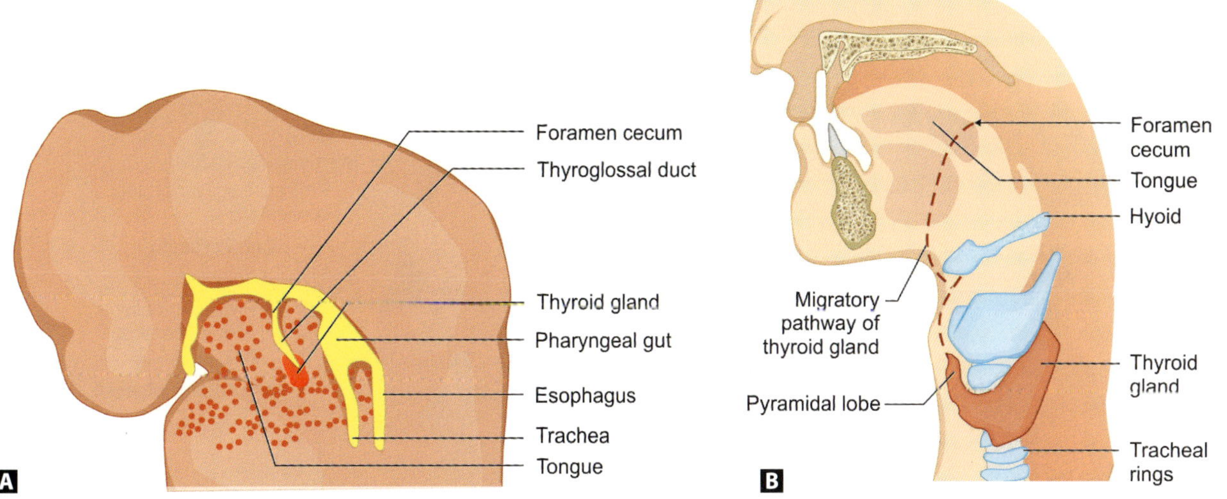

Figs. 1A and B: (A) The thyroid primordium arises as an epithelial diverticulum (thyroglossal duct) in the pharyngeal midline behind the tuberculum impar; (B) Position of the thyroid gland with its migratory pathway.

In the unilateral failure of formation, the left lobe is more commonly absent. This may be due to the mutation in the receptor for thyroid-stimulating hormone (TSH) in some cases.

Normally, the thyroglossal duct disappears, but foramen cecum persists in the proximal part of duct as a small pit in the dorsum of the tongue and the distal part becomes the pyramidal lobe.[1] Pyramidal lobe is approximately seen in 50% of the thyroid glands. The pyramidal lobe can be seen as a lateral extension in 30% cases and vertical extension from the isthmus in about 40% of the cases. Accessory thyroid tissue may be seen as a band of connective tissue or fibromuscular band, musculus levator glandular thyroideae extending from the pyramidal lobe to the hyoid bone.

The parts of the thyroglossal duct may persist in lingual, suprahyoid, retrohyoid, or infrahyoid positions. They may form ectopic masses of thyroid tissue, cysts, fistulae, or sinuses, usually located anywhere in the path of thyroid glandular descent in the midline of the neck. The thyroglossal duct and epithelium may form thyroglossal cysts, which are mostly located in the subhyoid region (approximately 50% of cysts) or close to the thyroid cartilage. Thyroglossal cysts are usually observed at the age of 5 years. Rupture of the thyroglossal duct cyst results in a fistula connected to the exterior, a thyroglossal fistula.[5]

The most common aberrant thyroid is found in the base of the tongue (lingual thyroid tissue; as many as 10% of autopsies), just behind the foramen cecum. Only one in 4,000 persons with thyroid disease is clinically relevant.[3] Aberrant glandular tissue with nodules may be seen anywhere in the inferior part of the thyroid, posterolateral part of sternocleidomastoid, on the thyrohyoid muscle, lateral to thyroid cartilage up to the pericardium, and the periaortic region in the superior mediastinum apart from the midline of the neck. The ectopic intrathoracic thyroid tissue will receive its blood supply from intrathoracic vessels. Intrathoracic thyroid tumors require a median sternotomy.

It is clinically important to differentiate an aberrant thyroid tissue from the thyroglossal cysts by radioisotope scanning in order to prevent the accidental surgical removal of the thyroid tissue. Failure to do so may leave the person to depend on lifelong thyroid medication.[3,6]

GROSS ANATOMY OF THE THYROID GLAND

The thyroid gland comprises two lateral lobes on either side connected in the midline by the isthmus and is highly vascular. The gland is present around the larynx and upper tracheal rings through a dense connective tissue called the posterior suspensory or Berry's ligament. Thyroid is covered by a thin false capsule, which has multiple fibrous septa dividing the gland into lobes and lobules. There is an external second true capsule, which is formed by the pretracheal layer of the deep cervical fascia.

The gland weighs about 25 g, but this varies. In females, the gland enlarges during menstruation and pregnancy. The size of the thyroid gland is clinically important in the thyroid disorders evaluation and management and can be measured by the diagnostic ultrasound. The anterolateral (superficial) part of the lobe is covered by sternothyroid and sternohyoid. Lateral extension of the thyroid onto the thyrohyoid is prevented by the attachment of sternothyroid to the oblique line of thyroid cartilage. If the sternothyroid and sternohyoid muscles are to be cut transversely, the surgeon must cut at a high level (cricoid level), to preserve their motor nerve, the ansa hypoglossi. Larynx, tracheal rings, and esophagus are located medially; the carotid sheath and sternocleidomastoid are located posterolaterally[1,4,6] **(Fig. 2)**.

The arterial supply of the thyroid gland consists of the superior and inferior thyroid arteries and sometimes an arteria thyroidea ima which is unpaired and appears in ~10% of people. It arises directly from the aorta or the internal thoracic artery or the brachiocephalic trunk. The isthmus is

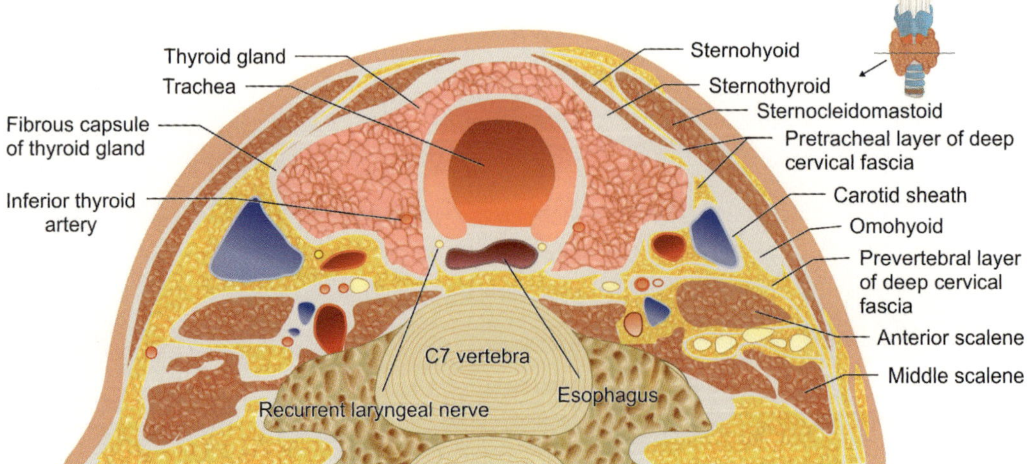

Fig. 2: Relationship of the thyroid gland.

supplied by the arteria thyroidea ima after its ascent on the anterior surface of the trachea.

Above the thyroid cartilage, the external carotid artery gives rise to the superior thyroid artery. The other variable origins are the common carotid artery or the bifurcation of the common carotid artery.[7] It branches out as the superior laryngeal artery and then descends deep to the sternothyroid muscle to reach the superior pole of the thyroid gland, pierces the thyroid fascia, dividing into anterior and posterior branches. The anterior surface of the gland is supplied by the branch of the superior thyroid artery medially, which gives a branch to the pyramidal lobe and isthmus. The posterior branch of the superior thyroid artery descends along the posterior border of the lobe and its anastomosis with the inferior thyroid artery to supply the lateral and medial surface of the gland **(Fig. 3)**.

The superior pole of the gland has an intricate relationship with both the superior thyroid artery and the external (motor) branch of the superior laryngeal nerve. The variations in the relationship of the nerve could be either with the superior thyroid artery or around its branches. Therefore, this nerve is highly vulnerable to injury while ligating the superior thyroid artery in thyroid surgeries. In 20% of the cases, the nerve is not located in the surgically accessible area, around the superior thyroid pole with the superior thyroid artery. In this type of variations, to locate the nerve, the dissection into or through the fibers of the pharyngeal constrictor muscles is necessary. This motor nerve supplies cricothyroid muscle, which tenses the vocal cord and produces high-pitched voice. Injury to this nerve (e.g., during thyroidectomy) results in a monotonous voice due to paralysis of the cricothyroid muscle failing to lengthen or tense the vocal cord. This injury could be critical for singers and orators but may not bother people who do not utilize a wide range of variation of tone in their speech.

The recommendation is to identify the branches of the artery to avoid ligation of its main trunk when ligating the superior thyroid artery in order to avoid damaging the external branch of the superior laryngeal nerve. The artery should be ligated and sectioned close to the superior pole of the gland, since the nerve is placed far away. The space of Reeve's between the superior pole and the cricothyroid muscle is dissected to push the vessels away from the nerve. This dissection needs a strong downward and outward traction of the superior pole of the gland from the medial side. The nerve is seen transversely between the cricothyroid or the pharyngeal constrictor and the superior thyroid vessels.

At the level of the cricoid cartilage, the thyrocervical trunk branches into the inferior thyroid artery trunk that runs superomedially posterior to the carotid sheath, reaches posterior aspect of the inferior pole of the thyroid, and then runs upward again to reach the gland's midportion. The artery gives rise to inferior, posterior, and internal branches supplying the different portions of the gland after piercing the pretracheal fascia. An inferior branch or the major trunk of the inferior thyroid artery supplies the inferior parathyroid gland (PIII). The superior and inferior thyroid arteries anastomose along the posterior border of the gland with their posterior branches.

At the lower and middle parts of the thyroid gland, the recurrent laryngeal nerve is located in close relation to the inferior thyroid artery. After a good retraction of the thyroid, the inferior thyroid artery becomes clearly obvious for the surgeon and the carotid artery with the internal jugular vein much laterally. It is easier to identify the recurrent laryngeal nerve this way since it puts tension on the inferior thyroid artery. Neck surgery puts a substantial risk on recurrent laryngeal nerves which attaches a lot of clinical importance on their identification. The recurrent laryngeal nerves can be dissected successfully with the markers of the tracheoesophageal groove, inferior thyroid artery, and/or angle under the thyroid cartilage.[5]

The position of the right recurrent laryngeal nerve near the inferior pole of thyroid runs more oblique and is closely related to the inferior thyroid artery and its branches.

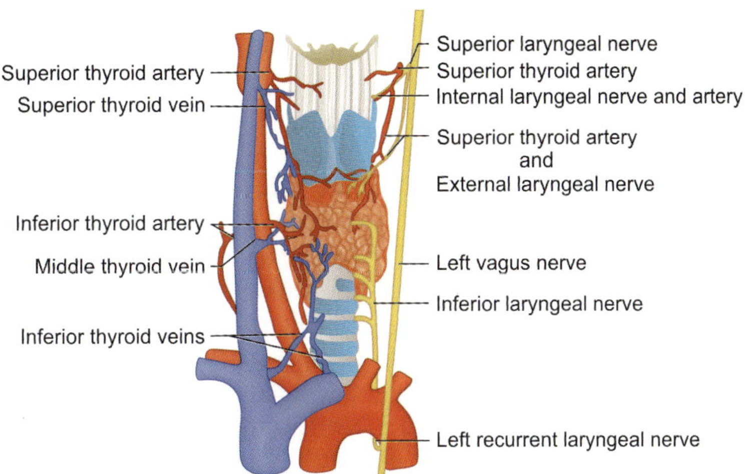

Fig. 3: Neurovascular relation to the thyroid gland.

Variable anatomical positions of this nerve may be between the branches or anterior or posterior to the branches of the inferior thyroid artery. Recurrent laryngeal nerve is most prone to injuries in these sites. The left recurrent laryngeal nerve may ascend vertically lateral to the tracheoesophageal groove or at the depth from the superior mediastinum. Usually, it crosses deep or superficial (rarely) to the inferior thyroid artery or it may pass between the terminal branches of the artery. The possibility of injuring the left recurrent laryngeal nerve during thyroid surgery is very less because of its course and location in the tracheoesophageal groove.

It is considered safe to look for the recurrent laryngeal nerve below the inferior thyroid artery while performing thyroidectomies. An exemplary way to safeguard the nerve and the inferior parathyroid gland is to ligate the inferior thyroid artery or its branches close to the gland after identification.[4] Sometimes, one of the terminal branches of the inferior thyroid artery, particularly the inferior laryngeal artery, may be mistaken as the recurrent laryngeal nerve. But the nerve is somewhat irregular, rounded, and cord-like structure as compared to the artery. A small, red, sinuous vessel, a vasa nervorum, is always observed on it. Sometimes, the nerve gives branches below the artery.

In a few cases of pathologically enlarged thyroid glands, the recurrent laryngeal nerves may appear to penetrate the thyroid gland itself before entering the larynx.

The enlarged thyroid gland (goiter) may compress the laryngeal nerves and lead to laryngeal muscles paralysis. The paralyzed vocal folds can be examined by the laryngoscopy before performing surgery in order to determine any preexisting nerve injury due to compression.

The thyroid gland is connected to the upper part of the trachea and esophagus by a whitish connective tissue band called— Berry's ligament. The classical location of the recurrent laryngeal nerve is posterolateral to Berry's ligament by not penetrating it neither is it found medial to the ligament. The nerve is posterior to the ligament and has an inferior laryngeal artery accompanying it before its entry into the larynx. The artery has a branch that crosses the nerve and is also posterior to the nerve while entering the gland making it a critical site of bleed. This area is critical to avoid injury to the nerve due to the bleed that is caused unnecessarily at Berry's ligament. Therefore, until the nerve has been successfully identified, the blood vessels in the corresponding portion of the ligament should never be clamped, as it may injure the recurrent laryngeal nerve.[8]

Medial retraction of the thyroid gland makes the recurrent laryngeal nerve more prone to injury during the thyroid lobectomy by displacing the nerve anterior to the trachea. This also creates tension on the inferior thyroid artery and its branches and on Berry's ligament. The posterior fibers of Berry's ligament press the nerve against the tracheal rings snugly on the lateral aspect, thereby increasing the complexity of dissection for the surgeons. Hence, a good retraction of the lobe will make the nerve straight and easier to trace till the entry point into larynx after inferior pole ligation. The recurrent laryngeal nerve innervates majority of the laryngeal muscles and specifically is responsible for abduction (opening) of the vocal cords. Injury to this nerve can result in a weakened voice (hoarseness) or loss of voice (aphonia) due to paralysis of vocal cord muscles and may cause difficulty in breathing (dyspnea). Vocal cord paresis or paralysis due to an iatrogenic injury of the recurrent laryngeal nerve is a major preventable complication in thyroid surgery. Although many procedures have been introduced to prevent the nerve injury, still the incidence of recurrent laryngeal nerve palsy varies between 1.5 and 14%.[9,10]

In general, the origin of the nonrecurrent laryngeal nerve is cervical. Depending upon its level of origin, the nerve makes a downward curve as it runs down along the vagus nerve and across the jugulocarotid groove. It always runs posterior to the common carotid artery. It has not been proved that the nonrecurrent laryngeal nerve really originates from the vagus nerve or from the sympathetic system (e.g., the stellate ganglion).[11] The incidence of the nonrecurrent laryngeal nerve is low, only occurring in 0.57% of people and most commonly found posterior to the inferior thyroid artery.[12] A rare anatomic variant is a right nonrecurrent laryngeal nerve (NRLN—0.3–0.8%) and 0.004% left NRLN. This nerve has been observed with concurrent variants of the great vessels. Aberrant right subclavian artery (ARSA) or arteria lusoria arising from the aortic arch is required to be identified for the presence of a right NRLN. The most common vascular variant with a right NRLN is an ARSA (97%), an intrathyroidal right common carotid artery (0.9%), and associated with normal vascular anatomy (1.9%). The left NRLN comprises an extremely rare variant and, if present, it is usually associated with situs inversus or right aortic arch.[13]

In the thyroid gland surgeries, sometimes the recurrent laryngeal nerve may not be identified in the regular location, at the crossing of the inferior thyroid artery and its branches, where it must be identified transversely between the medially retracted thyroid lobe and the laterally retracted carotid sheath. The other anomalous courses for the recurrent laryngeal nerve are documented only with pathologically enlarged thyroid glands and especially with large posterior nodules and substernal multinodular goiters. The nerve could also be sought superiorly at its entry point into the larynx at the level of the cricoid cartilage. A previous dissection of the superior pole of the thyroid gland or an "inside out" approach would be mandated after sectioning the isthmus of the thyroid.

The venous drainage of the thyroid is highly variable compared to the arteries with three pairs of the thyroid veins. The anterior part of the trachea and the surface of the thyroid will have a formed plexus of veins, which need to be cauterized during surgery. The superior thyroid veins run anterior and lateral to the superior thyroid arteries and the middle or lateral thyroid veins are greatly variable and do not accompany and pass on the thyroid lobe from the anterolateral side. The internal jugular vein forms the main drainage area directly or indirectly from both the superior and the lateral thyroid veins. Careful lateral retraction of the carotid sheath will help the middle thyroid veins' identification and their ligation. The inferior thyroid veins leaving the isthmus and the inferior pole of the gland drain either into the brachiocephalic vein after forming a plexus behind the manubrium sternum or directly into the internal jugular vein. Previous identification of the recurrent laryngeal nerve will enable safe ligation of the inferior thyroid veins.

The lymphatic vessels of the thyroid may run in all directions and may even cross-communicate with the isthmus and opposite lateral lobe. So, it is practically very difficult to remove all the potential lymph node metastases in thyroid carcinomas. However, the surgeon must consider two areas of lymphatic drainage for the thyroid gland. The first (medial) lymphatic area is the paraglandular space or medial visceral compartment of the neck which is bounded by the carotid sheath medially and the posterior surface of the prethyroid muscles and sometimes few lymph nodes, particularly just above the isthmus (Delphian nodes) anteriorly. The second (lateral) lymphatic area is the lateral cervical region and located lateral to the carotid sheath **(Fig. 4)**.

In the medial visceral compartment, there are two groups: (1) the pretracheal and the prelaryngeal and (2) the paratracheoesophageal. The thyroid isthmus drains into pretracheal lymph nodes located right below the isthmus, further collects and drains inferiorly to the anterior and superior mediastinal lymph nodes. The upper part of the isthmus drains into lateral cervical lymph nodes via the prelaryngeal and paralaryngeal lymph nodes present anterolateral to isthmus. The paratracheoesophageal lymph nodes located along the lateral and posterior aspects of the thyroid gland and along the course of the recurrent laryngeal

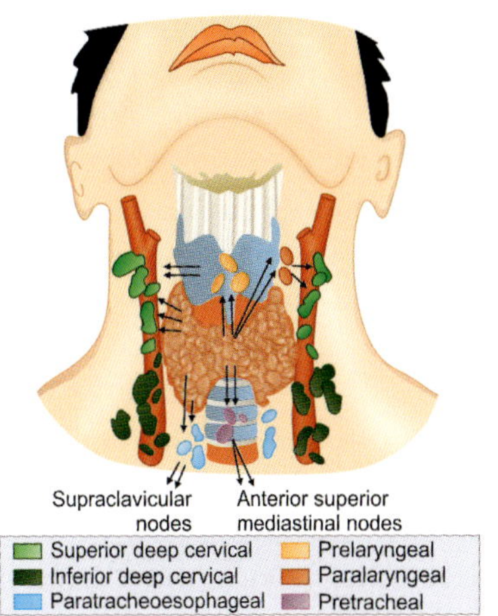

Fig. 4: Lymphovascular supply of the thyroid gland.

nerves collect the lymph from the central and lower parts of the lateral thyroid lobes and drain laterally into the supraclavicular lymph nodes and posteriorly with those around and behind the trachea, the larynx, the pharynx, and the esophagus.

The superior pole of the thyroid drains into superficial and deep groups of lateral cervical lymph nodes which run along the superior thyroid vessels superolaterally. This explains that in two-third of cases of the papillary thyroid cancers, the metastatic lateral cervical lymph nodes are identified in the superior pole of thyroid.[14] Therefore, the medial visceral compartment (central neck) is the primary area of lymphatic drainage for all thyroid cancers, especially papillary and medullary thyroid cancers, except those located in superior poles of the glands. Lateral neck areas (internal jugular chains and posterior triangles) are secondary areas of lymphatic drainage. Some of the involvement of lateral neck nodes may be brought about by the retrograde extension resulting from obstruction of the lymph flow route in the medial visceral compartment.[15]

PARATHYROID GLAND

◇ EMBRYOLOGY AND DEVELOPMENTAL ANOMALIES

During development of the head and neck in the fourth week, the mesenchymal tissue surrounds the pharynx to form the pharyngeal arches. The ectoderm lines the external aspects of the pharyngeal arches to form the pharyngeal clefts. The endoderm lines the internal aspects of the pharyngeal arches and penetrates it to form the pharyngeal pouches. In the 5th week, there is a proliferation of the endodermal epithelium in the third and fourth pharyngeal pouches. The development of the parathyroid glands is influenced by the FGF signaling pathways through FGF receptor substrate-2 (*FRS-2*) gene. The human embryo has four pairs of well-defined endodermal lining pharyngeal pouches. The fifth pouch is rudimentary or absent. Each pouch expands laterally and develops a dorsal and ventral region. The dorsal regions of the third pharyngeal pouch differentiate into the inferior parathyroid glands (PIII) while the ventral regions form the thymus gland. Superior parathyroid glands (PIV) arise from the dorsal part of the fourth pharyngeal pouch while ultimobranchial body comes from the ventral regions. The parafollicular cells of the thyroid originate from this ultimobranchial body.

Inferior parathyroid glands and thymus separate out from the pharyngeal wall while there is a caudal and medial migration of the thymus with the inferior parathyroid glands. These separated inferior parathyroid glands from the thymus migrate and rest on the dorsal surface of the thyroid lobes. The thymus moves down further to reach its fixed position in the anterior part of the thorax where it fuses with the opposite side. The superior parathyroid glands separate out from the fourth pharyngeal pouches and again migrate to the upper part of dorsal surface of thyroid lobes **(Figs. 5A and B)**.

Most of the humans have two pairs of parathyroid glands. Ectopic parathyroid glands or remnants of the parathyroid tissue may be found anywhere along the pathway, near or within the thyroid gland or thymus. Superior parathyroids are more consistent in their location when compared to the inferior parathyroid glands. The variations described are the location of the inferior parathyroid glands to the inferior thyroid poles, or their migration along with the thymus into the superior mediastinum (1–5%) or descent to the common carotid artery bifurcation or no descent at all. It is uncommon in few individuals to they have no parathyroid or more than four parathyroid to eight supernumerary glands (2.5–22%) that probably result from the division of primordia of parathyroid glands.[1-3]

GROSS ANATOMY OF THE PARATHYROID GLAND

The parathyroid glands have their own capsule and are located posterior to the thyroid lobes and vary in color, size, and shape. They are small, spherical, ovoid, or flat whose shapes are changed by the surrounding structures. Superior and inferior glands are two each in number on either side of the thyroid gland. There is evidence of supernumerary parathyroids—maybe smaller and scattered in the nearby connective tissue. In neonates, the parathyroid has variable size and position. The parathyroid glands will double in size between birth and puberty. The size of each gland is approximately 4–6 mm long, 3–4 mm wide, and 1–2 mm from front to back. The average size of the gland is about $5 \times 3 \times 1$. The average weight of a single gland is about 35–50 mg and may range from 10 to 70 mg.

The color of the parathyroid glands varies with age. They look gray in newborn, light pink in children, and yellow in adults as their adipose content increases and finally they turn darker in older adults.

All four parathyroid glands are symmetrical in approximately 60% of the cases. While the superior parathyroids are found to be symmetrical 80% of the times, the inferior ones are symmetrical only in 70% cases. The symmetry is less noted when the glands are found in an uncommon location.

The superior parathyroid glands are usually constant in position and lie on the posterior aspect of the thyroid gland, at the level of the inferior border of the thyroid cartilage in the tracheoesophageal groove >1 cm above to the point of entry of the inferior thyroid artery. They are usually seen within 2 cm area, about 1 cm above the intersection of the inferior thyroid artery and the recurrent laryngeal nerve. If the gland is located on the posterior part of the upper pole of the thyroid, the gland is invariably underneath the thyroid-investing facial sheath. At the cricothyroid junction, the parathyroid may be covered by a pad of fat and has a small pedicle as supply. The glands can also be located farther down, sometimes covered or hidden by the recurrent laryngeal nerve or the inferior thyroid artery. The true intrathyroidal superior parathyroids are rarely identified. An unusual location for the superior parathyroids may be in the posterior part of the neck, above the upper pole of the thyroid lobe, and the retroesophageal or retropharyngeal space.[4,6]

The location of the inferior parathyroid glands could be variable due to its migration with the thymus as part of the development. They are seen in the posterior part of the inferior pole slightly >1 cm below to the point of entry of the inferior thyroid artery, although the gland may be identified anterior, lateral, or inferior to the inferior pole of the thyroid gland **(Fig. 6)**. This is covered by a pad of fat too. Some of the inferior parathyroid glands are found above or below the thyroid lobe, within the cervical part of the thymus or close to the thyrothymic ligament.

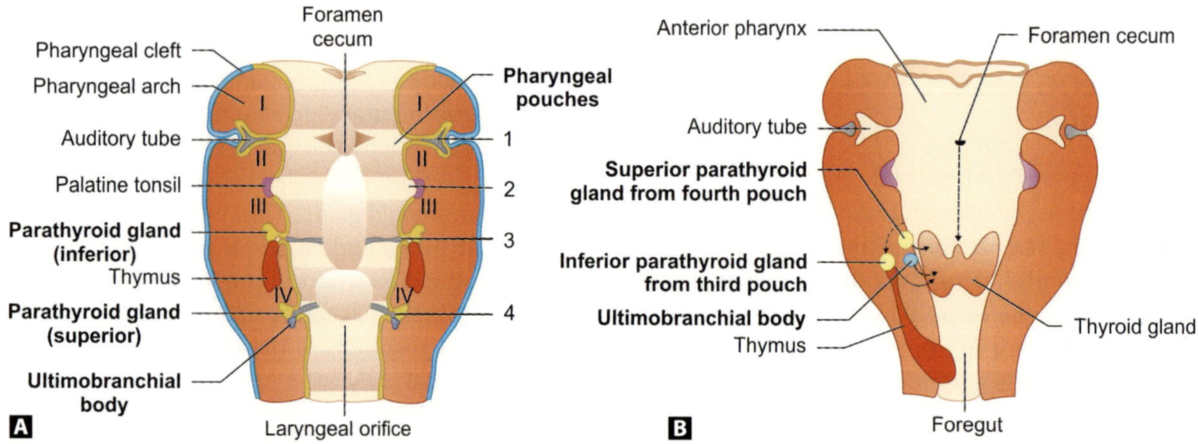

Figs. 5A and B: Development of the pharyngeal pouches. (A) The superior and inferior parathyroids formed by the dorsal portion of third and fourth pharyngeal pouches; (B) Migration of the inferior parathyroid gland alongside thymus gland and the superior parathyroid gland with the ultimobranchial body.

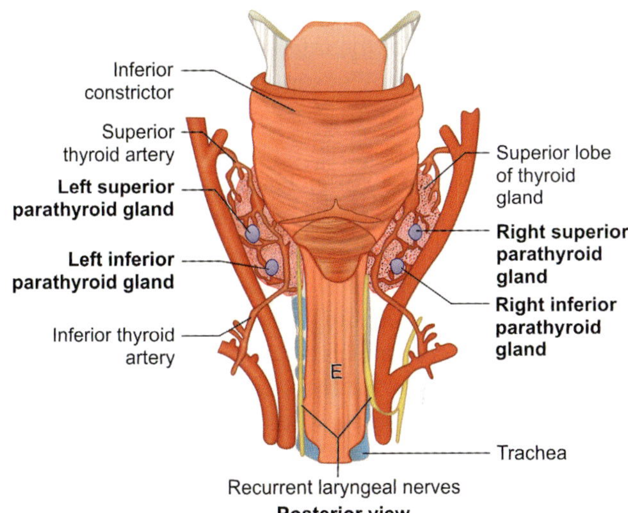

Fig. 6: The superior and inferior parathyroid glands are embedded in the fibrous capsule on the posterior surface of the thyroid gland with their depicted relationship with the superior and inferior thyroid arteries.

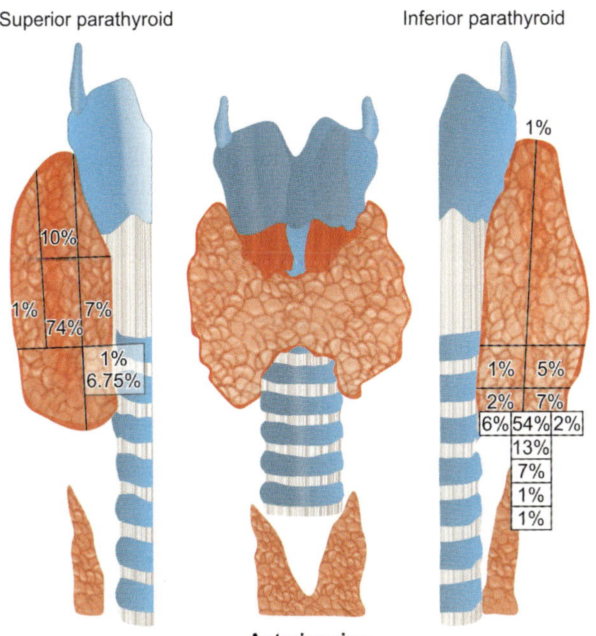

Fig. 7: The anatomical location of the superior and inferior parathyroid glands as reported by Gilmour.[17]

The inferior parathyroid gland may fail to descend during its development resulting in change in location of the gland (usually with thymic remnant) above the superior thyroid lobe or even much higher in the neck. The inferior parathyroid glands can also be located intrathyroidally, farther down in the thymus gland, adipose tissue of the anterior superior mediastinum, or at the carotid bifurcation. The true intrathyroid parathyroids are found in 3% of the cases.[16] If intrathyroid parathyroid glands are identified, they are all found in the lower third of the thyroid lobe. The frequency of anatomical locations of inferior and superior parathyroid glands is reported by Gilmour in a study on 428 autopsies[17] **(Fig. 7)**.

The parathyroid glands can be located either extracapsular or intracapsular to the thyroid gland. This anatomical feature has great surgical importance. When there is an intracapsular parathyroid gland disease, its size increases locally within the thyroid gland tissue, deep to the thyroid gland capsule, and stays in its place. On the other hand, when there is an extracapsular parathyroid gland disease, its size increases outside the thyroid gland tissue, superficial to the thyroid gland capsule and tends to be displaced to the area of the least resistance. Thus, an extracapsular parathyroid gland disease within the thymus gland is pushed behind the clavicle and enters the superior–anterior mediastinum whereas an extracapsular parathyroid gland disease at the level of cricothyroid junction falls into the posterior mediastinum.

There is a rare finding that two parathyroid glands are closely related to each other and seem to be combined. These kissing parathyroids could have a sperate capsule and are separated by a cleavage plane.

The identification of anastomosis of superior and inferior parathyroid arteries at the posterior surface of thyroid could help to trace the parathyroid glands. The various physical characteristics may help to differentiate the parathyroid from the other adjacent structures such as nodules of thyroid tissue, adipose lobule, and even lymph nodes. The parathyroid glands are vascular and slightly rounded structures that are softer in consistency.

The parathyroid gland looks like a small "body" that moves inside its own adipose capsule when gentle pressure is applied on its surface. On biopsy, diffuse bleeding can be seen on the cut surface. The above said physical properties are lacking in the nodules of thyroid tissue, adipose lobule, and lymph nodes. The thyroid nodules are harder, more reddish, and less comparable than the parathyroid glands. The fat lobules are softer with lack of consistency and do not have the blood vessels on the surface. The lymph nodes are rounded and more adherent to the surrounding tissues.

The significant importance has been placed on the relationship between the parathyroid glands and the recurrent laryngeal nerve. A rectangular area can be imagined visually with the medial retraction of lateral lobe of the thyroid gland. The rectangle area has the following imaginary boundaries—anteriorly by the trachea and the thyroid surface, posteriorly by the esophagus, the cranial part of the thyroid superiorly, and the point on trachea 4 cm below the inferior pole of the thyroid gland inferiorly. The usual course of the recurrent laryngeal nerve should divide this rectangle into a posterosuperior triangle being dorsal to the nerve and the anteroinferior triangle being ventral to the nerve. The superior parathyroid glands are generally dorsolateral to the recurrent laryngeal nerve and the inferior parathyroid glands are inferomedial in relation to the nerve. A study conducted on 100 autopsy specimens confirmed that 93% of parathyroid glands were in a predictable relation to the recurrent laryngeal nerve (i.e., the superior parathyroid glands are lying in the posterosuperior triangle and the inferior parathyroid glands are lying in the anteroinferior triangle).[18] This supports the reliability of the recurrent laryngeal nerve as a guide for locating the parathyroid glands.

The thyroid arteries give rise to superior and inferior parathyroid arteries which supply the parathyroid glands. Any of these could supply the parathyroid glands: the inferior thyroid artery, branches from the anastomosis between inferior and superior thyroid arteries, the arteria thyroidea ima (thyroid artery of Neubauer), or the laryngeal, tracheal, or esophageal arteries. Approximately one-third of human parathyroid glands have two or more parathyroid arteries. A study on 357 parathyroid gland pedicles found that a single artery supplies the parathyroid gland in 80% of the cases. The two noticeable arteries were found in 15% of the cases, three distinct arteries in 4%, and even four separate arteries in 1% of the cases. This single artery was simple in 65% of the cases, divided into two branches before its entry in 30%, and divided into three branches in 5%.[19]

The length of the parathyroid artery ranges from 8 to 12 mm. The pedicles of the inferior parathyroid are longer and tortuous in course. The superior parathyroid pedicles are shorter and hold the superior parathyroid hard against its vessel of origin.

Inferior thyroid artery branches usually supply both the parathyroid glands. The inferior thyroid artery supplies the superior parathyroids 80% of the times, the superior thyroid artery in 15% of the cases and by anastomoses between the superior and inferior thyroid arteries 5% of the times. The inferior thyroid artery supplies the inferior parathyroid glands in 90% of the cases, superior thyroid artery in 10% of the cases, and lastly by anastomoses between the superior and inferior thyroid arteries, or the arteria thyroidea ima (1–6%).

Thyroid plexus around the trachea forms the major venous drainage. The lymph vessels from the parathyroid glands are received by the lymph vessels of the thyroid gland (deep cervical and paratracheal lymph nodes).

ADRENAL GLANDS

◇ EMBRYOLOGY OF ADRENAL GLAND AND DEVELOPMENTAL ANOMALIES

The adrenal gland develops from two different components—cortex and medulla.[1] Mesoderm gives rise to the cortex and neuroectoderm to the medulla. Cortex develops from the coelomic epithelium and merges into the mesenchyme between root of mesentery and the urogenital ridge (mesonephros and the developing gonads) during the 5th week of development. This is the reason for the location of ectopic adrenal tissue below the kidney and in association with ovaries and testes. The proliferating adrenal tissue extends from the level of sixth to twelfth thoracic segments and differentiates into large acidophilic cells of the adrenal cortex.[2] Within a short time, the small-sized mesothelial cells penetrate and surround the original acidophilic cells and form the definitive cortex of the adrenal gland. Three zones—glomerulosa, transitory, and the dominant fetal zone—are organized in the adrenal cortex toward the end of gestation.[3,4,6] The fetal cortex regresses rapidly except its outermost layer after birth. The fetal cortex volume decreases from 70 to 3% of the total adrenal volume. The process slows down subsequently and some of its elements may persist up to the end of the 2nd year of life.[20,21] Neural crest is formed with the fetal cortex as a portion of the neuroectoderm remnant between the neural tube and the ectoderm. These neural crest cells migrate ventrally near the adrenal primordia to form the chromaffin cells of adrenal medulla or move to the dorsal aorta to form the sympathetic neurons after aggregation from the somite levels 18–24.[22,23] The adrenal medulla stains yellow–brown with chrome salts and is called chromaffin cell.

In embryonic life, chromaffin cells are scattered throughout the embryo, especially in the paravertebral sympathetic chain or the preaortic abdominal sympathetic plexus. All the chromaffin cells eventually degenerate postnatally only to persist as adrenal medullary chromaffin cells (**Figs. 8A to C**).

Development of venous sinusoids in the adrenal gland, adjoined by the capillaries of adjacent mesonephric arteries, and penetration into the adrenal cortex radially happen in the 8th gestational week. Initial branches arise from the aorta, the vessels to the septum transversum (later, the central part of the diaphragm), and the mesonephric arteries. Fetal adrenal glands are supplied by the inferior phrenic artery majorly.[24,25]

The fetal adrenal cortex begins to function as early as the 7th week of gestation, and steroidogenesis in the outer layers begins toward the end of the second trimester and is maximal by the third trimester. The rate of steroid secretion by the fetal adrenal glands may be fivefold higher than the adrenal glands of adults at rest.

It is generally being considered that the major role of the primate placenta is to convert the biologically active cortisol into its inactive metabolite cortisone (which does not bind to the glucocorticoid receptor) and protect the fetus from the relatively high concentrations of steroids present in the maternal circulation. The placenta plays a pivotal role in this sequence of events culminating in fetal adrenal development and function.

At the end of the 2nd week of development, the average weight of both adrenal glands is 5 g and becomes 4 g by 3 months. At birth, the adrenal glands are relatively large, 0.2% of the entire body weight and about one-third of the kidney size.

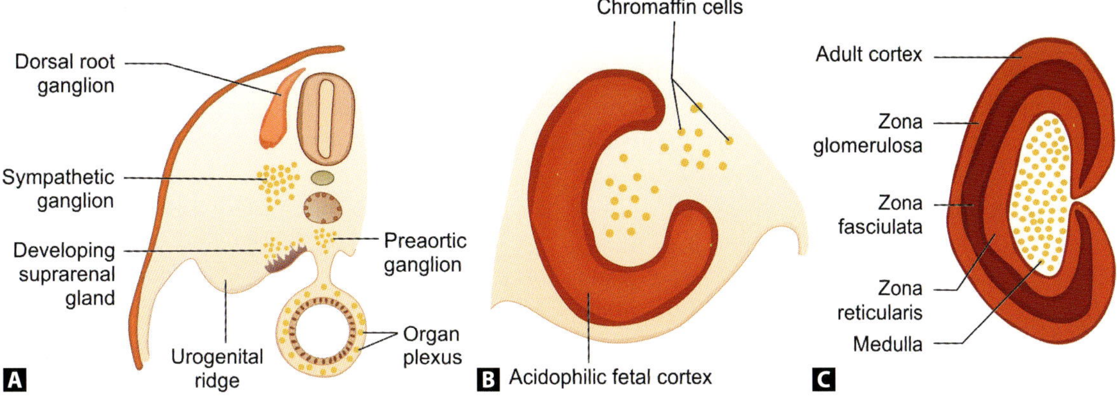

Figs. 8A to C: (A) The sympathetic neuroblasts migrate toward the proliferating mesothelium to constitute the adrenal medulla; (B) Chromaffin (sympathetic) cells penetrate the acidophilic fetal adrenal cortex; (C) The definitive cortex surrounds the medulla of the adrenal gland completely.

The accessory adrenal cortical tissues are found in the areolar tissue around the main adrenal glands. Sometimes, they are also found in relation to the sympathetic plexus and to the structures derived from the urogenital ridge—epididymis, vas deferens, broad ligament of the uterus, ovarian pedicle, or within the ovary or testis. Adrenocortical rests may occur in 50% of newborn infants and tend to degenerate after a few weeks. The ectopic medullary tissues also occur occasionally in conjunction with cortical tissue but more often as isolated masses along the abdominal aorta or in association with the sympathetic chain and the retroperitoneal celiac plexus. These have been described by Zuckerkandl, whose name is associated with an especially large mass that may occur anterior to the aorta and distal to the superior mesenteric arterial origin.[26] Extra-adrenal pheochromocytomas (also called paragangliomas) develop in "accessory" sites, particularly in ganglia in front of the inferior aorta (at the level of the organ of Zuckerkandl), around the aorta at the level of the kidney, in the mediastinum, or in the urinary bladder. Occasionally, the extra-adrenal pheochromocytomas have been reported in the neck, sacrococcygeal, anal, or vaginal areas. The incidence of extra-adrenal pheochromocytoma is higher in children than in adults.

◇| GROSS ANATOMY OF ADRENAL GLANDS

The adrenal glands are retroperitoneal organs resting on the superior and slightly anterior part of the corresponding kidney and crura of the diaphragm, at the level of T11–12 vertebrae. The perinephric fat and the renal fascia enclose the adrenal glands. There is a thick fibrous capsule, which allows them to easily separate from the kidneys. Fibrous bands and vasculature keep the adrenal glands in position.

The adrenal glands are golden yellow due to the presence of lipoid substances and firm in consistency compared with the surrounding perirenal fat. Each gland consists of two structural and functional areas—an outer thick cortex forming about nine-tenths of the gland and one-tenth forming the inner thinner medulla. The adrenal cortex has three zones—zona glomerulosa, zona fasciculata, and zona reticularis. Mineralocorticoids are produced in the zona glomerulosa, e.g., aldosterone, which is responsible for electrolyte and water balance; glucocorticoids in the zona fasciculata, e.g., cortisol which maintains carbohydrate balance; and sex hormones in the zona reticularis. The adrenal medulla consists of rounded clusters or short cords of pheochromocytes (chromaffin cells) supported by a network of reticular fibers and separated by the venous sinusoids. These cells are large, irregularly shaped polyhedrons with acidophilic cytoplasm and pale vesicular nuclei. They synthesize both adrenaline and noradrenaline.

At birth, the adrenal glands are approximately one-third of the ipsilateral kidney size. Postnatally, at the end of the second month, the weight of the adrenal has reduced by 50%. After 2 months of birth, its weight is half of what it was at birth. The gland slowly increases in size over 2 years and reaches birth weight at or before puberty. There is little further weight increase in adult life. In adults, each adrenal gland measures about 50, 30, and 10 mm in vertical, transverse, and anteroposterior dimensions and with a weight of about 4–5 g irrespective of age, sex, and bodyweight, but the weight could be 22 g at autopsy. The mean dimensions of the body of the adrenal gland are 0.79 cm (left) and 0.61 cm (right).[27,28] Adrenal glands are in the central and posterior position of the abdominal cavity. Normally, the glands cannot be felt; few tumors grow large enough to be palpated.

The topographic anatomical relations are important for understanding the radiologic anatomy. Each adrenal gland has two surfaces—anterior and posterior—and a medial border. The adrenal gland on the right is pyramidal shaped and a base touching the kidney with well-developed lower projections (limbs). The anterior surface on its medial aspect has the inferior vena cava (IVC) as its relation which is separated by the fascia and the connective tissue (not covered by peritoneum). The anterior surface on its lateral aspect has the right lobe of the liver as its relation where its upper part (superiorly) is in close proximity to the bare area of liver and the lower part may have a peritoneal covering. Its posterior surface on the upper part rests on the diaphragmatic right crus whereas the lower area of the posterior surface rests on the superior pole of right kidney. The right inferior phrenic artery with the right celiac ganglion is related to the adrenal at its medial border. If the inferior layer of the right triangular or coronary ligament of the liver lies at a high level, the right adrenal gland may reside partially in the upper part of the right paracolic gutter (pouch of Morison) where it is in contact with the peritoneum. The hilum of the right adrenal gland lies below the apex, near the anterior border, where a single adrenal vein arises to join the IVC.

The semilunar-shaped left adrenal gland is flattened in the anteroposterior plane. The upper part of the anterior surface has a peritoneal covering from the omental bursa that serves to segregate it from the stomach and sometimes the spleen. The stomach may be in approximation with the left adrenal gland. Its lower area of the anterior surface is a nonperitoneal area, which is in close approximation with the pancreatic tail and splenic artery. The left adrenal is largely sheltered anteriorly by the lesser sac peritoneum. Its medial area of the posterior surface is in close approximation to the diaphragmatic left crus. Its lateral area on the posterior surface is close to the left kidney. The medial border of the left adrenal gland is related to left celiac ganglion, left inferior phrenic artery, and left gastric arteries. The left adrenal hilum lies at the inferior part of the anterior surface and a single right adrenal vein originates inferomedially to join the left renal vein.

The adrenal glands are closely invested by a true connective tissue capsule, that dips in as septa carrying blood vessels into the interior of the adrenal. It is also enclosed by the perirenal fascia (fascia Gerota) of the kidneys. Superiorly, the Gerota fascia disappears on the abdominal surface of the diaphragm, whereas inferiorly, it is open and merges with the iliac fossa. The perirenal space is located between Gerota fascia and the true capsules of the adrenals and the kidneys.[29] The inclusion of the adrenal glands within the Gerota fascia is surgically important because the adrenals may be dissected from within the perirenal fat without compromising the peritoneum or the midline structures. Outside the perirenal fascia of Gerota lies the pararenal fat, anterior to which is the fascia of Zuckerkandl. It limits the retroperitoneum anteriorly.

The adrenal glands are very rich in vascular. Arterial supply is from superior, middle, and inferior suprarenal arteries, which may have multiple or duplicated branches. The superior suprarenal artery originates from the inferior phrenic artery which in turn originates from the abdominal aorta. They may sometimes be deficient. The middle suprarenal artery originates laterally from the abdominal aorta, at the superior mesenteric artery level and just above renal artery origin. The middle suprarenal artery runs over the diaphragmatic crus to the adrenal gland, where it anastomoses freely with adrenal branches of renal and inferior phrenic arteries. Right middle suprarenal artery, usually multiple in number, passes posterior to the IVC and right celiac ganglion. The left middle suprarenal artery is closely related to the celiac ganglion, upper border of the pancreas, and splenic artery. One or more inferior adrenal arteries from the renal arteries supply the adrenal gland. In addition to these three superior, middle, and inferior suprarenal arteries, other arteries in close proximity to the adrenal gland may also supply the gland. The source of these branches may be from the intercostal, the left ovarian/left internal spermatic arteries. The number of arteries entering the adrenal gland may vary. This anatomical detail is important when the surgeon plans to dissect within the perirenal fat, encounters these small arteries and veins herald proximity of the adrenal gland and the supplying arteries bleed in an irritating manner unless the branches are treated with diathermy or clip ligature **(Fig. 9)**.

Usually, the branches of the suprarenal arteries arborize forming a subcapsular plexus just before entering the adrenal. Short cortical arteries arising from the subcapsular plexus give rise to an extensive network of fenestrated sinusoids. These sinusoids pass around the clusters of the zona glomerulosa and run between the columns of the zona fasciculata and then form a deep plexus in the zona reticularis. The fenestrated capillary (sinusoidal) pores range in size from 100 nm in the outer glomerulosa to 250 nm in the inner fasciculata and reticularis. There is no direct arterial supply to the zona fasciculata and zona reticularis.[30] From the deep plexus of

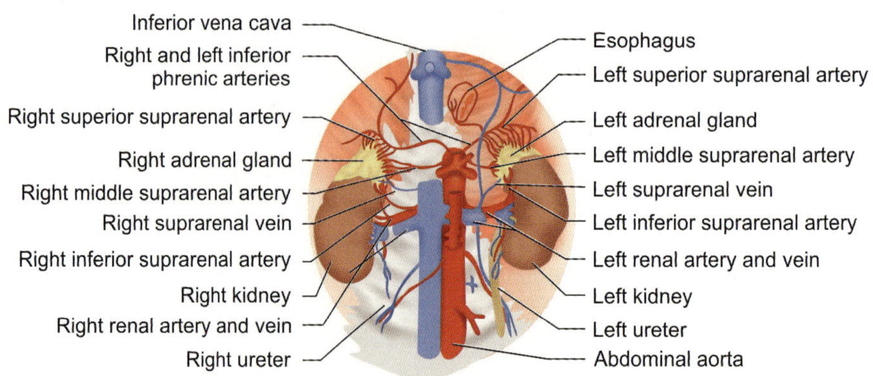

Fig. 9: The normal relationships of the right and left adrenal glands with the arterial supply and venous drainage.

the zona reticularis, venules pass between the medullary chromaffin cells and the medullary veins. The venules enter between the bundles of the longitudinally arranged smooth muscle fibers which are located around the chromaffin cells. These smooth muscle bundle fibers regulate the blood flow at the corticomedullary junction (at the deep aspect of the zona reticularis). The smooth muscle bundle fibers would control the rate of the blood flow through the zona reticularis and the zona fasciculata; it could provide part of a control mechanism for the availability of corticotropin to the secretory cells of these regions. Sometimes, relatively large arteries bypass this indirect route of arterial supply described previously and pass directly to supply the medullary region of the adrenal. So, the adrenal glands receive their arterial supply through indirect and direct routes. The arterial inflow of the adrenal gland at rest is approximately 10 mL/min. Under stress, corticotropin [adrenocorticotropic hormone (ACTH)] produces an immediate increase in blood flow to the adrenal glands.

The medullary veins emerge from the hilum of the suprarenal gland to form a single large suprarenal (central) vein. The right suprarenal vein is short (0.5 cm), runs horizontally, and drains directly into the IVC posteriorly. Due to its short length, there will be difficulty in ligation and individual anatomical variations can sometimes require the surgeon to side clamp the IVC. An accessory vein of the right suprarenal gland may be occasionally present and runs from the superomedial part of the hilum of the suprarenal gland to drain into the IVC. The left adrenal vein is around 2 cm long, descends medially, anterolateral to the celiac ganglion, and runs a retropancreatic course to drain into the left renal vein. The left adrenal vein joins the inferior phrenic vein before draining together into the left renal vein. Since a solitary suprarenal vein drains each adrenal, the damage to this vein is likely to cause infarction of that gland than damage to one of the suprarenal arteries. The suprarenal vein has up to four visible longitudinal smooth muscle bundles, the function of which is unknown. Probably, the smooth muscles cause venoconstriction and may increase cortical cell exposure to systemic factors (corticotropin) and the medullary cells to cortisol.

Each suprarenal gland is drained by two lymphatic plexuses. One lies deep to the capsule and the other is medullary. Many lymphatics leave the adrenal gland and end in the lateral aortic and the para-aortic lymph nodes, close to crus of the diaphragm and the origin of the renal artery **(Fig. 10)**. Few lymphatic vessels pierce the diaphragm and empty into the thoracic duct or the posterior mediastinal lymph nodes, which help to understand the development of local and distant metastases of the adrenal cortical cancers.

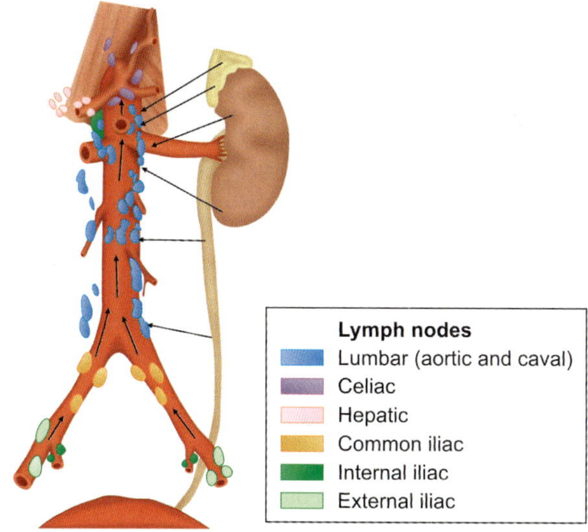

Fig. 10: The lymph vessels from the adrenal gland drain to the lumbar (the lateral aortic and the para-aortic) lymph nodes along with lymph vessels from the kidney and the ureter.

In malignant adrenal tumor surgeries, removal of local lymph nodes (para-aortic and paracaval nodes proximal to renal vessels) is recommended in order to achieve improved local control of the disease and facilitate more accuracy in classifying the extent of spread of the cancer.

The adrenal gland has a larger autonomic supply than any other organ. The adrenal medulla transforms the nervous signal (encoded electrically as action potentials) into an endocrine signal (chemically encoded), the neuroendocrine transducer. The sympathetic myelinated cholinergic fibers are preganglionic, arising from neuron cell bodies of the intermediolateral column between T3 and L3 spinal segments, pass through the hilum of the adrenal gland, and synapse with the cells in the medulla (pheochromocytes), which are synonymous with postganglionic sympathetic nerve fibers. Greater proportion of innervation (myelinated cholinergic preganglionic sympathetic fibers) reaches adrenal glands via the ipsilateral greater thoracic splanchnic nerves (T5 to T9). The acetylcholine is released into the systemic circulation on stimulation of the greater splanchnic nerves, which acts on muscarinic receptors on the pheochromocytes' membranes, alters their permeability, and permits the influx of calcium, which triggers exocytosis of the catecholamines. The adrenal cortex exclusively has a vasomotor innervation. The subcapsular arteriolar plexus has a sympathetic innervation. Also, the glomerulosa region cells and the subcapsular plexus contain innervation mediated by vasoactive intestinal polypeptide and neuropeptide Y. These axons are centrifugal and mostly serve to control steroidogenesis by the paracrine method.

PANCREAS

◇ EMBRYOLOGY OF PANCREAS AND DEVELOPMENTAL ANOMALIES

The pancreas is derived from the caudal part of the primitive foregut. Duodenal lining of endoderm gives rise to the dorsal and the ventral pancreatic buds, which appear at days 26 and 32 of the fetal development. The dorsal pancreatic bud from the dorsal part of the duodenum proliferates into the dorsal mesogastrium. The ventral pancreatic bud from the ventral duodenum proliferates between the layers of the ventral mesentery near the bile duct entry into the duodenum. Ventral pancreatic bud migrates with bile duct more dorsally with the differential growth of the duodenal wall and its rotation to the right. Finally, it fuses with the dorsal pancreatic bud after lying below it. The dorsal pancreatic bud gives rise to the head, the body, the tail of the pancreas, and the uncinate process. The dorsal part of the uncinate process and the head of the pancreas come from the ventral pancreatic bud **(Figs. 11A to C)**.[1-4,6]

The ventral pancreatic bud does not extend anterior to the superior mesenteric vein but it remains located to its right side. Initially, the body of the pancreas is in the dorsal mesoduodenum and then moves cranially into the dorsal mesogastrium. As the stomach, duodenum, and the ventral mesentery rotate, the pancreas becomes mainly retroperitoneal.

The distal part of the ventral and the dorsal pancreatic duct join to form the main duct of Wirsung in the developing exocrine pancreas. The dilated part of hepatoduodenal ampulla of Vater is formed by the fusion of the main pancreatic duct of Wirsung with the common bile duct, which drains into the second part of the duodenum through the major duodenal papilla. Accessory pancreatic duct of Santorini opens into the minor papilla just 2 cm proximal to the major duodenal papilla, which is formed by the persistent proximal part of the dorsal pancreatic duct without involution. A mechanism which involves the fibroblast growth factor-2 (FGF-2) produced by the developing heart also plays a vital role in the development of the pancreas. The development of the dorsal pancreatic bud depends on the notochord secreting activin (a TFG-β family member) and FGF-2 which block the expression of *SHH* gene in the duodenal endoderm. The PDX1 (pancreatic and duodenal homeobox 1) transcription factor is expressed in the duodenum to develop the ventral pancreatic bud.

Endodermal pancreatic buds proliferate and form the pancreatic parenchyma during 12th–16th week of the fetal development. The distal part of the proliferating pancreatic buds gives rise to the exocrine pancreatic acini and the ductal tributaries develop from the proximal portion of the proliferating pancreatic buds, which in turn drain into the second part of the duodenum as the hepatoduodenal ampulla of Vater. The pancreatic ductal branching pattern and the acinar structure are determined by the pancreatic mesenchyme. The chemokine *SDF-1* (stromal cell-derived factor) expressed in the mesenchyme regulates the formation and branching of the pancreatic ducts and buds. This pancreatic mesenchyme gives rise to the connective tissue sheath and the interlobular septa of the pancreas that are important in stimulating pancreatic proliferation and maintaining the relative proportions of acinar, alpha, and beta cells during development. The angiogenic mesenchyme invades the developing pancreas to produce the blood and the lymph vessels.

The endocrine pancreatic islet cells are initially located in the duct walls or in the pancreatic buds developing from them. Later, these endocrine cells separate from the duct or bud system and lie between the pancreatic acini. The pancreatic endocrine gland consists of beta, alpha, delta, polypeptide-producing, and clear cells. The beta cells account

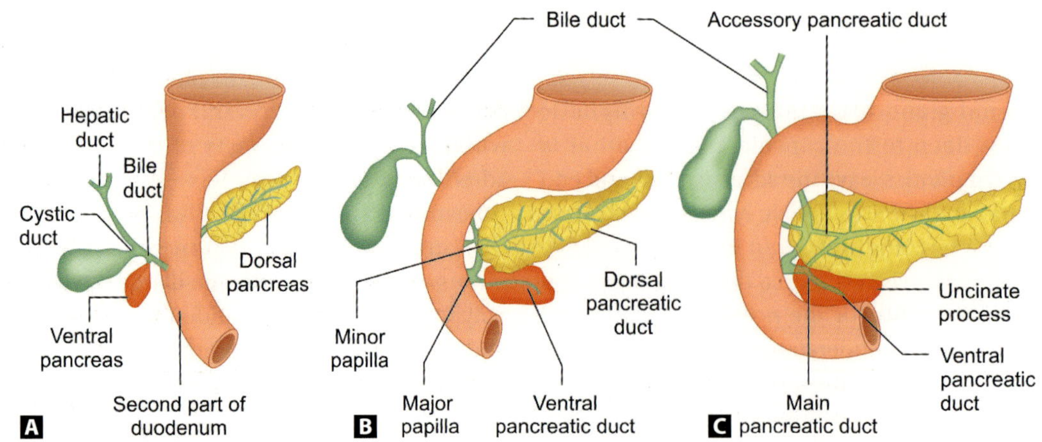

Figs. 11A to C: Stages in development of the pancreas. (A) The ventral pancreatic bud lies close to the liver bud; later, it moves posteriorly around the duodenum toward the dorsal pancreatic bud (5th week); (B) The ventral bud is in close contact with the dorsal pancreatic bud (6th week); (C) Fusion of the pancreatic buds and the ducts.

for approximately 70% of the islet cells, producing insulin and amylin, developing from the pancreatic duct epithelium. The alpha cells producing glucagon that constitutes 20% of islet cells and the pancreatic polypeptide-producing cells develop from the dorsal pancreatic bud. The insulin and glucagon secretion from the islets begins as early as the 15th week of the fetal development. Rest of the 5–10% of the islet cells are the delta cells, which produce somatostatin, gastrin, and pancreatic polypeptide seen only after 30 weeks. <5% of all the islet cells are clear cells with no described functional significance. The transcription factor Ngn-3 (neurogenin-3) expression is required for the differentiation of the pancreatic islet endocrine cells.

The malrotation of the ventral pancreas may result in an annular pancreas, which is a congenital malformation characterized by a ring of normal pancreatic tissue that encircles the second part of the duodenum. Sometimes, the annular pancreas constricts the second part of the duodenum and causes partial or complete obstruction in it. Hence, the annular pancreas probably results from the growth of a bifid ventral pancreatic bud and is common in females than males.

The fusion of the pancreatic ducts takes place late in the development of embryo or in the early postnatal period. In approximately 5–10% of individuals, the pancreatic ducts fail to join each other and remain as two separate pancreatic duct systems, called pancreatic divisum.

The ectopic or aberrant pancreatic tissues have been reported in 2% of the cases.[31] The ectopic pancreatic tissue in the form of nodular submucosal masses may be found in the stomach, duodenum, or jejunum.

◇ GROSS ANATOMY OF THE PANCREAS

The pancreas is a mixed endocrine and exocrine gland of the retroperitoneum that occupies the epigastric and left upper quadrant of the abdomen. Its extent is defined medially by the second part of the duodenum to the splenic hilum laterally, with the posterior extension across the L1 and L2 vertebrae on the posterior abdominal wall with relative mobility.

The adult pancreas weighs about 80–90 g. It is approximately 1–1.5 cm thick and 15–20 cm long with 3 cm width. IVC, portal vein, aorta, superior mesenteric and splenic vessels are anteriorly related to pancreas while the posterior relations are formed by the stomach and lesser sac, the spleen on the left, and the duodenum on the right. Pancreas is generally divided into five parts—head, neck, body, tail, and uncinate process. The C-loop of the duodenum shelves the expanded head of the pancreas. The pylorus of the stomach and the upper horizontal part of the duodenum form the anterior relation of the head of the pancreas as mentioned earlier. The medial border of the right kidney with the vasculature, IVC, and left renal vein lies posterior to the head of the pancreas. The terminal portion of the common bile duct courses posterior

to the head of the pancreas. The head of the pancreas and the C-shaped duodenum (descending, upper, and lower horizontal parts) share a common blood supply through the superior and inferior pancreaticoduodenal vessels from the gastroduodenal and the superior mesenteric vessels. So, the complete pancreatic head resection requires removal of the descending and most of the upper and lower horizontal portions of the duodenum.[32]

Head of the pancreas has an inferior projection called the uncinate process, which extends medially anterior to the IVC, left renal vein, and abdominal aorta, posterior to the superior mesenteric vessels and the portal vein. Numerous tiny superior mesenteric arterial branches course through the uncinate process to reach the head of the pancreas. This is referred to as the retroperitoneal margin of the pancreas, which is a very important concern when pancreaticoduodenectomy is performed for the malignancy due to the high rate of positive margins at this site.[33] Therefore, it is important to ascertain and clearly delineate the lateral margin of superior mesenteric artery in order to remove all the areolar, fibrous connective tissue in this retroperitoneal region.

The confluence of the superior mesenteric and splenic veins, which forms the portal vein, is anterior and flushes with the neck of the pancreas and is a short segment (1.5–2 cm). Pylorus of the stomach and the peritoneum covers the anterior part of the neck. There are no venous branches leaving the pancreatic neck into the superior mesenteric or portal veins. Usually, the presence of a cleavage plane between the neck of the pancreas and the underlying veins is noted, which can be separated by the simple blunt dissection. This is clinically important for the assessment of pancreatic resection. Identification of the superior mesenteric vein or the gastroduodenal artery and common bile duct or a combination of both of these methods is critical before the blunt dissection from the inferior or upper part of the neck of pancreas. During this maneuver, if the superior mesenteric or portal veins are cut, it is necessary to divide the neck of the pancreas to allow adequate space for the lateral venorrhaphy.

The portion of the pancreas to the left of the superior mesenteric vessels, overlying the L2 vertebra, is the pancreatic body. Peritoneum covers the anterior surface while posterior stomach bed is formed by the omental bursa and posterior part of the stomach. There is a nonperitoneal part of the posterior surface of the body of the pancreas, which has the splenic vessels lining the upper border with the aorta, left kidney, and left adrenal gland posteriorly. The body of the pancreas is closely associated with the lumbar vertebral bodies. So, the blunt trauma to the lumbar vertebral bodies may cause transaction to the pancreatic body. The short veins draining into the splenic vein constitute a major source of bleed in the body of the pancreas in a spleen-preserving distal pancreatectomy. Transverse colon forms the anterior attachment of the body of the pancreas. The middle colic artery is a branch of the superior mesenteric artery, runs beneath the body of the pancreas, and emerges between the peritoneal leaves of the transverse mesocolon **(Figs. 12A and B)**.

The pancreatic tail is relatively mobile, in front of the left kidney, and has its vessels at the level of T12 or L1 vertebra. It is found within the lienorenal ligament along with the splenic vessels at the splenic hilum. During splenectomy, the pancreatic tail may be at risk for the injury at the hilum of the spleen due to its relationship with the splenic vessels.

As discussed in the development section, the pancreas has a main pancreatic duct of Wirsung and an accessory pancreatic duct of Santorini. The main pancreatic duct, during its course from the tail to the pancreatic head, traverses through the pancreatic parenchyma close to its posterior surface and receives multiple small ductal tributaries. The main pancreatic duct receives the ductal tributaries from the uncinate process and then joins with the common bile duct that drains into a dilated, short, and common opening known as the ampulla of Vater. The smooth muscle sphincter around the intramural portion of the common bile duct and the main pancreatic duct is known as the sphincter of Oddi or the sphincter of Boyden. The ampulla of Vater passes through the major duodenal papilla, which is located in the second part of duodenum in the posteromedial wall, an average of 10.6 cm distal to the pylorus of the stomach.[33] Occasionally, the major duodenal papilla can be found in the third part of the duodenum.[34] A study showed that a true ampulla of Vater was found in 64%, and the common bile duct and main pancreatic duct entered the duodenum through separate openings in 14% of the cases.[35]

The ampulla of Vater length varies from 1 to 14 mm and is ≤5 mm length in 75% of the cases.[36] The main pancreatic duct length is generally between 15 and 20 cm. The diameters of the main pancreatic duct at different segments have been noted using the endoscopic retrograde cholangiopancreatography and vary from 0.9 to 2.4 mm in the tail, 2 to 4 mm in the body, and 3.1 to 5.3 mm in the pancreatic head.[37] The accessory duct of Santorini is smaller and is formed from the persistent proximal part of the duct from the embryonic dorsal pancreas. It drains the anterosuperior part of the head of pancreas and opens into the duodenum through the minor papilla, in the classical location in 70% of the cases. The minor duodenal papilla is usually located posterior to the gastroduodenal artery and thus is at risk for injury during surgery for the peptic ulcer disease. In case of peptic ulcer surgery, the duodenal dissection should end proximal to the gastroduodenal artery. Variations in the pancreatic ductal anatomy are common and specifically, the absence of a minor papilla in 30%, disconnected accessory and main pancreatic ducts in 10% of the cases was determined.[37]

Most of the arterial and the venous channels of the pancreas are situated posterior to the main pancreatic duct. The superior and the inferior pancreaticoduodenal arteries and tortuous splenic artery branches form the major arterial supply of the pancreas. The splenic artery traverses the superior border of the pancreas. The transverse pancreatic artery is a unique branch of the dorsal pancreatic artery, which may originate from the splenic artery in 37%, the celiac artery (33%), the superior mesenteric artery (21%), and the hepatic artery (8%).[38]

The pancreatic head and the C-loop of duodenum receive their arterial supply from an arterial arcade, formed by the confluence of the anterosuperior and the posterosuperior pancreaticoduodenal arteries of the gastroduodenal artery with the anteroinferior and posteroinferior pancreaticoduodenal arteries of the superior mesenteric artery. The supply of the uncinate process is mainly by the inferior pancreaticoduodenal artery collaterals and the perforators of the superior mesenteric artery. The head and uncinate process of the pancreas receive an additional arterial supply directly from a right branch of the dorsal pancreatic artery, anastomosing with the posterosuperior pancreaticoduodenal arterial arcade. The neck, body, tail, and the main pancreatic duct are supplied by the transverse pancreatic artery, which course inferiorly and posteriorly through the pancreas. The transverse pancreatic artery also anastomoses with small branches of the splenic artery. The tail of the pancreas receives an additional arterial supply from a caudal pancreatic artery, which may arise from the left gastroepiploic artery or the splenic artery at the hilum of the spleen **(Figs. 12A and B)**.

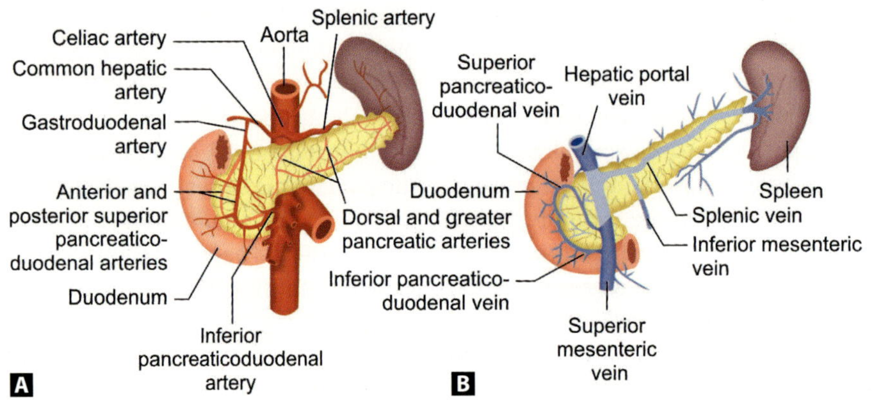

Figs. 12A and B: Relationships of the pancreas. (A) Arterial supply of the pancreas; (B) Venous drainage.

The important pancreatic arterial anomalies are reported in the literature. The surgeon must be able to identify the arterial anomalies to avoid injury during pancreatic surgery. The pancreatic arterial anomalies from the superior mesenteric artery pass anterior or posterior to or directly through the head of the pancreas.[37] The most common arterial anomaly is an aberrant right hepatic artery, arising from the superior mesenteric artery in 26% of the cadavers.[36] This aberrant right hepatic artery may run behind the head of the pancreas and be at risk for injury during pancreaticoduodenectomy. This aberrant right hepatic artery may be visible on preoperative computed tomographic (CT) scan in many cases. If an aberrant right hepatic artery is present, the palpable pulse can be felt from this artery within the posterolateral aspect of the porta hepatis. Dissection of the portal vein in the lateral aspect will typically help to identify this right hepatic artery, allow for its isolation and protection throughout the surgical procedure, especially important during removal of the uncinate process. The aberrant common hepatic artery may arise from the superior mesenteric artery in 2–4.5% of the cases. This aberrant common hepatic artery courses the pancreatic head posteriorly, before dividing into right and left hepatic arteries.[35] Injury to this aberrant common hepatic artery may result in both hepatic and duodenal ischemia and necrosis. The aberrant middle colic artery, originating from the superior mesenteric artery, may course directly through the head of the pancreas and be at risk for injury during pancreaticoduodenectomy.[35] If the aberrant middle colic artery is ligated proximally, the marginal artery of Drummond is typically present in most of the cases to prevent the colic ischemia.

The veins draining the pancreas are superficial to the pancreatic arteries. The uncinate process and head of the pancreas are drained by the venous arcade of the four pancreaticoduodenal veins.[35] The anterosuperior pancreaticoduodenal and both inferior (anterior and posterior) pancreaticoduodenal veins drain into the superior mesenteric vein, whereas the posterosuperior pancreaticoduodenal vein empties into the portal vein. The above veins and other tributaries from the pancreatic head terminate in the lateral or posterior part of the superior mesenteric and portal veins. They may be injured with traction on the head of the pancreas. These veins are thin, delicate, and variable with respect to the number and exact location. So, careful dissection is necessary to avoid their accidental avulsion and resultant bleeding. If bleeding occurs, it can be repaired using digital pressure rather than clamping to prevent further damage and perfuse bleeding. The neck, body, and tail of the pancreas are drained by many small veins that drain into either the splenic vein superiorly or the transverse pancreatic vein inferiorly. Splenic vein forms the drainage of the transverse pancreatic vein after emptying into the inferior mesenteric vein. Ligation of the splenic vein during distal pancreatectomy requires splenectomy whereas ligation of the

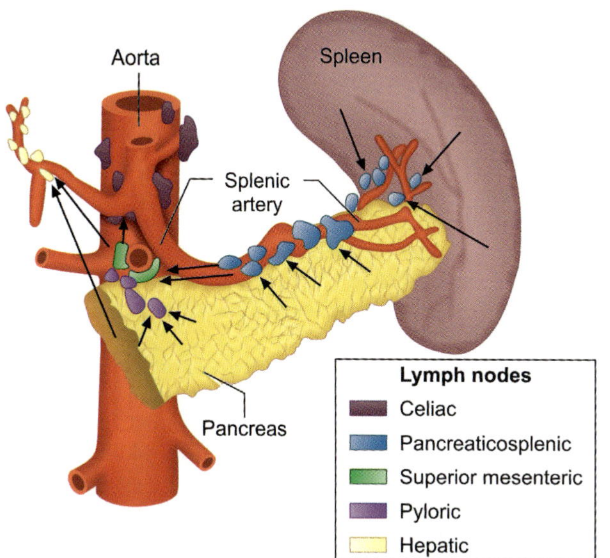

Fig. 13: Lymphatic drainage of the pancreas. The arrows signify flow of lymph into the lymph nodes.

splenic artery does not require resection of the spleen because the spleen still receives blood from the left gastroepiploic artery through the short gastric arteries. If ligation of the inferior mesenteric vein is mandatory during pancreatic mobilization, it may be undertaken with an exemption.

The pancreatic lymph vessels accompany the pancreatic vasculature. The lymph vessels from the uncinate process and head of the pancreas drain into the pyloric and the pancreaticoduodenal group of the lymph nodes. The neck, body, and pancreatic tail drain into the pancreaticosplenic group of the lymph nodes. The pyloric, pancreaticoduodenal, and superior pancreaticosplenic lymph nodes empty into the celiac nodes. The inferior pancreaticosplenic nodes empty into the superior mesenteric and the preaortic nodes. Based on the studies of metastatic drainage of the pancreas, there are five pancreatic groups of the lymph nodes—superior, inferior, anterior, posterior, and splenic.[38] The hepatic nodes form the drainage of the anterior, superior, and splenic lymph vessels after draining into the celiac nodes. The posterior and the inferior nodes empty into the superior mesenteric and preaortic nodes. Finally, the entire pancreatic lymphatic pathways subsequently drain through the thoracic duct and serve as a potential source for the supraclavicular nodal metastasis **(Fig. 13)**.

◇| REFERENCES

1. Standring S, Gray H. Gray's anatomy: The anatomical basis of clinical practice, 41st edition. Edinburgh: Churchill Livingstone/Elsevier; 2015.
2. Sadler TW, Thomas W, Langman J. Langman's Medical Embryology, 11th edition. Philadelphia: Wolters Kluwer Lippincott Williams & Wilkins; 2010.
3. Moore KL, Persaud TVN, Torchia MG. The developing human: clinically oriented embryology, 10th edition. Philadelphia: Saunders; 2015.

4. Clark OH, Duh QY, Gosnell JE, Kebebew E, Shen WT. Textbook of endocrine surgery, 3rd edition. New Delhi: Jaypee Bothers Medical Publishers; 2016.

5. Chen W, Liu Y, Wu K, Asmundo A, Sapienza D, Gianlorenzo D. Experience of the laryngeal recurrent nerve dissection in difficult thyroid surgery. Lin Chung Er Bi Yan Hou Tou Jing Wai Ke Za Zhi. 2014;28:318-21.

6. Keith ML, Dalley AF, Agur AMR. Clinically Oriented Anatomy, 8th edition. Philadelphia: Lippincott Williams & Wilkins; 2018.

7. Esen K, Ozgur A, Balci Y, Tok S, Kara E. Variations in the origins of the thyroid arteries on CT angiography. Jpn J Radiol. 2018;36:96-102.

8. Sasou S, Nakamura S, Kurihara H. Suspensory ligament of Berry: its relationship to recurrent laryngeal nerve and anatomic examination of 24 autopsies. Head Neck. 1998;20:695-8.

9. Zakaria HM, Al Awad NA, Al Kreedes AS, Al-Mulhim AMA, Al-Sharway MA, Hadi MA, et al. Recurrent laryngeal nerve injury in thyroid surgery. Oman Med J. 2011;26:34-8.

10. Shen C, Xiang M, Wu H, Ma Y, Chen L, Cheng L. Routine exposure of recurrent laryngeal nerve in thyroid surgery can prevent nerve injury. Neural Regen Res. 2013;8:1568-75.

11. Raffaelli M, Iacobone M, Henry JF. the false nonrecurrent inferior laryngeal nerve. Surgery. 2000;128:1082-7.

12. Ling XY, Smoll NR. A systematic review of variations of the recurrent laryngeal nerve. Clin Anat. 2016;29:104-10.

13. Bakalinis E, Makris I, Demesticha T, Tsakotos G, Skandalakis P, Filippou D. Non-recurrent laryngeal nerve and concurrent vascular variants: a review. Acta Med Acad. 2018;47:186-92.

14. Park JH, Lee YS, Kim BW, Chang HS, Park CS. Skip lateral node metastases in papillary thyroid carcinomas. World J Surg. 2012;36:743-7.

15. Noguchi S, Noguchi A, Murakami N. Papillary carcinoma of the thyroid: I. Developing pattern of metastasis. Cancer. 1970;2:1053-6.

16. Thompson NW, Eckhauser FE, Harness JK. The anatomy of primary hyperparathyroidism. Surgery. 1982;92(5):814-21.

17. Gilmour JR. The gross anatomy of the parathyroid glands. J Pathol. 1937;46:133-49.

18. Pyrtek L, Painter RL. An anatomic study of the relationship of the parathyroid glands to the recurrent laryngeal nerve. Surg Gynecol Obstet. 1964;119:509-12.

19. Filament JB, Delattre JF, Pluot M. Arterial blood supply to the parathyroid glands: implications for thyroid surgery. Anat Clin. 1982;3:279-287.

20. Bocian-Sobkowska J, Woźniak W, Malendowicz LK. Postnatal involution of the human adrenal fetal zone: stereologic description and apoptosis. Endocr Res. 1998;24(3-4):969-73.

21. Bocian-Sobkowska J. Morphometric study of the human suprarenal gland in the first postnatal year. Folia Morphol (Warsz). 2000;58(4):275-84.

22. Huber K, Karch N, Ernsberger U, Goridis C, Unsicker K. The role of Phox2B in chromaffin cell development. Dev Biol. 2005;279(2):501-8.

23. Pérez-Alvarez A, Hernández-Vivanco A, Albillos A. Past, present and future of human chromaffin cells: role in physiology and therapeutics. Cell Mol Neurobiol. 2010;30(8):1407-15.

24. Ishimoto H, Jaffe RB. Development and function of the human fetal adrenal cortex: a key component in the fetoplacental unit. Endocr Rev. 2011;32(3):317-55.

25. Pityński K, Skawina A, Polakiewicz J, Walocha J. Extraorganic vascular system of adrenal glands in human fetuses. Ann Anat. 1998;180(4):361-8.

26. Zuckerkandl E. The development of the chromaffin organs and the suprarenal glands. Manual of Human Embryology, volume 2. Philadelphia: JB Lippincott; 1912.

27. Russell RP, Masi AT, Richter ED. Adrenal cortical adenomas and hypertension. A clinical pathologic analysis of 690 cases with matched controls and a review of the literature. Medicine (Baltimore). 1972;51(3):211-25.

28. Neville AM, O'Hare MJ. Histopathology of the human adrenal cortex. Clin Endocrinol Metab. 1985;14(4):791-820.

29. Wood MA, Hammer GD. Adrenocortical stem and progenitor cells: unifying model of two proposed origins. Mol Cell Endocrinol. 2011;336(1-2):206-12.

30. Kikuta A, Murakami T. Microcirculation of the rat adrenal gland: a scanning electron microscope study of vascular casts. Am J Anat. 1982;164(1):19-28.

31. Pearson S. Aberrant pancreas: review of the literature and report of three cases, one of which produced common and pancreatic duct obstruction. Arch Surg. 1951;63:168.

32. Quinlan RM. Anatomy and embryology of the pancreas. In: Zuidema GD (Ed). Shackelford's Surgery of the Alimentary Tract. Philadelphia: WB Saunders; 1991.

33. Baldwin WM. The pancreatic ducts in man, together with a study of the microscopical structure of the minor duodenal papilla. Anat Rec. 1911;5:197-228.

34. Michels MA. Blood supply and anatomy of the upper abdominal organs. Philadelphia: JB Lippincott; 1955.

35. Skandalakis LJ, Rowe JS, Gray SW, Skandalakis JE. Surgical embryology and anatomy of the pancreas. Surg Clin North Am. 1993;73:661.

36. Pansky B. Anatomy of the pancreas. Emphasis on blood supply and lymphatic drainage. Int J Pancreatol. 1990;7:101.

37. Skandalakis JE, Gray SW, Rowe JS, Skandalakis LJ. Anatomical complications of pancreatic surgery. Contemp Surg. 1979;15: 17-50.

38. Angst E, Kim-Fuchs C, Kuruvilla Y, Inderbitzin D, Montani M, Candinas D, et al. How to counter the problem of R1 resection in duodenopancreatectomy for pancreatic cancer. J Gastrointest Surg. 2012;16:673.

Endocrine System Physiology

Sabaretnam M, Poongkodi K, Uma Devi, Prateek Mehrotra

INTRODUCTION AND THYROID PHYSIOLOGY

Sabaretnam M

◇ INTRODUCTION

The bodily activities of cells, tissues, and organs are coordinated by the interplay of several types of messengers.

- Neurotransmitters
- Endocrine hormones
- Neuroendocrine hormones
- Paracrine
- Autocrine
- Cytokines

◇ HORMONES

Hormones are released by glands or specialized cells into the circulation and they influence the function of target cells in another location.

The general class of hormones includes:

- Proteins and polypeptides
- Steroids
- Amino acid tyrosine derivatives

General characteristics of hormone secretion, duration of action, concentration, feedback, and transport have been explained in **Flowchart 1**.

Flowchart 1: General characteristics of hormone secretion, duration of action, concentration, feedback, and transport.

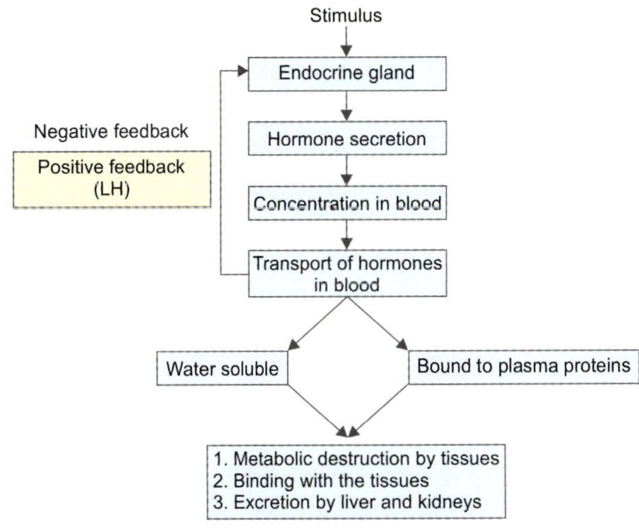

(LH: luteinizing hormone)

Hormones classified are also based on their receptors:

- *Hormones having intracellular receptors (cytoplasm or nucleus)*: Thyroid hormone and steroids
- *Hormones having cell-membrane receptors*:
  - Second messages cyclic adenosine monophosphate (cAMP)
  - Cyclic guanosine monophosphate (cGMP)
  - Calcium or phosphatidylinositol or both
  - Kinase or phosphate cascade

Measurement of Hormone Concentration in the Blood

Hormones are present in extremely minute quantities sometimes as low as 1 billionth of a milligram (1 picogram) per milliliter. Radioimmunoassay using antibody specific for the hormone and mixed with the radioactive isotope and the quantity of hormone is measured. Enzyme-linked immunosorbent assay used to measure any proteins including hormones using specific antibodies without radioactive isotopes.

◇ THYROID GLAND PHYSIOLOGY

Thyroid gland is a highly vascular ductless alveolar gland; infront of trachea located in the anterior neck and has two lobes right and left connected by the isthmus. The cellular composition includes follicular (epithelial) cells involved in thyroid hormone synthesis endothelial cells living the capillaries that provide blood supply to the follicles.

Parafollicular or "C" cells involved in production of calcitonin fibroblasts, lymphocytes, and adipocytes.

Thyroid Hormones

The thyroid secretes two significant hormones, the thyroxine and tri-iodothyroxine commonly called T4 and T3, respectively. About 93% of the metabolically active hormone secreted by the thyroid gland is thyroxine and 7% tri-iodothyroxine. However, almost all the thyroxines are eventually converted to tri-iodothyroxine in the tissues.

Physiologic Anatomy of the Thyroid Gland

The secretory or functional unit of the thyroid gland is the thyroid follicle (100–300 cm in diameter), consisting of a layer of epithelial cells arranged around central cavity filled with colloid. Colloid makes up to 30% of the thyroid gland weight and contains a protein called thyroglobulin (Tg). Tg plays a crucial role in the synthesis and storage of thyroid hormone.

Iodine

1 mg/week of iodine is needed for the formation of thyroid hormones. The ingested iodides are absorbed from the gastrointestinal tract into the blood. One-fifth of the absorbed iodides are selectively removed from the circulation by the cells of the thyroid gland for synthesis of thyroid hormones.

Iodide Pump and Iodide Trapping

The first stage in the formation of thyroid hormone is the transport of iodides from the blood into the thyroid glandular cells and follicles. The basal membrane of the thyroid cell has the specific ability to pump the iodide actively into the cell which is known as iodide trapping.

In a normal gland the iodide pump concentrates iodide to about 30 times of its concentration in the blood and when maximally active on rise up to 250 times. The rate of iodide trapping is influenced by thyroid stimulating hormone (TSH).

Formation of Thyroglobulin

The endoplasmic reticulum and Golgi apparatus synthesis are a large glycoprotein with a molecular weight of 335,000 and each molecule contains about 70 tyrosine amino acid residues which are the major substrate that combine with iodine to form thyroid hormones.

Oxidation of Iodine Ion

It is done by enzyme peroxidase which is located in the apical membrane of the cell.

Organification of Thyroglobulin

The binding of iodine with thyroglobulin is called organification. Oxidized iodine will bind directly to tyrosine slowly but iodinase enzyme makes this process to occur in seconds or minutes **(Flowchart 2)**.

Tyrosine is oxidized to monoiodotyrosine and then to di-iodotyrosine and finally the two important hormones thyroxine and tri-iodothyroxine forms.

Storage of Thyroglobulin

The thyroid gland has the ability to store large amount of hormone and can supply about 2–3 months requirements.

Release of Thyroxine and Tri-iodothyroxine

The apical surface has pseudopod extensions around small portion of colloid to form pinocytic vesicles that enter the apex of the thyroid cell. Then lysosomes in the cell cytoplasm will fuse to form digestive vesicles containing digestive enzymes from the lysosomes mixed with the colloid **(Fig. 1)**.

Multiple proteinases digest the thyroglobulin molecules and release thyroxine and tri-iodothyroxine in free form.

Transport and Tissue Delivery of Thyroid Hormones

Once thyroid hormones are released into circulation, they circulate bound to protein. Approximately 70% of T4 and T3 is bound to thyroid binding globulin. A small fraction 0.03% of T4 and 0.3% of T3 circulates in its free form. This fraction of the circulating hormone pool is bioavailable and can enter the cell to bind to the thyroid receptor. T4 binds more tightly compared to T3 and thus has a lower metabolic clearance rate and a longer half-life (7 days) than T3 (1 day). The kidneys readily excrete free T4 and T3.

Thyroid Hormone Metabolism

Thyroid release T4 and very small amounts of T3, yet T3 has grater thyroid activity than T4. The main source of circulating T3 is peripheral deiodination of T4 by deiodinases **(Flowchart 3)**.

Type I deiodinase catalysis outer and inner ring deiodination of T4 and rT3 predominantly found in liver, kidney, and thyroid. Type II is expressed in brain, pituitary, and placenta and only has outer ring activity and Type III deiodinase is expressed in brain and only has inner ring activity.

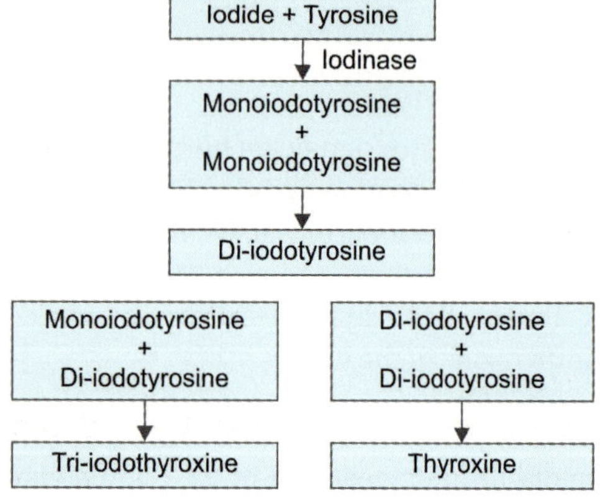

Flowchart 2: Oxidation of iodine ion.

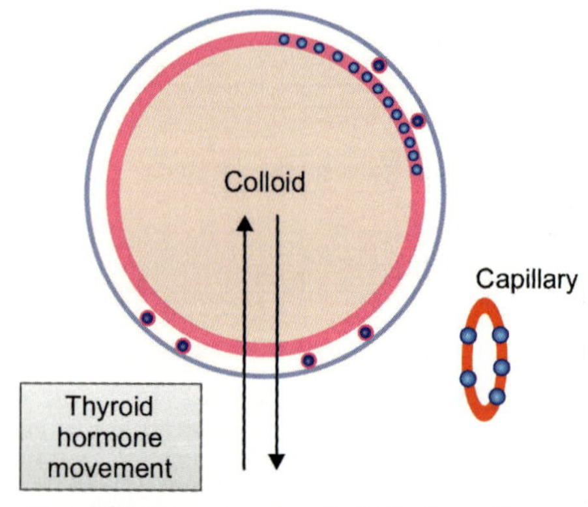

Fig. 1: Thyroid hormone synthesis—follicullar cell.

Flowchart 3: Deiodination of thyroid hormone.

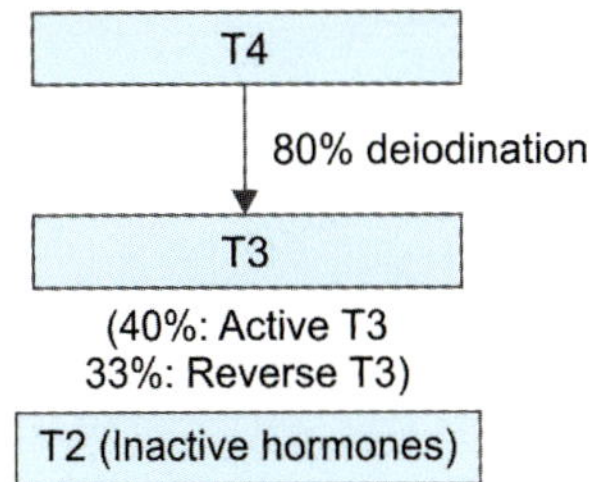

Biologic Effects of Thyroid Hormones

Receptors are expressed in virtually all tissues and affect multiple cellular events. The effects are medicated by transcriptional regulation of target genes and are known as genomic effects. Thyroid hormone has nongenomic effects which include stimulation of activity of Ca^{2+}-ATPase at the plasma membrane and sarcoplasmic reticulum.

Thyroid Hormone Receptors

Thyroid hormone receptors are nuclear receptors intimately associated with chromatin. They bind thyroid hormones with high affinity and specificity. Thyroid hormone receptors are DNA-binding transcription factors that function as molecular switches in response to hormone binding.

Organ—specific effects of thyroid hormone: Thyroid hormones are essential for normal growth and development, they control the rate of metabolism and hence the function of practically every organ.

Bone—essential for bone growth activates osteoclast and osteoblast activities.

Cardiovascular system—has cardiac ionotropic and chronotropic effects, increases cardiac output and blood volume, and decreases vascular resistance.

Fat—induces white adipose tissue differentiation lipogenic enzymes, intracellular lipid accumulation, and adipocyte proliferation.

Liver—regulates cholesterol and triglyceride metabolism.

Pituitary—regulates synthesis of pituitary hormones, stimulates growth hormones production, and inhibits TSH.

Brain—controls expression of genes involved in myelination, cell differentiation, and migration and signaling.

Disease of thyroid hormone overproduction and undersecretion: The widespread distribution of thyroid hormone receptors and multitude of physiologic effects, hormone overproduction and undersecretion results in multitude of effects.

Dysfunction can result from three factors:
1. Alternations in the circulating levels of thyroid hormones
2. Impaired metabolism of thyroid hormones in the periphery
3. Resistance to thyroid hormone actions at the tissue level

Hypersecretion and hyposecretion of thyroid hormones and their various metabolic effects are discussed in concerned chapters.

◇| SUGGESTED READING

1. Davies TF, Yin X, Latif R. The genetics of the thyroid stimulating hormone receptor: history and relevance. Thyroid. 2010;20(7):727-36.
2. Kundra P, Burman KD. The effect of medications on thyroid function tests. Medical Clinics. 2012;96(2):283-95.
3. Lamb MR, Janevic T, Liu X, Cooper T, Kline J, Factor-Litvak P. Environmental lead exposure, maternal thyroid function, and childhood growth. Environmental Research. 2008;106(2): 195-202.
4. Mihai R. Physiology of the pituitary, thyroid and adrenal glands. Surgery (Oxford). 2011;29(9):419-27.
5. Pearce EN. The relationship between serum TSH and free T4 is not log-linear and varies by age and sex. N Engl J Med. 1987;316:764-0.
6. Stathatos N. Anatomy and physiology of the thyroid gland. The Thyroid and its Diseases. 2019 (pp. 3-12). Springer, Cham.
7. Stathatos N. Thyroid physiology. Medical Clinics of North America. 2012;96(2):165.

PHYSIOLOGY OF PARATHYROID GLAND AND CALCIUM HOMEOSTASIS

Poongkodi K

◇| FUNCTIONAL ANATOMY

In 1880, the Swedish anatomist Victor Sandstorm first described a small gland in the vicinity of thyroid and named it glandulae parathyroidea. Humans usually have four parathyroid glands: two embedded in the superior poles of the thyroid and two in its inferior poles. Each parathyroid gland is a richly vascularized disk, about 3×6×2 mm, containing two distinct types of cells. The abundant *chief cells*, which contain a prominent Golgi apparatus, endoplasmic reticulum and secretory granules, synthesize and secrete *parathyroid hormone (PTH)*. The less abundant and larger *oxyphil cells* contain oxyphil granules and large numbers of mitochondria in their cytoplasm. In humans, few are seen before puberty, and thereafter they increase in number with age.

◇| PARATHYROID HORMONE

Human PTH is a linear polypeptide with a molecular weight of 9,500 that contains 84 amino acid residues (**Fig. 2**).

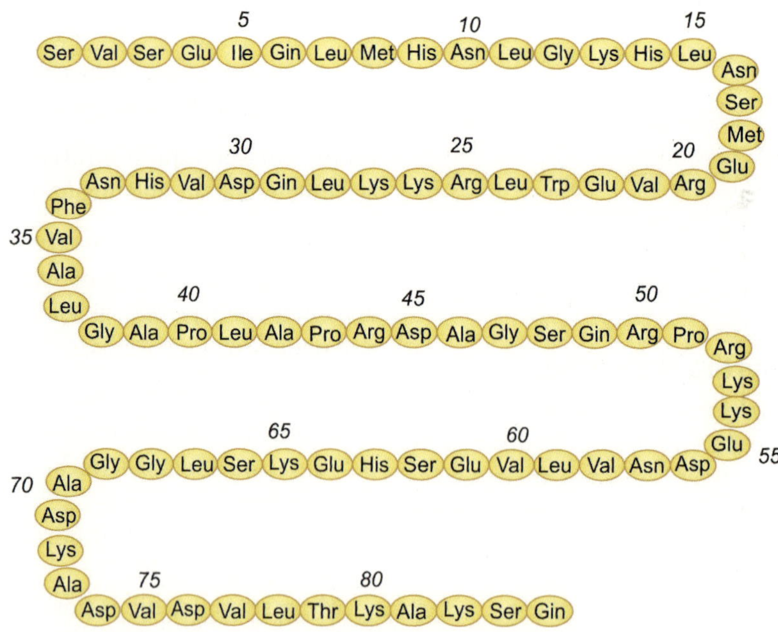

Fig. 2: Amino acid sequence of human parathyroid hormone.

PTH plays critical roles in calcium homeostasis and bone biology. First discovered as a calcium-regulating hormone in the 1920s, PTH is produced almost exclusively by the chief cells of parathyroid glands in mammals.

THE HUMAN PARATHYROID HORMONE GENE AND ITS MESSENGER RIBONUCLEIC ACID

The human *PTH* gene consists of three exons located on chromosome 11p15. The first exon is 85 nucleotides in length and is noncoding. Exon 2 (90 bp) encodes most amino acids of the prepropeptide sequence, whereas the third exon (612 bp) encodes the remainder of the propeptide sequence and all amino acids of the mature peptide, and it constitutes the 3′ noncoding region. Two messenger ribonucleic acids (mRNAs) that are 822 and 793 bp in length are derived in the human gene from the two transcriptional start sites, which follow two different functional TATA boxes that are separated by 29 bp.

PARATHYROID HORMONE BIOSYNTHESIS AND INTRAGLANDULAR PROCESSING

During the synthesis of the preproPTH molecule (115 amino acid residue), the signal sequence, which comprises the 25-amino-acid-containing "pre" sequence, is cleaved off after entry of the nascent peptide chain into the intracisternal space bounded by the endoplasmic reticulum. Subsequently, the pro-peptide (90 residue) is transported to the trans-Golgi network, where the prosequence (amino acid residues –6 through –1) is removed. This latter process may involve furin (paired basic amino acid cleaving enzyme) and/or proprotein convertase-7 (PC-7), which are both expressed in parathyroid tissue; their expression levels do not appear to be regulated by either calcium or $1,25(OH)_2D_3$. After removal of the basic prosequence, the mature polypeptide, PTH (84 amino acid residue), is packaged into secretory granules. This intact PTH (1–84) is the biologically active major secretory product of the parathyroid gland. Two proteases, cathepsins B and H, are subsequently involved in the intraglandular generation of carboxyl-terminal PTH fragments from the intact hormone; little amino-terminal PTH fragments appear to be released from the gland. Since small or intermediate-size carboxyl-terminal fragments of PTH are unlikely to be involved in the regulation of calcium homeostasis, the intraglandular degradation of intact PTH represents inactivating pathway. The pool of stored, intracellular PTH is small, and the parathyroid cell must therefore have mechanisms to increase hormone synthesis and release in response to sustained hypocalcemia. One such adaptive mechanism is to reduce the intracellular degradation of the hormone, thereby increasing the net amount of intact, biologically active PTH that is available for secretion. During hypocalcemia, the bulk of the hormone that is released from the parathyroid cell is intact PTH (1–84). As the level of extracellular Ca^{2+} (Ca^{2+}_o) increases, a greater fraction of intracellular PTH is degraded, and with overt hypercalcemia, most of the secreted immunoreactive PTH consists of biologically inactive C-terminal fragments and a few aminoterminus truncated species (7–84) having hypocalcemic properties. PTH synthesis is continuous. Its release is also continuous, with about 6–7 superimposed pulses each hour. Most PTH release (70%) occurs during the continuous or tonic phase, and approximately 30% can be attributed to pulsatile secretion. PTH is metabolized by the high capacity degradative systems (including kupffer cells) in the liver and kidney. Hepatic clearance of intact

PTH (40–75%) predominates over renal clearance of 20–30%. Rapid clearance of intact hormone contributes to short half-life of 2–4 minutes. Evidence regarding the renal clearance and metabolism of intact PTH (as distinct from C-terminal fragments) indicates a peritubular uptake process. Furthermore, other studies indicate that megalin, a multifunctional endocytic receptor expressed in the proximal renal tubules, can mediate the reuptake and subsequent degradation of the fraction of PTH that is subject to glomerular filtration. Megalin-mediated uptake depends on an intact N-terminus of PTH; C-terminal fragments that are eliminated by glomerular filtration are not recognized by megalin. Biologically active N-terminal fragments of PTH (1–34), if found in the circulation at all, are likely to circulate only at extremely low concentrations (<10–13 to 10–14 mol/L). In contrast, the inactive carboxy-terminal fragments having a longer half-life constitute 80% of the circulating PTH species and intact hormone accounts for 10% of the circulating PTH-related peptides. The normal plasma value of iPTH is 10–65 pg/mL. Newer immunoradiometric assays for PTH have N-terminal epitopes at extreme aminoterminus to detect only the intact PTH (1–84) and not these fragments in order to obtain an accurate measure of "bioactive" PTH.

◇ REGULATION OF PARATHYROID HORMONE GENE EXPRESSION

A reduction in Ca^{2+}_o increases, whereas an elevation in Ca^{2+}_o reduces the cellular levels of PTH mRNA by affecting both its stability and the rate of gene transcription. Phosphate ions also regulate, directly or indirectly, *PTH* gene expression. Hypophosphatemia and hyperphosphatemia, respectively, lower and raise the levels of mRNA for PTH through a mechanism that is independent of changes in Ca^{2+}_o or $1,25(OH)_2D_3$. Thus, elevated phosphate levels in renal failure results in secondary hyperparathyroidism.

Metabolites of vitamin D, principally $1,25(OH)_2D_3$, exerts long-term control on parathyroid function at several levels: by affecting the secretion of PTH and regulation of its gene; by regulating transcriptional activity of the genes encoding the calcium-sensing receptor (CaSR) and the vitamin D receptor (VDR); as well as by regulating parathyroid cellular proliferation. $1,25(OH)_2D_3$ acts through a nuclear receptor, the VDR, often in concert with other such receptors (i.e., those for retinoic acid or glucocorticoids), on DNA sequences upstream from the *PTH* gene. $1,25(OH)_2D_3$-induced upregulation of VDR and CaSR expression in the parathyroid could potentiate its inhibitory action(s) on PTH synthesis and secretion. Noncalcemic or less calcemic analogs of $1,25(OH)_2D_3$ inhibit PTH secretion while producing relatively little stimulation of intestinal calcium absorption and bone resorption and may thus be attractive candidates for treating the hyperparathyroidism of chronic renal insufficiency.

◇ REGULATION OF PARATHYROID HORMONE SECRETION BY Ca^{2+}_o AND OTHER FACTORS: THE OVERALL SECRETORY RESPONSE OF THE PARATHYROID CELL TO ALTERATIONS IN Ca^{2+}_o

The main physiologic effect of PTH is to maintain Ca^{2+} homeostasis. Its release is controlled in a tight feedback system by plasma Ca^{2+} concentrations. Small changes in the levels of Ca^{2+}_o are detected by the parathyroid Ca^{2+}-sensing receptor. The parathyroid cell manifests a temporal hierarchy of responses to decreases in Ca^{2+}_o that permits a progressively larger PTH secretory response that is appropriate for the rapidity, magnitude, and duration of the hypocalcemic stress. The most rapid response is the release of preformed PTH stored within secretory granules. This response occurs within seconds and can persist for as long as 60–90 minutes before these stores are completely depleted. This immediate secretory response exhibits a steep inverse sigmoidal relationship between PTH secretion and the level of Ca^{2+}_o **(Fig. 3)**. Four parameters of the curve are: parameter A, maximal secretory rate at low Ca^{2+}_o; parameter B, slope at the midpoint; parameter C, midpoint or "set point" (the level of Ca^{2+}_o half-maximally suppressing PTH); and parameter D, minimal secretory rate at high Ca^{2+}_o. Parameter A is the sum of the maximal rates of PTH release from all individual parathyroid chief cells, as reflected by the resultant, maximally stimulated level of circulating PTH. The steepness of the curve contributes importantly to the nearly constant level of Ca^{2+}_o. Indeed, parathyroid cells can readily detect reductions in Ca^{2+}_o of a few percentage points, and the

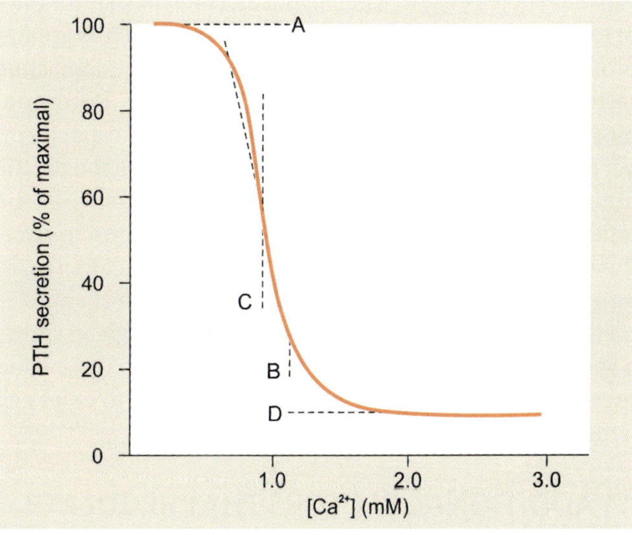

Fig. 3: Inverse sigmoid curve that shows the relationship between plasma calcium levels [Ca^{2+}] and parathyroid hormone (PTH) secretion rate in human parathyroid cells. *Point A:* Highest PTH secretion rate at low Ca^{2+}; *Point D:* Lowest PTH secretion rate at high Ca^{2+}; *Point B:* midpoint of slope of the curve; and, *Point C:* Ca^{2+} level half maximally suppressing PTH.

percent coefficient of variation in Ca^{2+}_0 in humans is <2%. The set point of the parathyroid gland is the key determinant of the level at which Ca^{2+}_0 is "set," thereby serving as one of the body's key "thermostats" for Ca^{2+}_0, or "calciostats". Thus, for a given Ca^{2+}_0, there is an optimal PTH level in the circulation which may be altered in diseased state. Thus, the parathyroid cell is normally more than half-maximally suppressed at normal levels of Ca^{2+}_0 and has a large secretory reserve for responding to hypocalcemic stress. Nevertheless, PTH levels fall dramatically (e.g., by 80%) when Ca^{2+}_0 rises to frankly hypercalcemic levels. In addition, elevated Ca^{2+}_0 increases intraglandular PTH degradation into inactive fragments, thereby decreasing the proportion of secreted intact PTH. Even with severe hypercalcemia, however, some residual release of intact PTH (1–84) still occurs and persists at a level approximately 5% of that observed with a maximal hypocalcemic stimulus. This nonsuppressible basal component of PTH release may contribute to the hypercalcemia caused by hyperparathyroidism when the mass of abnormal parathyroid tissue is very great (e.g., in patients with renal failure).

The PTH levels *depend* not only on Ca^{2+}_0 *per se,* but also on the rate of change of Ca^{2+}_0. This "rate-dependence" is apparent when Ca^{2+}_0 is falling rapidly, which elicits a more vigorous secretory response than when Ca^{2+}_0 decreases slowly. There is also direction dependence or hysteresis manifested by higher levels of PTH that are observed when Ca^{2+}_0 is falling than when it is rising. With sustained low levels of Ca^{2+}_0 over hours to days, the parathyroid cell also exhibits graded greater expression of the PTH gene, resulting from both increased transcription and enhanced stability of the mRNA encoding preproPTH. The resultant increase in the mRNA level for preproPTH is also accompanied by a more general increase in the parathyroid cell's biosynthetic capacity. In particular, when hypocalcemia persists for days or longer, it induces morphologic alterations such as greater prominence of organelles (such as the rough endoplasmic reticulum and Golgi apparatus) involved in hormonal biosynthesis, thereby increasing their secretory capacity on *per* cell basis. Finally, over several days to weeks or longer, the initiation of parathyroid cellular proliferation increases the total number of parathyroid chief cells and, as a consequence, the total secretory capacity for PTH by manyfold. Increases rather than decreases in Ca^{2+}_0 produce opposite changes in parathyroid cell function. However, parathyroid gland shows a sluggish and rather an incomplete capacity to rid itself of excess parathyroid chief cells once a stimulus to chief cell hyperplasia has abated.

ADDITIONAL FACTORS THAT REGULATE PARATHYROID HORMONE RELEASE

In addition to Ca^{2+}_0, several other factors, including vitamin D metabolites (especially $1,25(OH)_2D_3$), catecholamines and other biogenic amines, prostaglandins and peptide hormones, and phosphate and monovalent cations (e.g., potassium and lithium), also modulate PTH secretion. Of these, the most physiologically relevant are probably $1,25(OH)_2D_3$ and phosphate. $1,25(OH)_2D_3$ is thought to play an important role in the long-term (over days or longer) control of parathyroid function, tonically reducing PTH secretion, diminishing expression of the PTH gene, and probably inhibiting parathyroid cellular proliferation. Thus, actions of PTH on its target tissues produce negative-feedback regulation of parathyroid cellular function not only by raising Ca^{2+}_0 but also by enhancing the synthesis of $1,25(OH)_2D_3$, which then directly exerts negative feedback actions on parathyroid function **(Fig. 4)**. A rise or fall in plasma phosphate concentration will increase or decrease, respectively, PTH secretion, PTH gene expression, and parathyroid cellular proliferation. Also, novel factors involved in phosphate homeostasis, namely FGF-23 (a phosphaturic hormone) and α-klotho (a coreceptor for FGF receptors), inhibit and enhance parathyroid function, respectively. Plasma Mg^{2+} levels also regulate PTH secretion in a similar manner to that of calcium. PTH release can be stimulated by a decrease in plasma Mg^{2+}. Magnesium depletion or deficiency is frequently associated with hypocalcemia. This combined decrease in Mg^{2+} and Ca^{2+} leads to impairment in the individual's ability to secrete PTH. Moreover, severe hypomagnesemia not only impairs the PTH release but also decreases the target organ responsiveness to PTH. Adrenergic agonists have been shown to increase PTH release through β-adrenergic receptors on parathyroid cells.

PARATHYROID Ca²⁺ SENSING RECEPTOR

The Ca^{2+} sensor is a G protein ($G_{q/11}$ and G_i)–coupled receptor located on the plasma membrane of the parathyroid chief cells; it is also found in kidney tubule cells and thyroid C cells. Elevations in plasma Ca^{2+} concentrations lead to activation of CaSR and consequently, inhibition of PTH release. Activation of the CaSR initiates a signaling cascade involving phospholipases C, D, and A_2. The phosphorylation and activation of phospholipase A_2 activate the arachidonic acid cascade and increase leukotriene synthesis. The active leukotriene metabolites inhibit PTH secretion. Interestingly, the inhibition of PTH secretion by elevated Ca^{2+} levels is not due to an alteration in the rate of PTH synthesis, but due to increased degradation of preformed hormone into inactive fragments. The amino acids released during degradation of the formed PTH inside the parathyroid cells are reused in the synthesis of other proteins. In contrast, inhibition of PTH release by the active form of vitamin D ($1,25$-dihydroxyvitamin D_3; $1,25(OH)_2 D_3$) is the result of a decrease in PTH gene expression. During hypocalcemia, the parathyroid Ca^{2+} receptor is relaxed, not restrained. The rapid secretion of preformed PTH elicited by acute hypocalcemia is followed by increased stability of PTH mRNA and subsequently, the synthesis of new hormone on persistent hypocalcemia.

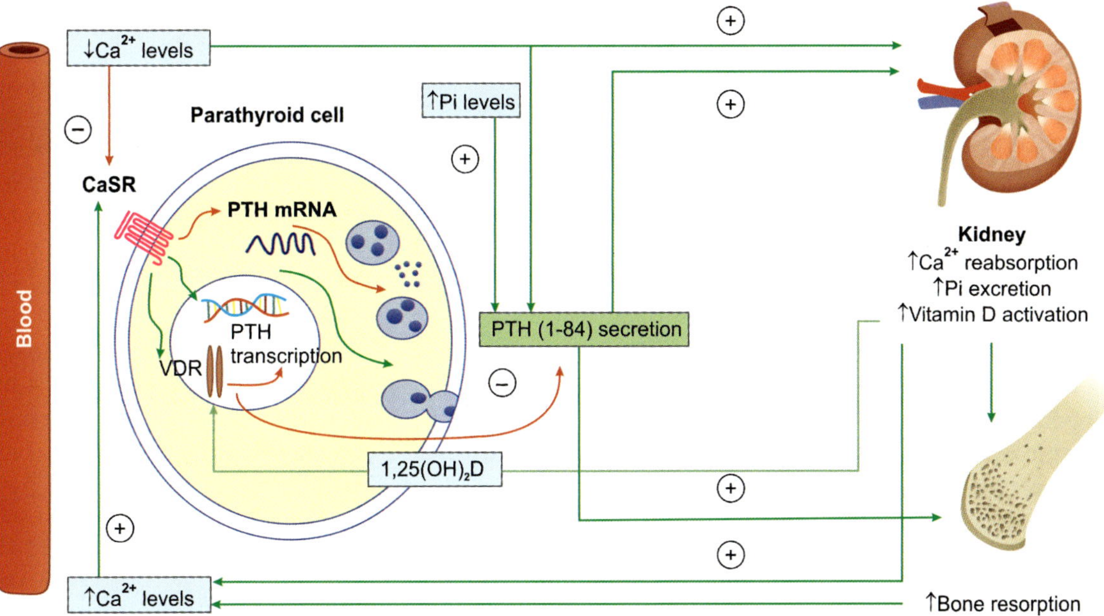

Fig. 4: Regulation of parathyroid hormone (PTH) release. A sudden fall in plasma calcium (Ca²⁺) levels stimulates PTH release from parathyroid gland. PTH increases calcium reabsorption and phosphate (Pi) excretion in urine. In addition, PTH increases vitamin D activation through increased renal 1-hydroxylase activity and indirectly enhances intestinal calcium and phosphate absorption. The rise in vitamin D and plasma calcium levels, in turn, exert negative feedback inhibition of PTH release. Elevations in plasma phosphate levels stimulate the PTH release. (mRNA: messenger ribonucleic acid; VDR: Vitamin D receptor)

◇ PARATHYROID HORMONE TARGET ORGANS AND PHYSIOLOGIC EFFECTS

The primary target organs for the physiologic effects of PTH are kidney and bone. The main physiologic response elicited by PTH is to increase plasma calcium levels by increasing renal Ca²⁺ reabsorption, bone resorption, and intestinal absorption indirectly (via vitamin D_3 activation). PTH also increases 1α-hydroxylase activity and renal phosphate excretion. As with other peptide hormones, the effects of PTH are mediated by binding to a cell membrane receptor in target organs. Three types of PTH receptors (PTHRs) have been identified (PTHR-1, PTHR-2, and PTHR-3), all of which are G protein-coupled receptors. The important physiologic effects of PTH are mediated by hPTH/PTHrP or PTHR-1; a second receptor, PTH-2 (hPTH2-R), does not bind PTHrP and is found in the brain, placenta, and pancreas. In addition, there is evidence for a third receptor, CPTH, which reacts with the carboxyl terminal rather than the amino terminal of PTH. The first two receptors are coupled to Gs, and via this heterotrimeric G protein they activate adenylyl cyclase, increasing intracellular cAMP. The hPTH/PTHrP receptor also activates PLC via Gq, increasing intracellular Ca²⁺ and activating protein kinase C.

Parathyroid Hormone Receptor 1 or hPTH/PTHrP Receptor and Mechanism of Signal Transduction

Parathyroid hormone receptor 1 (PTHR-1) is expressed in bone osteoblasts and kidney, where it binds PTH and PTH-related protein (PTHrP). PTHrP is important because it mimics the physiologic effects of PTH in the bone and kidney. Unlike PTH, PTHrP is expressed in multiple adult and fetal tissues, encoded by chromosome 12p12.1–11.2. PTHrP was recently discovered as the humoral factor inducing hypercalcemia of malignancy. Thus, PTH/PTHrP receptor (PTHR 1) not only mediates the endocrine effects of PTH, but also mediates autocrine/paracrine effects of PTHrP. PTH binding to the G protein-coupled PTHR-1 initiates a cascade of intracellular processes primarily by signaling through the α-subunit of the stimulatory G-protein, $G_{\alpha s}$ leading to an increased synthesis of cAMP and activation of protein kinase A and phosphorylation of target proteins at serine residues. The result is the activation of preformed proteins as well as the induction of gene transcription. Other pathways include: Gαq-phospholipase C (PLC) β-inositol triphosphate-cytoplasmic Ca²⁺-protein kinase C; $G\alpha_{12/13}$-phospholipase D-transforming protein RhoA; and β-arrestin-extracellular signal-regulated kinase 1/2 (ERK-1/2).

◇ CELLULAR EFFECTS OF PARATHYROID HORMONE IN KIDNEY

As mentioned earlier, PTH directly stimulates Ca²⁺ reabsorption in the kidney, it decreases the reabsorption of phosphate, and it stimulates the activity of 1-α-hydroxylase, the enzyme responsible for formation of the active form of vitamin $D(1,25(OH)_2 D_3)$. Approximately 10 g of calcium is filtered at the glomerulus daily. The bulk of Ca²⁺ reabsorption (65%) occurs via passive, paracellular mechanisms in the proximal tubules and to a lesser extent (20%) in the thick ascending limb of Henle's loop, and (10%) the distal convoluted tubule.

The calcium-sensing receptor plays an important PTH-independent role in the adjustment of renal calcium reabsorption in the cortical thick ascending limb (CTAL). The physiologically important PTH-mediated renal calcium reabsorption (8–10%) occurs almost entirely in the distal nephron.

Ca²⁺ reabsorption in the proximal tubule is closely coupled to the bulk transport of solutes, such as sodium and water, and PTH has little effect on Ca²⁺ transport in this segment of the nephron. Perhaps, PTH modestly inhibits proximal tubular Ca²⁺ absorption by decreasing sodium conductance. It exerts this effect, similar to its other biologic actions in the kidney, by interacting with its own G-protein-coupled receptor that is linked to activation of both adenylate cyclase and phospholipase C. cAMP appears to play the dominant role in mediating PTH-induced alterations in renal Ca²⁺ handling. In the CTAL, PTH increases the overall activity of the Na/K/2Cl cotransporter that drives transcellular NaCl reabsorption in this nephron segment. This increased transcellular salt transport elevates the lumen-positive, transepithelial potential difference that drives paracellular transport of Ca²⁺ and Mg²⁺ in the CTAL through paracellin 1 responsible for Cl⁻ conductance. In contrast, CaSR present along the basolateral membrane of the same epithelial cells of the CTAL decreases overall cotransporter activity, probably both by inhibiting the cotransporter as well as by reducing the activity of an apical potassium channel that recycles K⁺ back into the tubular lumen. The resultant decrease in the transepithelial potential gradient diminishes the paracellular reabsorption of both Ca²⁺ and Mg²⁺.

The calcium-sensing receptor probably also inhibits adenylate cyclase, which decreases hormone- and cAMP-stimulated divalent cation transport.

In the distal convoluted tubule, Ca²⁺ absorption is entirely transcellular and is regulated by PTH, vitamin D, and calcitonin; it can also be affected by Ca²⁺-sparing drugs such as thiazide diuretics. PTH stimulates the insertion and opening of the epithelial Ca²⁺ channel type 1 (ECaC-1 or transient receptor potential vanilloid type 5, TRPV-5) on the apical/brush border membrane, facilitating the entry of Ca²⁺ into the cell. These epithelial cells, such as the thyroid follicular epithelial cells, are polarized; that is, they permit unidirectional flux of the ion from the apical to the basolateral membrane as illustrated in **Figure 5**. Inside the tubular epithelial cell, Ca²⁺ binds to calbindin-D$_{28K}$ and then diffuses out through the basolateral membrane. Calbindin-D$_{28K}$ is a vitamin D-dependent calcium-binding protein that is present in the cytosol of cells lining the distal part of the nephron. Calbindin is thought to act as either a transport protein or a buffer to prevent excess elevation of cytosolic Ca²⁺ levels; it facilitates the cytosolic diffusion of Ca²⁺ from the apical influx to the basolateral efflux sites. Transport of Ca²⁺ out of the cell into the interstitial space is mediated by a Na⁺/Ca²⁺ exchanger and a Ca²⁺ adenosine triphosphatase (ATPase).

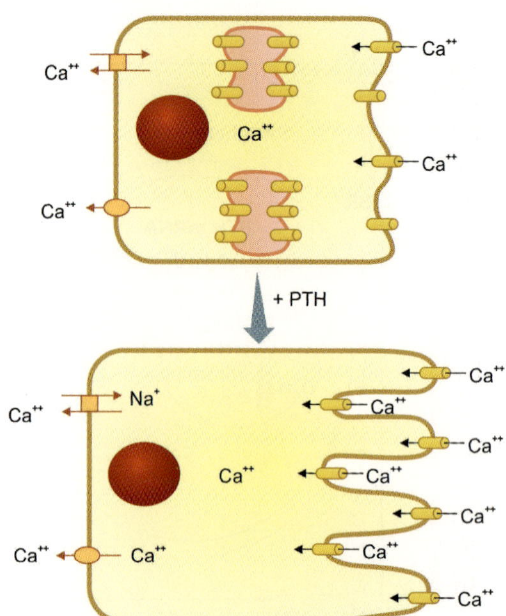

Fig. 5: Parathyroid hormone (PTH) mediated transepithelial calcium transport in renal distal tubular cells. PTH stimulates the translocation of preformed voltage-dependent calcium channels from intracellular sequestration sites to luminal brush border membrane, which also increases several folds increasing its surface area. Calbindin facilitates cytosolic diffusion of Ca²⁺ from apical influx to the basolateral efflux sites, via enhanced sodium-calcium exchange, supported by high affinity Ca ATPase.

Parathyroid hormone decreases the renal reabsorption of Pi by decreasing the expression of the type II Na⁺/Pi cotransporters. In the kidney, PTH acutely (in minutes to hours) decreases the expression of the Na⁺/Pi IIa cotransporters by stimulating their internalization via coated vesicles. PTH binding to its receptor initiates signaling pathways (that are still not well understood) leading to membrane retrieval followed by lysosomal degradation of this transporter. Thus, this is an irreversible internalization. On the other hand, Na⁺/Pi IIc cotransporters which is internalized, is recycled back to the membrane upon cessation of stimulus. The decreased expression of the transporter results in decreased Pi reabsorption.

◇ REGULATION OF 1α- AND 24-HYDROXYLASE ACTIVITY

Parathyroid hormone is a major inducer of the activity of proximal tubular 1α-hydroxylase, a microsomal cytochrome P-450 enzyme that synthesizes biologically active 1,25(OH)₂D from the substrate 25(OH)D. This effect of PTH on synthesis of the renal enzyme shows longer lag times than its effect on renal Ca²⁺ transport and is mediated, at least in part, by the protein kinase A (PKA) signaling pathway of the PTH/PTHrP receptor. Hypophosphatemia is, similar to PTH, a major inducer of 1α-hydroxylase, whereas hypercalcemia, as would be generated by sustained increases in circulating levels of PTH or PTHrP, suppresses synthesis of the enzyme, thus limiting overall $1,25(OH)_2D_3$ synthesis in a homeostatic manner. Hydroxylation of $25(OH)D_3$ and $1,25(OH)_2D_3$ by the 24-hydroxylase produces metabolites $24,25(OH)_2D_3$ and $1,24,25(OH)_3D_3$, respectively with no biological activity. PTH has an inhibitory effect on the 24-hydroxylase, thus reducing the inactivation of $1,25(OH)_2D_3$; in contrast, $1,25(OH)_2D_3$ stimulates the synthesis of 24-hydroxylase, thereby inducing its own metabolism.

Control of Gastrointestinal Ca²⁺ Absorption

Ca^{2+} absorption is the result of both passive diffusions across the intestinal mucosa via the paracellular route and active, transcellular transport. The passive, paracellular diffusion of Ca^{2+} is concentration dependent and nonsaturable; it accounts for absorption of approximately 10–15% of dietary Ca^{2+} (i.e., 100–150 mg/day of ingested Ca^{2+} when dietary Ca^{2+} is 1,000 mg/day). The active transcellular component of Ca^{2+} absorption is a saturable, carrier-mediated mechanism regulated by $1,25(OH)_2D$. It involves apical uptake of calcium by a Ca^{2+}-permeable channel(s) (TRPV6), transcellular movement that likely involves the intracellular Ca^{2+}-binding protein, calbindin D_{9K}, and then eventual extrusion of calcium at the basolateral cell surface by the Ca^{2+}-ATPase and, perhaps, the Na^+-Ca^{2+} exchanger. The highest density of sites of active Ca^{2+} absorption is in the proximal small intestine, i.e., duodenum. There is vitamin D-responsive Ca^{2+} absorption in more distal segments of the intestine as well, including both the small intestine (ileum > jejunum) and the proximal large bowel. Because these segments of the GI tract are much longer than the duodenum, they may well contribute significantly to overall Ca^{2+} absorption. PTH indirectly increases intestinal calcium absorption through activation of vitamin D-mediated transcellular uptake.

◇ PARATHYROID HORMONE—CELLULAR EFFECT ON BONE

In the skeletal system, PTH binds to receptors found in osteoblasts resulting in a cascade of events culminating in an increase in bone turnover, leading to a rapid release of Ca^{2+} from the bone matrix into the extracellular compartment, where it enters the systemic circulation. These receptor-mediated effects of PTH in osteoblasts are mediated through the synthesis or activity of several proteins, including *osteoclast-differentiating factor (ODF)*, also known as receptor activator of nuclear factor B ligand (RANKL) or osteoprotegerin ligand. In bone, the overall effects of PTH are osteoblast activation and stimulation of genes vital to the processes of degradation of the extracellular matrix and bone remodeling (collagenase-3), production of growth factors (insulin-like growth factor-I), and stimulation and recruitment of osteoclasts (RANKL and interleukin-6).

Parathyroid Hormone Mobilization of Bone Ca²⁺

For a better understanding, the basics of bone structure and cells involved in PTH-mediated mobilization of calcium will be described. Bone consists of an extracellular matrix, the organic phase that is composed of type I collagen, proteoglycans, and noncollagenous proteins. This extracellular bone matrix also contains growth factors and cytokines that have an important regulatory role in bone remodeling, or formation of new bone. The inorganic phase of bone matrix is composed mainly of calcium hydroxyapatite, which functions as a reservoir of calcium and phosphate ions and plays a major role in the homeostasis of these minerals. Most of the skeleton (80%) is composed of *cortical bone,* found mainly in the shafts of long bones and the surfaces of flat bones. Cortical bone consists of compact bone surrounding central canals (haversian systems) that contain blood vessels, lymphatic tissue, nerves, and connective tissue.

Trabecular bone, found mainly at the ends of long bones and within flat bones, consists of interconnecting plates and bars, inside which lies hematopoietic or fatty bone marrow.

Three cell types are found in bone.
1. *Osteoblasts*—Osteoblasts are responsible for bone formation and mineralization and express PTHRs. They are derived from pluripotent mesenchymal stem cells, which can also differentiate into chondrocytes, adipocytes, myoblasts, and fibroblasts. Several hormonal and nonhormonal molecules stimulate the differentiation of osteoblasts from stem cell precursors.
2. *Osteoclasts*—Osteoclasts are large multinucleated bone-resorbing cells derived from hematopoietic precursors of the monocyte-macrophage lineage. They are formed by the fusion of mononuclear cells and are characterized by a ruffled border, which consists of an infolding of the plasma membrane, and a prominent cytoskeleton. Osteoclasts are rich in lysosomal enzymes.
3. *Osteocytes*—Osteocytes, the most numerous cells in bone, are small, flattened cells within the bone matrix. They are connected to one another and to osteoblastic cells on the bone surface by an extensive canalicular network that contains the bone's extracellular fluid (ECF). These cells are terminally differentiated from osteoblasts and ultimately undergo apoptosis or phagocytosis during osteoclastic resorption. Their function and their contribution to osteoclastic bone resorption are not completely understood.

Mechanism of Bone Resorption

Bone remodeling involves the continuous removal of bone (bone resorption) followed by synthesis of new bone matrix and subsequent mineralization (bone formation). This coupling of the functions of osteoblasts and osteoclasts is central not only for the hormonal regulation of bone turnover, but also for the evaluation of their altered function. During skeletal development and throughout life, cells from the osteoblast lineage synthesize and secrete molecules that in turn initiate and control osteoclast differentiation. Osteoclasts are stimulated hormonally and locally by growth factors and cytokines. Osteoclastic activity induced by PTH is indirectly mediated through osteoblast activation **(Fig. 6)**.

Osteoclastic bone resorption requires the recruitment and differentiation of osteoclast precursors from the granulocyte-macrophage colony-forming unit (CFU) into preosteoclasts followed by fusion of preosteoclasts to form multinucleated functional osteoclasts. PTH binding to PTH receptor 1 on osteoblasts triggers the synthesis of RANKL also known as osteoclast differentiation factor (ODF) and as osteoprotegerin ligand. RANKL (expressed in the osteoblasts) binds to RANK in the osteoclast precursors and stimulates their differentiation into functional osteoclasts. The initial event in bone degradation is the attachment of osteoclasts to the bone surface. The mature and activated osteoclast is characterized by the formation of the ruffled membrane under which bone resorption occurs.

Osteoclasts attach to the bone surface through β-integrins generating an isolated extracellular microenvironment. Acidic intracellular vesicles fuse to the cell membrane facing the bone matrix forming the scalloped or ruffled border. Hydrogen ions generated by carbonic anhydrase II are delivered across the plasma membrane by H^+-ATPases recruited into the cell's ruffled membrane. The acidification of this isolated extracellular microenvironment to a pH of about four favors the dissolving of hydroxyapatite and provides optimal conditions for the action of the lysosomal proteases including collagenase and cathepsins to dissolve bone mineral. The products of bone degradation are endocytosed by the osteoclast and transported to and released at the cell's antiresorptive surface providing ionized Ca^{2+}, inorganic phosphate, and alkaline phosphatases, into

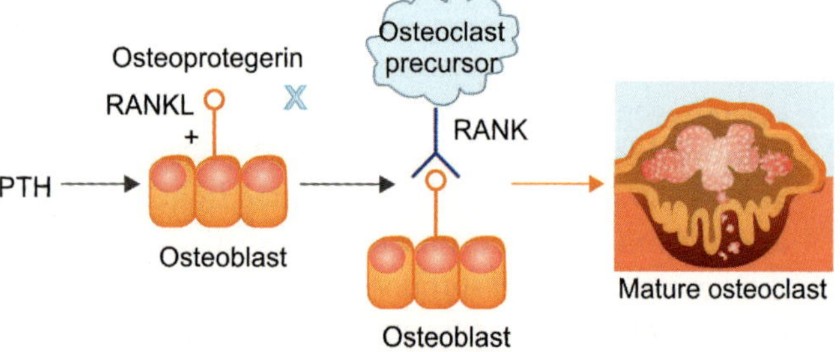

Fig. 6: Parathyroid hormone (PTH) mediated bone resorption. Binding of PTH to PTHR1 receptor in osteoblasts stimulates the surface expression of receptor activator of nuclear factor B ligand (RANKL). RANKL binds to receptor activator of nuclear factor B (RANK), a cell surface protein expressed on osteoclast precursors, which in turn, activates their differentiation into functional osteoclasts. Activated and mature osteoclast with ruffled border attaches to the bone surface and mediates bone resorption.

circulation. Osteoprotegerin is a soluble protein secreted by osteoblasts that serves as a decoy ligand for RANKL, preventing binding of RANKL to RANK, thereby inhibiting the process of osteoclastic bone resorption. As a result, there is a decrease in the differentiation of precursor cells into oscteoclasts and decreased bone resorption. Production of osteoprotegerin is increased by estrogen and decreased by glucocorticoids. PTH inhibits the production of osteoprotegerin.

◁ CALCIUM HOMEOSTASIS

The human body contains approximately 1,100 g of calcium, 99% of which is deposited in bones and teeth. The small amount found in plasma is divided into three fractions: ionized calcium (50%), protein-bound calcium (40%), and calcium complexed to citrate and phosphate forming soluble complexes (10%). The complexed and ionized Ca^{2+} fractions (about 60% of plasma Ca^{2+}) can cross the plasma membrane. The majority (80–90%) of protein-bound Ca^{2+} is bound to albumin, and this interaction is sensitive to changes in blood pH. Acidosis leads to a decrease in protein binding of Ca^{2+} and an increase in "free" or ionized Ca^{2+} in the plasma. Alkalosis results in increased Ca^{2+} binding and a decrease in ionized Ca^{2+} in the plasma. A smaller fraction (10–20%) of protein-bound Ca^{2+} is bound to globulins.

The resting intracellular (cytosolic) calcium concentration is about 100 nM, but this can increase to 1 M by the release of Ca^{2+} from intracellular stores or by uptake of extracellular Ca^{2+} in response to cellular activation. In contrast, the extracellular ionized calcium concentration is approximately 10,000-fold higher than the intracellular calcium concentration and remains virtually constant at approximately 1 mM. Ca^{2+} is an essential intracellular messenger and cofactor for various enzymes. Ca^{2+} also has diverse extracellular functions (e.g., in the clotting of blood, maintenance of skeletal integrity, and modulation of neuromuscular excitability). Thus, calcium plays critical role in both intra- and extracellular spaces. Ultimately, all Ca^{2+} are derived from extracellular fluid (ECF). Therefore, it is vital to maintain the near constancy of level of extracellular Ca^{2+} (Ca^{2+}_o) for critical intracellular functions. For example, Na^+ channel voltage-gating is dependent on the extracellular Ca^{2+} concentration. Decreased plasma Ca^{2+} concentrations reduce the voltage threshold for the action potential firing, resulting in neuromuscular hyperexcitability. This can result in numbness and tingling of fingertips, toes, and the perioral region or muscle cramps. Clinically, neuromuscular irritability can be demonstrated by mechanical stimulation of the hyperexcitable nerve leading to tetanic-like muscle contraction by eliciting Chvostek's (ipsilateral contraction of facial muscles elicited by tapping the skin over the facial nerve) or Trousseau's (carpal spasm induced by inflation of the blood pressure cuff to 20 mm Hg above the patient's systolic blood pressure for 3–5 minutes) sign.

Normal plasma concentrations of Ca^{2+} range between 8.5 and 10.5 mg/dL. The two key components of the system that maintains Ca^{2+} homeostasis are: (1) cell types that sense changes in extracellular calcium and release calcium-regulating hormones, PTH, calcitonin (Ctn), and 1,25-dihydroxyvitamin D namely, the chief cells of the parathyroid glands, thyroidal parafollicular C cells, and proximal tubular cells of the kidney, respectively and (2) the target organs of these hormones, including the kidneys, bones, and intestine, that respond with changes in calcium mobilization, excretion, or uptake.

Interaction of Bone, Kidney, and Intestine in Maintaining Calcium Homeostasis

Bone

Calcium in bone is distributed in a readily exchangeable pool and a stable pool. The readily exchangeable pool is involved in maintaining Ca^{2+} plasma levels by the daily exchange of 550 mg of calcium between the bone and ECF. The stable Ca^{2+} pool is involved in bone remodeling. Bone is metabolically active throughout life. After skeletal growth is complete, remodeling of both cortical and trabecular bone continues with an annual turnover rate of about 10% of the adult skeleton.

Kidney

In the kidney, virtually all filtered Ca^{2+} is reabsorbed. About 40% of the Ca^{2+} that is reabsorbed is under hormonal regulation by PTH. Most filtered Ca^{2+} is reabsorbed in the proximal tubules, mainly by passive transport processes independent of hormonal regulation. Ca^{2+} reabsorption in the CTALs is mediated by a combination of active and passive absorption. Ca^{2+} reabsorption in the distal convoluted tubules is mediated by active transcellular route, which is stimulated by PTH binding to PTHR-1. Transcellular transport of Ca^{2+} is facilitated by vitamin D through the increase in the Ca^{2+}-binding protein calbindin-D_{28K} and in the expression of Ca^{2+} transporters in the basolateral membrane.

Intestine

The availability of dietary calcium is a critical determinant of calcium homeostasis. Dietary intake of calcium averages 1,000 mg/day, of which only 30% is absorbed in the intestinal tract. This percentage of dietary Ca^{2+} that is absorbed is significantly enhanced by vitamin D during growth, pregnancy, and lactation. During growth, there is a net bone accretion. After completion of the growth phase in the young and healthy individual, there is no net gain or loss of Ca^{2+} from bone despite a continuous turnover of bone mass; the amount of Ca^{2+} lost in urine is approximately equal to net Ca^{2+} absorption.

Intestinal absorption of Ca^{2+} occurs by a saturable, transcellular process and a nonsaturable, paracellular pathway. The paracellular pathway predominates when dietary Ca^{2+} is abundant. The active transcellular pathway is vitamin D-dependent and plays a major role in absorption when the Ca^{2+} supply is limited.

Intestinal transepithelial Ca^{2+} transport, similar to that in the distal tubule, is a three-step process consisting of passive entry across the apical membrane, cytosolic diffusion facilitated by vitamin D-dependent calcium-binding proteins (calbindins), and active extrusion of Ca^{2+} across the opposing basolateral membrane mediated by a high-affinity Ca^{2+}-ATPase and Na^+/Ca^{2+} exchanger.

Complex Interplay of Parathyroid Hormone, Vitamin D and Calcitonin in Calcium Homeostasis

As explained previously, a slight decrease in the free ionized Ca^{2+} level is sensed through the Ca^{2+} sensor in parathyroid chief cells, resulting in an increased release of PTH. PTH binds to receptors in osteoblasts leading to the recruitment of preosteoclasts and their maturation to active osteoclasts, which are responsible for increased bone resorption and release Ca^{2+} and Pi into the circulation. In the kidney, PTH promotes Ca^{2+} reabsorption and Pi excretion in urine. In addition, PTH stimulates the hydroxylation of 25-hydroxyvitamin D_3 at the 1-position, leading to the formation of the active form of vitamin D (calcitriol). Vitamin D increases intestinal absorption of dietary Ca^{2+} and renal reabsorption of filtered Ca^{2+}. In bone, vitamin D increases the number of osteoclasts and stimulates bone resorption, with a resulting increase in the release of Ca^{2+} into the circulation. An increase in free ionized Ca^{2+} levels decreases the release of PTH from the parathyroid gland, decreases the activation of vitamin D in the kidney, and stimulates parafollicular cells of the thyroid gland to release the hormone calcitonin.

Calcitonin counteracts the effects of PTH. Calcitonin inhibits osteoclast activity, decreasing bone resorption and increasing renal Ca^{2+} excretion; the result is a decrease in free ionized Ca^{2+} levels. Overall, PTH, calcitriol, and calcitonin work together to maintain plasma Ca^{2+} levels within a narrow normal range.

◇ ADDITIONAL REGULATORS OF Ca^{2+} AND BONE METABOLISM

Although PTH and vitamin D play central roles in the regulation of bone metabolism, the contribution of other hormones cannot be ignored. Sex steroids (androgens and estrogens) have been shown to increase 1-hydroxylase activity, decrease bone resorption, and increase osteoprotegerin synthesis. Estrogen stimulates the proliferation of osteoblasts and the expression of type I collagen and alkaline phosphatase; influences the expression of receptors for vitamin D, growth hormone, and progesterone; and modulates responsiveness of bone to PTH. Estrogen decreases the number and activity of osteoclasts as well as the synthesis of cytokines affecting bone resorption. Growth hormone and insulin-like growth factor-I both exert effects on bone metabolism. Growth hormone stimulates the proliferation and differentiation of osteoblasts and bone protein synthesis and growth. Insulin-like growth factors, produced by the liver and by bone cells, stimulate bone formation by increasing the proliferation of osteoblast precursors and by enhancing the synthesis and inhibiting the degradation of type I collagen. Normal thyroid function is required for physiological bone remodeling. However, excess thyroid hormone levels result in increased bone resorption. Prolactin increases Ca^{2+} reabsorption and 1-hydroxylase activity. Glucocorticoids play an overall catabolic role in bone metabolism by increasing bone resorption and decreasing bone synthesis, resulting in an increase in the risk of fractures. The mechanisms by which glucocorticoids exert their effects are not fully understood, but inhibition of osteoprotegerin may help stimulate osteoclastic bone resorption. The cytokines tumor necrosis factor-α, interleukin-1, and interleukin-6 increase the proliferation and differentiation of osteoclast precursors and their osteoclastic activity and are therefore potent stimulators of bone resorption in vitro and in vivo. The overall interaction of these various factors during health and disease plays an important role in maintaining bone mass. Their specific contributions may vary depending on the disease and on the prevailing hormone and cytokine levels in bone.

CLINICAL PEARLS

- Parathyroid hormone release is under negative feedback regulation by Ca^{2+} and vitamin D.
- The main physiologic effects of PTH are mediated by the PTHR-1 expressed in bone and kidney.
- Parathyroid hormone receptor-1 binds PTH and PTHrP, a peptide responsible for the pathophysiologic elevation of Ca^{2+} in some malignancies.
- In the kidney, PTH increases renal Ca^{2+} reabsorption, increases the activity of 1-hydroxylase (which mediates

the final activation step in the synthesis of vitamin D), and decreases Pi reabsorption.

- In bone, PTH increases osteoclast-mediated bone resorption indirectly through stimulation of osteoblast activity.
- Calcitonin decreases bone resorption and lowers plasma Ca^{2+} levels.
- Vitamin D increases bone resorption, renal Ca^{2+} reabsorption, and intestinal Ca^{2+} absorption.
- In the intestine, PTH indirectly enhances calcium absorption through vitamin D activation.

SUGGESTED READING

1. Molina PE. Endocrine Physiology, 3rd Edition. [online] Available from http://www.accessmedicine.com. [Last accessed April, 2020].
2. Barrett K, Brooks H, Boitano S, Barman S. Ganong's Review of Medical Physiology, 23rd Edition. New York, NY: McGraw-Hill Medical; 2009.
3. Bilezikian JP, Marcus R, Levine MA. The Parathyroid: Basic and Clinical Concepts, 2nd Edition. San Diego: Academic Press; 2001. pp. 399-409.
4. Cozzolino M, Galassi A, Conte F, Mangano M, Di Lullo L, Bellasi A. Treatment of secondary hyperparathyroidism: the clinical utility of etelcalcetide. Therap Clin Risk Manage. 2017;13: 679-89.
5. Jameson JL, De Groot LJ. Endocrinology: Adult and Pediatric, 6th Edition. United States: Elsevier Saunders; 2010. p. 3064.
6. Brown EM, MacLeod RJ. Extracellular calcium sensing and extracellular calcium signaling. Physiol Rev. 2001;81: 239-97.
7. Canalis E, Giustina A, Bilezikian JP. Mechanisms of anabolic therapies for osteoporosis. N Engl J Med. 2007;357:905-16.
8. Jones G, Strugnell SA, DeLuca HF. Current understanding of the molecular actions of vitamin D. Physiol Rev. 1998;78: 1193-231.
9. Khosla S. Mini review: the OPG/RANKL/RANK system. Endocrinology. 2001;142:5050-5.
10. Gensure RC, Gardella TJ, Juppner H. Parathyroid hormone and parathyroid hormone-related peptide, and their receptors. Biochem Biophys Res Commun. 2005;328:666-78.
11. Marx SJ. Medical progress: hyperparathyroid and hypoparathyroid disorders. N Engl J Med. 2000;343: 1863-75.
12. Murer H, Hernando N, Forster L, Biber J. Molecular mechanisms in proximal tubular and small intestinal phosphate reabsorption. Mol Membr Biol. 2001;18:3-11.

ADRENAL GLAND PHYSIOLOGY

Uma Devi

INTRODUCTION

The two adrenal glands each of them weighs about 4 g consists of two parts *adrenal medulla* and *adrenal cortex*. The adrenal medulla, the central 20%, secretes epinephrine and norepinephrine related to sympathetic stimulation. These

hormones cause almost same effect as direct stimulation of sympathetic nervous system.

The adrenal cortex secretes corticosteroids which are produced from steroid cholesterol. All they have similar chemical formulas but slight different in molecular structural difference gives them different and important functions.

◇| CORTICOSTEROIDS

Mineralocorticoids, Glucocorticoids, and Androgens

Two major types of adrenocortical hormones are mineralocorticoids and glucocorticoids are secreted by adrenal cortex. In addition, sex hormones are also secreted especially androgens.

Mineralocorticoids gained their name because they especially affect the minerals such as sodium and potassium in extracellular fluids. Glucocorticoids gained their name because they increase the blood glucose levels. They also have additional effects on fat and protein metabolism. More 30 steroids are identified from adrenal cortex and of which two of them are the most important, aldosterone and cortisol.

Synthesis and secretion of adrenocortical hormones

Adrenal cortex has three layers:

1. *Zona glomerulosa*, thin layer of cells underneath the capsule, which constitutes around 15% of adrenal cortex, only cells in adrenal which secrete aldosterone because they contain aldosterone synthase. Secretion is regulated by angiotensin II and potassium.
2. *Zona fasciculata*, middle part, constitutes about 75% of adrenal cortex and secretes glucocorticoids cortisol and corticosterone. It also secretes small amounts of adrenal androgens and estrogens. Secretion of these is controlled by hypothalamic-pituitary-adrenocortical axis (HPA) via adrenocorticotropic hormone (ACTH).
3. *Zona reticularis*, deeper layer of cortex, secrets androgens dehydroepiandrosterone (DHEA) and androstenedione as well as small amount of glucocorticoids and estrogens. ACTH also regulates secretion of these cells.

The aldosterone and the cortisol are regulated by independent mechanisms. Factor such as angiotensin-II that specifically increases the output of aldosterone and causing hypertrophy of zona glomerulosa.

Factors such as ACTH that increase secretion of cortisol and adrenal androgens and cause hypertrophy of the zona fasciculata and zona glomerulosa.

Synthetic pathway for adrenal steroids

Principal steps in adrenal steroids synthesis occur in two organelles of the cell mitochondria and endoplasmic reticulum. Each step is catalyzed by a specific enzyme. A change in a single enzyme in this can cause vastly different types and relative portions of hormones to be formed.

Mineralocorticoids

- Aldosterone (very potent, accounts for about 90% of all mineralocorticoid activity)
- Desoxycorticosterone (1/30 as potent as aldosterone, but very small quantities secreted)
- Corticosterone (slight mineralocorticoid activity)
- 9α-fluorocortisol (synthetic, slightly more potent than aldosterone)
- Cortisol (very high mineralocorticoid activity)
- Cortisone (synthetic, slight mineralocorticoid activity)

Glucocorticoids

- Cortisol (very potent, accounts for 95% of glucocorticoid activity)
- Corticosterone (less potent than cortisol, 4% of total glucocorticoids)
- Cortisone (almost as potent as cortisol, synthetic)
- Prednisolone (four times as potent than cortisol, synthetic)
- Methylprednisolone (five times as potent than cortisol, synthetic)
- Dexamethasone (30 times more potent than cortisol, synthetic)

Adrenocortical hormones are bound to plasma proteins, especially to globulin called cortisol-binding globulin. 90–95% cortisol binds to globulin, so the half-life of cortisol is around 60–90 minutes.

Only about 60% of aldosterone are bound to plasma protein so that half-life of aldosterone is about 20 minutes.

Adrenal steroids are degraded mainly in the liver and conjugated to glucuronic acid and lesser extent to sulfates. 25% of conjugates are excreted in bile and then in feces. Remaining conjugates formed in the liver enter the circulation and are highly soluble in plasma. These are readily filtered in kidney and excreted through urine. Conjugated forms are inactive forms. So in patients with liver disease, inactivation is markedly decreased, and in renal disease, it reduces the excretion of inactivated conjugates.

The normal concentration of aldosterone in blood is 6 ng/100 mL and that of cortisol is 12 µg/100 mL.

Functions of mineralocorticoid hormones: Mineralocorticoids deficiency causes severe renal sodium chloride wasting with hyperkalemia. Total loss of adrenal corticoid steroid synthesis can cause death in 3–14 days unless with excessive salt intake or mineralocorticoid injection. Aldosterone exerts 90% mineralocorticoid activity, but cortisol also provides mineralocorticoid activity. Aldosterone's mineralocorticoids activity is 3,000 times more than cortisol, but plasma concentration of cortisol is almost 2,000 times than that of aldosterone.

Aldosterone increases renal tubular reabsorption of sodium with secretion of potassium. A high concentration of aldosterone in plasma causes decrease in sodium transiently, as loss in urine as little as milliequivalents per day. Potassium loss in urine is increased severalfold causing hypokalemia. Excess aldosterone increases extracellular fluid volume and arterial pressure but only a small effect on sodium concentration in plasma. When sodium is reabsorbed in the tubule, there is simultaneous absorption of water occurs.

Even though aldosterone is one of body's most powerful sodium retaining hormones, only transient sodium retention occurs with high aldosterone levels. Aldosterone-mediated increase in ECF volume lasting for >1–2 days leads to increase in arterial pressure. The rise in arterial pressure then increases kidney excretion of both salt and water called pressure natriuresis and pressure diuresis.

After the ECF increases 5–15% above normal, arterial pressure also increases up to 15–25 mm Hg. This elevated blood returns the renal output of salt and water to normal. This is called "aldosterone escape".

Excess aldosterone causes hypokalemia and muscle weakness. When the potassium ion concentration falls below one-half normal muscle weakness occurs because of alteration of electrical excitability of the nerve and muscle fiber membranes.

Excess aldosterone increases tubular hydrogen secretion in exchange for sodium in collecting duct causes mild alkalosis.

Regulation of aldosterone secretion has been shown in **Figure 7.**

The major stimulus for aldosterone synthesis is angiotensin II. Angiotensinogen, the ~55 kDa precursor glycoprotein for angiotensin II, is synthesized and released by the liver. Angiotensinogen in serum is cleaved to form angiotensin I (a 10-amino acid peptide) by renin, a very specific protease synthesized by the juxtaglomerular apparatus of the kidney. Angiotensin I is then converted to the active octapeptide angiotensin II by angiotensin converting enzyme. *Cleavage by renin is the rate limiting step for the production of angiotensin II.* Because the normal serum concentration of angiotensinogen is close to the Km for the renin cleavage

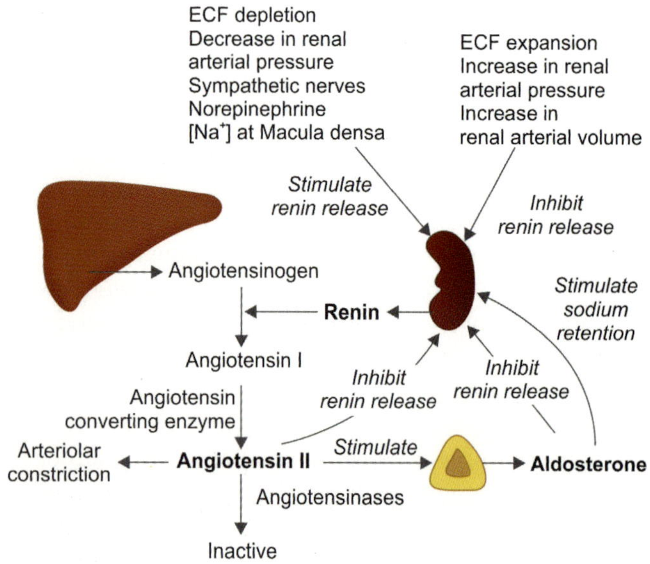

reaction, the rate of angiotensin II production depends on both the concentration of renin and the concentration of angiotensinogen. The release of angiotensinogen from the liver is constitutive, but can be stimulated by cortisol, by estrogens, and by angiotensin II. Renin release from the kidney is stimulated by ECF depletion, by low serum sodium concentrations, and by decreases in blood pressure; renin release is inhibited by angiotensin II, aldosterone, and by elevated blood pressure. The zona glomerulosa responds to increases in serum potassium levels by increasing aldosterone synthesis. While decreases in serum sodium levels also stimulate aldosterone synthesis, the effect of sodium is almost certainly mediated by increased angiotensin II secondary to increased renin release from the kidney. In contrast, the regulation by increased potassium appears to be due to a direct effect of high serum potassium levels on the adrenal; recent evidence suggests that it may be mediated by intra-adrenal production of angiotensin-II.

A peptide hormone released by the heart, atrial natriuretic peptide (ANP), is the only known inhibitor of aldosterone production. ANP is released in response to elevated atrial pressure. The actions of ANP appear to be mediated by both inhibition of renin released by the kidney and by direct effect on the adrenal to inhibit aldosterone synthesis. ANP is a vasodilator and has additional effects related to reduction of blood pressure.

Functions of glucocorticoids:
- Stimulation of gluconeogenesis
- Decreased utilization of glucose
- Reduction in cellular protein
- Cortisol increases liver and plasma proteins
- Cortisol mobilizes amino acids from extrahepatic tissues
- Mobilization of fatty acids
- Cortisol causing obesity
- Resisting stress and inflammation
- Prevents development of inflammation by stabilizing lysosome
- Cortisol causes resolution of inflammation
- Cortisol blocks inflammatory effects to allergic reaction

Regulation of cortisol by ACTH from anterior pituitary (**Fig. 8**): Secretion of cortisol is almost entirely by ACTH secreted by anterior pituitary. This hormone is also known as corticotropin or adrenocorticotropin. ACTH secretion is controlled by a releasing factor from hypothalamus known as "corticotropin releasing hormone". ACTH stimulates adrenocortical cells by activating adenylyl cyclase in the cell membrane. This induces the formation of cAMP in the cytoplasm. This cAMP further activates the intracellular enzymes for the formation of adrenocortical hormones. ACTH stimulates protein kinase A which causes conversion of cholesterol to pregnenolone. This is the rate limiting step of all adrenocortical hormones

Fig. 7: Regulation of aldosterone secretion.
(ECF: extracellular fluid)

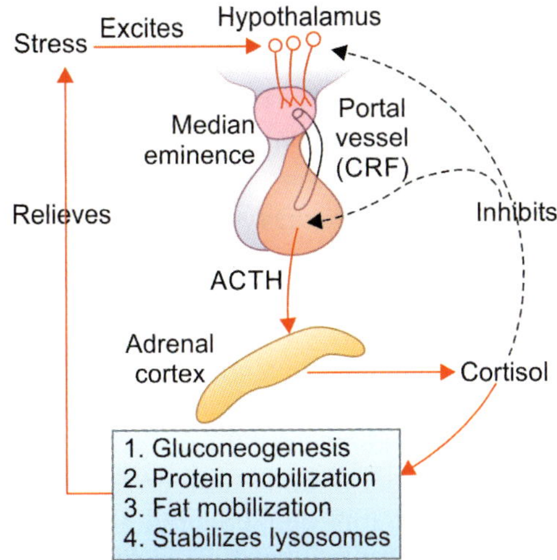

Fig. 8: Regulation of cortisol by adrenocorticotropic hormone (ACTH) from anterior pituitary.
(CRF: corticotropin-releasing factor)

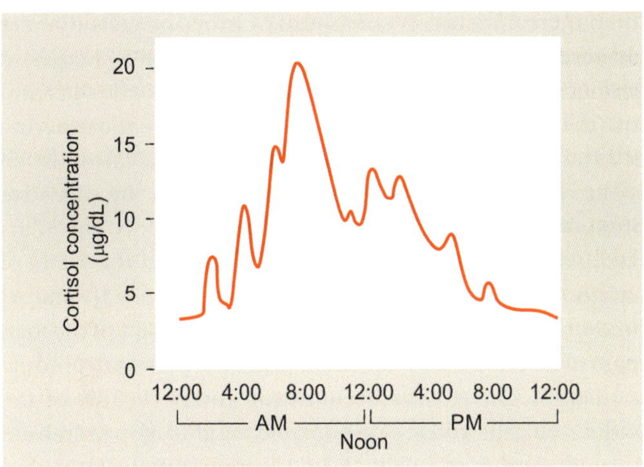

Fig. 9: *Circadian rhythm of cortisol*: Cortisol concentration.

synthesis, that is why ACTH is normally needed for any adrenocortical hormone synthesis.

*Circadian rhythm of cortisol (**Fig. 9**):* The secretory rates of corticotropin-releasing hormone (CRH)-ACTH and cortisol are high in the early morning but low in the late evening. Plasma cortisol level ranges between a high of about 20 µg/ L an hour before arising in the morning and a low of about 5 µg/dL around midnight. This affects results from a 24-hour cyclical alteration in the signals from the hypothalamus that causes cortisol secretion. When a person changes daily sleeping habits, the cycles change correspondingly.

Adrenal Androgens

Several moderately active male sex hormones are called "adrenal androgens", most important dehydroepiandrosterone (DHEA), are continually secreted by the adrenal cortex especially during fetal life.

◇ SUGGESTED READING

1. Chan LF, Metherell LA, Clark AJ. Effects of melanocortins on adrenal gland physiology. European Journal of Pharmacology. 2011;660(1):171-80.
2. Corander MP, Coll AP. Melanocortins and body weight regulation: glucocorticoids, Agouti-related protein and beyond. European Journal of Pharmacology. 2011;660(1): 111-8.
3. Dutt M, Wehrle CJ, Jialal I. Physiology, adrenal gland. StatPearls [Internet]. 2020, May 29.
4. Imperiale A, Elbayed K, Moussallieh FM, Reix N, Piotto M, Bellocq JP, Goichot B, Bachellier P, Namer IJ. Metabolomic profile of the adrenal gland: from physiology to pathological conditions. Endocr Relat Cancer. 2013;20(5):705-16.

ENDOCRINE PANCREAS

Prateek Mehrotra

◇ INTRODUCTION

The pancreas is a mixed exocrine and endocrine gland that plays a central role in digestion and in the metabolism, utilization, and storage of energy substrates. Normal pancreatic function involving the production and release of the hormones insulin and glucagon is essential for the physiologic control of glucose homeostasis.

The endocrine function of the pancreas through the release of insulin and glucagon and the mechanisms by which these hormones regulate events central to maintaining glucose homeostasis. In the case of glucose, the process involves a regulated balance among hepatic glucose release (from glycogen breakdown and gluconeogenesis), dietary glucose absorption, and glucose uptake and disposal from skeletal muscle and adipose tissue. The pancreatic hormones insulin and glucagon play central roles in regulating each of these processes and their overall effects are in part modified by other hormones such as growth hormone, cortisol, and epinephrine. In addition to secreting insulin and glucagon, the endocrine pancreas also secretes somatostatin, amylin, and pancreatic polypeptide.

◇ FUNCTIONAL ANATOMY

The pancreas is a retroperitoneal gland divided into a head, body, and tail and is located near the duodenum. Most of the pancreatic mass is composed of exocrine cells that are clustered in lobules (acini) divided by connective tissue and connected to a duct that drains into the pancreatic duct and into the duodenum. The product of the pancreatic exocrine cell is an alkaline fluid rich with digestive enzymes, which is secreted into the small intestine to aid in the digestive process. Embedded within the acini are richly vascularized, small clusters of endocrine cells called the islets of Langerhans, in which two endocrine cell types (β and α) predominate. The β-cells constitute about 73–75% of the total mass of endocrine cells and their principal secretory product is insulin. The α-cells account for about 18–20% of the endocrine cells and are responsible for glucagon secretion. A small number of δ-cells (4–6%) secrete somatostatin, and an even smaller number of cells (1%) secrete pancreatic polypeptide. The localization of these cell types within the islets has a particular pattern, with the β-cells located centrally, surrounded by α- and δ-cells. This arrangement plays a role in the cell-to-cell paracrine regulation of hormone release.

Parasympathetic, sympathetic, and sensory nerves richly innervate the pancreatic islets, and the respective neurotransmitters and neuropeptides released from their nerve terminals exert important regulatory effects on pancreatic endocrine hormone release. Acetylcholine, vasoactive intestinal polypeptide, pituitary adenylate cyclase-activating polypeptide, and gastrin-releasing peptide are released from the parasympathetic nerve terminals. Norepinephrine, galanin, and neuropeptide-Y are released from sympathetic nerve terminals. Vagal nerve activation stimulates the secretion of insulin, glucagon, somatostatin, and pancreatic polypeptide. Sympathetic nerve stimulation inhibits based and glucose-stimulated insulin secretion and somatostatin release and stimulates glucagon and pancreatic polypeptide secretion.

The arterial blood supply to the pancreas is derived from the splenic artery and the superior and inferior pancreaticoduodenal arteries. Although islets represent only 1–2% of the mass of the pancreas, they receive about 10–15% of the pancreatic blood flow. The rich vascularization by fenestrated capillaries allows ready access to the circulation for the hormones secreted by the islet cells. The direction of blood flow is preferentially from the center of the islet to the periphery. Therefore, α- and δ-cells are exposed to high concentrations of hormones produced by the β-cells (i.e., insulin), contributing to the inhibition of glucagon release by high local insulin concentrations. Venous blood from the pancreas drains into the hepatic vein. Therefore, the liver, principal target organ for the physiologic effects of pancreatic hormones, is exposed to the highest concentrations of pancreatic hormones. Following first-pass hepatic metabolism, the pancreatic endocrine hormones are distributed to the systemic circulation.

◇ PANCREATIC HORMONES INSULIN SYNTHESIS

The process involved in the synthesis and release of insulin, a polypeptide hormone, by the β-cells of the pancreas is similar to that of other peptide hormones. Preproinsulin undergoes cleavage of its signal peptide during insertion into the endoplasmic reticulum, generating proinsulin. Proinsulin consists of an amino-terminal β-chain, a carboxy-terminal α-chain, and a connecting peptide in the middle known as the C-peptide. C-peptide links the α- and β-chains, allowing proper folding of the molecule and the formation of disulfide bonds between the two chains. In the endoplasmic reticulum, proinsulin is processed by specific endopeptidases known as prohormone convertases, which cleave the C-peptide to generate the mature from of insulin. Removal of the C-peptide exposes the end of the insulin chain that interacts with the insulin receptor. Insulin and the free C-peptide are packaged into secretory granules in the Golgi apparatus and are released together. These secretory granules accumulate in the cytoplasm. About 5% of the granules are stored in a readily releasable pool. Most of the granules (>95%) belong to a reserve pool and need to be chemically modified, or even physically translocated, to become immediately available for release. This release of insulin granules from different pools leads to a biphasic pattern of insulin release in response to stimulation of the β-cell by glucose. Only a small proportion of the cellular stores of insulin is released even under maximal stimulatory conditions.

◇ SUGGESTED READING

1. Bakhti M, Böttcher A, Lickert H. Modelling the endocrine pancreas in health and disease. Nature Reviews Endocrinology. 2019;15(3):155-71.
2. Engelking LR. Physiology of the endocrine pancreas. In Seminars in Veterinary Medicine and Surgery (small animal) 1997 Nov 1 (Vol. 12, No. 4, pp. 224-229).
3. Woods SC, Porte Jr DA. Neural control of the endocrine pancreas. Physiological Reviews. 1974;54(3):596-619.

CHAPTER 3

Thyroid Function Tests and their Interpretation

Sushil Gupta, Rekha Singh

INTRODUCTION

Thyroid disorders are common in population but the symptoms of hypothyroidism are nonspecific and hence cannot be used for making diagnosis of thyroid hormone disorders. A series of blood test are used to assess the functionality of the thyroid gland. Thyroid function tests are used to differentiate normal thyroid functioning called as euthyroid state from hyperthyroidism or hypothyroidism. The commonly available thyroid function tests include thyroid stimulating hormone (TSH), total thyroxine (T4), free T4, total triiodothyronine (T3) and free T3. Understanding of the physiology of thyroid hormone secretion and regulation is important for interpreting the results of thyroid function tests.

In normal physiology, thyroid hormone concentration homeostasis is maintained by pituitary and hypothalamus through the hormone TSH and thyrotropin releasing hormone (TRH) respectively. Through TRH, hypothalamus regulates TSH secretion by stimulating its secretion from pituitary. TSH primarily and predominantly regulates the functioning of thyroid gland and its activity. In turn, the thyroid hormones in circulation are the major regulator of TSH secretion from pituitary by their inhibitory effect on thyrotropes of pituitary.[1] T3 directly through nuclear receptors in thyrotropes of pituitary and T4 indirectly by local conversion to T3 inhibit the synthesis and release of TSH.[2] In addition, T3 and T4 indirectly regulate TSH secretion by their inhibitory effect on TRH. Thyroid hormones are regulated very tightly. TSH level is very sensitive to changes in thyroid hormone level as TSH has a log linear relationship to circulating thyroid hormone levels. Very tight control of TSH secretion allows to maintain thyroid hormones within very narrow limits in normal homeostasis.[2,3]

THYROID HORMONE PHYSIOLOGY AND METABOLISM

T3 and T4 are the two biologically active thyroid hormones. Both T4 and T3 are secreted by thyroid gland. T4 is solely a product of the thyroid gland, whereas T3 is a product of the thyroid and of many other tissues, in which it is produced by deiodination of T4. Almost 80% of T3 is produced by extrathyroidal conversion of T4 in peripheral tissue. Approximately, 85 µg of T4 is produced daily by thyroid gland.

Liver and kidney are the major source of T3 from extrathyroidal conversion of T4, although most other tissues also convert T4 locally.[4] Nutrition, other hormones, and illness-related factors regulate the extrathyroidal conversion of T4 to T3.

Approximately, 99.95% of the T4 and 99.5% of the T3 in serum are bound to several serum proteins, thyroxine-binding globulin (TBG), transthyretin (TTR), albumin, and lipoproteins. Roughly, 0.02% of T4 is free (2 ng/dL) while 75% is bound to TBG, 10% to TTR, 12% to albumin and 3% to lipoproteins. For T3, approximately 80% is bound to TBG, 5% to TTR, and 15% to albumin and lipoproteins.[5] Approximately 0.5% of T3 is free (0.4 ng/dL) while 80% is bound to TBG, 5% to TTR and 15% to albumin and lipoproteins. Many drugs and diseases can affect the concentration of the binding proteins in circulation and thereby influence the serum total T4 and T3 levels. However, the protein changes do not alter free hormone concentrations or the absolute rate of metabolism of these hormones.

The biological function of thyroid hormones is determined by serum free T4 and free T3. The binding proteins acts as storage and buffer of these hormones in circulation, thereby maintain the serum free T4 and free T3 in narrow limits. These binding proteins of thyroid hormones in circulation protect tissues from sudden increases in thyroid secretion or extrathyroidal T3 production.

LABORATORY ASSESSMENT OF THYROID FUNCTION TEST

Serum Thyroid Stimulating Hormone

Thyroid function test is best screened both for hypothyroid and hyperthyroid state by TSH level estimation, if subject is in steady state condition and pituitary and hypothalamic disorders are ruled out. However, measurement of T4 in hypothyroidism and T3 and T4 in thyrotoxicosis is still important in many subjects where pituitary and hypothalamic dysfunction cannot be ruled out or patient has critical illness where only TSH levels estimation may be misleading.

The normal TSH level is 0.4–4.5 mIU/L. Multiple factors influence the normal range of serum TSH, e.g., sex, age, pregnant or nonpregnant state, ethnicity, iodine intake, body mass index, etc. The interpretation of TSH level should be based on age-specific reference range especially in the young and elderly population. Ideally, a reference range of serum TSH should be derived from each population. The reference range of serum TSH in pregnancy is trimester specific. If population and trimester specific range are not available in the laboratory, the following reference range is recommended by American Thyroid Association guideline: 1st trimester 0.1–2.5 mIU/L; 2nd trimester 0.2–3.0 mIU/L; and 3rd trimester 0.3–3.0 mIU/L. Twin pregnancy is associated with a higher concentration of human chorionic gonadotropin compared to a singleton pregnancy. Therefore, serum TSH may be less than 0.1 mIU/L physiologically in 1st trimester with twin pregnancy.[6]

Currently used third generation chemiluminescence assay is used for estimation of serum TSH with lower detection limit of 0.01 mIU/L. The currently used third generation assays are sufficiently sensitive for clinical diagnosis purposes as they can differentiate low TSH level seen in thyrotoxicosis form low normal TSH levels. With very few exceptions, TSH is low to undetectable range in thyrotoxicosis, whereas euthyroid state has normal range TSH. Previous generations of TSH assays did not have enough sensitivity to differentiate low TSH level of thyrotoxicosis from low normal TSH levels.

As we understood from thyroid pituitary axis physiology, TSH is very sensitive to the thyroid hormone levels change due to inverse log linear relationship. This sensitivity of TSH to thyroid level changes makes serum TSH as the most reliable screening measure of thyroid function. Serum TSH is used as the first-line test to confirm or screen for the diagnosis of hyperthyroidism. However, there are exceptions to this, e.g., pituitary disorders, hypothalamic disorders, and nonthyroidal illness.

Normally, TSH exhibits a diurnal variation with a peak shortly after midnight and a nadir in the late afternoon. TSH values can be expected to vary by as much as 20% between measurements without any change occurring in thyroid status. However, these variations do not affect the interpretation of results significantly as mostly the tests are done between 8 AM and 4 PM and the reference intervals for TSH has been typically established using samples collected at similar timings. Hence, TSH test may be measured anytime of the day without fasting. There is no need to withhold LT4 therapy on the day of blood testing for serum TSH.[6] Serum TSH level is used to monitor therapy in primary hypothyroidism.

Serum Total T4 and Total T3, and Free T4 and Free T3

Serum total T4 (TT4) and total T3 (TT3) are the free hormones in circulation bound to binding proteins and in unbound form found in nanomolar concentration. The estimation of total hormone is easier compared to free thyroid hormones estimation. As we know the free hormone of T4 and T3 are the one actually available for functioning. The level of free hormones T4 (fT4) and T3 (fT3) corresponds to the TT4 and TT3 if all the patients had similar binding proteins concentration. However, in clinical practice, the variation in the binding proteins distorts the proportionality of the total to free thyroid hormones. TT4 reference intervals range from 4.5 to 12.5 µg/dL approximately depending on assay method used. During pregnancy, TT4 level is approximately 1.5 times of normal range due to increased TBG elevations.[7] TT3 reference intervals range from 80 to 180 ng/dL approximately. Total hormones are preferred test compared to free hormones estimation in pregnancy and sometimes in non-thyroidal illness.[4] In central hypothyroidism, TT4 or fT4 is used to monitor therapy on follow-up. Serum TT4 levels or fT4 levels must be measured before levothyroxine intake or 6 hours after LT4 intake.

Free T4 and T3 hormones assay are difficult test considering these hormones need to be displaced from the protein binding step prior to measurement step.

◇| DIAGNOSIS OF HYPOTHYROIDISM

Hypothyroidism symptoms lack specificity. Therefore, the diagnosis of hypothyroidism is primarily laboratory investigation based. As serum TSH has inverse log linear relationship with thyroid hormones, hypothyroidism is characterized by high serum TSH and low TT4 and fT4 concentration.[1-3] Change in the serum TSH level is the first abnormality to appear in thyroid disease even before thyroid hormones level decreases due to the high sensitivity of TSH to thyroid hormones level change. Dysfunction at the level of thyroid is called as primary hypothyroidism and is associated with elevated serum TSH levels.[8] Subclinical hypothyroidism is characterized by high serum TSH level but normal TT4 and fT4 concentration. While overt primary hypothyroidism is characterized by high serum TSH level and low TT4 and fT4 concentrations.

Central hypothyroidism is caused by pituitary disorders (secondary hypothyroidism) or hypothalamic disorders (tertiary hypothyroidism).[8] As the thyroid pituitary axis is knocked down in pituitary and hypothalamic disorders, there is a discrepancy in expected response of serum TSH to the thyroid hormones level. The diagnosis of central hypothyroidism is based on low TT4 or fT4 concentration with inappropriately normal, low or mildly raised serum TSH level. Similarly, nonthyroidal illness and some drugs affect the thyroid pituitary axis and cause discrepancies between TSH levels and thyroid hormones level. The discordant serum TSH and thyroid hormones level must be interpreted in the clinical context.

◇| HYPERTHYROIDISM

Hyperthyroidism develops due to excessive presence of thyroid hormones in circulation. As we know, TSH level has inverse log linear relationship with thyroid hormones level, thereby serum TSH level is suppressed below normal reference range or undetectable in case of hyperthyroidism. In overt hyperthyroidism, serum thyroid hormones level is elevated and serum TSH level is undetectable, while in subclinical hyperthyroidism serum TSH level is suppressed with normal thyroid hormones level. Rarely only T3 can be elevated with suppressed serum TSH levels and normal T4 levels in early stages of Graves' disease and is called "T3 toxicosis".

Exceptions of hyperthyroidism with normal or high serum TSH level include pituitary TSH secreting adenoma or thyroid hormone resistance syndrome. Rarely spurious assays due to presence of heterophile antibodies TSH level may be normal with thyrotoxicosis. Excluding these rare exceptions, serum TSH level has the best sensitivity and specificity for diagnosis of hyperthyroidism. Serum TSH has the highest sensitivity and specificity as single blood test in the evaluation of thyrotoxicosis. Diagnostic accuracy improves with addition of thyroid hormones assessment with serum TSH estimation.

DISEASES AFFECTING THYROID HORMONES LEVEL WITH EUTHYROID STATE

Inherited conditions such as X-linked trait of TBG excess can increase TT4 and TT3 with normal free thyroid hormones and normal serum TSH levels due to increase pool of TBG bound thyroid hormones in circulation. Other clinical conditions, which can increase TBG, include pregnancy, hepatitis, and acute intermittent porphyria.[9]

INTERPRETATION OF THYROID FUNCTION TEST IN PREGNANCY

Normal physiology of pregnancy is associated with changes such as an increase in renal iodine excretion, an increase in thyroxine binding proteins, an increase in thyroid hormone production, and very high levels of hCG seen in 1st trimester of pregnancy has mild stimulatory effect on TSH hormone receptor causing TSH like stimulatory effect on thyroid. These physiological changes alter the normal serum thyroid hormone level and bound thyroid hormone levels.

The increase in TBG level is estrogen induced and results in approximately 150% increase in TT3 and TT4 levels as compared to the nonpregnant state. Free thyroid hormone levels usually remain normal in pregnancy, but are not reliable for clinical interpretation. In pregnancy, TT4 and TT3 of pregnancy ranges are used for clinical decision making. The high hCG level in 1st trimester causes subclinical hyperthyroidism such as picture which resolves spontaneously after 12 weeks of pregnancy.

DIFFICULT AREAS IN INTERPRETATION OF THYROID FUNCTION TEST

Drugs and Thyroid Hormone Function

Many drugs interfere with thyroid hormones homeostasis. These pharmacological agents may influence thyroid hormone homeostasis at multiple levels. Drugs can affect at pituitary or hypothalamic level and influence TSH secretion, e.g., dopamine frequently used in critical care set-up, dopamine agonist such as cabergoline, glucocorticoids, and octreotide used for variceal bleed can suppress TSH secretion; rexinoids a subclass of retinoids used in lung and breast cancers reduce serum TSH levels. Heparin is known to cause artifactual elevation of fT3 and fT4 by displacing thyroid hormones from their binding sites in vitro. Hence, for patients on heparin TT3 and TT4 is measured as not affected by heparin. Drugs can alter the serum TT3 and TT4 without affecting fT4 and fT3 by changing the protein binding. TT3 and TT4 levels are increased with normal free thyroid hormones by estrogen, 5-fluorouracil, tamoxifen, clofibrates, heroin, mitotane, etc. by increasing TBG concentration. In contrast, drugs can decrease TT3 and TT4 levels with normal free thyroid hormones by decreasing TBG concentration, e.g., androgen, asparaginase, glucocorticoids, high-dose salicylates, phenytoin, carbamazepine, etc.[9]

Nonthyroidal Illness

Nonthyroidal illness is associated with change in the thyroid hormone metabolism and hypothalamic-pituitary-thyroid axis, collectively known as the nonthyroidal illness syndrome or sick euthyroid syndrome. Within few hours of acute stress, serum T3 concentration decreases and is called as low T3 syndrome. Acute phase of illness is often associated with rise in serum TSH and fT4 and decrease in fT3. In chronic illness, serum TT3 and, often, fT3 are low. In mild-to-moderate nonthyroidal illness serum TSH and free T4 stay normal. In critically ill patients, low TSH and low serum T4 are associated with poor prognosis. Similar changes in thyroid hormones are seen in fasting and malnutrition states. During recovery from illness, a rapid rise in serum T4 and TSH is seen but TSH levels usually do not exceed 10 mIU/L. Serum T3 levels also rise following TSH rise. Hence, interpretation of thyroid function in nonthyroidal illness is difficult and needs to be interpreted in the clinical context.[8] Administration of T4 or T3 to these patients does not improve outcome.

Psychiatric Illness

Acute psychiatric illness transiently increases the thyroid hormone levels, usually in depression and acute psychosis.

LABORATORY ARTIFACTS AFFECTING THYROID FUNCTION TEST

The thyroid hormone assays results may be affected by factors in laboratory, and it is important to identify these artifacts. The commonly used immunoassays for TSH may be affected by the presence of antianimal human antibodies causing falsely raised or high serum TSH readings. Currently the commonly used immunoassays are biotin-based assays. Biotin is a common component of multivitamins supplements.

Excessive ingestion of biotin in form of medicine can falsely show low levels of serum TSH and high free T4 levels. With these results a person may falsely be treated as thyrotoxicosis. Although total T4 levels are not affected. As discussed before, heparin use in patient can affect the in vitro tests especially if sample is stored before testing. Hence, these factors must be considered when clinically correlating the hormone assays results.[10]

Other specific test used for thyroid disorders is mentioned here.

Thyroglobulin

Thyroglobulin is synthesized and stored in thyroid follicles and normally secreted in circulation along with the thyroid hormones. Thyroglobulin is specific to thyroid and in biopsy, specimen's presence of thyroglobulin confirms the thyroid origin of the tissue. In absence of functioning thyroid tissue, serum thyroglobulin is expected to be undetectable in circulation. This specificity of thyroglobulin to thyroid is used to assess the presence or absence of residual tissue or recurrence or metastasis in patient with differentiated thyroid cancer. The values in normal subjects with intact thyroid in most laboratories range from 1 to 30 ng/mL approximately. Serum thyroglobulin should be tested using a sensitive assay. Currently immunoassays are used for the assessment. Thyroglobulin is serially measured in post total thyroidectomy cases with differentiated thyroid cancers. It is recommended to use the same assay for serial measurements due to substantial variability in results with different assays, despite a trend toward assay standardization. Using thyroid stimulation either by thyroid hormone withdrawal or by recombinant TSH use, the sensitivity of serum thyroglobulin detection is increased.[11]

In the new sensitive thyroglobulin assays, serum thyroglobulin concentrations measured while receiving levothyroxine suppression therapy correlate with recombinant TSH stimulated thyroglobulin concentrations. Patients with a TSH-suppressed serum thyroglobulin concentration < 0.1 ng/mL (measured with an assay with a functional sensitivity of 0.05 ng/mL) were unlikely to have a recombinant TSH stimulated thyroglobulin above 2.0 ng/mL.

Antithyroglobulin antibodies should be measured with each measurement of serum thyroglobulin. Antithyroglobulin antibodies presence falsely decreases the levels of thyroglobulin by interfering with the assays. Post total thyroidectomy and ablation of residual tissue by radioiodine ablation, serum antithyroglobulin antibodies usually fall to undetectable levels over 3–5 years, while levels remain detectable or rise in patient with persistent disease. After total thyroidectomy and radioiodine ablation, serum thyroglobulin levels is low (<1–2 ng/mL), on levothyroxine and stimulated recombinant TSH, if the patient is cured. A serial follow-up serum thyroglobulin appears to be useful to detect progression of thyroid cancer and should lead to a search for the disease.

◇ REFERENCES

1. Spencer CA, LoPresti JS, Patel A, Guttler RB, Eigen A, Shen D, et al. Applications of a new chemiluminometric thyrotropin assay to subnormal measurement. J Clin Endocrinol Metab. 1990;70(2):453-60.
2. Hoermann R, Eckl WA, Hoermann C, Larisch R. Complex relationship between free thyroxine and TSH in the regulation of thyroid function. Eur J Endocrinol. 2010;162:1123-9.
3. Hoermann R, Midgley JEM, Giacobino A, Eckl WA, Wahl HG, Dietrich JW, et al. Homeostatic equilibria between free thyroid hormones and pituitary thyrotropin are modulated by various influences including age, body mass index and treatment. Clin Endocrinol (Oxf). 2014;81:907-15.
4. Engler D, Burger AG. The deiodination of the iodothyronines and of their derivatives in man. Endocr Rev. 1984;5(2): 151-84.
5. Bartalena L. Recent achievements in studies on thyroid hormone-binding proteins. Endocr Rev. 1990;11(1):47-64.
6. Soldin OP, Chung SH, Colie C. The use of TSH in determining thyroid disease: how does it impact the practice of medicine in pregnancy? J Thyroid Res. 2013, Article ID 148157, 8 pages.
7. Alexander EK, Pearce EN, Brent GA, Brown RS, Chen H, Dosiou C, et al. 2017 Guidelines of the American Thyroid Association for the diagnosis and management of thyroid disease during pregnancy and the postpartum. Thyroid. 2017;27(3):315-89. Erratum in: Thyroid. 2017;27(9):1212.
8. Garber JR, Cobin RH, Gharib H, Hennessey JV, Klein I, Mechanick JI, et al. Clinical practice guidelines for hypothyroidism in adults: cosponsored by the American Association of Clinical Endocrinologists and the American Thyroid Association. Endocr Pract. 2012;18(6):988-1028. Erratum in: Endocr Pract. 2013;19(1):175.
9. Koulouri O, Moran C, Halsall D, Chatterjee K, Gurnell M. Pitfalls in the measurement and interpretation of thyroid function tests. Best Pract Res Clin Endocrinol Metab. 2013;27(6):745-62.
10. Després N, Grant AM. Antibody interference in thyroid assays: a potential for clinical misinformation. Clin Chem. 1998;44(3):440-54.
11. Haugen BR. 2015 American Thyroid Association Management Guidelines for adult patients with thyroid nodules and differentiated thyroid cancer: what is new and what has changed? Cancer. 2017;123(3):372-81.

CHAPTER 4

History Taking and Clinical Examination of Goiter

Anand Kumar Mishra, Kul Ranjan Singh, Loreno E Enny, Surabhi Garg

INTRODUCTION

Pathologies of the thyroid are associated with many symptoms and signs, some of which are quite specific. A thorough elucidation of history and examination of patient is of prime importance in guiding the further management of presenting patients. History comprises presenting symptoms, details of development of symptoms, and significant personal or family history.[1]

AGE

Age of the patient has a significant effect on reaching the probable diagnosis. Dyshormogenetic goiters and thyroglossal cyst are usually evident in the first decade of life. Physiological goiters occur in pubertal age group and childbearing age. Multinodular goiters, solitary nodule, or colloid goiters can occur at any age but are common in second and third decades. The probability of nodule harboring a malignancy is higher in children and older adults. Anaplastic cancers are usually diagnosed in older individuals. Graves' disease is more common in younger individuals. Hashimoto's thyroiditis is commonly encountered in middle-aged women.

SEX

Majority of endocrine disorders occur in women and so do thyroid disorders. Thyroid nodules in males are more likely to be malignant but overall thyroid cancers are more common amongst women.

OCCUPATION

Radiation exposure, stressful jobs, mining industry, and those exposed to perchlorates are amongst the more common occupational hazards associated with thyroid disorders and should be enquired for.[2]

RESIDENCE

Gangetic plains, mountainous regions, and coastal regions of our country have a higher incidence of goiter. This has been attributed to low iodine in the food chain due to deficiency of iodine in soil and water of the region. Higher radiation from thorium-containing sands of Kerala has been told to be responsible for increasing incidence of thyroid cancer in the region but no causative role has been proven till date.[3] Increased autoimmunity to thyroid antigens resulting in thyroiditis has occasionally attributed to increasing iodine in the diet.

Symptoms of thyroid hormone excess or deficiency: A detailed history regarding presence of symptoms of hypo- or hyperthyroidism should be elicited. Each individual symptom has varying incidence, sensitivity, and specificity for suspecting altered thyroid function. Many of them are very subjective and presence of more than one discriminatory symptom of thyroid hormone deficiency/excess are likely to clinch the diagnosis. History of urticaria, pruritis, vitiligo, eczema, and connective tissue disorders may be seen in autoimmune thyroid diseases.

LOCAL SYMPTOMS AND SIGNS

Swelling

Onset, duration, pattern of progress, associated pain and cervical lymph nodes, and swelling elsewhere in the body should be probed in detail as they provide important clues to the diagnosis. Onset of diffuse thyroid swelling with symptoms of thyrotoxicosis points toward Graves' disease or thyroiditis. Concomitant appearance of eye signs would help clinch the diagnosis of Graves' disease. The rate of progress in size of thyroid nodule is usually misleading. A malignant nodule increases in size more rapidly, but a significant proportion are notorious for gradual increase in size and often remain static in size for variable periods. Poorly differentiated thyroid carcinoma (PDTC) and anaplastic thyroid carcinoma (ATC) are usually characterized by extremely rapid progress.

Association with Pain

Thyroid swellings are usually painless; however, a painful diffuse swelling is likely to be because of thyroiditis. A rapidly progressing painful thyroid swelling may be because of bleed into a thyroid nodule, a de novo ATC or transformation into anaplastic variant of thyroid carcinoma. Thyroid abscess though extremely rare presents with swelling, pain, and fever.

Compressive Features

Compression on the trachea, esophagus, and recurrent laryngeal nerves (RLNs) may occur during the course of thyroid pathology. The compressive features may not correlate with the size of the thyroid mass. A large mass that is located anteriorly may be totally asymptomatic whereas a small nodule that is located posteriorly may cause symptomatic compression on the RLN and esophagus. A malignant mass is more likely to have compressive features.

- *Recurrent laryngeal nerve*: Voice changes are not uncommon in thyroidal illnesses and are important clinical pointers. A recent change in voice quality should raise the suspicion of malignant etiology or transformation. Benign nodules/goiters because of their location or sheer size may cause voice changes.

  Voice changes may occur because of alterations in functional status of thyroid. Hoarseness with or without loss of range of voice is an important feature of hypothyroidism. Thyroid hormone excess may result in hoarseness due to abnormal movements of vocal cords.[4]
- *Esophagus*: Globus pharyngeus and progressive difficulty in swallowing may be encountered in many patients. This is said to be more common in left-sided pathology. Often the patient may not appreciate the symptoms distinctly as the changes occur gradually and are subtle.
- *Tracheal compression*: A greater than two-thirds luminal compromise of the trachea is required to have significant respiratory complaints or stridor. Many describe it as a choking sensation. Presence of a retrosternal component is likely making the patient more symptomatic and very often the symptoms have a positional variation.

◇ RISK FACTORS

The location of thyroid gland predisposes to it increased ill effects of radiation exposure. Increased radiation exposure from the environment or diagnostic procedures has been linked to increased incidence of thyroid cancer albeit in a small number.[2] The effect is more pronounced if the exposure occurred at a young age.

Level of iodine intake affects thyroid function. Deficiency of iodine association is an established cause of goiter. A few epidemiological studies have shown temporal association with iodine excess and thyroid carcinoma and autoimmune thyroid disorders.[5] More follicular carcinomas are seen in iodine deficient areas and papillary subtypes in iodine-rich areas.

Prospective cohort studies and observational studies have shown association between obesity, diabetes, and thyroid cancer. Women account for almost three-fourths of all thyroid cancer patients; however, there is no evidence that links thyroid cancer to estrogen.

Hashimoto's thyroiditis has been associated with increased incidence of thyroid cancers (PTC and lymphomas); however, a causal relationship has not been proven. An association of thyroid cancer and hepatitis C virus (HCV) and hepatitis B virus (HBV) has been seen of late.

Past History

Eliciting relevant past history gives relevant information about the course of the disease and its response to treatment received till date. Certain drugs have been classified as goitrogens. Information on previous hospitalizations/surgery/response to anesthesia, and presence of chronic conditions such as asthma, hypertension, ischemic heart disease, tuberculosis, etc., give us important information on perioperative risk assessment and help plan better.

Family History[6]

Differentiated thyroid carcinomas (DTCs) account for >85–90% and <5% are familial but medullary thyroid carcinomas (MTC) account for <5% of all thyroid cancers but 25% are familial. There is a 2–10-fold higher risk of sporadic DTC in presence of family history of thyroid cancer. MTCs are associated with MEN 2a/MEN 2b and familial MTC. Familial adenomatous polyposis (FAP), PTEN hamartoma tumor syndrome, Cowden's syndrome, Carneys complex, Pendred's syndrome, and Werner syndrome have predominance of no thyroidal syndromes with minimal increase in incidence of thyroid lesions. Familial syndromes characterized by predominance of papillary thyroid carcinoma (PTC) also occur such as pure familial PTC (fPTC), fPTC associated with papillary renal cell carcinoma, and fPTC with multinodular goiter. Hashimoto's thyroiditis, Graves' disease, and benign goiters also have shown familial association and same should be enquired for.

Personal History

Information regarding presence of alcohol, tobacco, and smoking should be sought in all patients.[7] No causal associations have been proven till date. Alcohol causes direct cellular toxicity in thyroid gland and also affects the neuroendocrine axis bringing about complex poorly understood changes. Moderate alcohol consumption has been associated with reduce in incidence of autoimmune thyroid diseases, goiter, and thyroid carcinoma.

Smoking increases the serum concentration of thiocyanates and has shown to increase the thyroid volume. Thiocyanates have a T1/2 of >5 days and inhibits iodine uptake by the thyroid, interferes with organification process, and increases iodine excretion by the kidney. However, it has not shown to affect the rate of progression of thyroid nodule growth. The adverse effects of smoking in thyroid has been more pronounced in iodine deficient population. Smoking has surprisingly shown association with reduced incidence of DTC.

Dietary History[8]

Many food items have been said to act as goitrogens if it forms a staple part of the diet. Hence, a detailed dietary history may give information about the probable etiology. Cassava (tapioca), lima beans (sem), sorghum, flax seeds, and sweet potato (shakarkand) are popular foods in our country which have cyanogenic glucosides which interferes with iodine uptake. Glucosinolates found in cruciferous vegetables like cabbage, cauliflower, broccoli, turnips, and rapeseeds also interfere with iodine uptake by the thyroid. Peroxidase activity is compromised by soy products and millets. Deficiency of iron, vitamin A, selenium, and increased dietary nitrates also predisposes to goiter formation by various mechanisms, if severe.

◇| EXAMINATION[9]

Examination of the patient starts with inspection followed by palpation. A normal thyroid gland is often difficult to see or palpate. A swelling in the region of thyroid that moves with deglutition is likely to be a thyroid or arising from the thyroid barring a few exceptions like central compartment lymph node, etc.

The entire gland is palpated from the front and standing behind the patient. Palpation from behind is useful in those with a heavy neck. Turning the patients head to the side of palpation relaxes the sternocleidomastoid and increases the accuracy of palpatory findings. The act of swallowing during palpation elevates the gland upward against the fingers and small nodules become more evident and helps define the lower border and rule out retrosternal extension.

Inspection

With the patient seated upright and the neck in slight extension, the anterior and lateral aspect of neck is observed. A normal thyroid is butterfly shaped and is normally not visualized or palpated unless the individual is of very thin built. A normal-sized thyroid but high lying in a thin individual with long neck is often perceived as a goiter. Other causes of pseudogoiter include lipomas and pharyngeal diverticula. Rarely, a normal thyroid in an individual with increased lordosis of cervical spine may be visible or palpable. This has been termed Modigliani syndrome.

- *Size, shape, and location*: The thyroid swelling is described as diffuse/localized, uninodular/multinodular. Uninodular or solitary and multinodular swellings can be unilateral/bilateral. The sternocleidomastoids are used as lateral landmarks and hyoid prominence and suprasternal notch as superior and inferior landmarks, respectively to describe the extent of mass. A note should be made on the presence of swelling on the lateral side of the neck which are likely to be lymph nodes.
- *Surface*: The surface is typically smooth in a diffuse goiter (physiological goiter, Graves' disease, thyroiditis) or a uninodular goiter. A multinodular goiter is characterized by nodular/bosselated surface.
- *Border*: Benign swellings usually have well-defined borders whereas malignant lesions are often characterized by irregular/indistinct borders.

- *Skin over the neck*: Redness and edema of overlying skin may denote an inflammatory etiology. A scar may suggest a previous intervention. Sinuses in the anterior aspect of neck with history of swelling that burst open may suggest a thyroglossal cyst and sinus. Dilated veins over the swelling and in neck and anterior chest wall may suggest a malignant etiology. Ulceration and fungation of overlying skin may occur due to pressure necrosis in large benign masses or skin involvement in malignancy.
- *Movement with deglutition and protrusion of tongue*: A thyroid swelling or any node attached to it would move with swallowing at the thyroid gland is attached to the laryngeal framework by the ligament of berry which is a condensation of the pretracheal fascia and attaches to the cricoid and first tracheal ring. A note should be made to visualize the lower border of the thyroid on deglutition. The movement of the swelling with protrusion of tongue should be ascertained to rule out thyroglossal cyst/fistula because of its attachment with thyroglossal tract and base of the tongue.

Palpation

The inspectory findings are confirmed on palpation. Thyroid can be palpated from front and back but is best palpated from the back with the neck slightly flexed using the pulps of fingers **(Fig. 1)**. The neck can be tilted to the side of palpation to relax the ipsilateral sternocleidomastoid muscle. Occasionally, additional palpation of a nodule in an extended neck may be more informative. Temperature and tenderness are looked for followed by size, shape, extent of swelling, borders, surface, fixity of skin, mobility, and consistency. The thyroid surface appears smooth in physiological goiters and primary thyrotoxicosis. Surface is bosselated in multinodular goiter. Consistency of the nodule can be deceiving. Malignant nodules feel hard to touch but benign tense cystic nodules of long-standing calcified benign goiter may feel hard. Follicular carcinomas are usually not

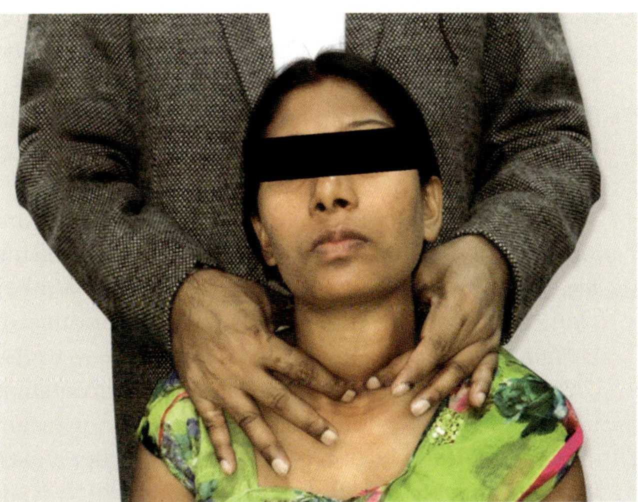

Fig. 1: Palpation of thyroid gland.

hard on palpation. Restricted mobility of the thyroid mass is suggestive of infiltrative pathology due to malignancy or inflammation. Inability to palpate the lower border of thyroid suggests the possibility of retrosternal extension of the thyroid mass.

Cervical lymph nodes: A sequential spread of thyroid cancers like PTC/MTC occurs to various lymph node stations in the neck. Level 6 (central compartment) is the first lymph node basis followed by level 2/3/4 to be involved. Levels 1 and 5 are rarely involved. Lymph nodal spread in follicular thyroid carcinoma (FTC) is rare. The lymph node stations, number, size, margin, consistency, mobility, tenderness, and matting should be described. Additional lymph nodal basins like axillary and inguinal should be examined also. Delphian lymph node lies anterior to cricothyroid ligament. This node may be involved in thyroid cancer, thyroiditis, etc.

Examination of trachea: The lower part of cervical trachea is palpable in the suprasternal notch. This may be shifted to one side by unilateral swellings or may be central in bilateral involvement of the thyroid. This test is performed by standing in front of the patient with the index and ring fingers on the sternoclavicular joints and running down the trachea with the middle finger **(Fig. 2)**.

Additional maneuvers in inspection and palpation:
- *Pizzillo's method*: Thyroid can be made more prominent for inspection in obese and short-necked individuals by asking them to extend the neck against their hand placed behind the head **(Fig. 3)**.
- *Lahey's method*: This maneuver is performed from the front of the patient. To palpate the right lobe, the thyroid gland along with the laryngotracheal complex is pushed to the right with the left hand and simultaneously palpating the right lobe with left hand **(Fig. 4)**.
- *Crile's method*: Subtle enlargements of thyroid or smaller nodule/nodules can be appreciated by placing the thumb on the thyroid gland and asking the patient to swallow. The nodule moves against the thumb. The method is more useful for small nodules located in the tracheoesophageal groove. The examiner needs to sit in front of the patient and place both thumbs on either side of the airway and asked the patient to deglutition **(Figs. 5A and B)**.
- *Kocher's test*: This test is done by fixing the thyroid and laryngotracheal complex with one hand and compressing the thyroid lobe with the opposite hand on the other side. Development of stridor signifies presence of incipient critical tracheal narrowing because of the thyroid swelling. Scabbard trachea is the approximation of the lateral walls of the trachea due to compression and is a radiological sign. A positive Kocher's sign is not synonymous with tracheomalacia which is an intraoperative finding **(Fig. 6)**.

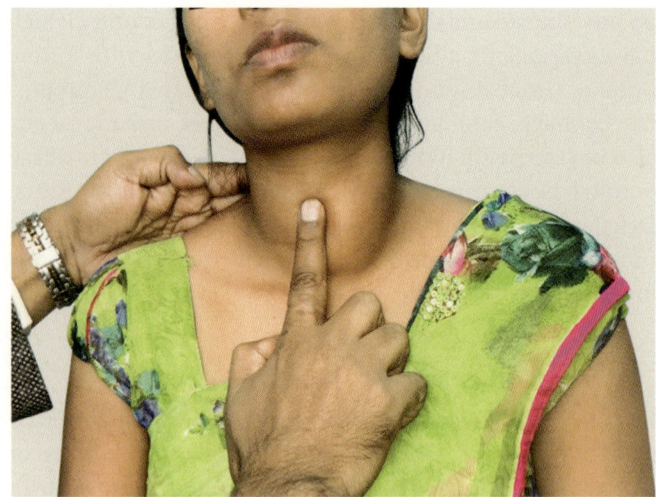

Fig. 2: Palpation of trachea.

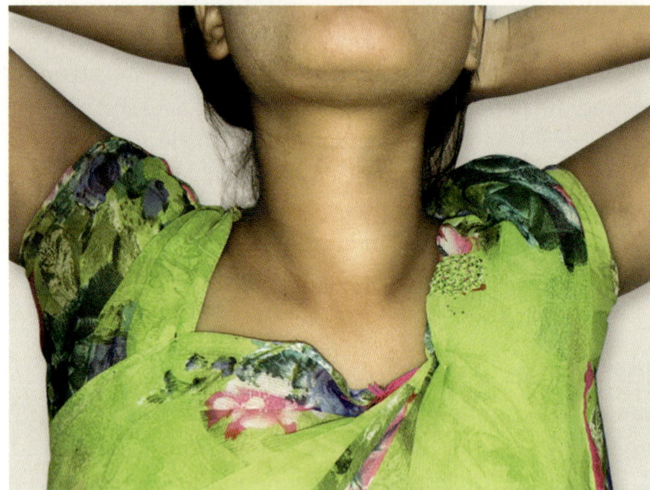

Fig. 3: Pizzillo's method.

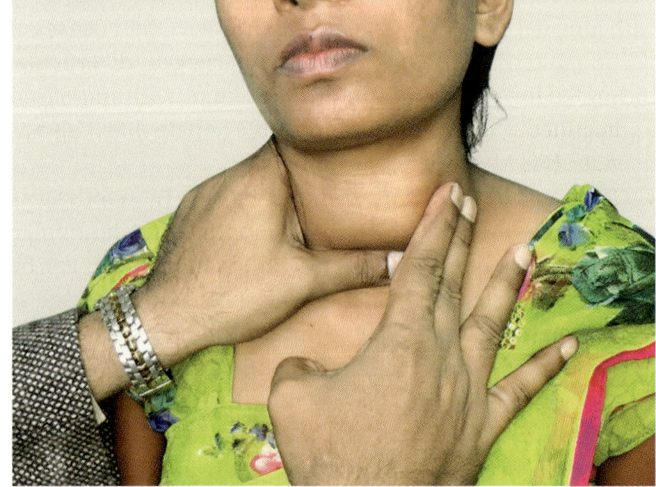

Fig. 4: Lahey's method.

- *Berry's sign*: Palpate for the carotid pulsation. It is normally felt in the anterior triangle against the transverse process of the cervical vertebrae one at a time. The common carotid artery usually divides at the level of upper border of the lamina of the thyroid cartilage (C4). This may be

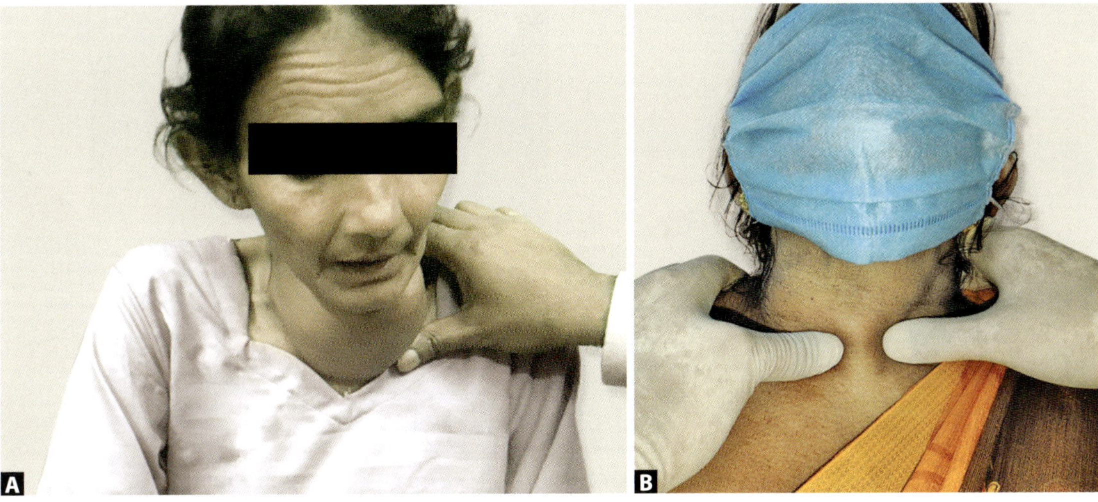

Figs. 5A and B: Crile's method.

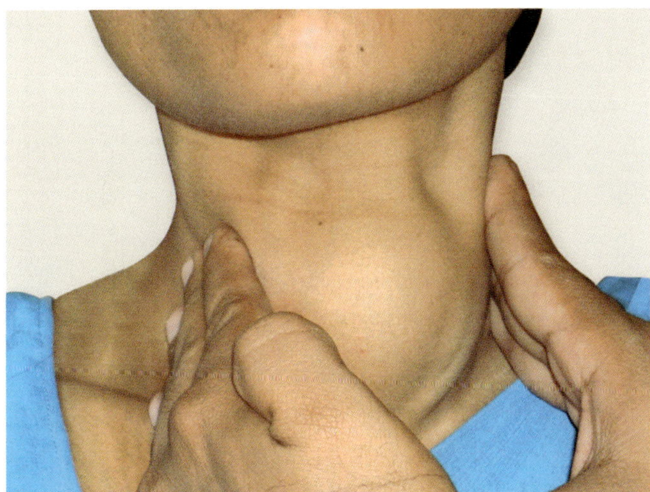

Fig. 6: Kocher's test.

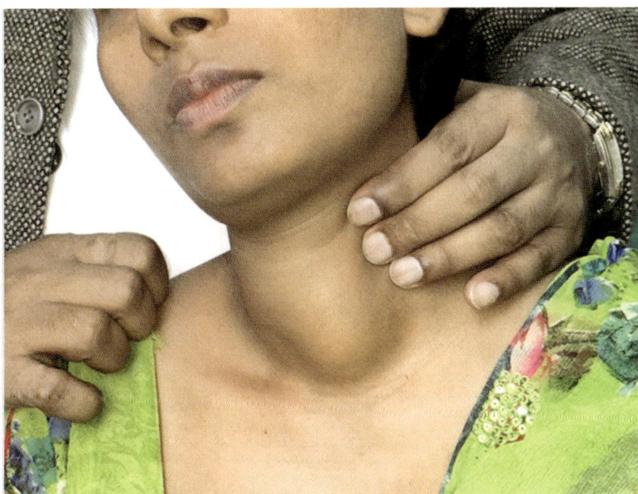

Fig. 7: Berry's sign.

shifted laterally in large benign goiters or may be absent if engulfed/encased by a malignant lesion (Positive Berry's sign) **(Fig. 7)**.

- *Horner's syndrome*: Thyroid masses may compress or infiltrate the cervical sympathetic chain resulting in Horner's syndrome which is characterized by ipsilateral miosis, enophthalmos, ptosis, and anhidrosis (absence of sweating on the affected side of the face). These findings can be elicited as a part of history/inspection.

Percussion over Manubrium Sterni

Percussion over the manubrium sterni normally has a tympanic note. A dull note on percussion suggests retrosternal extension of the thyroid mass/lymph nodes. An individual in whom the lower extent of thyroid mass can be palpated but percussion over manubrium sterni is dull should raise the suspicion of possibility of coexisting detached thyroid nodule, coexistent mediastinal goiter, or enlarged superior mediastinal nodes **(Fig. 8)**.

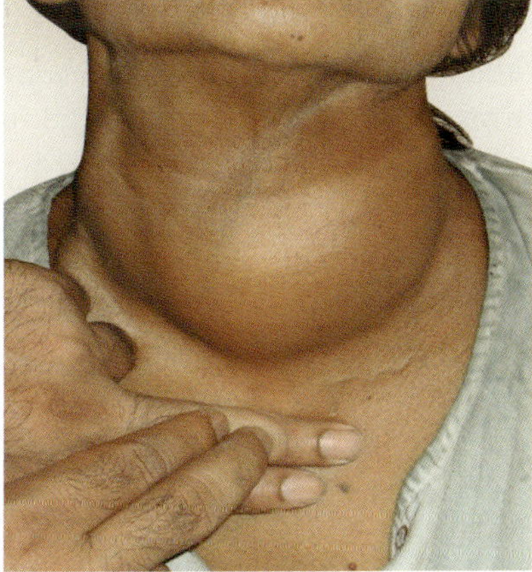

Fig. 8: Percussion over manubrium sterni.

Thrill and Bruit

Thyroid is a very vascular organ and its vascularity is increased manifolds in toxicity and malignancy. The increased vascularity can be appreciated by a palpable thrill and an

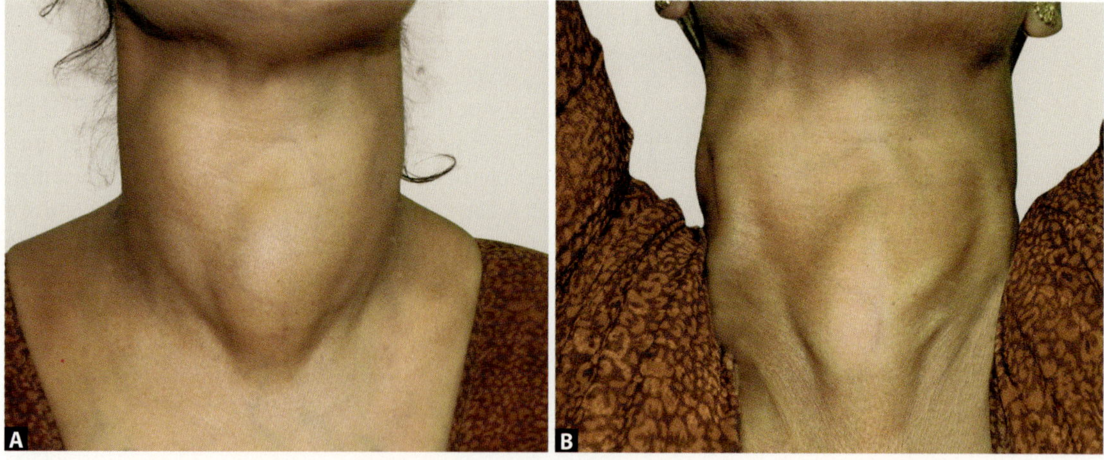

Figs. 9A and B: Pemberton's sign.

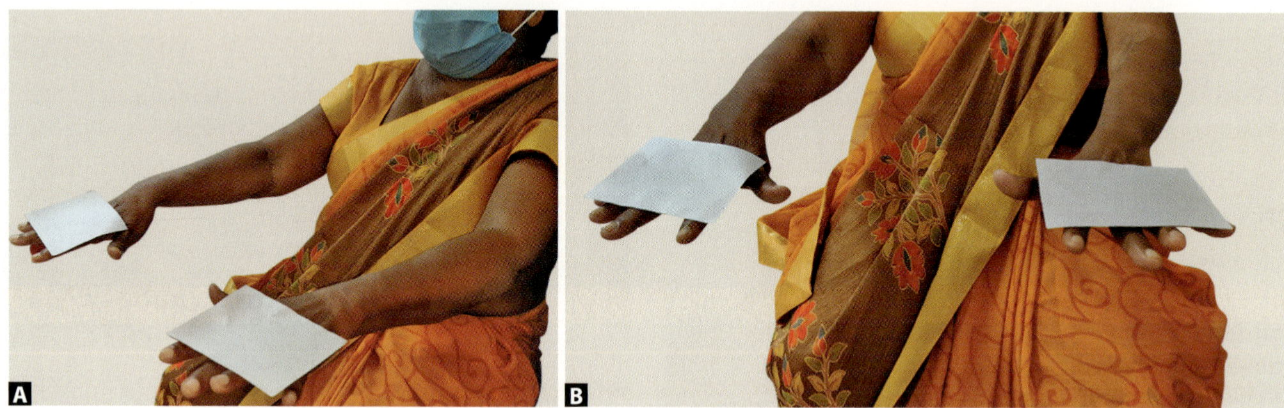

Figs. 10A and B: Examination for hand tremors.

auscultatory bruit in the region of superior pole of the thyroid gland.

Pemberton's Sign[10]

This sign is elicited in case of a goiters with retrosternal extension by asking the patient to raise both his arms overhead with at the arms touching the sides of head for a minute. A positive Pemberton's sign is characterized by the appearance of facial plethora, vascular engorgement, cyanosis, or distress. The vascular compression occurs has been shown to occur because of the medial and inferior movement of lateral (acromial) end of clavicle rather than cork effect brought about by the craniocaudal movement of the thyroid or upward movement of the thoracic inlet **(Figs. 9A and B)**.

◇ GENERAL EXAMINATION

Thyroid Dermopathy[11]

Skin changes (dermopathy) can occur in those with Graves' disease with ophthalmopathy and rarely in chronic autoimmune thyroiditis. Classical pretibial myxedema is characterized by diffuse nonpitting pedal edema with orange peel appearance most commonly in the anterior aspect of shin but can occur elsewhere. Plaques and nodules can also occur.

Thyroid acropachy is a rare manifestation of autoimmune thyroid disorders and consists of clubbing and swelling of digits along with periosteal reaction of extremity bones.

Skin and hair changes commonly occur in both hypo- and hyperthyroidism and should be looked for.

Cardiovascular System

This is of great importance in toxic patients. Pulse rate and character should be examined. A collapsing pulse which may be of water hammer in character due to wide pulse pressure is seen. A sleeping pulse rate gives more accurate information. Hyperdynamic apex along with apical systolic murmur is often seen in toxic patients. Atrial fibrillation should be looked for.

Tremors

This is checked in outstretched hands with fingers widely spaced. A small sheet of paper may be placed on the hand to make it more obvious. The tremors in hyperthyroidism are typically low amplitude with a high frequency often described as fine tremors. This can also be elicited in the tongue **(Figs. 10A and B)**.

Table 1: Clinical signs of Graves' orbitopathy.	
Sign	*Description*
Dalrymple's	Upper eyelid is at a higher than normal position (upper sclera visible)
Von Graffe's	Upper eyelid cannot keep pace with downward gaze
Joffroy's	Absence of forehead creases on upward gaze
Stellwag's	Incomplete and infrequent blinking
Moebius	Failure of convergence of eyeballs
Becker's	Abnormal intense pulsation of retinal arteries
Boston's	Jerky movements of upper eyelid on downward gaze
Cowen's	Extensive hippus of consensual pupillary reflex
Enroth's	Upper eyelid edema
Gifford's	Difficulty of upper eyelid eversion
Griffith's	Lower lid lag on upward gaze
Hertoghe's	Loss of lateral eye brows
Jellinek's	Hyperpigmentation of superior eyelid folds
Kocher's	Spasmatic retraction of upper eyelid on gaze fixation
Riesman's	Bruit over the eyelid
Suker's	Inability to maintain fixation on fixation in extreme lateral gaze

Ophthalmopathy

The symptoms of hypothyroidism are usually distinct from hyperthyroidism but occasionally patients of hyperthyroidism may present with weight gain due to excessive eating.

Older patients of hyperthyroidism may present with symptoms like apathy/depression, breathlessness, worsening angina, and congestive heart failure which are not very characteristics of hyperthyroidism. This has been often referred to apathetic hyperthyroidism.

Eye involvement is common in thyrotoxicosis. Presence of diffuse goiter with ophthalmopathy is pathognomonic of Graves' disease and this combination obviates the need of specialized tests for diagnosis. Certain signs like staring look and lid retraction which are caused by sympathetic overactivity can be seen in any case of thyrotoxicosis. However, orbitopathy is limited to cases of Graves' disease and this leads to irritation, excessive tearing, eye/retro-orbital discomfort, conjunctival injection, blurred vision, diplopia, proptosis, and loss of vision in neglected cases. Symptoms of orbitopathy are subjective whereas signs are often objective. These subjective symptoms and signs of Graves' ophthalmopathy can be graded as NO SPECS, Clinical Activity Score (CAS), VISA (vision, inflammation, strabismus, appearance), and EUGOGO (European Group of Graves' Orbitopathy) classifications.

The various clinical signs of Graves' orbitopathy are as shown in **Table 1**.

Trousseau's and Chvostek's sign: This should be elicited preoperatively in any patient likely to undergo total thyroidectomy as these important clinical signs of hypocalcemia may be present in some individuals in normocalcemia also.

◇ CONCLUSION

The importance of elaborate history and detailed examination is of prime importance in management of patients with a thyroid pathology. It helps us to formulate an appropriate diagnostic and treatment algorithm for a patient.

◇ REFERENCES

1. Das S. Examination of thyroid gland. A Manual on Clinical Surgery, 12th edition. Kolkata: S Dass Publishers; 2008.
2. Aschebrook-Kilfoy B, Ward MH, Della Valle CT, Friesen MC. Occupation and thyroid cancer. Occup Environ Med. 2014;71(5):366-80.
3. Aravindam KP. Papillary thyroid cancer: Why the increase and what can be done? Indian J Cancer. 2017;54(3):491-2.
4. Hari Kumar KV, Garg A, Ajai Chandra NS, Singh SP, Datta R. Voice and endocrinology. Indian J Endocrinol Metab. 2016;20(5):590-4.
5. Zimmermann MB, Galetti V. Iodine intake as a risk factor for thyroid cancer: a comprehensive review of animal and human studies. Thyroid Res. 2015;8:8.
6. Nosé V. Familial thyroid cancer: a review. Mod Pathol. 2011;24(2):S19-S33.
7. Liu Y, Su L, Xiao H. Review of factors related to the thyroid cancer epidemic. Int J Endocrinol. 2017;2017:5308635.
8. Choi WJ, Kim J. Dietary factors and the risk of thyroid cancer: a review. Clin Nutr Res. 2014;3(2):75-88.
9. Sreeharan V. Examination of the thyroid gland and thyroid status. J Clinical Exam. 2007;3:1-7.
10. De Filippis EA, Sabet A, Sun MR, Garber JR. Pemberton's sign: exlained nearly 70 years later. J Clin Endocrinol Metab. 2014;99(6):1949-54.
11. Singla M, Gupta A. Nodular thyroid dermopathy: not a hallmark of Graves' disease. Am J Med. 2019;132(3):e521-2.

Solitary Thyroid Nodule

Ranil Fernando

◇ INTRODUCTION

Nodules of the thyroid are one of the most common problems encountered in surgical endocrinology world over. Thyroid nodules have been defined by the American Thyroid Association (ATA) as "discrete lesions within the thyroid gland, radiologically distinct from surrounding thyroid parenchyma."[1] A nodule may also be defined as a discrete lesion, within the thyroid gland, due to an abnormal and focal growth of thyroid cells.

A solitary nodule of the thyroid (STN) has a special significance in that the most common presenting feature of a thyroid cancer is a STN. The STN in a child is of special concern as the incidence of cancer in such a setting is higher.[2] In addition, the STN may cause thyroid dysfunction and, if big, give rise to features of compression. These concerns and clinical aspects need to be addressed when managing the STN. The diagnosis and management of these nodules is beset by several contentious issues. Evidence-guided management strategies will enable the surgeon/endocrinologist to offer the best possible treatment for the patients.

◇ PREVALENCE OF THYROID NODULES

The prevalence of thyroid nodules varies with the modality employed to detect nodules. When clinical methods are used for detection the prevalence is around 4–7%.[3] This may be higher in areas of iodine deficiency.[4] The prevalence rates in image-based studies and postmortem studies are much higher and exceed 50%.[5-8] There appears to be an increasing prevalence of thyroid nodules world over. It is debatable whether this is a true increase or a reflection of sophisticated and highly sensitive diagnostic method. The latter is the more likely reason for the increase. There is an increase in the prevalence of nodules with age.[9] While most of the detected nodules are truly solitary, it must be remembered that some of the STNs may be the early stage of a multinodular goiter (MNG), dominant nodule of an MNG or the emergence of nodules in Hashimoto thyroiditis. Even though fear of cancer is a concern only about 5–15% of thyroid nodules are truly malignant.[10]

◇ CLINICAL EVALUATION OF A SOLITARY THYROID NODULE

Clinical evaluation remains a cornerstone in decision making in the management of an STN. Most patients are likely to be asymptomatic. The nodule may have been detected on routine examination or on the basis of an ultrasound (US) scan of the neck, done for another indication. This is not uncommon due to the increasing awareness among patients and the easy availability of imaging modalities. The main contentious issue regarding image-based detection of a very small nodule would be the possibility of over diagnosis and risks involved in overtreatment of these patients.

In the history, special attention must be given to the age <20 years or >70 years old, male sex, the presence of a family history of thyroid disease especially thyroid cancer, possible prior exposure to radiation and other features such as compression in the case of a large STN. On examination, even though traditionally the thyroid gland is examined from behind, it is necessary to emphasize that examinations *both* from the front and back are mandatory. Some characteristics such as asymmetry, visible nodules, and consistency of a nodule are much better assessed from the front. Eye signs can properly be assessed, only from the front.

While firm consistency is more suggestive of a possible malignancy; care is needed in making a judgment as the assessment is subjective. Most authors would agree features such as change in voice, fixity to adjacent structures, associated lymphadenopathy and a size of >4 cm are definitive indicators of the possibility of malignancy.[11]

There is general consensus that a nodule must be around 1 cm (10 mm) for it to be palpable clinically. Even though bigger lesions are thought to have a greater propensity to be malignant, the size of the lesion may not predict possibility of malignancy.[8,12,13] There is a debate about the relevance of treating lesions < 10 mm (1 cm) as it does not appear to offer any health benefit apart from relieving anxiety. Follow-up will definitely be needed in such patients. They can be offered definitive treatment if there is any change which will be of concern to the clinician and the patient.

◇ IMAGING OF A SOLITARY THYROID NODULE—US SCAN

The US scan remains the main mode of imaging for an STN. Nodules as small as 2–3 mm can be detected on US scan. The US scan will provide information about the size, shape, solid or cystic nature of the nodule, and if a flow study is added, the blood flow and vascularity of the STN can also be assessed. Features such as absence of a halo, solid appearance, increased vascularity, irregular margins, and microcalcifications are recognized as constant features associated with malignancy.[14]

The US scan supplemented by clinical findings and a fine-needle cytology will be sufficient in majority of patients to offer or differ definitive treatment. US-scan imaging alone cannot be relied on to make accurate prediction about malignancy in a thyroid nodule. However, appearances such as a true cyst or spongiform pattern are more likely to predict a benign lesion.[15]

CT SCAN AND OTHER IMAGING MODALITIES

These will only be needed in a few patients where specific issues need to be addressed and should be done after discussion at a multidisciplinary team (MDT) meeting. There is no indication to undertake these investigations unless there is a clear indication such as involvement and fixity to vessels, retrosternal extension, etc. CT scan, MRI or fluorodeoxyglucose positron emission tomography (FDG-PET) scan may be indicated in some patients before a definitive decision is made.

FINE-NEEDLE CYTOLOGY

Fine-needle cytology (FNC) is the main diagnostic tool in the assessment of an STN. FNC can be performed with or without aspiration. While some authors claim that fine-needle nonaspiration cytology (FNNAC) is better.[16] There is no clear evidence or consensus that nonaspiration technique provides a diagnostically superior yield.[17] This is probably due to individual variation in the techniques performed at different centers. The diagnostic accuracy of FNC in predicting malignancy varies from center to center and the sensitivity, specificity, and positive and negative predictive values too have a wide range of variation in different parts of the world.[18-20] This can be explained by the experience of the persons undertaking the technique and also the system of reporting used to provide the results of the FNC. One of the problems with FNC is the interpretation and obtaining a clear diagnosis in some patients. There are several systems of classification for thyroid cytology. The commonly used classifications are: The Bethesda System for Reporting Thyroid Cytology (TBSRTC) introduced by Cibas and Ali[21] and the Thy Classification of the British Thyroid association.[22] These classifications have made reporting of FNC more uniform world over. Other systems of reporting such as the 2014 Italian Reporting System for Thyroid (TIR) Cytology[23] are available in the literature. All the classification systems have a 4–6 levels of diagnosis. The second and the last levels (2, 5 and 6) usually do not cause issues as they are either clearly benign (2) or clearly malignant (5 and 6). The difficulties are with intermediate levels that cause management dilemmas.

Fine-needle cytology quality of the aspirate belongs to three categories namely satisfactory, unsatisfactory, and indeterminate. Unsatisfactory smears (5–10%) result from hypocellular specimens, cystic fluid, bloody smears, or unsatisfactory preparation of the smears.[20] In the unsatisfactory category repeat FNC is essential to determine the management of these patients. The indeterminate group is about 10–20% of patients. Overall risk of malignancy in the indeterminate group is generally believed to be around 10–15% but some studies have shown that it may range from 15–60%, depending on the specifics of the report.[20]

It has been noted, in addition, that with the increase of the size of the nodule the predicative accuracy of malignancy decreases.[24] This is understandable as the needle may easily miss a malignant focus in a larger lesion. To make the diagnostic accuracy better the current trend is to perform FNC under US scan guidance. This should enable more accurate sampling. Yet the studies do not show much better diagnostic yield with US scan guidance.[25] As in all techniques there is a learning curve and individual variation. But if the initial "blind FNC" produces a doubtful result, then a US-scan-guided FNC will be the best next option.

The indeterminate lesions (Bethesda 3–4) include poor quality specimens as well as an atypia of undetermined significance/follicular lesion of undetermined significance (AUS/FLUS) category of lesions as determined by the Bethesda system. The decision making in these lesions becomes difficult and complex.

ATYPIA OF UNDETERMINED SIGNIFICANCE AND FOLLICULAR LESION OF UNDETERMINED SIGNIFICANCE LESIONS

Atypia of undetermined significance and follicular lesion of undetermined significance are acronyms for atypia of unknown significance (AUS) and follicular lesion of unknown significance (FLUS). When faced with an AUS/FLUS lesion the clinician must decide on what to do next. Several tests are likely to be needed to exclude a malignancy. What can be done will depend on expertize and the facilities available. Easiest is to perform a repeat FNC. The timing of the repeat FNC is a matter of debate but there is no clear evidence to suggest that doing the repeat assessment 3 months after the initial FNC gives a better diagnostic yield as suggested previously.[26] The timing should be decided by the need to minimize discomfort to the patient and relieving the anxiety of the patient. Repeat FNC in about 4–6 weeks appears a good compromise.

This may or may not produce the desired result. Various centers have developed and utilized other methods including the use of molecular markers to determine the likelihood of malignancy. The cheapest option is to have a predictive scoring system such a "Radiomics Score" for thyroid nodules.[27] Radiomics (rad-score) is a new tool used in oncology, which extracts large amount of quantitative features from medical images using data-characterization algorithms enabling the development of a score. The McGill Thyroid Nodule Score (MTNS) utilizes clinical, laboratory imaging, and cytological data to predict the chances of malignancy.[28] For a resource poor healthcare system, scoring systems appear to offer a good way of reducing unnecessary surgery. In addition each country/region must try to develop its own score/system based on facilities and expertize available. Some centers have used the US findings, repeat biopsy, and immunocytochemistry. Immunohistochemical markers such as galectin-3, 7 HBME-1, 8 fibronectin-1, CITED-1, and cytokeratin-19 have yielded suboptimal results.[29] Molecular genetics using BRAFV-600E mutation in cytological specimens have helped to resolve the issue in some patients.[30]

It is likely that, in the future, better imaging modalities and genetic markers will evolve. The only issue of contention then is the universal availability of such modalities. Despite best efforts, in some patients, ultimately the clinician and the patient will have to make a combined decision whether close observation or hemithyroidectomy is the preferred option. Following surgery and histology if the AUS/FLUS lesion proves to be benign, the patient is cured but if it turns out to be malignant then another decision about completion thyroidectomy needs to be taken based on evidence-guided management of thyroid cancer.

◇ CORE NEEDLE BIOPSY OF THYROID

Fine-needle cytology remains the main tool for tissue diagnosis in dealing with nodules of the thyroid, but due to the difficulties alluded to above in the interpretation other techniques such as core biopsy has been practiced in some centers.[31] The concept of core biopsy of thyroid seems a bit drastic as the possible complications of bleeding and injury to neighboring structures are distinct possibilities. In general core biopsy of thyroid must not be done. The only indication that is universally accepted, for core biopsy of the thyroid, is the clinical suspicion of a thyroid lymphoma, where the cell type of the lymphoma is critical in deciding the treatment options.[32] Core biopsy should only be practiced in specialized centers with expert operators. The biopsy is done under strict recommendations.[33] These must be followed diligently. The advantage of core needle biopsy of thyroid (CNB) is that it provides better specimens not only for histology but also for ancillary tests such as immunocytochemistry and molecular genetics. This procedure may be fine-tuned in the future and may become a very useful adjunct especially in follicular lesions but it must be performed only by experts in centers of excellence.

◇ HORMONE ASSAY

Every patient with a thyroid nodule must have a hormone assay done. Most patients would be asymptomatic and euthyroid, but some are likely to have dysfunction which may be subclinical. In a resource poor setting of initial assessment of a thyroid stimulating hormone (TSH) would suffice even as dysfunction without alteration in TSH is very rare. Though some may not agree with this policy, it is a useful guide in resource limited setting. In the case of suppressed TSH the possibility of autonomously functioning thyroid nodule (AFTN) needs to be considered.

◇ AUTONOMOUSLY FUNCTIONING THYROID NODULE

In 1918, Emil Goetsch proved that AFTNs can cause hyperthyroidism and described the pathophysiology of AFTNs. A series of publications between 1967 and 1980 confirmed Goetsch's findings and AFTN was recognized as a clinical entity.[34] AFTN constitutes about 5% of all thyroid nodules. They are also called autonomous thyroid adenoma. AFTN is characterized by a single thyroid adenoma which is functioning autonomously and independently of pituitary stimulation or any other extrathyroidal stimulator. The thyroid hormone secreted by the nodule has a negative feedback on the production of TSH. By this mechanism, the function of the TSH-dependent extranodular tissue is suppressed to a variable degree. This gives the thyroid gland the typical appearance on Scintiscan. Two types of monoclonal autonomously functioning nodules have been reported. Both are due to somatic mutations. One involves the TSH receptor (TSHR) gene and the other involves the Gs-α protein gene mutations of the TSHR gene play a major (principal) role in the pathogenesis of AFTN. The Gs-α gene has a much lower prevalence.[35]

Many patients with a solitary AFTN are euthyroid. Progression to persisting hyperthyroidism occurs in only a small number of patients (5–10%). Patients with hyperfunctioning adenomas who are euthyroid initially develop hyperthyroidism at a rate of about 4% per year. This depends on the size of the adenoma, iodine intake, and the age of the patient.[36] Toxicity rarely develops in nodules <2.5 cm in diameter.[36] Spontaneous degeneration of the nodule is also documented.

The natural history of AFTN also suggests that a small number of patients become hypothyroid no matter what form of therapy is chosen. Therefore, nontoxic autonomous thyroid nodules are regularly left untreated. AFTNs with a normal TSH value are diagnosed only rarely. Cognizance and clinical suspicion will facilitate a diagnosis of AFTN. TSH is not a screening tool for AFTN. The diagnosis of AFTN is considered when concentration of the radionuclide tracer is greater or equal to that of the extranodular tissue (hot nodule).

Treatment consists mainly of surgery or radiotherapy[37] with other less invasive options such as ethanol injection, radiofrequency ablation (RFA), high-intensity focused ultrasound (HIFU) and laser as alternatives in selected individuals.[38] Surgery (hemithyroidectomy) is offered mainly for patients below 50 years of age, those with compressive features and when malignancy is suspected or is diagnosed during assessment. The other options are offered for other patients especially older patients.

ISOTOPE SCANNING

[99m]Tc, ^{123}I, and ^{131}I are the isotopes commonly used for thyroid isotope scanning. They provide information about the function of the thyroid gland. Historically cold (hypoactive) nodules were considered to indicate a possible malignancy. Due to the very low diagnostic accuracy and the advent of far more sensitive FNC, there is consensus that the role of the isotope is very limited in the initial assessment of a thyroid nodule.[39] The specific indication for an isotope scan is the suspicion of an AFTN. It is one indication where a Scintiscan is essential when evaluating an STN.

OTHER ASSESSMENTS

Other investigations such as, thyroid antibodies, serum calcitonin assessment, thyroid-stimulating antibody level (TSAb), thyroglobulin, etc. will be needed only for specific indications and do not form part of the initial assessment of an STN.

MOLECULAR GENETICS

In an effort to resolve problems associated with indeterminate cytology, molecular testing has been used in several centers around the world to reduce the diagnostic uncertainty of cytological indeterminate thyroid nodules. Several genetic markers have been used. There is some success with BRAFV-600E mutation in cytological specimens.[29] Some centers have used gene expression classifiers (GEC) to assess malignancy risk in indeterminate lesions. The GEC has been useful as a negative predictor of malignancy.[30] Overall the results of molecular testing have been modest so far. Different classifiers appear to give varying results.[30] Further development of molecular genetics with improvement in multiplex molecular techniques will assist in resolving difficult diagnostic issues in the future. Large cohort of studies with long follow-up is needed to establish the role of molecular genetics in the routine assessment of an STN. Molecular testing needs significant amount of resources and in resource poor settings molecular testing must be used judiciously.

MANAGEMENT STRATEGIES FOR SOLITARY NODULE OF THE THYROID

Once the diagnostic assessment is completed, several possibilities will be encountered as listed here. Each category will need a different approach of management and more than one treatment method may have to be used. There are numerous algorithms available in the literature.[8,40,41]

- *Nondiagnostic on initial assessment*: Nondiagnostic smears are the result of aspiration of insufficient material or poor material (blood) to make a cytological diagnosis. Repeat FNC should be done after a time gap to minimize the influence of inflammation and bleeding from the initial FNC. Satisfactory smears can be obtained in 50% of cases.[8] Definitive therapy can then be offered based on the findings. Very rarely if repeated aspirations fail to provide the answer and a clinical suspicion exists, surgery may have to be considered if the matter cannot be resolved by nonsurgical methods. The benefits must be carefully balanced against the risks in such a situation.
- *Benign euthyroid STN—Cystic*: If the diagnosis is a benign thyroid cyst then the best option is to aspirate under the US guidance. Many patients will only require follow-up after that. If the cyst recurs then respiration or hemithyroidectomy may be considered if the cyst is large. This will be a minority.[41]
- *Benign euthyroid STN—Solid*: If the lesion is solid and small it will only need close follow-up as some of the nodules may resolve spontaneously. If the nodule is large (>3 cm) a decision must be made whether intervention is needed or it needs to be observed with close follow-up. Six monthly clinical evaluation and imaging must be done initially. If there is any change an FNC is indicated. If the lesion increases in size, causing compressive features of diagnostically indeterminate then surgery must be considered.[40,41] The role of thyroxine in reducing nodule size has been debated for many years. While there is some reduction in size initially it is not sustainable and the nodule tends to grow soon after the stoppage of the thyroxine. The dose required is a suppressive dose and the optimal duration is unknown. The cardiovascular, skeletal and other side effects of thyroxine such as iatrogenic hyperthyroidism have prompted many authors who recommend abandoning the use of thyroxine to reduce the size of thyroid nodules.[42] Several guidelines discourage the use of thyroxine to reduce nodule size of STN. There is an urgent need to stop the indiscriminate use of thyroxine in general.
- *Benign hyperthyroid—(AFTN or Hashimoto Thyroiditis, early toxic MNG or rarely Graves' disease):* If the nodule is hyperfunctioning in the initial assessment then the four possibilities listed above need to be considered. Other diagnostic methods will assist in defining which disease entity it is and the management appropriate for that entity must be instituted. There will be a need to suppress hormone production using antithyroid drugs initially in all, entities except Hashimoto disease where there is no excess hormone production.

Once the patient is euthyroid what further treatment is required will need to be decided. This will vary depending on the age of the patient, general status of the patient, the expertise available, and the wishes of the patient. Some patients will require at least a hemithyroidectomy, e.g., large AFTN. Others may need total thyroidectomy, e.g., Graves' disease.

- *Indeterminate and AUS/FLUS lesions*: Management of these lesions has been discussed previously. This is the category that raises several issues as discussed. The management strategies must be evidence-guided to avoid inappropriate or overtreatment. It must be borne in mind the good prognosis and slow progression of most thyroid cancers.

- *Malignant euthyroid*: If the final conclusion in the assessment is a malignancy, the most appropriate treatment for the malignancy must be instituted. If the lesion is >1 cm there is no issue in dealing with the lesion as there are clear guidelines on management and the guidelines must be followed. But if the lesion is <1 cm then a dilemma arises regarding the best course of action. It has been shown clearly that subcentimeter tumors do not progress to clinically manifest cancers in many patients and that they follow an indolent course.[43,44] The main argument is that these small cancers are unlikely to cause morbidity or mortality due to their indolent nature and offering treatment early is overtreatment and may involve unnecessary risks to the patients. In addition patient can be offered treatment if there is any worrying change in the lesion.

Adoption of a policy of observation and surveillance needs to be done cautiously and only in centers with experience and expertise.

- *Malignant hyperthyroid*: The first priority in such a patient is to control the toxicity with antithyroid drugs. Patient can then be offered stage appropriate treatment for the thyroid cancer guided by evidence.

Should you screen for thyroid nodules?

The imaging modalities such as US scan are easily available at low cost nowadays. Some patients will request screening tests for thyroid cancer. A US scan combined with a fine-needle aspiration appears to be the obvious method to detect early thyroid cancer. There have been seminal studies on this. The evidence completely negates such an approach. The authors of the much quoted Korean study on screening ultrasonography made an earnest plea that "Concerted efforts are needed at a national level to reduce unnecessary thyroid ultrasound examinations in the asymptomatic general population".[45] This advice must be heeded to by all endocrinologists, endocrine surgeons, and any doctor dealing with a thyroid nodule. It must be remembered that thyroid cancer has very good prognosis. It has been clearly demonstrated that detecting small cancer does not improve survival. If worldwide epidemics of detection are to be prevented, screening must not be done.[45,46]

CONCLUSION

Solitary thyroid nodules are a common clinical problem in endocrinology and endocrine surgery. The main concern both for the doctor and the patient is the possibility that the nodule represents cancer, as STN is the most common presenting feature of a thyroid cancer. Fortunately only about 10–15% of STNs are truly malignant. Even if the STN turned out to be a thyroid malignancy, the prognosis is very good.

In most patients arriving at a diagnosis in the STN poses no problems as the combination of clinical examination, US scan, FNC, and hormone assay will provide the answer and direct the clinician toward an evidence-guided management plan. FNC report remains the main arbiter of a management strategy as it differentiates between a benign and malignant nodule but in about 15–20% of patients the FNC is unable to determine whether it is benign or malignant and the report is that of an indeterminate lesion. These patients are the ones that cause several dilemmas in the management of STNs. AUS/FLUS lesions belong to the indeterminate category. Every effort should be made to reach a diagnosis before management decisions are made. While clinical evaluation has an important role in such patients' methods such as scoring systems, immunocytochemistry, and molecular genetics have contributed to an increased diagnostic yield although the contribution of these ancillary methods remains modest. It is likely that better imaging modalities and genetic markers will evolve in the future. The onus is on the clinician to offer the best evidence-guided treatment and to avoid overtreatment and unnecessary morbidity. Being cognizant of entities such as AFTN is also important in the management of STNs. Once a diagnosis is reached management must be evidence-guided and individualized.

The modalities of treatment for STN include surgery, radioactive iodine therapy, ethanol injection, and laser therapy. The best modality for each patient must be decided after considering all factors including the patient's wishes, expertise and facilities available, cost considerations and the strategy must be guided by evidence. There is no role for blind therapy with suppressive dose of thyroxine as the risks outweigh the benefits. It should not be part of a treatment strategy in the management of STN. In the future, better imaging modalities, scoring systems, and molecular genetics will make the diagnosis of the STN easier and exciting. STN is an entity where majority of patients will have an excellent outcome if treatment is offered appropriately and wisely.

REFERENCES

1. Cooper DS. Revised American Thyroid Association management guidelines for patients with thyroid nodules and differentiated thyroid cancer. Thyroid. 2009;19(11):1167-214.
2. Francis Gary L, Waguespack Steven G, Bauer Andrew J, Angelos P, Benvenga S, Cerutti Janete M, et al. Management Guidelines for Children with Thyroid Nodules and Differentiated Thyroid Cancer. Thyroid. 2015;25(7):716-59.
3. Vanderpump Mark PJ. The epidemiology of thyroid disease. The epidemiology of thyroid disease. Brit Med Bulletin. 2011;99(1):39-51.
4. Belfiore A, La Rosa GL, La Porta GA, Giufridda D, Milazzo G, Lupo L, et al. Cancer risk in patients with cold thyroid nodules: relevance of iodine intake, sex, age, and multinodularity. Am J Med. 1992;93:363-9.

5. Hegedüs L. The thyroid nodule. N Engl J Med. 2004;351:1764-71.

6. Ezzat S, Sarti DA, Cain DR, Braunstein GD. Thyroid incidentalomas. Prevalence by palpation and ultrasonography. Arch Intern Med. 1994;154(16):1838-40.

7. Jiang H, Tian Y, Mu Y. The Prevalence of thyroid nodules and an analysis of related lifestyle factors in Beijing communities. Int J Environ Res Public Health. 2016;13(4):442.

8. Yeung Meei J, Serpell Jonathan Wl. Management of the Solitary Thyroid Nodule. The Oncologist. 2008;13:105-12.

9. Mazzaferri Ernest L. Managing small thyroid cancers. JAMA. 2006;295(18):2179-82.

10. Siegel R, Naishadham D, Jemal A. Cancer statistics, 2012. CA Cancer J Clin. 2012;62:10-29.

11. Papini E, Guglielmi R, Bianchini A, Crescenzi A, Taccogna S, Nardi F, et al. Risk of malignancy in non-palpable thyroid nodules: Predictive value of ultrasound and color-Doppler features. J Clin Endocrinol Metab. 2002;87:1941-6.

12. Nam-Goong IS, Kim HY, Gong G, Lee HK, Hong SJ, Kim WB, et al. Ultrasonography-guided fine needle aspiration of thyroid incidentaloma: Correlation with pathological findings. Clin Endocrinol (Oxf). 2004;60:21-8.

13. Bomeli Steven R, Le Beau Shane O, Ferris Robert L. Evaluation of a thyroid nodule. Otolaryngol Clin North Am. 2010;43(2): 229-38.

14. Brito JP, Gionfriddo MR, Al Nofal A, Boehmer Kasey R, Leppin Aaron L, Reading C, et al. The accuracy of thyroid nodule ultrasound to predict thyroid cancer: systematic review and meta-analysis. J Clin Endocrinol Metab. 2014;99(4):1253-63.

15. Maurya AK, Mehta A, Mani NS, Nijhawan VS, Batra R. Comparison of aspiration vs. non-aspiration techniques in fine-needle cytology of thyroid lesions. J Cytol. 2010;27(2):51-4.

16. Song H, Wei C, Li D, Hua K, Song J, Maskey N, et al. Comparison of fine needle aspiration and fine needle nonaspiration cytology of thyroid nodules: a meta-analysis. Biomed Res Int. 2015;2015:796120.

17. Keelawat S, Rangdaeng S, Koonmee S, Jitpasutham T, Bychkov A. Current status of thyroid fine-needle aspiration practice in Thailand. J Pathol Transl Med. 2017;51(6):565-70.

18. Shipra A, Deepali J. Thyroid cytology in india: contemporary review and meta-analysis. J Pathol Transl Med. 2017;51(6):533-47.

19. Schmidt Robert L, Factor Rachel E, Witt Benjamin L, Layfield Lester J. Quality appraisal of diagnostic accuracy studies in fine-needle aspiration cytology: a survey of risk of bias and comparability. Arch Pathol Lab Med. 2013;137(4):566-75.

20. Dean Diana S, Gharib H, Feingold KR, Anawalt B, Boyce A, Chrousos G, et al. Fine-needle aspiration biopsy of the thyroid gland. Endotext [Internet]. South Dartmouth (MA): MDText. com, Inc.; 2000-15.

21. Cibas ES, Ali SZ. The Bethesda system for reporting thyroid cytopathology. Am J Clin Pathol. 2009;132:658-65.

22. British Thyroid Association, Royal College of Physicians. Guidelines for the management of thyroid cancer, 2nd edition. Report of the Thyroid Cancer Guidelines Update Group. London: RCP; 2007.

23. Guido F, Diana Rossi E. The 2014 Italian Reporting System for Thyroid Cytology: Comparison with the National Reporting Systems and Future Directions. J Basic Clin Med. 2015;4(2):46-51.

24. Rohaizak M, Aman Fuad Y, Naqiyah I, Saladina JJ, Shahrun Niza AS. Accuracy of fine needle aspiration cytology in solitary or dominant nodular goitre: a single centre study. Med J Malaysia. 2017;16(2):85-8.

25. Lee YH, Baek JH, Jung SL, Kwak JY, Kim JH, Shin JH, et al. Ultrasound-guided fine needle aspiration of thyroid nodules: a consensus statement by the Korean society of thyroid radiology. Korean J Radiol. 2015;16(2):391-401.

26. Singh RS, Wang HH. Timing of repeat thyroid fine-needle aspiration in the management of thyroid nodules. Acta Cytologica. 2011;55:544-8.

27. Liang J, Huang X, Hu X, Liu Y, Zhou Q, Cao Q, et al. Predicting Malignancy in Thyroid Nodules: Radiomics Score Versus 2017 American College of Radiology Thyroid Imaging, Reporting and Data System. Thyroid. 2018;28(8):1024-33.

28. Sands NB, Karls S, Amir A, Tamilia M, Gologan O, Rochon L, et al. McGill Thyroid Nodule Score (MTNS): "Rating the Risk," a Novel Predictive Scheme for Cancer Risk Determination. J Otolaryngol Head Neck Surg. 2011;40:S1-S13.

29. Ming Z, Oscar L. Molecular testing of thyroid nodules: a review of current available tests for fine-needle aspiration Specimens. Arch Pathol Lab Med. 2016;140(12):1338-44.

30. Jinih M, Foley N, Osho O, Houlihan L, Toor A, Khan JZ, et al. BRAFV600E mutation as a predictor of thyroid malignancy in indeterminate nodules: a systematic review and meta-analysis. Eur J Surg Oncol. 2017;43(7):1219-27.

31. Baek JH, Na DG, Lee JH, Jung SL, Kim JH, Sung JY, et al. Core needle biopsy of thyroid nodules: consensus statement and recommendations. J Korean Soc Ultrasound Med. 2013;32:95-102.

32. Buxey K, Serpell J. Importance of core biopsy in the diagnosis of thyroid lymphoma. ANZ J Surg. 2012;82(1-2):90.

33. Kim TH, Jeong Dae J, Hahn Soo Y, Shin Jung H, Oh Young L, Ki CS, et al. Triage of patients with AUS/FLUS on thyroid cytopathology: effectiveness of the multimodal diagnostic techniques. Cancer Med. 2016;5(5):769-77.

34. Hamburger Joel I. The autonomously functioning thyroid nodule: Goetsch's disease. Endocr Rev. 1987;8(4):439-47.

35. Nishihara E, Amino N, Maekawa K, yoshida H, Ito M, kubota S, et al. Prevalence of TSH Receptor and Gs-α Mutations in 45 Autonomously Functioning Thyroid Nodules in Japan. Endocr J. 2009;56(6):791-8.

36. Corvilain B. The natural history of thyroid autonomy and hot nodules. Ann Endocrinol (Paris). 2003;64(1):17-22.

37. Burch Henry B, Farzana S, Fitzsimmons Thomas R, Jaques David P, Shriver Craig D. Diagnosis and Management of the Autonomously Functioning Thyroid Nodule: The Walter Reed Army Medical Center Experience, 1975-1996. Thyroid. 1998;8(10):872-80.

38. Yukiko Y, Kiminori S, Junko A. Treatment of autonomously functioning thyroid nodules at a single institution: radioiodine therapy, surgery, and ethanol injection therapy. Ann Nucl Med. 2011;25:749-54.

39. Cases JA, Surks MI. The changing role of scintigraphy in the evaluation of thyroid nodules. Semin Nucl Med. 2000;30(2):81-7.

40. Laszlo H. The Thyroid Nodule. N Engl J Med. 2004;351:1764-71.

41. Desforges JF, Mazzaferri EL. Management of a solitary thyroid nodule. N Engl J Med. 1993;328(8):553-59.

42. Maria P, Haymart Megan R. Inappropriate use of suppressive doses of thyroid hormone in thyroid nodule management: Results from a nationwide survey. Endocr Pract. 2016;22(11):1358-60.

43. Yasuhiro I, Akira M. Nonoperative management of low-risk differentiated thyroid carcinoma. Curr Opin Oncol. 2015;27(1):15-20.

44. Gong Y, Li G, Lei J, You J, Jiang K, Li Z, et al. A favorable tumor size to define papillary thyroid microcarcinoma: an analysis of 1176 consecutive cases. Cancer Manag Res. 2018;10:899-906.

45. Park S, Oh CM, Lee JS. Association between screening and the thyroid cancer "epidemic" in South Korea: evidence from a nationwide study. BMJ. 2016;355:i5745.

46. Hyeong SA, Jung KH, Gilbert WH. Korea's Thyroid-Cancer "Epidemic"—Screening and Over diagnosis. N Engl J Med. 2014;71:1765-67.

Muthukumar S, Mohamed Salmon M, Ravikumar

Euthyroid Multinodular Goiter

INTRODUCTION

Enlargement of thyroid gland is referred to as "goiter." A goiter may be diffuse or nodular. A nodular goiter may be classified based on anatomy or functionality. Based on anatomy, a goiter may be solitary or multinodular. Based on functionality, it may be classified into nontoxic or toxic goiters **(Figs. 1A and B)**. Sporadic nontoxic multinodular goiter (NMNG) develops in areas of iodine sufficiency with normal thyroid functions. Endemic goiters occur in places of iodine deficiency.

DEFINITION

Presence of more than one nodule in an otherwise normal thyroid gland is termed "multinodular goiter." Any thyroid nodule can be termed "adenoma" only if it is encapsulated (histology), whereas that without a capsule is termed "hyperplasia."

ETIOLOGY

There are many factors which play a vital role in the formation of NMNG. These factors may be modifiable or nonmodifiable. Nonmodifiable factors include age, genetic susceptibility, and female gender. Modifiable etiological factors include body weight, smoking habits, alcohol consumption, and environmental factors.[1-3] With age, the nodularity in thyroid increases and old age people tend to harbor many nodules of different sizes and textures.[2]

Genetic Susceptibility

Occurrence of goiter in families suggests a strong evidence of genetic predisposition with a dominant pattern of inheritance. A proportional higher incidence of goiter in females also acknowledges the importance of genes in the occurrence of goiters. Recent studies have found a locus on chromosome 14q for familial NMNG. Other rare causes of familial NMNG include thyroid hormonal resistance due to mutation in thyroid-stimulating hormone (TSH) receptor. In addition, some somatic mutations may also play a role in the formation of NMNG.

Personal Habits

Smoking is one of the etiological factors for the development of NMNG. This is mainly mediated through thiocyanates which competitively inhibit the iodide transport into the thyroid gland.[1] In contrast, there exists an inverse relationship between alcohol consumption and thyroid size, leading to thyroid fibrosis.[4,5]

Dietary Factors

Globally, iodine deficiency is considered the most important environmental factor in the formation of endemic NMNG.[2,6] With time, iodine deficiency may result in an increase of

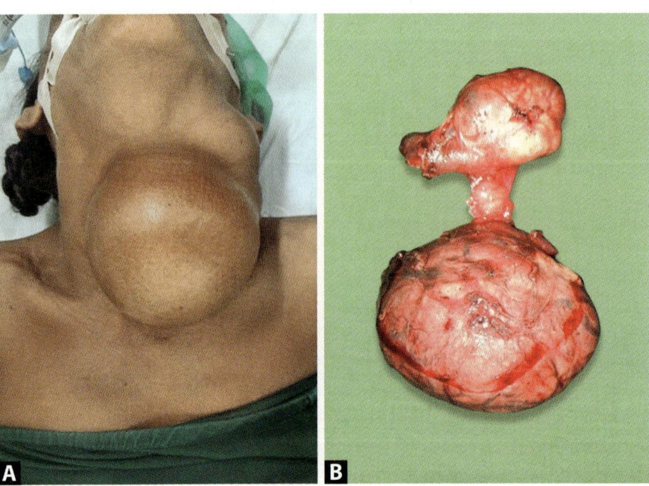

Figs. 1A and B: Grossly enlarged multinodular goiter—nontoxic. (A) Preoperative; (B) Postoperative.

serum TSH, which acts as a growth stimulus for thyroid gland resulting in the formation of NMNG.

PATHOPHYSIOLOGY

The formation of thyroid nodules increases with age. At around 60–70 years of age nearly 70% of people harbor nodules, though many are subcentimetric and clinically will not be detectable. During periods of increased demand and intermittent TSH stimulation, thyroid glands tend to increase in size. With repeated periods of waxing and waning of demand for thyroid hormones, the gland tends to become nodular, when their blood supply is outgrown.

Another mechanism is the gland may undergo diffuse hyperplasia due to many factors such as iodine deficiency or goitrogens. At this stage, mutations may occur due to increased proliferation of cells along with deoxyribonucleic acid (DNA) damage leading onto cells with mutational defects. These mutations may activate cyclic adenosine monophosphate (cAMP) cascade [e.g., thyroid stimulating hormone receptor (TSHR) and Gsα mutations] which stimulates growth and function.[7] In a proliferating thyroid, with increasing growth factor expression most cells divide and form small clones. After increased growth factor expression ceases, small clones with activating mutations will further proliferate with self-stimulation. These self-stimulated small foci could form as autonomously functioning thyroid nodules (AFTNs).

CLINICAL FEATURES

At least around 80% of NMNGs are asymptomatic at diagnosis. Most NMNGs are detected incidentally by the patient relatives or by the consulting physician during routine examination or by neck imaging for non-thyroid purposes.

If at all symptoms should occur, the most common would be a globus sensation in the throat. Most of the symptoms are due to the compression caused by the NMNG. Others include pain, difficulty in swallowing, sticky sensation in throat, cough, voice alterations, respiratory distress, and choking sensation. Majority of patients come to out-patient department (OPD) because of fear of cancer and cosmesis.[8] Pain as a symptom is less common unless there is a hemorrhage into the nodule or a cyst embedded in the goiter. Pain may also occur if there is coexisting thyroiditis. Due to the location of NMNG in the neck, it may cause compression of the vital structures such as trachea, esophagus, nerves, and blood vessels **(Fig. 2)**.

Upper airway obstruction resulting in dyspnea though can occur is a rare phenomenon. Usually, the trachea is displaced, but in certain patients, it may encircle the trachea causing compression resulting in respiratory difficulty. Dyspnea usually occurs only when the goiter extends retrosternally causing compression on the trachea or if it undergoes malignant change causing infiltration into the trachea or recurrent laryngeal nerve palsy.

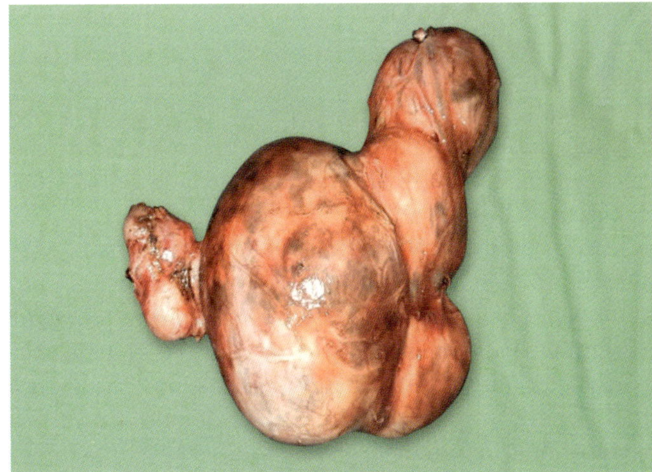

Fig. 2: Postoperative specimen of multinodular goiter—left lobe with multiple enlarged nodules.

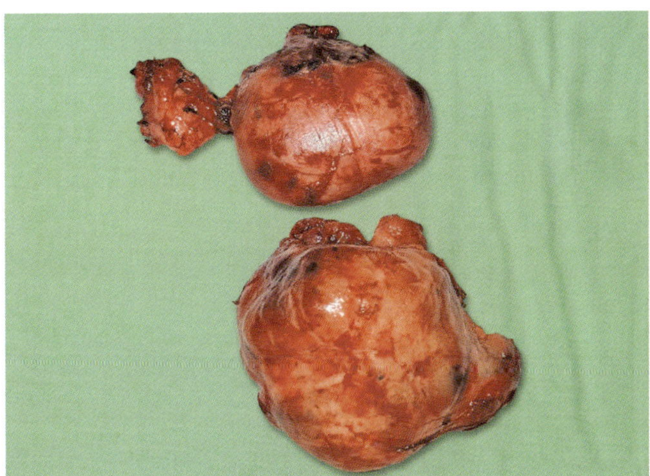

Fig. 3: Multinodular goiter with grade 4 thyrothymic rest.

Dysphagia as a symptom is present in >70% of patients with NMNG. It is more common in patients with a coexisting thyroiditis where they experience an apparent dysphagia. Dysphagia caused by direct compression of the esophagus is rare. It is the motility disturbances which are more common and cause swallowing difficulty because of anatomical dislocation of esophagus.[9,10]

Patients with NMNG may also present with phonatory symptoms, such as hoarseness, vocal fatigue, and vocal straining due to direct compression **(Fig. 3)**.

DIAGNOSIS

The first laboratory investigation for a NMNG is evaluation of TSH to determine whether the patient is euthyroid, hypothyroid, or hyperthyroid. Obviously, measurement of serum TSH should be the initial biochemical test, and if the level of TSH is outside the reference range, assessments of serum-free thyroxine (T4) and free tri-iodothyronine (T3) should follow, though in most of the cases they are within the range or mildly hypothyroid. Measurement of thyroid antibodies to thyroid peroxidase, thyroglobulin, and TSHR in serum should be considered in patients who have TSH outside the normal range.

X-ray of neck is done to look for compression of trachea, calcification, curvature of cervical spine, and retrosternal extension.

Any patient with NMNG should be first evaluated with ultrasound (USG) using 7.5 MHz. Thyroid appears fine, homogeneous, and hyperechoic compared to adjacent muscles and has prominent capsule and very little identifiable internal structure. USG facilitates identification of additional nodules, differentiate cystic and solid nodules, identifies nodules that have sonographic features of malignancy, guides precise fine needle aspiration (FNA) of suspicious lesion, and assesses cervical lymph node basin for presence of metastasis. The features of benign nodule are honeycomb appearence, well-defined regular cyst, presence of halo, hyperechoic to isoechoic, and comet tail sign. No single USG sign independently is fully predictive of a malignant lesion. To report USG features linking to malignancy a system called "thyroid imaging reporting and data system" (TIRADS) has been developed. Disadvantages of USG include operator dependency, the inability to access retrosternal goiters and difficult inaccurate volume estimation of very large goiters.

There is no role for computed tomography (CT) or magnetic resonance imaging (MRI) in a case of NMNG, unless there is a suspicion of retrosternal extension, recurrence, or a strong suspicion of malignancy to know about the infiltration into surrounding structures **(Figs. 4A and B)**.

The next investigation in a NMNG is fine needle aspiration cytology (FNAC). All patients with a nodule >2 cm should be evaluated with FNAC. Any patient with normal or elevated TSH with USG features suggestive of malignancy or a rapidly progressing nodule or a complex nodule should undergo a FNAC evaluation. Any patient with lymphadenopathy, history of head and neck irradiation, and history of thyroid cancer in one or more first-degree relatives should undergo FNAC. A USG-guided FNAC is always preferred over a conventional FNAC. But in certain circumstances, USG-guided FNAC is absolute. Those indications include nodules that are not palpable, predominantly cystic/complex, located posteriorly, palpation-guided FNAC is non-diagnostic and cervical nodes with suspected metastasis. The limitations include inadequate samples and follicular neoplasia. A satisfactory specimen in FNAC is one that has at least six groups of benign follicular

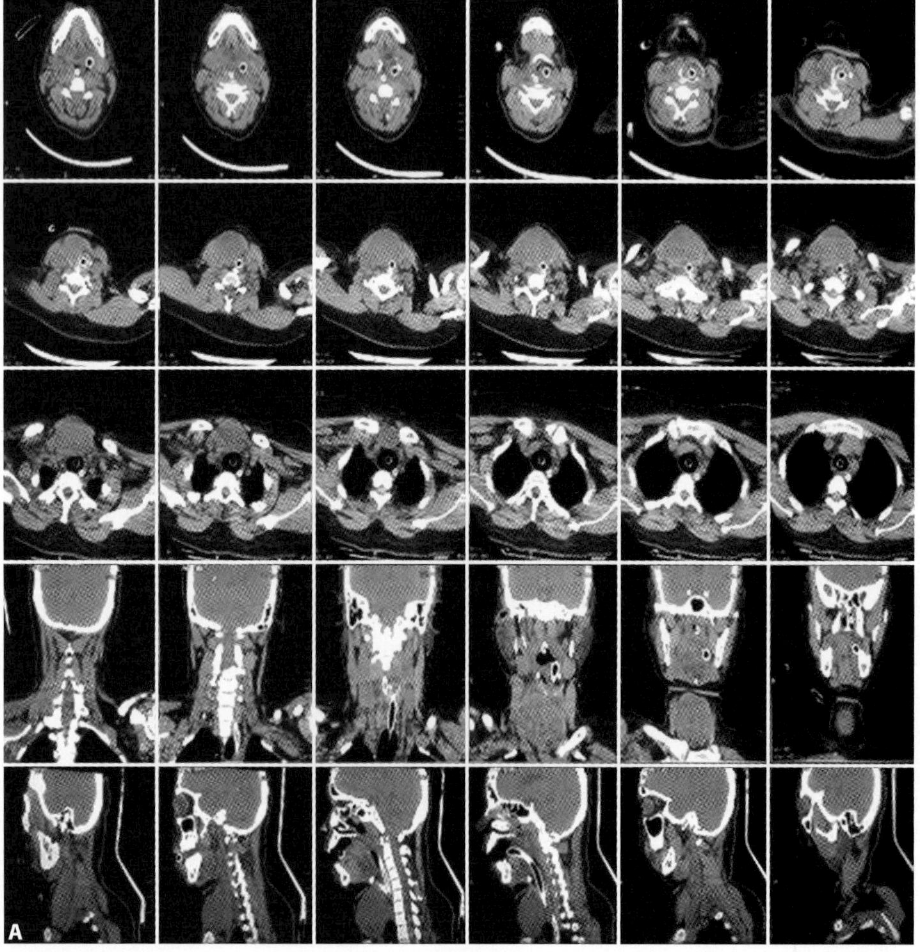

Fig. 4A

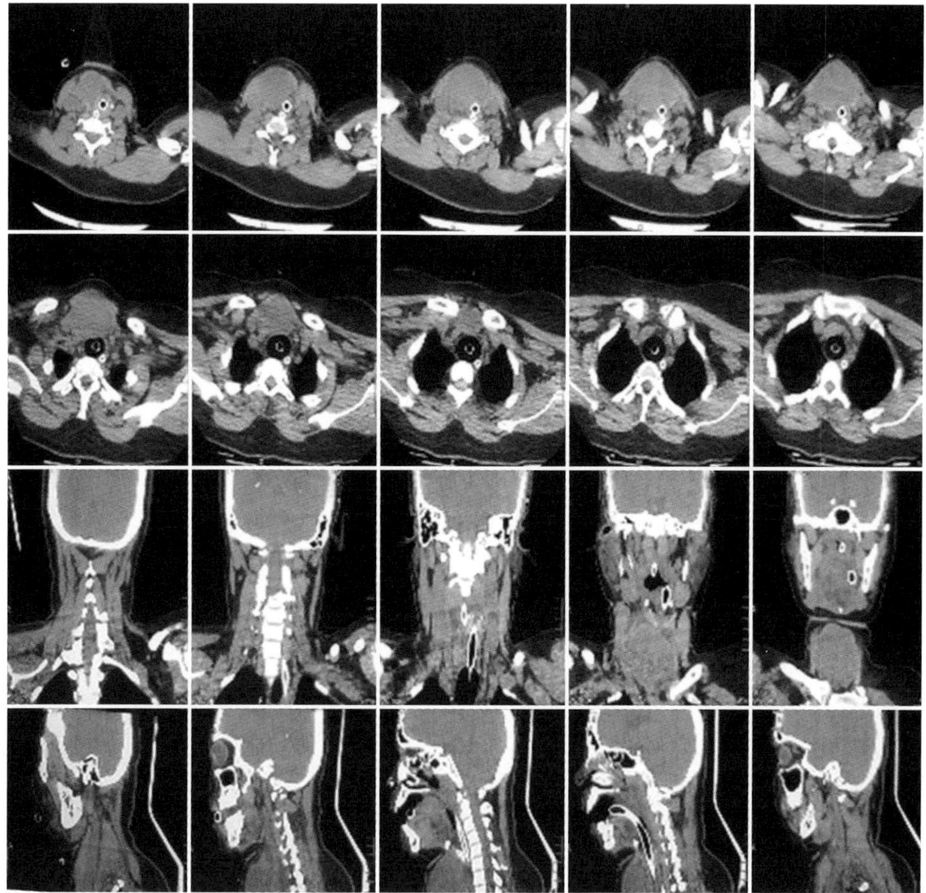

Fig. 4B

Figs. 4A and B: Computed tomography (CT) of the neck showing right side recurrent MNG, after left hemithyroidectomy.

cells, each group composed of at least 10–15 cells from at least two aspirates.

Growth of a nodule is an indication for repeat FNAC. A nodule is considered grown when there is 20% increase in nodule diameter with a minimum increase in two or more dimensions of at least 2 mm or >50% change in volume. In mixed cystic–solid nodules, the indication should be based upon growth of the solid component.

The Bethesda classification of FNAC is based on six cytological diagnostic categories. They are nondiagnostic, benign, atypia of undetermined significance, follicular lesion of undetermined significance, suspicious for malignancy, and malignant. When FNAC shows indeterminate nodules, molecular markers such as BRAF, GALECTINS, HMBE 1, RET/PTC, PAX8-PPARGamma and micro-RNA can be used.

There is no routine role for scintigraphy in a multinodular goiter unless toxicity is suspected.

◇| TREATMENT

The main goals of treatment in a NMNG include relief of compressive symptoms such as cosmesis, suspicion of coexistent malignancy, and patients' preferences. Patients with small nodules and incidentally detected asymptomatic nodules can be followed up safely, if there are no suspicious features.

In small-to-moderate NMNG with iodine deficiency, iodine supplementation may have a small but significant effect. Levothyroxine therapy is also useful in patients with iodine deficiency and subclinical hypothyroidism. This therapy is particularly useful in patients with small nodules. The rationale for this treatment is to decrease serum TSH which is the main growth stimulator. But this therapy can induce cardiovascular dysfunction and osteoporosis in the vulnerable population.

Radioiodine therapy is not routinely used in the treatment of NMNG, though certain centers across the globe use it as a treatment modality. It is used in patients with poor surgical risk and it produces 40–50% reduction in size over 2 years.

Surgery is reserved in certain patients. The indications include suspicion of cancer, large NMNG, presence of cold nodules, need for rapid relief, need of treatment during pregnancy, and severe compressive symptoms. A total thyroidectomy (TT) is preferred over other surgeries in case of NMNG. In experienced hands, the rate of complications is the same for TT compared to any other surgeries. The perioperative mortality risk is <1%, and other complications include pre- and postoperative bleeding, infection, vocal cord paralysis, and hypoparathyroidism, the latter two being either transient or permanent.[11]

There are other minimally invasive therapies which overcome the potential complications associated with surgeries. Noninvasive interventional therapy includes injection therapy, which targets only the symptomatic nodule and results in its shrinkage. Complications may include leakage of the ethanol into the surrounding tissue, with necrosis and scarring of healthy tissue. The major advantages of these techniques are their minimally invasive nature and avoidance of general anesthesia and morbidity associated with surgery. Some of the adverse effects include pain, recurrent laryngeal nerve damage, and possibility of extrathyroidal fibrosis which may render further surgery difficult.[12]

◇| REFERENCES

1. Brix TH, Hansen PS, Kyvik KO, Hegedüs L. Cigarette smoking and risk of clinically overt thyroid disease: a population-based twin case-control study. Arch Intern Med. 2000;160(5):661-6.
2. Carlé A, Krejbjerg A, Laurberg P. Epidemiology of nodular goitre: influence of iodine intake. Best Pract Res Clin Endocrinol Metab. 2014;28(4):465-79.
3. Knudsen N, Brix TH. Genetic and non-iodine-related factors in the aetiology of nodular goitre. Best Pract Res Clin Endocrinol Metab. 2014;28(4):495-506.
4. Hegedüs L, Rasmussen N, Ravn V, Kastrup J, Krogsgaard K, Aldershvale J. Independent effects of liver disease and chronic alcoholism on thyroid function and size: the possibility of a toxic effect of alcohol on the thyroid gland. Metabolism. 1988;37(3):229-33.
5. Knudsen N, Bülow I, Laurberg P, Perrild H, Ovesen L, Jørgensen T. Alcohol consumption is associated with reduced prevalence of goitre and solitary thyroid nodules. Clin Endocrinol (Oxf). 2001;55(1):41-6.
6. Fiore E, Tonacchera M, Vitti P. Influence of iodization programmes on the epidemiology of nodular goitre. Best Pract Res Clin Endocrinol Metab. 2014;28(4):577-88.
7. Krohn K, Führer D, Bayer Y, Eszlinger M, Brauer V, Neumann S et al. Molecular pathogenesis of euthyroid and toxic multinodular goiter. Endocr Rev. 2005;26(4):504-24.
8. Abdul-Sater L, Henry M, Majdan A, Mijovic T, Franklin JH, Brandt MG, et al. What are thyroidectomy patients really concerned about? Otolaryngol Head Neck Surg. 2011;144(5):685-90.
9. Sørensen JR, Hegedüs L, Kruse-Andersen S, Godballe C, Bonnema SJ. The impact of goitre and its treatment on the trachea, airflow, oesophagus and swallowing function: a systematic review. Best Pract Res Clin Endocrinol Metab. 2014;28:481-94.
10. Glinoer D, Verelst J, Ham HR. Abnormalities of esophageal transit in patients with sporadic nontoxic goitre. Eur J Nucl Med. 1987;13:239-43.
11. Bonnema SJ, Hegedüs L. Radioiodine therapy in benign thyroid diseases: effects, side effects, and factors affecting therapeutic outcome. Endocr Rev. 2012;33(6):920-80.
12. Papini E, Pacella CM, Misischi I, Guglielmi R, Bizzarri G, Døssing H, et al. The advent of ultrasound-guided ablation techniques in nodular thyroid disease: towards a patient-tailored approach. Best Pract Res Clin Endocrinol Metab. 2014;28(4):601-18.

CHAPTER 7

Retrosternal Goiter

Han Boon Oh, Rajeev Parameswaran

INTRODUCTION

The most common cause of goiters worldwide is due to iodine deficiency, especially in the low socioeconomic regions. The term "goiter" is derived from the Latin word *tumidumguttur*, also known as swollen throat, defining the thyroid to be big. Several authors have sought to define goiter, either by their diameter or the weight of the thyroid gland. This was previously estimated by means of clinical examination to preoperative imaging to postoperative measurement of the surgical specimens. In a normal healthy adult thyroid gland, the weight ranges between 10 and 20 g. Definition of goiter in terms of weight varied anywhere between 80 and 200 g, with most studies defining it to be significant with a weight of >100 g.[1-3]

The first descriptions of retrosternal goiter date back as far as 1749 by Haller and clinically described by Lingl in 1830. However, the value of X-ray in the diagnosis of such a goiter was defined by Schieff in 1899. When a goiter extends beyond the cervical zone to the thoracic inlet, or with the presence of >50% of its volume below this level is defined to be retrosternal. However, there appear to many definitions of a retrosternal goiter **(Table 1)**. Several other terms such as substernal, intrathoracic, and mediastinal or infraclavicular goiters have been used to define extension of the thyroid gland beyond the thoracic inlet. The importance of establishing extension beyond the thoracic inlet preoperatively helps to determine whether mediastinal dissection is required and the extent of dissection.

Based on the site of origin, retrosternal goiters may be classified as primary or secondary,[4] with secondary type accounting for majority of the cases **(Figs. 1A and B)**. Secondary goiters commonly descend into the anterior mediastinum usually sitting in a position anterior to the recurrent laryngeal nerve (RLN) and anterolateral to the trachea. A small proportion however descends into the posterior mediastinum, usually in a position posterior to the carotid sheath and the RLN.[5] The posterior retrosternal goiters are usually right sided because the aortic arch and subclavian and carotid arteries impede descent into the left chest.

The primary mediastinal goiters are rare in occurrence, with an incidence of 1% of all retrosternal goiters.[6] These goiters usually arise in ectopic thyroid tissue located in the mediastinum and have no connection with the cervical thyroid.[7,8] These goiters may be located either in the anterior or posterior mediastinum and receive their blood supply from the mediastinal vessels.[5] Three possible explanations for the origins of primary intrathoracic goiter include: embryologic fragmentation of thyroid anlagen with hyperdescent, formation as an exophytic nodule through progressive attenuation of the nodule-thyroid stalk and as a parasitic nodule (thyroid tissue fragment implant in the upper mediastinum from past goiter surgery).

Keywords: Retrosternal, goiter, thyroidectomy, airway, VATS

PREVALENCE

The prevalence of multinodular goiters is estimated to be 4% of the US population and 10% of the British population.[9] However, in endemic countries such as Bangladesh, as high as 47% of the population was thought to be afflicted in a report from 1994.[10] The majority is due to iodine deficiency. In most developed countries, nowadays, goiters from iodine deficiency is much less common given the iodine-rich diet. The more likely cause of goiters in developed countries is due to Hashimoto's thyroiditis or Graves' disease. The prevalence of retrosternal goiters estimated to be present in 0.02% of

Table 1: Various definitions of retrosternal goiter in the literature.

Authors	Year	Definition
Lahey and Swinton	1934	Gland in which the greatest diameter of the intrathoracic component by X-ray is well below the upper aperture of the thoracic inlet
Crile	1939	Thyroid gland extending to the aortic arch
DeCourcy and Price	1944	More than one-third of the thyroid gland in the thorax
Johnston and Twente	1956	Largest diameter of the thyroid lies well below the thoracic inlet
Lindskog and Goldenberg	1957	Goiter whose lower border radiographically reaches the transverse process of the fourth thoracic vertebra or lower
Katlic, Grillo, and Wang	1985	When >50% of the goiter is present retrosternally
Sanders et al.	1992	Goiters which require mediastinal exploration and dissection for removal

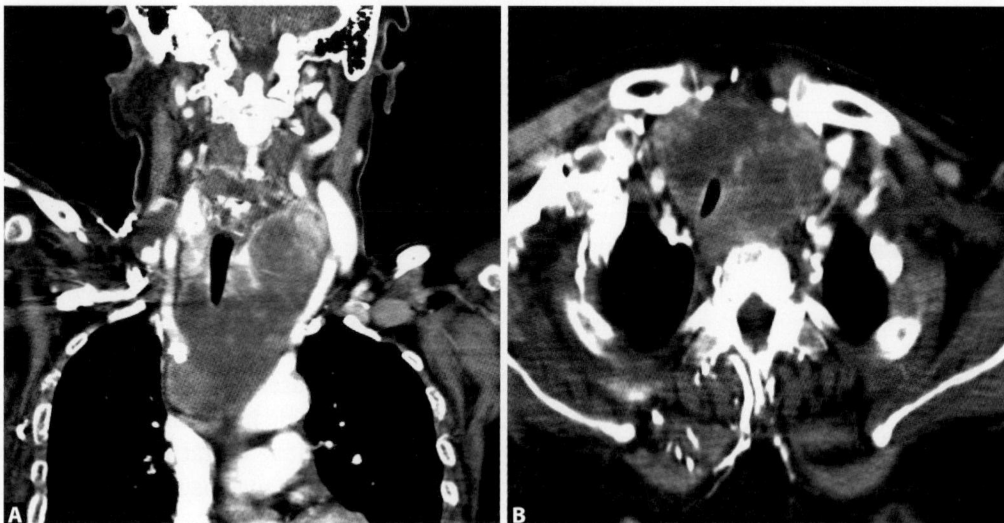

Figs. 1A and B: A case of large retrosternal goiter of the secondary type with tracheal and mediastinal compression.

general population and 0.05% of females above the age of 40 years.[11] The incidence appears to increase with age with 60% of goiters occurring in patients over the age of 60 years. However, the incidence appears to be decreasing and this may be due to iodization of salt, thyroid hormone suppressive therapy, use of radioiodine in selective cases, and earlier detection and intervention.[12] Most retrosternal goiters are in the anterolateral mediastinum while around 10% are in the posterior mediastinum. The overall prevalence of retrosternal goiters excised range anywhere from 2 to 19%.[13]

PATHOPHYSIOLOGY

Iodine deficiency or chronic Hashimoto's thyroiditis results in an increase in the thyroid stimulating hormone (TSH) cause a stimulation of the thyroid follicular cells resulting in goiters. Iodine deficiency is mainly due to low dietary intake in areas of iodine-deficient regions such as the Himalayas, Andes, and coastal regions. Goitrogens such as thiocyanate found in the brassica family of vegetables including cabbage, cauliflower, mustard, and cassava. In patients with Graves' disease, autoimmunity from the TSH receptor antibodies (TRAb) stimulate the TSH receptor to cause growth and excess thyroxine secretion. This results in diffuse and subsequently multinodular thyroid disease later in life. Some of the nodules become autonomous from activating mutations in the TSH receptor or G proteins within the follicular cells and is supported by the following observations:[14]

- The volume of goiter is larger in the older age group.
- The longer the duration of the disease, the larger the goiter.
- The larger the goiter, the lower the serum TSH levels.

The general predictable pattern is a slow growth of the thyroid gland, reported by Berghout to be 10–20% volume increase per year.[15] Other stimulants of growth include pregnancy, consumption of goitrogens or change in antithyroid dosages. Hyperthyroidism can also exist in up to 10% of patients with goiters. Hemorrhage into a nodule can also result in acute pain or obstructive symptoms.

CLINICAL PRESENTATION

Most patients with retrosternal goiters are asymptomatic. These patients are usually diagnosed either on physical examination for unrelated conditions or picked up incidentally on neck imaging. The symptoms of retrosternal goiters are due to compression. The most common compressive symptom is exertional dyspnea.[16] Stridor or wheeze can be present especially during activity due to increase in oxygen demand. This happens when the trachea diameter is <8 mm. The classic Pemberton's sign, which was first published in 1921, showed that symptoms can be reproduced on positional change. Symptoms may be provoked by positions such as raising one's arms, extreme neck extension or flexion or even when lying supine such as during sleep.[17] Other symptoms include change in phonation, sensation of globus or dysphagia. Superior vena caval (SVC) obstruction from a posterior mediastinal goiter can also elicit the similar positional symptoms. Patients may also complain of symptoms and signs of obstructive sleep apnea and thyroidectomy and may improve their symptoms. Patients with Hashimoto's or Graves' diseases can also have symptoms of hypo- or hyperthyroidism associated with their goiters. Other less common symptoms include phrenic nerve paralysis, Horner's syndrome from compression of the cervical sympathetic chain, jugular vein thrombosis or hoarseness from RLN compression.

INVESTIGATING THE RETROSTERNAL GOITER

As with all goiters, the complete evaluation includes clinical assessment, thyroid hormonal status, imaging, and cytology. All patients should have their serum TSH measured together with serum free thyroxine (T4) and total triiodothyronine (T3). In patients with low TSH signifying clear or subclinical hyperthyroidism, Graves' disease or toxic goiter is the most likely diagnosis. In these patients, the cause of hyperthyroidism should also be subjected to 24-hour radioiodine uptake scans, serum levels of TSH receptor antibodies (TRAb) and measurement of vascularity on ultrasonography.

If TSH is high, then Hashimoto's disease is the most likely diagnosis, followed by goiter from iodine deficiency. Patients with suspected Hashimoto's disease associated with goiters should also have serum levels of thyroid peroxidase antibiotics (anti-TPO) checked as well. Even if anti-TPO levels are not raised, seronegative Hashimoto's thyroiditis can occur as well. Other rare causes of hypothyroidism and goiters include infiltrative diseases of the thyroid, or partial biosynthetic defects in thyroid hormone synthesis or iodine utilization.

In all patients with goiters, ultrasound of the thyroid should be obtained to assess each nodule in nodular goiters. The sonographic texture of the goiter and Doppler flows can also contribute to the possible diagnoses. Additional information such as cervical lymphadenopathy and assessing the inferior border of the thyroid during ultrasonography with the patient's neck extended may also aid in surgical planning.

For patients with retrosternal goiters, additional imaging should also be obtained to evaluate the extent of the goiter and the surrounding structures either from CT or MRI scans. Some incidental retrosternal goiters are also picked up from chest radiographs causing tracheal deviation, tracheal narrowing or superior mediastinal widening. CT scans are done for most patients in our practice with retrosternal goiters. Noncontrast CT scans of the neck and thorax are as good as contrasted scans to assess for the extent of the goiters. Care must be taken when evaluating goiters with CT, as the entire length of the thyroid gland should be imaged, and some centers may specify CT scanning of both the neck and thorax. Additionally, CT scanning is usually performed with the patient supine with neck slightly flexed and this may exaggerate the retrosternal extension of the goiter. We do not routinely require iodinated contrast for CTs as the contrast may exacerbate hyperthyroidism in patients with hyperthyroidism. MRI of the neck is a suitable alternative but not all surgeons are as proficient in reading MRIs compared to CTs.

Other than the extent of the goiter, other useful information can also be obtained from cross-sectional imaging as compared to ultrasound. These include the relationship of the blood vessels to the goiter, and the state of the trachea. Any antero-posterior compression of the trachea from the goiter may signify risk of tracheomalacia. The diameter of the trachea to preclude tracheal stenosis can also be assessed with both CT and MRI.

FINE-NEEDLE ASPIRATION BIOPSY

Fine-needle aspiration (FNA) biopsy is indicated for all suspicious nodules picked up on ultrasound. While total thyroidectomy is indicated for all retrosternal goiters, FNA helps to guide the need for lymphadenectomy in proven cancers. Any rapid growth or suspicious features on ultrasonography is also an indicated for FNA, particularly to rule out thyroid lymphoma or anaplastic cancer. However, FNA may not be feasible in nodules located in the substernal components of retrosternal goiters, even with dynamic maneuvers such as extension of the neck.

FLOW-VOLUME LOOP STUDIES

Flow volume loop (FVL) studies have been used to identify tracheal compression in both symptomatic and asymptomatic patients. In a study by Miller et al. tracheal compression was found in a third of patients using FVL, with symptoms improving following thyroidectomy[3] and has subsequently recommended that FVL be used routinely in all patients with compressive goiters.[18] While FVL appears to be beneficial in documenting significant airway obstruction, they do not correlate well with airway symptoms and weight of the goiter, and hence, currently not recommended for routine work up in patients with retrosternal goiter.[19] Only about a third to half of patients with FVL abnormalities have symptoms and those with normal with FVL, about 60% have symptoms. Compared to FVL, cross-sectional imaging such as computed tomography appears to be a better and sensitive investigation for tracheal compression.[16,20] Nasoendoscopy or laryngoscopy is also essential in patients with retrosternal goiters to assess for airway compromise as well as to document the function of the vocal cords. This is especially relevant in patients who are symptomatic from airway obstruction or compressive symptoms such as hoarseness.

CLASSIFICATION OF RETROSTERNAL GOITERS

Attempts have been made to classify retrosternal goiters to aid in the surgical approach. This is generally classified according to their location within the mediastinum and the extent of extension of the goiter in relation to the thoracic structures by Randolph.[21] Most retrosternal goiters are classified as Type I goiters which are located in the anterior mediastinum, accounting for approximately 85% of all retrosternal goiters. These Type I goiters extend anterior to the subclavian and innominate vessels and lie anterior to the RLN. As per usual goiters, the RLN lies deep and posterior to the goiter in Type I goiters. Generally, transcervical incision as with usual thyroidectomies should suffice unless the intrathoracic diameter is greater than the thoracic inlet diameter, in which case a sternotomy or partial manubriotomy may be indicated.

The next most common retrosternal goiters are the Type II goiters, which are in the posterior mediastinum. These occur when the goiter extends posterior to the trachea, great vessels and RLN thus displacing these structures anteriorly. It is of the utmost importance to the thyroid surgeon to identify a Type II retrosternal goiter as the RLN may be stretched or cut during dissection as it runs anterior to the goiter. The Type II goiter's anatomy can also be variable, and may be bounded by the azygous vein, vertebral column, phrenic nerves, SVC and even the first rib. Type II goiters can be further subdivided into the following categories: ipsilateral extension (Type IIA), contralateral extension (Type IIB), extension posterior to both tracheal and esophagus (Type IIB1), extension between trachea and esophagus (Type IIB2). Most type IIA goiters can be managed by transcervical incision with possible sternotomy, or right posterolateral thoracotomy in the cases of type IIB goiters. Lastly, retrosternal goiters may present as a Type III isolated mediastinal goiter, where they may exist without any connection to the orthotopic cervical thyroid. Other terms that have been used to describe these goiters include ectopic mediastinal goiter or aberrant mediastinal goiters. These goiters represent only 0.2–3% of all goiters.[22,23] Blood supply can be from mediastinal arteries, direct branches from the aorta, subclavian, internal mammary, thyrocervical trunk or innominate arteries. Hence, it is important to identify such anatomy prior to surgical resection in order to plan the approach. Thoracic access is often inevitable in Type III goiter resections.

◇ MANAGEMENT OF RETROSTERNAL GOITERS

While suppressive therapy and radioiodine can be offered as part of the treatment for retrosternal goiters, the authors strongly recommend surgery for all retrosternal goiters. The rationale for offering thyroidectomy even in asymptomatic patients are that the goiters will progressively grow and increase in size. The growth can cause airway obstruction that is often unpredictable and may be rapid. A "watch and wait" approach will result in increase in operative risks once the patient is symptomatic or in crisis. In the modern era, thyroidectomy can also be safely offered with low morbidity in a high-volume center. At the same time, thyroidectomy can rule out malignancy which is otherwise inaccessible to the usual FNA for cervical goiters. In patients with concurrent hyperthyroidism, thyroidectomy also "cure" patients of hyperthyroidism unlike antithyroid medications which can have variable results. Surgery also has no risks of thyroxine induced atrial fibrillation or osteoporosis, and no risk of radioiodine-induced airway complications.

Strong indications for surgery include the following:
- Compressive symptoms from goiter including dysphagia or airway obstruction
- Radiological evidence of tracheal compression
- Masses >5 cm
- Goiters associated with hyperthyroidism
- When thyroid cancer is suspected
- All patients with retrosternal extension

◇ INTUBATION AND ANESTHESIA

In most patients with a retrosternal goiter, even in the large ones, intubation is usually straightforward as the laryngeal opening is generally in the normal position. It is generally preferable to use a smaller tube for intubation. Most intubations can be easily performed under a general anesthesia and paralysis. Awake fiberoptic intubation may rarely be necessary but is often a struggle and can cause considerable distress to the patient. Where there is an anticipation of a difficult intubation, a joint multidisciplinary approach with the surgeon, anesthesiologist, and nurse anesthetist is required.[24]

Large retrosternal goiters can result in difficult intubation at anesthesia when there is significant compression of the trachea or significant mediastinal extension. The risk posed to the airway by a large retrosternal goiter can be anticipated in most patients with preoperative axial imaging and it is very rare that there will be a situation of unanticipated tracheal intubation necessitating an emergency surgical access. There is evidence to suggest that compression of the airway by >50% can result in life-threatening respiratory complications.[25] The incidence of difficult intubation in thyroid surgery is reported to be around 5%.[26]

There is a considerable variation in practice when it comes to managing a difficult airway secondary to a large retrosternal goiter.[27] Some experts preferred to do an awake intubation, some opted for spontaneous ventilation, and some preferred advanced techniques such as jet ventilation; and most drew their opinions on their own personal experience of difficult cases.[27] An algorithm for difficult airways has been proposed by the difficult airway society as shown in **Flowchart 1**. In patients with a large goiter with compressive symptoms and overlying the trachea surgical cricothyroidotomy or an emergent tracheostomy may not be possible and may require salvage with extracorporeal membrane oxygenation (ECMO).

In cases where intubation may not be possible or failed with multiple attempts, veno-venous or veno-arterial ECMO may be an option.[28-30] Also known as extracorporeal life support, ECMO achieves gas exchange with intubation and ventilation and can provide support for severe respiratory and cardiac failure. ECMO has several advantages over cardiopulmonary bypass as it can be used for a longer period, less red blood cells damage, blood loss and heparin use.[31] In our institution, three patients required ECMO as a salvage for failed intubation in patients with a large retrosternal goiter with successful outcomes in two patients. Following surgery, patients with difficult airway is best managed on the intensive care unit for close monitoring, especially for tracheomalacia or laryngeal edema.

◇ POSITIONING

As with cervical thyroidectomy, the patient is placed supine with both arms tucked in by the sides. A shoulder roll using

Flowchart 1: Strategies for difficult airway in retrosternal goiter.

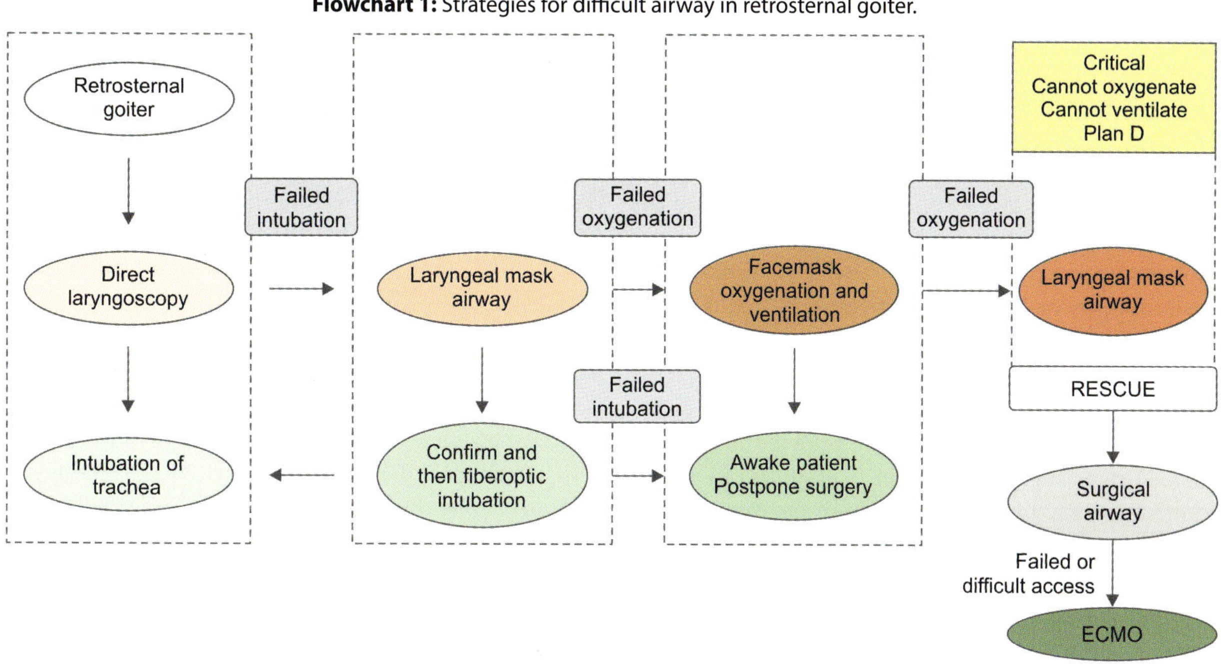

(ECMO: extracorporeal membrane oxygenation)

a gel support or reinforced by surgical towels can be used to hyperextend the neck. In cases where possible manubriotomy or sternotomy may be expected, cleansing and draping is until the upper abdomen.

◇| **SURGICAL APPROACH**

A typical skin crease collar incision as for cervical thyroidectomy is appropriate. Mini-incisions or remote access approaches are inappropriate for the cervical component. Lateral extensions to the lateral borders of the sternocleidomastoid is often needed to allow for appropriate exposure. Superior and inferior subplatysmal flaps are also developed in the usual fashion and are held in place with Joll's retractors or skin sutures. Strap muscles are sometimes required to be divided in order to allow exposure of the goiter. It is our practice to apply stay sutures to either side of the strap muscles before dividing as they tend to retract to allow for repair at the end of surgery. Energy-sealing devices such as the "Ligasure" or "Harmonic" are employed during division of straps to allow for hemostasis. Lateral dissection is then performed using blunt, sweeping motions either with a "peanut" or thyroid dissector until the carotid sheath is identified. It is recommended to do this using a subcapsular dissection approach. The superior thyroid vessels are then isolated by dissecting in the avascular space of Reeves and ligated at the level of the superior thyroid pole to avoid injury to the external branch of the superior laryngeal nerve (EBSLN). Care should also be taken to identify the superior parathyroid glands and preserve them on their pedicles. As per routine cervical thyroidectomy, the middle thyroid vein is ligated thereafter. Care is noted to ensure that the RLN

is not stretched anteriorly to the goiter especially in Type II retrosternal goiters. The nerve should be carefully identified and dissected off before delivering the thyroid gland through the cervical incision.

The inferior thyroid vessels may not be evident in the case of retrosternal goiters, but once identified, should be ligated close to the thyroid capsule to avoid devascularizing the inferior parathyroid glands. Once the blood supply of the goiter is secured, as with most goiters, the retrosternal component can be easily delivered out through the cervical incision in the hyperextended position. Drains can be placed in cases where heavy hemorrhage is encountered or in extirpation of large goiters to decrease seroma formation.

◇| **APPROACHING THE RETROSTERNAL COMPONENT**

Sternotomy is only required in approximately 1% of all retrosternal goiters.[32] Whenever possible, cases which may necessitate sternotomy or manubriotomy should have the involvement of a thoracic surgeon to be on a standby after assessing the CT scan preoperatively. In general, once the bloody supply of the goiter is secured, finger dissection along the capsular border, while continuously being aware of the location of the RLN, can easily deliver the intrathoracic component out superiorly via the cervical incision. It may be necessary to mobilize the contralateral cervical component first to allow for more mobility of the gland to extirpate the ipsilateral retrosternal component. Other adjuncts to help deliver the retrosternal component include the use of a spoon to deliver the goiter by Kocher or a Foley's catheter as in the case of Sanders.[33]

THORACIC EXPOSURE

Rarely is a sternotomy or even a thoracotomy is required in most retrosternal goiters. However, cases which the thyroid surgeon should be aware of the need of chest incisions include those Type IIB and Type III goiters, recurrent retrosternal goiters, known carcinomas extending into the mediastinum and those which have a larger intrathoracic diameter as compared to the thoracic inlet. Manubriotomy, partial sternotomy or full sternotomy may be required for cases above. For most cases, manubriotomy to a level just beyond the angle of Louis is all that is required for most cases. This can be performed by extending a vertical incision from the midpoint of the collar incision down to the angle of Louis. A finger sweep maneuver is essential to sweep the innominate vein and pleura free from the manubrium. Once the manubrium is isolated free from the innominate and pleura, access can be performed by an electric saw or a Lebsche knife and mallet in the midline. This would be enough to allow access to the superior mediastinum in most cases. However, if further exposure is required, partial sternotomy can be performed more inferiorly beyond the manubrium. In rare cases where nodal involvement or large intrathoracic goiters are encountered, a full sternotomy may be required to access the mediastinum. The division of the sternum is in the midline all the way to the xiphoid process, taking care to free the diaphragmatic and pericardial sac free from the sternum.

VIDEO-ASSISTED APPROACHES

With the advent of minimally invasive surgery, video-assisted thoracoscopic surgery (VATS) is increasingly popular to help mobilize the mediastinal components, thereby avoiding a manubriotomy or sternotomy. Not only has it been utilized in retrosternal goiters, this technique has also gained popularity in resection of mediastinal parathyroid adenomas or for thymectomies.[34] Cases should be planned together with the anesthetist as well as the thoracic surgeon. A double-lumen endotracheal tube (ETT) is required to allow for collapse of the lungs in VATS. In general, most thoracic surgeons would prefer a right-sided approach as it makes identification of the innominate vein easier using the SVC as a landmark. The patient can be placed in a left lateral decubitus position, and this necessitates a change in position intraoperatively. It is our practice to perform the cervical thyroidectomy and secure the blood supply at least in the superior pole vessels to decrease blood supply to the goiters. VATS mobilization of the mediastinal components can be done using an energy device and care is taken to identify the RLN as it courses into the chest. The port site can then be extended in cases whereby the diameter of the goiter is greater than the thoracic inlet, thus allowing for specimen retrieval from the thoracoscopic site rather than from the cervical incision.[35]

POSTOPERATIVE CARE

It is essential to manage patients post-total thyroidectomy for retrosternal goiters in a monitored care setting such as ICU or HDU for signs of airway obstruction. In cases where tracheomalacia is confirmed intraoperatively, intubation overnight may be required or prophylactic tracheostomy may be performed. In cases of straightforward bilateral vocal cord paralysis, or intraoperative nerve monitoring shows failure of integrity of bilateral vagus or RLN nerves, tracheostomy should be consented for preoperatively. Thankfully, incidence tracheomalacia has been found to be low between 0.001 and 1.5%.[36,37] Calcium and parathyroid hormone levels should also be assessed postoperatively as iatrogenic hypoparathyroidism can be as high as 8% in such patients. 25-OH vitamin D levels should also be checked and replaced accordingly.

COMPLICATIONS OF RETROSTERNAL SURGERY

The complications of retrosternal goiter surgery are similar to that of standard thyroid surgery and include those of bleeding, RLN injury, hoarseness of voice, inability to raise the voice, and temporary or permanent hypoparathyroidism. However, the incidence of some of these complications appear to be higher due to the size of the large goiters and extensive dissection required in most cases, especially hypoparathyroidism and neuropraxia of the RLN.[38,39] Where parathyroid glands have been inadvertently removed, they must be autotransplanted into the neck. Wound infection and hematoma are also not uncommon. Rarely, pneumothorax have also been described.[40]

One of the more serious complications well-described in long-standing retrosternal goiter with tracheal compression is that of tracheomalacia.[41,42] However, the condition is more associated with anteroposterior compression of the trachea and at surgery this is seen as loss of the tracheal scaffolding. This is rarely seen in clinical practice, and if seen, the patient may be kept intubated for another 24 hours, following which a leak test may be performed to assess if a tracheostomy is required. The need for special interventions such as silastic rings or tracheopexy is rarely necessary in patients with large goiters.

ROLE OF RADIOIODINE AND THYROXINE SUPPRESSIVE THERAPY IN RETROSTERNAL GOITER

Radioiodine therapy has been used to treat nontoxic multinodular goiter and has been shown to reduce the size of the goiter with a 40–60% reduction in volume within 2 years of therapy.[43] Most of the shrinkage occurs within the first few months of treatment. The modality has been preferred for patients not considered fit for surgery.[44] The effect of radioiodine has only been shown in a few studies with very large goiters with a mean reduction in volume of about 30% and have shown improvement in respiratory symptoms.[45] Side effects of radioactive iodine (RAI) treatment in the treatment of retrosternal goiter include increased growth in up to 25%, radiation thyroiditis and risk of developing Grave's disease. The efficacy of treatment is unpredictable in the treatment of retrosternal goiter, with failure of treatment seen in a fifth of patients.[46]

Thyroxine therapy has limited role in the treatment of nodular goiter and does not have any effect in reducing the size of the goiter.[47] Suppressive therapy is also associated with risks, especially atrial fibrillation and osteoporosis in elderly women. Current guidelines do not mandate the use of suppressive therapy in the treatment of retrosternal goiter.[48]

◁| CONCLUSION

Retrosternal goiter is not uncommonly encountered in clinical practice and where seen is usually of the secondary type. Most retrosternal goiters are asymptomatic and where symptomatic usually is associated with tracheal compression. Long-standing retrosternal goiters are associated with slightly increased risk of malignancy, tracheomalacia and tracheostomy. Thyroxine suppression and radioiodine treatment are generally not beneficial. More than 98% of patients can be treated with a transcervical thyroidectomy but is associated with an increased risk of RLN palsy and hypoparathyroidism. Minimally invasive video-assisted thoracoscopic surgery is a promising adjunct along with a cervical incision obviating the need for a manubrectomy or sternotomy.

◁| REFERENCES

1. McHenry CR, Piotrowski JJ. Thyroidectomy in patients with marked thyroid enlargement: airway management, morbidity, and outcome. Am Surg. 1994;60(8):586-91.
2. Torre G, Borgonovo G, Amato A, Arezzo A, Ansaldo G, De Negri A, et al. Surgical management of substernal goiter: analysis of 237 patients. Am Surg. 1995;61(9):826-31.
3. Miller MR, Pincock AC, Oates GD, Wilkinson R, Skene-Smith H. Upper airway obstruction due to goitre: detection, prevalence and results of surgical management. Quarterly J Med. 1990;74(274):177.
4. Hashmi SM, Premachandra DJ, Bennett AMD, Parry W. Management of retrosternal goitres: results of early surgical intervention to prevent airway morbidity, and a review of the english literature. J Laryngol Otol. 2006;120(8):644-9.
5. Mack E. Management of patients with substernal goiters. Surg Clin North Am. 1995;75(3):377-94.
6. Foroulis CN, Rammos KS, Sileli MN, Papakonstantinou C. Primary intrathoracic goiter: a rare and potentially serious entity. Thyroid. 2009;19(3):213-8.
7. Hall TS, Caslowitz P, Popper C, Smith GW. Substernal goiter versus intrathoracic aberrant thyroid: a critical difference. Ann Thorac Surg. 1988;46(6):684-5.
8. Rives JD. Mediastinal aberrant goiter. Ann Surg. 1947;126(5):797-810.
9. Gittoes NJ, Miller MR, Daykin J, Sheppard MC, Franklyn JA. Upper airways obstruction in 153 consecutive patients presenting with thyroid enlargement. BMJ. 1996;312(7029):484.
10. Yusuf HKM, Rahman AM, Chowdhury FP, Mohiduzzaman M, Banu CP, Sattar MA, et al. Iodine deficiency disorders in Bangladesh, 2004-05: ten years of iodized salt intervention brings remarkable achievement in lowering goitre and iodine deficiency among children and women. Asia Pac J Clin Nutr. 2008;17(4):620.
11. Reeve TS, Rubinstein C, Rundle FF. Intrathoracic goitre: its prevalence in Sydney metropolitan mass radiography surveys. Med J Aust. 1957;44(5):149-56.
12. Fritts L, Thompson NW. The surgical treatment of substernal goiter. Operat Tech Otolaryngol—Head Neck Surg. 1994;5(3):179-88.
13. White ML, Doherty GM, Gauger PG. Evidence-based surgical management of substernal goiter. World J Surg. 2008;32(7):1285-300.
14. Elte JW, Bussemaker JK, Haak A. The natural history of euthyroid multinodular goitre. Postgraduate Med J. 1990;66(773):186-90.
15. Berghout A, Wiersinga WM, Touber JL, Smits NJ, Drexhage HA. Comparison of placebo with L-thyroxine alone or with carbimazole for treatment of sporadic non-toxic goitre. Lancet. 1990;336(8709):193-7.
16. Mackle T, Meaney J, Timon C. Tracheoesophageal compression associated with substernal goitre. Correlation of symptoms with cross-sectional imaging findings. J Laryngol Otol. 2007;121(4):358-61.
17. Resende PN, de Menezes MB, Silva GA, Vianna EO. Pemberton sign: a recommendation to perform arm elevation spirometry with flow-volume loops. Chest. 2015;148(6):e168-e70.
18. Krishan Thusoo T, Gupta U, Kochhar K, Singh Hira H. Upper airway obstruction in patients with goiter studied by flow volume loops and effect of thyroidectomy. World J Surg. 2000;24(12):1570-2.
19. Stevens JL, Constantinides V, Todd J, Meeran K, Christakis I, Tolley NS, et al. Do flow volume loops alter surgical management in patients with a goitre? Clin Endocrinol. 2014;81(6):916-20.
20. Cooper JC, Nakielny R, Talbot CH. The use of computed tomography in the evaluation of large multinodular goitres. Ann R Coll Surg Engl. 1991;73(1):32-5.
21. Randolph G. Surgery of the thyroid and parathyroid glands, 2nd edition. Philadelphia, PA: Saunders/Elsevier; 2013.
22. Katlic MR, Grillo HC, Wang CA. Substernal goiter. Analysis of 80 patients from Massachusetts General Hospital. Am J Surg. 1985;149(2):283-7.
23. Higgins CC. Intrathoracic goiter. Arch Surg. 1927;15(6):895-912.
24. Shaha AR. Difficult airway and intubation in thyroid surgery. Ann Otol Rhinol Laryngol. 2015;124(4):334-5.
25. Bechard P, Letourneau L, Lacasse Y, Cote D, Bussieres JS. Perioperative cardiorespiratory complications in adults with mediastinal mass: incidence and risk factors. Anesthesiology. 2004;100(4):826-34.
26. Bouaggad A, Nejmi SE, Bouderka MA, Abbassi O. Prediction of difficult tracheal intubation in thyroid surgery. Anesth Analg. 2004;99(2):603-6.
27. Cook TM, Morgan PJ, Hersch PE. Equal and opposite expert opinion. Airway obstruction caused by a retrosternal thyroid mass: management and prospective international expert opinion. Anaesthesia. 2011;66(9):828-36.

28. De Piero ME, Bergamini C, Costa A, Artusio D, Livigni S. Venovenous-ECMO as a tool in airway management in a patient with large retrosternal goiter. Trends Anaesth Crit Care. 2018;23:48.

29. Lee PK-GMF, Gerard Booth AWMF, Lloyd BSMF. When cardiopulmonary bypass is not an option—a case of massive retrosternal goiter with severe tracheal compression in an extremely obese patient. J Cardiothor Vasc Anesth. 2017;32(2):956-9.

30. De Piero ME, Fontana D, Quaglino F, Attisani M, Baroncelli F, Cavallo A, et al. Extracorporeal Membrane Oxygenation (ECMO)-Assisted Surgery for Mediastinal Goiter Removal. J Cardiothor Vasc Anesth. 2018;32(1):448-51.

31. Shao YMD, Shen MMD, Ding ZMDP, Liang YMD, Zhang SMD. Extracorporeal membrane oxygenation-assisted resection of goiter causing severe extrinsic airway compression. Ann Thoracic Surg. 2009;88(2):659-61.

32. Randolph GW, Shin JJ, Grillo HC, Mathisen D, Katlic MR, Kamani D, et al. The surgical management of goiter: Part II. Surgical treatment and results. Laryngoscope. 2011;121(1): 68-76.

33. Sanders LE, Rossi RL, Shahian DM, Williamson WA. Mediastinal goiters: the need for an aggressive approach. Arch Surg. 1992;127(5):609-13.

34. Shigemura N, Akashi A, Nakagiri T, Matsuda H. VATS with a supraclavicular window for huge substernal goiter: an alternative technique for preventing recurrent laryngeal nerve injury. Thorac Cardiovasc Surg. 2005;53(4):231-3.

35. Gupta P, Lau KKW, Rizvi I, Rathinam S, Waller DA. Video-assisted thoracoscopic thyroidectomy for retrosternal goitre. Ann Royal Coll Surg Engl. 2014;96(8):606-8.

36. Green WE, Shepperd HW, Stevenson HM, Wilson W. Tracheal collapse after thyroidectomy. British J Surg. 1979;66(8): 554-7.

37. Mayer JEC. Tracheal collapse, during thyroidectomy; a case report. Curr Res Anesth Analges. 1951;30(4):238.

38. Sancho JJ, Kraimps JL, Sanchez-Blanco JM, Larrad A, Rodríguez JM, Gil P, et al. Increased mortality and morbidity associated with thyroidectomy for intrathoracic goiters reaching the Carina Tracheae. Arch Surg. 2006;141(1):82-5.

39. Testini M, Gurrado A, Avenia N, Bellantone R, Biondi A, Brazzarola P, et al. Does mediastinal extension of the goiter increase morbidity of total thyroidectomy? A Multicenter Study of 19,662 Patients. Ann Surg Oncol. 2011;18(8):2251-9.

40. Khan MN, Goljo E, Owen R, Park RCW, Yao M, Miles BA. Retrosternal goiter: 30-day morbidity and mortality in the transcervical and transthoracic approaches. Otolaryngology–Head Neck Surg. 2016;155(4):568-74.

41. Bennett AM, Hashmi SM, Premachandra DJ, Wright MM. The myth of tracheomalacia and difficult intubation in cases of retrosternal goitre. J Laryngol Otol. 2004;118(10):778-80.

42. Agarwal A, Agarwal S, Tewari P, Gupta S, Chand G, Mishra A, et al. Clinicopathological profile, airway management, and outcome in huge multinodular goiters: An institutional experience from an endemic goiter region. World J Surg. 2012;36(4):755-60.

43. Bonnema SJ, Hegedüs L. Radioiodine therapy in benign thyroid diseases: effects, side effects, and factors affecting Therapeutic Outcome. Endocr Rev. 2012;33(6):920-80.

44. Bonnema SJ, Hegedüs L. A 30-year perspective on radioiodine therapy of benign nontoxic multinodular goiter. Curr Opin Endocrinol, Diab, Obes. 2009;16(5):379-84.

45. Bonnema SJ, Bertelsen H, Mortensen J, Andersen PB, Knudsen DU, Bastholt L, et al. The feasibility of high dose iodine 131 treatment as an alternative to surgery in patients with a very large goiter: effect on thyroid function and size and pulmonary function. J Clin Endocrinol Metabol. 1999;84(10):3636-41.

46. Fast S, Nielsen VE, Bonnema SJ, Hegedus L. Time to reconsider nonsurgical therapy of benign non-toxic multinodular goitre: focus on recombinant human TSH augmented radioiodine therapy. Eur J Endocrinol. 2009;160(4):517-28.

47. Wesche MFT, Tiel-v Buul MMC, Lips P, Smits NJ, Wiersinga WM. A randomized trial comparing levothyroxine with radioactive iodine in the treatment of sporadic nontoxic goiter. J Clin Endocrinol Metabol. 2001;86(3):998-1005.

48. Cooper DS, Doherty GM, Haugen BR, Hauger BR, Kloos RT, Lee SL, et al. Revised American Thyroid Association Management Guidelines for patients with thyroid nodules and differentiated thyroid cancer. Thyroid: Official J Am Thyroid Assoc. 2009;19(11):1167.

◇ INTRODUCTION

Thyroiditis is inflammation of the thyroid gland. Thyroiditis can be acute, subacute, or chronic thyroiditis. Acute is usually due to bacterial infection; subacute is due to viral etiology; and chronic is a part of autoimmune disease. The classification of thyroiditis is provided in **Table 1**. Subacute thyroiditis is also known as de Quervain's thyroiditis, nonsuppurative thyroiditis, granulomatous, pseudotuberculous thyroiditis, or strauma granulomatosa. Painless/silent thyroiditis occurs after pregnancy in about 3.9–10% of the pregnancies. Thyroiditis with pain can be observed in acute thyroiditis, de Quervain's thyroiditis, post-traumatic thyroiditis, and the radiation-induced thyroiditis whereas the postpartum thyroiditis and chronic thyroiditis are painless.

◇ ETIOLOGY (TABLE 1)

Acute Thyroiditis

Immunocompromised patients, and also those with pre-existing diseases of the thyroid like carcinoma, multinodular goiter, and Hashimoto's thyroiditis are predisposed. The common symptoms of patients with acute thyroiditis include neck pain, difficulty in swallowing, fever, redness over the neck swelling, and infrequently an abscess formation. The thyroid function may be normal with elevated white blood cell (WBC) count and raised erythrocyte sedimentation rate (ESR). Technetium 99m pertechnetate scans will demonstrate the lack of uptake and cold areas in region of abscess. To confirm the infection further testing like fine needle aspiration with gram/fungal/acid–fast bacilli (AFB) staining is done.

A computed tomography (CT) scan or magnetic resonance imaging (MRI) is done in selected cases where a fistula is suspected. The treatment includes antibiotics based on culture and sensitivity and incision and drainage of the abscess if present.

Subacute Thyroiditis

Neck pain is the most common symptoms. Fever, difficulty in swallowing, body ache, fatigue, anxiety, and sweating are the other associated symptoms. The patients complain of constant dull pain which increases on movement of the neck and on swallowing. On examination of the thyroid gland it will appear to be tender. The gland is mildly enlarged and nodular in a few cases. The clinical course is of thyrotoxicosis initially (3–6 weeks), progressing to transient hypothyroidism (4–6 months). Laboratory investigations often reveal elevated ESR, C-reactive protein, and serum thyroglobulin. Radioactive iodine uptake (RAIU) shows decreased/no uptake. In patients who take exogenous thyroxine, the thyroglobulin levels will be normal. Thyroid autoantibodies are negative or low in titer. Ultrasound of the thyroid gland usually reveals hypoechogenicity with low/normal vascularity. In 95% of these cases, patients become euthyroid by 6–12 months since the disease is self-limiting. The relapse rate is <5%.

Autoimmune Thyroiditis

Autoimmune thyroid disease (AITD) is one of the most common organ-specific autoimmune disorders. AITD includes Graves' disease, Hashimoto's thyroiditis, postpartum thyroiditis, silent thyroiditis, and the atrophic thyroiditis. The diagnosis is based on the elevated antibodies against thyroglobulin antibody (TgAb), thyroid peroxidase antibody (TPOAb) and/or thyroid-stimulating hormone-receptor antibody (TSH-R Ab). Middle age women are commonly affected. The incidence of AITD increases with age and above the age of 75 years, 10% of the population is affected with AITD. The clinical features aided by antibody status, ultrasound, and fine needle aspiration cytology (FNAC) establish the diagnosis.

Mechanism of Autoimmune Thyroid Disorders

Thyroid autoimmunity: The activation of thyroid antigen-specific helper T cells initiates the immune response.

Table 1: Classification of thyroiditis.		
Acute	*Subacute*	*Chronic*

• *Radiation-induced*: I¹³¹
• *Drug-induced*:
  – Amiodarone
  – Interferon therapy
• *Infective*:
  – Bacterial
    (*Staphylococcus*)
  – Fungal
    (*Aspergillus*)
	• *Silent thyroiditis*:
	  Postpartum thyroiditis
	• *Infective origin*:
	  – Mumps
	  – Influenza
	  – Coxsackie
		• *Autoimmune*:
		  – Hashimoto's thyroiditis
		  – Focal thyroiditis
		  – Atrophic thyroiditis
		• Riedel's thyroiditis
		• *Infective parasitic*:
		  – Echinococcosis
		  – Cysticercosis

The activation can be due to multiple factors including viral infection.[1] Activated helper cells induce B cells to produce thyroid antibodies. This results in thyroid cell damage with lymphocytic inflammatory destruction of the thyroid gland which results in hyperthyroidism inflammation.

Genetic susceptibility: Association of Hashimoto's thyroiditis and painless postpartum thyroiditis with human leukocyte antigen (HLA)-DR-3, HLA-DR-4, and HLA-DR-5 is reported. The *CTLA-4* gene region is associated with some familial Hashimoto's thyroiditis. Higher incidence of subacute thyroiditis is reported with HLA-Bw35 haplotype.[1]

Environmental factors: Increased risk for thyroiditis is reported in smokers. Dietary iodine insufficiency is said to be protective against acute infectious thyroiditis (AIT) diseases.[2]

◇ CLINICAL COURSE OF THYROIDITIS[1]

The initial thyrotoxicosis phase is seen in painless sporadic thyroiditis, postpartum thyroiditis, and painful subacute thyroiditis. As the thyroid hormone stores are depleted there is progression to euthyroid and later hypothyroid state. The initial biochemical change in thyroiditis is raised in serum thyroglobulin levels. Biochemical evaluation reveals suppressed TSH with elevated T4 and T3. In thyroiditis the T4 levels are proportionately higher than in Graves' and toxic multinodular goiters where T3 is higher than T4. All types of thyroiditis can progress to chronic hypothyroidism. Initially, there is subclinical hypothyroidism which later becomes florid hypothyroidism.

The clinical, demographic, and biochemical findings are depicted in **Table 2**.

◇ TREATMENT[3]

In the hyperthyroid phase, beta blockers play an important role in controlling the symptoms. Once the patient becomes euthyroid/progresses to hypothyroid phase this is discontinued. During hypothyroid phase levothyroxine is used and dose titrated targeting a normal TSH (0.3–5 mIU/L). However, if associated pain is present it is controlled with nonsteroidal anti-inflammatory drug (NSAID).[4] Steroids are occasionally used to control the inflammation which is not responding to the NSAID (prednisolone 40 mg/day). Glucocorticoids, mycophenolate, and tamoxifen are tried in Riedel's thyroiditis to decrease the fibroblast proliferation.[5,6]

◇ LONG-TERM PROGNOSIS

In chronic lymphocytic thyroiditis the hypothyroidism is usually permanent. In postpartum thyroiditis, Riedel's thyroiditis, painless sporadic thyroiditis, and subacute thyroiditis the incidence of permanent hypothyroidism approximately is 25%, 30%, 11%, and 15%, respectively.[2]

◇ MALIGNANCY AND THYROIDITIS

The risk of lymphoma is increased by 67% in patients with Hashimoto's thyroiditis. Patients with thyroiditis and nodule should undergo FNAC to rule out lymphoma and thyroid carcinoma (usually papillary carcinoma thyroid). Thyroid carcinoma with lymphocytic thyroiditis usually has better prognosis when compared to those without lymphocytic thyroiditis.[1]

Table 2: The clinico-biochemical findings in various thyroiditis.[1]

Patient characteristics	Hashimoto's thyroiditis	Postpartum painless thyroiditis	Sporadic painless thyroiditis	Subacute painful thyroiditis	Riedel's thyroiditis	Suppurative thyroiditis
Age	30–50 years	Child-bearing age	30–40 years	20–60 years	30–60 years	Children, 20–40 years
F:M	9:1	–	2:1	5:1	3:1	1:1
Etiology	Autoimmune	Autoimmune	Autoimmune	Unknown	Unknown	Infection
Thyroid status	Hypothyroidism	Thyrotoxicosis hypothyroidism	Thyrotoxicosis hypothyroidism	Thyrotoxicosis hypothyroidism	Euthyroid	Euthyroid
Thyroid peroxidase antibody	Positive	Positive	Positive	Low/absent	Positive	Absent
Erythrocyte sedimentation rate	Normal	Normal	Normal	Increased	Normal	Increased
I^{123} Uptake	Variable	<5%	<5%	<5%	Low/normal	Normal
Pathology	Lymphocytic infiltration and fibrosis, germinal centers +	Lymphocytic infiltration	Lymphocytic infiltration	Granulomas and giant cells are present	Dense fibrosis	Abscess formation

◇| DRUGS AND THYROIDITIS (TABLE 3)[3]

Table 3: Drugs with uses, effect, and mechanism.

Drug	Current uses	Effect on thyroid function	Mechanism of interference
Lithium	Depression/bipolar disorders	Hypothyroidism occasionally hyperthyroidism	Autoimmune
Interleukin-2	Renal cell carcinoma and melanoma	Hypothyroidism occasionally hyperthyroidism	Autoimmune
Interferon alpha	Kaposi sarcoma, leukemia, lymphoma, and chronic hepatitis B and C	Hypo- or hyperthyroidism	Autoimmune
Kinase inhibitors	Gastrointestinal stromal tumors and renal cell carcinoma	Hypothyroidism	Inhibition of iodine uptake by thyroid
Amiodarone	Atrial fibrillation and ventricular arrhythmia	Hypo- or hyperthyroidism	• *Type 1*: Increased synthesis of thyroid hormones (in patients with pre-existing goiters). Treated with antithyroid drugs + beta blockers • *Type 2*: Increased release of thyroid hormones due to destructive thyroiditis • Treated with beta-blockers

◇| REFERENCES

1. Pearce NE, Farwell AP, Braverman LE. Thyroiditis. N Engl J Med. 2003;348(26):2646-55.
2. Laurgerg P, Pedersem KM, Hreidarsson A, Sigfusson N, Iversen E, Knudsen PR. Iodine intake and the pattern of thyroid disorders: a comparative epidemiological study of thyroid abnormalities in the elderly in Iccland and in Jutland, Denmark. J Clin Endocrinol Metab. 1998;83(3):765-9.
3. Sweeney LB, Stewart C, Gaitonde DY. Thyroiditis: an integrated approach. Am Fam Physician. 2014;90(6):389-96.
4. Agarwal NK. Thyroiditis. J Assoc Physicians India. 2011;59:46-50.
5. Few J, Thompson NW, Angelos P, Simeone D, Giordano T, Reeve T. Riedel's thyroiditis: treatment with tamoxifen. Surgery. 1996;120(6):993-8.
6. Vaidya B, Harris PE, Barret P, Kendall-Taylor P. Corticosteroid therapy in Riedel's thyroiditis. Postgrad Med J. 1997;73(866): 817-9.

Toxic Goiter-Toxic Multinodular Goiter and Toxic Adenoma

Ravikumar, Muthukumar S

◇ INTRODUCTION

Hyperthyroidism is defined as the clinical symptoms caused by the excessive secretion of thyroid hormones, the source being the thyroid gland itself. Thyrotoxicosis refers to the clinical syndrome caused by excessive thyroid hormone secretion secreted by extrathyroid sources [e.g., struma ovarii, gestational trophoblastic diseases, pituitary adenoma-secreting thyroid-stimulating hormone (TSH]. The cause of hyperthyroidism should be clearly distinguished between the disorders which produce increase in thyroid hormone secretion per se and the disorder causing excess release of preformed thyroid hormones. The differentiation is characterized by radioactive iodine uptake (RAIU) scan in which the former shows increased uptake and the latter shows decreased uptake.

The three most common causes of hyperthyroidism are Graves' disease, toxic multinodular goiter, and toxic adenoma (TA). Of these three, Graves' disease is the most common hyperthyroid condition which is characterized by thyrotoxicosis, ophthalmopathy, dermopathy, thyroid acropachy, and elevated antibodies directed against thyroid hormone receptor.

◇ TOXIC MULTINODULAR GOITER

Toxic multinodular goiter (TMNG) is considered to be the second most common cause of hyperthyroidism following Graves' disease. Multinodular goiter refers to the presence of one or more nodules in a palpable thyroid gland. TMNG arises from the nontoxic multinodular goiter, wherein over time, enough thyroid nodules become autonomous secreting thyroid hormones independently, to cause hyperthyroidism.[1]

This condition is also named Plummer disease, named after Henry Plummer. TMNG occurs in older individuals belonging to 50 years and above. It is more prevalent in iodine-deficient geographical areas and more commonly manifesting as cardiovascular abnormalities such as atrial fibrillation or congestive heart failure since it occurs more commonly in the elderly. Hyperthyroidism can also be precipitated by administration of iodine-containing contrast agents or drugs (e.g., amiodarone) in TMNG. This effect is called Jod–Basedow thyrotoxicosis.

The nodules in TMNG gain their autonomy due to the somatic mutations in the TSH receptor gene.[2] This is discussed separately below in mutagenesis of autonomous nodules. The "warm" or "hot" nodules as observed in nuclear scintigraphy are rarely malignant and they do not require any biopsy. These nodules can exist with other nodules, which can harbor malignancy, and evaluation of those nodules should be done separately.

The diagnostic work-up of TMNG consists of physical, biochemical, and radiological examination. Physical examination reveals multiple nodules in an enlarged thyroid gland. The biochemical picture in TMNG will be suppressed TSH levels and elevated free T_3 and free T_4. In addition, thyroid receptor antibodies should be done to rule out Graves' disease and autoimmune thyroiditis. The RAIU scan will show increased uptake in autonomous nodules surrounded by diminished activity indicating suppressed neighboring thyroid tissue.[3] RAIU is the first line of imaging in TMNG. The RAIU scan helps in identifying the number and location of autonomously functioning nodules and/or regions **(Fig. 1)**.

The clinical features of TMNG are similar to Graves' disease without the extrathyroid features.[4] These include weight loss despite adequate calorie intake and facial flushing. The skin is warm and moist on touching. The patients will have heat intolerance, anxiety, insomnia, tremors (fine), irritability, and increased gastrointestinal (GI) motility. Since TMNG is common among older individuals, they will present with atrial fibrillation and congestive heart failure. Sometimes, it may progress to cardiovascular collapse and death. The management of TMNG involves three options discussed below.

◇ TOXIC ADENOMA

Toxic adenoma is defined as a single autonomously functioning nodule in an otherwise normal thyroid gland. The single nodule undergoes autonomy and secretes thyroid hormones independent of TSH stimulus. This is also attributed to the constitutively activated mutations in *TSHR* gene. TA is more common in women and among the younger patients. They notice a growth of a long-standing nodule with symptoms of hyperthyroidism.

The diagnosis of TA is similar to TMNG. The physical examination of thyroid gland reveals a solitary nodule and

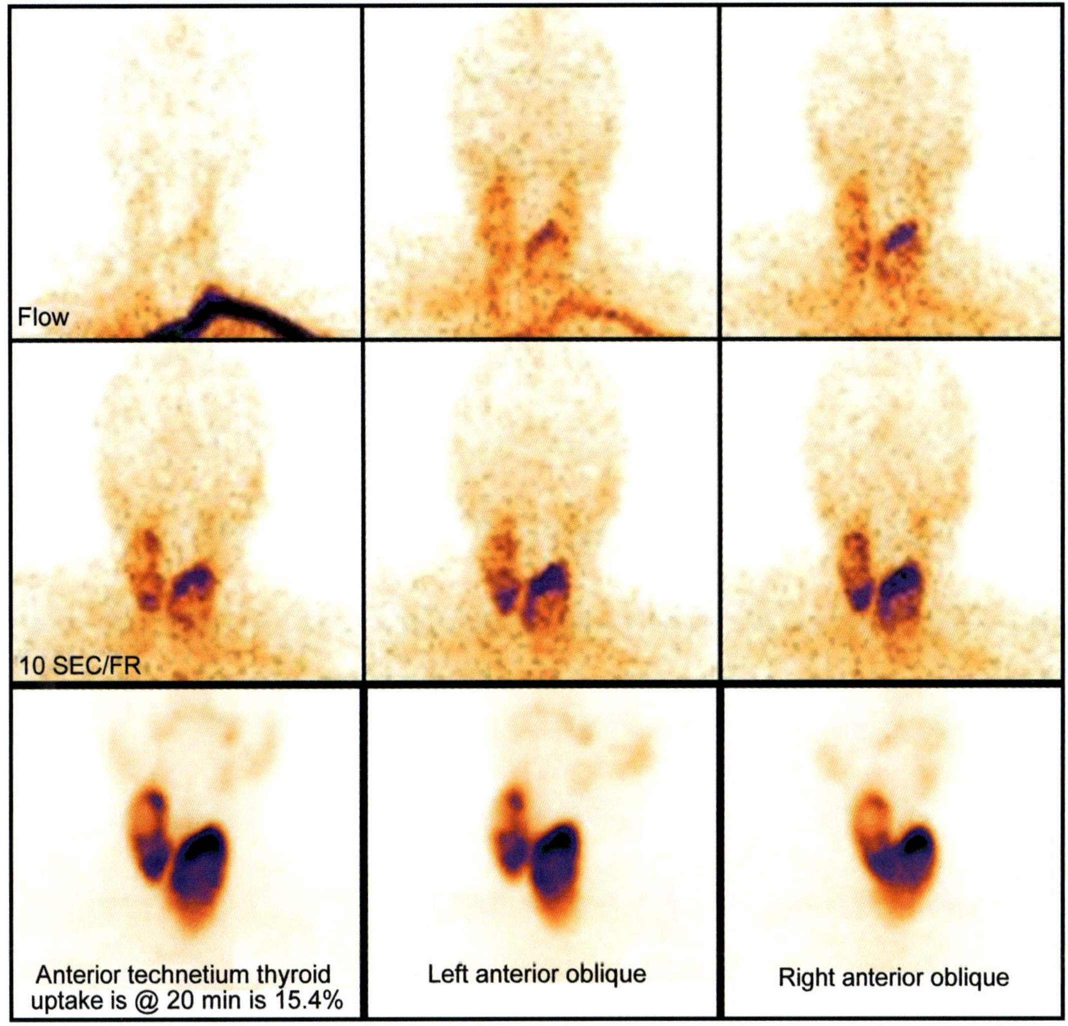

Fig. 1: Technetium scan of thyroid showing toxic multinodular goiter with increased uptake in nodules.

otherwise impalpable thyroid. The biochemical screening reveals elevation of free T_3 and free T_4 and suppressed TSH. Sometimes, only T3 is elevated and T4 is normal with suppressed TSH. This condition is termed T3 toxicosis. Solitary TA is the frequent cause of T3 toxicosis. The RAIU scan reveals a single hot nodule with remaining gland activity suppressed **(Fig. 2)**. These nodules are rarely malignant.[3]

The clinical features and management of TA are similar to TMNG.

Mutagenesis

The chief cause which results in the formation of autonomous nodules is the constitutively activating mutations in the *TSHR* gene. The *TSHR* gene is located on the long arm of chromosome 14 and encodes a 764 amino acid. The TSH receptor belongs to the glycoprotein hormone family of G-protein-coupled receptor. It consists of N-terminal end encoded by the first nine exons and carboxylate terminal encoded by exon 10. The long N-terminal end helps in binding TSH with high affinity.[5]

The *TSHR* gene initiates signaling by activating G proteins that regulate the activity of effector molecules the Gs protein; this leads to the activation of cAMP cascade. Somatic mutations of TSHR and Gs α proteins activate the cAMP pathway and result in clonal expansion and hyperfunction of the thyroid follicular cells. Cells expressing these mutations also have increased expression of sodium iodide symporter, which results in "hot nodule" on thyroid scintigraphy scans.[5]

Once a somatic mutation has occurred, the thyroid cell will undergo successful division to form a clinically apparent adenoma with autonomous activity. It has been estimated that it takes at least 5–7 such divisions in adults and 30 divisions in children to reach a critical size (~3 cm). The cause of rapid proliferation in TA and TMNG may be attributed to the loss of negative feedback control and telomere shortening.

Radioactive Iodine Uptake Scan

Radioactive iodine uptake is the first-line imaging in hyperthyroidism. Both I^{131} and I^{123} are used. The latter is preferred because of its shorter half-life, 12–14 hours (whereas the former has longer 8–10 days of half-life).

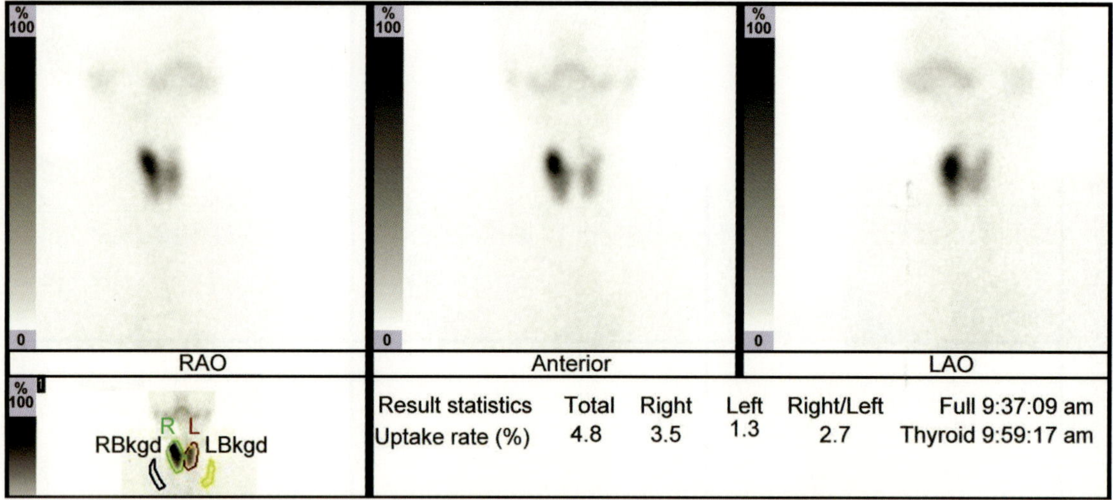

Fig. 2: RAIU scan showing toxic nodule in right lobe with increased uptake.

The amount of radiation exposure is also lesser with I^{123}. They provide information about the size and shape of the gland and also the functional activity. Glands with nodules showing increased activity are termed "hot" and less radioactivity is termed "cold." The comparison is made with the surrounding structures. The risk of malignancy is high in cold" lesions (20%) compared with "hot" lesions (<5%). The autonomous function of the nodules can be demonstrated by giving T3 in suppressive doses. This does not affect the hyperfunctioning nodules but suppresses the activity of normal gland, thereby making the autonomous nodule more apparent.

MANAGEMENT OF TOXIC ADENOMA AND TOXIC MULTINODULAR GOITER

There are three main methods in the treatment of hyperthyroidism: antithyroid drugs, RAI ablation, and surgery. Antithyroid medications are not much accepted as a definitive treatment for TMNG/TA because they are less effective and needed for longer duration. They are used as an adjunct to control hyperthyroidism and for preparation for more definitive treatment. Prior to surgery, patients are made euthyroid by giving antithyroid medications such as propylthiouracil 100–300 mg three times daily or methimazole 10–30 mg three times daily, and the tachycardia is managed by propranolol 20–40 mg three times/day. Propylthiouracil is preferred to methimazole in pregnant women during the first trimester because the latter may result in serious adverse effects such as congenital aplasia.

Radioactive iodine can also be offered to patients with TMNG/TA, if surgery is contraindicated. The goal of this therapy is the destruction of autonomous tissues resulting in euthyroidism. The main disadvantage of RAI is that 20% of

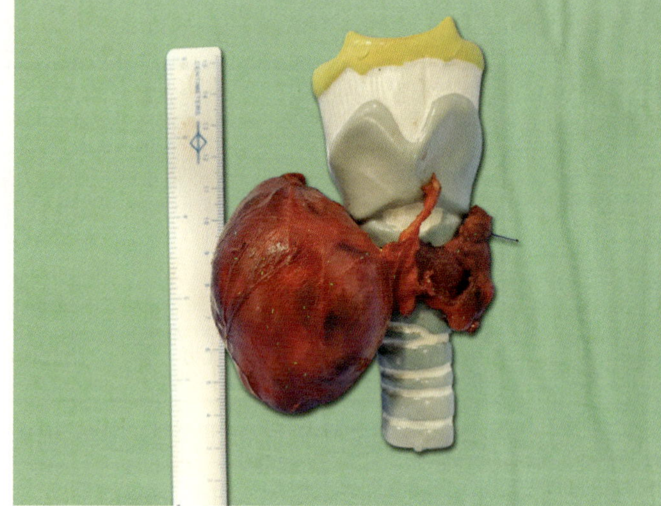

Fig. 3 : Gross specimen showing toxic multinodular goiter predominantly right lobe.

patients required second treatment and the doses required are higher than those of Graves' disease. Almost twice the doses are needed.[6]

Surgery is the preferred treatment for TA and TMNG. Patients with single functioning adenoma are best managed with hemithyroidectomy. In case of TMNG, total or near-total thyroidectomy is considered to avoid the risk of recurrent hyperthyroidism **(Figs. 3 and 4)**. The patients must be made euthyroid before surgery with antithyroid drugs. Surgery should be done in case of large goiter causing pressure symptoms or if there is a possibility of carcinoma. The incidence of cancer in a TMNG is 3–5%.

CONCLUSION

Toxic MNG occurs in <5% of population in iodine-sufficient areas, but it is more common in places with iodine

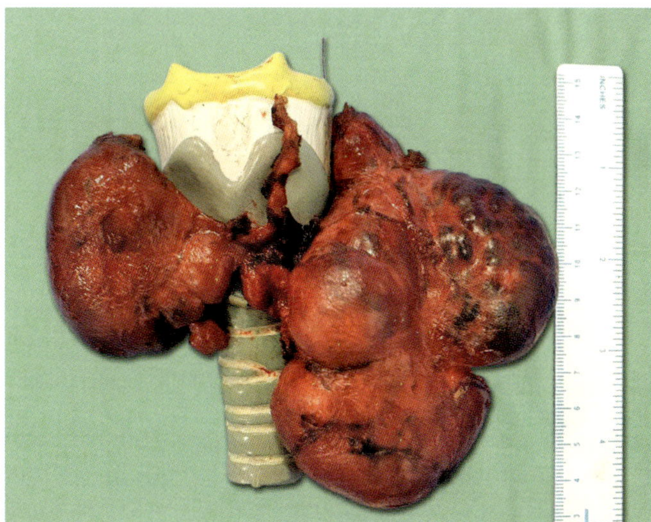

Fig. 4 : Specimen showing toxic multinodular goiter involving both the lobes, clinically causing pressure symptoms.

deficiency. Since most of the times remission is not possible with antithyroid drugs as in Graves' disease, surgery forms the central role in management with RAI therapy. Total or near-total thyroidectomy for TMNG has largely replaced subtotal thyroidectomy and resulted in lesser recurrence. Antithyroid drugs are used in preparation for surgery.

◇| REFERENCES

1. WM McConahey, DS Pady. Henry Stanley Plummer. Endocrinology. 1991;129(5):2271-3.
2. Siegel RD, Lee SL. Toxic nodular goiter. Toxic adenoma and toxic multinodular goiter. Endocrinol Metab Clin North Am. 1998;27(1):151-68.
3. Lal G, Clark OH. Chapter 38: Thyroid, Parathyroid, and Adrenal. In: Brunicardi FC, Andersen DK, Billiar TR, Dunn DL, Kao LS, Hunter JG, Matthews JB, Pollock RE (Eds). Schwartz Principles of Surgery, 11th edition. New York: McGraw Hill; 2019. pp. 1637-8.
4. Porterfield JR, Thompson GB, Farley DR, Grant CS, Richards ML. Evidence-based management of toxic multinodular goitre. World J Surg. 2008;32(7);1278-84.
5. Grob F, Deladoëy J, Legault L, Spigelblatt L, Fournier A, Vassart G, et al. Autonomous adenomas caused by somatic mutations of the thyroid-stimulating hormone receptor in children. Horm Res Paediatr. 2014;81(2):73-9.
6. Kang AS, Grant CS, Thompson GB, van Heerden JA. Current treatment of modular goitre with hyperthyroidism (Plummer's disease): Surgery versus Radioiodine. Surgery. 2002;132(6):916-23; discussion 923.

CHAPTER 10

Graves' Disease

Supriya Sen, Deepak Abraham, Maruthu Pandian, Kamaludeen, S Babu

INTRODUCTION

Thyrotoxicosis was first described by Caleb Parry, an English physician, in 1786 but it was reported after his death in 1825. Graves' disease got its name in the English speaking world from Sir Robert James Graves an Irish physician. However, in Europe, is known as Basedow's disease after the German physician, Carl Adolph von Basedow.[1,2]

RELEVANT ANATOMY

Macroscopically, the thyroid gland is diffusely enlarged and soft with increased vascularity. Microscopically, both hypertrophy and hyperplasia of the thyroid follicles are seen. The follicles are small with scanty colloid and the follicular epithelium presents a columnar aspect with pseudopapillary appearance.

DEFINITION

Thyrotoxicosis is defined as inappropriately high thyroid hormone action in the tissues due to inappropriately high tissue thyroid hormone levels.

CAUSES OF THYROTOXICOSIS

- Excessive stimulation of gland by trophic factors
- Increased synthesis and secretion causing increase in hormone release.
- Passive release of preformed thyroid hormone in excessive amounts.
- Exposure to extrathyroidal sources of thyroid hormone which may be endogenous or exogenous.

Hyperthyroidism is defined as a type of thyrotoxicosis in which there is inappropriately high synthesis and secretion of thyroid hormones.

Graves' disease, toxic multinodular goiter, and toxic adenoma are common causes of hyperthyroidism.[3]

INCIDENCE

The incidence of Graves' disease is 1.2–1.6% of which about 0.5–0.6% is overt and 0.7–1% is subclinical. It accounts for 60–80% of hyperthyroidism in iodine sufficient areas. This occurs more in fifth to seventh decade and is 4–6 times more common in females as compared to males.[3,4]

PATHOPHYSIOLOGY

Graves' disease is caused by thyroid-stimulating hormone (TSH) receptor autoantibodies (TRAbs) on the thyroid follicular cell. This further leads to increase in cyclic adenosine monophosphate (cAMP) which stimulates synthesis of thyroid hormones resulting in thyroid gland growth and increased function. Thyroid hypersecretion causes both hypertrophy and hyperplasia of thyroid follicles.

Inflammatory mediators like interleukin-1 (IL-1), tumor necrosis factor-α (TNF-α), and interferon-α are upregulated which in turn activate local inflammatory cells. These inflammatory mediators bind to and stimulate follicular cells including human leukocyte antigen (HLA) class I antigen and further increase TRAb.[2,4,5]

Autoimmune process can be triggered by environmental factors like infections (e.g., *Yersinia enterocolitica*), stress, and iodine exposure.

In Graves' ophthalmopathy, orbital fibroblasts in orbital fat have increased expression of TSH receptor. Once the TSH receptor on fibroblast is activated, it is internalized and degraded by antigen-presenting cell (APC) which helps activate helper T cells. Helper T cells secrete cytokines which differentiate B cells into plasma cells which further increase TRAb. This leads to production of hyaluronan, prostaglandin E2, and IL-8 which accumulate in orbital fat **(Fig. 1)**.[2,4-6]

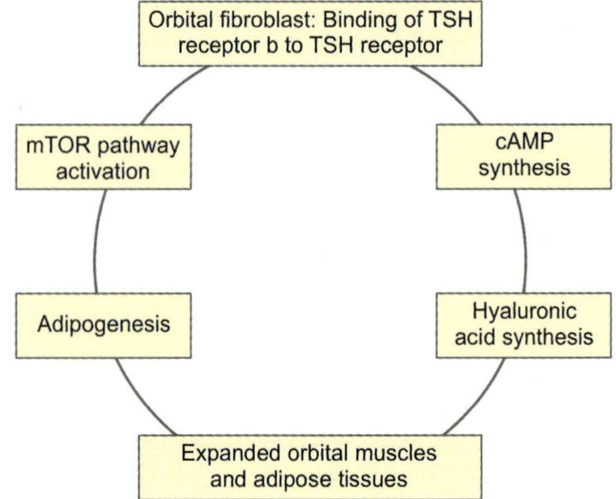

Fig. 1: Pathophysiology in Graves' ophthalmopathy. (cAMP: cyclic adenosine monophosphate; mTOR: mammalian target of rapamycin; TSH: thyroid-stimulating hormone)

In pretibial myxedema, there are high levels of TSH receptors in pretibial spaces, suggesting an immunologic and inflammatory process. Specifically, skin thickening and myxedema are caused by accumulation of glycosaminoglycans in dermis and subcutaneous tissue as a result of fibroblast proliferation.[2,7]

CLINICAL MANIFESTATIONS

- Goiter
- Hyperthyroidism
- Ophthalmopathy
- Dermopathy
- Thyroid acropachy

Goiter is often firm, diffuse, and tender. In the patients aged <50 years, the goiter is present in 90% while in older patients 75% present with goiter. The elderly may present with symptoms of Graves' without goiter.

The common hyperthyroid symptoms in Graves' are nervousness, fatigue, irritability, palpitations, heat intolerance, weight loss, tremors, or menstrual irregularities in women. The less common manifestations of hyperthyroidism are greying of hair, vitiligo, onycholysis, and alopecia.[3-5]

The severity of Graves' ophthalmopathy can be evaluated by using scoring systems. Two commonly used scoring systems are "NOSPECS" and "clinical activity score (CAS)."

NOSPECS

Refer **Box 1**.

Clinical Activity Score

Clinical activity score, first examination[1-7] is shown in **Box 2**.

There are numerous eponymous eye signs in Graves' disease. Some of the commonly used ones are shown in **Table 1**.

Thyroid dermopathy is a rare manifestation of Graves' disease characterized by localized thickening of the skin commonly seen in the pretibial area. It is almost always associated with ophthalmopathy (96%) and sign and symptoms of hyperthyroidism **(Figs. 2A and B)**.[8]

Thyroid acropachy is a rare extrathyroid manifestation which affects about 0.3% of patients with Graves' disease. It may occur within weeks to many years after treatment of original thyrotoxicosis. It is almost always associated with thyroid ophthalmopathy and dermopathy. It manifests as soft tissue swelling with digital clubbing and periosteal reaction of the extremities.[9]

INVESTIGATIONS

Biochemical Investigations

Serum TSH is the most sensitive and specific test to detect hyperthyroidism. Additionally, free T4 and total T3 should be measured as both are elevated in overt hyperthyroidism. The ratio of total T3 to total T4 is usually >20 in Graves' disease, as T3 is synthesized relatively more.[3]

Thyroid-stimulating hormone receptor autoantibody assay is specific for Graves' disease which aids in confirmation of diagnosis.

Box 2: Clinical activity score, first examination.

- Spontaneous retrobulbar pain
- Pain on attempted upward or downward gaze
- Swelling of eyelids
- Redness of eyelids
- Redness of conjunctiva
- Swelling of conjunctiva (chemosis)
- Swelling of caruncle or plica

Monitoring after 1–3 months, point 8–10:
- Increase in measured proptosis >2 mm
- Decrease in eye movement limit of >8° in any direction
- Decrease in visual acuity equal to 1 Snellen chart line

Note:
- Active GO = CAS ≥3/7 in first examination or >4/10 on monitoring
- Inactive GO = CAS <3/7 in first examination or ≤4/10 on monitoring[6]

Box 1: NOSPECS

N	No signs or symptoms
O	Only signs (lid retraction, stare with or without lid lag)
S	Soft tissue involvement (conjunctival and lid erythema and edema)
P	Proptosis
E	Eye muscle involvement
C	Corneal involvement
S	Sight loss

Table 1: Eye signs in Graves' disease.

Von Graefe's sign	Lid lag in downward gaze
Joffroy's sign	Absence of wrinkling of forehead on superior gaze
Grove's sign	Resistance to pulling down the retracted eyelid
Stellwag's sign	Incomplete and infrequent blinking
Boston sign	Jerky irregular movement on downward gaze
Dalrymple's sign	Widened palpebral fissure during fixation
Kocher's sign	Eye globe lag in upgaze
Möbius sign	Poor convergence
Ballet sign	Restriction of one or more extra ocular muscles
Gifford sign	Difficulty in everting upper lid
Griffith sign	Lower lid lag on downgaze
Jellinek's sign	Increased pigmentation on the lids

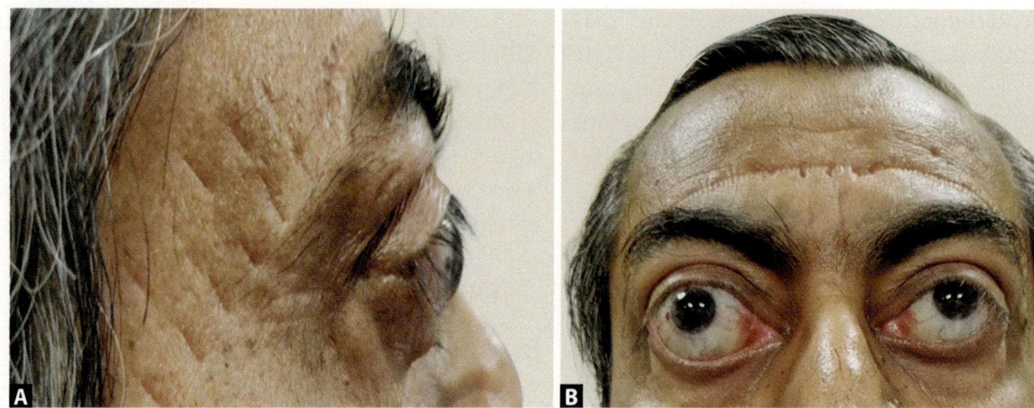

Figs. 2A and B: Graves' ophthalmopathy.

Radiological Investigations

Ultrasound of thyroid gland usually shows a diffuse gland with increased flow on Doppler. It may also be beneficial to detect any suspicious areas within the gland to rule out malignancy which may be present along with Graves' disease.

Ultrasound with color Doppler flow can distinguish thyroid hyperactivity from destructive thyroiditis.

Quantitative Doppler measures peak systolic velocity from intrathyroidal arteries or the inferior thyroidal artery. This test may be particularly useful when radioactive iodine (RAI) is contraindicated during pregnancy or breastfeeding.[4,10]

Functional Imaging

Radioactive iodine uptake (RAIU) shows a diffuse uptake in thyroid gland.[3,4]

◇ TREATMENT

The aim of treatment in Graves' disease is to:
- Return to and maintenance of euthyroid state
- Control of disease manifestation
- Minimal morbidity
- Reasonable cost

There are multiple factors which may be taken into consideration while planning a specific modality of treatment including patient's age, size of thyroid gland, any suspicious nodules within the gland, any compressive symptoms or retrosternal extension due to goiter, severity of ophthalmopathy if present, and any contraindications to antithyroid drugs or RAI. Most often the patient's choice also plays a crucial role in planning final management for the disease.[3,4,10-12]

The treatment of Graves' disease can be broadly classified as:
- Antithyroid medications
- Radioactive iodine ablation
- Surgery

Antithyroid Drugs

This modality is preferred in those who have a higher chance of remission (especially women, mild disease, small goiter, negative, or low TRAb titers), pregnancy, elderly in whom surgical risk is high due to coexisting comorbidities.

The treatment with antithyroid drugs may have a role in immunosuppression, either by primarily decreasing thyroid specific autoimmunity or secondarily by ameliorating the hyperthyroidism state which may restore dysregulated immune system back to normal.[3]

Thionamides

Methimazole, carbimazole, and propylthiouracil (PTU) are the main drugs used in Graves' disease. Carbimazole which gets converted to methimazole is widely used.

Mechanism of action: They inhibit the synthesis of thyroid hormone by acting against iodide organification and also inhibit complexing of iodotyrosines. They also have immunosuppressive action.

Methimazole (MMI) is 10 times more potent than PTU and is the drug of choice in adults, children, and in pregnancy. However, in first trimester of pregnancy PTU is preferred.

The dose of carbimazole or methimazole should be titrated to normalize thyroid functions while have least adverse effects. The initial MMI daily dosing may be adjusted as follows:
- 5–10 mg if free T4 is 1–1.5 times the upper limit of normal
- 10–20 mg if free T4 is 1.5–2 times the upper limit of normal
- 30–40 mg if free T4 is 2–3 times the upper limit of normal

Propylthiouracil has a shorter duration of action and has to be administered as 50–150 mg twice or thrice a day depending on severity of disease.[3]

Adverse Drug Reactions

- *Mild side effects*: Pruritic rash and arthralgia
- *Severe side effects*: Agranulocytosis, hepatotoxicity amounting to fulminant hepatic necrosis, vasculitis, and teratogenicity if given in first trimester like choanal atresia and aplasia cutis.[11]

Monitoring of Patients on Antithyroid Drugs

- Free T4 and total T3 should be monitored 2–6 weeks after initiation of therapy to ensure normalization of thyroid function tests. It is essential to check free T3 as sometimes free T4 may normalize but T3 may be raised causing toxicity.

- Once thyroid function tests (TFTs) are normalized, antithyroid drugs should be decreased by 30–50% and biochemical testing repeated every 4–6 weeks. Once euthyroid levels are attained at minimal dose, biochemical testing can be repeated every 2–3 months.

Remission is defined as normal TSH, free T4, and total T3 1 year after discontinuation of antithyroid drugs. The remission rate following antithyroid drugs varies between 30 and 50% depending on various geographical areas. A meta-analysis showed no increased benefit in treating with antithyroid drugs for more than 18 months.[3,4]

Beta-Blockers

Mechanism of action: They block the response to catecholamines at the receptor site and reduce tremors, palpitations, excessive sweating, eyelid retraction, and heart rate. They also block conversion of T4 to T3.

Commonly used drugs are:
- *Atenolol*: 25–100 mg qid/bd
- *Metoprolol*: 25–50 mg od
- *Propranolol*: 40–160 mg qid

  Beta-blockers should be used cautiously in patients with asthma, congestive heart failure, bradyarrhythmias, and Raynaud phenomenon. In these patients, calcium channel blocker therapy is an alternative to β-blockers for heart rate control.[3,10,11]

Radioactive Iodine Therapy

Radioactive iodine is incorporated into thyroid hormone, releasing beta particles that cause ionizing damage to thyroid follicular cells. This causes gradual destruction of the gland.

The onset of hypothyroidism occurs depends on the size of the thyroid, the RAIU, the degree of thyrotoxicosis, and the activity of RAI administered.

Some contraindications to RAI therapy are pregnancy, lactation, in children (due to radiation exposure), and in possibility of malignant disease.

Due to the risk of transient worsening of thyrotoxicosis after RAI, patients who are older or have comorbidity such as coronary artery disease may benefit from pretreatment with antithyroid drugs. In those patients pretreated with antithyroid drugs, they should be stopped 2–3 days prior to RAI to enable incorporation of RAI in thyroid hormone, and can be restarted 4–5 days post RAI administration.

In patients with Graves' orbitopathy, corticosteroids can be given in mild category. RAI is avoided in case of active and moderate to severe sight-threatening orbitopathy.[9,10]

Surgery

Surgery, i.e., total thyroidectomy, is a definitive treatment in Graves' disease. The following are the common indications for surgery in Graves' disease:
- Large goiter with compressive symptoms
- Suspicious thyroid nodules
- Patients with active or severe Graves' orbitopathy
- Patient's choice
- Women with Graves' disease who want to plan pregnancy in 6 months
- Patient who cannot tolerate antithyroid drugs or cannot take RAI.

Lugol's iodine (LS) or super saturated potassium iodide (SSKI) is still used at many centers in preoperative setting to decrease vascularity of the gland and decrease intraoperative blood loss. It is typically started 10 days prior to surgery. Classically, LS is prescribed in a dose of 5–10 drops thrice daily with each drop containing 5–8 mg/drop and SSKI is given as 1–2 drops thrice daily with each drop being 50 mg/drop.[3,13] Typically, antithyroid drugs should be continued till surgery and stopped postoperatively while β-blockers should be continued postoperatively and tapered and stopped postoperatively.[3]

Due to advances in surgical techniques, total thyroidectomy is surgery of choice over bilateral subtotal thyroidectomy. Total thyroidectomy minimizes the chance of recurrence with low morbidity when performed in high volume centers.[3,4] Total thyroidectomy has the lowest relapse rate of 10% when compared to RAI with a relapse rate of 15% and antithyroid drug with a relapse rate of 52% as showed in a recent meta-analysis including eight studies.[13,14] The complications of total thyroidectomy includes a slightly higher incidence of hypoparathyroidism (usually temporary) and recurrent laryngeal nerve injury.[9]

In pregnancy, surgery is usually performed in second trimester.

Thus to summarize surgical management:
- *Preoperative management*:
  - Aim is to make patient euthyroid as far as possible with antithyroid drugs.
  - Use β-blockers to control sympathetic overactivity.
  - Use of Lugol's iodine or SSKI immediately before surgery to decrease vascularity of gland especially in large goiters.
  - It may be beneficial to correct vitamin D preoperatively if low.
- *Operative management*:
  - Total thyroidectomy is the preferred treatment of choice as it minimizes risk of recurrence.
  - In high volume centers, the risk of hypocalcemia (usually temporary) and recurrent laryngeal nerve injury is not high.

Hence, when feasible total thyroidectomy is the preferred surgical management as opposed to subtotal thyroidectomy.

Flowchart 1: Biochemistry of TSH.

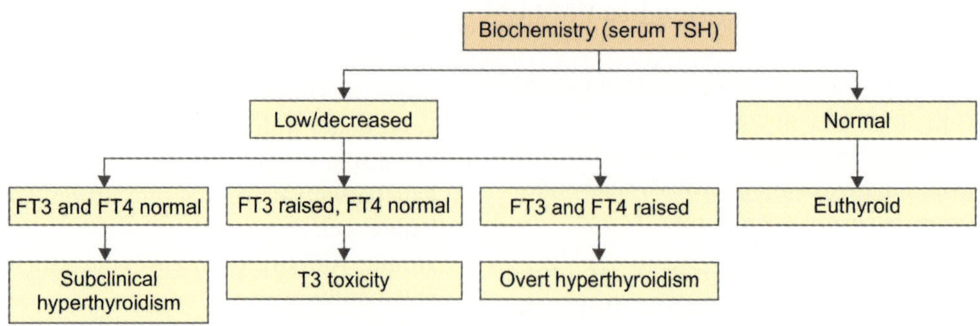

(FT3: free T3; TSH: thyroid-stimulating hormone)

Flowchart 2: Serology of TSH.

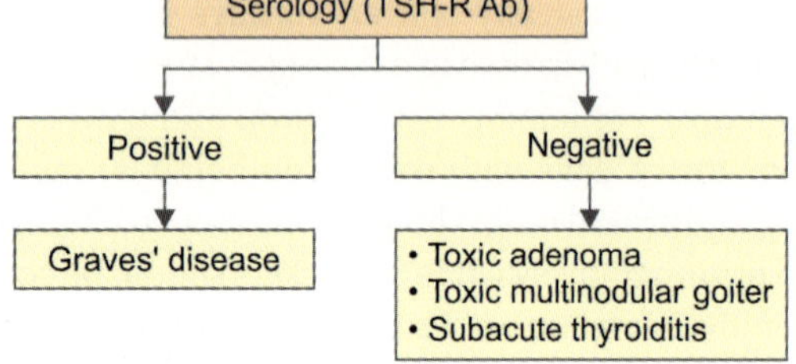

(TSH-R Ab: thyroid-stimulating hormone receptor antibody)

- *Postoperative management*:
  - Antithyroid drugs should be stopped postoperatively. β-blockers are tapered postoperatively and stopped.
  - Thyroid replacement is usually started a week after surgery.
  - Postoperative hypocalcemia can be managed with calcium supplements and activated vitamin D postoperatively.
  - Hungry bone syndrome may be seen in those who are hyperthyroid prior to surgery. This can also be treated with calcium supplements.[3,4,10,11,13]

◇ MANAGEMENT ALGORITHM

Flowchart 1 shows the biochemistry of TSH and **Flowchart 2** depicts the serology of TSH.

◇ SPECIAL SCENARIOS

Thyroid Storm

- Presentation is usually with high-grade fever, profuse diaphoresis, tachycardia, arrhythmias, congestive cardiac failure, tachypnea, tremors, severe agitation, altered sensorium which may progress to coma, severe diarrhea, and abdominal pain.
- Early diagnosis and treatment are most essential to avoid fatal outcome.
- Biochemical investigations suggest hyperthyroidism.

- "Burch and Wartofsky's diagnostic criteria" helps to arrive at diagnosis. A score of 25–44 is suggestive of impending storm and >45 is suggestive of thyroid storm.[3,4]

Graves' Disease in Children

- PTU should be avoided in children and adolescents.
- Carbimazole is the choice of antithyroid drug which can be given with monitoring.
- RAI is avoided in children.
- Surgery is the definitive treatment option.[3,4]

Graves' Disease in Pregnancy

- As mentioned before, pregnancy is a contraindication for RAI treatment.
- Carbimazole is avoided in first trimester due to teratogenic side effects. Propylthiouracil is considered safer in first trimester.
- Surgery is usually performed in second trimester.
- It is safer, if women with Graves' disease are euthyroid prior to planning pregnancy.[3,4]

Apathetic Hyperthyroidism

- Elderly usually presents with mild symptoms of mood changes, weight loss, and breathlessness.
- Some may present with atrial fibrillation, congestive cardiac failure, and acute coronary syndrome. These patients may benefit from RAI therapy.
- Elderly patients with mild Graves' disease and multiple comorbidities can be managed with antithyroid drugs.[3,4]

Immune Reconstitution

- First seen in patients with multiple sclerosis who were put on alemtuzumab. It is also seen in human immunodeficiency virus (HIV) patients on antiretroviral therapy and bone marrow transplant patients.
- Graves' disease precipitated by immunomodulatory therapy can be managed conservatively with antithyroid drugs or may rarely need definitive treatment with RAI or surgery.

- It may be transient and can be easily managed conservatively and followed with serial measurement of TRAb.[3,4]

CLINICAL PEARLS

Graves' disease is an autoimmune disease triggered by a variety of etiological factors like infection, stress, and exposure to iodine. It is usually self-limiting and medical therapy is the first line of management. In those where definitive therapy is required, surgical or RAI ablation can be chosen for the appropriate patient. The choice for the definitive treatment is best selected after appropriate counseling.

REFERENCES

1. Taylor S. Graves of Graves' disease, 1796-1853. JR Coll Physicians Lond. 1986;20(4):298-300.
2. Weetman AP. Graves' disease. N Engl Med. 2000;343(17): 1236-48.
3. Ross DS, Burch HB, Cooper DS, Greenlee MC, Laurberg P, Maia AL, et al. 2016 American Thyroid Association Guidelines for Diagnosis and Management of Hyperthyroidism and Other Causes of Thyrotoxicosis. Thyroid. 2016;26(10):1342-421.
4. Kahaly GJ, Bartalena L, Hegedüs L, Leenhardt L, Poppe K, Pearce SH. 2018 European Thyroid Association Guideline for the Management of Graves' Hyperthyroidism. Eur Thyroid J. 2018;7(4):167-86.
5. Cooper DS. Hyperthyroidism. Lancet. 2003;362(9382):459-68.
6. Subekti I, Soewondo P, Soebardi S, Darmowidjojo B, Harbuwono DS, Purnamasari D, et al. Practical guidelines management of Graves' ophthalmopathy. Acta Med Indones. 2019;51(4):364-71.
7. Cooper DS. (2003). Hyperthyroidism. [online] Available from https://reader.elsevier.com/reader/sd/pii/S014067360314073 1?token=B912723F6B1D5A7D344B8F631BF1D63F0681F2FFB BA674FF60F7E21C82B8B19C8347BBB8C723015D3F82FC3B3 E0D085A [Last accessed June, 2021].
8 Dhali TK, Chahar M. Thyroid dermopathy-a diagnostic clue of hidden hyperthyroidism. Dermatoendocrinol. 2015;6(1):e981078.
9. Jadidi J, Sighary M, Efendizade A, Grigorian A, Lehto SA, Kolla S. Thyroid acropachy: A rare skeletal manifestation of autoimmune thyroid disease. Radiol Case Rep. 2019;14(8): 917-9.
10. DeGroot LJ. Diagnosis and treatment of Graves' disease. MDText.com, Inc.; 2000-2016.
11. Burch HB, Cooper DS. Management of Graves disease: a review. JAMA. 2015;314(23):2544-54.
12. Sjölin G, Holmberg M, Törring O, Byström K, Khamisi S, de Laval D, et al. The long-term outcome of treatment for Graves' Hyperthyroidism. Thyroid. 2019;29(11):1545-57.
13. Smithson M, Asban A, Miller J, Chen H. Considerations for thyroidectomy as treatment for Graves disease. Clin Med Insights Endocrinol Diabetes. 2019;12:1179551419844523.
14. Sundaresh V, Brito JP, Wang Z, Prokop LJ, Stan MN, Murad MH, et al. Comparative effectiveness of therapies for Graves' hyperthyroidism: a systematic review and network meta-analysis. J Clin Endocrinol Metab. 2013;98(9): 3671-7.

Thyroglossal Duct Cyst and Fistula

Mohanty Biswa N, Kailash C Mohapatra, Mohanty Arun K

INTRODUCTION

Thyroglossal duct cyst (TDC) takes its origin from the epithelial remnants of the thyroglossal duct that forms during descent of the thyroid gland from the foramen cecum to its final destination in the anterior neck. TDC constitutes the most common congenital anomaly of the neck in childhood.[1] Still then half of these cases are diagnosed in the second decade of life and even some cases are encountered later in adulthood.[2]

EMBRYOLOGY

The thyroid gland develops as an invagination of the endoderm lining the ventral floor of the primitive pharynx between the copula and the tuberculum impar.[3] This median structure descends caudally and bifurcates into a bilobed diverticulum. During its descent, the gland leaves behind an epithelial tract known as the thyroglossal duct or thyroglossal tract (TT). In the usual course of events, the connection between the cervical thyroid and the base of the tongue gets obliterated and disappears between 5th and 10th gestational week[3] **(Fig. 1)**.

Thyroglossal tract traverses down in the midline of the neck passing anterior (at times through the substance or posterior) to the developing hyoid bone. As the hyoid bone matures and rotates to assume its adult position, the TT moves around the inferior edge of the bone and then turns to lie behind its concavity on the posterior surface, before descending down close to the thyrohoid membrane.[4] Such tortuous course of the TT makes its remnants to present either anterior or posterior to the hyoid bone.

The thyroglossal tract remnant (TTR) may persist as an ectopic thyroid or may clinically present as a cyst, sinus and fistula later in life.[5]

ANATOMY

The thyroglossal cyst can occupy any position along the developmental tract from the foramen cecum in the tongue to the suprasternal region but it is mostly near or in the midline of the neck.[6] Thus, it may be described as lingual, suprahyoid, subhyoid, and suprasternal. Most of the thyroglossal cysts occupy a position in close proximity to the thyroid cartilage. In about 60% of patients it occupies thyrohyoid (subhyoid) position[3] **(Fig. 2)**.

PATHOLOGY

Thyroglossal duct cysts are usually unilocular but may be multilocular. The content is usually mucoid. Infected cysts contain mucopurulent material or pus **(Fig. 3)**. The histological diagnosis is based on the presence of either respiratory epithelium (pseudostratified ciliated columnar

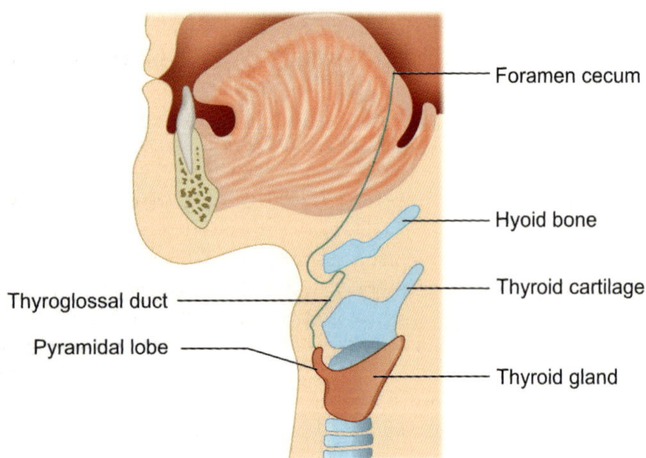

Fig. 1: Thyroglossal duct during embryological development.

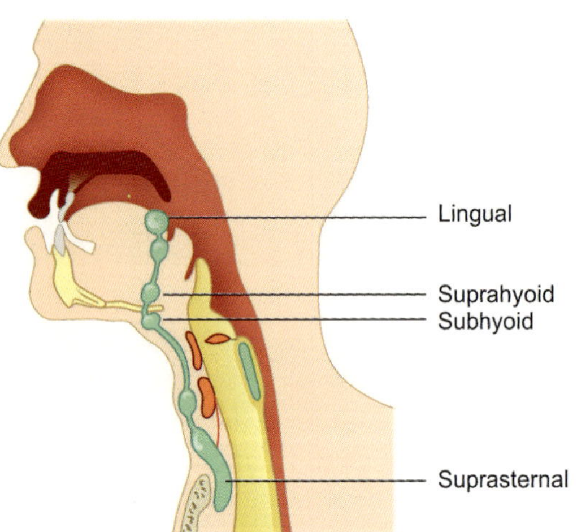

Fig. 2: Thyroglossal duct cyst locations.

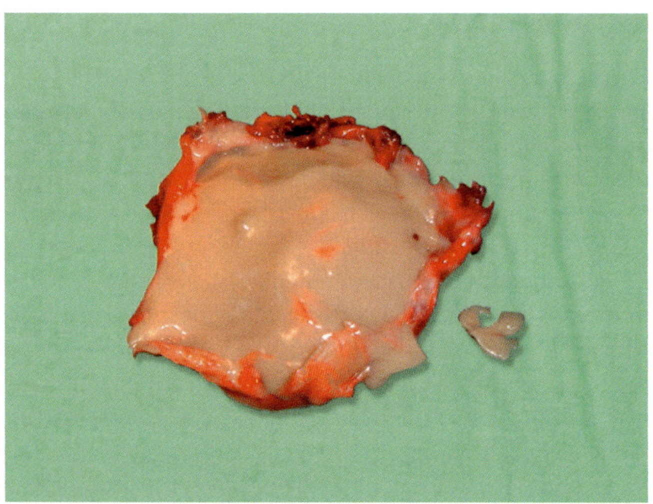

Fig. 3: Mucopurulent content of a thyroglossal duct cyst.

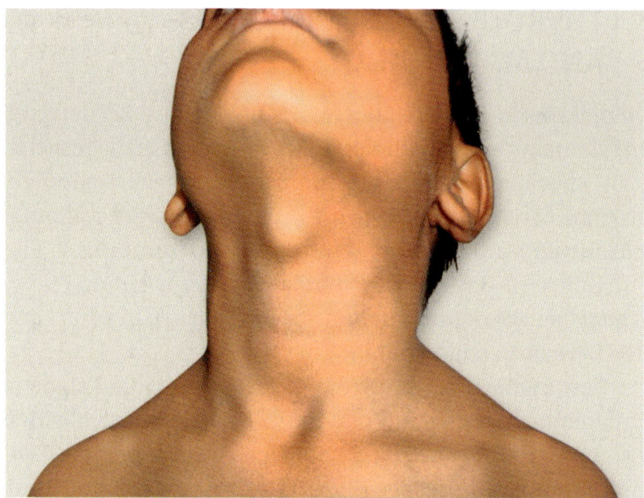

Fig. 4: Thyroglossal duct cyst presenting as a midline neck swelling.

or low cuboidal cells) or squamous epithelium. Squamous epithelium when present is predominantly nonkeratinizing.[7]

Thyroid follicles may be present in the wall of the cyst.[3] The follicles are even found at times in the close vicinity of the perichondrium of the hyoid bone.[8]

ETIOLOGY

Incomplete involution of the TT results in formation of the thyroglossal cyst. Mentioned below are some theories postulated to explain the development of the cyst from the TTR:

- *The most commonly supported one is the inflammatory theory*: Lymphoid tissue closely associated with the duct hypertrophies in response to repeated upper respiratory tract infection, which then causes occlusion of the duct resulting in cyst formation.[3]
- Retention of secretion as a result of blocked thyroglossal duct may give rise to cyst formation.[3]
- Rarely patients may present with familial TDC which can be detected by routine genetic testing.[9]

CLINICAL FEATURES

The usual clinical presentation of TDC is a midline neck swelling situated in proximity to the hyoid bone (**Fig. 4**). About 25% of cysts may not be present in the midline, these swellings are usually present to the left side.[10] The TDC is usually soft, nontender and mobile on palpation, unless it is infected.[6] A male preponderance is observed in children with female preponderance in adults.[11]

The cyst may occupy a position anywhere between foramen cecum and the suprasternal notch along the thyroglossal duct tract. However, the most common position is just below the hyoid bone. Usual size of the TDC is 2–4 cm in diameter. The cysts generally move during deglutition and with protrusion of the tongue because of thyroglossal tract attachment to the hyoid bone and to foramen cecum.[12]

Inflammation of the cyst may result in a painful tender mass. The patient may present in such a situation with fever, dysphagia, dysphonia and/or a discharging sinus.[13]

Large TDCs when located at the base of the tongue may cause airway obstruction[14] manifesting clinically with dyspnea, rasping respiration, and periodic cyanosis.[14,15]

INVESTIGATIONS

History and physical examination are adequate to make a diagnosis of TDC. The investigative modalities used for preoperative evaluation are imaging studies, viz., thyroid ultrasonography, CT, magnetic resonance imaging (MRI) and radioisotope scan.[16]

On USG imaging, a TDC can have variable appearance. A simple cyst will be anechoic and well circumscribed. Pseudo-solid appearance of a cyst is due to proteinaceous fluid, cholesterol crystals and keratin contained in it. Cysts with previous infection or hemorrhage will have a heterogeneous pattern with internal echoes. Most TDCs in children have a pseudo-solid appearance in US.[16] However, presence of a solid lesion with or without microscopic calcification raises the suspicion of malignancy.[17] Enlargement and other characteristics of neck nodes can be assessed by US.

CT and MRI are useful to delineate the anatomy of large cysts and MRI may help in detecting a residual fistulous tract in recurrent disease.[16]

Preoperative radioisotope scanning in these patients is not necessary, if USG indicates a normal thyroid gland in its usual position.[6,16]

Fine-needle aspiration differentiates a cystic lesion from an ectopic thyroid gland. It is a useful investigation to diagnose malignancy. US-guided fine-needle aspiration cytology (FNAC) would be required to aspirate solid component of cystic masses. Papillary TD carcinoma should be suspected if large, atypical squamous cells or psammoma bodies are found in the FNAC material.[18]

THYROGLOSSAL DUCT CYSTS AND MALIGNANCY

Neoplasms in TDC are uncommon and are usually detected incidentally during pathological examination of the resected TDC specimen. The most common malignancy is papillary thyroid carcinoma followed by mixed papillary follicular carcinoma and then squamous cell carcinoma.[19] The incidence of primary carcinoma in TTRs is about 1%.[19,20] The mean age of presentation is fourth decade in adults and 12–13 years in children.[21]

Fast increase in the size of a TDC, absence of signs of inflammation, detection of a mural mass, and calcification on thyroid ultrasonography are signs of malignancy. TDC carcinoma may be suspected in a cyst that appears hard, fixed, and irregular on palpation with recent change in size of the swelling. FNAC or imaging is essential in making a diagnosis.

THYROGLOSSAL FISTULA AND SINUS

Thyroglossal fistula is rarely encountered. Here the cyst in neck communicates through a channel with the foramen of cecum; hence, content of the cyst can be expressed in to the oral cavity by pressure over the cyst.[22]

Thyroglossal sinuses, on the other hand, are secondary to spontaneous rupture of infected thyroglossal cyst or sequelae of surgical drainage. The cutaneous opening is around 1–3 mm in diameter. The location of the opening may be anywhere in the anterior neck from the suprasternal notch to the hyoid bone **(Fig. 5)**. Drops of mucoid, clear or purulent fluid can be made to escape from these openings. One may be able to feel a tract running from the skin lesion proximally to the hyoid bone.[3,10]

Ultrasonography and MRI are useful investigations in evaluation of thyroglossal sinus or fistula. Thyroglossal fistulography is rarely necessary to demonstrate a fistulous communication with foramen cecum.[23]

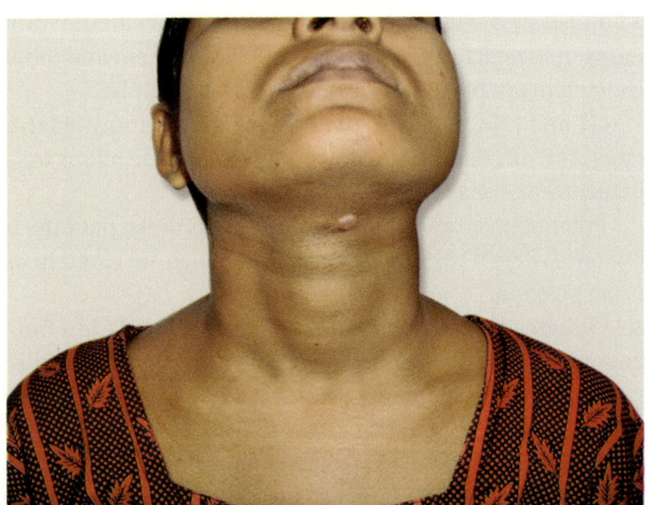

Fig. 5: Thyroglossal sinus.

TREATMENT

Thyroglossal duct cysts were treated before the year 1893 with simple incision and drainage. This had resulted in recurrence rates reaching almost 50%.[24] A procedure that entailed removal of the mid-portion of the hyoid bone along with the TDC was described first by Schlange in 1893.[25] This caused a fall in the recurrence rate down to 20%.[24]

Subsequently in 1920 Walter Ellis Sistrunk demonstrated that excision of a cylinder of tissue following the embryologic course of the thyroglossal duct between the hyoid bone and the foramen cecum added to removal of TDC in continuity with mid portion of the hyoid bone reduced the recurrence rate up to 5%.[26,27]

Over time this remained as the most appropriate surgical procedure for treatment of thyroglossal cyst and was designated as the Sistrunk's procedure. In a later published communication, Sistrunk reported that entering the oral cavity is not necessary and that tongue muscle can be resected without opening the mucous membrane of the mouth.[28]

Various modified Sistrunk's procedures were described subsequently where a deep core of tissue was not removed because of nonavailability of convincing evidence in the literature that such excision offers greater benefit. Majority of these cases are now cured whether core is removed or not. Hence, additional operating time and higher morbidity by deeper dissection may not be justified.[12]

In patients where malignancy can be excluded, percutaneous ethanol injections may be tried as a modality of treatment particularly in TDCs with compromised cardiovascular status rendering them unsuitable for surgery under general anesthesia.[29]

Patients presenting with an abscess of the TDC should have the abscess aspirated first than undertaking incision and drainage so as to make subsequent surgery easier and also to reduce recurrence.[12]

The treatment for lesions of thyroglossal system whether cyst, sinus or fistula consists of complete removal of the tract to the foramen cecum with removal of the central portion of the hyoid bone.

The optimal management strategy for TDC carcinoma remains controversial, with differing views as regards management of the thyroid gland. Some authors recommend Sistrunk's operation to be adequate and curative in most cases, while others consider total thyroidectomy should be combined with the former procedure in view of high incidence of associated papillary or mixed carcinoma in the thyroid the gland.[30] The rationale for combining total thyroidectomy in all patients with thyroglossal duct carcinoma is to eliminate concomitant thyroid malignancy if present in the main thyroid gland, to permit use of radioactive iodine as an adjuvant therapy and to allow long-term patient follow-up by using serum thyroglobulin as a tumor marker for thyroid cancer.[31]

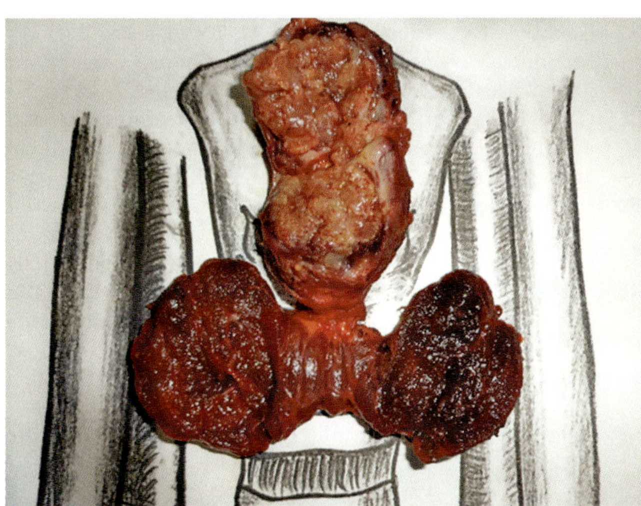

Fig. 6: Sistrunk's operation combined with total thyroidectomy for a patient with thyroglossal duct cyst carcinoma (Papillary).

The etiology of TDC carcinoma is not clear, although the proposed theories are either metastatic disease from an occult primary in thyroid gland or de novo development of neoplastic lesion from ectopic thyroid tissue found within the TDC wall.[32]

The choice of surgical approach may be based on risk group stratification. Hence, Sistrunk's operation may be considered as a stand-alone procedure in patients with clinically and radiologically normal thyroid gland with low risk tumors, i.e., for patients who are <45 years of age, no history of radiation exposure, no soft tissue invasion, no aggressive tumor histology and absence of spread to lymph nodes or to distant sites.[33] Other patients with tumors in the cyst >1 cm in diameter or presence of concomitant thyroid malignancy in the main thyroid gland should be considered for additional total thyroidectomy[34] **(Fig. 6)**. Lymph node dissection should be performed in patients with clinically positive nodes.

◇ SUMMARY

Thyroglossal duct cyst is the most common congenital anomaly of the neck in childhood. In majority of cases, it occupies a subhyoid position. Inflammation of the cyst may result in a painful tender mass. Thyroglossal sinuses result from spontaneous rupture of infected thyroglossal cysts or as sequelae of surgical drainage. The investigative modalities used for preoperative evaluation are imaging studies, viz., thyroid ultrasonography, CT, MRI, and radioisotope scan. The incidence of primary carcinoma in the cyst is about 1%. The treatment for lesions of thyroglossal system whether cyst, sinus or fistula consists of complete removal of the tract to the foramen cecum with removal of the central portion of the hyoid bone. As regard TDC carcinoma some authors recommend Sistrunk's operation to be adequate and curative, while others consider total thyroidectomy to be combined with the former procedure in view of high incidence of associated papillary or mixed carcinoma in the thyroid gland.

◇ REFERENCES

1. Hsieh YY, Hsueh S, Hsueh C, Lin JN, Luo CC, Lai JY, et al. Pathological analysis of congenital cervical cysts in children: 20 years of experience at Chang Gung Memorial Hospital. Chang Gung Med J. 2003;26:107-13.
2. Türkyilmaz Z, Sönmez K, Karabulut R, Demirgoullari B, Sezer C, Basaklar AC, et al. Management of thyroglossal duct cysts in children. Pediatr Int. 2004;46:77-80.
3. Allard RHB. The thyroglossal cyst. Head Neck Surg. 1982;5:134-46.
4. Ellis PD, van Nostrand AW. The applied anatomy of thyroglossal tract remnants. Laryngoscope. 1977;87:765-70.
5. Wenglowski R. Fistulae and cysts of neck. Arch F Klin Chir. 1912;98:151.
6. Organ GM, Organ CH. Thyroid gland and the surgery of the thyroglossal duct: Exercise in applied embryology. World J Surg. 2000;24:886-90.
7. Chandra RK, Maddalozzo J, Kovarik P. Histological characterization of the thyroglossal tract: implications for surgical management. Laryngoscope. 2001;111:1002-5.
8. Sprinzl GM, Koebke J, Wimmers-Klick J, Eckel HE, Thumfart WF. Morphology of the human thyroglossal tract: a histologic and macroscopic study in infants and children. Ann Otol Rhinol Laryngol. 2000;109:1135-9.
9. Brousseau VJ, Solares CA, Xu M, Krakovitz P, Koltai PJ. Thyroglossal duct cysts: presentation and management in children versus adults. Int J Pediatr Otorhinolaryngol. 2003;67:1285-90.
10. Deane SA, Telander RL. Surgery for thyroglossal duct and branchial cleft anomalies. Am J Surg. 1978;136(3):348-53.
11. Thompson LDR, Herrera HB, Lau SK. A Clinicopathologic Series of 685 Thyroglossal Duct Remnant Cysts. Head Neck Pathol. 2016;10(4):465-74.
12. Vanni M, Alfio F, Enrico M, Carl ES, Johannes JF, Kenneth OD, et al. Thyroglossal duct cyst: personal experience and literature review. Auris Nasus Larynx. 2008;35:11-25.
13. Ostlie DJ, Burjonrappa SC, Snyder CL, Watts J, Murphy JP, Gittes GK, et al. Thyroglossal duct infections and surgical outcomes. J Pediatr Surg. 2004;39:396-9.
14. Purdom E, Robitschek J, Littlefield PD, Cable B. Acute airway obstruction from a thyroglossal duct cyst. Otolaryngol Head Neck Surg. 2007;136:317-8.
15. Kanawaku Y, Funayama M, Sakai J, Nata M, Kanetake J. Sudden infant death: lingual thyroglossal duct cyst versus environmental factors. Forensic Sci Int. 2006;156:158-60.
16. Ahuja AT, Wong KT, King AD, Yuen EH. Imaging for thyroglossal duct cyst: the bare essentials. Clin Radiol. 2005;60(2):141-8.
17. Glastonbury C, Harnsberger HR. Thyroglossal duct calcifications. Neuroradiology. 2001;43:1015.
18. Bardales RH, Suhrland MJ, Korourian S, Schaefer RF, Hanna EY, Stanley MW. Cytologic findings in thyroglossal duct carcinoma. Am J Clin Pathol. 1996;106:615-9.
19. Motamed M, McGlashan JA. Thyroglossal duct carcinoma. Curr Opin Otolaryngol Head Neck Surg. 2004;12:106-9.
20. Peretz A, Leiberman E, Kapelushnik J, Hershkovitz E. Thyroglossal duct carcinoma in children: case presentation and review of literature. Thyroid. 2004;14:777-85.
21. Doshi SV, Cruz RM, Hilsinger RL Jr. Thyroglossal duct carcinoma: a large case series. Ann Otol Rhinol Laryngol. 2001;110:734-8.
22. Clute HM, Cattell RB. Thyroglossal cysts. Ann Surg. 1930; 92:57.

23. Massoud TF, Schnetler JF. Case report: taste of success in thyroglossal fistulography. Clin Radiol. 1992;45:281-3.

24. Wagner G, Medina JE. Excision of thyroglossal duct cyst: the Sistrunk procedure. Oper Tech Otolaryngol. 2004;15: 220-3.

25. Schlange H, Ueber die. Fistula Colli Congenita. Arch Klin Chir. 1893;46:390-2.

26. Gross E, Sichel JY. Congenital neck regions. Surg Clin N Am. 2006;86:383-92.

27. Galluzzi F, Pignataro L, Gaini RM, Hartley BEJ. Risk of recurrence in children operated for thyroglossal duct cysts: a systematic review. J Paediatr Surg. 2013;48(1):222-7.

28. Sistrunk WE. Technique of removal of cysts and sinuses of the thyroglossal duct. Surg Gynecol Obstet. 1928;46:109-12.

29. Baskin HJ. Percutaneous ethanol injection of thyroglossal duct cysts. Endocr Pract. 2006;12:355-7.

30. Gebbia V, Di Gregorio C, Attard M. Thyroglossal duct cyst carcinoma with concurrent thyroid carcinoma: a case report. J Med Case Rep. 2008;2:132.

31. Carter Y, Yeutter N, Mazeh H. Thyroglossal duct remnant carcinoma: beyond the Sistrunk procedure. Surg Oncol. 2014;23(3):161-6.

32. Underwood HJ, Williams DM, Kundel A. Papillary thyroid carcinoma within thyroglossal duct cyst: case report and review of literature. JSM Head Neck Cancer Cases Rev. 2016;1(2):1006.

33. Bakkar S, Biricotti M, Stefanini G, Ambrosini CE, Materazzi G, Miccoli P. The extent of surgery in thyroglossal cyst carcinoma. Langenbecks Arch Surg. 2017;402(5):799-804.

34. Dan D, Rambally R, Naraynsingh V, Maharaj R, Hariharan S. A case of malignancy in a thyroglossal duct cyst—recommendations for management. J Natl Med Assoc. 2012;104(3,4):211-4.

CHAPTER 12

Differentiated Thyroid Cancer

Roma Pradhan, Amit Agarwal

INTRODUCTION

The incidence of thyroid cancer continues to rise worldwide, mostly as a result of the widespread use of ultrasound and aspiration of thyroid nodules. Thyroid cancer is the fifth most common cancer in women in the USA, while in India it does not figure in the top 10 cancers in women. Interestingly despite the rising incidence, mortality from thyroid cancer has changed minimally over the past five decades. The broad heterogeneity of thyroid cancer represents one of the most amazing examples of variability amongst all solid malignancies. Thyroid cancers range from a papillary thyroid microcarcinoma which may not even merit any treatment to anaplastic thyroid carcinoma (ATC), one of the deadliest malignancies, which is fatal in the vast majority of cases even if radically resected at an early stage. Even within the differentiated thyroid carcinoma (DTC) group, heterogeneity is seen with most DTCs being rather indolent tumors characterized by a good response to standard treatment with a 10-year survival rate reaching 90%[1] to aggressive cancers with 10-year survival of only 40%. Thus, the challenge faced by physicians who treat thyroid cancers is to balance the therapeutic approach so that patients with lower risk disease are not overtreated and at the same time, they need to recognize those patients with more high-risk disease, who need a more aggressive treatment approach.

CLINICAL PRESENTATION

A physician may pick up DTC in various scenarios such as:

- As an incidentally discovered palpable or nonpalpable thyroid nodule which is highly suspicious/positive for malignancy on ultrasonography (USG) and fine needle aspiration cytology (FNAC; most common presentation)
- Reported to be DTC on a lobectomy specimen done for a Bethesda category 2, 3, 4 or 4 lesion
- As a thyroid incidentaloma on a positron emission tomography (PET) scan done for an unrelated reason
- Detected on aspiration of a deep cervical lymph node (LN) with no palpable lesion in thyroid
- Patients may sometime present with advanced or aggressive features such as a fixed thyroid mass with or without vocal cord palsy (uncommon).

EVALUATION

Clinical Assessment

Important elements in the patient's history or physical examination which are pointers toward the presence of malignancy in a thyroid nodule or goiter are as follows:

- History of radiation in childhood
- Recent rapid growth
- Dyspnea, dysphagia
- Presentation in extreme of ages (<20 years, >70 years)
- Fixation to adjacent structures
- Presence of deep cervical lymphadenopathy (LAP)
- Vocal cord immobility

Laboratory Studies

Serum thyroid-stimulating hormone (TSH) is cost-effective. If below normal, as happens only in 10%, then free T3 and T4 are ordered.

High-resolution Ultrasonography and Elastography

Before asking for fine needle aspiration (FNA), the nodule should undergo high-resolution USG with Doppler study to characterize the nodules and select them for guided aspiration. USG is usually performed with a 5–12-MHz linear array transducer. US features of each thyroid nodule are recorded in following categories:[2]

- *Composition*: Solid, predominantly solid, predominantly cystic
- *Echogenicity*: Hyper-, iso-, or hypoechoic
- *Margin*: Circumscribed or microlobulated/irregular
- *Calcification*: Microcalcification, macrocalcification, or mixed calcification
- *Shape*: Parallel or nonparallel (i.e., taller than wide)

Features suggestive of malignancy include marked hypoechogenicity, noncircumscribed margin, micro or mixed calcification, and taller than wide. It should be kept in mind that a single USG feature has poor sensitivity for predicting malignancy which is better predicted by a combination of USG features. This is the basis of the development of TI-RADS system.

TI-RADS is a risk-stratification system for classifying thyroid nodules based on USG features. It is an objective system which considers a group of ultrasound features rather than depending upon a single USG feature to make a prediction of thyroid malignancy. It is similar to the BIRADS system used for breast lesions. The following categories are used in TI-RADS **(Table 1)**.

ACR-TIRADS

Scoring is determined from five categories of ultrasound findings. The higher the cumulative score, the higher the TR (TI-RADS) level and the likelihood of malignancy.

One score is assigned from each of the following categories:
- *Composition* (choose one):
  - Cystic or completely cystic: 0 points
  - Spongiform: 0 points
  - Mixed cystic and solid: 1 point
  - Solid or almost completely solid: 2 points
- *Echogenicity* (choose one):
  - Anechoic: 0 points
  - Hyper- or isoechoic: 1 point
  - Hypoechoic: 2 points
  - Very hypoechoic: 3 points
- *Shape* (choose one) (assessed on the transverse plane):
  - Wider than tall: 0 points
  - Taller than wide: 3 points
- *Margin* (choose one):
  - Smooth: 0 points
  - Ill-defined: 0 points
  - Lobulated/irregular: 2 points
  - Extrathyroidal extension: 3 points

Any and all findings in the final category are also added to the other four scores.
- *Echogenic foci* (choose one or more):
  - None: 0 points
  - Large comet-tail artifact: 0 points
- Macrocalcifications: 1 point
- Peripheral/rim calcifications: 2 points
- Punctate echogenic foci: 3 points
- Highly suspicious

Among the initial studies, a prospective study by Horvath et al.[3] of 210 patients with 502 nodules comparing TI-RADS to pathology reported a risk of malignancy among TI-RADS 2, 3, 4, and 5 to be 0, 1.8, 76.1, and 98.9%, respectively. Using TI-RADS 4–5 to perform FNA, the authors reported a sensitivity, specificity, positive predictive value (PPV), and negative predictive value (NPV) of 99.6, 74.35, 82.1, and 99.4%, respectively.[1,4] In the study, Friedrich-Rust et al.[4] showed a high NPV (92–100%) for TI-RADS 4 and 5 in excluding malignancy. Similarly, a retrospective analysis[5] of 100 consecutive cases comparing single-surgeon-performed ultrasonographic TI-RADS findings to cytopathology, including all Bethesda categories, found a concordance rate of 83% with a sensitivity, specificity, and NPV of 70.6, 90.4, and 93.8%, respectively.

There are at least five systems of TI-RADS. Among them, the ACR-TI-RADS had the highest interobserver agreement, a trend to have highest sensitivity and NPV for the diagnosis of malignant thyroid nodules.[6]

Ultrasound Elastography (Fig. 1)

This technique purposes to differentiate the tissues according to their stiffness or elasticity. The principle of elastography is based on the fact that the pathologic processes alter the structure of the tissues and ultimately their elasticity. The malignant tissues are therefore stiffer than normal or benign tissue. Elastography compares the stiffness of the then thyroid nodule with stiffness of adjacent normal thyroid parenchyma and thus can predict malignancy in a given thyroid nodule. There are two approaches to elastography: strain elastography (SE) and shear wave elastography (SWE).

Table 1: Categories used in TI-RADS.				
TI-RADS Category	**Scoring**	**Classification**	**Risk of malignancy**	**Recommendations**
TR1	0 points	Benign	0.3%	No FNA required
TR2	2 points	Not suspicious	1.5%	No FNA required
TR3	3 points	Mildly suspicious	4.8%	≥1.5 cm follow-up, ≥2.5 cm FNA Follow-up: 1, 3, and 5 years
TR4	4–6 points	Moderately suspicious	9.1%	≥1.0 cm follow-up, ≥1.5 cm FNA Follow-up: 1, 2, 3, and 5 years
TR5	≥7 Points	Highly suspicious	35%	≥0.5 cm follow-up, ≥1.0 cm FNA annual follow-up for up to 5 years

(FNA: fine needle aspiration)

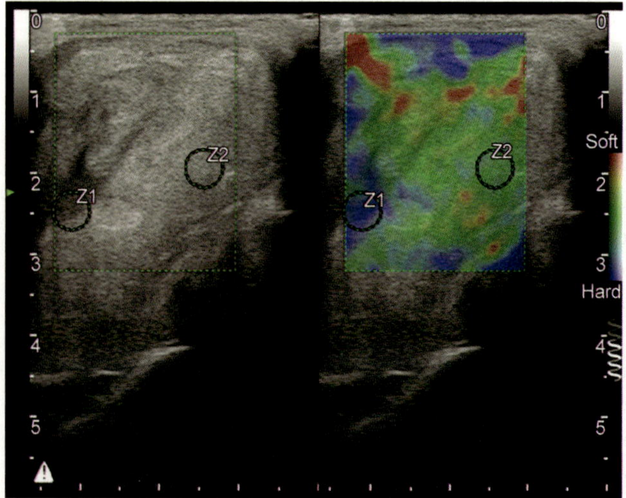

Fig. 1: Ultrasound elastography (USE). A 39-year-old woman with a solitary thyroid nodule with FNAC of Bethesda 2, with EUS showing hard areas; underwent total thyroidectomy and HPE revealed PTC.

Strain elastography (SE): This assesses the elastic properties of tissues by analyzing tissue strain, that is, tissue deformation produced by the applied force. Malignant tissues are hard and therefore are not deformed or strained whereas benign or normal tissue would displace or deform more. Deformation may be induced by a pure mechanic force (which can be either external force of a transducer or internal force of carotid pulsations) or by ultrasound [using acoustic force radiation impulse (AFRI)]. The tissue stiffness is displayed either in gray scale or in a continuum of colors from red to green to blue representing soft (high strain), intermediate (equal strain), and hard (no strain). Semiquantitative elastographic measurement is done either by visual scoring systems or by strain ratio (SR).

Strain ratio: The most common technique is the semiquantitative SE with external force—either on the reference image (Q-elastography) or on a representative image selected by the operator from the video sequence; a strain ratio or strain rate (SR) is computed. This is, usually, the ratio of the strain of normal parenchyma to the strain of the nodule or area under analysis. There is some disagreement on the critical cutoff value to differentiate between benign and malignant nodules. Cutoffs of >4 and >3.79 have been suggested with different sensitivities.[7] Briefly, the technique is as follows: on pressing the elastography option two boxes appear on the screen, one for the B-mode ultrasound and another for elastography. Constant repetitive pressure is applied with the transducer on nodule in a perpendicular direction till the machine identifies that the applied pressure and acquired image are appropriate for analysis by giving green signal [thus obviating the subjectivity of applied pressure in earlier models of ultrasound elastography (USGE)]. This image is then fixed on the screen and colorimetric score noted. After this, the strain ratio button on the keypad is pressed and two circles pop up on the screen. One circle is placed over normal thyroid tissue (Z1) and another on our targeted area (Z2). The machine then automatically calculates the SR (Z2/Z1). Various studies have evaluated the diagnostic performance of SE[8–10] but with varying sensitivities and specificities.

Shear wave elastography: In this technique, the transducer sends pulses into the tissues that sets up transverse shear waves which are conducted through the tissues at a speed which is related to the stiffness of the tissues—stiffer tissues (malignant) conduct shear waves faster. This speed is then measured and computed to reflect the stiffness of the thyroid nodule.

In clinical practice, USE should be performed as a tool which is complimentary to conventional USG. In fact, it has been shown that a combination of USG and USE resulted in better sensitivity and specificity as compared to that of each technique alone.[11] The advantage of USE is that it can be useful for selecting nodules that need to be aspirated and to follow-up nodules that have been found to be negative on FNA and hence not operated.

Table 2: Bethesda cytology categories.

Diagnostic category	Cytological diagnosis	Risk of malignancy, %	Recommended management
I	Nondiagnostic or unsatisfactory	1–4	Repeat FNA with ultrasound guidance
II	Benign	0–3	Clinical follow-up
III	AUS/FLUS	5–15	Repeat FNA
IV	FNS/SFN	15–30	Surgical lobectomy
V	Suspicious for malignancy	60–75	Near-total thyroidectomy or surgical lobectomy
VI	Malignancy	97–99	Near-total thyroidectomy

(AUS/FLUS: atypia of undetermined significance/follicular lesion of undetermined significance; FNS/SFN: follicular neoplasm or suspicious for follicular neoplasm)

Cytology of thyroid nodules: FNAC gives a diagnostic information about thyroid nodules which helps in decision-making. It is a safe, simple, reliable, and cheap diagnostic test. Reporting of the result of FNAC was standardized a decade back using the Bethesda system and more recently the updated Bethesda system.[12,13] The advantage of the six-tiered Bethesda System for Reporting Thyroid Cytopathology (TBSRTC) is the standardization of reporting of cytology and another advantage being the added information given by each category about the implied risk of malignancy that translates into a recommendation for clinical decision-making. Over the last decade or so, TBSRTC has shown consistent and high sensitivity as well as high NPV in almost all centers all around the world **(Table 2)**.[14]

Diagnostic categories 2, 5, and 6 provide high NPV and PPV; however, DC 3 and 4 comprising about 20–30% of all FNAC are together clubbed as an indeterminate category with a risk of malignancy of 10–40% and usually require additional evaluation.[15] The recent updated TBSRTC system also takes into account the recently identified noninvasive follicular thyroid neoplasm with papillary-like nuclear features (NIFTP) entity.[12]

Cytological picture of papillary thyroid carcinoma (PTC): The various cytologic features of classical PTC are high cellularity, papillary fronds, enlarged oval nucleus with longitudinal intranuclear grooves, nuclear crowding and overlapping, cellular swirls, and chewing gum colloid.

Method and adequacy: A specimen is labeled as adequate if there are at least six groups of follicular cells in total on the D-K (Diff-Quik) stained smears on two slides with a minimum of 10 cells in each group. Usually, four to six passes are made from the thyroid nodule.[16,17] After each pass, a drop is put on a plain slide and smeared by a positively charged slide. One smear is air-dried with D-Q and immediately evaluated. Other smears are quickly fixed with 95% alcohol and later stained with Papanicolaou stain.

Two cytopreparatory techniques are used for FNA—conventional smear (CS) and monolayer technique (MT). The computed tomography (CT) is more accurate than MT.

In the CS technique, two smears are obtained as follows:
1. *Air-dried (D-Q/M-GG method)*: This tells about the background colloid, cell architecture, and cytoplasm.
2. *Alcohol-fixed smear (Papanicolaou stain)*: It is a wet smear that is fixed immediately with 95% alcohol and enhances the nuclear architecture such as intranuclear inclusions and grooving.

An inadequate or nondiagnostic smear may occur as a result of sampling error or lack of cellular component or poor processing.

Aspiration technique: FNAC is usually performed with a 22-gauge needle with either of these two methods:
1. *Suction technique*: The needle is attached to a 10-mL syringe, which is inserted into the target nodule and moved back and forth within the nodule. Suction is already applied when the needle is advanced into the nodule and then suction is halted just before the needle is removed from the nodule.
2. *Capillary method (nonaspiration method)*: Here, the needle is introduced into the nodule without the syringe and is move back and forth within the thyroid nodule and also angled in different directions; the needle is then withdrawn when the sample material appears in the hub of needle.

Molecular testing in FNAC: Bethesda categories 3, 4, and 5 have been labeled as indeterminate because they have an intrinsic limitation in predicting malignancy and such patients will undergo thyroid surgery with a resultant malignant histology only in 20% cases. Thus, molecular testing in FNA samples was thought of to compensate for this inherent limitation of FNAC. Broadly, the molecular tests can be divided into two types: rule-out test and rule-in test.

Rule-out tests: These aim to rule out malignancy in indeterminate nodules and thus avoid unnecessary surgery. The rule-out test was developed by the name of Afirma Gene Expression Classifier (GEC). In this, the expressions of 25 gene transcripts (first step) and 142 genes (second step) are analyzed. The samples are subsequently classified as either benign or suspicious. The reported NPV of the initial study was 95% [atypia of undetermined significance/follicular lesion of undetermined significance (AUS-FLUS)], 94% [follicular neoplasm or suspicious for follicular neoplasm (FN-SFN)], and 85% (suspicious for malignancy). However, subsequent independent studies brought out some lacunae in the founder study:[18-21]

- These later studies had a lower PPV (16%) from the initial 44–47%.
- These independent studies projected only 25% reduction in surgery as compared to 74% projected by the initial founder study.
- Much less cost-effective than suggested in initial study.
- Pretest risk of malignancy as determined by a cyto-pathologist of a particular center influences the NPV.

In Alexander et al.'s study,[22] a pretest probability of <23% achieved an NPV of >95%, but this may not be true for many other institutions.

- This method requires two extra passes in addition to that required for routine FNA.
- Postoperative follow-up data published for nodules classified as benign by Afirma GEC are limited to 8.5 months;[22] thus, definitely a much longer longitudinal follow-up is needed to detect false-negative results.

However, many of these lacunae have been addressed in second-generation GEC tests.

Rule-in tests: For this, a seven-gene panel is used—*BRAF, NRAS, KRAS, HRAS, RET, PAX8,* and *PPARG*. The sensitivity and specificity range widely in different studies from 18 to 100%, respectively.[19,23,24] However, the advantage of gene testing is that it can be performed on routine air-dried FNA or residual liquid cytology material, so there is no need for additional FNA passes. The lower specificity in molecular studies is perhaps due to prevalence of *RAS* and *PAX8-PPARG* mutations in benign nodules. The inter- and intraobserver variability even in the histology which is considered to be the gold standard further creates difficulty;[25] another issue is of low prevalence of malignancy in FN-SFN category which results in low PPV in indeterminate category.

Recent improvements in molecular testing: Limitations of both rule-in and rule-out tests have been addressed by next-generation sequencing (NGS)-based assays (ThyroSq v. 2.0 and 2.1) which have much improved sensitivity and specificity.[26] The updated Afirma genomic sequencing classifier (GSC) is an improvement over GEC as it further reduces surgery in indeterminate thyroid nodules by improving the specificity of Afirma system without compromising the sensitivity, and this improvement is due to improvement in specificity of oncocytic fine needle aspiration biopsy (FNAB) aspirates.[27,28]

Other molecular tests: ThyGen X/ThraMIR (Interpace Diagnostics, Parsippany, NJ) incorporates the seven-gene mutation panel along with *PIK3CA* mutation. In Bethesda 3 and 4, it has a sensitivity of 89%, specificity of 85%, PPV of 68%, and NPV of 97%.[19]

RosettaGX Reveal is an miRNA-based assay. miRNAs are an important class of noncoding RNAs implicated in gene expression regulation, and their expression profiles have been associated with thyroid cancer.[29]

Ancillary Investigations

- *Radioisotope scan*: In the initial work-up of thyroid nodule, there is no place for radioactive iodine (RAI) scan except when TSH is below normal.
- *CECT*: It is not indicated in the initial workup; however, it is useful in locally advanced thyroid cancers for better delineation of airway and vessels for operability. CECT is also useful in suspected retrosternal extension. Despite general thinking, recent studies have shown that the

contrast used in CECT does not interfere with RAI studies after thyroidectomy if more than 4 weeks have elapsed.

- *PET scan*: 18-Fluorodeoxyglucose (FDG) PET scan does not play a role in the initial workup of thyroid nodule; however, any thyroid incidentaloma discovered on an 18-FDG PET scan deserves a thorough workup, especially if there is focal uptake because of 30% risk of malignancy if uptake is focal. Unfortunately, unlike other solid cancers where SUVmax can be used to differentiate between benign and malignant tumors, in thyroid cancers such a distinction cannot be made based on SUVmax.

Pathology of DTC

- *PTC:*
  - Conventional papillary carcinoma
  - Follicular variant of PTC
  - Encapsulated variant of PTC
  - Papillary microcarcinoma
  - Columnar cell variant of PTC
  - Oncocytic variant of PTC
- *Follicular thyroid carcinoma (FTC):*
  - Minimally invasive FTC
  - Encapsulated angioinvasive FTC
  - Widely invasive
- *Hurthle (oncocytic) cell tumors:*
  - Hurthle cell carcinoma

Morphological picture of classical PTC **(Figs. 2A to H):** The pathological diagnosis of classical PTC is relatively straightforward. The stoma has a papillary architecture and the characteristic nuclear changes of PTC include nuclear enlargement and overlap, nuclear elongation, irregular nuclear

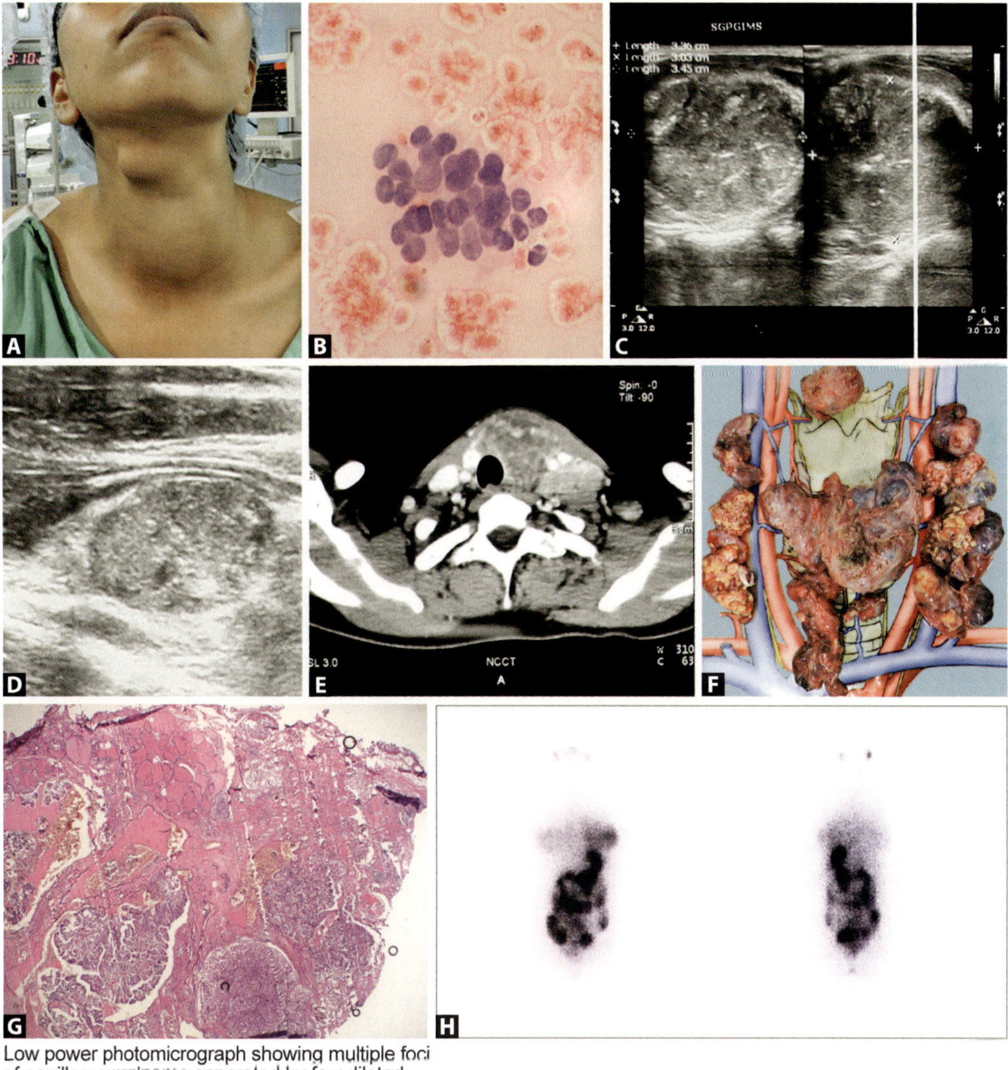

Low power photomicrograph showing multiple foci of papillary carcinoma separated by few dilated colloid filled follicles (arrow) [H&E, 4X Magnification]

Figs. 2A to H: Multifocal PTC. A 22-year-old lactating lady presented with painless swelling of anterior neck for 1 year, gradually, progressive increase in size. On examination: 6*4 cm, oval-shaped swelling in the anterior neck, well-defined, smooth surface, firm in consistency, and moving with deglutition, along with level II lymph node (A); FNAC revealed cystic papillary neoplasm with ipsilateral cervical lymph node metastasis (B); USG showed presence of microcalcification in thyroid lobe (C) and LN (D); *CECT neck*: Heterogeneously enhancing mass noted replacing left lobe of thyroid gland, showing specifications of internal calcification (E); She underwent total thyroidectomy+CCLND+B/L SLND (IIA to VB) (F); HPE showed multifocal PTC (G); WBRAI revealed no abnormal uptake in neck or elsewhere (H).

contours, nuclear pseudoinclusions or prominent longitudinal grooves, and empty appearance of the nucleoplasm described as optically clear or ground glass nuclei. Psammoma bodies (lamellated calcifications) occur in about 50% cases. Multifocal diseases may be present in 20–40% cases.

Follicular variant of PTC (Figs. 3A to C)—Variants of PTC: In recent times, histological variants of classical PTC are well recognized and documented. They can be broadly divided into (**Table 3**):

- *Aggressive variants*: These show a more aggressive behavior as compared to the classical PTC but are less aggressive than poorly differentiated thyroid cancer.
- *Less aggressive variants*: These are closer to the conventional PTC.
- *Aggressive variants*: These show a higher rate of extra-thyroidal extension (ETE), distant metastases (DMs), local recurrence, and loss of RAI avidity and poorer survival. Preoperative diagnosis by cytology is difficult in all of them.

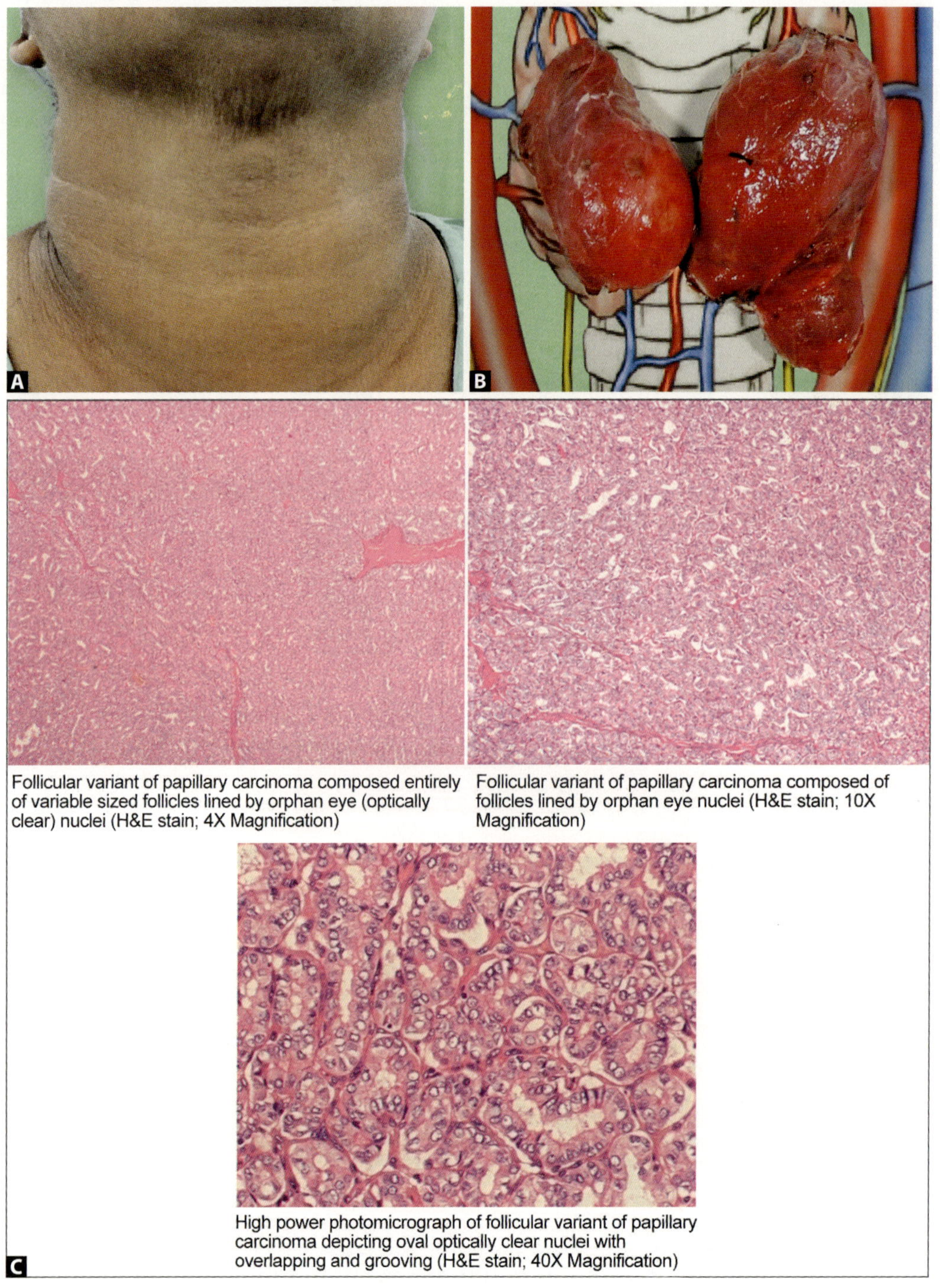

Follicular variant of papillary carcinoma composed entirely of variable sized follicles lined by orphan eye (optically clear) nuclei (H&E stain; 4X Magnification)

Follicular variant of papillary carcinoma composed of follicles lined by orphan eye nuclei (H&E stain; 10X Magnification)

High power photomicrograph of follicular variant of papillary carcinoma depicting oval optically clear nuclei with overlapping and grooving (H&E stain; 40X Magnification)

Figs. 3A to C: Follicular variant of papillary thyroid carcinoma (FVPTC). Euthyroid MNG for 1 year with recent change in voice (A); FNAC reported as follicular neoplasm (Bethesda IV); underwent total thyroidectomy (B); HPE reported as follicular variant of FVPTC (C).

Table 3: Aggressive variants of PTC.

Variant	Incidence (%)	Morphology	M:F	Aggressive features	Age	Recurrence rate	Distant metastases	Survival	Molecular signature	Ref	USG
DSV	6	Classical nuclear feature of PTC	1:1.75	Multifocal, ETD, LNM; however, primary is small in size	<30	40%	10%	96% 5-year survival	Lacks BRAF but shows RET/PTC rearrangement	30, 31	Mimics Hashimoto's thyroiditis
TCV (Figs. 4A to E)	5–11	Predominantly of cells whose heights are at least three times their width	–	Primary is usually >4 cm, RAI refractory, LNM	>50	35%	8%		High expression of MUC-1 and BRAF mutation (77)	32–35	
ITV	0.3	Presence of nests or insulae of tumor cells and resemble widely invasive FTC	1:1	Large tumors >6 cm, ETC, LNM	>60	30%	30%	72% 5-year survival	Only *RAS* mutations	32, 36	

(DSV: diffuse sclerosing variant; ETD: extranodal tumor deposit; LNM: lymph node metastasis; PTC: papillary thyroid carcinoma; RAI: radioactive iodine; TCV: tall cell variant; USG: ultrasonography)

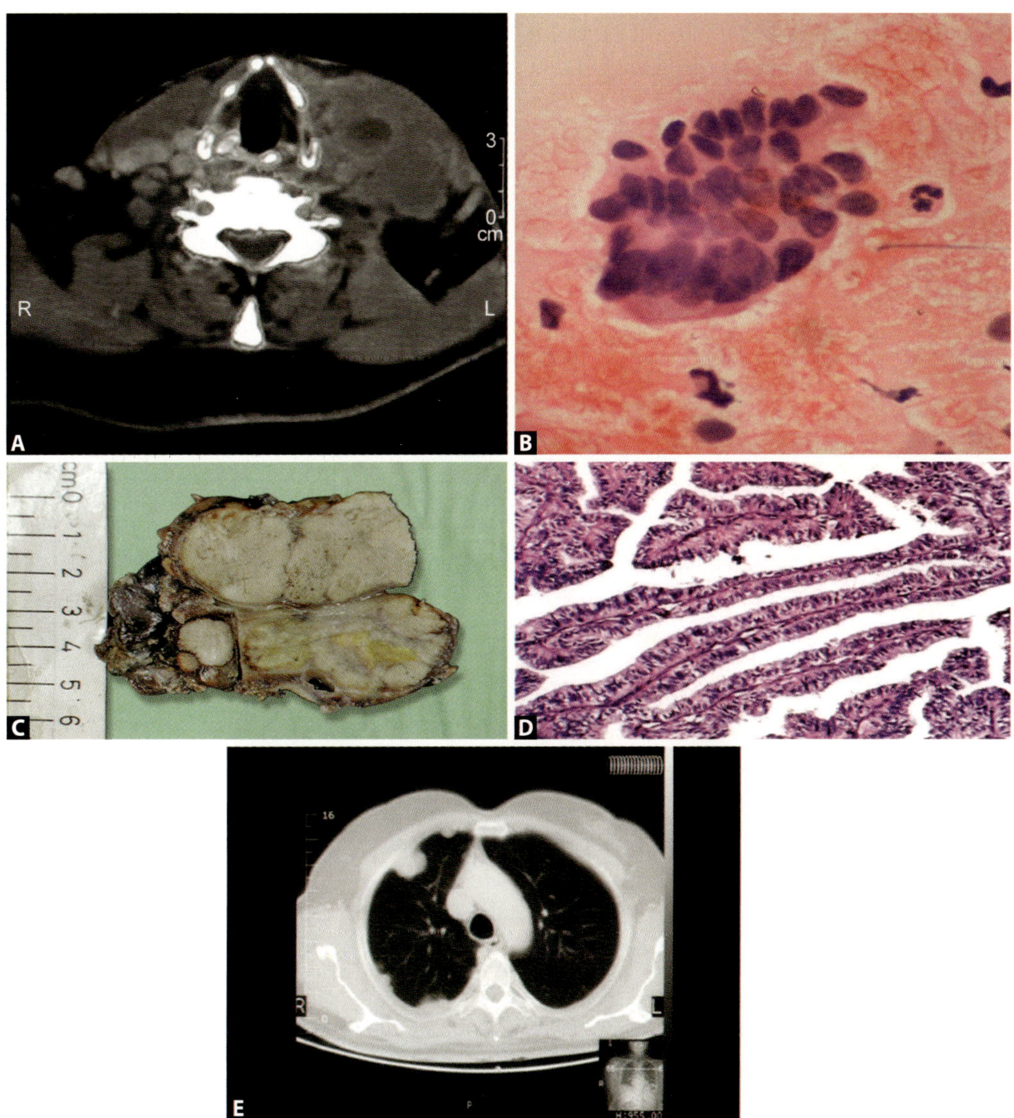

Figs. 4A to E: Tall cell variant of PTC. A 67-year-old male presented with swelling in left side of neck for 3 months, solitary thyroid nodule with matted LN mass palpable in the left upper deep cervical region 3 × 2 cm in size (A); FNAC (LN)—metastatic PTC (B); Total thyroidectomy with left radical neck dissection with CCLND was done with sacrifice of IJV as it was infiltrated by LN mass (C); HPE was reported as Tall cell variant of PTC (D); Developed recurrent LN and elevated Tg and CT throax revealed multiple neck nodes, mediastinal nodes and lung metastasis (E). He finally succumbed to florid metastases.

They include:
- Diffuse sclerosing variant (DSV)
- Tall cell variant (TCV)
- Insular thyroid variant (ITV)

- *Less aggressive variants include:*
  - *Warthin-like variant* **(Fig. 5)**: The key histopathological feature is oncocytic follicular epithelium arranged in papillae with nuclear features of PTC and a brisk infiltrate of plasma cells with lymphocytes in the core of the papillary fronds.
  - *Macrofollicular variant*: It is a follicular variant of PTC that is entirely composed of large colloid-filled follicles, i.e., macrofollicular growth pattern. It can be mistaken for a macrofollicular adenoma or hyperplastic/adenomatous goiter.
  - *Cribriform-morular variant* (CMV): CMV is described in families of familial adenomatous polyposis (FAP). It almost exclusively occurs in females. It is multifocal and growth pattern is either cribriform solid or spindle cell. It usually exhibits beta-catenin mutation and thus shows strong nuclear immunoreactivity for beta-catenin.
  - *Solid variant:* It is associated with radiation and seen in the children affected by "Chernobyl nuclear disaster." It shows a solid growth pattern in at least 50% with nests of tumor cells with nuclear features of PTC; true papillary formation is absent.
  - *Encapsulated columnar cell variant:* It shows papillae lined by tumor cells with pseudostratification but with a thick capsule.
  - *Hyalinizing trabecular neoplasm (HTN):* It is composed of elongated cells arranged around capillaries in a background of hyaline matrix with tumor cells showing features of PTC.
  - *Hobnail variant:* The cells show a high nuclear/cytoplasmic ratio and apically placed and grooved nuclei that produce a surface bulge leading to a hobnail or matchstick appearance.

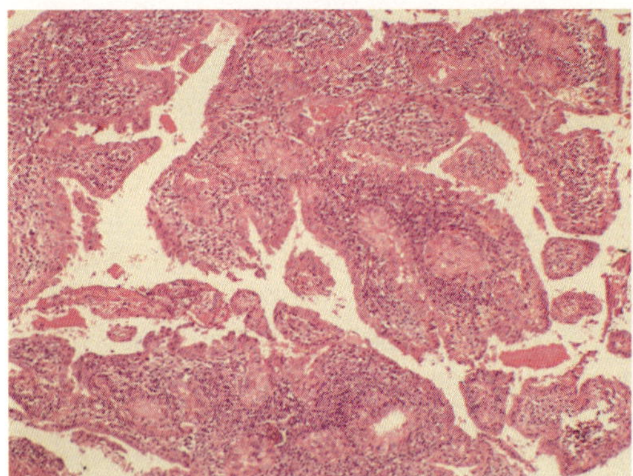

Low power view of Warthin variant of papillary carcinoma showing heavy lymphomononuclear cell infiltrate in the cores of papillae lined by tumor epithelial cells (H&E stain; 10X Magnification)

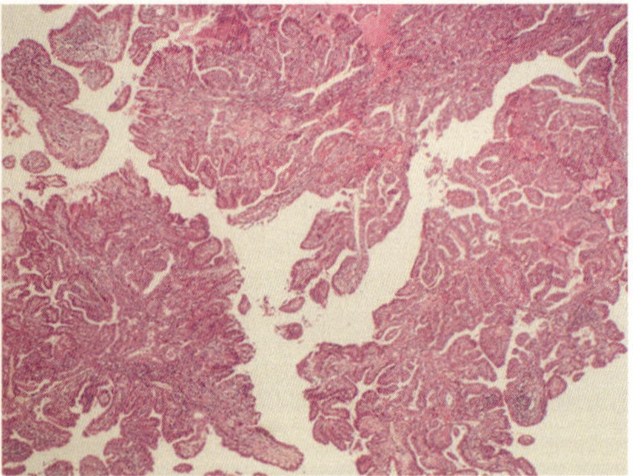

Low power view of Warthin variant of papillary carcinoma showing heavy lymphomononuclear cell infiltrate in the cores of papillae lined by tumor epithelial cells (H&E stain; 4X Magnification)

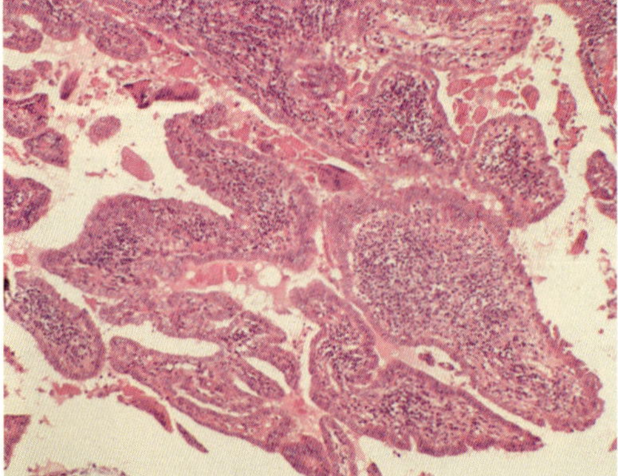

Low power view of Warthin variant of papillary carcinoma showing heavy lymphomononuclear cell infiltrate in the cores of papillae lined by tumor epithelial cells [H&E stain; 20X Magnification]

Fig. 5: Warthin variant of PTC. A 42-year-old female was being evaluated for generalized weakness and found to have a diffusely enlarged thyroid with nodule of size 3 × 2 cm in left lobe and 2 × 2 cm in right lobe. FNAC was done which was s/o PTC. Total thyroidectomy with CCLND was done; strap muscles found densely adherent to thyroid, and were excised. On HPE, the key histopathological feature was oncoytic follicular epithelium arranged in papillae with nuclear features of PTC and a brisk infiltrate of plasma cells with lymphocytes in the core of the papillary fronds suggestive of Warthin variant of PTC.

Table 4: Arguments for lobectomy vs total thyroidectomy.

Procedure	Views in favor of lobectomy	References	Counter view: Views in favor of total thyroidectomy	References	Counter counter-view: Views in favor of lobectomy	References
Lobectomy vs total thyroidectomy	1. With proper selection (i.e., excluding ETE, LNM and mulifocality, locoregional rates <1–4% and completion thyroidectomy rates <10% can be achieved following lobectomy alone as the initial procedure 2. Since RAI is now recommended more selectively the argument in favor of TT facilitating use of RAI becomes less significant 3. Post-thyroidectomy surveillance for recurrence is now more dependent upon USG and TG rather than RAI scan findings	37, 38	1. Proper selection can be difficult; USG is a subjective and examiner-dependent study and shows only 2-dimensional images and hence cannot perfectly assess ETE preoperatively, Also difficult to pick up multifocality by USG 2. RAI has survival advantage 3. Tg levels after lobectomy are affected by various factors such as amount of residual cancer or normal thyroid issue, anti-Tg levels and time elapsed since thyroid lobectomy and therefore it is more difficult to determine the Tg cut-off values to differentiate each response to therapy (# excellent, indeterminate, biochemically incomplete and structurally incomplete)	39-41	Status of minimal ETE as an independent prognostic factor in PTC has recently been questioned *Similarly, multifocality was not an independent risk factor of structural recurrence*	42, 43

(RAI: radioactive iodine; Tg: thyroglobulin; TT: total thyroidectomy)

- *Clear cell variant*: It is characterized by cells showing clear cytoplasm and nuclear features of PTC.
- *Oncocytic variant*: It displays papillae composed of cells with large oncocytic granular cytoplasm with nuclear features of PTC.
- *PTC with spindle cell metaplasia*: There is a spindle cell proliferation in association with PTC. It can be confused with spindle cell variety of anaplastic thyroid cancer.

Papillary thyroid carcinoma *with nodular fasciitis–like stroma variant*: It has a stromal component similar to that seen in nodular fasciitis and is composed of spindle cells arranged in fascicles with a vascularized fibromyxoid stroma. It can be confused with Riedel's thyroiditis or Hashimoto's thyroiditis.

◇| MANAGEMENT

The management of differentiated thyroid cancer involves three elements.
1. Surgical management
2. Adjuvant RAI therapy
3. TSH suppression

Surgical Management

This involves two elements:
1. Management of the primary thyroid tumor
2. *Management of lymph nodes*: Central nodes and lateral neck nodes

Management of the Primary Thyroid Tumor

This is based on the risk stratification and the size of the primary: For tumors <1 cm and tumors between 1 and 4 cm **(Table 4)**.

Management of Central Compartment Lymph Nodes (Figs. 6A and B)

The central compartment is designated as Level VI and lies between the two common carotids laterally, the hyoid bone superiorly, and the suprasternal notch inferiorly. It is important to remember that the rate of CNM is high in most studies though it ranges from 20 to 80%[44] as shown in the meta-analysis.

Nomenclature: Central compartment lymph node dissection (CCLND) may be required in three situations: (1) *Therapeutic CCLND*: Dissection is done when there is preoperative (either clinical or imaging) or intraoperative evidence of enlarged central nodes. There is no controversy on this indication; (2) *Prophylactic CCLND:* Central compartment is dissected in a clinically negative neck, cN0. This is a hugely controversial topic; (3) *Prophylactic converted to therapeutic*: Central compartment is dissected only when enlarged central nodes are found intraoperatively after opening the deep cervical fascia. Only some surgeons follow this approach.

Common practices followed: There are basically six types of practices that are followed by endocrine/thyroid surgeons all over the world with regard to central node dissection:

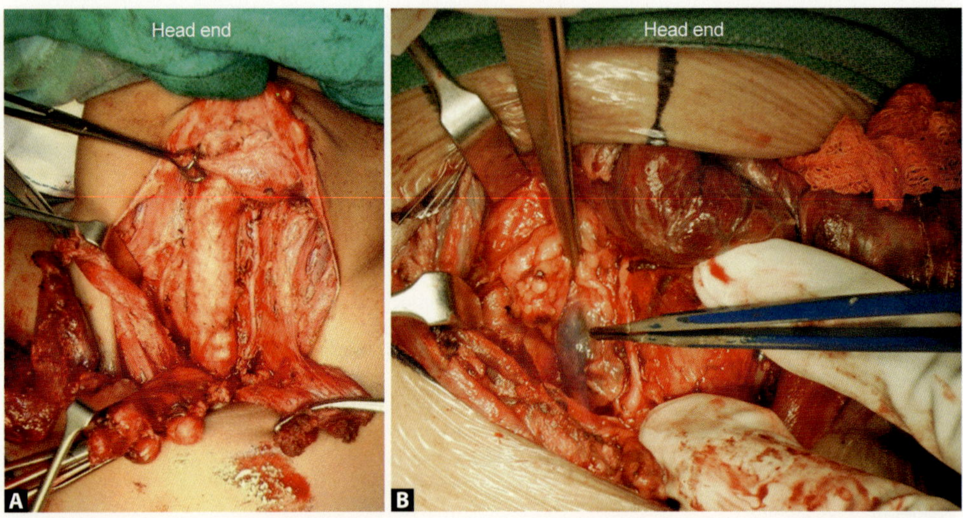

Figs. 6A and B: Central compartment lymph node dissection (CCLND). (A) Multiple LN of central compartment; (B) Black LN of the central compartment, lateral to the RLN.

1. Some surgeons perform prophylactic CCLND routinely.
2. Some surgeons perform only therapeutic CCLND.
3. Some surgeons perform CCLND only if lateral nodes are positive.
4. Some surgeons rely on intraoperative assessment.
5. Some surgeons do only unilateral CCLND. Some will also do frozen section (FS) and if positive a bilateral dissection is done.
6. As per American Thyroid Association (ATA) guidelines of 2015, prophylactic CCLND is done only for T3/T4 tumors.

Arguments in favor of prophylactic CCLND:
- It is difficult to evaluate both preoperatively and intraoperatively the status of central LN.
- It decreases thyroglobulin (Tg) levels and is therefore thought to be associated with a greater biochemical cure rate.[45-48]
- It decreases recurrence by upstaging the patients to make them eligible to receive RAI ablation therapy.[49]
- In high-volume endocrine/thyroid surgeons, the complication rates are acceptable.
- Two meta-analyses have shown that though there may be increased rate of transient hypocalcemia; nevertheless, there is no difference in rates of recurrent laryngeal nerve (RLN) injury or permanent hypocalcemia.[50,51]

Arguments against routine prophylactic CCLND:
- There is greater risk of postoperative complications, especially if performed by low-volume surgeons.[52,53]
- There is no real decrease in recurrence rate following prophylactic CCLND.[54,55]

Risk factors: Some risk factors have been identified which can predict central node metastasis, such as multifocality, extracapsular extension, histological variant of PTC,[56] and size of thyroid primary.

Unilateral CCLND: This is a more limited approach to obviate the presumed high rate of surgical complications following CCLND and at the same time taking care of the involved central LN. Some surgeons who favor unilateral CCLND also do an FS of removed nodes and if found metastatic, then unilateral CCLND is converted to bilateral CCLND.[57]

Intraoperative assessment of central LN in a cN0 neck: Although many strategies are adopted by surgeons for intraoperative assessment of central nodes, nonetheless strategies like inspection and palpation may have poor sensitivity and specificity because central LN lie deep to deep cervical fascia and unless the fascia is opened it will be difficult to evaluate the nodes and it will require some extent of dissection to see the LN lying posterior to the RLN which in some cases may be the only enlarged node. According to one study,[58] the number of LN in central compartment ranges from 2 to 42 and most common is the pretracheal LN (67%). Also, it is proposed by some surgeons that precricoid LN (also known as Delphian LN) must be looked for as it predicts the status of the remainder of the central compartment, and if this node is enlarged then it would mandate proceeding with the central dissection.[59]

Management of Lateral Neck Nodes (Figs. 7A to G)

Papillary thyroid carcinoma frequently metastasizes to lateral LN (LND) and micrometastases can be found in as much as 90% cases.[60,61] Aggressive features of the carcinoma such as ETE, larger size, presence of *BRAF* mutation, and higher age are associated with more frequent LN metastases.[62,63] Even though conventionally lateral LNM (lymph node metastases) has not been considered important enough to affect survival, recently it has been shown that lateral LNM may affect recurrence and survival rates, especially in elderly.

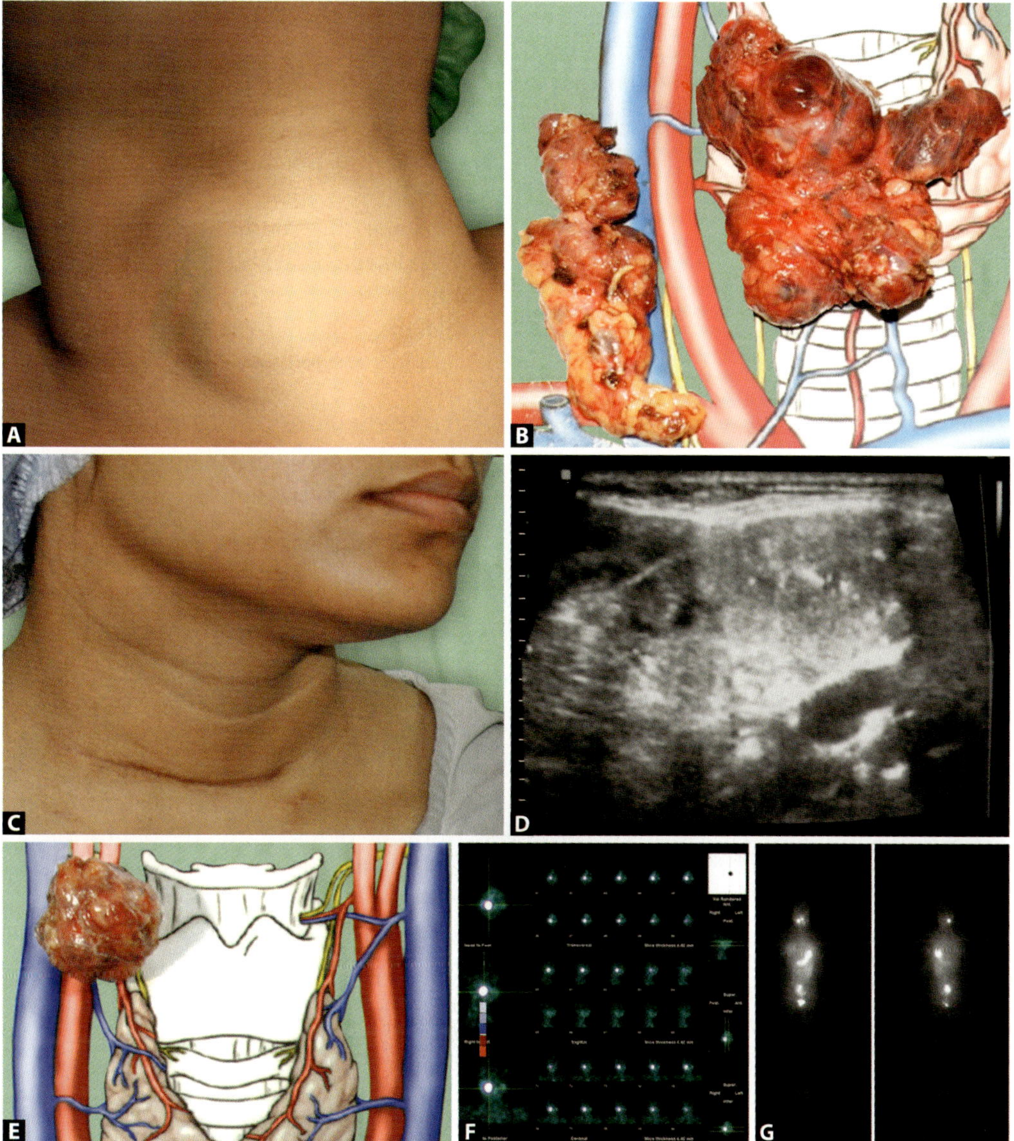

Figs. 7A to G: Recurrent PTC. A 29-year-old woman presented with a solitary thyroid nodule of 1 year duration (A); On examination right, STN with multiple hard deep cervical LN on left side. FNAC was suggestive of PTC; underwent total thyroidectomy with left SLND (B); HPE revealed PTC with LN metastases (CCLND; 13/13, right SLND: 4/11); 2 months later developed recurrent right level 2 LN (arrow, C) which showed calcification on USG (D) and was excised (E) and was positive for PTC. Postoperative Tg was 15.7 ng/mL and WBRAI revealed uptake in right level 2 LN (F) and was treated with 125 mCi (G).

Preoperative assessment of lateral neck: Physical examination is unacceptably unreliable for excluding metastatic lateral nodes. Routine preoperative imaging of the lateral neck changes the extent of surgery in as much as 40% of the patients.[64] The most common imaging modality recommended for lateral neck is the high-resolution USG. CECT is not routinely used to assess the lateral neck and may have a slightly lower sensitivity (60–80%) for detecting metastatic LND,[65,66] as compared to USG and also as compared to the sensitivity in detecting LNM in squamous cell carcinoma, because in PTC it is usually micrometastases which does not alter the appearance of the LN on CT. Various features on USG are used to predict metastases in lateral neck nodes such as long axis > 1 cm, loss of fatty hilum, cystic appearance, and hyperechoic punctate calcification.

Ultrasonography-guided FNAC: The suspected lateral neck node has a high sensitivity (85%) and almost 100% specificity. Measurement of Tg in FNA aspirate fluid can further help to increase the sensitivity to 85–100%.[67]

Management: Compartment-based dissection of the lateral neck is the recommended procedure to improve both recurrence and survival rates.[68] Selective LN removal, also called "berry-picking," is not recommended. Further, only therapeutic lateral neck dissection is recommended in clinically apparent or FNA-proved LN metastases or if the enlarged lateral neck node found intraoperatively is positive on frozen section. Despite a high rate of micrometastases, there is no role of prophylactic lateral neck dissection in PTC.

Anatomy of lateral neck levels and extent of dissection: Although there is complete agreement on therapeutic lateral neck dissection, it is the extent of surgery that is a matter of controversy. Most authors recommend dissection of levels IIA, III, IV, and VB; there is controversy regarding the exclusion of levels IIB and VA. The incidence of metastases according to the levels is as follows:

- *Level IIA*: 53%
- *Level IIB: 16%*
- *Level III*: 71%
- *Level IV*: 66%
- *Level VA: 8%*
- *Level VB*: 22%

The authors who recommend exclusion of these two levels argue that these levels are infrequently involved in PTC and also that unnecessary dissection of these levels places XI cranial nerve at risk of injury.[69] ATA guidelines also recommend that it is left to the discretion of the surgeons. As compared to a super-selective neck dissection (III-IV) which results in a very high persistent/recurrent disease (71%), a formal SLND (II, III, IV, V) has better regional control.

Impact of LND on survival and recurrence: Various studies have shown that formal LND reduces recurrence and improves survival.[68,70] Factors that impact nodal recurrence are:
- N1a disease
- Extranodal extension (ENE) (24% recurrence rate)
- Number of nodes [<5 nodes—RR 4%, >5 nodes—RR 19%]

Surgical excision is the treatment of choice for recurrent lateral LN. Recurrence in a previously dissected lateral compartment which has had a formal compartment-based dissection should be retreated by only a focused or selective dissection of the region containing the nodal recurrence.[71]

Complications: Increased risk of recurrence and poor survival in undissected lateral neck outweigh the risks of complications from LND. The most common complication is shoulder dysfunction, especially if level V is dissected. However, at 1 year postoperatively, there is no difference in health-related quality of life (QOL) secondary to shoulder dysfunction between modified radical neck dissection (MRND) and selective neck dissection.[72,73]

Radioiodine Treatment

In the past years, almost every patient of PTC was being offered RAI ablation following thyroidectomy. However, it is only recently that clinicians are being selective and patients are being subjected to RAI ablation based on their risk category. The recent ATA guidelines[74] have defined three risk categories based on the initial prognostic factors (patient and tumor factors), serum Tg and USG findings following surgery. The risk categories are as follows:

American Thyroid Association High-risk Category

DTC patients are defined at high risk if they have:
- Macroscopic invasion of tumor into the perithyroidal soft tissues
- Incomplete tumor resection
- DMs
- Postoperative serum Tg suggestive of DMs
- Pathologic N1 with any metastatic LN = 3 cm in largest dimension
- Follicular thyroid cancer with extensive vascular invasion (>4 foci of vascular invasion)

ATA Intermediate-risk Category

DTC patients are defined at intermediate risk, if they have:
- Microscopic invasion of tumor into the perithyroidal soft tissues
- RAI-avid metastatic foci in the neck on the first post-treatment whole-body scan (WBS)
- Aggressive histology (e.g., tall cell, hobnail variant, columnar cell carcinoma)
- PTC with vascular invasion
- Clinical N1 or >5 pathologic N1 with all involved LNs <3 cm in largest dimension
- Multifocal papillary microcarcinoma with microscopic invasion of tumor into the perithyroidal soft tissues and BRAFV600E mutation (if known)

ATA Low-risk Category

DTC patients are defined at low risk if they have:
- Intrathyroidal PTC without vascular invasion, with or without small-volume LN metastases (clinical N0 or =5 pathologic N1 micrometastases, <0.2 cm in largest dimension)
- Intrathyroidal encapsulated follicular variant of papillary thyroid cancer or intrathyroidal well-differentiated follicular cancer with capsular or minor vascular invasion (less than four vessels involved)
- Intrathyroidal papillary microcarcinomas that are either *BRAF* wild type or *BRAF* mutated

It is also important to know the *goals of RAI therapy in DTC*:
- As an adjunct therapy, the goal of RAI is to destroy microscopic or occult persistent disease following surgery.
- It helps to restage the patient by revealing possible metastatic disease on post-treatment scan (in presence of thyroid remnant, the pretreatment thyroid scan does not reveal metastatic disease).
- By destroying the thyroid remnant, RAI therapy greatly facilitates follow-up by serum Tg measurement which then truly reflects recurrence if high as the recurrent disease then becomes the sole source of Tg.

Published literature strongly suggests that overall RAI ablation improves disease-free survival (DFS) and disease-specific mortality (DSM) for high-risk category patients[75] while the advantages are not so clear for intermediate-risk (IR) patients and definitely not advantageous in the low-risk (LR) patients.

Rationale for not Using RAI in IR and LR Category Patients

- Neck USG and Tg levels are equivalent or even superior in detecting and localizing residual disease compared to RAI therapy and scanning.
- In such patients who do not receive RAI therapy, USG is the investigation of choice for early postoperative follow-up (because in this period Tg levels fluctuate and thus assays are difficult to interpret) while in the late follow-up period, Tg values become stable and are thus more reliable.
- The evidence of efficacy of RAI therapy as adjuvant treatment in reducing DSM is less clear.

Evidence in Low-risk Patient Category

In low-risk category, DSM and persistent/recurrent disease is so low that it is unlikely to be improved further by giving RAI therapy. In a retrospective series of >900 patients and with a follow-up of >10 years, no impact of RAI therapy was seen on overall survival (OS) or DFS.[76] There is even prospective data which have provided evidence that overall mortality or DSM are not improved by RAI therapy.[77,78] As expected, in microcarcinoma as well, RAI therapy is unlikely to improve outcome in the absence of high-risk factors.[79] However, in LR patients if Tg levels are between 5 and 10 ng/mL, then RAI therapy can be considered.

Evidence in Intermediate-risk Category

These are those LR patients who have at least one of these additional factors: minimal ETE, aggressive histology [tall cell variant (TCV), diffuse sclerosing variant (DSV), columnar cell variant (CCV)], vascular invasion, RAI uptake outside thyroid bed, and nodal disease. Existing data suggest that the greatest potential benefit of RAI therapy may be observed only with aggressive histology,[34] increased number and size of LN,[80,81] and lateral LN and age >45 years.[82] For other risk factors, postoperative USG findings can be used to select out IR patients for RAI therapy.

Evidence in High-risk (HR) Category

A meta-analysis of 79 studies supports the use of RAI ablation for higher-risk category patients.[83]

Additional Information about RAI Therapy

- *Diagnostic RAI scanning before RAI therapy*: Recently, there has been an increasing trend to avoid diagnostic RAI scanning because of the fear of causing stunning of thyroid remnant and even DMs by I-131; another concern is that such imaging does not induce any significant modification in management. However, proponents of diagnostic scanning argue that 1–3 mCi of I-131 in unlikely to cause stunning and also that pretherapy scan contributes in appropriate dose selection.[84,85] One study[84] found that WBS prior to ablation detected unsuspected regional metastases in 35% of patients and DMs in 8% of patients. The alternative pharmaceutical I[121] does not cause stunning but is expensive and not readily available and also has a short half-life. Although ATA guidelines of 2015 recommend that WBS may be useful, it has C rating (expert opinion).
- *Preparation for RAI ablation*: It is desirable that before RAI therapy, TSH should be >30 mU/L in order to induce robust uptake of RAI in thyroid follicular cells (both normal and cancerous cells). For this, one of the following three approaches can be used:
  - Stop levothyroxine (LT4) for 3–4 weeks prior to scanning and therapy, or
  - Switch from LT4 to liothyronine (LT3) for few weeks and then stop LT3 for 2 weeks, or
  - Administer recombinant human TSH (rhTSH). It has been a matter of debate whether rhTSH administration is better than endogenous thyroid hormone withdrawal. Most studies, including a randomized trial, have shown that ablation rates are similar with either approach.[86-88] Both approaches were found to be equally effective at both 50 and 100 mCi dose of RAI and also equally effective in both low-risk and IR category patients.[89] Nonetheless, administration of rhTSH does help maintain QOL and reduces hospitalization time as well as reduce radiation exposure. Thus, the use of rhTSH is approved with any I-131 activity in USA, Europe, and India.
- *Dose of I-131 for remnant ablation*: This has also been a matter of debate, but both retrospective and prospective studies have shown that ablation rates were comparable between 30 and 100 mCi.[90-92] Even in IR category patients, authors found no difference in ablation rates between low and high RAI activity. The doses that are recommended are given in **Table 5**.[93,94]
- *Low-iodine diet (LID)*: Using LID of <50 µg/day of iodine for 1–2 weeks may result in increase in RAI uptake but does not necessarily increase ablation rates.[95] But it is recommended to avoid iodine contamination (caused by IV contrast agents, amiodarone, or iodine-containing drugs); such contamination can be detected by measuring urinary iodine just before ablation.
- *Adverse effects of RAI therapy*: Most frequent side effects with 30–100 mCi are nausea, transient sialoadenitis, and transient change in smell and taste.[96,97] Uncommon side effects are abnormalities in complete blood count (CBC), lacrimal function, and gonadal function.[97] A very significant side effect is the increased risk of second malignancy, both solid cancers and leukemia.[97] It has been observed that second primary is more likely to develop

Table 5: Recommended doses for remnant ablation.

Risk class	Indication for remnant ablation	Activity of I-131 when indicated	Preparation
Low	Not routinely recommended	30 mCi	rhTSH
Intermediate	May be considered	• 30 mCi (if low-volume central neck nodal metastases with no other known residual disease are present) • 30–150 mCi (if extensive lymph node disease, multiple clinically involved LN, or suspected or documented microscopic residual disease are present)	rhTSH
High	Routinely recommended	100–150 mCi	Thyroid hormone withdrawal or rhTSH

in younger patients and within first 5 years of therapy.[97,98] Furthermore, higher activity is more likely to result in the second malignancy and hence this is the reason that higher activities of RAI should be avoided more so because it has been shown that higher activity has no benefit beyond that achieved with 30–50 mCi.[99]

- *Effect on quality of life:* Thyroid hormone withdrawal for remnant ablation has been shown to be associated with worsening of health-related QOL issues.[100] RAI scanning and therapy have been shown to be associated with negative disease perception.[101]
- *Patients who can be spared RAI therapy:*
  - LR and select IR category patients
  - Where diagnostic WBS is negative
  - When serum Tg is undetectable

Summary

- Selective use of RAI therapy; avoid in LR and select IR category patients.
- Patients should be informed and proper counseling should be done.
- Low activity (30 mCi) and rhTSH should be preferred or minimize side effects and QOL impairment.

Thyroid-stimulating Hormone Suppression

All patients treated with total thyroidectomy and some who have had lobectomy are put on long-term TSH suppression by giving supranormal doses of thyroxine. This is because TSH is thought to act as a growth factor for thyroid follicular cells and can stimulate growth of thyroid cancer.[102] Evidence for this also comes from studies which have shown that serum TSH concentration seems to be an independent predictor for the development of DTC[103] and secondly, TSH levels > 2.26 mU/L are associated with threefold increase in thyroid cancer.[104,105]

Level of Suppression

This varies with risk status of the patient as recommended by ATA **(Table 6)**.

- There is enough evidence in literature, including a meta-analysis that TSH suppression improves disease-specific survival in high-risk cases.[83,106,107]

Table 6: Level of suppression as recommended by ATA.

	TSH levels
High-risk patients	<0.1 mU/L
Intermediate-risk patients	0.1–0.5 mU/L
Low risk with remnant ablation and undetectable Tg	0.5–2 mU/L
Low risk with remnant ablation and low Tg	0.1–0.5 mU/L
Low risk with lobectomy	0.5–2 mU/L

(ATA: American Thyroid Association; Tg: thyroglobulin; TSH: thyroid-stimulating hormone)

- Use of TSH suppression during the time between surgery and initial postoperative disease assessment (usually 6–18 months) appears to have no significant effect on the structural disease recurrence detected 1–3 years after primary treatment in LR and IR patients as well as in those HR patients whose stimulated Tg level prior to RAI treatment ablation was <1 ng/mL.[108]

Risks of TSH Suppression

The adverse effects of TSH suppression can impact the following:

- *Cardiovascular system*: TSH suppression, especially if continued for long, can result in atrial fibrillation, tachycardia, diminished cardiac reserve, and diastolic failure.[109] The effects are more pronounced in elderly >65 years and those with hypertension and diabetes mellitus.
- *Skeletal system*: TSH suppressive therapy of >5 years duration is associated with bone loss and increased fracture risk, especially in men/women >50 years and postmenopausal women of any age.[110]
- *Quality of life*: TSH suppressive therapy can diminish QOL in all its domains—psychological, social, and physical particularly when TSH levels are kept undetectable.

Thus, the ATA recommends a graded algorithm in which potential benefits of therapy are carefully weighed against its skeletal and CVS side effects.[74]

Initial Follow-up from Postoperative Surveillance to 2 Years

This includes the following:

- Initial risk stratification
- Voice assessment within 2 weeks postoperatively to 4 weeks

- High-resolution cervical USG
- Serum Tg with Tg Ab
- WBS as and when indicated

Initial Risk Stratification

This can be done either by using the various scoring systems or by considering various clinical, operative, and pathological features. Disease staging systems are necessary, first to allow the caregivers to estimate the prognosis for a particular patient and to make a reliable estimate of the expected benefits from therapy and second to provide common criteria (usually clinicopathologic) that enable different clinicians in different institutions to communicate about any given patient. For thyroid carcinoma, several staging systems have been proposed; however, none of these have been able to achieve the said purposes of a staging system either because they were not found to be reproducible or because of poor prediction of mortality. This may be partly due to inherent limitations of the clinicopathological factors and noninclusion of other potentially important criteria such as molecular markers. Nonetheless, several studies have demonstrated that AJCC/UICC TNM (tumor, node, metastasis) systems and MACIS system were the most accurate when predictability was measured by PVE (proportion of variance explained).

Common Staging Systems

- *AMES* (developed by Lahey Clinic, USA): It is a binary classification which divided patients into low-risk and high-risk groups[87]. It takes into account *Age*, *Distant Metastases*, *Extent*, and *Size*.
- *AGES* (developed by Mayo Clinic, USA): It considers Age, Grade, Extent, and Size. Application of this classification system was found to be infrequent across institutions because of limited reporting of histologic grade in reports of most institutions.
- *MACIS* (Mayo Clinic, USA): It includes metastases, age, *completeness of resection, invasion,* and size. It is a scoring system and it excludes the need of grading of the earlier system of AGES. According to this system, 20-year DSM is: stage I (score <6) 1%; stage II (score 6–6.99) 11%; stage III (score 7–7.99) 44%, and stage IV (score >8.0) 76%.
- *DeGroot's or University of Chicago classification*: It divides into four classes:
  1. *Ohio State University classification*: It has four stages.
  2. European Organization of Research and Treatment of Cancer (EORTC)
  3. National Thyroid Cancer Treatment Cooperative Study (NTCTCS) Registry
  4. ATA

According to 2015 ATA guidelines, the risk-stratification system recommended by ATA 2009 is useful in predicting the risk of disease recurrence and/or persistence. Further, several studies have shown that the ATA risk stratification system can be applied in HR category[111,112] as well as in IR and LR categories.[76,113] Risk stratification is usually done once the histology is available.

Follow-up for Initial 2 Years

After initial risk stratification, the most appropriate tests to be performed are the Tg with thyroglobulin antibody (TgAb) and USG. Tg will reach nadir by 3–4 weeks after the surgery and so the earliest it should be tested is 6 weeks postoperatively. Usual protocol is to do Tg (and TgAb from the same laboratory assay) and USG every 6–12 months. In high-risk patients, more frequent Tg measurement can be done. If TSH-suppressed Tg is <0.2–0.3 ng/mL, then there is no need for stimulated Tg. In fact, TSH-suppressed Tg measurement is good enough because TSH-suppressed Tg value <1 ng/mL is associated with a 1% risk of recurrence.[114,115] Therefore, in patients with a low Tg level after initial treatment, there may be little added value to obtaining a stimulated Tg level. However, if TSH-suppressed Tg is undetectable, then TSH-stimulated Tg should be done with or without recombinant TSH.

A stimulated Tg 0.5–1.0 ng/mL (without anti-TgAbs) has been shown to have a 98–99.5% chance of no disease recurrence and follow-up can be lessened in these patients.[84-89] Stimulated Tg levels of 0.2–2 ng/mL should undergo serial Tg levels to detect increases or short doubling times that indicate progressive disease, if there is no other evidence of disease clinically or on imaging.[116,117] Stimulated Tg levels > 2 ng/mL correlate with recurrent or residual disease and further imaging and/or treatment is often indicated.[118]

Subsequent Follow-up

As patient progresses through the first 2 years of postoperative period, restratification is done based on response to initial therapy. *Concept of dynamic FUP*: Mike Tuttle from MSKCC conceptualized the system of dynamic risk stratification whereby it is recommended that the initial risk stratification should not be considered to be rigid or absolute and they should be continuously modified during the follow-up. This concept takes into account the biology of the disease (i.e., response to initial therapy, development of recurrence) and thus the intensity of FUP can be individualized in terms of labeling the patient as cured or prescribing particular biochemical or imaging tests and their timing.[119]

- *Excellent response to therapy*: Negative imaging and either suppressed Tg <0.2 ng/mL or TSH-stimulated Tg <1 ng/mL. Recommended TSH suppression is 0.1–0.5 mU/L.
- *A biochemical incomplete response* is considered suppressed Tg >1 ng/mL, stimulated Tg >10 ng/mL, or increasing anti-TgAbs with negative imaging. Up to 30% of these patients will spontaneously achieve a disease-free state, but 20% will need additional therapy and another

20% will develop structural disease. Tg levels should be evaluated every 6 months with annual neck US for several years. Patients with stable or decreasing Tg levels can convert to routine surveillance, but rising Tg or anti-TgAbs should initiate further imaging or consider additional therapy. Recommended TSH suppression is 0.1–0.5 mU/L.

- *Structural incomplete response* in high-risk patients may have variable Tg or TgAbs levels but shows persistent or newly identified locoregional or DMs. Such cases may undergo additional therapy or close observation based on size, location, histology, RAI avidity, rate of growth, and specific pathologies of persistent or recurrent lesions. Unfortunately, up to 50–85% of patients will continue to have persistent disease regardless of additional therapies. Recommended TSH suppression is 0.1–0.5 mU/L.

- *Indeterminate responses* are those with nonspecific imaging findings, mild RAI uptake on WBS, or low Tg levels (suppressed <1 ng/mL or stimulated <10 ng/mL. These patients are recommended to continue surveillance with Tg every 6–12 months and annual neck USG for 2–3 years and then rerisk stratified. Recommended TSH suppression is 0.1–0.5 mU/L.

Aggressive DTC (Figs. 8A to F)

Ten percent of DTC behave aggressively and have a very high mortality unlike the innocuous DTC. Aggressive DTC behave more aggressively than the high-risk category cancers and the presence of major ETE particularly differentiates such aggressive DTCs from the innocuous or the garden variety of the high-risk cases. Unlike the innocuous DTC, the aggressive ones have *different histology* (they have lesser areas of differentiated tumor), *different phenotype* (increasing patient age and size, DM, ETE, intensity of PET positivity, impairment of Tg production, RAI resistance, higher recurrence, and disease-specific mortality rates), and *different biology and genetic landscape* (accumulation of common mutations such as BRAF, RAS, TERT, etc.). Management of such cancers require a different approach starting from the time the patient is first seen:

- *History taking and examination*: There will be signs and symptoms suggestive of local invasion such as hoarseness of voice, hemoptysis, restricted mobility, etc.

- *Evaluation*: Tissue biopsy is more often required to rule out ATC or lymphoma or sarcoma and the pathologist must comment on the histologic type and grade unlike the innocuous DTC. More detailed evaluation of structure and function of laryngotracheal complex is needed with a low threshold for direct laryngoscopy, upper gastrointestinal (GI) endoscopy, CECT/magnetic resonance imaging (MRI), and PET scanning.

- *Management:* Different options are the following:
  - *Surgery*: Even though surgery is the mainstay of treatment, sometimes upfront surgery is not the best option and one can explore neoadjuvant tyrosine kinase inhibitor (TKI) before operating. Further, surgery for aggressive cancers should be performed in a high-volume center because it involves more than just a standard total thyroidectomy. Unlike innocuous DTC, neck dissection of potentially involved neck levels is paramount both electively and therapeutically in aggressive DTC. Also, the guiding principle in such cases is to maintain a balance between complete tumor clearance and acceptable postoperative functional outcome. The minimum outcome requirement after radical thyroidectomy should be an airway that permits laminar, nonturbulent flow; normal or near-normal upper GI tract patency; and at least a single functionally intact RLN.
  - *RAI therapy*: Even though the efficacy of RAI is limited in aggressive DTC, nonetheless residual well-differentiated areas are still there and retain some RAI avidity.
  - *External beam radiation therapy (EBRT)*: Unlike typical high-risk cancers, aggressive thyroid cancers should be more frequently treated by EBRT along with doxorubicin.
  - *TKI*: Various TKIs such as sorafenib (works on RAS pathology) and lenvatinib [works on vascular endothelial growth factor (VEGF) pathology]

Radioiodine Refractory DTC (Figs. 9A to D)

Two-thirds of the 10% patients of DTC who develop metastases will become refractory to RAI treatment and such patients have only <10% 10-year survival.

RAI refractory tumors are defined as those with:[120-124]

- Metastatic disease that does not take up RAI at the time of the first I^{131} treatment
- Ability to take up RAI lost after previous evidence of uptake
- RAI uptake retained in some lesions but not in others
- Metastatic disease that progresses despite substantial uptake of RAI
- Absence of complete response to treatment after >600 mCi of cumulative activity of RAI
- High uptake of 18-FDG on PET/CT scan
- Advanced disease and unfeasible thyroidectomy

Management

The mainstay of treatment of RAIR is use of multityrosine kinase (MKI). However, the real challenges in the use of MKIs are issues such as when to start, which agents to use, and when to stop the MKIs. Patient selection is important because these medications cause life-threatening adverse side effects and also cause substantial decrease in QOL.

- *Prerequisite:* Good overall performance status and acceptable life expectancy, absence of comorbidities or contraindications, and good compliance to treatment

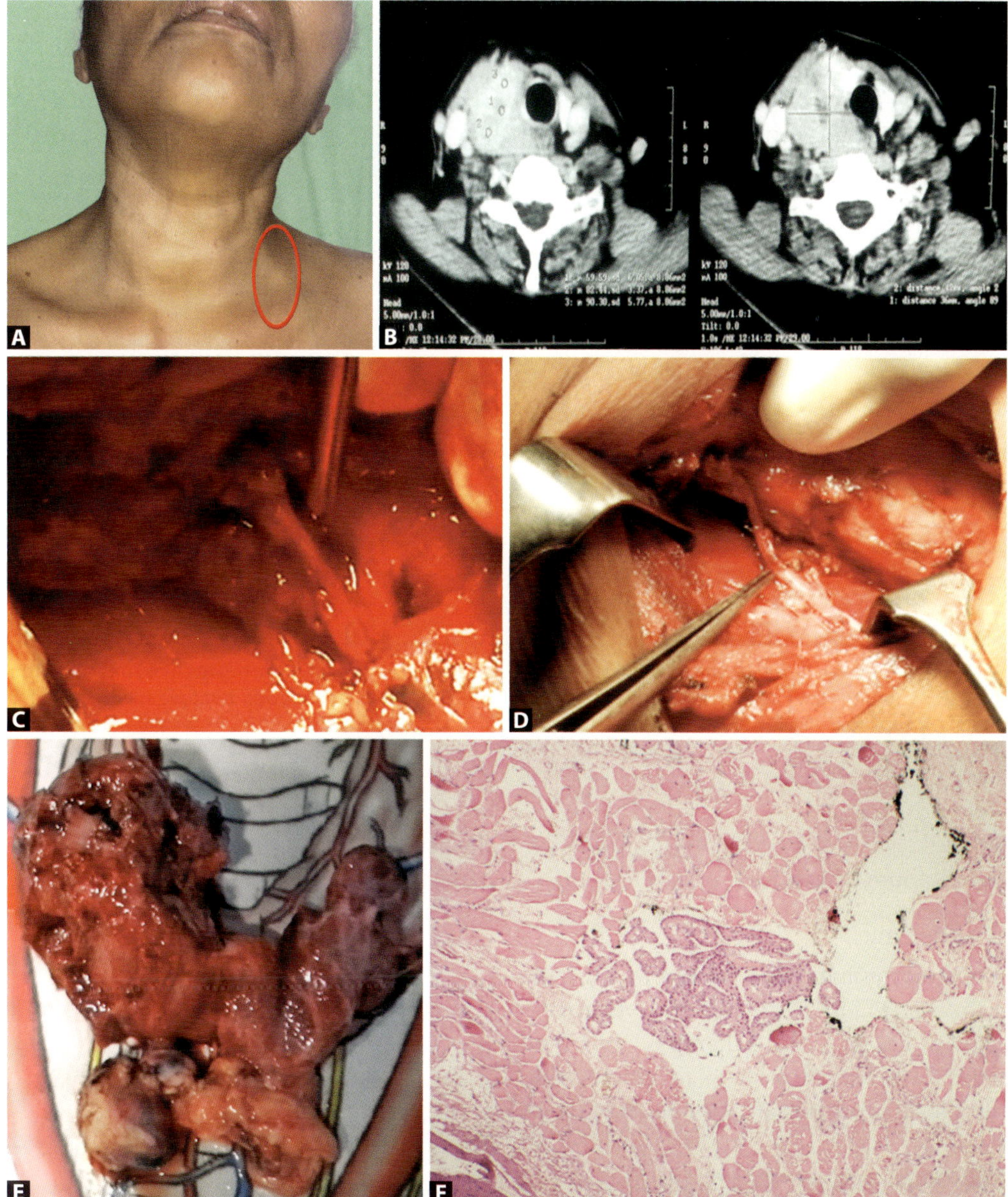

Figs. 8A to F: Locally advanced PTC. A 45-year-old lady presented with solitary thyroid nodule with restricted mobility (A); FNAC was suggestive of PTC. CT scan suggesting infiltration into strap muscles and tumor reaching up to T-0 groove indicating possibility of RLN invasion (B); Intraoperative CCLN was found to be infiltrating RLN (C); Saved by sharp dissection (D); Total thyroidectomy done; (E) HPE showing muscle infiltration by tumor cells (F); Tg was elevated (13.1 ng/mL). pre-therapy scan showed uptake in thyroid bed and right level V lymph node; 75 mCi[131] RAI given.

■ *When to start MKI*: The possible indications to start MKI are rapidly progressive disease (reflected by a thyroglobulin doubling time of <1 year or a significant increase in tumor volume on imaging) and large tumor burden, symptomatic disease which cannot be handled by local treatments and the risk of local complications.

■ *Which agents to start*:
  • *Multikinase inhibitors*: Sorafenib, lenvatinib, pazopanib, cabozantinib, motesanib, axitinib, nintedanib, sunitinib, vandetanib
  • *Selective BRAF inhibitors*: Vemurafenib (and dabrafenib), everolimus, crizotinib, selumetinib
  • *Combined therapy*[125,126]

■ *When to stop these medications*: Though adverse events (AEs) are the most common among them do not necessitate withdrawal and dose reduction is enough. Discontinuation becomes necessary in case of development of nephrotic syndrome (lenvatinib) or prolonged QTc (vandetinib).

Metastatic DTC

In 10% patients who develop metastases, the most common organs involved are the lungs and bones: <5% metastasize to liver, skin, and brain.[127] The treatment options are as follows:

■ TSH-suppressive therapy
■ Radioiodine treatment
■ Locoregional and adjuvant/adjunctive treatments

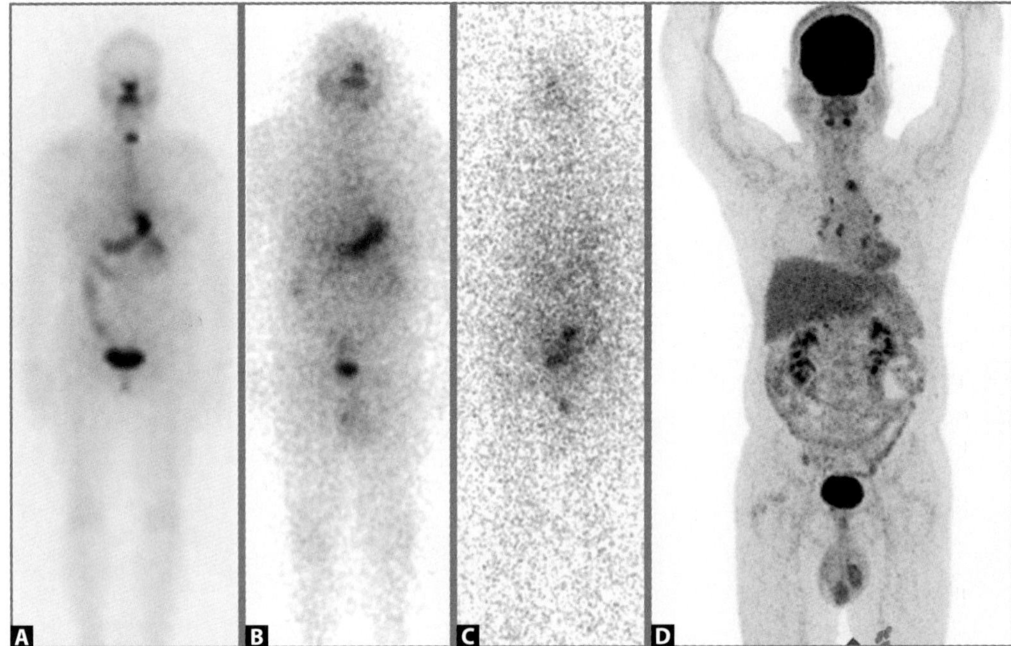

Figs. 9A to D: *Case of TENIS:* PTC treated by total thyroidectomy, WBRAI revealed thyroid bed remnant; (A) treated by 65 mCI; 6 months later scan showed no uptake but Tg >22 (B); 9 months later scan showed no uptake but Tg >223 (C); FDG pet showed multiple mediastinal, hilar and pulmonary metastases (D).

- Targeted systemic treatment
- Redifferentiation
- Novel therapeutic approaches

TSH-suppressive Therapy

TSH-suppressive therapy has been shown to prolong progression-free survival (PFS).[83,128] The dose of levothyroxine should be adjusted to obtain a TSH value of 0.1 mU/L or slightly below, since further suppression to an undetectable level has not been shown to provide any further benefit.

Radioiodine Treatment

Radioiodine therapy is the mainstay of the treatment of the metastasized DTC, in fact curative at times with acceptable side effects. If tumor deposits take up radioiodine, this treatment is possibly curative. In one study, the OS after diagnosis of metastatic disease in patients with radioiodine uptake in the tumor was 56% at 10 years, 45% at 15 years, and 40% at 20 years, compared with 10% at 10 years, and 6% at 15 years in patients without iodine uptake.[129] If the metastases can be completely cured by radioiodine therapy, the overall 10-year survival is 92%, compared with 29% in patients with residual disease. Possibility of complete response is higher in younger age, well-differentiated histology, limited tumor size (e.g., diffuse micronodular lung metastases visible only on RAI scan and not on X-ray) and extent of metastases, and high ^{131}I uptake.

In most centers, radioiodine treatments are performed with a fixed dose. In cases of widespread DMs, usually an empiric dose of 3.7–7.4 GBq of I-131 is applied. It should be kept in mind that it is logical that the higher the dose is to the metastatic deposit, the more effective will be the expected response. Sublethal dosing may lead to the survival of the more radioiodine-resistant tumor cell clones and reduce the effect of subsequent therapies.

Locoregional and Adjuvant/Adjunctive Treatments

In cases of oligometastatic disease, local treatment such as surgery, radiotherapy, thermal/ethanol ablation/cryoablation, and embolization can be tried. Local interventions are usually just palliative and the guiding principle is that it should be limited to either addressing the pacemaker lesion, that is, a single rapidly progressive metastasis, or to obtaining control in an area at risk for tumor-associated complications, such as the neck/back (impending quadriplegia/paraplegia and especially near vulnerable structures such as large vessels, esophagus, and trachea).

External-beam radiotherapy is sometimes helpful for painful bone metastasis.[130] Brain metastases should, if not radioiodine avid, be treated by resection or external-beam radiotherapy. Antiresorptive therapy should be considered in patients with bone metastases, especially the use of denosumab, a receptor activator of nuclear factor-κB ligand (RANKL) inhibitor.[131,132]

Targeted systemic treatment: Use of TKI and MKI

Redifferentiation Therapy

More effective redifferentiation therapies are now possible once the underlying mitogen-activated protein kinase (MAPK) pathway was better understood. The *BRAFV600E* mutation is the most common genetic alteration in PTC, being a major driver for developing RAIR through suppression of key iodine metabolizing genes involved in iodine uptake and metabolism.[133,134] Additionally, *RAS* mutations are found in approximately 10–20% of PTCs and 40–50% of FTCs, which are responsible for suppression of these genes as well, resulting in dedifferentiation.[135] Both preclinical[136,137] and clinical studies have shown that the inhibition of MAPK signaling can be pharmacologically performed through inhibition of *BRAF* or downstream of *BRAF* resulting in upregulation of iodine metabolism–related genes and, consequently, that these tumors become sensitive to radioiodine treatment. Two agents selumetinib and dabrafenib[138,139] have been investigated with modest results.

Novel Therapies

Immunotherapy: Some tumors evade immunosurveillance, through an inhibition of T-cell function by expressing molecules such as cytotoxic T-lymphocyte associated antigen-4 (CTLA-4), programmed cell death-1 (PD-1), or programmed death-ligand 1 (PD-L1).[140,141] Treatment with antibodies directed against checkpoint inhibitors (e.g., PD-1/PD-L1) has shown promise in other solid cancers and is being investigated in advanced RAI-refractory and metastatic thyroid cancer, used either alone or in combination with a multikinase inhibitor (MKI) or an RAI.[142]

Follicular Thyroid Cancer

It differs from PTC in all aspects. In many countries, dietary iodine supplementation has increased the PTC to FTC ratio,[143] resulting in a reported decreasing incidence of FTC over time.

Clinical Presentation

It usually presents with a solitary thyroid nodule but since FTC spreads hematogenously, DMs at presentation (M1) may be seen in 15–25% of patients[144,145]—thus patients may present with a sternal mass, skull bone metastases, or even soft-tissue metastases like eye/scalp. Cervical LN metastases are much less common, only seen in 2–8%.[146,147]

USG Features

These are very different from PTC. Presence of features such as hypoechoic nodule, absent/discontinuous halo, and irregular margins are more predictive of FTC as compared to follicular adenoma (FA).[148] K-TI-RADS classification systems are not useful for differentiating FA from FC. The only USG finding that differentiates FA from FTC is presence of tumor protrusion in a highly vascularized FTC, but this is a rare presentation.

Cytology

Unlike PTC, FTC cannot be diagnosed by FNAC because the distinction between FTC (which shows capsular and/or vascular invasion) and FA (which does not show invasion) requires pathological examination of tumor capsule after thyroidectomy. Follicular patterned lesions include FA, FTC, follicular variant of papillary thyroid carcinoma (FVPTC), and noninvasive follicular thyroid neoplasm with papillary-like nuclear features (NIFTP). On cytology, all these lesions will be categorized as either Bethesda class III (rate of malignancy being 5–15%) or class IV (rate of malignancy being 15–30%).[149]

Genetic Landscape

Unlike PTC where *BRAF* is the most common oncogenic mutation, in FTC the primary mutations are the *RAS* point mutations (40–50%; *NRAS*, *HRAS*, and less commonly *KRAS*) as well as the PAX8PPARy rearrangements (30–40%[150]). However, these mutations are not diagnostic of malignancy and they are also detected in FA.

Molecular Testing

Novel genetic approaches are now available as commercial assays. However, these assays have been validated mostly with PTC. These assays are marketed mainly as rule-out tests with the objective of identifying benign nodules for avoiding lobectomy. These assays are:[19,151-153] ThyroSeq V2 (sensitivity/specificity 70 and 77%), GEC (Afirma), NPV of 94–95%, PPV of 37–38%, ThyraMIR and ThyGenX (sensitivity and specificity—n 89 and 85%).

Histology

Unlike the classical PTC, where the histopathological diagnosis is straightforward, the pathological diagnosis of FTC is rather difficult because of the need of examination of multiple sections/whole of the capsule, because of lack of standardized definition of types of FTC, and because of significant inter- or intraobserver variations.

Definitions: Capsular invasion (CI)—WHO defines presence of capsular invasion when a tumor completely transgresses the tumor capsule, often mushrooming beyond the capsule.[154] True vascular invasion (VI) is defined as invasion into veins with tumor cells adherent to vessel wall, either covered by endothelium or within a thrombus or fibrin. Number of sections—the diagnosis of CI or VI requires examination of multiple sections of tumor; some recommend at least 10 sections[155] while others recommend examination of the entire tumor capsule while still others recommend a minimum of at least four blocks/cm.[156]

Categories of FTC: The WHO divided FTC into three main pathological categories:[154]

- *Minimally invasive*: Tumor with only CI **(Figs. 10A to F)**
- *Encapsulated angioinvasive*: Without reference to the number of blood vessels
- *Widely invasive*: Gross invasion **(Figs. 11A to G)**

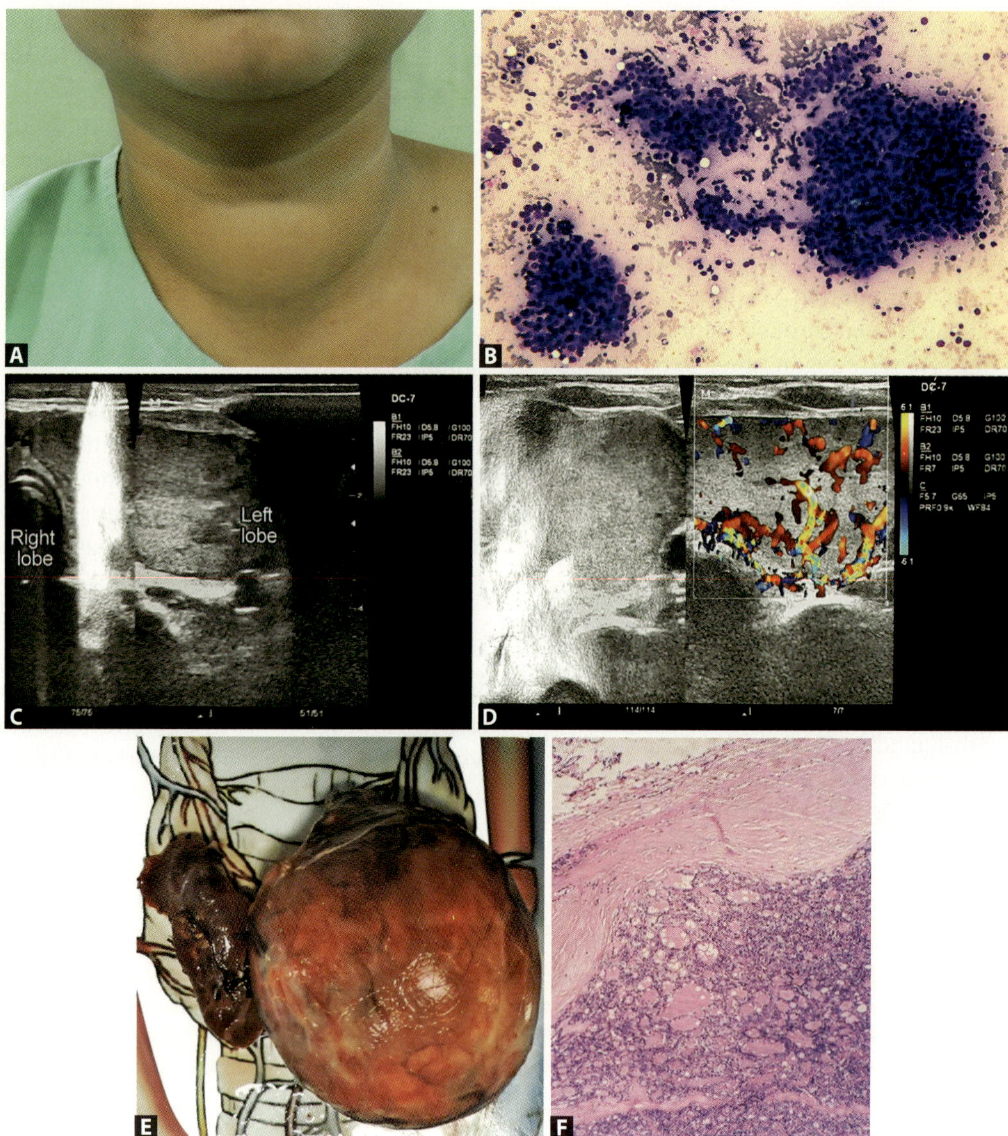

Figs. 10A to F: Minimally invasive follicular thyroid cancer (MIFTC). A 25-year-old lady presented with a 6 × 6.5 cm solitary thyroid nodule (A) which was reported as follicular neoplasm (Bethesda IV) on FNAC (B); USG revealed a solid, hypoechoic, homogeneous lesion (C) with increased peripheral and central vascularity (D); underwent total thyroidectomy (E); HPE was reported as minimally invasive follicular carcinoma as the tumor did not invade the full thickness of the capsule (F).

ATA 2015 guidelines recommend:

- FTC with CI only
- FTC with minimal VI (<4 blood vessel invasion)
- FTC with extensive VI (>4 blood vessel invasion)

Other authors like Daniels[157] *have recommended using the criteria*: CI alone, minimal VI (<4) ± CI, extensive VI (>4), or extensive ETE.

It should be remembered that minimally invasive follicular thyroid cancer (MIFTC) is much more common (85%) than widely invasive follicular thyroid carcinoma (WIFTC) (15%).

FTC are usually larger than PTC—The SEER (Surveillance, Epidemiology, and End Results) database reported FTC with a median diameter of 3.0 cm as against the median diameter of 1.8 cm for PTC.[158] Similarly, multifocality and lymphatic invasion are rare in FTC. In fact, if the histopathologist finds lymphatic invasion, then the diagnosis is likely to be FVPTC rather than FTC. It is unknown whether insular or solid/trabecular areas in FTC are signs of a more aggressive tumor and possible transition to poorly differentiated thyroid carcinoma (PDTC).

Prognostic Factors

The following factors have been identified as independent predictors of recurrence, survival, and DMs: older age, large tumor size, advanced stage, angioinvasion, DM, ETE, and presence of *TERT* mutations. In fact, follicular thyroid cancer histotype itself is thought to be an independent predictor of poorer survival.[159]

Staging Systems

Neither AJCC/TNM (8th edition) nor ATA risk categories have been validated specifically for FTC. Interestingly, even though

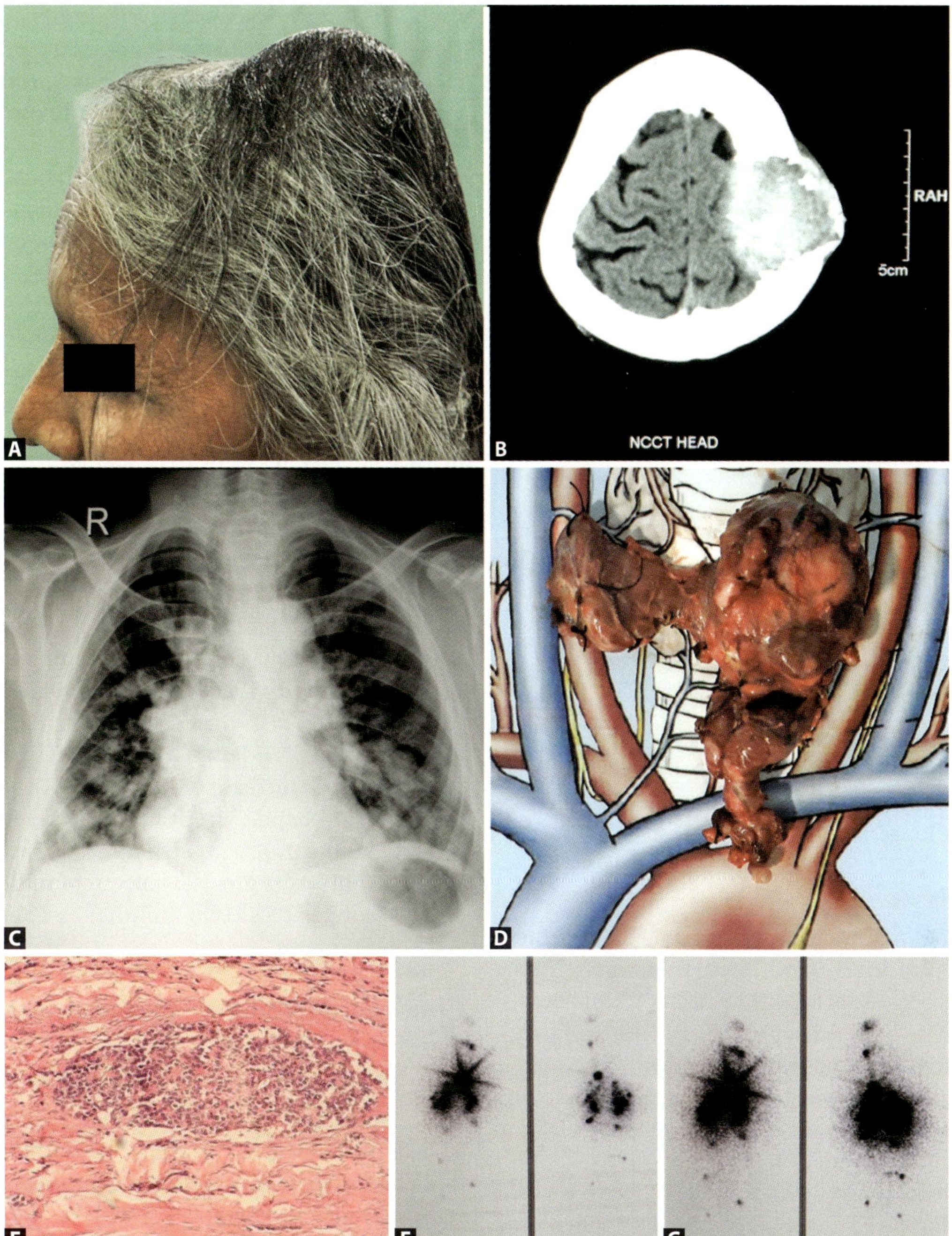

Figs. 11A to G: Widely invasive FTC. A 65-year-old lady presented with a scalp swelling (A) along with a goiter. CT brain showed expansile lesion in the parietal region with intra- and extra-cranial extension (B); Chest X-ray revealed cannon-ball secondaries (C); Underwent total thyroidectomy (D); HPE was suggestive of widely invasive FTC (capsular invasion) (E); Diagnostic WBRAI scan revealed, multiple skeletal (F); and lung metastases (G).

most studies on FTC consider the presence and extent of VI as an important risk factor for DM and DSM, yet it is not included in the AJCC/TNM 8th edition classification. It should be kept in mind that the 8th edition of AJCC/TNM classification has increased the age cutoff for stage I disease to 55 years to prevent potential overtreatment.

Primary Treatment and Extent of Surgery

A diagnosis of FTC is rarely confirmed prior to surgery. Usually, the patients with the Bethesda category III or IV cytology result would have undergone hemithyroidectomy with the pathology

report of FTC. According to some authors,[160-163] hemithyroidectomy is considered sufficient if histopathological examination (HPE) is MIFTC with

- Only CI with no VI
- <45 years old
- Tumor <4 cm
- No LNM, no DM

All others should undergo completion thyroidectomy. In the study done at Mayo Clinic,[161] determination of cause-specific mortality (CSM) was the presence of DM at diagnosis and VI.

RAI Therapy

Radioactive iodine for FTC is generally administered to treat or discover DM and not to treat local recurrence or persistent local disease. In the study by Sugino et al.[164] posttherapeutic scintigraphy showed that 57% of the included patients had RAI uptake in their metastases. RAI is strongly recommended for FTC patients who fall into ATA high-risk category (MI, M2, VI with >4 foci, extensive ETE)

Metastatic FTC

Multiple metastases are best treated by RAI and sometimes with EBRT; multiple RAI doses can be given every 6 months along with suppressive thyroxine therapy. Spinal metastatic disease and spinal cord compression are the major causes of morbidity and mortality.[164] The treatment of metastatic disease of spine requires surgical decompression, reconstruction, and stabilization of spine in addition to EBRT.[164] Patients with multiple brain metastases can be treated with EBRT or gamma knife. For single, demonstrable, resectable metastasis, in long bones or brain, surgical resection should be considered.

Follow-up and Recurrence

Recurrence rates in FTC vary from 3 to 40%.[165,166] Local recurrence (thyroid bed/LNM) are rare in FTC while DM are more common (lungs, bones, brain, soft tissues).

Rare Clinical Scenario

Uncommonly but not rarely, it may be difficult to achieve high TSH despite total thyroidectomy and thyroxine withdrawal. It is because of hyperthyroidism (thyrotoxicosis) produced by DMs. The mechanism is as follows:

- Activating TSH mutations when DM grow[167,168]
- Some patients with concomitant Graves' disease and FTC develop hyperthyroidism as TRAb drives the DMs to produce thyroid hormone.[169,170]
- 3,5,3' Triiodothyronine thyrotoxicosis (T3 thyrotoxicosis) may also occur in FTC with bulky DM due to increased conversion of administered levothyroxine to T3 by type II iodothyronine deiodinase.[171,172] In this scenario, elevated (or high normal) serum T3 occurs when levothyroxine is administered, and profound hypothyroidism occurs when levothyroxine is discontinued. Because a fully suppressed serum TSH is often the therapeutic goal in FTC patients with DM, unless serum T3 (or free T3) is measured, deiodinase-induced hyperthyroidism will be missed.

◇| HURTHLE CELL CARCINOMA

It is a variant of FTC and its biological behavior is similar to FTC; hence, they are studied together. They are primarily composed of Hurthle cells (also known as oncocytic or oxyphilic cell) which are large cells with increased granular cytoplasm (reflecting increased and enlarged mitochondria) along with large, hyperchromatic nuclei with an increased cytoplasmic/nuclear ratio. Thus, for cytological diagnosis of Hurthle cell neoplasm, the following are needed: presence of abundant Hurthle cells (>50–75%) along with a group of cytological features like scant colloid, small cell dysplasia, and dyshesion (single cells). On histopathology, capsular and vascular invasion is necessary for diagnosis of Hurthle cell carcinoma (HCC). However, LNM and soft-tissue DMs are more common than FTC. The genetic landscape of HCC is different from FTC—it shows mitochondrial DNA mutation in complex 1 of electron transport chain.[173] *RAS* mutations and PAX8PPARy fusions are much less common in HCC as compared to FTC. Unlike FTC, upfront total thyroidectomy is more acceptable for Hurthle cell neoplasm. Two studies concluded that total thyroidectomy was the only independent factor for improved cancer-specific survival.[174,175] Unfortunately, HCC is much less likely to be RAI avid and in fact RAI uptake studies in HCC may give false-positive results. On the contrary, 18FDG-PET is particularly useful in follow-up of patients with HCC because of its particular avidity for this tracer.[176] 18FDG-PET in HCC has a sensitivity of 95.8% and a specificity of 95%. Further, 18FDG-PET has a prognostic value—for each increase of 1 SUV of FDG, a 6% increase in mortality was found.[176] In HCC, TKIs are the best approach to systemic RAIR progressive disease[177] as shown by the SELECT trial where a reasonable proportion of HCC (18%) showed longer PFS (18.8 months) as compared to PTC (16.4 months).

Childhood Papillary Thyroid Carcinoma (Figs. 12A to E)

Amongst the thyroid cancers in children, PTC is the most common malignancy seen in childhood with an incidence of 1.8% as per SEER data.[178] It is also the second most common malignancy seen in children with prior history of having received radiation therapy.[179] Low-level radiation doses to thyroid <30 Gy increase the risk for thyroid cancer, especially in ages <10 years.[180-182] PTEN syndrome and FAP are amongst the genetic predisposition syndromes where children may develop DTC.[183,184] The characteristic distinguishing features of childhood PTC include high incidence of LN metastases (50%) and high incidence of lung metastases at presentation (20%)[185-187] and high incidence of multifocal disease (40%).[188-190]

The genetic landscape of pediatric PTC is characterized by high incidence of RET/PTC 1 and 2 rearrangement seen in 72% of children exposed to radiation in Chernobyl nuclear disaster.[191] RET/PTC3 expression has been associated with an aggressive solid PTC variant while RET/PTC 1 has been thought to be associated with less aggressive classical PTC.[192,193] *BRAF* mutation is seen less commonly (in 17–63%).[194] However, *BRAF* mutation is associated with less aggressive disease

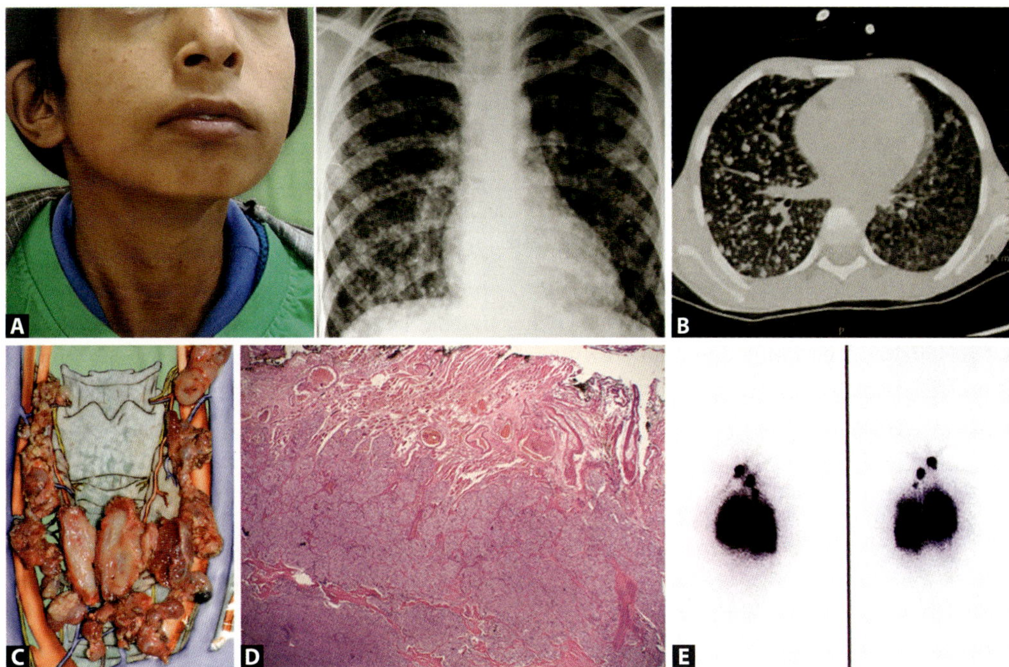

Figs. 12A to E: Childhood PTC. An 11-year-old boy presented with progressively increasing anterior neck swelling × 4 years. History of occasional cough with breathlessness on exertion. On examination, solitary thyroid nodule with multiple bilateral deep cervical LN; positive for PTC on FNAC; Chest X-ray and CECT suggestive of lung metastases (A and B); underwent total thyroidectomy with bilateral MRND (C); HPE was reported as solid variant of PTC (D) (Tumor composed of solid nest and trabecular pattern separated by a thin fibrovascular septa and occasional papillary areas (2%); I[131] scan showed uptake in thyroid bed, right level II lymph node and bilateral lung metastases (E). 100 mCi I[131] therapy given under steroid cover.

as compared to those with RET/PTC rearrangement. *RAS* mutations are less common. In fact, none of the Chernobyl-related PTC had RAS mutations.[195] NTRK rearrangement may be seen in children with more extensive disease [196]

Management: Very few pediatric PTC are low risk. Standard of care is total thyroidectomy with lateral LN dissection in positive LN metastases, followed by selective use of RAI therapy.[197]

RAI therapy: Almost all guidelines recommend RAI treatment for iodine-avid residual nodal/locoregional disease not amenable to surgery and/or distant metastatic disease.[198] Studies have shown complete (in 47.32%) or partial response (38.39%).[199] The method of calculation of RAI activity and the need for continued use of RAI therapy for children with residual pulmonary metastases are controversial areas. There are three approaches for calculating the activity of I-131.

Calculation is based on bone-marrow toxicity, using dosimetry and giving a fixed dose known as empiric dosing. Empiric dosing is simpler and widely used but may result in under-/overtreatment and hence reserved for children with pulmonary metastases. It must be kept in mind that much higher doses are needed for ablating the residual thyroid remnant (300 Gy) as compared to LN/distant metastatic foci (80 Gy). Some researchers would give repeated activities of I-131 till the pulmonary metastases disappear and Tg normalizes,[129,200] but in this approach there is a risk of

pulmonary fibrosis due to repeated doses of RAI. In contrast, Biko et al.[201] showed that it may not be essential to give repeated doses in children with lung metastases as children showed a continual decline of Tg in the years even after I-131 therapy has been stopped before complete remission. Some special points to be remembered with respect to RAI therapy in children are thyroid hormone withdrawal (THW) for 14 days is enough, they should be advised a LID prior to therapy, constipation should be avoided, and in children with lung metastases, frequent pulmonary function test (PFT) studies should be done. Short-term side effects of RAI therapy include gonadal dysfunction and xerostomia. Long-term effects include permanent dysfunction of salivary glands, secondary salivary malignancy, dental caries, pulmonary fibrosis, second malignancy, and hematological malignancies.

The ATA recommendations are:[197]

Survival: 98% 10-year survival.[202] Even in the presence of metastatic disease, 30-year survival rates of 90–99% for children with DTC are possible.[203-205]

Thyroid Cancer and Pregnancy

Important issues that need to be addressed are:

- Impact of pregnancy on outcome/prognosis of survivors of PTC
- Magnitude of increased levothyroxine requirement in pregnant women who have been treated for thyroid cancer
- Management of thyroid cancer diagnosed during pregnancy

Impact of pregnancy on the outcome/prognosis of survivors of PTC: Since it is known that increased levels of human chorionic gonadotropin (HCG) and estrogen during the first trimester of pregnancy have a stimulatory effect on thyroid, there has been some speculation that this may result in recurrence or progression of thyroid cancer. However, recent studies have confirmed that pregnancy does not cause thyroid cancer recurrence in PTC survivors who have had no structural or biochemical evidence of disease persistence at the time of conception. Further, the authors also postulated that a nonsuppressed TSH during pregnancy does not stimulate disease progression.[206,207] Hirsch et al.[207] have defined thyroid cancer progression during pregnancy as 20% or more increase in serum Tg from the prepregnancy level, consistent increase of 20% in serum TgAb, a new metastatic lesion on neck USG performed within 1 year of delivery, or an increase in size of a prepregnancy lesion on neck USG.

Magnitude of increased levothyroxine requirement in pregnant women who have been treated for thyroid cancer: The interpretation of thyroid function tests during pregnancy in a thyroid cancer survivor is a challenge because of three reasons. In patients who have had thyroidectomy, unlike in women with intact thyroid glands in whom elevated levels of HCG stimulate the release of T4 without causing increase of TSH, this feedback loop does not exist and therefore thyroidectomized patients have a different TSH level. Secondly, during pregnancy there is a rise in T4-binding globulin (TBG) as well as expansion of plasma volume which results in increased LT4 requirement to maintain normal FT4 levels. In thyroidectomized patients, this can only be met be increasing the dose of thyroxine. Thirdly as the pregnancy progresses and placenta grows, its type 3 deiodinase activity increases, resulting in inactivation of T4 and again in a patient who is thyroidectomized, increase in thyroxine dosage would be needed. Previous studies have shown that patients with thyroid cancer on an average required a 9% increase in LT4 dose in the first trimester, 21% increase in the second trimester, and a 26% increase in the third trimester.[208-211]

The recommendations are as follows:

- Individuals who have undergone lobectomy should be screened for hypothyroidism during pregnancy, because of the increased demand for thyroid hormone during pregnancy.
- Interpretation of thyroid function studies is challenging in pregnancy due to the effects of physiologic changes on test results. There is no consensus yet on a trimester-specific normal range for these hormone values, and the society recommends that normal ranges for each trimester of pregnancy should be developed by individual laboratories.
- Thyroid function should be monitored every 6–8 weeks during pregnancy. If an adjustment in levothyroxine dose is made, then the next blood tests should be performed in 30 days. A dose increase over the course of pregnancy of as much as 30–50% may be needed. In the month following parturition, the levothyroxine dosage should be adjusted back down to the prepregnancy dose.

However, the study by Loh et al.[210] have shown that patients with thyroid cancer required smaller, less frequent adjustments to LT4 dosage during pregnancy as expected and as compared to those patients who have had thyroidectomy for benign diseases. This may be because of patients with thyroid cancer being on a higher prepregnancy LT4 dosages with suppressed TSH. In fact, it may be feasible to reduce TSH suppression during pregnancy without any adverse effect on DSF or recurrence rates. Thus, patients with a suppressed prepregnancy TSH may be allowed to have a TSH within the normal range by reducing their LT4 doses.

Management of thyroid cancer diagnosed during pregnancy: Endocrine society guidelines for care of pregnant patients who are diagnosed with thyroid nodules or thyroid cancer are as follows:

- Thyroid nodules measuring 1 cm or larger should be evaluated by FNA biopsy.
- Individuals with nodules that are malignant or show rapid growth should be offered surgery in the second trimester of pregnancy.
- It may be appropriate for patients with follicular neoplasia or early stage papillary thyroid cancers to wait until postpartum for thyroidectomy as these lesions are not expected to progress rapidly, and the risk of surgery may outweigh benefits of immediate intervention.
- Patients with known thyroid cancer should maintain a low but measurable TSH and normal thyroxine (T4) values on levothyroxine during pregnancy.
- RAI therapy should not be provided to women who are breastfeeding.
- After RAI therapy, women should wait 6–12 months before becoming pregnant.

Locally Invasive PTC

Locally advanced thyroid cancer occurs when there is either extrathyroidal extension from the primary tumor in thyroid or from extracapsular extension from involved LNs into the surrounding structures. The incidence of invasive disease depends on the pathology of the thyroid cancer. The structures which are in close association with the thyroid gland have more chances of invasion like the strap muscles, RLN, trachea, great vessels, vagus nerve, esophagus, and larynx. Therefore, even though the surgical treatment of thyroid lesions that invade adjacent structures is controversial, the basic principles remain the same: removing as much abnormal tissue as possible and maintaining the functional integrity of the neck structures. The type of thyroid cancer is also an important criterion, which decides the extent of operation. For aggressive thyroid cancers such as anaplastic and medullary when present with airway compromise, palliative management is the treatment of choice because of poor prognosis, in contrast to the differentiated thyroid cancer where extensive resection with curative intent is the best option. The strap muscles (sternohyoid, sternothyroid, and omohyoid) are the most common structures involved in locally advanced thyroid cancer, but recently it has been shown by a study from MD Anderson[212] that gross strap muscle invasion may not be an important survival prognostic factor for staging purposes. Invasion of the aerodigestive tract including the larynx, trachea, hypopharynx, and esophagus can be found in 1–8% of all patients with thyroid cancer.[213-215] Due to anatomical proximity, the respiratory tract invasion can be found in 50%, while esophagus invasion is in 25% of locally advanced thyroid cancers.[7] It should be kept in mind that because of intramural spread, the area of tumor invasion is very often much larger than expected from intraluminal assessment. Management of differentiated thyroid cancer invading the trachea depends on depth of invasion into the wall and horizontal and vertical extent of invasion. McCaffrey[216] and Nishida et al.[217] advocated shave excision for Shin stage I. The advocates of shave excision favor it because it avoids morbidity associated with tracheal resection and also its complications such as tracheal stenosis. Deeper invasions, however, require complete wall resections. A primary anastomosis can be performed with a maximum resection of 5–6 cm of trachea or —seven to eight tracheal rings. To ensure a tension-free repair in such circumstances, various procedures can be performed.

- Supralaryngeal release to gain extra 2 cm
- Division of suprahyoid muscle
- Hilar mobilization of trachea through sternotomy

For esophageal involvement of only the muscular layer, no repair or simple suture repair is all that is required, if an intact submucosal layer can be maintained. Full-thickness invasion may require partial resection and immediate repair.

CONTROVERSIES IN THYROID CANCER

- *The rising incidence of differentiated thyroid cancer*: Is it due to "overdiagnosis" or due to environmental factors, which thus far remain uncertain?
- Is active surveillance a reasonable strategy for small papillary thyroid cancers and whether it is reproducible across all institutions?
- Role of less invasive therapies (e.g., radiofrequency ablation, laser)?
- For low-risk disease, is lobectomy a reasonable option?
- Whether postoperative RAI therapy should be routinely recommended after total thyroidectomy for patients with differentiated thyroid cancer?
- *Newer therapies with MKIs and redifferentiation strategies*: When to start, which agents to start and how long and whether they unequivocally demonstrate improved OS?

CONCLUSION

The management of low-risk and high-risk thyroid cancer, as well as approaches to thyroid nodules, has changed markedly in the past decade. Advances in imaging, particularly ultrasound and elastography, and availability of commercial molecular test of indeterminate thyroid nodules is beginning to influence disease management by being incorporated in the initial evaluation even though no test has so far been able to discriminate malignant from benign nodules reliably. Compartment-based LN dissection has reduced recurrence rates. Risk stratification had led to a more conservative surgical approach, has also led to reduced use of RAI, and relax TSH-suppressive treatment in appropriately selected patients. Dynamic risk stratification has led to more patients being labeled as cured and liberated them from battery of frequent testing and also objectivizing the outcome of initial treatment so that further follow-up is tailored according to the response to initial treatment. Also cutting-edge treatments are being explored for aggressive, RAIR, and metastatic DTCs like tyrosine kinase inhibitors, redifferentiation therapy, and novel treatments like immunotherapy, thus moving toward a more personalized approach for care of patients with thyroid cancer.

CLINICAL PEARLS

- Even within the group of DTC, there is a lot of heterogeneity—both intrapatient and interpatient.
- Clinicians can use modern tools such as elastography and molecular/genetics tests for making a better preoperative prediction of DTC in a solitary thyroid nodule.
- The ATA guidelines may help to decide the extent of thyroidectomy, but each center should develop its own protocols.
- Proper and repeated counseling should be done.
- Surgery for thyroid cancer should preferably be performed by high-volume thyroid surgeons.
- Lateral neck dissection should be compartment based and thorough dissection is advisable to avoid recurrence; there is controversy regarding exclusion/inclusion of excision of levels IIB and VA.
- Policy of selective use of RAI therapy should be followed.
- Clinicians should adopt dynamic risk stratification for following up their thyroid cancer patients.
- FTC differs in many aspects from PTC.
- HCC is an aggressive malignancy and early PET scan is advisable with use of TKI in progressive disease.
- For advanced thyroid cancer, clinicians should use the two angiogenic drugs that have been approved—sorafenib and lenvatinib.

- Treatment of childhood PTC should be by an experienced thyroid surgeon, and repeated RAI therapy should be avoided.
- Pregnant thyroid cancer survivors may require decrease in thyroxine dosage in the first trimester if they are on suppressive doses of thyroxine.
- Extensive resection can be offered to locally invasive PTC with intention to cure. Thyroid surgeons must be trained in tracheal resections.

◇ REFERENCES

1. Sosa JA, Hanna JW, Robinson KA, Lanman RB. Increases in thyroid nodule fine-needle aspirations, operations, and diagnoses of thyroid cancer in the United States. Surgery. 2013;154:1420-6.
2. Kim EK, Park CS, Chung WY, Oh KK, Kim DI, Lee JT, et al. New sonographic criteria for recommending fine needle aspiration biopsy of nonpalpable solid nodules of the thyroid. Am J Roentgenol. 2002;178(3):687-91.
3. Horvath E, Majlis S, Rossi R, Franco C, Niedmann JP, Castro A, et al. An ultrasonogram reporting system for thyroid nodules stratifying cancer risk for clinical management. J Clin Endocrinol Metab. 2009;94:1748-51.
4. Friedrich-Rust M, Meyer G, Dauth N, Berner C, Herrmann E, Zeuzem S, et al. Interobserver agreement of Thyroid Imaging Reporting and Data System (TIRADS) and realtime elastography for the assessment of thyroid nodules. Ultraschall Med. 2013;34:WS_SL11_01.
5. Sahli ZT, Karipineni F, Hang J-F, Canner JK, Mathur A, Prescott JD, et al. The association between the ultrasonography TIRADS classification system and surgical pathology among indeterminate thyroid nodules. Surgery. 2019;165(1): 69-74.
6. Phuttharak W, Boonrod A, Klungboonkrong V, Witsawapaisan T. Interrater Reliability of Various Thyroid Imaging Reporting and Data System (TIRADS) classifications for differentiating benign from malignant thyroid nodules. Asian Pac J Cancer Prev. 2019;20(4),1283-8.
7. Cosgrove D, Barr R, Bojunga J, Cantisani V, Chammas MC, Dighe M, et al. WFUMB guidelines and recommendations on the clinical use of ultrasound elastography: part 4. Thyroid. Ultrasound Med Biol. 2017;43(1):4-26.
8. Sebag F, Vaillant-Lombard J, Berbis J, Griset V, Henry JF, Petit P, et al. Shear wave elastography: a new ultrasound imaging mode for the differential diagnosis of benign and malignant thyroid nodules. J Clin Endocrinol Metab. 2010;95:5281-8.
9. Xu JM, Xu XH, Xu HX, Zhang YF, Zhang J, Guo LH, et al. Conventional US, US elasticity imaging, and acoustic radiation force impulse imaging for prediction of malignancy in thyroid nodules. Radiology. 2014;272:577-86.
10. Bojunga J, Dauth N, Berner C, Meyer G, Holzer K, Voelkl L, et al. Acoustic radiation force impulse imaging for differentiation of thyroid nodules. PLoS One. 2012;7:e42735.
11. Trimboli P, Guglielmi R, Monti S, Misischi I, Graziano F, Nasrollah N, et al. Ultrasound sensitivity for thyroid malignancy is increased by real-time elastography: a prospective multicenter study. J Clin Endocrinol Metab. 2012;97:4524-30.
12. Baloch ZW, Cooper DS, Gharib H, Alexander EK. Overview of diagnostic terminology and reporting. In: Ali SZ, Cibas ES (Eds). The Bethesda System for Reporting Thyroid Cytopathology: Definitions, Criteria, and Explanatory Notes. New York, NY: Springer; 2017.
13. Ali SZ, Cibas ES. The Bethesda System for Reporting Thyroid Cytopathology. Definitions, Criteria and Explanatory Notes. New York, NY: Springer; 2010.
14. Bongiovanni M, Spitalea A, Faquin WC, Mazzucchelli L, Baloch ZW. The Bethesda system for reporting thyroid cytopathology: a meta-analysis. Acta Cytologica. 2012;56:333-9.
15. Lundgren CI, Zedenius J, Skoog L. Fine-needle aspiration biopsy of benign thyroid nodules: an evidence-based review. World J Surg. 2008;32(7):1247-52.
16. McHenry CR, Walfish PG, Rosen IB. Non-diagnostic fine needle aspiration biopsy: a dilemma in management of nodular thyroid disease. Am Surg. 1993;59:415-9.
17. Chow LS, Gharib H, Goellner JR, van Heerden JA. Nondiagnostic thyroid fine-needle aspiration cytology: management dilemmas. Thyroid. 2001;11:1147-51.
18. Nikiforova MN, Chiosea SI, Nikiforov YE. MicroRNA expression profiles in thyroid tumors. Endocr Pathol. 2009;20:85-91.
19. Labourier E, Shifrin A, Busseniers AE, Lupo MA, Manganelli ML, Andruss B, et al. Molecular testing for miRNA, mRNA, and DNA on fine-needle aspiration improves the preoperative diagnosis of thyroid nodules with indeterminate cytology. J Clin Endocrinol Metab. 2015;100:2743-50.
20. Nikiforov YE, Ohori NP, Hodak SP, Carty SE, LeBeau SO, Ferris RL, et al. Impact of mutational testing on the diagnosis and management of patients with cytologically indeterminate thyroid nodules: a prospective analysis of 1056 FNA samples. J Clin Endocrinol Metab. 2011;96:3390-7.
21. Najafian A, Noureldine S, Azar F, Atallah C, Trinh G, Schneider EB, et al. RAS mutations and RET/PTC and PAX8/PPAR-gamma chromosomal rearrangements are also prevalent in benign thyroid lesions: implications thereof and a systematic review. Thyroid. 2017;27:39-48.
22. Alexander EK, Schorr M, Klopper J, Kim C, Sipos J, Nabhan F, et al. Multicenter clinical experience with the Afirma gene expression classifier. J Clin Endocrinol Metab. 2014;99:119-25.
23. Beaudenon-Huibregtse S, Alexander EK, Guttler RB, Hershman JM, Babu V, Blevins TC, et al. Centralized molecular testing for oncogenic gene mutations complements the local cytopathologic diagnosis of thyroid nodules. Thyroid. 2014;24:1479-87.
24. Eszlinger M, Böhme K, Ullmann M, Görke F, Siebolts U, Neumann A, et al. Evaluation of a two-year routine application of molecular testing of thyroid fine needle aspirations (FNA) using a 7 gene-panel in a primary referral setting in Germany. Thyroid. 2017;27:402-11.
25. Eszlinger M, Piana S, Moll A, Bösenberg E, Bisagni A, Ciarrocchi A, et al. Molecular testing of thyroid fine needle aspirations (FNA) improves pre-surgical diagnosis and supports the histological identification of minimally invasive follicular thyroid carcinomas. Thyroid. 2015;25:401-9.
26. Nikiforov YE, Carty SE, Chiosea SI, Coyne C, Duvvuri U, Ferris RL, et al. Highly accurate diagnosis of cancer in thyroid nodules with follicular neoplasm/suspicious for a follicular neoplasm cytology by ThyroSeq v2 next-generation sequencing assay. Cancer. 2014;120:3627-34.
27. Wei S, Veloski C, Sharda P, Ehya H. Performance of the Afirma genomic sequencing classifier versus gene expression classifier: an institutional experience. Cancer Cytopathol. 2019;127:720-4.
28. Mack Harrell R, Eyerly-Webb SA, Golding AC, Edwards CM, Bimston DN. Statistical comparison of Afirma GSC and Afirma GEC outcomes in a community endocrine surgical practice: early findings. Endocr Pract. 2019;25(2):161-4.

29. Song YS, Lim JA, Choi H, Won J-K, Moon JH, Cho SW, et al. Prognostic effects of TERT promoter mutations are enhanced by coexistence with BRAF or RAS mutations and strengthen the risk prediction by the ATA or TNM staging system in differentiated thyroid cancer patients. Cancer. 2016;122:1370-9.

30. Koo JS, Hong S, Park CS. Diffuse sclerosing variant is a major subtype of papillary thyroid carcinoma in the young. Thyroid. 2009;19:1225-31.

31. Regalbuto C, Malandrino P, Tumminia A, Moli RL, Vigneri R, Pezzino V. A diffuse sclerosing variant of papillary thyroid carcinoma: clinical and pathologic feature and outcomes of 34 consecutive cases. Thyroid. 2011;21:383-9.

32. Silver C, Owen R, Rodrigo J, Rinaldo A, Devaney KO, Ferlito A. Aggressive variants of papillary thyroid carcinoma. Head Neck. 2011;7:1052-9.

33. Choi Y, Shin J, Kim J, Jung SL, Son EJ, Oh YL, et al. Tall cell variant of papillary thyroid carcinoma: sonographic and clinical findings. J Ultrasound Med. 2011;30:853-8.

34. Kazaure HS, Roman SA, Sosa JA. Aggressive variants of papillary thyroid cancer: incidence, characteristics and predictors of survival among 43,738 patients. Ann Surg Oncol. 2012;19: 1874-80.

35. Chan JK, Rosai J. Tumors of the neck showing thymic or related branchial pouch differentiation: a unifying concept. Hum Pathol. 1991;22(4):349-67.

36. Kazaure HS, Roman SA, Sosa JA. Insular thyroid cancer: a population-level analysis of patient characteristics and predictors of survival. Cancer. 2012;118:3260-7.

37. Nixon IJ, Ganly I, Patel SG, Palmer FL, Whitcher MM, Tuttle RM, et al. Thyroid lobectomy for treatment of well differentiated intrathyroid malignancy. Surgery. 2012;151:571-9.

38. Vaisman F, Shaha A, Fish S, Michael TR. Initial therapy with either thyroid lobectomy or total thyroidectomy without radioactive iodine remnant ablation is associated with very low rates of structural disease recurrence in properly selected patients with differentiated thyroid cancer. Clin Endocrinol (Oxf). 2011;75:112-9.

39. Kwak JY, Kim EK, Youk JH, Kim MJ, Son EJ, Choi SH, et al. Extrathyroid extension of well-differentiated papillary thyroid microcarcinoma on US. Thyroid. 2008; 18(6): 609-14.

40. Ishigaki S, Shimamoto K, Satake H, Sawaki A, Itoh S, Ikeda M, et al. Multi-slice CT of thyroid nodules: comparison with ultrasonography. Radiat Med. 2004; 22(5):346-53.

41. Iacobone M, Jansson S, Barczyński M, Goretzki P. Multifocal papillary thyroid carcinoma—a consensus report of the European Society of Endocrine Surgeons (ESES). Langenbecks Arch Surg. 2014;399(2):141-54.

42. Leboulleux S, Rubino C, Baudin E, Caillou B, Hartl DM, Bidart JM, et al. Prognostic factors for persistent or recurrent disease of papillary thyroid carcinoma with neck lymph node metastases and/or tumor extension beyond the thyroid capsule at initial diagnosis. J Clin Endocrinol Metab. 2005;90:5723-9.

43. Wang F, Yu X, Shen X, Zhu G, Huang Y, Liu R, et al. The prognostic value of tumor multifocality in clinical outcomes of papillary thyroid cancer. J Clin Endocrinol Metab. 2017;102 3241-50.

44. Liang J, Li Z, Fang F, Yu T, Li S. Is prophylactic central neck dissection necessary for cN0 differentiated thyroid cancer patients at initial treatment? A meta-analysis of the literature. Acta Otorhinolaryngol Ital. 2017;37:1-8.

45. Shaha AR. Prophylactic central compartment dissection in thyroid cancer: a new avenue of debate. Surgery. 2009;146: 1224-7.

46. Hughes DT, White ML, Miller BS, Gauger PG, Burney RE, Doherty GM. Influence of prophylactic central lymph node dissection on postoperative thyroglobulin levels and radioiodine treatment in papillary thyroid cancer. Surgery. 2010;148:1100-6.

47. Carling T, Carty SE, Ciarleglio MM, Cooper DS, Doherty GM, Kim LT, et al. American Thyroid Association design and feasibility of a prospective randomized controlled trial of prophylactic central lymph node dissection for papillary thyroid carcinoma. Thyroid. 2012;22(3):237-44.

48. Popadich A, Levin O, Lee JC, Smooke-Praw S, Ro K, Fazel M, et al. A multicenter cohort study of total thyroidectomy and routine central lymph node dissection for cN0 papillary thyroid cancer. Surgery. 2011;150(6):1048-57.

49. Wang TS, Cheung K, Farrokhyar F, Roman SA, Sosa JA. A meta-analysis of the effect of prophylactic central compartment neck dissection on locoregional recurrence rates in patients with papillary thyroid cancer. Ann Surg Oncol. 2013;20(11):3477-83.

50. Chisholm EJ, Kulinskaya E, Tolley NS. Systematic review and meta-analysis of the adverse effects of thyroidectomy combined with central neck dissection as compared with thyroidectomy alone. Laryngoscope. 2009;119(6):1135-9.

51. Zetoune T, Keutgen X, Buitrago D, Aldailami H, Shao H, Mazumdar M, et al. Prophylactic central neck dissection and local recurrence in papillary thyroid cancer: a meta-analysis. Ann Surg Oncol. 2010;17(12):3287-93.

52. Giordano D, Valcavi R, Thompson GB, Pedroni C, Renna L, Gradoni P, et al. Complications of central neck dissection in patients with papillary thyroid carcinoma: results of a study on 1087 patients and review of the literature. Thyroid. 2012;22: 911-7.

53. Sancho JJ, Lennard TW, Paunovic I, Triponez F, Sitges-Serra A, et al. Prophylactic central neck dissection in papillary thyroid cancer: a consensus report of the European Society of Endocrine Surgeons (ESES). Langenbecks Arch Surg. 2014;399:155-63.

54. Shen WT, Ogawa L, Ruan D, Suh I, Duh Q-Y, Clark OH, et al. Central neck lymph node dissection for papillary thyroid cancer: the reliability of surgeon judgment in predicting which patients will benefit. Surgery. 2010;148:398-403.

55. Zuniga S, Sanabria A. Prophylactic central neck dissection in stage N0 papillary thyroid carcinoma. Arch Otolaryngol Head Neck Surg. 2009;135:1087-91.

56. Blanchard C, Brient C, Volteau C, Sebag F, Roy M, Drui D, et al. Factors predictive of lymph node metastasis in the follicular variant of papillary thyroid carcinoma. Br J Surg. 2013;100: 1312-7.

57. Raffaelli M, De Crea C, Sessa L, Fadda G, Bellantone C, Lombardi CP. Ipsilateral central neck dissection plus frozen section examination versus prophylactic bilateral central neck dissection in cN0 papillary thyroid carcinoma. Ann Surg Oncol. 2015;22:2302-8.

58. Tavares MR, da Cruz JAS, Waisberg DR, de Almeida Toledo SP, Takeda FR, Cernea CR, et al. Lymph node distribution in the central compartment of the neck: an anatomic study. Head Neck. 2014;36(10):1425-30.

59. Oh EM, Chung YS, Lee YD. Clinical significance of Delphian lymph node metastasis in papillary thyroid carcinoma. World J Surg. 2013;37(11):2594-9.

60. Baldini E, Sorrenti S, Di Gioia C, De Vito C, Antonelli A, Gnessi L, et al. Cervical lymph node metastases from thyroid cancer: does thyroglobulin and calcitonin measurement in fine needle

aspirates improve the diagnostic value of cytology? BMC Clin Pathol. 2013;13:7.

61. Baldini E, Sorrenti S, Catania A, Guaitoli E, Prinzi N, Mocini R, et al. Diagnostic utility of thyroglobulin measurement in the fine needle aspirates from cervical lymph nodes: a case report. G Chir. 2012;33:387-91.

62. Bonnet S, Hartl D, Leboulleux S, Baudin E, Lumbroso JD, Al Ghuzlan A, et al. Prophylactic lymph node dissection for papillary thyroid cancer less than 2 cm: implications for radioiodine treatment. J Clin Endrocrinol Metab. 2009;94: 1162-7.

63. Ulisse S, Baldini E, Sorrenti S, Barollo S, Prinzi N, Catania A, et al. In papillary thyroid carcinoma BRAFV600E is associated with increased expression of the urokinase plasminogen activator and its cognate receptor, but not with disease-free interval. Clin Endocrinol (Oxf). 2012;77:780-6.

64. Kouvaraki MA, Shapiro SE, Fornage BD, Edeiken-Monro BS, Sherman SI, Vassilopoulou-Sellin R, et al. Role of preoperative ultrasonography in the surgical management of patients with thyroid cancer. Surgery. 2003;134(6):946-54 [discussion: 954-5].

65. Soler ZM, Hamilton BE, Schuff KG, Samuels MH, Cohen JI. Utility of computed tomography in the detection of subclinical nodal disease in papillary thyroid carcinoma. Arch Otolaryngol Head Neck Surg. 2008;134(9):973-8.

66. Kim E, Park JS, Son K-R, Kim J-I, Jeon SJ, Na DG. Preoperative diagnosis of cervical metastatic lymph nodes in papillary thyroid carcinoma: comparison of ultrasound, computed tomography, and combined ultrasound with computed tomography. Thyroid. 2008;18(4):411-8.

67. Jeon MJ, Kim WG, Jang EK, Choi YM, Lee Y-M, Sung T-Y, et al. Thyroglobulin level in fine-needle aspirates for preoperative diagnosis of cervical lymph node metastasis in patients with papillary thyroid carcinoma: two different cutoff values according to serum thyroglobulin level. Thyroid. 2015;25(4):410-6.

68. Scheumann GF, Gimm O, Wegener G, Hundeshagen H, Dralle H. Prognostic significance and surgical management of locoregional lymph node metastases in papillary thyroid cancer. World J Surg. 1994;18(4):559-67 [discussion: 567-8].

69. Sturgeon C, Yang A, Elaraj D. Surgical management of lymph node compartments in papillary thyroid cancer. Surg Oncol Clin N Am. 2016;25(1):17-40.

70. Lee J, Sung TY, Nam KH, Chung WY, Soh EY, Park CS. Is level IIb lymph node dissection always necessary in N1b papillary thyroid carcinoma patients? World J Surg. 2008; 32:716-21.

71. Tuttle R, Haddad R, Ball DW, Byrd D, Dickson P, Duh Q-Y, et al. Thyroid carcinoma v.2.2014. J Natl Compr Canc Netw. 2014;12:1671-80.

72. Cappiello J, Piazza C, Giudice M, De Maria G, Nicolai P. Shoulder disability after different selective neck dissections (levels II-IV versus levels II-V): a comparative study. Laryngoscope. 2005;115:259-63.

73. Prim MP, De Diego JI, Verdaguer JM, Sastre N, Rabanal I. Neurological complications following functional neck dissection. Eur Arch Otorhinolaryngol. 2006;263:473-6.

74. Haugen BR, Alexander EK, Bible KC, Doherty GM, Mandel SJ, Nikiforov YE, et al. American Thyroid Association management guidelines for adult patients with thyroid nodules and differentiated thyroid cancer: The American Thyroid Association Guidelines Task Force on Thyroid Nodules and Differentiated Thyroid Cancer. Thyroid. 2016;26(1):1-133.

75. Jonklaas J. Role of radioactive iodine for adjuvant therapy and treatment of metastases. J Natl Compr Canc Netw. 2007;5(6):631-40.

76. Schvartz C, Bonnetain F, Dabakuyo S, Gauthier M, Cueff A, Fieffé S, et al. Impact on overall survival of radioactive iodine in low-risk differentiated thyroid cancer patients. J Clin Endocrinol Metab. 2012;97(5):1526-35.

77. Rosário PW, Borges MA, Valadão MM, Vasconcelos FPJ, Rezende LL, Padrão EL, et al. Is adjuvant therapy useful in patients with papillary carcinoma smaller than 2 cm? Thyroid 2007;17:1225-8.

78. Nixon IJ, Ganly I, Patel SG, Palmer FL, Di Lorenzo MM, Grewal RK, et al. The results of selective use of radioactive iodine on survival and on recurrence in the management of papillary thyroid cancer, based on Memorial Sloan-Kettering Cancer Center risk group stratification. Thyroid. 2013;23:683-94.

79. Sugitani I, Kasai N, Fujimoto Y, Yanagisawa A. A novel classification system for patients with PTC: addition of the new variables of large (3 cm or greater) nodal metastases and reclassification during the follow-up period. Surgery. 2004;135:139-48.

80. Adam MA, Pura J, Goffredo P, Dinan MA, Reed SD, Scheri RP, et al. Presence and number of lymph node metastases are associated with compromised survival for patients younger than age 45 years with papillary thyroid cancer. J Clin Oncol. 2015;33:2370-5.

81. Randolph GW, Duh QY, Heller KS, LiVolsi VA, Mandel SJ, Steward DL, et al. The prognostic significance of nodal metastases from papillary thyroid carcinoma can be stratified based on the size and number of metastatic lymph nodes, as well as the presence of extranodal extension. Thyroid. 2012;2:1144-52.

82. Sacks W, Fung CH, Chang JT, Waxman A, Braunstein GD. The effectiveness of radioactive iodine for treatment of low-risk thyroid cancer: a systematic analysis of the peer-reviewed literature from 1966 to April 2008. Thyroid. 2010;20:1235-45.

83. Jonklaas J, Sarlis NJ, Litofsky D, Ain KB, Bigos ST, Brierley JD, et al. Outcomes of patients with differentiated thyroid carcinoma following initial therapy. Thyroid 2006;16: 1229-42.

84. Van Nostrand D, Aiken M, Atkins F, Moreau S, Garcia C, Acio E, et al. The utility of radioiodine scans prior to iodine 131 ablation in patients with well-differentiated thyroid cancer. Thyroid. 2009;19:849-55.

85. Chen MK, Yasrebi M, Samii J, Staib LH, Doddamane I, Cheng DW. The utility of I-123 pretherapy scan inI-131 radioiodine therapy for thyroid cancer. Thyroid. 2012;22:304-9.

86. Pak K, Cheon GJ, Kang KW, Kim SJ, Kim IJ, Kim EE, et al. The effectiveness of recombinant human thyroid-stimulating hormone versus thyroid hormone withdrawal prior to radioiodine remnant ablation in thyroid cancer: a meta-analysis of randomized controlled trials. J Korean Med Sci. 2014;29:811-7.

87. Elisei R, Schlumberger M, Driedger A, Reiners C, Kloos RT, Sherman SI, et al. Follow-up of low-risk differentiated thyroid cancer patients who underwent radioiodine ablation of postsurgical thyroid remnants after either recombinant human thyrotropin or thyroid hormone withdrawal. J Clin Endocrinol Metab. 2009;94:4171-9.

88. Rosario PW, Mineiro Filho AF, Lacerda RX, Calsolari MR. Long-term follow-up of at least five years after recombinant human thyrotropin compared to levothyroxine withdrawal for thyroid remnant ablation with radioactive iodine. Thyroid. 2012;22:332-3.

89. Hugo J, Robenshtok E, Grewal R, Larson S, Tuttle RM. Recombinant human thyroid stimulating hormone assisted radioactive iodine remnant ablation in thyroid cancer patients at intermediate to high risk of recurrence. Thyroid. 2012;22:1007-15.

90. Bal C, Padhy AK, Jana S, Pant GS, Basu AK. Prospective randomized clinical trial to evaluate the optimal dose of 131 I for remnant ablation in patients with differentiated thyroid carcinoma. Cancer. 1996;77:2574-80.

91. Pilli T, Brianzoni E, Capoccetti F, Castagna MG, Fattori S, Poggiu A, et al. A comparison of 1850 (50 mCi) and 3700 MBq (100 mCi) 131-iodine administered doses for recombinant thyrotropin-stimulated postoperative thyroid remnant ablation in differentiated thyroid cancer. J Clin Endocrinol Metab. 2007;92:3542-6.

92. Maenpaa HO, Heikkonen J, Vaalavirta L, Tenhunen M, Joensuu H. Low vs. high radioiodine activity to ablate the thyroid after Thyroidectomy for cancer: a randomized study. PLoS One. 2(3):e1885.

93. Schlumberger M, Catargi B, Borget I, Deandreis D, Zerdoud S, Bridji B, et al. Strategies of radioiodine ablation in patients with low-risk thyroid cancer. NEJM. 2012;366:1663-73.

94. Mallick U, Harmer C, Yap B, Wadsley J, Clarke S, Moss L, et al. Ablation with low-dose radioiodine and thyrotropin alfa in thyroid cancer. NEJM. 2012;366:1674-85.

95. Sawka AM, Ibrahim-Zada I, Galacgac P, Tsang RW, Brierley JD, Ezzat S, et al. Dietary iodine restriction in preparation for radioactive iodine treatment or scanning in well-differentiated thyroid cancer: a systematic review. Thyroid. 2010;20:1129-38.

96. Van Nostrand D, Neutze J, Atkins F. Side effects of "rational dose" iodine-131 therapy for metastatic well-differentiated thyroid carcinoma. J Nucl Med. 1986;27(10):1519-27.

97. Lin WY, Shen YY, Wang SJ. Short-term hazards of low-dose radioiodine ablation therapy in postsurgical thyroid cancer patients. Clin Nucl Med. 1996;21(10):780-2.

98. Brown AP, Chen J, Hitchcock YJ, Szabo A, Shrieve DC, Tward JD. The risk of second primary malignancies up to three decades after the treatment of differentiated thyroid cancer. J Clin Endocrinol Metab. 2008;93:504-15.

99. Berthe E, Henry-Amar M, Michels JJ, Rame JP, Berthet P, Babin E, et al. Risk of second primary cancer following differentiated thyroid cancer. Eur J Nucl Med Mol Imaging. 2004;31:685-91.

100. Husson O, Haak HR, Oranje WA, Mols F, Reemst PH, van de Poll-Franse LV. Health-related quality of life among thyroid cancer survivors: a systematic review. Clin Endocrinol (Oxf). 2011;75(4):544-54.

101. Hirsch D, Ginat M, Levy S, Benbassat C, Weinstein R, Tsvetov G, et al. Illness perception in patients with differentiated epithelial cell thyroid cancer. Thyroid. 2009;19(5): 459-65.

102. Haymart MR, Repplinger DJ, Leverson GE, Elson DF, Sippel RS, Jaume JC, et al. Higher serum thyroid stimulating hormone level in thyroid nodule patients is associated with greater risks of differentiated thyroid cancer and advanced tumor stage. J Clin Endocrinol Metab 2008;93(3):809-14.

103. Kim HK, Yoon JH, Kim SJ, Cho JS, Kweon SS, Kang HC. Higher TSH level is a risk factor for differentiated thyroid cancer. Clin Endocrinol (Oxf). 2013;78(3):472-7.

104. Golbert L, de Cristo AP, Faccin CS, Farenzena M, Folgierini H, Graudenz MS, et al. Serum levels as a predictor of malignancy in thyroid nodules: a prospective study. PLoS One. 2017;12(11): e0188123.

105. Tam AA, Ozdemir D, Aydin C, Bestepe N, Ulusoy S, Sungu N, et al. Association between preoperative thyrotrophin and clinicopathological and aggressive features of papillary thyroid cancer. Endocrine. 2018;59(3):565-72.

106. Mazzaferri EL, Jhiang SM. Long-term impact of initial surgical and medical therapy on papillary and follicular thyroid cancer. Am J Med. 1994;97(5): 418-28.

107. McGriff NJ, Csako G, Gourgiotis L, Lori CG, Pucino F, Sarlis NJ. Effects of thyroid hormone suppression therapy on adverse clinical outcomes in thyroid cancer. Ann Med. 2002;34(7-8): 554-64.

108. Tian T, Huang R, Liu B. Is TSH suppression still necessary in intermediate- and high-risk papillary thyroid cancer patients with pre-ablation stimulated thyroglobulin <1 ng/mL before the first disease assessment? Endocrine. 2019;65: 149-54.

109. Pajamaki N, Metso S, Hakala T, Ebeling T, Huhtala H, Ryodi E, et al. Long-term cardiovascular morbidity and mortality in patients treated for differentiated thyroid cancer. Clin. Endocrinol (Oxf). 2018;88(2):303-10.

110. Yoon BH, Lee Y, Oh HJ, Kim SH, Lee YK. Influence of thyroid-stimulating hormone suppression therapy on bone mineral density in patients with differentiated thyroid cancer: a meta-analysis. J Bone Metab. 2019;26(1):51-60.

111. Tuttle RM, Tala H, Shah J, Leboeuf R, Ghossein R, Gonen M, et al. Estimating risk of recurrence in differentiated thyroid cancer after total thyroidectomy and radioactive iodine remnant ablation: using response to therapy variables to modify the initial risk estimates predicted by the new American Thyroid Association staging system. Thyroid 2010;20:1341-9.

112. Vaisman F, Momesso D, Bulzico DA, Pessoa CH, Dias F, Corbo R, et al. Spontaneous remission in thyroid cancer patients after biochemical incomplete response to initial therapy. Clin Endocrinol (Oxf). 2012;77:132-8.

113. Pitoia F, Bueno F, Urciuoli C, Abelleira E, Cross G, Tuttle RM. Outcomes of patients with differentiated thyroid cancer risk-stratified according to the American Thyroid Association and Latin American Thyroid Society risk of recurrence classification systems. Thyroid. 2013;23:1401-7.

114. Ronga G, Filesi M, Ventroni G, Vestri AR, Signore A. Value of the first serum thyroglobulin level after total thyroidectomy for the diagnosis of metastases from differentiated thyroid carcinoma. Eur J Nucl Med. 1999;26:1448-52.

115. Lin JD, Huang MJ, Hsu BR, Chao TC, Hsueh C, Liu FH, et al. Significance of postoperative serum thyroglobulin levels in patients with papillary and follicular thyroid carcinomas. J Surg Oncol. 2002;80:45-51.

116. Nascimento C, Borget I, Troalen F, Al Ghuzlan A, Deandreis D, Hartl D, et al. Ultrasensitive serum thyroglobulin measurement is useful for the follow-up of patients treated with total Thyroidectomy without radioactive iodine ablation. Eur J Endocrinol. 2013;169:689-93.

117. Rosario PW, Xavier AC, Calsolari MR. Value of postoperative thyroglobulin and ultrasonography for the indication of ablation and ^{131}I activity in patients with thyroid cancer and low risk of recurrence. Thyroid. 2011;21:49-53.

118. Giovanella L, Suriano S, Ceriani L, Verburg FA. Undetectable thyroglobulin in patients with differentiated thyroid carcinoma and residual radioiodine uptake on a postablation whole-body scan. Clin Nucl Med. 2011;36:109-12.

119. Vaisman F, Tuttle RM. Clinical assessment and risk stratification in differentiated thyroid cancer. Endocrinol Metab Clin N Am. 2019;48:99-108.

120. Schlumberger M, Brose M, Elisei R, Leboulleux S, Luster M, Pitoia F, et al. Definition and management of radioactive iodine-refractory differentiated thyroid cancer. Lancet Diabetes Endocrinol. 2014;2(5):356-8.

121. Sabra MM, Grewal RK, Tala H, Larson SM, Tuttle RM. Clinical outcomes following empiric radioiodine therapy in patients with structurally identifiable metastatic follicular cell-

derived thyroid carcinoma with negative diagnostic. Thyroid. 2012;22(9):877-82.

122. Sgouros G, Kolbert KS, Sheikh A, Pentlow KS, Mun EF, Barth A, et al. Patient-specific dosimetry for 131I thyroid cancer therapy using 124I PET and 3-dimensional-internal dosimetry (3D-ID) software. J Nucl Med. 2004;45(8):1366-72.

123. Wang W, Larson SM, Tuttle RM, Kalaigian H, Kolbert K, Sonenberg M, et al. Resistance of [18F]-fluorodeoxyglucose-avid metastatic thyroid cancer lesions to treatment with high-dose radioactive iodine. Thyroid. 2001;11(12): 1169-75.

124. Vaisman F, Tala H, Grewal R, Tuttle RM. In differentiated thyroid cancer, an incomplete structural response to therapy is associated with significantly worse clinical outcomes than only an incomplete thyroglobulin response. Thyroid. 2011;21(12):1317-22.

125. Dadu R, Devine C, Hernandez M, Waguespack SG, Busaidy NL, Hu MI, et al. Role of salvage targeted therapy in differentiated thyroid cancer patients who failed first-line sorafenib. JCEM. 2014;99(6):2086-94.

126. Massicotte M-H, Brassard M, Claude-Desroches M, Borget I, Bonichon F, Giraudet A-L, et al. Tyrosine kinase inhibitor treatments in patients with metastatic thyroid carcinomas: a retrospective study of the TUTHYREF network. Eur J Endocrinol. 2014;170(4):575-82.

127. Schlumberger M, Challeton C, De Vathaire F, Travagli JP, Gardet P, Lumbroso JD, et al. Radioactive iodine treatment and external radiotherapy for lung and bone metastases from thyroid carcinoma. J Nucl Med. 1996;37:598-605.

128. Pujol P, Daures J-P, Nsakala N, Baldet L, Bringer J, Jaffiol C. Degree of thyrotropin suppression as a prognostic determinant in differentiated thyroid cancer. J Clin Endocrinol Metab. 1996;81:4318-23.

129. Durante C, Haddy N, Baudin E, Leboulleux S, Hartl D, Travagli JP, et al. Long-term outcome of 444 patients with distant metastases from papillary and follicular thyroid carcinoma: benefits and limits of radioiodine therapy. J Clin Endocrinol Metab. 2006;91:2892-9.

130. Ford D, Giridharan S, McConkey C, Hartley A, Brammer C, Watkinson JC, et al. External beam radiotherapy in the management of differentiated thyroid cancer. Clin Oncol (R Coll Radiol). 2003;15:337-41.

131. Vitale G, Fonderico F, Martignetti A, Caraglia M, Ciccarelli A, Nuzzo V, et al. Pamidronate improves the quality of life and induces clinical remission of bone metastases in patients with thyroid cancer. Br J Cancer. 2001;84:1586-90.

132. Mazziotti G, Formenti AM, Panarotto MB, Arvat E, Chiti A, Cuocolo A, et al. Real-life management and outcome of thyroid carcinoma-related bone metastases: results from a nationwide multicenter experience. Endocrine. 2018;59(1):90-101.

133. Durante C, Puxeddu E, Ferretti E, Morisi R, Moretti S, Bruno R, et al. BRAF mutations in papillary thyroid carcinomas inhibit genes involved in iodine metabolism. J Clin Endocrinol Metab. 2007;92:2840-3.

134. Liu D, Hu S, Hou P, Jiang D, Condouris S, Xing M. Suppression of BRAF/MEK/MAP kinase pathway restores expression of iodide-metabolizing genes in thyroid cells expressing the V600E BRAF mutant. Clin Cancer Res. 2007;13:1341-1349.

135. De Vita G, Bauer L, da Costa VMC, De Felice M, Baratta MG, De Menna M, et al. Dose-dependent inhibition of thyroid differentiation by RAS oncogenes. Mol Endocrinol. 2005;19: 76-89.

136. Chakravarty D, Santos E, Ryder M, Knauf JA, Liao X-H, West BL, et al. Small-molecule MAPK inhibitors restore radioiodine incorporation in mouse thyroid cancers with conditional BRAF activation. J Clin Invest. 2011;121:4700-11.

137. Nagarajah J, Le M, Knauf JA, Ferrandino G, Montero-Conde C, Pillarsetty N, et al. Sustained ERK inhibition maximizes responses of BrafV600E thyroid cancers to radioiodine. J Clin Invest. 2016;126:4119-24.

138. Ho AL, Grewal RK, Leboeuf R, Sherman EJ, Pfister DG, Deandreis D, et al. Selumetinib-enhanced radioiodine uptake in advanced thyroid cancer. N Engl J Med. 2013;368:623-32.

139. Rothenberg SM, McFadden DG, Palmer EL, Daniels GH, Wirth LJ. Redifferentiation of iodine-refractory BRAF V600E-mutant metastatic papillary thyroid cancer with dabrafenib. Clin Cancer Res. 2015;21:1028-35.

140. French JD. Revisiting immune-based therapies for aggressive follicular cell–derived thyroid cancers. Thyroid. 2013;23(5): 529-42.

141. Cunha LL, Marcello MA, Ward LS. The role of the inflammatory microenvironment in thyroid carcinogenesis. Endocr Relat Cancer. 2014;21(3):85-103.

142. Bernet V, Smallridge R. New therapeutic options for advanced forms of thyroid cancer. Expert Opin Emerg Drugs. 2014;19(2):225-41.

143. Rego-Iraeta A, Perez-Mendez LF, Mantinan B, Garcia-Mayor RV. Time trends for thyroid cancer in northwestern Spain: true rise in the incidence of micro and larger forms of papillary thyroid carcinoma. Thyroid. 2009;19: 333-40.

144. McLeod DS, Jonklaas J, Brierley JD, Ain KB, Cooper DS, Fein HG, et al. Reassessing the NTCTCS staging systems for differentiated thyroid cancer, including age at diagnosis. Thyroid. 2015;25:1097-105.

145. Alfalah H, Cranshaw I, Jany T, Arnalsteen L, Leteurtre E, Cardot C, et al. Risk factors for lateral cervical lymph node involvement in follicular thyroid carcinoma. World J Surg. 2008;32:2623-66.

146. Parameswaran R, Shulin Hu J, Min En N, Tan WB, Yuan NK. Patterns of metastasis in follicular thyroid carcinoma and the difference between early and delayed presentation. Ann R Coll Surg Engl. 2017;99:151-4.

147. Zaydfudim V, Feurer ID, Griffin MR, Phay JE. The impact of lymph node involvement on survival in patients with papillary and follicular thyroid carcinoma. Surgery. 2008;144: 1070-77.

148. Kobayashi K, Hirokawa M, Yabuta T, Masuoka H, Fukushima M, Kihara M, et al. Tumor protrusion with intensive blood signals on ultrasonography is a strongly suggestive finding of follicular thyroid carcinoma. Med Ultrason. 2016;18:25-9.

149. Cibas ES, Ali SZ. The Bethesda system for reporting thyroid cytopathology. Am J Clin Pathol. 2009;132:658-65.

150. Nikiforov YE. Molecular diagnostics of thyroid tumors. Arch Pathol Lab Med. 2011;135:569-77.

151. Wu JX, Young S, Hung ML, Li N, Yang SE, Cheung DS, et al. Clinical factors influencing the performance of gene expression classifier testing in indeterminate thyroid nodules. Thyroid. 2016;26:916-22.

152. Ghossein R. Update to the College of American Pathologists reporting on thyroid carcinomas. Head Neck Pathol. 2009;3:86-93.

153. Franc B, de la Salmoniere P, Lange F, Hoang C, Louvel A, de Roquancourt A, et al. Interobserver and intraobserver reproducibility in the histopathology of follicular thyroid carcinoma. Hum Pathol. 2003;34:1092-100.

154. 2017 WHO Classification of Tumours of Endocrine Organs (4th edition). Lyon: IRAC; 2017.

155. Lang W, Georgii A, Stauch G, Kienzle E. The differentiation of atypical adenomas and encapsulated follicular carcinomas in the thyroid gland. Virchows Arch Pathol Anat Histol. 1980;385:125-41.

156. Lang BH, Shek TW, Wu AL, Wan KY. The total number of tissue blocks per centimetre of tumor significantly correlated with the risk of distant metastasis in patients with minimally invasive follicular thyroid carcinoma. Endocrine. 2017;55:496-502.

157. Daniels GH. Follicular thyroid carcinoma: a perspective. Thyroid. 2018;28(10):1229-42.

158. Kuo EJ, Roman SA, Sosa JA. Patients with follicular and Hürthle cell microcarcinomas have compromised survival: a population level study of 22,738 patients. Surgery. 2013;154:1246-53; discussion 1253-44.

159. Goffredo P, Sosa JA, Roman SA. Differentiated thyroid cancer presenting with distant metastases: a population analysis over two decades. World J Surg. 2013; 37: 1599-605.

160. Huang CC, Hsueh C, Liu FH, Chao TC, Lin JD. Diagnostic and therapeutic strategies for minimally and widely invasive follicular thyroid carcinomas. Surg Oncol 2011;20(1):1-6.

161. Van Heerden JA, Hay ID, Goellner JR, Salomao D, Ebersold JR, Bergstralh EJ, et al. Follicular thyroid carcinoma with capsular invasion alone: a non-threatening malignancy. Surgery. 1992;112:1130-6.

162. Collini P, Sampietro G, Pilotti S. Extensive vascular invasion is a marker of risk of relapse in encapsulated non-Hürthle cell follicular carcinoma of the thyroid gland: a clinicopathological study of 18 consecutive cases from a single institution with an 11-year median follow-up. Histopathology. 2004;44(1):35-9.

163. Harness JK, Thompson NW, McLeod MK, Eckhauser FE, Lloyd RV. Follicular carcinoma of the thyroid gland: trends and treatment. Surgery. 1984;96(6):972-80.

164. Sugino K, Kameyama K, Ito K, Nagahama M, Kitagawa W, Shibuya H, et al. Outcomes and prognostic factors of 251 patients with minimally invasive follicular thyroid carcinoma. Thyroid. 2012;22(8):798-804.

165. Asari R, Koperek O, Scheuba C, Riss P, Kaserer K, Hoffmann M, et al. Follicular thyroid carcinoma in an iodine-replete endemic goiter region: a prospectively collected, retrospectively analyzed clinical trial. Ann Surg. 2009;249:1023-31.

166. Mueller-Gaertner HW, Brzac HT, Rehpenning W. Prognostic indices for tumor relapse and tumor mortality in follicular thyroid carcinoma. Cancer. 1991;67:1903-11.

167. Niepomniszcze H, Suarez H, Pitoia F, Pignatta A, Danilowicz K, Manavela M, et al. Follicular carcinoma presenting as autonomous functioning thyroid nodule and containing an activating mutation of the TSH receptor (T620I) and a mutation of the Ki-RAS (G12C) genes. Thyroid. 2006;16:497-503.

168. Spambalg D, Sharifi N, Elisei R, Gross JL, Medeiros-Neto G, Fagin JA. Structural studies of the thyrotropin receptor and Gs alpha in human thyroid cancers: low prevalence of mutations predicts infrequent involvement in malignant transformation. J Clin Endocrinol Metab. 1996;81:3898-901.

169. Ishihara T, Ikekubo K, Shimodahira M, Iwakura T, Kobayashi M, Hino M, et al. A case of TSH receptor antibody-positive hyperthyroidism with functioning metastases of thyroid carcinoma. Endocr J. 2002;49:241-5.

170. Stathatos N, Gaz R, Ross DS, Daniels GH. High radioactive iodine uptake despite a fully suppressed TSH in a patient with thyroid cancer. J Clin Endocrinol Metab. 2011;96:589.

171. Kim BW, Daniels GH, Harrison BJ, Price A, Harney JW, Larsen PR, et al. Overexpression of type 2 iodothyronine deiodinase in follicular carcinoma as a cause of low circulating free thyroxine levels. J Clin Endocrinol Metab. 2003;88:594-8.

172. Miyauchi A, Takamura Y, Ito Y, Miya A, Kobayashi K, Matsuzuka F, et al. 3,5,3'-Triiodothyronine thyrotoxicosis due to increased conversion of administered levothyroxine in patients with massive metastatic follicular thyroid carcinoma. J Clin Endocrinol Metab. 2008;93:2239-42.

173. Gasparre G, Porcelli AM, Bonora E, Pennisi LF, Toller M, Iommarini L, et al. Disruptive mitochondrial DNA mutations in complex I subunits are markers of oncocytic phenotype in thyroid tumors. Proc Natl Acad Sci U S A. 2007;104:9001-6.

174. Mills SC, Haq M, Smellie WJ, Harmer C. Hurthle cell carcinoma of the thyroid: retrospective review of 62 patients treated at the Royal Marsden Hospital between 1946 and 2003. Eur J Surg Oncol. 2009;35:230-4.

175. Oluic B, Paunovic I, Loncar Z, Djukic V, Diklic A, Jovanovic M, et al. Survival and prognostic factors for survival, cancer specific survival and disease free interval in 239 patients with Hurthle cell carcinoma: a single center experience. BMC Cancer. 2017;17:371.

176. Pryma DA, Schoder H, Gonen M, Robbins RJ, Larson SM, Yeung HWD, et al. Diagnostic accuracy and prognostic value of 18F-FDG PET in Hurthle cell thyroid cancer patients. J Nucl Med. 2006;47:1260-6.

177. Bulotta S, Celano M, Costante G, Russo D. Emerging strategies for managing differentiated thyroid cancers refractory to radioiodine. Endocrine. 2016;52:214-21.

178. Howlader N, Noone AM, Krapcho M, et al. SEER Cancer Statistics Review, 1975–2014. Bethesda, MD: National Cancer Institute; 2017.

179. Turcotte LM, Neglia JP. Subsequent malignant neoplasms in the survivor of childhood cancer: where we have been and where we are going? Future Oncol. 2017;13:23.

180. Sigurdson AJ, Ronckers CM, Mertens AC, Stovall M, Smith SA, Liu Y, et al. Primary thyroid cancer after a first tumour in childhood (the Childhood Cancer Survivor Study): a nested case-control study. Lancet. 2005;365:2014-23.

181. Dolphin GW. The risk of thyroid cancers following irradiation. Health Phys. 1968;15:219-228

182. Ron E, Lubin JH, Shore RE, Mabuchi K, Modan B, Pottern LM, et al. Thyroid cancer after exposure to external radiation: a pooled analysis of seven studies. Radiat Res. 1995;141:259-277.

183. Tan MH, Mester JL, Ngeow J, Rybicki LA, Orloff MS, Eng C. Lifetime cancer risks in individuals with germline PTEN mutations. Clin Cancer Res. 2012;18(2):400-7.

184. Fenton PA, Clarke SE, Owen W, Hibbert J, Hodgson SV. Cribriform variant papillary thyroid cancer: a characteristic of familial adenomatous polyposis. Thyroid. 2001;11(2):193-7.

185. Chow SM, Law SC, Mendenhall WM, Au S-K, Yau S, Mang O, et al. Differentiated thyroid carcinoma in childhood and adolescence-clinical course and role of radioiodine. Pediatr Blood Cancer. 2004;42(2):176-83.

186. Welch Dinauer CA, Tuttle RM, Robie DK, McClellan DR, Svec RL, Adair C, et al. Clinical features associated with metastasis and recurrence of differentiated thyroid cancer in children, adolescents and young adults. Clin Endocrinol. 1998;49(5):619-28.

187. Ren PY, Liu J, Xue S, Chen G. Pediatric differentiated thyroid carcinoma: the clinicopathological features and the coexistence of Hashimoto's thyroiditis. Asian J Surg. 2019;42(1):112-9.

188. Handkiewicz-Junak D, Wloch J, Roskosz J, Krajewska J, Kropinska A, Pomorski L, et al. Total thyroidectomy and

adjuvant radioiodine treatment independently decrease locoregional recurrence risk in childhood and adolescent differentiated thyroid cancer. J Nucl Med. 2007;48(6):879-88.

189. Grigsby PW, Gal-or A, Michalski JM, Doherty GM. Childhood and adolescent thyroid carcinoma. Cancer. 2002;95(4): 724-9.

190. Nanapragasam A. Papillary thyroid cancer. 2019. Available from https://radiopaedia. org/articles/papillary-thyroid-cancer. Accessed May 20, 2019.

191. Unger K, Zitzelsberger H, Salvatore G, Santoro M, Bogdanova T, Braselmann H, et al. Heterogeneity in the distribution of RET/PTC rearrangements within individual post-Chernobyl papillary thyroid carcinomas. J Clin Endocrinol Metab. 2004;89(9):4272-79.

192. Nikiforov YE, Rowland JM, Bove KE, Monforte-Munoz H, Fagin JA. Distinct pattern of ret oncogene rearrangements in morphological variants of radiation-induced and sporadic thyroid papillary carcinomas in children. Cancer Res. 1997;57(9):1690-94.

193. Thomas GA, Bunnell HA, Cook HA, Williams ED, Nerovnya A, Cherstvoy ED, et al. High prevalence of RET/PTC rearrangements in Ukrainian and Belarussian post-Chernobyl thyroid papillary carcinomas: a strong correlation between RET/PTC3 and the solid-follicular variant. J Clin Endocrinol Metab. 1999;84(11):4232-38.

194. Givens DJ, Buchmann LO, Agarwal AM, Grimmer JF, Hunt JP. BRAF V600E does not predict aggressive features of pediatric papillary thyroid carcinoma. Laryngoscope. 2014;124(9):389.

195. Suchy B, Waldmann V, Klugbauer S, Rabes HM. Absence of RAS and p53 mutations in thyroid carcinomas of children after Chernobyl in contrast to adult thyroid tumours. Br J Cancer. 1998;77:952-5.

196. Prasad ML, Vyas M, Horne MJ, Virk RK, Morotti R, Liu Z, et al. NTRK fusion oncogenes in pediatric papillary thyroid carcinoma in northeast United States. Cancer. 2016;122(7):1097-107.

197. Francis GL, Waguespack SG, Bauer AJ, Angelos P, Benvenga S, Cerutti JM, et al.; American Thyroid Association Guidelines Task Force. Management guidelines for children with thyroid nodules and differentiated thyroid cancer. Thyroid. 2015;25(7):716-59.

198. Jarzab B, Handkiewicz-Junak D, Wloch J. Juvenile differentiated thyroid carcinoma and the role of radioiodine in its treatment: a qualitative review. Endocr Relat Cancer. 2005;12(4):773-803.

199. Pawelczak M, David R, Franklin B, Kessler M, Lam L, Shah B. Outcomes of children and adolescents with well-differentiated thyroid carcinoma and pulmonary metastases following 131-I treatment: a systematic review. Thyroid. 2010;20(10):1095-101.

200. Bal CS, Kumar A, Chandra P, Dwivedi SN, Mukhopadhyaya S. Is chest X-ray or high-resolution computed tomography scan of the chest sufficient investigation to detect pulmonary metastasis in pediatric differentiated thyroid cancer? Thyroid. 2004;14:217-25.

201. Biko J, Reiners C, Kreissl MC, Verburg FA, Demidchik Y, Drozd V. Favourable course of disease after incomplete remission on 131I therapy in children with pulmonary metastases of papillary thyroid carcinoma: 10 years follow-up. Eur J Nucl Med Mol Imaging. 2010;38:1269-302.

202. Sugino K, Nagahama M, Kitagawa W, Shibuya H, Ohkuwa K, Uruno T, et al. Papillary thyroid carcinoma in children and adolescents: long-term follow-up and clinical characteristics. World J Surg. 2015;39(9):2259-65.

203. O'Gorman CS, Hamilton J, Rachmiel M, Gupta A, Ngan BY, Daneman D. Thyroid cancer in childhood: a retrospective review of childhood course. Thyroid. 2010;20:375-80.

204. Rachmiel M, Charron M, Gupta A, Hamilton J, Wherrett D, Forte V, et al. Evidence-based review of treatment and follow up of pediatric patients with differentiated thyroid carcinoma. J Pediatr Endocrinol Metab. 2006;19:1377-93.

205. Powers PA, Dinauer CA, Tuttle RM, Robie DK, McClellan DR, Francis GL. Tumor size and extent of disease at diagnosis predict the response to initial therapy for papillary thyroid carcinoma in children and adolescents. J Pediatr Endocrinol Metab. 2003;16:693-702.

206. Leboeuf R, Emerick LE, Martorella AJ, Tuttle M. Impact of pregnancy on serum thyroglobulin and detection of recurrent disease shortly after delivery in thyroid cancer survivors. Thyroid. 2007;17:543-7.

207. Hirsch D, Levy S, Tsvetov S, Weinstein R, Lifshitz A, Singer J, et al. Impact of pregnancy on outcome and prognosis of survivors of papillary thyroid cancer. Thyroid. 2010;20(10):1179-85.

208. Oken E, Braverman LE, Platek D, Mitchell ML, Lee SL, Pearce EN. Neonatal thyroxine, maternal thyroid function, and child cognition. J Clin Endocrinol Metab. 2009;94:497-503.

209. Holt EH. Care of the pregnant thyroid cancer patient. Curr Opin Oncol. 2010;22:1-5.

210. Loh JA, Wartofsky L, Jonklaas J, Burman KD. The magnitude of increased levothyroxine requirements in hypothyroid pregnant women depends upon the etiology of the hypothyroidism. Thyroid. 2009;19(3):269-75.

211. Abalovich M, Amino N, Barbour LA, Cobin RH, De Groot LJ, Glinoer D, et al. Management of thyroid dysfunction during pregnancy and postpartum: an Endocrine Society Clinical Practice Guideline. J Clin Endocrinol Metab. 2007;92 (8 Suppl):S1-S47.

212. Amit M, Boonsripitayanon M, Goepfert RP, Tam S, Busaidy NL, Cabanillas ME, et al. Extrathyroidal extension: does strap muscle invasion alone influence recurrence and survival in patients with differentiated thyroid cancer? Ann Surg Oncol. 2018;25(11):3380-8.

213. Dralle H, Brauckhoff M, Machens A, Gimm O. Surgical management of advanced thyroid cancer invading the aerodigestive tract. In: Clark OH, Duh QY, Kebebew E (Eds.). Textbook on Endocrine Surgery, 2nd edition. Philadelphia, PA: Elsevier Saunders; 2005. pp. 318-33

214. Brauckhoff M, Dralle H. Extrathyroidal thyroid cancer: results of tracheal shaving and tracheal resection. Chirurg. 2011;82: 134-40.

215. Brauckhoff M, Dralle H. Cervicovisceral resection in invasive thyroid tumors. Chirurg. 2009;80:88-98.

216. McCaffrey JC. Aerodigestive tract invasion by well-differentiated thyroid carcinoma: diagnosis, management, prognosis, and biology. Laryngoscope. 2006;116:1-11.

217. Nishida T, Nakao K, Hamaji M. Differentiated thyroid carcinoma with airway invasion: Indication for tracheal resection based on the extent of cancer invasion. J Thorac Cardiovasc Surg. 1997;114:84-92.

Follicular Neoplasm of the Thyroid Gland

Natarajan Dorairajan, Poongkodi K

◇ INTRODUCTION

Tumors of the thyroid gland most often arise from the thyroid follicle, which constitutes the basic functional unit of the thyroid gland. These follicular cell-derived tumors include follicular neoplasm (FN) and papillary thyroid carcinoma (PTC). The thyroid follicle is composed of sphere of single-layered thyroid follicular epithelial cells (TFCs), around a central space filled with colloid. Each follicle, about 100–300 μm in size, is surrounded by a network of capillaries, supporting fibrous stroma, nerves, and parafollicular cells. The TFCs are derived from embryonic endometrium of the floor of primitive pharynx; whereas, the parafollicular cells or C cells secreting calcitonin are of neural crest origin, which migrates through the ultimobranchial bodies to be distributed predominantly at the junction of upper and middle third of the lateral lobes of thyroid gland. The primary function of the thyroid follicle is thyroid hormone synthesis and its release under the stimulation of thyroid-stimulating hormone (TSH). TFCs exhibit marked polarity such that the sodium iodide symporter (NIS) and TSH receptor are expressed along the basolateral membrane while pendrin with thyroperoxidase and dual oxidase enzyme complex are along the apical membrane. By the virtue of high expression of the NIS, these TFCs selectively take up iodine and conjugate iodine to produce triiodothyronine (T3) and thyroxine (T4). NIS expression by follicular-derived cancers provided the opportunity for the first and to date, the most effective targeted therapy for cancer, radioactive iodine 131-I therapy. Thyroglobulin (Tg) is exclusively synthesized by TFCs and, therefore, can be used as a tumor marker for prognostication of these TSH-dependent well-differentiated cancers including PTC and follicular thyroid carcinoma (FTC). In contrast, medullary thyroid carcinoma arising from calcitonin-secreting parafollicular cells are neither TSH dependent nor iodine avid. This chapter focuses on an FN of the thyroid gland. The term FN refers to the new growth of follicular-derived cells including both the benign follicular adenoma (FA) and malignant follicular carcinoma of thyroid. PTC and Hürthle cell tumors will be described elsewhere in the text.

◇ INCIDENCE AND PREVALENCE OF FOLLICULAR NEOPLASM

Follicular thyroid carcinoma is the second most common thyroid malignancy after PTC. FTC constitutes 10–15% of all the thyroid malignancies. Depending on environmental factors including dietary habits, iodine intake, and ethnicity, the registered incidence of FTC varies widely from 10 to 32% of differentiated thyroid carcinoma (DTC) or even higher, up to 40% in iodine-deficient areas. With the turn of the century and advent of high-frequency ultrasonography, increasing incidence of DTC, including subcentimeter PTC, was reported. Although it was initially attributed to surveillance bias, recent data suggests that a true rise is likely due to the increasing incidence rates of DTC across all sizes and stages. On the contrary, more recently, an Italian cohort study comprising 4,187 patients reported a decline in FTC prevalence rate from 19.5 to 9% in patients diagnosed with DTC before and after 1990. Similarly, the French Thyroid Cancer registry registered an annual decline rate of 2.2% among men and 0.5% among women in the FTC incidence from the year 1983 to 2000. The decline in FTC incidence may be explained partly by the use of strict histologic criteria [e.g., exclusion of atypical FA, identification of follicular variants of PTC, and noninvasive follicular thyroid neoplasm with papillary-like nuclear features (NIFTP)] and also to iodine supplementation programs. Epidemiological data suggests that transition from increased risk of FTC to PTC is associated with increased iodine intake (either due to national iodine supplementation program or immigration from iodine-deficient to iodine-replete zones).

◇ ETIOPATHOGENESIS

The important risk factors for DTC are exposure to ionizing radiation during childhood and the presence of family history of thyroid cancer. Chernobyl nuclear outbreak resulted in the development of PTCs associated with RET/PTC rearrangements, and a few cases of FTC. Iodine deficiency and endemic goiter increase the risk of development of FTC. Iodine supplementation has resulted in the decline of FTC but relative rise in PTC incidence rate worldwide. Molecular studies have revealed various oncogene activation and genetic alteration in an FN. *Rat sarcoma (RAS)* gene mutations or a *paired box gene 8/peroxisome proliferator-activated receptor gamma (PAX8-PPARγ)* gene rearrangement is found in 80% of FTC cases. The *RAS* gene codes for multiple G proteins that are involved in intracellular signaling through the Raf-MEK-MAPK kinase pathway. Point mutations in the *N-RAS*, *H-RAS*, and *K-RAS* gene cause constitutive activation of signaling proteins involved in mitogen activated protein kinase pathways, leading to uncontrolled growth. *RAS* mutations occur in 40–49% of FTC cases. The *PAX8-PPAR* gene rearrangement occurs exclusively in an FN, about 4–13% in FAs and 29–56% in FTCs. *PAX8* is a gene that codes for a nuclear protein product of a thyroid-specific transcription factor that is involved in follicular cell differentiation. *PAX8-PPAR* gene rearrangement results from chromosomal translocation t(2;3) (q13; p25), which in turn impairs PPAR function, leading to loss of growth inhibitory controls. Micro-RNAs (miRNAs) are small noncoding segments of RNA containing about 25 nucleotides. miRNAs negatively regulate gene transcription by binding to gene promoters, thereby affecting apoptosis and cell proliferation. The expression of many miRNAs including miR-192, miR-197, miR-328, and miR-346 is reported to be significantly higher in FTC compared to FA. Mutations in the *phosphatase* and *tensin homolog suppressor* gene and the phosphatidylinositol 3-kinase-Akt pathway appear to be important pathway in the development of FTC, compared to mitogen-activated protein kinase (MAPK) pathway, which is more common in PTC. Recently, telomerase reverse transcriptase (TERT) promotor mutations are frequently seen in FTCs, and more common in aggressive variants. Gene mutations in p53, c-myc, c-fos, thyrotropin (TSH) receptor and loss of heterozygosity for *HGF* have also been implicated in the pathogenesis of follicular thyroid cancer. Activating mutations in the *TSH receptor* gene and less frequently in the adenylate cyclase-stimulating *G-alpha protein* gene that results in increased thyroid hormone secretion independent of TSH can result in monoclonal expansion of TFCs and hence, functioning FAs. Whereas, about 20% of patients with nonfunctioning FAs possess *N-RAS* and *K-RAS* mutations, which may play a role in the evolution of FA to FTC.

◇ CLINICAL PRESENTATION AND EVALUATION OF FOLLICULAR NEOPLASM

The most common presentation of an FN, including both FA and FTC, is a solitary thyroid nodule and may be associated with thyroiditis or nodular hyperplasia. Most patients are asymptomatic. But large tumors compressing the trachea, esophagus, or recurrent laryngeal nerve can cause difficulty in breathing, swallowing, coughing or choking spells, and hoarseness. Sudden increase in size or pain may occur due to intratumoral hemorrhage or cystic degeneration. Rarely, patients may present with hyperthyroidism. Every thyroid nodule identified by the patient or directed physician's examination or detected as incidentaloma should be carefully evaluated with high-frequency neck ultrasound, thyroid function tests, and fine-needle aspiration cytology (FNAC) as per the American Thyroid Association (ATA) recommendations.

High-frequency Ultrasound of the Neck

Cervical ultrasound with high-frequency probe of 7–10 MHz is the best available noninvasive modality for the evaluation of thyroid nodules. Sonographic features associated with high risk of malignancy include solid nature, hypoechogenicity, presence of punctate microcalcification, indistinct or irregular margins/microlobulations, absent halo sign, taller than wide configuration in transverse axis, chaotic intranodular vascularity, break in egg-shell calcifications, and lymph node with metastatic deposits. Rounded configuration, lack of fatty hilum, punctate calcification, and peripheral vascularity should raise the suspicion of malignant lymph node. Assessment of blood flow in an FN with Duplex Doppler ultrasonography has shown a high negative predictive value (NPV) of 96% for carcinoma, but low positive predictive value (PPV) of only 15%, implying that malignancy is unlikely in an FN lacking intranodular blood flow. Ultrasound evaluation of contralateral lobe has important clinical implications and can detect nonpalpable nodules in 60–70% of the cases.

Fine-needle Non-aspiration Cytology

Fine-needle aspiration cytology is a well-established diagnostic tool for the preoperative evaluation of thyroid nodules. It is performed manually by simply passing a 25-G or 27-G needle to and fro into the thyroid nodule without any suction device or piston mounted on it. The cytologic material is collected in the hub of the needle by capillary action and is extruded onto the slide for on-site examination. Hence, referred as fine-needle capillary cytology (FNCC) or fine-needle nonaspiration cytology (FNNAC), wherein, the yield is cellular and adequate. This cytopuncture technique is less painful and hemorrhagic, compared to aspiration with larger-bore needle (23 or 24 G) mounted with suction device. Air-dried smears prepared by Romanowsky-modified methods (Hemacolor, May–Grünwald–Giemsa or Diff-Quik method) give information on cellular architecture (monolayer sheets, papillary, trabecular, and macro- and microfollicular pattern); cell types (TFCs, Hürthle cells, and lymphocytes); and background (watery colloid and hemorrhage). Wet smears detail the nuclear features (enlargement, grooves, inclusions, etc.) necessary to make a diagnosis of PTC. Adequacy of smear is defined by the presence of at least six cluster of 10–20 well-preserved follicular epithelial cells and may require as many as six passes into a nodule. FNNAC under ultrasound guidance is recommended for the following: (1) nodules located posteriorly, (2) complex cyst/partially cystic nodules to direct on the solid component/wall of the lesion, and (3) small or nonpalpable nodules having sonographic features suspicious for malignancy. The ATA and European Thyroid Association have recommended uniform reporting of FNNAC using *The Bethesda System for Reporting of Thyroid Cytopathology* (TBSRTC). TBSRTC uses standard terminology and morphologic criteria for thyroid cytopathology to facilitate clear communication, epidemiological data collection, and comparison across international borders. TBSRTC is a six-tiered categorization of cytopathology that indicates escalating risk of malignancy and appropriate clinical management. However, FNNAC cannot distinguish benign FA from malignant FTC. The gold standard histopathologic examination of formalin-fixed paraffin-embedded tissue is necessary to demonstrate the presence of capsular and/or vascular invasion to confirm malignancy. Thus, follicular lesions or nodules with indeterminate cytology are included in the Bethesda category III (atypia of undetermined significance or follicular lesion of undetermined significance) and Bethesda category IV (an FN or suspicious for an FN).

Bethesda Category IV: Follicular Neoplasm or Suspicious for a Follicular Neoplasm

This diagnostic category helps to identify a nodule that might be an FTC and triages it for surgical lobectomy. The limitation of FNNAC is its inability to distinguish FA from FTC. Hence, these cytologic smears are reported as "follicular neoplasm". Thus, FNNAC only functions as a screening test in follicular lesions of thyroid and definitive diagnosis often requires surgical resection and a complete histopathological examination (HPE). The terminology *suspicious for an FN* is preferred over an *FN* since more than one-third of the lesions included under this category turn out to be hyperplastic proliferations of TFCs from multinodular goiter rather than neoplasm. This diagnostic category is further subdivided into two subcategories, namely, (1) lesions that are likely benign and (2) lesions that are suspicious for neoplasm and possibly malignant. The cytologic criteria that distinguish benign from potentially malignant thyroid lesions include the follicular group architecture, amount of colloid, and cytologic atypia. The thyroid aspirates from benign lesion exhibit a predominance of macrofollicles and flat orderly honeycomb sheets of TFCs in a background of colloid. In contrast, thyroid aspirates composed of microfollicles (small follicular groups of 6–12 follicular cells with or without a small amount of central colloid or crowded trabeculae and groups of overlapping follicular cells) are features of FTC as well as some adenomas. Other cytologic features predicting malignancy include transgressing vessels, anisokaryosis, nuclear pleomorphism, increased cellularity with crowding, greater percentage of single cells, and a fewer macrofollicular formations. This FN/SFN category accounts for 20% of all FNNACs and has a

15–30% risk of malignancy. Surgical removal of the lesion is generally warranted in this group. Many of FN/SFN lesions prove to be FAs or adenomatoid nodules of multinodular goiter, both of which are more common than FTC. Majority of the lesions that prove to be malignant are FTCs, but follicular variants of papillary carcinoma constitute a significant proportion of cases and occasionally classical PTC.

Bethesda Category III: Atypia of Undetermined Significance or Follicular Lesion of Undetermined Significance

The atypia of undetermined significance or follicular lesion of undetermined significance (AUS/FLUS) category is reserved for specimens "that contain follicular, lymphoid, or other cell types with architectural and/or nuclear atypia that is not sufficient to be classified as suspicious for an FN, suspicious for malignancy, or malignant. Whereas, the atypia is more markedly seen than that of benign lesions." Interpretation as AUS is appropriate under the following circumstances.

- An aspirate that contains a prominent population of microfollicles which does not otherwise fulfill the criteria for an "FN/suspicious for an FN." Such a scenario is likely when the aspirate is sparingly cellular with predominance of microfollicles and scant colloid. On the other hand, in a moderately or markedly cellular aspirate, a more prominent than usual population of microfollicles may occur, but the overall proportion of microfollicles is not sufficient for a diagnosis of an FN/suspicious for an FN.
- A sparsely cellular aspirate with predominance of Hürthle cells and scant colloid.
- Presence of sample preparation artifact, which hinders the interpretation of follicular cell atypia, e.g., (1) air-drying technique can cause artifacts which include cytoplasmic and nuclear enlargement, smudgy and pale chromatin, and/or mildly irregular nuclear contours and (2) crowding due to clotting artifact.
- Presence of a virtually exclusive population of Hürthle cells in a moderately or markedly cellular aspirate, but the clinical setting is suggestive of benign Hürthle cell nodule, e.g., (1) chronic lymphocytic thyroiditis or Hashimoto's thyroiditis and (2) multinodular goiter.

An AUS/FLUS accounts for 3–18% of all thyroid FNNAC and has a 5–15% risk of malignancy. This category warrants a repeat FNA in 3–6 months. A repeat FNA provides more definitive interpretation in most cases but a repeat AUS occurs in 20% of the cases. In such a situation, patient is kept under observation or taken up for surgery in view of risk factors, and concerning clinical and sonographic features.

Molecular testing on FNA samples could possibly increase the diagnostic accuracy of cytologically indeterminate lesion and, hence, decrease the need for diagnostic lobectomy. Recently, a seven-gene mutation testing panel has been proposed to test for *BRAF*, *NRAS*, *HRAS*, and *KRAS* point mutations, as well as *RET/PTC1* and *RET/PTC3*, with or without *PAX8/PPARγ* rearrangements. Owing to the high rate of specificity (86–100%) and high PPV (84–100%), they can be useful as a *rule-in test*. However, a negative test result does not definitely rule out malignancy in this population. On the other hand, high sensitivity and NPV (of 92% and 93%, respectively) of 167 gene expression classifier (GEC) identifying mRNA expression of 167 genes make it a useful *rule-out test*. The relatively low specificity of the 167 GEC test (mean values 48–53% in indeterminate nodules subject to histopathologic confirmation) suggests that the test cannot definitely rule-in malignancy in indeterminate nodules. Other tests include immunohistochemical staining with galectin-3, Hector Battifora mesothelial-1 (HBME-1), and cytokeratin-19 (CK19); molecular markers such as mRNA and miRNA; and finally, peripheral blood TSH receptor mRNA assay. However, no single test can definitely rule in or rule out malignancy in these cytologically indeterminate lesions and the ATA guidelines have no evidence-based recommendation for or against the use of these methods.

CLINICAL FEATURES OF FOLLICULAR ADENOMA

Follicular adenoma usually presents as a solitary thyroid nodule in an euthyroid patient and can occur at any age, though common in young adults. Adenomas tend to grow slowly, be unchanged over the years, and rarely become symptomatic. Tumors can grow >3 cm in size and cause local symptoms such as dysphagia, voice change, pain, or stridor. Bleeding or necrosis of the central portion of the nodule may cause sudden increase in size and pain. The vast majority of FAs is hypofunctional on radioiodine (RAI) scan and is seen as "cold" or "warm" (the same as normal thyroid) nodules. A small proportion of these nodules may be hyperfunctional, concentrating iodine very avidly, which may suppress function in the remainder of the thyroid. They may occasionally produce thyrotoxicosis (toxic adenoma) and are seen as "hot" nodules. Few evidences suggest transformation of FA to invasive carcinoma. Rarely, a stepwise progression from hyperplasia to adenoma and to invasive carcinoma is seen in some patients with congenital goitrous hypothyroidism. The indications for surgical removal of FA include—(1) evaluation for possible carcinoma; (2) treatment of toxic adenoma; and (3) resolution of local compressive symptoms.

CLINICAL FEATURES OF FOLLICULAR THYROID CARCINOMA

Although FTC can occur at any age, median age at presentation is typically in the 6th decade of life, which is higher than in patients with PTC. Like FAs, follicular thyroid cancer also most commonly presents as solitary thyroid nodule and may be associated with thyroiditis and nodular hyperplasia.

The generally accepted risk of thyroid cancer in a nodule is 10–15%, including nodules that are noticed by the patient, by directed physician examination, or incidentalomas on imaging procedures (chest computed tomography scan, carotid ultrasound, etc.) for evaluation of other diseases. Recent rapid increase in size, hard texture, and fixity of the thyroid nodule/s, presence of family history of thyroid cancer or childhood exposure to ionizing radiation or radiotherapy to head and neck, voice change, and difficulty in breathing or swallowing are concerning clinical features implying increased risk of malignancy. High-frequency ultrasound of the neck is recommended to define the characteristics of thyroid nodule, any additional nodules, and lymph node metastases. Ultrasound alone cannot differentiate between FA and FTC, but larger lesion size, lack of a sonographic halo, hypoechoic appearance, and absence of cystic change favor an FTC diagnosis. FTC has a propensity for vascular invasion and often metastasizes through hematogenous pathways to the lung, bone, liver, and brain in the decreasing order of frequency. Bone metastasis is most often osteolytic and commonly occurs in the body of vertebrae followed by the pelvis, femur, skull, and ribs. Rarely, FTC metastasizes to cervical lymph nodes (10%), which is more typical of PTC. FNA of these distant metastases may demonstrate relatively benign appearing follicular tumor; however, by its invasive malignant behavior, it has defined itself as FTC. Most of the thyroid nodules that harbor malignancy appear as "cold" (reduced radiotracer uptake than the surrounding normal thyroid tissue)/hypofunctioning nodule in ^{123}I radioiodine scan or ^{99m}TcO$_4$ technetium pertechnetate scintigraphy scan. Occasionally, FTC may appear as "warm" nodule with radiotracer uptake and activity similar to the normal thyroid tissue and rarely as "hot" nodules with increased radiotracer concentration with a little or no uptake in the surrounding thyroid tissue. Hypofunctioning nodule diagnosed as an FN harbors a greater risk of malignancy of 20% versus <1% in a hyperfunctioning nodule. Such a rare "functional" thyroid cancer is nearly always an FTC rather than a papillary tumor.

TREATMENT OF A PATIENT WITH A FOLLICULAR NEOPLASM

Diagnostic lobectomy or hemithyroidectomy is the minimum procedure recommended in patients having FNNAC consistent with an FN. Total thyroidectomy should be considered in patients with an FN having concerning clinical and sonographic features or contralateral thyroid disease.

Role of Frozen Section

Frozen section examination has limited utility in distinguishing between FA and FTC and rarely helps in making correct intraoperative decision. The assessment of capsular invasion by frozen-section examination is time consuming, cumbersome, and limited by sampling error. Furthermore, the diagnosis of capsular invasion is difficult with varying thickness of an irregular capsule. Also, vessel distortion and collapse associated with frozen sectioning make the diagnosis of vascular invasion difficult. Additionally, sectioning artifacts can cause "dragging" of tumor cells into thyroid vessels mimicking vascular invasion. Inter- and intraobserver variations are other limitations. Recently, immunohistochemistry staining for *PAX8/PPARγ* mutation in frozen section specimens of an FN has shown an increase in sensitivity to from 84 to 96% but a decline in the specificity from 100 to 90% and also time consuming.

Surgical Procedure of Choice

Surgery is the mainstay of treatment for an FN. Hemithyroidectomy is the definitive treatment for patients with a benign FA and patients with minimally invasive follicular cancer. The consensus report developed at the 2013 Workshop of the European Society of Endocrine Surgeons devoted to minimally invasive follicular thyroid carcinoma (MI-FTC) includes the following conclusions: (1) Candidates for hemithyroidectomy are MI-FTC with exclusive capsular invasion, patients <45 years old at presentation, tumor size < 4 cm, without vascular invasion, and without any node or distant metastases, (2) Candidates for total thyroidectomy are MI-FTC in patients ≥ 45 years at presentation, tumor size ≥4 cm, presence of vascular invasion, regional nodal, and distant metastases. Invasive FTC has a more aggressive behavior with a propensity for systemic metastases and a worse prognosis. Total thyroidectomy is the initial procedure of choice for patients with invasive FTC. The advantages of total thyroidectomy as an initial procedure are as follows: Allows more complete eradication of the disease; decreases the incidence of hypoparathyroidism and injury to laryngeal nerves compared to revision surgery; facilitates 131-radioactive iodine ablation; facilitates the use of serum Tg levels as prognostic indicators; improves the sensitivity of diagnostic radioactive iodine whole-body scans and post-therapy scans; and improves the therapeutic effects of 131-radioactive iodine therapy for metastases. Prophylactic central neck dissection is not a consideration in patients with FTCs, due to <10% incidence of lymph node metastases. Central and modified neck dissections are reserved for patients with clinically evident and/or biopsy-proven lymph node metastases. The timing of completion thyroidectomy is preferably within the 1st week of initial surgery or 3 months later to avoid operation during the period of maximal scarring. Delay in performing completion thyroidectomy by >6 months after the initial surgery may increase the risk of metastases and decrease the survival rate. Patients with a solitary toxic nodule, which is most often a functioning FA, may be treated with radioiodine-131 therapy or hemithyroidectomy. Surgical management of toxic adenoma allows prompt resolution of thyrotoxic and compressive symptoms, avoids radiation exposure to the normal thyroid tissue, and occasionally removal of the functional tumor treats rare cases of carcinoma.

PATHOLOGY OF FOLLICULAR ADENOMA

Follicular adenomas are benign tumors of the thyroid gland, which grow in glandular or follicular patterns. The lesions tend to grow slowly within a capsule of surrounding compressed thyroid glandular tissue. The capsule becomes dense over a period of time and the lesion becomes palpable when they are 5–10 mm in size. On cut section, they vary from a soft grayish white tissue, which bulges out above the cut surface to brown gelatinous tissue. On histologic examination, the FA is composed of bland-appearing TFCs, often exhibiting marked variability and predominantly in microfollicular formations with scant colloid. FAs are subdivided into microfollicular, macrofollicular, and other variants. Colloid nodules are made of extremely large dilated glandular structures with abundant colloid and only a very scant stroma. Embryonal adenomas are composed of nearly solid cords of tumor cells with rudimentary acinar formation. Fetal adenomas are composed of small well-formed acini very similar to normal thyroid tissue with large amount of hyaline cholangitis fibrous tissue separating the follicles. Finally, adenomas composed of follicles containing large polygonal cells with granular eosinophilic cytoplasm, hyperchromatic nuclei with prominent nucleolus, and large number of mitochondria are called oncocytic/Hürthle cell variant. When Hürthle cells constitute 75% or more of tumor cells, in the absence of macrophages, lymphocytes, or plasma cells, they are called Hürthle cell neoplasm (HCN).

PATHOLOGIC FEATURES OF FOLLICULAR THYROID CARCINOMA

Histologically, follicular lesions of the thyroid are classified into three types, namely, FA, FTC, and the follicular variant of PTC. FTCs are the malignant counterparts to FA. The salient feature is capsular and/or vascular invasion, which could be demonstrated only in the histologic sections of the permanent paraffin-fixed tissues **(Figs. 1A to C)**. Capsular invasion is defined as tumor extension through the entire thickness of the capsule. An FN with tumor invasion partially into the capsule (capsular disruption) but not complete penetration through the entire capsule is considered an FA. Vascular invasion is defined as tumor penetration into a large-caliber vessel within or outside the capsule. Tumor invasion of a large vessel with an identifiable wall and an endothelial lining is definitive morphologic evidence of vascular invasion. Mere presence of tumor plugs in vascular spaces within the tumor mass did not qualify as vascular invasion. Angioinvasion is the most reliable sign of malignancy. FTC is subdivided into minimally invasive and invasive variants based on morphologic criteria. MI-FTC is an encapsulated tumor with microscopic penetration of the tumor capsule without vascular invasion. Minimally invasive FTC is a less aggressive tumor associated with excellent prognosis and a disease-free survival similar

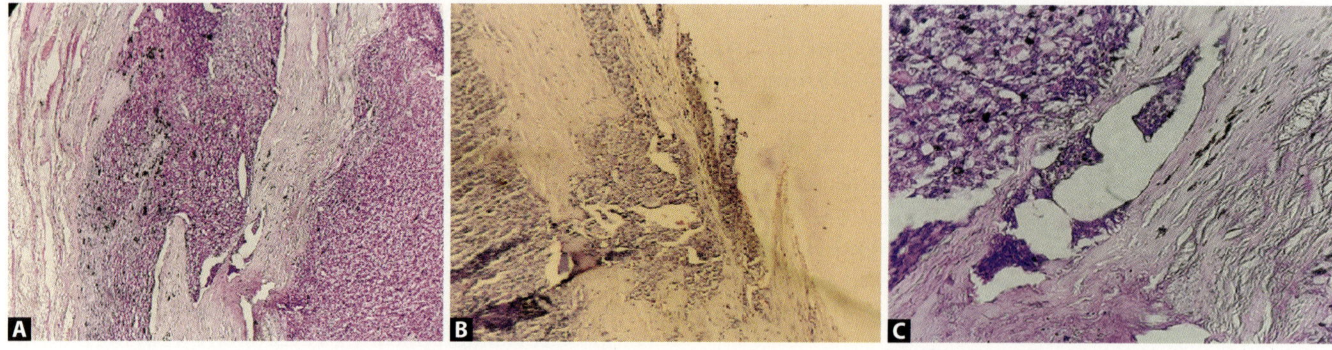

Figs. 1A to C: Follicular thyroid carcinoma. (A) Scanner view (4X); (B) Low power view (10X) showing capsular invasion; (C) High power view (40X) showing vascular invasion (H & E).

to that of a benign FA. However, there are a few reports of distant metastasis and mortality in a small subset of MI-FTC. Patients with minimally invasive FTC tend to be younger compared to patients with invasive FTC, and it has been suggested that minimally invasive FTC may be a precursor to its invasive counterpart. Invasive FTC is defined as an FTC with vascular invasion, extrathyroidal extension into adjacent soft tissues, locoregional spread, and systemic metastases. It is associated with a worse prognosis. It has been subdivided into moderately invasive (angioinvasion < four foci) and widely invasive variants based on the extent of angioinvasion with or without capsular invasion versus extensive invasion of the capsule and the thyroid parenchyma. Van Heerden et al. reported a 10-year disease-specific mortality of 15–28% in patients with invasive FTC. Histologically, these tumors are adenocarcinomas with substantial range in the size and differentiation of the acinar follicles. Some carcinomas have only small incomplete gland formation with very little colloid. These resemble the embryonal pattern of FA. The follicular variant of papillary thyroid carcinoma (FVPTC) is a follicular-patterned tumor with nuclear features of PTC. They may contain papillary structures, psammoma bodies, or optically clear nuclei (Orphan Annie nuclei). FVPTC is a unique entity with a propensity for lymph node metastases, similar to PTC. Oncocytic variant of follicular thyroid cancer contains cells that are large and have an abundant acidophilic cytoplasm with small pyknotic central nuclei. Hürthle cell carcinoma is discussed elsewhere. A subgroup of follicular tumors that contains solid, trabecular pattern, or insular component is associated with aggressive clinical behavior and worse prognosis. This insular component is composed of solid nests of cells separated by capillaries with a few follicular formations inside the nests and scant colloid.

◇ HÜRTHLE CELL NEOPLASM

Hürthle cell neoplasms composed of Hürthle/oxyphilic cells show histologic patterns similar to classic FN. FNNAC cannot distinguish Hürthle cell adenoma from Hürthle cell carcinoma in an HCN, as it is based on the presence of capsular and vascular invasion on histologic sections or evidence of extrathyroidal extension, regional nodal or distant metastasis. The World Health Organization defines HCN as an encapsulated lesion with a predominance of Hürthle cells, constituting >75% of the cell population. Individual Hürthle cells have abundant granular eosinophilic cytoplasm, large number of mitochondria, medium-to-large round nucleus, and a prominent nucleolus. Colloid is typically absent or scant and features of prior hemorrhage (hemosiderin-laden histiocytes) may be present. Occasionally, fire-flare cells (detected in hyperfunctioning lesions or in juvenile thyroiditis) and small thyrocytes can be detected suggesting a benign lesion with an oxyphilic component. Unlike their follicular counterpart, Hürthle cells may feature nuclear enlargement and pleomorphism, either in benign neoplasms or even in hyperplastic lesions. Atypia of the Hürthle cells and presence of transgressing vessels may correlate with the risk of malignancy. A diagnosis of HCN means a 15–30% likelihood of malignancy.

◇ NONINVASIVE FOLLICULAR THYROID NEOPLASM WITH PAPILLARY-LIKE NUCLEAR FEATURES

Revision of Tumor Nomenclature

Based on the recent clinical evidence and pathological parameters, a consensus panel has offered to rename noninvasive encapsulated follicular variant of PTC with the following characteristics: (1) main morphological features, i.e., the follicular growth pattern and nuclear features of PTC; (2) lack of invasion, which separates this tumor from invasive encapsulated follicular variant of papillary thyroid carcinoma (EFVPTC); (3) clonal origin determined by finding a driver mutation, which indicates that the lesion is biologically a neoplasm; and (4) a very low risk of adverse outcome when the tumor is noninvasive. The new nomenclature "noninvasive follicular thyroid neoplasm with papillary-like nuclear features" (NIFTP) conveys histologic features of this lesion and also reflects the indolent course of this tumor. NIFTP has stringent histopathologic diagnostic criteria established by the panel. First, being "noninvasive," the entire capsule or tumor/normal interface must be completely examined microscopically to rule out invasion as capsular or vascular invasion would exclude the tumor from a NIFTP classification. Second, a follicular growth pattern defined as <1% papillae, <30% of the lesion composed of a solid, trabecular, or insular growth pattern, and a lack of psammoma bodies helps to classify this lesion as "follicular." Follicular growth patterns including microfollicular, macrofollicular, and normofollicular with colloid are acceptable. "Papillary-like nuclear features" must be present, with an overall qualifying score of 2–3 based upon a consensus grading system. Include 1 point each for the presence of either (1) nuclear enlargement/overlapping/ crowding or elongation, (2) nuclear membrane irregularities, grooves, or pseudoinclusions, or (3) glassy nuclei/cleared chromatin with margination. Finally, there must be no tumor necrosis and mitoses must be <3 per 10 high-power fields. The immunohistochemical stains apart from hematoxylin and eosin are not required for the diagnosis of NIFTP; however, HBME-1, galectin-3, and CK19 are positive in follicular-patterned tumors which could support a differential diagnosis including NIFTP and EFVPTC. From a molecular standpoint, NIFTP is often characterized by RAS-type mutations, similar to other follicular-patterned lesions. On the contrary, *BRAF* mutations are commonly associated with conventional PTC as well as 50% of the cases of invasive FVPTC. However, the presence of BRAF mutation is not compatible with a diagnosis of NIFTP. Treatment recommendation for NIFTP is surgical lobectomy/hemithyroidectomy. Neither radioactive iodine therapy nor a prophylactic central neck lymph node staging is considered as NIFTP is nonmalignant.

◇| POSTOPERATIVE FOLLOW-UP

Several risk-stratification systems have been described to guide postoperative management and follow-up surveillance of these well-differentiated tumors, which are associated with low risk for recurrence and mortality. In patients with FTC, age > 45 years and the presence of metastases at presentation are associated with worse prognosis and poor 5-year survival. Other important prognostic factors include the size of the primary tumor > 4 cm, degree of invasion (microinvasive vs. widely invasive), the degree of tumor cell differentiation, and completeness of resection. Low-risk follicular cancer is defined as a tumor <4 cm in size that is confined to the thyroid gland without metastases in a patient <45 years of age. High-risk follicular cancer is defined by a widely invasive FTC, aggressive histology, tumor size > 4 cm, extrathyroidal extension, systemic metastases, or age of the patient 45 years or more. Patients with a final diagnosis of FA or minimally invasive FTC warrant no additional therapy. Thyrotropin-suppressive therapy is not necessary. Alternatively, supplementary doses of levothyroxine shall be given when hypothyroidism develops, which usually occurs in 22% of cases after hemithyroidectomy. Radioactive iodine ablation and whole-body scanning are not indicated for minimally invasive FTC. Annual neck examination, cervical ultrasound examination, and a screening serum TSH level are recommended for follow-up.

Postoperatively, in patients with invasive FTC, serum TSH levels are raised above 30 µIU/mL, either by thyroid hormone withdrawal for 3–6 weeks (iatrogenic hypothyroidism) or administration of recombinant human TSH 0.9 mg intramuscularly on two consecutive days (and a baseline stimulated Tg level is obtained). An ablation dose of 30 mCi of 131-radioactive iodine (RAI) is given as an outpatient procedure to destroy residual thyroid tissue or microscopic malignancy, thereby reducing the risk of recurrence. 131-I post-therapy whole-body scan is recommended 5–7 days later to detect the hidden metastases, which become apparent in 25% of the cases. RAI ablation eliminates normal thyroid tissue as a source for Tg and iodine uptake, enhancing the sensitivity of serum Tg monitoring, and iodine whole-body scanning for detection of recurrent disease. Patients with invasive FTC are treated with suppressive doses of levothyroxine to prevent TSH-induced growth of residual cancer cells and improve disease-free survival. In patients with low-risk follicular cancer who are free of disease, serum TSH levels are maintained between 0.3 and 2.0 µIU/mL. In patients with high-risk FTC, serum TSH levels are maintained between 0.1 and 0.5 µIU/mL. In patients with persistent or metastatic disease, serum TSH levels are maintained <0.1 µIU/mL. An estimated risk of recurrence is 11–39% among FTC patients, which mostly develops within the first 2 years after surgery. The follow-up surveillance with history, physical examination, and serum TSH, Tg, and antithyroglobulin antibody levels (anti-Tg) is recommended at 3–6-month intervals for the first 2 years and annually thereafter. High-frequency neck ultrasound is performed at 6 and 12 months after surgery and yearly thereafter for 3–5 years depending on the patient's risk for recurrent disease and results of Tg monitoring. An unstimulated Tg < 2 ng/mL is indicative of absence of disease. Alternatively, Tg levels > 2 ng/mL may be indicative of recurrent disease, and necessitate screening for TSH-stimulated Tg level. A stimulated Tg level > 10 ng/mL is suggestive of recurrence. Routine iodine whole-body scanning is unnecessary for patients without clinical evidence of disease who have an undetectable serum Tg level, a negative ultrasound of the neck, and a prior negative iodine whole-body scan. Repeat whole-body scanning is obtained when a patient has an elevated serum Tg level and a negative cervical ultrasound. Computed tomography (CT) of the head, neck, and chest; magnetic resonance imaging (MRI) of the spine, pelvis, and femurs; and positron emission tomographic imaging with 2-deoxy-2-[fluorine-18] fluoro-D-glucose (^{18}F-FDG PET) are reserved for patients with elevated Tg levels, a negative ultrasound of the neck, and a negative iodine-131 whole-body scan. Thin-cut or spiral CT is the best imaging modality for identifying pulmonary metastases.

An MRI is the best modality for identifying bone metastases. As the disease transforms from differentiated cancers to de-differentiated cancer, there is progressive decrease in the NIS expression, ability to trap iodine and later, Tg production. Hence, these tumors become noniodine avid and are negative in iodine-131 whole-body scan but are readily detected in FDG-PET/CT scans, owing to their high metabolic activity. This is referred as flip-flop phenomenon. FDG-PET positive but noniodine avid lesions are associated with a worse prognosis. Thus, FDG-PET/CT imaging has both a diagnostic and prognostic role.

TREATMENT OF LOCAL RECURRENCE AND METASTATIC DISEASE

Surgical resection with tumor-free margins is the mainstay of therapy for local recurrence along with removal of any remaining thyroid tissue. Macroscopic lymph-node metastases are treated with compartment-oriented neck dissection. Central compartment neck dissection entails complete removal of lymph nodes and fibrofatty tissues from the hyoid bone superiorly to innominate vessels inferiorly and between carotid sheath on either side, without compromising vascularity of parathyroid glands. This includes prelaryngeal, pretracheal, paratracheal, and retropharyngeal nodes of level IV and VII. Functional neck dissection or modified radical neck dissection type III entails complete removal of all fibrofatty and nodal tissues of levels II-V with preservation of ipsilateral internal jugular vein, sternomastoid, and spinal accessory nerve.

Macroscopic solitary metastases isolated to the lung, bone, or brain that are amenable to surgery are best resected with improved survival. Diffuse and multiple metastases are treated with high doses of 131-RAI therapy. Surgery is indicated for bone metastases involving the spine or weight-bearing joints and for palliation of neurological sequelae. Patients with vertebral body metastases and neurological compromise are candidates for spine stabilization with tumor resection with or without adjuvant radioiodine therapy or radiation. Microscopic metastases are treated with high doses of radioiodine. Metastases from FTC will concentrate radioiodine in 75% of patients. The appropriate doses of 131-RAI for the treatment of microscopic metastases to the lymph nodes, lungs, and bone are 150 mCi, 200 mCi, and 250 mCi, respectively or calculated as per dosimetry. The cycle of radioiodine scan and therapy is repeated at every 6–9-month interval (not exceeding a cumulative dose of 1 Curie) as appropriate for the given patient's physiological status and tumor response. Radioiodine therapy is most effective in young patients with iodine-avid micronodular pulmonary metastases that are not detected in chest X-rays and are associated with 90% 10-year survival. Whereas,

macronodular pulmonary metastases that are identified on chest X-ray are less responsive to radioiodine therapy and are associated with a 10-year patient survival of only 11%. Unlike pulmonary metastases, bone metastases do not readily concentrate radioiodine and are associated with a worse prognosis. External radiation therapy may play a role in palliation of bone pain and control of tumor growth of metastases that is refractory to radioiodine therapy. Periodic intravenous infusions of bisphosphonate drugs may help to reduce pain, pathologic fractures, and progression of bone metastases. Patients with asymptomatic bone metastases that do not concentrate radioiodine can be observed with suppressive dose of levothyroxine therapy alone. Brain metastases account for <1% of the systemic metastases from FTC. They are associated with a poor prognosis and a median survival of only 1 year. When surgical resection is not possible, whole-brain irradiation can be used for palliation. Radioiodine therapy has the potential to cause cerebral edema, which may be prevented with corticosteroid therapy. Patients with progressive radioiodine-refractory metastases may be considered for clinical trial with tyrosine kinase inhibitor such as sorafenib or sunitinib.

OUTCOME

D'Avanzo et al. reported that overall 10-year survival rate was 97.8% for MI-FTC, 80% for moderately invasive, and only 37% for widely invasive variants of FTC. The cause of death is most commonly from progression of distant metastases.

CONCLUSION

FNs of the thyroid gland include benign FA and malignant FTC. Currently, an FTC cannot be distinguished from an FA based on cytologic, sonographic, or clinical features. Iodine deficiency, certain oncogene, and/or miRNA activation have been implicated in the pathogenesis of FTC. Advances in molecular testing for genetic mutations may enable preoperative differentiation of an FTC from an FA in the future. Currently, a patient having FNNAC diagnosis consistent with an FN warrants surgical resection to make definitive diagnosis as capsular and/or vascular invasion can be demonstrated only in the histologic section of paraffin-embedded tissues. Diagnostic lobectomy or hemithyroidectomy would be a definitive treatment for a benign FA or a minimally invasive follicular cancer. Completion thyroidectomy is necessary for invasive FTC. Total thyroidectomy as an initial procedure for invasive FTC allows more complete eradication of the disease, decreases the incidence of hypoparathyroidism and injury to laryngeal nerves compared to revision surgery, facilitates 131-radioactive iodine ablation, facilitates the use of serum Tg levels as prognostic indicators, improves the sensitivity of diagnostic radioactive iodine whole-body scans and post-therapy scans, and improves the therapeutic effects of

131-radioactive iodine therapy for metastases. Adjunctive TSH suppressive therapy with levothyroxine is recommended for these TSH-dependent well-differentiated thyroid cancers. A compartment-oriented neck dissection is reserved for clinically apparent/biopsy-proven lymph node metastases, which occurs in <10% of cases with FTC. FTC metastasizes through hematogenous route, most commonly to lungs and bone, less commonly to brain and liver. Diffuse systemic metastases are treated with high doses of 131-radioactive iodine. Isolated solitary metastasis and recurrence are best resected with improvement in survival. The follow-up surveillance includes history and physical examination, serial monitoring with neck ultrasound, serum TSH and Tg levels. In addition, rising titers of antithyroglobulin antibody may serve as surrogate tumor marker. Other imaging studies are reserved for patients with an elevated serum Tg level and a negative cervical ultrasound. Patients with MI-FTC have excellent prognosis with overall 10-year survival of 98%, while it drops to 37% in patients with widely invasive FTC.

◇ SUGGESTED READING

1. Haugen BR, Alexander EK, Bible KC, Doherty GM, Mandel SJ, Nikiforov YE, et al. 2015 American Thyroid Association Management Guidelines for Adult Patients with Thyroid Nodules and Differentiated Thyroid Cancer: The American Thyroid Association Guidelines Task force on Thyroid nodules and differentiated Thyroid Cancer. Thyroid. 2016;26:1-33.

2. Bychkov A, Jung CK, Liu Z, Kakudo K. Noninvasive follicular thyroid neoplasm with papillary-like nuclear features in Asian practice: perspectives for surgical pathology and cytopathology. Endocrine Pathology. 2018;29(3):276-88.

3. Clarke OH, Duh QY, Kebebew E, Gosnell JE, Shen WT. Textbook of Endocrine Surgery, 3rd edition. New Delhi: Jaypee Brothers Medical Publishers; 2016.

4. D'Avanzo A, Treseler P, Ituarte PH, Wong M, Streja L, Greenspan FS, et al. Follicular thyroid carcinoma: histology and prognosis. Cancer. 2004;100:1123-9.

5. Dionigi G, Kraimps JL, Schmid KW, Hermann M, Sheu-Grabellus SY, De Wailly P, Beaulieu A, Tanda ML, Sessa F. Minimally invasive follicular thyroid cancer (MIFTC)—a consensus report of the European Society of Endocrine Surgeons (ESES). Langenbeck's Archives of Surgery. 2014;399:165-84.

6. Jug R, Jiang X. Noninvasive follicular thyroid neoplasm with papillary-like nuclear features: an evidence-based nomenclature change. Pathology research international. 2017:1057252.

7. King-Yin LA. Pathology of Endocrine Tumors Update: World Health Organization New Classification 2017—Other Thyroid Tumors. AJSP: Rev Rep. 2017;22:209-16.

8. McHenry CR, Phitayakor R. Follicular adenoma and carcinoma of the thyroid gland. The Oncologist. 2011;16:585-93.

9. Paschke R, Cantara S, Crescenzi A, Jarzab B, Musholt TJ, Sobrinho SM. European Thyroid Association Guidelines regarding Thyroid Nodule Molecular Fine-needle Aspiration Cytology Diagnostics. Eur Thyroid J. 2017; 6: 115–29.

10. Xu B, Ghossein R. Evolution of the histologic classification of thyroid neoplasms and its impact on clinical management. Eur J Surg Oncol. 2018;44:338-47.

CHAPTER 14

Hürthle Cell Neoplasm and Carcinoma

R Dayananda Babu, Deepak Paul

DEFINITION

Hürthle cell neoplasm may be benign (adenoma) or carcinoma. The diagnosis of carcinoma is by capsular and vascular invasion. Hürthle cell cancer is defined as a tumor composed of >75% Hürthle cells with a trabecular or follicular pattern with complete vascular and capsular invasion.[1] According to Bronner et al. and Cannon et al., it is defined as solitary masses in thyroid comprised of at least 50% Hürthle cells found in a gland not otherwise overcome by chronic thyroiditis.[2,3] For practical purposes, presence of Hürthle cells along with absence of lymphocytes will make a pathological diagnosis of Hürthle cell neoplasm. Hürthle cell carcinoma has been classified by the World Health Organization (WHO) as a variant of follicular cancer and is included in differentiated thyroid cancer.[1]

HISTORICAL BACKGROUND

In 1894, Hürthle described the parafollicular cells of thyroid of a dog as Hürthle cells.[4] True Hürthle cells were initially described in 1898 in a patient with thyrotoxicosis by Askanazy. Langhans reported the first Hürthle cell tumor in 1907.[5] These tumors are synonymously called Askanazy cell tumor, Langhans tumors, and Hürthle cell tumors.

WHAT IS A HÜRTHLE CELL?

Hürthle cell is a large polygonal cell with abundant eosinophilic granular cytoplasm with a large hyperchromatic round nucleus and prominent nucleolus. It also contains numerous mitochondria which are responsible for eosinophilic staining. Hürthle cells can secrete thyroglobulin similar to thyroid follicular cells. They are also seen in inflammatory diseases of the thyroid. However, Hürthle cell cancers are less likely to trap radioactive iodine as compared to follicular cancers.[6] Therefore, it is suggested that Hürthle cells tumors should be classified as a distinct category.

INCIDENCE

Hürthle cell cancers account only 3% of thyroid cancers having a variable biological behavior and having lymph node metastases from 2.7 to 56% and distant metastases in 5–50%.[7] Hürthle cell cancers are more aggressive in clinical behavior compared to the rest of the differentiated thyroid cancers. As reported by Lopez Penabad, there was multifocality in 33%.[8]

RISK FACTORS

- Previous childhood and head and neck radiation[9]
- Male gender
- Larger tumor size

CLINICAL PRESENTATION

Hürthle cell neoplasms usually present with a solitary thyroid nodule or a dominant nodule. About 15–45% of Hürthle cell neoplasms are carcinomas.[10-12] They may also rarely present with palpable cervical lymph nodes or lung metastases. Patients with Hürthle cell carcinoma are usually in their 5th decade with a male preponderance.[13] 11% of patients will have lymph node metastases in Hürthle cell carcinoma and 15% will have metastases to bone or lung.[14,15]

DIAGNOSIS

Ultrasound

There is scanty available data for the sonographic appearance of Hürthle cell neoplasm.[16] In Hürthle cell carcinoma, the lesions are more hypoechoic and larger than benign tumors.[17] The risk of malignancy is directly correlated with tumor size.[18] The Hürthle cell subgroup is more likely to be older with a median age of 64 years and they are less likely to contain calcifications.

Fine-needle Aspiration Cytology

Hürthle cells are metaplastic thyroid follicular cells with an oncocytic appearance characterized by hyperchromatic nuclei with prominent nucleoli and granular eosinophilic cytoplasm. They are observed in many thyroid conditions such as Hashimoto's thyroiditis and other thyroid malignancies. The presence of Hürthle cells in cytology specimens increases the risk of malignancy.[19] Hürthle cell neoplasms composed entirely of Hürthle cells can be benign (Hürthle cell adenoma) or malignant (Hürthle cell carcinoma) according to the presence of capsular and vascular invasion. The cytological criteria apart of abundance of Hürthle cells include Hürthle cells >50–75%, scanty colloid, cell dysplasia, transgressing vessels, and dyshesion (single cell).[20]

Five cytological criteria are reported to predict Hürthle cell carcinoma.[21] They are:

1. Predominant Hürthle cells
2. Scanty colloid
3. Either small-cell dysplasia (cytoplasmic diameter less than twice the nuclear diameter with often quite bland cells—benign appearing cells) or large-cell dysplasia (more than twice the variation in nuclear diameter, large cells typically have prominent nucleoli and irregular nuclear outlines).
4. Crowding (nuclei touching)
5. Dyshesion

They are associated with nuclear pleomorphism, nuclear enlargement, and absence of macrophages, plasma cells, or lymphocytes.[22] However, the cornerstone of diagnosis of Hürthle cell carcinoma remains careful histological evaluation.

Staging

The AJCC Cancer Staging Manual, 8th edition is used for staging of Hürthle cell carcinoma.

Histopathology

Several studies reveal that histologic criteria can differentiate Hürthle cell adenoma and carcinoma.[23] Histopathological diagnosis of Hürthle cell carcinoma is by capsular and vascular invasion, invasion of adjacent structures, lymph node metastases, and distant metastases. The College of American Pathologists clarified the definition of substantial capsular invasion and vascular invasion as the diagnostic feature of Hürthle cell carcinoma and suggested that capsular irregularities and incomplete capsular penetration could be classified as adenoma.[24] Carcangiu et al. grouped Hürthle cell neoplasms into three categories—benign, intermediate, and malignant.[25] Malignant lesions are identified by full-thickness capsular invasion, vascular invasion, or invasion of adjacent structures. The intermediate lesions had minimal capsular invasion, marked nuclear atypia, and extensive necrosis. As in the case of follicular carcinoma, intermediate lesions are termed minimally invasive meaning they will not penetrate the entire thickness of the capsule.[26,27] Ghossein et al. found that even minimally invasive tumors can recur provided there were more than four foci of vascular invasion.[28] Sine qua non of Hürthle cell carcinoma is full-thickness capsular and/or vascular invasion. The presence of nonencapsulated Hürthle cells does not signify a neoplastic process because they are commonly associated with thyroiditis, nodular goiters, and Graves' disease.

Molecular Testing

The molecular tests available are classified into the following:

- *Immunohistochemical*: The panels of immuno-histochemistry (IHC) markers are cyclin D1 and cyclin D3. They are used in fine-needle aspiration (FNA) samples suspicious for Hürthle cell neoplasm. Positive staining for cyclin D3 in combination with D1 is having highest sensitivity and specificity for carcinoma.[29]
- *Polymerase chain reaction (PCR) identification of specific genetic mutation*:
  - *PAX8* (paired boxed gene 8) and *PPARγ* (peroxisome proliferator activated receptor gamma rearrangement mutation).
  - *PAX8* is part of a gene family that encodes for nuclear proteins involved in follicular cell development. *PPARγ* encodes for nuclear receptor protein that is a regulator of adipocyte differentiation. When fused together, *PAX8/PPARγ* oncogene was found in 68% of follicular carcinoma. Cases of Hürthle cell carcinoma that stained positive had more favorable prognosis.[30]
- *RAS* mutations are common in follicular thyroid cancer. Hürthle cell tumors are less likely to harbor *RAS* mutation (11% of Hürthle cell carcinoma and 8% of Hürthle cell adenoma) compared to 52% of follicular thyroid cancer and 48% of follicular adenomas.[31]
- *RET/PTC* rearrangement is present in some Hürthle cell adenomas and carcinomas but not in hyperplastic lesions with Hürthle cell metaplasia.[32]
- DNA aneuploidy is associated with distant metastases in patients with Hürthle cell carcinoma. However, Hürthle cell adenomas are also often aneuploid.[9] Mitochondrial DNA mutations and micro-RNAs are other techniques to distinguish Hürthle cell neoplasm from carcinoma.[33,34]

A high rate of false-positive results was reported in Hürthle cell predominant nodules by gene expression analysis.[35]

◇ MANAGEMENT

Surgery

About 20–25% of the Hürthle cell neoplasms are malignant and they usually present as solitary thyroid nodules. In some series, up to 60% are cancers.[36-38] Therefore, it is preferable to do a minimum surgery of hemithyroidectomy (ipsilateral lobectomy with isthmusectomy) as the initial procedure. In patients with contralateral nodules, nodules >4 cm, history of radiation exposure, family history of thyroid cancer, and patients with suspicious ultrasound features, the initial surgery should be a total thyroidectomy.

During surgery, one should carefully look for features of malignancy such as adjacent structure involvement and metastatic nodes. When there is history of head and neck irradiation, there is 50% chance for concomitant papillary thyroid cancer and multifocality.[39] The recurrence rate of Hürthle cell carcinoma will depend on the extent of original surgery.[25] In a cohort of 62 patients with Hürthle cell carcinoma proved by pathology, total thyroidectomy was the only independent predictor of improved cancer-specific survival.[40] In another retrospective study in 239 patients of Hürthle cell carcinoma, total thyroidectomy was independently associated with improved outcome in terms of cancer-specific survival whereas reoperation for tumor relapse was an independent predictor of poor cancer-specific survival.[41] When there is invasion of the surrounding structures or lymph node involvement, resection of all gross and microscopic disease is to be performed. Surgical resection is the only curative treatment for Hürthle cell carcinoma. More radical surgery may be required for involvement of trachea, larynx, esophagus, soft tissues, and skin.

Role of Frozen Section Examination

The diagnosis of Hürthle cell carcinoma is by the presence of capsular and vascular invasion. In a review of 125 patients, it was found that frozen section evaluation was of minimal value rendering no additional diagnostic information in 87% of the time.[42] Diagnostic information was provided only in 13% of patients and only in 3.3%, the frozen section correctly modified the surgical procedure. In a study of 309 follicular neoplasms, intraoperative pathological examination had a positive predictive value of 100%, a negative predictive value of 85.9%, an accuracy of 86.7%, and a sensitivity of 29.6%.[43] Intraoperative pathological examination is more effective in widely invasive tumors than minimally invasive tumors.[44] It may not be useful in minimally invasive Hürthle cell carcinomas.

Completion Thyroidectomy

In patients undergoing hemithyroidectomy whose final pathology is Hürthle cell carcinoma, a completion thyroidectomy must be done except in low-risk minimally invasive tumors. However, in such patients, a close clinical follow-up and thyroid suppression are recommended. If the pathology report is Hürthle cell adenoma, no further intervention is required.

Radioactive Iodine

Only 5–38% of Hürthle cell carcinomas will concentrate iodine.[3,8,45] The role of radioactive iodine in Hurtle cell carcinoma is controversial. Therefore, aggressive surgical resection is the management for Hürthle cell tumors. There have been reports of resolution of pulmonary metastases with radioactive iodine. However, it is important to note that uptake does not always correlate with tumor responsiveness.[46]

Thyroglobulin

Hürthle cell adenomas and carcinomas are able to secrete thyroglobulin.[47] Some centers therefore perform ^{131}I scans in patients with elevated thyroglobulin after 4–6 weeks after total thyroidectomy and recommend ^{131}I ablation if a residual uptake is present. This has got the advantage of screening for recurrence by thyroglobulin levels. After ablation, thyroglobulin should be checked every 6 months. If it is elevated ultrasound of the neck, radioiodine uptake scan, CT, or fluorodeoxyglucose-positron emission tomography (FGD-PET) is done to identify metastatic disease/recurrence. If the imaging is positive, the patient should undergo treatment with ^{131}I or external beam radiation or surgery depending on the situation.

Other Modalities of Treatment

External Beam Radiation

External beam radiation to the neck has shown no effect on survival. However, there is a definite role for pain relief and disease control in bone metastases.[3,25]

Targeted Therapy

Tyrosine kinase inhibitors are used to treat radioiodine refractory progressive disease. Improvement in disease-free survival of such patients with sorafenib and lenvatinib is reported.[48,49] The number of Hürthle cell carcinomas included is too small to make any definite conclusion.

◁| PROGNOSIS AND FOLLOW-UP

After total thyroidectomy, ^{131}I is recommended to destroy the remnants so that screening for recurrence is possible by measurement of thyroglobulin levels. Thyroglobulin should be checked at 6-month interval initially. If thyroglobulin is elevated, further imaging by neck ultrasound radioiodine uptake scan or CT is carried out. FDG-PET (fluorodeoxyglucose-positron emission tomography) is useful for the follow-up of Hürthle cell carcinoma because of the avidity of oncocyte for this tracer. It has a sensitivity of 95.8%, specificity of 95%, accuracy of 95.5%.[50] However, false-positive and false-negative findings can occur.[50] FDG-PET uptake also has prognostic significance. For each increase of one standardized uptake value unit of FDG, a 6% increase in mortality was found.[50]

The 10-year survival of papillary cancer is 95%, follicular is 85%, and Hürthle cell carcinoma ranges from 75 to 80%.[51-53] The recurrence rates for Hürthle cell carcinoma range from 14 to 44%.[28,54-56]

◁| CONCLUSION

Hürthle cell tumors are rare tumors comprising 3–10% of thyroid tumors. Hürthle cell cancers make up 1–3% of thyroid cancers. Fine-needle aspiration cytology can identify Hürthle cell neoplasm but cannot differentiate cancer because the diagnosis is by capsular and vascular invasion. The value of per operative frozen section is doubtful. The primary modality of treatment is surgical. Treatment with ^{131}I may not be effective because of the poor uptake of the tracer by Hürthle cells. 10-year survival of Hürthle cell cancer is less than that of the other two differentiated thyroid cancers.

◇ REFERENCES

1. Du BC; Armed Forces Institute of Pathology. Third series, fascicle 6. Atlas of Tumor Pathology. Tumors of the Parathyroid. RA DeLellis. Washington, DC: Armed Forces Institute of Pathology; 1993.
2. Bronner MP, Clevenger CV, Edmonds PR, Lowell DM, McFarland MM, LiVolsi VA. Flow cytometric analysis of DNA content in Hürthle cell adenomas and carcinomas of the thyroid. Am J Clin Pathol. 1988;89(6):764-9.
3. Cannon J. The significance of Hürthle cells in thyroid disease. Oncologist. 2011;16(10):1380-7.
4. Machens A, Schneyer U, Holzhausen HJ, Dralle H. Prospects of remission in medullary thyroid carcinoma according to basal calcitonin level. J Clin Endocrinol Metab. 2005;90(4):2029-34.
5. Askanazy M. Pathologisch-anatomische Beiträge zur Kenntniss des Morbus Basedowii, insbesondere über die dabei auftretende Muskelerkrankung. Dtsch Arch Klin Med. 1898;61:118-86.
6. Hoos A, Stojadinovic A, Singh B, Dudas ME, Leung DHY, Shaha AR, et al. Clinical significance of molecular expression profiles of Hürthle cell tumors of the thyroid gland analyzed via tissue microarrays. Am J Pathol. 2002;160(1):175-83.
7. Hundahl SA, Fleming ID, Fremgen AM, Menck HR. A National Cancer Data Base report on 53,856 cases of thyroid carcinoma treated in the U.S., 1985-1995. Cancer [Internet]. 1998;83(12):2638-48.
8. Lopez-Penabad L, Chiu AC, Hoff AO, Schultz P, Gaztambide S, Ordonez NG, et al. Prognostic factors in patients with Hürthle cell neoplasms of the thyroid. Cancer. 2003;97(5):1186-94.
9. Thompson NW, Dunn EL, Batsakis JG, Nishiyama RH. Hürthle cell lesions of the thyroid gland. Surg Gynecol Obstet. 1974;139(4):555-60.
10. Machens A, Niccoli-Sire P, Hoegel J, Frank-Raue K, van Vroonhoven TJ, Roeher H-D, et al. Early malignant progression of hereditary medullary thyroid cancer. N Engl J Med. 2003;349(16):1517-25.
11. Moley JF, DeBenedetti MK. Patterns of nodal metastases in palpable medullary thyroid carcinoma: recommendations for extent of node dissection. Ann Surg. 1999;229(6):880.
12. Decker RA, Geiger JD, Cox CE, Mackovjak M, Sarkar M, Peacock ML. Prophylactic surgery for multiple endocrine neoplasia type IIa after genetic diagnosis: is parathyroid transplantation indicated? World J Surg. 1996;20(7):814-21.
13. Goffredo P, Roman SA, Sosa JA. Hürthle cell carcinoma: a population-level analysis of 3311 patients. Cancer. 2013;119(3):504-11.
14. McLeod MK, Thompson NW. Hürthle cell neoplasms of the thyroid. Otolaryngol Clin North Am. 1990;23(3):441-52.
15. Barnabei A, Ferretti E, Baldelli R, Procaccini A, Spriano G, Appetecchia M. Hürthle cell tumours of the thyroid. Personal experience and review of the literature. Acta Otorhinolaryngol Ital. 2009;29(6):305-11.
16. Lee SK, Rho BH, Woo SK. Hürthle cell neoplasm: correlation of gray-scale and power Doppler sonographic findings with gross pathology. J Clin Ultrasound. 2010;38(4):169-76.
17. Lee KH, Shin JH, Ko ES, Hahn SY, Kim JS, Kim JH, et al. Predictive factors of malignancy in patients with cytologically suspicious for Hürthle cell neoplasm of thyroid nodules. Int J Surg. 2013;11(9):898-902.
18. Sippel RS, Elaraj DM, Khanafshar E, Zarnegar R, Kebebew E, Duh QY, et al. Tumor size predicts malignant potential in Hürthle cell neoplasms of the thyroid. World J Surg. 2008;32(5):702-7.
19. Yang GCH, Goldberg JD, Ye PX. Risk of malignancy in follicular neoplasms without nuclear atypia: statistical analysis of 397 thyroidectomies. Endocr Pract. 2003;9(6):510-6.
20. Rossi ED, Martini M, Straccia P, Raffaelli M, Pennacchia I, Marrucci E, et al. The cytologic category of oncocytic (Hürthle) cell neoplasm mostly includes low-risk lesions at histology: an institutional experience. Eur J Endocrinol. 2013;169(5):649-55.
21. Pompili G, Tresoldi S, Primolevo A, De Pasquale L, Di Leo G, Cornalba G. Management of thyroid follicular proliferation: an ultrasound-based malignancy score to opt for surgical or conservative treatment. Ultrasound Med Biol. 2013;39(8):1350-5.
22. Herrera MF, Hay ID, Wu PS, Goellner JR, Ryan JJ, Ebersold JR, et al. Hürthle cell (oxyphilic) papillary thyroid carcinoma: a variant with more aggressive biologic behavior. World J Surg. 1992;16(4):665-9.
23. Grant CS, Barr D, Goellner JR, Hay ID. Benign Hürthle cell tumors of the thyroid: a diagnosis to be trusted? World J Surg. 1988;12(4):488-94.
24. Ghossein R. Update to the College of American Pathologists reporting on thyroid carcinomas. Head Neck Pathol. 2009;3(1):86-93.
25. Carcangiu ML, Bianchi S, Savino D, Voynick IM, Rosai J. Follicular Hürthle cell tumors of the thyroid gland. Cancer. 1991;68(9):1944-53.
26. Ito Y, Hirokawa M, Masuoka H, Yabuta T, Kihara M, Higashiyama T, et al. Prognostic factors of minimally invasive follicular thyroid carcinoma: extensive vascular invasion significantly affects patient prognosis. Endocr J. 2013;60(5):637-42.
27. Ghossein R. Encapsulated malignant follicular cell-derived thyroid tumors. Endocr Pathol. 2010;21(4):212-8.
28. Ghossein RA, Hiltzik DH, Carlson DL, Patel S, Shaha A, Shah JP, et al. Prognostic factors of recurrence in encapsulated Hürthle cell carcinoma of the thyroid gland: a clinicopathologic study of 50 cases. Cancer. 2006;106(8):1669-76.
29. Troncone G, Volante M, Iaccarino A, Zeppa P, Cozzolino I, Malapelle U, et al. Cyclin D1 and D3 overexpression predicts malignant behavior in thyroid fine-needle aspirates suspicious for Hürthle cell neoplasms. Cancer. 2009;117(6):522-9.
30. Sahin M, Allard BL, Yates M, Powell JG, Wang XL, Hay ID, et al. PPARgamma staining as a surrogate for PAX8/PPARgamma fusion oncogene expression in follicular neoplasms: clinicopathological correlation and histopathological diagnostic value. J Clin Endocrinol Metab. 2005;90(1):463-8.
31. Nikiforova MN, Lynch RA, Biddinger PW, Alexander EK, Dorn GW 2nd, Tallini G, et al. RAS point mutations and PAX8-PPAR gamma rearrangement in thyroid tumors: evidence for distinct molecular pathways in thyroid follicular carcinoma. J Clin Endocrinol Metab. 2003;88(5):2318-26.
32. Chiappetta G, Toti P, Cetta F, Giuliano A, Pentimalli F, Amendola I, et al. The RET/PTC oncogene is frequently activated in oncocytic thyroid tumors (Hürthle cell adenomas and carcinomas), but not in oncocytic hyperplastic lesions. J Clin Endocrinol Metab. 2002;87(1):364-9.
33. Maximo V, Soares P, Lima J, Cameselle-Teijeiro J, Sobrinho-Simoes M. Mitochondrial DNA somatic mutations (point mutations and large deletions) and mitochondrial DNA variants in human thyroid pathology: a study with emphasis on Hürthle cell tumors. Am J Pathol. 2002;160(5):1857-65.
34. Kitano M, Rahbari R, Patterson EE, Xiong Y, Prasad NB, Wang Y, et al. Expression profiling of difficult-to-diagnose thyroid histologic subtypes shows distinct expression profiles and identify candidate diagnostic microRNAs. Ann Surg Oncol. 2011;18(12):3443-52.

35. Wu JX, Young S, Hung ML, Li N, Yang SE, Cheung DS, et al. Clinical factors influencing the performance of gene expression classifier testing in indeterminate thyroid nodules. Thyroid. 2016;26(7):916-22.

36. Brandi ML, Gagel RF, Angeli A, Bilezikian JP, Beck-Peccoz P, Bordi C, et al. Guidelines for diagnosis and therapy of MEN type 1 and type 2. J Clin Endocrinol Metab. 2001;86(12): 5658-71.

37. Frilling A, Dralle H, Eng C, Raue F, Broelsch CE. Presymptomatic DNA screening in families with multiple endocrine neoplasia type 2 and familial medullary thyroid carcinoma. Surgery. 1995;118(6):1094-9.

38. Wells SAJ, Chi DD, Toshima K, Dehner LP, Coffin CM, Dowton SB, et al. Predictive DNA testing and prophylactic thyroidectomy in patients at risk for multiple endocrine neoplasia type 2A. Ann Surg. 1994;220(3):237-50.

39. Arganini M, Behar R, Wu TC, Straus F 2nd, McCormick M, DeGroot LJ, et al. Hürthle cell tumors: a twenty-five-year experience. Surgery. 1986;100(6):1108-15.

40. Mills SC, Haq M, Smellie WJB, Harmer C. Hürthle cell carcinoma of the thyroid: Retrospective review of 62 patients treated at the Royal Marsden Hospital between 1946 and 2003. Eur J Surg Oncol. 2009;35(3):230-4.

41. Oluic B, Paunovic I, Loncar Z, Djukic V, Diklic A, Jovanovic M, et al. Survival and prognostic factors for survival, cancer specific survival and disease free interval in 239 patients with Hürthle cell carcinoma: a single center experience. BMC Cancer. 2017;17(1):371.

42. Chen H, Nicol TL, Udelsman R. Follicular lesions of the thyroid. Does frozen section evaluation alter operative management? Ann Surg. 1995;222(1):101-6.

43. Monzani F, Caraccio N, Iacconi P, Faviana P, Dardano A, Basolo F, et al. Prevalence of cancer in follicular thyroid nodules: is there still a role for intraoperative frozen section analysis? Thyroid. 2003;13(4):389-94.

44. Dosen D, Turic M, Smalcelj J, Janusic R, Grgic MP, Separovic V. The value of frozen section in intraoperative surgical management of thyroid follicular carcinoma. Head Neck. 2003;25(7):521-8.

45. McHenry CR, Sandoval BA. Management of follicular and Hürthle cell neoplasms of the thyroid gland. Surg Oncol Clin N Am. 1998;7(4):893-910.

46. Bondeson L, Bondeson AG, Ljungberg O. Treatment of Hürthle cell neoplasms of the thyroid. Arch Surg. 1983;118(12):1453.

47. Caplan RH, Abellera RM, Kisken WA. Hürthle cell neoplasms of the thyroid gland: reassessment of functional capacity. Thyroid. 1994;4(3):243-8.

48. Brose MS, Nutting CM, Jarzab B, Elisei R, Siena S, Bastholt L, et al. Sorafenib in radioactive iodine-refractory, locally advanced or metastatic differentiated thyroid cancer: a randomised, double-blind, phase 3 trial. Lancet (London, England). 2014;384(9940):319-28.

49. Schlumberger M, Tahara M, Wirth LJ, Robinson B, Brose MS, Elisei R, et al. Lenvatinib versus placebo in radioiodine-refractory thyroid cancer. N Engl J Med. 2015;372(7):621-30.

50. Pryma DA, Schöder H, Gönen M, Robbins RJ, Larson SM, Yeung HWD. Diagnostic accuracy and prognostic value of 18F-FDG PET in Hürthle cell thyroid cancer patients. J Nucl Med. 2006;47(8):1260-6.

51. Cooper DS, Schneyer CR. Follicular and Hürthle cell carcinoma of the thyroid. Endocrinol Metab Clin North Am. 1990;19(3):577-91.

52. Sugino K, Ito K, Mimura T, Kameyama K, Iwasaki H, Ito K. Hürthle cell tumor of the thyroid: analysis of 188 cases. World J Surg. 2001;25(9):1160-3.

53. Nagar S, Aschebrook-Kilfoy B, Kaplan EL, Angelos P, Grogan RH. Hürthle cell carcinoma: an update on survival over the last 35 years. Surgery. 2013;154(6):1263-71; discussion 1271.

54. Chindris AM, Casler JD, Bernet VJ, Rivera M, Thomas C, Kachergus JM, et al. Clinical and molecular features of Hürthle cell carcinoma of the thyroid. J Clin Endocrinol Metab. 2015;100(1):55-62.

55. Petric R, Gazic B, Besic N. Prognostic factors for disease-specific survival in 108 patients with Hürthle cell thyroid carcinoma: a single-institution experience. BMC Cancer. 2014;14:777.

56. Sanders LE, Silverman M. Follicular and Hürthle cell carcinoma: predicting outcome and directing therapy. Surgery. 1998;124(6):967-74.

Medullary Thyroid Carcinoma

Radan Dzodic, Nada Santrac

INTRODUCTION

Medullary thyroid carcinoma (MTC) is a rare thyroid malignancy of C-cell origin, occurring in two forms: (1) sporadic, nonhereditary (75%) and (2) familial, hereditary (25%), based on the absence and presence of REarranged during Transfection (*RET*) proto-oncogene germline mutation, respectively. Hereditary MTC is inherited in an autosomal dominant pattern and is expressed within multiple endocrine neoplasia (MEN) type 2 syndromes (MEN2A and MEN2B).[1] Although sporadic MTC is a nonhereditary form, it was found to have genetic setting in somatic *RET*, *HRAS*, *KRAS*, and, rarely, *NRAS* mutations.[1]

Medullary thyroid carcinoma is characterized by the secretion of calcitonin, serotonin, chromogranin A, carcinoembryonic antigen (CEA), and other peptides. Diagnosis of MTC can be set based on symptoms (painful tumor, hoarseness, flushing, diarrhea, bone pain, "crying without tears", etc.), clinical or radiological examination, basal and stimulated calcitonin levels, fine-needle aspiration biopsy (FNAB), or genetic screening for germline RET mutations. Serum calcitonin level is a precise marker for initial diagnosis of MTC, while calcitonin and CEA measured concurrently give the best assessment of disease progression, if any.[1]

Medullary thyroid carcinomas have more aggressive behavior than differentiated thyroid carcinomas and tend to spread relatively early into regional lymph nodes (LNs).[2] Distant metastases occur by hematogenous spread to liver, lungs, and bones, usually in a fine miliary pattern that can be missed on imaging.[3] Reported cancer-specific 10-year survival rates vary from 69 to 89%,[4-6] depending mainly on the age at diagnosis and tumor stage, as well as biochemical and radiological remission.[7]

Lymphonodal burden of the disease can be assessed by preoperative imaging, calcitonin levels measurement, or intraoperative evaluation by the surgeon (palpation); however, neither of these methods is reliable enough.[1]

Given that it is not responsive to radioiodine therapy or thyroid-stimulating hormone (TSH) suppression, surgery is the only curative treatment for MTC, as a prophylactic surgery for RET mutation carriers, a primary surgery for established MTC (clinically, biochemically, or cytologically), a redo surgery for persistent or recurrent disease, and a palliative procedure.[3] The aim of the surgery is to achieve adequate tumor and LN clearance,[2,3,8,9] and, if possible, a biochemical cure.[10]

Publications on MTC treatment are setting of many debates regarding the most adequate approach for MTC management, with majority of concerns focused on undertreatment rather than overtreatment of patients. This chapter will not only enlighten the problem of surgical treatment of sporadic and hereditary MTCs by systematization of current surgical recommendations but also give a personal authors' perspective for primary surgery and persistent or recurrent disease management.

EMBRYOLOGY OF C CELLS

The discovery of thyroid C cells is related to 1876 and E. Cresswell Baber who described new parenchymatous cells in a thyroid of a dog, different than the previously known follicular cells.[11] These were named *parafollicular cells* in 1932 by Nonidez,[12] a term which was widely used in the literature for a long time, until it was discovered that C cells can also be located interfollicularly or intrafollicularly. Finally, in 1966 Pearse[13,14] proposed the most appropriate name, C cells, based on the specific expression of calcitonin.

From the discovery of the second epithelial component in the thyroid gland, there was a debate on its origin.[15] Nowadays, it is known that thyroid C cells derive from the ultimobranchial body, an embryological structure that arises from the ventral portion of the fourth pharyngeal (branchial) pouch. At the 5th week of gestation, the ultimobranchial body fuses with the posterior aspect of the medial thyroid primordia in the neck, at the site of Zuckerkandl's tubercle and C-cell precursors disseminate to the upper third of both lateral lobes.[16-18] Consequently, this is the site of MTC occurrence.

It was always believed that the neuroendocrine origin of C cells is attributed to neural crest cells that enter the ultimobranchial body before its mobilization toward medial thyroid primordium. However, later studies showed that they originate from endoderm, revealing the true epithelial nature of C cells, with the expression of E-cadherin.[15,18,19]

Other than very well-established theories on ultimobranchial origin of C cells, evidence exists that some C cells may also be derived directly from the progenitor cells of the midline thyroid primordium.[15] This is collaborated by several publications in which the presence of C cells was described in patients with the DiGeorge anomaly, where ultimobranchial bodies fail to develop,[20] or in lingual thyroid, although it is unlikely that the ultimobranchial body can fuse with undescended thyroid.[21,22]

◇| BIOLOGY OF C CELLS

There are several specific characteristics of C-cell biology that influence clinical behavior, diagnosis, and treatment of MTCs. One of the most important is the *absence of the sodium–iodide symporter* and inability to uptake iodine, so authors of German guidelines clearly indicate that any residual tumor, LN, or distant metastases cannot be treated with radioiodine therapy, unlike differentiated thyroid carcinomas.[23] This is an important fact and must be taken into consideration during the initial surgery, which must provide complete clearance of the tumor and affected LNs.

C cells are *not responsive to TSH suppression*, contrary to differentiated thyroid carcinomas, and the *expression of E-cadherin* on C-cell membrane is an important characteristic which is directly related to the pathogenesis of MTC and will be explained in detail in the corresponding section.

Secretory products of C cells are various (adrenocortico-tropic hormone, chromogranin, somatostatin, B-melanocyte-stimulating hormone, histamine, neurotensin, etc.); however, calcitonin and CEA are most valuable as tumor markers for MTC.[1]

- *Calcitonin (Ct)* is a 32-amino acid monomeric peptide that is derived from preprocalcitonin, through precursor procalcitonin (proCt).[24] Studies have shown equal or superior diagnostic accuracy of Ct compared to proCt[1]; however, there is a potentially useful predictive role of proCt in disease progression, since high proCt-Ct ratio was found to be associated with an increased risk of aggressive disease and shorter progression-free survival.[1,25]

  The *Ct* gene is switched on in embryonic C cells concomitantly with the thyroglobulin gene in prefollicular cells,[17] which is highly suggestive of a common mechanism of activation, although, so far, triggering factors for the functional differentiation toward endocrine or neuroendocrine phenotype have not been determined.[25] Nearly all C cells secrete Ct; however, in <1% of cases, calcitonin-negative sporadic MTC can be observed.[26] Ct can be measured as a basal value (without stimulation) or after pentagastrin- or calcium stimulation.[1,23] Stimulated Ct measurement can be useful for: (1) diagnostic distinction between C-cell hyperplasia and MTC, (2) detecting MTC in nodular goiter patients, (3) deciding time of prophylactic thyroidectomy in children who are RET proto-oncogene mutation carriers, and (4) evaluation of persistent or recurrent disease following surgery.[1,27,28]

Usually, basal Ct levels correlate with tumor mass and disease extent; however, it may not always be the case. Thus, Ct findings must be correlated with clinical and imaging evaluation to avoid undertreatment of patients [American Thyroid Association (ATA) 2015, Grade C recommendation].[1] Opposite to this, serum Ct levels may be increased without neoplastic C-cell process in various diseases such as autoimmune thyroiditis, hyperparathyroidism, chronic renal failure, mastocytosis, or some nonthyroid malignancies such as lung cancer, pulmonary or enteric neuroendocrine tumors, and prostate cancer.[1,29] Differentiating markers for nonthyroid malignancies are (1) absence of Ct increase after stimulation, which is, on contrary, observed in MTCs and (2) lower basal Ct values, given that, usually, extrathyroid tumors produce less Ct per gram of tissue, compared to MTCs.[1]

Interpretation of serum Ct values should be careful due to age-, gender- and assay-related variations (ATA 2015, Grade B recommendation). Namely, serum Ct is highly elevated under 3 years of life, with a peak in the first 6 months,[1,30] while it is indistinguishable from adults after the age of 3 years. Basal Ct levels are higher in men due to larger C-cell mass in the thyroid gland,[1,30,31] and some drug interactions can also be responsible for increased Ct levels.[23] Serum Ct has a half-life up to 30 hours. Its elimination from human body may take several weeks or even longer,[32] so interpretation of postoperative Ct values has to be careful. In addition to that, there is a variability of Ct measurements among commercial assays; thus, guidelines recommend evaluation of samples in the same assay prior to and after surgery.[1]

- *Carcinoembryonic antigen* is not a specific marker for MTC, i.e., serum CEA elevation can be observed in many benign conditions, including tobacco smoking, heterophilic antibodies, gastrointestinal inflammatory disease, and benign lung disease, as well as in earlier described nonthyroid malignancies.[1] Calcium or pentagastrin stimulation tests do not increase serum CEA levels, in contrast to Ct elevation. CEA is not routinely used for the initial diagnosis of MTC; however, it is useful for evaluating disease progression after surgery.[1,26,33-35]

Mendelsohn et al.[11] described back in 1984 that CEA and Ct are expressed in almost every MTC cell, especially in early and localized disease (C-cell hyperplasia, microscopic MTC, or palpable MTC limited to thyroid gland). In this study, simultaneous elevation of serum Ct and CEA levels suggested that a disease progression, while constantly increasing the CEA level, accompanied with stable or declining serum Ct levels, indicated a poorly differentiated MTC and aggressive disease course.[33] Other studies[26,34,35] showed that normal or low serum levels of both Ct and CEA in patients with advanced MTC disease indicate an advanced dedifferentiation and a very poor prognosis.

The lethal outcome in these patients with nonsecretory MTC can occur rapidly, even within the first 2 years after diagnosis.[26]

Given all these data, there is a recommendation that serum basal Ct and CEA should be analyzed at the same time for a more precise evaluation of disease progression after MTC treatment (ATA 2015, Grade B recommendation).[1]

Another important characteristic of C cells is the *expression of E-cadherin* on the membrane, which is directly related to pathogenesis of MTC.[19]

EPIDEMIOLOGY AND CLASSIFICATION OF MEDULLARY THYROID CARCINOMA

Medullary thyroid carcinoma is a rare malignancy, comprising 3% of all thyroid cancers in adults and 10% of pediatric thyroid carcinomas.[8] MTC occurs in two forms: sporadic, nonhereditary (75%) and familial, hereditary (25%), expressed within MEN2A and MEN2B syndromes.

According to the current classification, proposed by the ATA,[1] MEN2A syndromes include four variants: (1) classical variant: MTC, pheochromocytoma (PHEO), primary hyperparathyroidism (PHPT); (2) MEN2A with cutaneous lichen amyloidosis (CLA); (3) MEN2A with Hirschsprung's disease (HD); and (4) familial MTC (FMTC). Although FMTC was earlier an individual entity, now it is considered a part of the MEN2A syndrome spectrum, with MTC as the only clinical feature.[36]

Gender distribution of MTC in sporadic and hereditary forms is almost equal, while the age of occurrence differs. Sporadic MTCs have the highest incidence of detection in fourth to sixth decades of life,[1] while hereditary forms occur in early childhood in MEN2B, early adulthood in MEN2A, and middle age in FMTC.[1,23,37]

PATHOGENESIS OF MEDULLARY THYROID CARCINOMA

Although the etiology of MTC is largely demystified, the mechanisms of MTC pathogenesis are largely unknown. Studies on embryonic mice thyroid gland development gave some closer insight into this problem,[19] offering significant observations regarding factors that correlate with MTC tumor growth and invasion. Differentiated C cells co-express forkhead box transcription factors (Foxa1 and Foxa2) and calcitonin. Opposed to this, Foxa1 and Foxa2 are differentially expressed in embryonic and neoplastic C cells. Namely, coexpression of Foxa1 in Ki67+ embryonic and neoplastic C cells, lacking Foxa2 expression, indicates that nuclear Foxa1 promotes growth of neoplastic C cells. Foxa2, on the contrary, is normally expressed in nonproliferating (Ki67_) embryonic and differentiated C cells, while it is downregulated in neoplastic cells. This implies that tumor spreading (invasion) is a consequence of epithelial-to-mesenchymal transition of MTC cells, directed by loss of Foxa2 and E-cadherin.[19] Neoplastic C cells with diminished Foxa2 and E-cadherin expression are more prone to metastasize than clusters of Foxa2+ cells that are constrained by E-cadherin–based adhesion.[19]

GENOTYPE–PHENOTYPE CORRELATIONS IN MEDULLARY THYROID CARCINOMA

The RET oncogene was first discovered by Takahashi et al.[38] in 1985. It comprises 21 exons located on the long arm of chromosome 10 (10q11.2). RET is expressed in cells derived from the branchial arches [parathyroid glands (PTGs)], the neural crest (brain, parasympathetic and sympathetic ganglia, thyroid C-cells, adrenal medulla, and enteric ganglia), and the urogenital system.[39] RET encodes a single-pass transmembrane receptor of the tyrosine kinase family of proteins that is divided into three of the following domains: (1) N-terminal extracellular domain containing four cadherin-like regions, (2) cysteine-rich region with a transmembrane domain, and (3) cytoplasmic domain with tyrosine kinase activity.[40] Unlike most of the other hereditary cancer syndromes, which are usually associated with inactivation of tumor suppressor genes, MEN2 syndromes are associated with gain-of-function RET proto-oncogene mutations.[41]

More than 100 RET proto-oncogene mutations have been described in patients with MTC. RET germline mutations are present in all patients with hereditary disease,[1] while around 50% of patients with sporadic disease have RET somatic mutations in exons 11, 13, and 16.[42] In 18–80% of RET-negative sporadic MTCs, somatic mutations of *HRAS*, *KRAS*, or *NRAS* are reported.[43,44]

Genotype–Phenotype Correlations in Sporadic Medullary Thyroid Carcinoma

Patients with sporadic MTCs do not harbor RET germline mutations, but majority of them have some RET or RAS somatic mutation.[42-45]

Sporadic MTCs are usually diagnosed between the fourth and the sixth decades of life.[46] Among patients who initially present with a palpable tumor, 70% have cervical and 10% have distant metastases.[3] The clinical behavior of sporadic MTC is unpredictable, but age and disease stage at the time of diagnosis are distinguished as significant independent prognostic factors.[6,47] Reported 10-year survival rates in stages I, II, III, and IV are 100, 93, 71, and 21%, respectively.[47]

It was shown that sporadic MTCs with RET somatic M918T mutation in exon 16 have a higher growth rate, more aggressive clinical course, and poorer prognosis compared to MTCs with other RET mutations.[48] Opposed to this, there is a low prevalence of this mutation in micro-MTCs.

Genotype–Phenotype Correlations in Hereditary Medullary Thyroid Carcinoma

Hereditary MTCs occur as a part of MEN2A (95%) and MEN2B (5%) syndromes, both of whom are characterized with nearly 100% penetrance of MTC.[3] Its clinical course is expressed in a mutation-specific, age-related manner. Most aggressive MTC behavior is found in MEN2B syndrome, with invasive carcinoma expressed in the first months after birth. MTC in MEN2A syndrome associated with codon 634 mutations has a higher risk of LN metastases in adolescence. FMTC or MTC in MEN2A associated with noncodon 634 mutations tend to be least aggressive, presenting in second or third decade of life.[3] However, it was shown that many MEN2A families with the same RET mutation have significant variability in the clinical manifestation which might be a result of disease-modifying alleles.

MEN2A Syndrome

MEN2A syndrome is sporadic in 10% of cases, with de novo RET mutations[49] arising from paternally inherited allele,[50] while in 90% it occurs in families with manifestations of MEN2A.[1] As previously described, MEN2A phenotype is characterized with four variants: classical MEN2A, MEN2A with CLA, MEN2A with HD, and FMTC.

Classical MEN2A is the most common MEN2A variant, associated with germline mutations in RET exons 10 (codons 609, 611, 618, and 620) and 11 (codon 634) in >95% of cases.[1,40,41] MTC is expressed in all patients with classical MEN2A, while occurrence of PHEO and PHPT depends on the specific RET germline mutation.[1,41] The most frequent mutation in MEN2A is C634R mutation in exon 11. Patients with RET codon 634 mutations are associated with almost complete penetrance of MTC at young ages, 50% penetrance of PHEO,[50,51] and 30% penetrance of PHPT. On the other hand, exon 10 RET mutations are associated with a much lower penetrance of PHEO (4–26%) and PHPT (2–12%).[52,53] In very rare families that have all the features of classical MEN2A, without detectable RET germline mutation, the presence of characteristic phenotype in one or more first-degree relatives can support the diagnosis.[1]

MEN2A with CLA is mainly associated with RET codon 634 mutation (55), although it can occur in codon 804 mutation.[54] In addition to classical MEN2A variant phenotype, it is characterized by dermatological lesions in the scapular regions (corresponding to dermatomes T2–T6), that can have an early-onset, preceding MTC.[55]

MEN2A with HD occurs in approximately 7% MEN2A syndromes,[56] and it is associated with exon 10 RET point mutations in codons: 620 (50%), 618 (30%), 609 (15%), and 611 (5%)[1]—never with codon 634 mutations. HD is predominantly present just after birth. MTC penetrance is 100%, while penetrance of PHEO and PHPT is much lower, due to exon 10 codon mutations.[1]

FMTC is an MEN2A syndrome variant with MTC as the only clinical feature.[36] It can be manifested in families with MTC who develop neither PHEO nor PHPT, or in isolated individuals of MTC-negative families.[1] It is associated with an RET germline mutation in 88% of cases,[45] usually the same mutations as in MEN2A, with the exception of C634.[3] Double RET germline mutations on the same allele were also described in FMTC, with varying aggressiveness.[57]

MEN2B Syndrome

MEN2B syndrome is sporadic in 75% of cases, with de novo RET mutations[49] in paternally inherited allele,[50] while in 25%, it occurs in families with manifestations of MEN2B.[1]

MEN2B syndrome accounts for 5% of hereditary MTCs that have 100% penetrance and are almost always present in early infancy, with highly aggressive disease course, regarding both regional and distant metastases.[1] There is a 50% penetrance of PHEO in MEN2B, usually occurring in adolescence and early adulthood, but PHPT, CLA, or HD never occur.[1,23]

These patients have a very striking physiognomy due to numerous skeletal and ophthalmologic abnormalities. Most common clinical appearance includes narrow long face, thickened, everted eyelids with mild ptosis, high-arched palate, gingival and lingual ganglioneuroma, marfanoid habitus with scoliosis, pectus excavatum, pes cavus, and slipped capital femoral epiphyses. Infants are unable to make tears, while generalized mucosal ganglioneuromatosis leads to abdominal symptoms such as bloating, intermittent constipation, and diarrhea.[1]

Around 95% of MEN2B patients have RET codon M918T germline mutation in exon 16.[1] Codon A883F mutation in exon 15 is less frequent (up to 5%) and shows less aggressive MTC phenotype, compared to M918T.[58] Rare double RET germline mutations on the same allele present with atypical MEN2B, characterized with later age of onset (20–30 years of age) and varying aggressiveness.[41]

American Thyroid Association Risk Stratification of Medullary Thyroid Carcinoma

Genotype–phenotype correlations in MTCs were presented so far in several guidelines for MTC management, with many mutual differences. New, more unified risk stratification was proposed in 2015 by ATA Task Force,[1] classifying disease aggressiveness into three categories (instead of four, as previously suggested in 2009 guidelines[59]):

- "Highest risk" (former ATA D) category, including patients with MEN2B and the RET codon M918T mutation in exon 16
- "High-risk" (former ATA C) category, including patients with RET codon C634 mutations in exon 11 and RET codon A883F mutation in exon 15
- "Moderate-risk" (former ATA A and B) category, including patients with RET codon mutations other than M918T, C634, and A883F.

Table 1: Most common RET germline mutations in MEN2 syndromes and ATA risk categories based on clinical aggressiveness of MTC.

ATA risk category*	RET codon mutation	MTC onset age	Hereditary syndrome
Highest risk (former ATA D[†])	M918T	Early infancy, age of <1 year	MEN2B
High risk (former ATA C[†])	C634 A883F	Below age of 5 years	High-risk MEN2A MEN2B
Moderate risk (former ATA A and B[†])	321, 515, 531, 532, 533, 600, 603, 606, 635, 649, 666, 768, 777, 790, 791, 804, 819, 833, 844, 866, 891, 912 (Former ATA A); 609, 611, 618, 620, 630, 631, 633 (Former ATA B)	Second or third decade of life	Low-risk classical MEN2A, MEN2A with CLA, MEN2A with HD, FMTC

*Based on revised ATA management guidelines for MTC from 2015.[1]
[†]Based on ATA management guidelines for MTC from 2009.[59]
(ATA: American Thyroid Association; MTC: medullary thyroid carcinoma; RET: REarranged during Transfection)

Table 1 summarizes the most common RET germline mutations in MEN2 syndromes and ATA risk categories based on clinical aggressiveness of MTC.

◇ CLINICAL PRESENTATION OF MEDULLARY THYROID CARCINOMA

Sporadic MTC is usually diagnosed from fourth to sixth decade of life, with the highest incidence in the fifth decade.[45,46] Hereditary MTC can be present at birth (MEN2B) or very early in childhood (MEN2A with 634 codon mutation), but it can also be diagnosed later, in adulthood (MEN2A noncodon 634 mutation or FMTC), depending on the RET codon mutation and genetic screening possibility.[1,23]

Medullary thyroid carcinoma is multifocal and bilateral in 90% of patients with a hereditary and up to 20% of patients with a sporadic disease form.[3,60] It can be rarely presented as a subclinical disease, with elevation of basal Ct, or even diagnosed on pathology examination of a multinodular goiter specimen, without previous suspicion of MTC. However, the most common clinical presentation of sporadic and late-onset hereditary forms of MTC is a solitary, palpable thyroid tumor, or a lesion within thyroid goiter,[3] usually accompanied by elevation of serum Ct levels.

Approximately 15% of patients with palpable tumors have symptoms caused by local tumor growth or invasion of recurrent laryngeal nerve (RLN) or aerodigestive tract, such as pain, hoarseness, dysphagia, or respiratory difficulties.[1,3,45] Locally advanced disease, with gross neck and mediastinal LN metastases, may also cause symptoms and signs of superior vena cava syndrome.

Medullary thyroid carcinomas behave more aggressively than differentiated thyroid carcinomas,[3] with an early locoregional spread.[2] Data show that 80% of patients with palpable tumors have central compartment (CC) LN metastases at the time of diagnosis, while 75 and 47% have LN metastases in ipsilateral and contralateral jugulocarotid regions, respectively.[3] In addition, LN metastases are found in <35% of micro-MTCs.[61]

Distant metastases occur by hematogenous spread to liver, lungs, and bones, usually in a fine miliary pattern that can be missed on imaging.[3] Approximately 10–15% of patients have distant metastases at initial presentation.[3] These can be accompanied with symptoms like bone pain, vasomotor flushing, or diarrhea, due to hypercalcitoninemia and secretion of other peptides from neoplastic C cells.[8]

Medullary thyroid carcinoma-specific survival rates depend on (1) age and (2) disease stage at the time of diagnosis, as independent prognostic factors, and (3) biochemical and radiological remission.[6,7,47,48] Corroborating this (1) patients with early MTC onset in MEN2B or high-risk MEN2A syndrome have faster tumor growth, early onset of LN metastases, and poorer prognosis[48]; (2) 10-year survival rates in patients with MTCs are 100, 93, 71, and 21% in stage I, II, III, and IV, respectively[47]; and (3) patients in whom biochemical and radiological remission was not achieved with surgery had slightly reduced 10-year survival rates, to 73%.[7]

Serum Ct levels usually correlate with disease burden, both in preoperative and in postoperative setting. However, in <1% of cases, sporadic MTC can be calcitonin-negative.[26] Also, it is possible to have an advanced disease without elevation of Ct or CEA, which is highly suggestive of MTC dedifferentiation and poor prognosis.[26] Patients with nonsecretory MTCs have a variable survival, from 12.5 to only 1.75 years after diagnosis.[1]

◇ EVALUATION OF MEDULLARY THYROID CARCINOMA PATIENTS IN PREOPERATIVE AND POSTOPERATIVE SETTINGS

Patients can be initially suspected of having an MTC based on symptoms (flushing, diarrhea, "crying without tears"), elevation of serum Ct and CEA levels, physical or radiological examination; cytology finding after FNAB of single or multiple nodules in thyroid goiter, genetic screening; presence of MTC in patient's family, and previous treatment of PHEO in patient or family.

Every thorough evaluation of the patient with a suspicion of MTC should include the following steps: (1) medical history (anamnesis), (2) physical examination, (3) imaging methods, (4) FNAB with cytology, (5) functional evaluation, (6) genetic testing for RET germline mutations, and (7) laryngoscopy.

- *Medical history (anamnesis)* alone is sufficient to raise a suspicion of patient having an MTC, based on presence of symptoms (like "crying without tears", pain, hoarseness, dysphagia, and diarrhea) or based on evidence of prior or current diseases in patient or family (e.g., PHEO or MEN2). It should provide information on tumor growth, progression of symptoms, and prior diagnostics, so that further diagnostic can be planned.

- *Physical examination* can be a crucial examination method for suspecting of MTC. It should include evaluation of the tumor and regional LNs (for distant metastases it is rather irrelevant). Tumor, if palpable, should be assessed in the mater of its size, shape, position, mobility, multifocality, relation to surrounding neck structures, and its sensibility (MTC tend to be accompanied by pain!). Firm, rapidly growing, irregular tumor, fixed to surrounding structures, or a new onset of hoarseness, indicates a malignant nature of the tumor and possible infiltration of surrounding structures like RLN.[23,25] Absence of palpable thyroid mass should not exclude MTC by itself, since MTC tumors are most commonly localized in the posterior of the lobe and, if small, can be easily overlooked. In addition, MTC can occur in the form of multifocal, several millimeter tumors in the lobe(s), which might not be diagnosed by ultrasonography (US), let alone by physical examination. Patients with MTC have a high percentage of LN metastases in central and jugulocarotid regions at the initial presentation.[3] Experienced physicians can detect LN metastases in the neck by palpation; however, metastases can be very small, impalpable. Thus, absence of LN disease in central or lateral neck compartments by palpation cannot reliably exclude LN metastases. Central neck compartment might be especially challenging for palpation, depending on the patient's constitution.

- *Imaging methods* for the evaluation of patients with MTC should be applied rationally, with regard to the necessity, usefulness, and costs. If there is no reason to think of the metastatic disease, based on initial standard imaging (neck and abdominal US, chest X-ray, laryngoscopy, or computed tomography), Ct levels and clinical symptoms and signs, additional imaging might be omitted. However, if metastatic MTC is expected at the initial presentation, or if there is a suspicion of regional or distant MTC relapse, additional imaging procedures are indicated.[1,8] Unfortunately, none of the procedures by itself provides an optimal whole-body imaging.[1]

  - US, as a standard of care for evaluation of thyroid tumors and regional LNs, is an important imaging method for assessing the extent of thyroid cancer surgery and should be performed in all patients.[1,23,62]

    Irregular tumor margins, microcalcifications, and central hypervascularization are the most reliable sonographic characteristics of a thyroid malignancy (risk up to 80%).[45,63] US features that are most suggestive of malignant LNs are round shape, hyperechogenicity, calcifications, cystic changes, peripheral or chaotic vascularization, and loss of fatty hilum, even though reliability of the latter is debatable.[64]

    Preoperative US should provide more evidence to the clinical suspicion of tumor malignancy, but it is not suitable to rule out malignancy.[23] In addition, contribution of US evaluation of cervical LNs is disputable in the literature due to variable overall method's accuracy in the reported series. Namely, several authors reported a low US sensitivity in the preoperative evaluation of central neck compartment (9.5–61%), but high for assessment of lateral LNs (64–93.9%) in papillary thyroid carcinoma.[65] Opposed to this, other authors report a low US sensitivity in lateral neck compartments.[66] US elastography was proposed as a complementary method for cervical LN assessment, since metastatic LNs show greater stiffness than benign ones. Following this, score 1 or 2 suggests a benign LN, while score 3 or 4 implies a malignant one.[67]

    In a review from 2017 by Kim, it was discussed that several clinical factors might affect poor value of preoperative US staging in some patients.[64] For example, diffuse thyroid disease lowers the accuracy of CC evaluation, while it does not interfere with lateral LN assessment.[68,69] Similarly, obesity interferes with the detection of central LN metastases, with accuracy of 53.1 and 71.7% in patients with body mass index (BMI) ≥30 and BMI <30 kg/m^2, respectively.[70] In general, the rationale for poor US sensitivity in central neck compartment might be the small size of metastatic LNs and anatomical limitations (bones, fatty tissue).[71]

- Contrast-enhanced computed tomography (CE-CT) is a very useful imaging method for the evaluation of extrathyroidal tumor extension, regional and distant LN metastases in MTC,[1,3,8,62] with a high sensitivity for the central neck compartment, mediastinal region, lung, and liver metastases. It is recommended in patients with extensive neck disease and signs or symptoms of regional or distant metastases and should be done in all patients with Ct elevation >500 pg/mL (ATA 2015, Grade C recommendation).[1] It is of value for the persistent or recurrent MTC disease, as well.

- Contrast-enhanced magnetic resonance imaging (CE-MRI) is indicated if there is a suspicion of a locally advanced disease.[8,62] Along with CE-CT of liver, it is the most sensitive method for the detection of liver metastases[1] and should be done in patients with signs or symptoms of distant metastases, or in patients with Ct elevation >500 pg/mL at initial presentation (ATA 2015, Grade C recommendation).[1] It is also of value in the follow-up if liver metastases are suspected of.

- Axial MRI and bone scintigraphy are complementary and the most sensitive imaging methods to detect bone metastases, both at initial presentation and in the follow-up.[72]
- Fluorodeoxyglucose-positron emission tomography (FDG-PET)/CT and F-DOPA-PET/CT are less sensitive in detecting metastases, compared to other imaging procedures.[72] In the current ATA guidelines from 2015, there is a recommendation against using these methods for detection of distant metastases.[1] On the contrary, British guidelines from 2014 refer from its use in the initial setting, prior to the first surgery, while they do not disapprove of its application in the recurrent disease.[8]
- Scintigraphy with ^{131}I is not useful for the diagnosis of MTC. Due to the C-cell biology, MTC cells do not uptake radioiodine and consequently present as "cold", nonfunctional thyroid nodule on scintigraphy.[3] Imaging with anti-carcinoembryonic antigen (anti-CEA) antibodies and scintigraphy with metaiodobenzylguanidine (MIBG), dimercaptosuccinic acid, somatostatin analogs, and gastrin are of low sensitivity.[1]
- *FNAB with cytology* should be performed on thyroid tumors that are clinically/radiologically suspicious or on the suspicious LNs.[1,8,23,62] It is considered a safe and useful tool in the initial diagnosis of thyroid tumors; however, misinterpretations are possible and decision for surgical treatment cannot be made based on cytology alone.

Fine-needle aspiration biopsy of a tumor suspicious of MTC can be difficult, due to its posterolateral position in the junction of upper and middle third of the lobe. With regard to safety, local hemorrhage and RLN injury might rarely occur during FNAB, and needle tract metastases have also been described in the literature, but without affecting clinical outcome.[73] Usefulness, on the contrary, is debatable. One meta-analysis from 2015 showed the accuracy of only 50% in diagnosis of MTC by cytology.[74] Namely, MTCs have variable cytological presentations, like spindle-shaped, plasmacytoid, or epithelioid cells. Cytologically, it can be misdiagnosed for sarcomas, plasmacytomas, or follicular lesions, Hürthle cell neoplasms, anaplastic thyroid cancer, or achromatic melanoma.[1,45] Cytological criteria that are highly suggestive of MTC are dispersed polygonal or triangular cells, eccentrically placed nuclei with coarse granular chromatin and amyloid, and azurophilic cytoplasmic granules.[1,75] The diagnostic accuracy of FNAB in MTC tumor or metastatic LNs can be increased by (1) measuring Ct levels in the FNAB washout fluid and by (2) immunohistochemistry of FNAB sample to detect Ct, CEA, and chromogranin and confirm thyroglobulin absence.[1,76] Given this, ATA recommends these additional analyses for FNAB findings that are inconclusive or suggestive of MTC (ATA 2015, Grade B Recommendation).[1]

- *Functional evaluation* that is of importance for MTC implies measurement of serum Ct and CEA, as valuable clinical biomarkers for (1) initial MTC diagnosis, (2) deciding upon time of surgery in RET mutation carriers, and (3) clinical follow-up of MTC patients after surgery.[1,8,9,23]

Calcitonin can be measured as a basal serum value and as a stimulated value after calcium or pentagastrin injection.[1,23] Most commonly, serum Ct levels correlate with tumor mass and disease extent; however, these findings must always be interpreted along with physical examination and imaging findings, and with regard to age- and gender-related variations, to provide adequate decision on the treatment.[1] In order to reduce the risk of misinterpretation due to assay-related variations, it is mandatory to perform evaluation of patient samples in the same assay. Some clinical conditions, nonthyroid malignancies, and drug interactions can also be responsible for the increased basal Ct value. However, differentially, elevation of stimulated Ct is observed only in MTCs,[1] not in the above-mentioned cases. In addition to this, Ct stimulation tests are useful for the evaluation of certain RET mutation carriers, in terms of necessity for and timing of surgical treatment, as well as for assessment of persistent or recurrent MTC following surgery.[1,8,23,27,28] CEA per se is of no benefit for early MTC diagnosis or follow-up, but, if measured concurrently with basal Ct, it is of high value for disease follow-up.[1]

There are no unanimous recommendations on Ct screening in patients with thyroid goiters prior to surgery. Advocates argue benefits of early MTC diagnosis, prompt, adequate, one-step initial surgery, and potentially better outcome or biochemical cure.[8,23,77] Opponents argue cost-effectiveness and lack of benefit in terms of long-term outcome.[1,8] ATA 2015 guidelines[1] strongly recommend individual approach to Ct screening in the initial setting, based on the availability of secretagogues (calcium and pentagastrin), costs, and effectiveness. German 2013 guidelines,[23] on the contrary, recommend measurement of serum Ct in all patients in need for thyroid surgery, since early MTC diagnosis is thought to improve survival,[77] and US and FNAB cannot reliably rule out micro-MTC as additional finding in nodular or multinodular goiters. British 2014 guidelines[8] recommend US, FNAB, and basal Ct as initial evaluation of patients with suspected MTC but state that there is insufficient evidence for recommending Ct screening in all patients with thyroid disease. Japanese 2018 guidelines[78] did not discuss routine measurement of serum Ct for patients with thyroid nodules. However, at Kuma Hospital, whose results are one of the fundamentals of Japanese guidelines, serum Ct is measured only in patients with tumors that are suspicious of MTC on FNAB, not in patients with thyroid nodules or other thyroid carcinomas (personal communication with Professor Akira Miyauchi).

There were some indications that intraoperative serum Ct measurement can be of use in prediction of completeness of MTC surgical resection.[79] However, De Crea et al. showed that relying on this method, approximately 30% of the patients would be undertreated, with residual neck disease, and about 20% of cured patients would have unnecessary lateral neck dissection (LND).[80]

Normalization of serum Ct levels after surgery, most frequently addressed as "biochemical cure", is a favorable prognostic indicator of a long-term cure for MTC patients.[81] ATA guidelines from 2015 recommend measuring serum Ct levels not earlier than 3 months after surgery to assess the treatment outcome and timely identify patients with persistent disease by Ct elevation.[1] However, Machens et al. have shown in their recent study that Ct levels often normalize within just 1 week after surgery, particularly in node-negative patients, while Ct clearance may be delayed in node-positive disease.[82]

Authors of this chapter recommend routine Ct screening in all patients with nodular/multinodular goiter or thyroiditis, in patients with any symptoms that could be related to MTC (flushing or diarrhea), and in patients with hypercalcemia or suspicious PHEO (suggesting a hereditary disease form). This strategy is beneficial for earlier diagnosis of MTCs, especially microcarcinomas that can easily be overlooked on US or FNAB, and it is useful for the detection of C-cell hyperplasia which cannot be visually verified. Based on physical examination and serum Ct level at the initial presentation, additional imaging can be suggested for better evaluation of locally advanced disease, or distant metastases, if suspected. It is important to have in mind that LN and distant metastases can be found in lower preoperative CT values,[83] which can lead to undertreatment of patients. In some asymptomatic RET mutation carriers, with moderate risk MTC (*See* **Table 1**),[1] serum Ct levels can help decide on the optimal timing of surgery. We do not find intraoperative Ct measurement to be an adequate method for guiding extent of surgery or for early evaluation of the completeness or surgical resection, since serum Ct level is expected to decrease within several postoperative days, or even weeks. This decrease is prompt in lower preoperative Ct values and thyroid-limited disease, but it is expected to be prolonged in higher Ct levels prior to surgery and node-positive patients. We recommend the measurement of postoperative Ct at the earliest 2 days after surgery. Absence of decrease or normalization of postoperative Ct on the first measurement, especially in locally advanced disease with higher preoperative Ct values, should not be immediately contributed to the inadequate surgery, since decrease may occur in the upcoming weeks. However, if

decrease is not observed until 3 months after surgery, persistent disease has to be suspected and additional evaluation is necessary. It is of great value to assess simultaneously Ct and CEA, always in the same laboratory, for timely diagnosis of persistent or recurrent disease.

As a part of functional evaluation in the preoperative work-up, PHEO and PHPT should be excluded or confirmed in patients with suspected or proven hereditary MTC,[1,8,23,62] as well as in apparently sporadic disease form if genetic testing is unavailable. Investigation should include 24-hour metanephrines and catecholamine urinary analysis, plasma-free normetanephrines estimation for PHEO detection, and serum calcium and parathyroid hormone (PTH) evaluation for PHPT detection.[1,23,62]

- *Genetic counseling and genetic testing for RET germline mutation* is a very important step in the diagnosis and treatment of MTC. It was shown that up to 7% of patients with apparently sporadic disease in fact have a hereditary MTC.[84,85] Additionally, 75% of the patients with MEN2B and up to 10% of patients with MEN2A have de novo RET mutations.[49,86,87]

Genetic counseling and genetic testing for RET germline mutation are recommended to be done in the following cases[1,8,23,45]:

- In any patient with preoperatively suspected or proven MTC, even in the absence of a positive family history[8] or bilateral tumors[3,60] (apparently sporadic MTC)
- Postoperatively, in all cases when MTC is found incidentally on pathohistological analysis of a thyroid specimen, with or without positive family history[62]
- In the first-degree relatives (also other family members) of proven RET mutation carriers, ideally before the age of recommended prophylactic thyroid surgery[1,23,45]
- In a newborn with any previously described phenotype characteristics that could match MEN2B genotype (ophthalmologic abnormalities, skeletal malformations, or generalized mucosal ganglioneuromatosis) or in parents of infants or young children with MEN2B phenotype[1]
- In patients with CLA[1]
- In infants or young children with HD and exon 10 RET germline mutation[1]
- In adults with MEN2A and exon 10 RET germline mutation, who have symptoms suggestive of HD.[1]

At present, it is not a standard of care to analyze sporadic, non-RET germline MTC for the somatic RET mutation at codon M918T or somatic RAS mutations, although it might be of value.[1]

Revised ATA management guidelines from 2015 offer systematized evidence and precise recommendations for approach to RET germline testing. In families with hereditary MTC and known RET germline mutation, a targeted analysis can be performed in at-risk family members to detect the mutated RET allele,[1] with least possible costs. Opposed to this, in new families with hereditary MTC and unknown specific RET germline mutation, it is common to test most frequent mutations in exons 10 and 11 (C609, C611, C618, C620, C620, and C634), and then additional mutations in exons 13, 14, 15, and 16, sometimes exon 8.[1] This comprehensive approach guarantees detection of rare double or multiple RET mutations that would be omitted by a two-step approach;[88] however, costs of full RET sequencing are very high.[1] A two-step approach starts with analysis of the most commonly mutated "hotspot" exons (10 and 11), and if a specific RET mutation is not identified, or there is a discrepancy between phenotype and identified RET mutation, sequencing of the remaining RET exons should be performed (ATA 2015, Grade B Recommendation).[1] In families with negative genotype, but positive MEN2 phenotype, experts recommend screening of family members for MTC, PHEO, and PHPT by conventional methods at 1- to 3-year intervals.[1]

The recommended testing for MEN2A phenotype is a single- or multi-step analysis of exon 10 (codons 609, 611, 618, and 620); exon 11 (codons 630 and 634); and exons 8, 13, 14, 15, and 16, to detect RET mutations (ATA 2015, Grade B Recommendation).[1]

The recommended testing for MEN2B phenotype is a two-step analysis of M918T RET mutation in exon 16, and, if negative, A883F RET mutation in exon 15. If neither of these two mutations is identified, the entire RET coding region should be sequenced (ATA 2015, Grade B Recommendation).[1]

Screening with molecular methods for RET proto-oncogene mutations is becoming more affordable; unfortunately, it is not available in all parts of the world. If genetic testing is unavailable, imaging methods and functional evaluation should be used to confirm or exclude PHEO and PHPT in patients with MTC.

There are several ethical issues for genetic screening in adults and pediatric population, especially in prenatal context, which will not be discussed in this chapter, but readers should refer to revised ATA 2015 guidelines for further recommendations on this.[1]

- Laryngoscopy should be done in all patients as a part of preoperative work-up for thyroid surgery. By systematic examinations, preexisting vocal cord palsy can be verified in patients who are apparently asymptomatic.[89] Dysphonia at initial presentation or vocal cord dysfunction should suggest the MTC extrathyroidal extension, and possible infiltration or compression of RLN, in which case additional imaging (like CE-CT), and esophagoscopy should be done preoperatively. It is mandatory to do laryngoscopy before a redo surgery. If RLN palsy is verified, it is preferable to use intraoperative neuromonitoring.[1,23]

STAGING OF MEDULLARY THYROID CARCINOMA

The most frequently used staging system for MTC is the TNM (tumor, node, metastases) staging system by the American Joint Committee on Cancer (AJCC) Cancer Staging Manual, which has recently been updated in the 8th edition.[90]

There are several differences from the previous edition.[91] T category has been divided into two subcategories: T3a, defined as a tumor >4 cm, limited to the thyroid gland and T3b, defined as a tumor of any size with gross extrathyroidal extension to infrahyoid strap muscles.[64,90] N category has also been significantly reclassified. Namely, upper mediastinal LNs (level VII) that were previously addressed as N1b subcategory[91] are now referred to as N1a subcategory, along with level VI LNs, unilaterally or bilaterally.[90]

Evaluation of tumors, LNs, and distant metastases can be clinical (including all imaging methods and physical examination), which should be noted with the prefix "c", as well as pathological, which should be marked with prefix "p".

Suffix "s" in T category suggests a solitary tumor, while suffix "m" stands for multifocal tumors. In multifocal tumors, the largest tumor diameter determines the T category. In N category, suffix "sn" should be added if LN metastasis is identified only by sentinel LN biopsy, while suffix "f" suggests that LN metastasis is identified only by fine-needle or core-needle biopsy. It is strictly suggested that terms pM0 and Mx must not be used in classification of distant metastases. Terms cM0, cM1, and pM1 are eligible, and any of these categories may be used with pathological stage grouping.[90]

Current classifications of MTCs by T, N, and M categories, as well as grouped TNM stages, are adapted from the AJCC Cancer Staging Manual, 8th edition[90] and are given in **Tables 2 to 5**.

ANATOMICAL AND SURGICAL CLASSIFICATIONS OF CERVICAL LYMPH NODES

Anatomically, there are four compartments of cervical LNs: central, mediastinal, and two lateral,[92] which are further divided into LN groups.

- *Central compartment* is limited superiorly by hyoid bone, inferiorly by the brachiocephalic trunk on the right and left brachiocephalic vein on the left, and laterally by common carotid arteries. It includes prelaryngeal (Delphian) LNs, pretracheal LNs, paratracheal LNs on the right and left side of trachea, as well as suprabrachiocephalic part of the upper mediastinal LNs. Paratracheal regions, with regard to RLNs, include anterior and posterior LNs.[23]
- *Mediastinal compartment* (MC) is limited superiorly by the left brachiocephalic vein, inferiorly by the pericardium and tracheal bifurcation, and laterally by the mediastinal pleura. It includes anterior LN group around

Table 2: Tumor staging in medullary thyroid carcinoma by the American Joint Committee on Cancer, 8th edition.[90]

T category	Criteria
TX	Primary tumor cannot be assessed
T0	No evidence of primary tumor
T1	Tumor ≤2 cm in greatest dimension, limited to the thyroid
T1a	Tumor ≤1 cm in greatest dimension, limited to the thyroid
T1b	Tumor >1 and ≤2 cm in greatest dimension, limited to the thyroid
T2	Tumor >2 and ≤4 cm in greatest dimension, limited to the thyroid
T3	Tumor >4 cm limited to the thyroid, or any tumor with extrathyroidal extension to strap muscles
T3a	Tumor >4 cm in greatest dimension, limited to the thyroid
T3b	Tumor of any size with gross extrathyroidal extension to infrahyoid strap muscles (sternohyoid, sternothyroid, thyrohyoid, or omohyoid muscles)
T4	Advanced disease
T4a	Moderately advanced disease; tumor of any size with extrathyroidal extension and invasion of recurrent laryngeal nerve, larynx, trachea, esophagus, or subcutaneous soft tissue
T4b	Very advanced disease; tumor of any size with gross extrathyroidal extension toward prevertebral fascia, spine, and large blood vessels of the neck and mediastinum

Note: Prefix "c" indicates clinical evaluation of tumor by imaging methods and physical examination, while prefix "p" signifies pathological analysis. Suffix "s" suggests a solitary tumor, while suffix "m" stands for multifocal tumors (in multifocal tumors, the largest tumor determines the T category).

Table 3: Regional lymph node staging in medullary thyroid carcinoma by the American Joint Committee on Cancer, 8th edition.[90]

N category	Criteria
NX	Regional lymph nodes cannot be assessed
N0	No evidence of regional lymph node metastases
N0a	Cytological or histological confirmation of benign regional lymph nodes
N0b	No radiological or clinical evidence of regional lymph node metastases
N1	Metastases in regional lymph nodes
N1a	Metastases in levels VI and/or VII (Delphian/prelaryngeal, pretracheal, paratracheal, and upper mediastinal lymph nodes), unilaterally or bilaterally
N1b	Metastases in ipsilateral, contralateral or bilateral lateral neck lymph nodes (levels I, II, III, IV, and V), or metastases in retropharyngeal lymph nodes

Note: Regional lymph nodes for thyroid gland are lymph nodes of regions I to VII. Prefix "c" in N1 stage indicates that lymph node metastases are suspected on imaging methods and physical examination, while prefix "p" signifies pathological confirmation of lymph node metastases. Suffix "sn" should be added if lymph node metastasis is identified only by sentinel lymph node biopsy, while suffix "f" suggests that lymph node metastasis is identified only by fine-needle or core-needle biopsy.

Table 4: Distant metastases staging in medullary thyroid carcinoma by the American Joint Committee on Cancer, 8th edition.[90]

M category	Criteria
cM0	No clinical evidence of distant metastases
cM1	Clinical evidence of distant metastases
pM1	Pathological confirmation of distant metastases

Note: Prefix "c" in indicates that distant metastases are suspected on imaging methods and physical examination, while prefix "p" signifies pathological confirmation of distant metastases. Categories cM0, cM1, and pM1 may be used with pathological stage grouping.

Table 5: Stage groups in medullary thyroid carcinoma by the American Joint Committee on Cancer, 8th edition.[90]

TNM stage	T category	N category	M category
I	T1	N0	M0
II	T2/T3	N0	M0
III	T1/T2/T3	N1a	M0
IVA	T4a	Any N	M0
	T1/T2/T3	N1b	M0
IVB	T4b	Any N	M0
IVC	Any T	Any N	M1

Note: Regardless of the method of evaluation (clinical or pathological), all M categories may be combined with pathological T and N stages.

bone and subclavian vein, medially by common carotid artery, laterally by trapezius muscle, and posteriorly by posterior cervical fascia, which lies on the deep neck muscles and phrenic nerve. They include upper, middle, lower, and lateral jugular LNs.[23]

Surgically, four classifications are commonly used for reporting status of regional LNs in thyroid cancer.

- *Compartment classification* by Dralle et al.,[92] proposed in 1994, is based on four previously explained anatomical compartments. Compartment 1 refers to central LNs, with 1a being right and 1b as left cervicocentral group; compartment 2 implies right cervicolateral LN group; compartment 3 indicates left cervicolateral LN group; and compartment 4 includes infrabrachiocephalic upper mediastinal LNs, with 4a being right and 4b as left group. Compared to this, other surgical classifications do not include compartment 4 LNs and do not identify the side of LNs (right vs. left). German guidelines refer to compartment classification in their recommendations.

- *Japanese classification* by Qubain et al., proposed in 2002,[93] identifies seven LN groups: groups 1–4 in CC and groups 5–7 in LCs.

- *Union for International Cancer Control (UICC) classification*, proposed in 2003,[94] refers to eight LN groups. CC includes groups 1 (submental), 2 (submandibular), and 8 (central), while groups 2 and 3 (upper jugular), 4 (mid-jugular), 5 (lower jugular), 6 (posterior-lateral), and 7 (lateral-supraclavicular) appertain to each LC.

the thymus and preaortic nodes and a posterior group of paratracheoesophageal nodes.[23]

- *Lateral compartments* (LCs) are limited on each side superiorly by hypoglossal nerve, inferiorly by clavicular

American Head and Neck Society classification, proposed in 2008,[95] is the most frequently used classification in thyroid cancer reporting, and, as such, will be used further throughout this chapter. Based on this classification, LNs are divided into seven levels (I–VII). CC includes levels I (submental and submandibular), VI (central), and VII (lower central—suprabrachiocephalic upper mediastinal LNs). LC includes levels IIA and IIB (upper jugular), III (mid-jugular), IV (lower jugular), VA, and VB (lateral jugular).

SURGICAL APPROACHES AND SKIN INCISIONS IN THYROID CARCINOMA SURGERY

Lymphonodal dissections in thyroid carcinoma surgery can be performed via (1) cervical and (2) trans-sternal approaches or a combination of these two.

- All neck regions, except for infrabrachiocephalic upper mediastinal LN group, can be surgically managed via a cervical approach, including suprabrachiocephalic upper mediastinal LNs (level VII). After mobilization of level VI LNs with the surrounding fatty tissue, dissection can be extended to level VII, whose contents can be "pulled" cranially since there is no anatomical barrier between these two regions. Although this approach has some risks in less experienced hands, it is strongly encouraged not to leave metastatic LN tissue in the upper mediastinal region. Majority of surgeons make "hockcy stick" incisions for lateral LN dissection, which, in some patients, especially in bilateral procedures, can cause severe fibrosis and mutilation.[96] We perform dissections of all compartments via standard collar incision for thyroid surgery, placed in the natural skin line, between sternocleidomastoid muscles of both sides. If it is impossible to safely perform complete clearness of LN metastases in the regions IIA and IIB through this approach, another smaller incision can be made in the natural skin line of the level II, with good cosmetic effect.
- Transsternal approach is advised for pathological lymph-adenopathy in the infrabrachiocephalic mediastinal region on CE-CT or CE-MRI,[97] without evidence of distant metastases.[8] It is usually used as a combined approach with cervical incision to perform extensive dissections at initial surgery, but also if a redo surgery is indicated, especially after external beam neck irradiation (fibrosis increases the risk of severe vascular injuries). In case of disease relapse in mediastinal LNs only, it can be used as a single surgical approach.

SURGICAL PROCEDURES ON CERVICAL LYMPH NODES

Based on indications, LN dissection can be (1) *prophylactic (elective)*, in the absence of metastatic LNs on preoperative examinations, and (2) *therapeutical*, if LN metastases are verified clinically or confirmed pathologically.

With regard to the extent of resection of other structures, surgical procedures on LNs can be (1) *radical*, with resection of muscles/vessels/nerves due to tumor or metastatic LN infiltration, and (2) *modified radical*, functional, with muscle/nerve/vessel sparing.

In terms of the extent of LN dissection, surgery of LNs can be (1) *compartment-oriented*, with clearance of all LN groups of CC and/or LC, and (2) *selective*, with clearance of several LN groups.

Sentinel lymph node biopsy (SLNB) was proven to be a useful method for selecting clinically N0, but true positive patients for dissection in breast cancer and melanoma. It is also used for thyroid carcinoma staging by several teams in the world.[98-101]

Original Dzodic's method of SLNB with methylene blue dye (MBD) is used as a standard procedure in our National Cancer Research Center in Serbia *for intraoperative staging of lateral neck LNs in clinically N0 papillary and MTCs*, with high accuracy.[99,102-104] This original technique is performed in the following steps: (1) peritumoral injection of 0.2–0.5 mL of 1% MBD solution into the thyroid lobes, beneath thyroid capsule, with thermal coagulation of the injection site to avoid the leakage of the dye **(Fig. 1)**; (2) exploration of both jugulocarotid regions for colored afferent lymphatic vessels and LNs **(Fig. 2)**; (3) meticulous removal of colored, sentinel, LNs **(Fig. 3)** (if colored LNs cannot be found, a few noncolored LNs that are closest to the colored afferent lymphatic vessel are removed as sentinel LNs); and (4) frozen section analysis (FSA) of sentinel LNs. If sentinel LNs are malignant on FSA, in MTC surgery we perform one-time selective dissection of levels II to IV on the affected side. If sentinel LNs are benign on FSA, there is no need for further LND. This way, patients who are true negative can benefit from less extensive surgery, followed

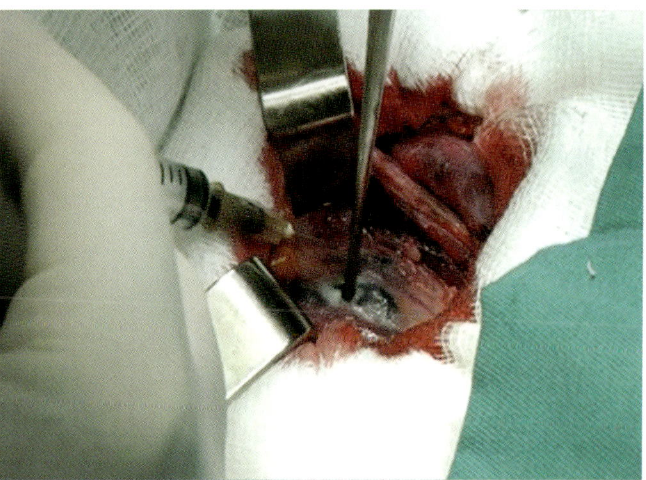

Fig. 1: Injection of 0.2–0.5 mL of 1%-methylene blue dye solution using a 27-gauge needle in thyroid lobe, beneath thyroid capsule, with thermal coagulation of the injection site through surgical tweezers, to avoid the leakage of the tracer.

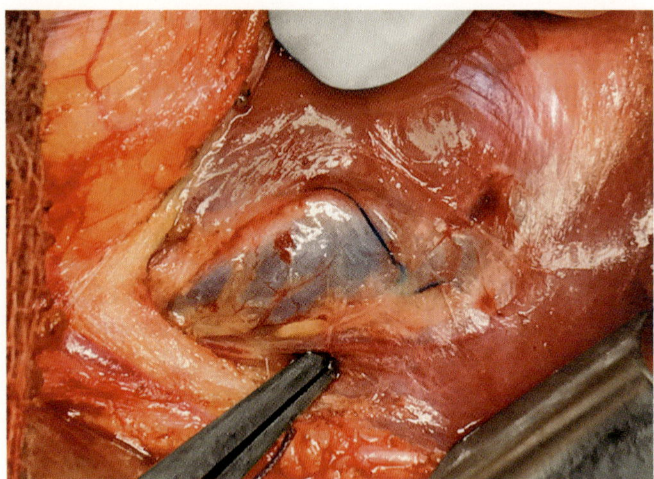

Fig. 2: Identification of blue-stained afferent lymphatic vessel in the jugulocarotid region.

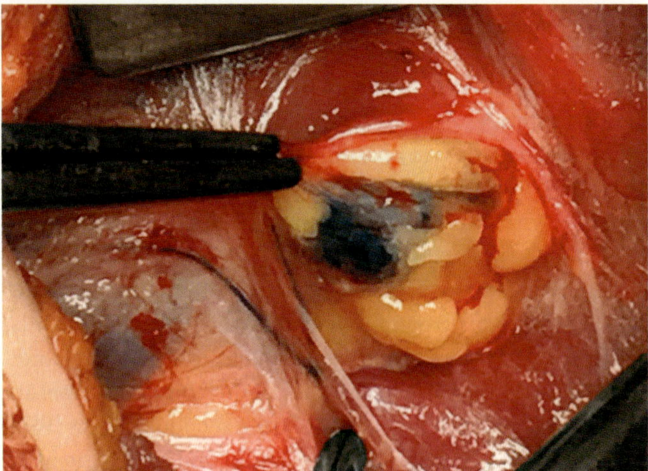

Fig. 3: Identification and extirpation of blue-stained, sentinel, lymph nodes from the jugulocarotid region.

by lower risk for complications and lifelong morbidity. On the contrary, patients who appear to be node-negative on preoperative evaluation, but have occult LN disease in LCs on frozen section, can be timely selected for one-time LND. Random removal of neck LNs (*"berry picking"* or *"node plucking"*)[105] is not advised in operable or resectable thyroid malignancy, only as a diagnostic biopsy.

◇ LYMPHONODAL DISSECTIONS: PITFALLS AND TIPS

Due to many important neural and vascular structures in the neck, LN dissections of CC and LC are technically challenging.[106] The following text will provide readers with tips for safe, but comprehensive, neck dissections.

Central Neck Dissection

Complete central neck dissection (CND) includes removal of level I, VI, and VII LNs, with preservation of the external branch of superior laryngeal nerves, RLNs, and PTGs.[106] However, level I is not routinely dissected in thyroid carcinomas since LN metastases are rarely found in this group.[8,105] Surgeons must actively search for LN metastases posterior to RLNs, especially on the right side, since they can be overlooked.

Major controversies on PTG management are related to in situ preservation versus PTG autotransplantation during CND for MTC, in matter of completeness and adequacy of CND if PTGs are preserved in situ as well as possible graft-dependent hyperparathyroidism in MEN2A.

Some authors suggest four-gland parathyroidectomy with autotransplantation, arguing that adequate CND is not possible if PTGs remain in situ.[107] Others make resection of two PTGs ipsilateral to the tumor and contralateral inferior PTG, while preserving on vascular pedicle the contralateral superior PTG.[97] Removed PTG tissue is then minced and implanted in the muscle pockets by the Wells technique.[108] However, reported outcomes of PTG autotransplantation differ in the referent publications.[109,110]

The ATA guidelines offer very clear recommendations for in situ preservation of normal PTGs on a vascular pedicle, or, if vascularization is compromised, autotransplantation (1) into the sternocleidomastoid muscle in sporadic MTC, FMTC, MEN2B, and MEN2A with RET mutation rarely associated with PHPT or (2) in the nondominant forearm muscle in MEN2A with RET mutation associated with a high incidence of PHPT, due to possible graft-dependent hyperparathyroidism.[1] Several publications have shown that in situ preservation of PTGs in MEN2A patients, who have no evidence of PHPT at the time of prophylactic or curative surgery for MTC, reduces postoperative morbidity and does not interfere with completeness of CND.[111-113]

The authors of this chapter encourage in situ preservation of all PTGs on their venous-arterial pedicles, regardless of the extent of surgery (with or without CND).[106,113] Application of MBD for SLNB is very useful if CND is performed, namely, MBD does not interfere with PTG lymphatic drainage. As a result, PTGs remain noncolored, opposed to blue-colored central LNs **(Figs. 4 A and B)**. This facilitates CND and reduces chance of PTG removal.[113] If blood supply is evidently compromised, PTG should be removed, minced, and implanted in a muscle pocket by Wells et al.[108] following the above-explained ATA recommendations.[1] In addition to this, we advise autotransplantation of at least one normal PTG in the brachioradialis muscle of nondominant arm in the locally advanced MTC patients who might benefit from adjuvant external beam neck radiation.

Lateral Neck Dissection

Complete LND includes removal of LNs of levels IIA to VB. However, levels IIB, VA, and VB are not routinely dissected in thyroid carcinomas, unless macroscopic LN metastases are found.[8] Dissection of upper jugular regions carries

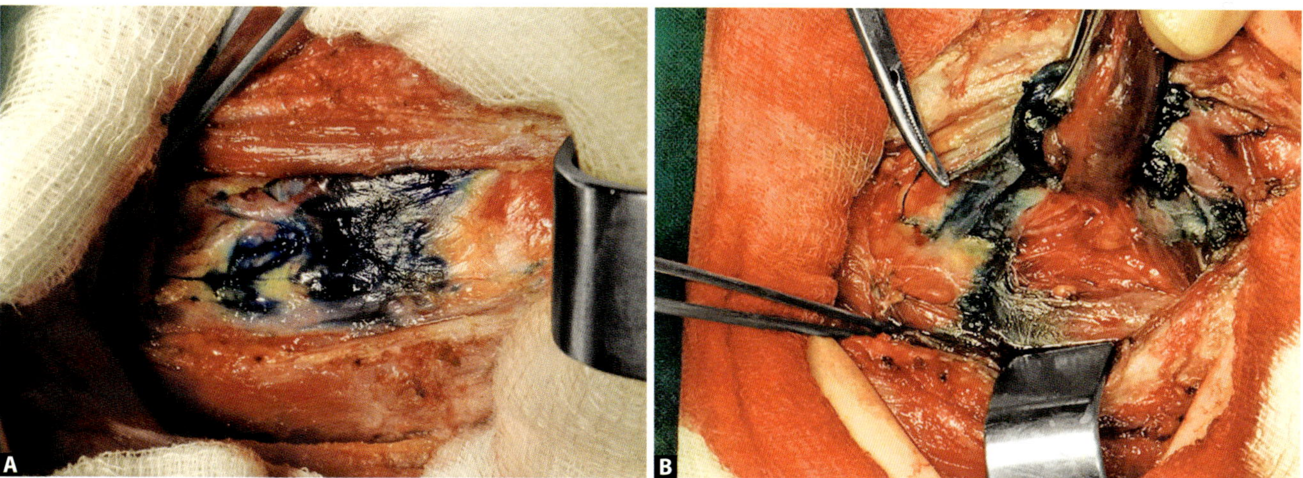

Figs. 4A and B: (A) Methylene blue dye affecting thyroid lobes, lymphatic vessels, and lymph nodes of central compartment; (B) Removal of thyroid lobe, with preservation of parathyroid glands that are not colored with methylene blue dye, while central lymph nodes uptake the vital dye.

the risk for injury of important neural structures,[106] most frequently (25–50%) spinal accessory nerve injury,[1] but also contusion of the marginal branch of facial nerve or lesion of the sympathetic plexus.[106] Supraclavicular and lower jugular dissection (especially on the left side) can lead to injury of major lymphatic vessels and lymphatic leakage, occurring in 0.5–8% of patients.[1,106]

SURGICAL TREATMENT OF MEDULLARY THYROID CARCINOMA

Surgery is the only curative treatment for MTC, with the aim to achieve biochemical cure by adequate clearance of tumor and LNs.[2,3,8-10] Other modalities, such as radioiodine therapy, external beam radiotherapy (EBRT), and chemotherapy, as well as thyroid-stimulating hormone suppression, are of no or limited value for MTC treatment. Surgery for MTC should be performed in referent tertiary care centers, and management of children with MTC should be trusted to experienced surgeons.[1]

In patients with sporadic or hereditary MTC, or MTC of unknown genetic setting, concurrent PHEO should be excluded, or, if diagnosed, it should be treated prior to MTC or PHPT surgery.[1,45,97] Laparoscopic or retroperitoneoscopic unilateral adrenalectomy is advised for unilateral tumor; however, contralateral PHEO is expected to occur within 10 years.[114] Due to high probability of bilateral adrenalectomies during lifetime in MEN2A/B patients, subtotal adrenalectomy with preservation of 10–15% of adrenal cortical tissue might be a more appropriate procedure. Corroborating this, majority of these patients will not need corticosteroid supplementation at all, and the risk of recurrent PHEO is 20% in 20 postoperative years.[1]

In MEN2A, concurrent PHPT should be excluded, or, if diagnosed, it should be treated simultaneously with MTC by removal of affected PTGs.[1,23] If all PTGs are enlarged, ATA

recommends subtotal parathyroidectomy with preservation of a part of one PTG in situ or total parathyroidectomy with heterotopic autograft. The same procedure needs to be followed if PHPT is detected after previous MTC treatment (ATA, Grade C recommendation).[1] If three PTGs have already been removed in previous surgeries, de novo enlarged remaining PTG should be partially preserved in situ or as a heterotopic autograft.[1]

Medullary thyroid carcinoma surgery has roles in several settings: (1) prophylactic setting, for RET germline mutation carriers without clinically evident disease; (2) primary curative setting, for clinically, biochemically, or cytologically suspected or proven MTC; (3) redo curative setting, for persistent or recurrent disease; and (4) palliative setting.[3] This section will summarize the indications and recommendations for all surgical settings.[1,8,9,23,45,62,78]

Prophylactic Surgery for Medullary Thyroid Carcinoma

The term "prophylactic" refers to thyroid surgery in RET germline mutation carriers before MTC occurs or for clinically unapparent MTC confined to the thyroid gland.[1] The exact timing of prophylactic surgery is determined by genotype (ATA risk category) and basal Ct levels.[1,23] Majority of guidelines recommend prophylactic total thyroidectomy (pTT) without CND for hereditary MTC with normal basal Ct levels, but if Ct is elevated, CND should be performed as well.

In MEN2B children who carry an M918T RET mutation (ATA highest risk), MTC has a very early onset, in infancy, and a very aggressive form; thus, pTT should be performed at the earliest, not later than 6 months to 1st year of life.[1,8,23,45,62] Since LN metastases are expected to occur in the first several months after birth, one-time prophylactic CND (pCND) can be advised, but only if PTGs can be adequately managed to avoid severe lifelong morbidity.[1,9,45,97] PTG preservation is especially difficult in these patients, being almost undistinguishable from fat and LN tissues, and MBD injection can be of great benefit during CND.

In high-risk MEN2A, with C634 or A883F RET mutations, pTT should be performed not later than the age of 5 years[1,8,9,62] or even earlier, with pCND, if Ct is elevated.[1,23,97]

Moderate-risk MTC carriers (MEN2A with RET mutations other than C634 and A883F, and FMTC) can have pTT around the age of 5 years or they can be monitored and surgically treated when Ct is elevated or there is US evidence of the disease.[1,8,23,62]

Japanese guidelines[78] are more conservative with regard to prophylactic surgery for MTC in RET gene carriers. They do not recommend surgery unless some feature of the MTC presence is observed, such as slightly elevated basal Ct.

Patients in ATA "high-risk" and "moderate-risk" categories should be screened for both PHEO and PHPT by the age of 11 and 16 years, respectively, while "highest-risk" category should be screened for PHEO by the age of 11 years (PHPT does not occur).[1]

Prophylactic surgery can also be performed in RET-negative patients with negative US findings, and unclear significance of basal Ct, but elevation of stimulated Ct, usually to reveal C-cell hyperplasia or micro-MTC.

Initial Surgery for Evident Medullary Thyroid Carcinoma

Medullary thyroid carcinoma is considered "evident" if it is clinically (physical examination and imaging methods), biochemically, or cytologically suspected or proven, regardless of the genetic setting (sporadic or hereditary). Surgical recommendations are based on many parameters (preoperative Ct levels, tumor size and bilaterality, clinical N status, and genetic component) and rather diverse in the view of neck dissections. Regardless, initial surgery aims to achieve a biochemical cure by complete removal of tumor and involved LNs. Function-preserving LN dissections are strongly advisable, unless there is a locally advanced disease, in which case more extensive resections are necessary to reduce the disease burden. Available guidelines for sporadic MTC treatment[1,8,9,23,45,62,78] will be briefly discussed in the following section.

National Comprehensive Cancer Network Guidelines in Medullary Carcinoma, 2010[45]

In cN0 patients, tumors ≥ 10 mm in size or bilateral tumors should be treated with TT and bilateral pCND (level VI), while unilateral disease with tumors < 10 mm in size can be managed with TT +/− pCND. Therapeutical dissections have to be performed in all affected compartments. Prophylactic ipsilateral LND (levels II to V) is advised in patients with CC metastases and should be considered for patients with tumors ≥10 or >5 mm in size for MEN2B syndrome.

German Association of Endocrine Surgeons Guidelines for the Surgical Management of Malignant Thyroid Tumors, 2013[9,23]

If there is clinical/biochemical/cytological evidence of MTC, TT has to be performed. Compartment-oriented dissections are indicated in clinically, biochemically, or cytologically suspected LN metastases. Correlations between basal CT values and extent of LN involvement form the basis of biomarker-based risk stratification, published by Machens and Dralle in 2010.[9] Based on this, LN metastases are usually not found in basal Ct level <20 pg/mL; thus, LN dissection is not necessary in these patients. In patients with basal Ct values from 20 to 200 pg/mL, complete pCND and ipsilateral LND are recommended, and basal Ct elevation >200 pg/mL requires consideration for contralateral LND, which should be discussed with patients with regard to benefits versus risks and one-stage versus two-stage surgery.[9]

British Thyroid Association Guidelines for the Management of Thyroid Cancer, 2014[8]

A minimum for cN0 MTC has to be TT and pCND (levels VI and VII), with exception of incidental, sporadic (RET negative), unifocal MTC, <5 mm in size, than can be treated with lobectomy, and monitored postoperatively for any increase of basal Ct, in which case completion thyroidectomy and CND should be done. Prophylactic ipsilateral LND levels IIA-VB (±contralateral LND) can be performed in cN0 patients based on tumor size or basal Ct level, and in cN0 patients with pathohistologically confirmed central LN metastases as well as in cN+ patients. RET mutation carriers with late presentation of MTC have to be treated in the same manner, based on radiological and biochemical findings.

American Thyroid Association Guidelines for the Management of Medullary Thyroid Carcinoma, 2015[1]

Generally, TT and CND (level VI) are recommended for cN0M0 MTC patients, although lobectomy can be considered for some sporadic MTCs. The necessity for LND (levels II–V) is decided based on the Ct level. Clinically, N+ compartments should be completely dissected. If ipsilateral LC is positive on imaging, while contralateral LC is clear, contralateral LND should be considered in Ct >200 pg/mL.

United Kingdom National Multidisciplinary Guidelines on the Management of Thyroid Cancer, 2016[62]

In MTCs over 5 mm in diameter, TT and CND should be performed (it is not explained what is the recommendation for tumors < 5 mm). LND (levels IIA–VB) is indicated in T2–T4 tumors (prophylactic bilateral LND), c/pN1a disease (prophylactic ipsilateral LND), and cN1b patients (therapeutical LND).

Japanese Clinical Guidelines for the Treatment of Thyroid Tumors, 2018

In Japanese, data were obtained from personal communication with Professor Akira Miyauchi.[78] TT is recommended for hereditary MTCs and sporadic, bilateral tumors, while hemithyroidectomy is indicated in sporadic, unilateral MTC. Complete pCND is recommended in all cases, while there are no clear recommendations for prophylactic LND. Kuma Hospital experts, however, reported good clinical outcomes if one-time prophylactic ipsilateral LND is performed.[115]

Authors' Recommendations for the Treatment of Evident Medullary Thyroid Carcinoma

In suspected or proven MTCs of any size, without clinical or radiological evidence of LN involvement, we perform TT, complete pCND, and bilateral SLNB for intraoperative assessment of LCs. As previously explained, one-time LND (levels II–IV) is done if sentinel LN is malignant on frozen section and/or definite histopathology, or in case there is intraoperative macroscopic evidence of metastases in LC, despite negative preoperative findings. If there is preoperative suspicion for LN metastases, complete dissection of affected compartments has to be done in a function-sparing manner. In patients with gross mediastinal disease and no distant metastases, a combined cervical and transsternal approach is advised for complete clearance of LN disease, if not in one, then in a two-step surgery.

If the extent of initial surgery was inadequate, it is hard to achieve a biochemical cure with another intervention.

Redo Surgery for Persistent or Recurrent Medullary Thyroid Carcinoma

Biochemical cure (normalization of Ct levels) is the indicator of complete surgical removal of tumor and affected LNs, i.e., adequate initial surgery.[10,23] Postoperative Ct is expected to decrease in a few weeks. However, evidence shows that normalization of postoperative Ct levels is less likely to be achieved if more LNs are involved with metastasis. Miyauchi et al.[116] reported a biochemical cure rate of 92% in pN0 patients, 75% in pN+ patients with 1–10 positive LNs, and only 14% in patients with more than 10 LN metastases. Machens et al.[82] recently published somewhat poorer findings on postoperative Ct normalization rates. In their series, 92% of patients without LN metastases achieved Ct normalization in 4.7 days in average, while in those with over 10 affected LNs only 5% achieve biochemical cure, within an average time of 57 days. Namely, LN metastases are commonly associated with the presence of systemic disease that precludes normalization of postoperative Ct even after appropriate surgery.[2]

For these reasons, ATA Task Force suggested in 2015 that quantitative assessment of LN metastases should be included into the AJCC staging system as an important prognostic classifier.[1] The current classification (*See* **Table 3**), with N1a and N1b categories, suggests only the quality of LN compartments,[90] while proposed categories N1, N2, and N3 should signify 1–10, 11–20, and more than 20 LN metastases, respectively,[117] which is of greater prognostic value.

If the initial postoperative values of Ct fail to normalize, it is necessary to repeat the analysis of Ct and CEA in the same assays that are used preoperatively. Serum Ct values that remain elevated 3 or more months after surgery are suggestive of persistent disease.[1] Recommendations for management of persistent disease are as follows:

- If postoperative Ct fails to normalize in the setting of complete initial surgery and lack of imaging evidence of persistent disease, redo surgery should not be performed.[23] Patients should be observed with Ct, CEA, and imaging methods for locoregional or distant disease.
- If postoperative Ct is elevated after complete initial surgery, but with imaging evidence of locoregional deposits, redo surgery should be done based on US and CT findings.[23]
- If postoperative Ct remains elevated after less than optimal extent of initial surgery, redo surgery is necessary for clearance of residual tumor or LNs while possible, to prevent future complications such as invasion of RLNs, aerodigestive tract, or lateral neck nerves.[1,118] The ATA limits the benefit of redo LN dissection only to patients with preoperative basal Ct levels <1,000 pg/mL and five or fewer metastatic LNs removed at the initial surgery.[1]
- If MTC is an incidental specimen finding after lobectomy (hemithyroidectomy), there is no indication for a redo completion surgery unless RET mutation is confirmed, or imaging studies suggest a residual disease, or there is an elevation of basal or stimulated serum Ct levels in the postoperative course.[1] If there are radiologically enlarged LNs, with normal serum Ct values, there are no indications for redo surgery.[1] Regular Ct and CEA check-ups are mandatory on a 6-month basis.[23,116]

Any increase of previously normal postoperative Ct values is indication for further imaging studies to diagnose local or distant relapse, so that surgery of locally recurrent disease can be performed on time.

It is hard to achieve biochemical cure after a redo surgery, especially if Ct levels are >1,000 pg/mL.[119] Even if Ct levels remain elevated after a reoperation, new surgery is not indicated if there is no visible relapse on US, CE-CT, CE-MRI, or PET/CT, and observation is justified.

Palliative Surgery

There are three indications for palliative MTC surgery:
1. Locally advanced MTC, suspicious of infiltration of surrounding structures, with no evident distant disease—surgery is performed with the intent to maximally reduce the disease burden, while preserving speech,

PTG function, swallowing, and arm and shoulder mobility.[1] This concept is different from papillary or follicular thyroid carcinoma management, due to worse prognosis and little or no benefit of extensive resections. The necessity and the extent of resections of infiltrated neck organs (larynx, trachea, esophagus, or thyroid cartilage) should be decided by an experienced multidisciplinary expert team, with an individual approach to every patient.[1]

2. MTC with distant metastases at initial presentation—surgery is performed with the intent to prevent compression or invasion of the RLNs, trachea, and esophagus and preserve patients' quality of life.[8,120]

3. Solitary, locally dominant, or symptomatic distant MTC metastasis in the mediastinum, lungs, or liver.[23]

Palliative surgery is usually performed along with systemic therapy, EBRT, and other nonsurgical adjuvant modalities, for local disease control.[1,120]

◇ NONSURGICAL MODALITIES FOR ADVANCED AND PROGRESSIVE MEDULLARY THYROID CARCINOMA TREATMENT

Nonsurgical modalities are not a standard of care for all MTC patients but are of great value for advanced or progressive MTC, with goals to provide locoregional disease control, to manage hormonal excess (diarrhea, Cushing's syndrome), to palliate symptomatic metastases (pain, bone fracture), and to control life-threatening metastases (asphyxiation, esophageal obstruction, bronchial obstruction, spinal cord compression).[1]

Adjuvant *radioiodine therapy* is not indicated in MTC, unless patients have regional or distant metastases of mixed type (MTC and differentiated thyroid carcinoma).[1,23,121]

EBRT is not a standard therapy for MTC adjunctive to surgery since it has not been shown to improve patients' survival[122-124]; however, adjuvant EBRT can be effective in achieving better locoregional control of the disease in patients with locally invasive MTC or regional metastatic MTC (presence of microscopic or macroscopic residual disease after surgical removal, extrathyroidal extension, or extensive LN metastases).[1,125,126] However, potential benefits of EBRT must be compared to possible acute and chronic EBRT-associated toxicity.[1] Also, EBRT should not be used to compensate inadequate initial surgery for operable MTC and, if a redo neck surgery is possible, it should be the first-line treatment, prior to introducing EBRT in these selected patients. Redo surgery after EBRT is more technically challenging and carries a significant risk of complications. Sometimes, it is not possible to perform sternotomy after EBRT due to severe fibrosis, and this can be considered a potential contraindication for surgery.[106] In patients with distant progression, EBRT can be used for painful bone metastases,[1,120,127] symptomatic brain metastases,[1,8,120,128] and lung or skin metastases.[1,120,129]

Chemotherapy is used for systemic treatment of persistent or recurrent MTC, but there are no recommendations of its administration as the first-line therapy. Namely, single-agent or combination cytotoxic chemotherapeutic regimens achieve low response rates (15–20%), with short duration. Combination therapy with doxorubicin and another agent, or 5-fluorouracil and dacarbazine was shown to be most effective.[1,8]

Systemic treatment with *radiolabeled molecules* or *pretargeted radioimmunotherapy* may be considered in selected patients.[1] There are no randomized controlled trials on application of radiolabeled molecules for MTC treatment, but limited effects (symptom palliation) have been observed in inoperable, metastatic MTC with use of 131I MIBG and 90Y/177Lu-labeled peptides.[8,130,131] Pretargeted radioimmunotherapy using bispecific monoclonal anti-CEA antibody and a 131I-labeled bivalent hapten increased the overall survival metastatic progressive MTC to 110 months (vs. 61 months in the historical controls).[132]

In patients with advanced and progressive MTC, *molecular targeted therapy* should be considered as a systemic therapy. In the past years, two tyrosine kinase inhibitors, vandetanib and cabozantinib, have been approved as molecular targeted therapy agents for first-line systemic therapy. Two phase III clinical trials showed high rates of disease control with durable responses and a highly significant improvement of progression-free survival with these agents, compared to placebo groups.[133,134] For vandetanib, it remains unknown if and how RET mutation status affects progression-free survival,[133] but it was shown that M918T-mutated tumors have increased sensitivity.[135] For cabozantinib, response rates were not affected by presence or absence of RET mutation,[134] but the benefits of this treatment in RET or RAS mutated tumors were observed.[136] Several more agents have been evaluated in phase I and II clinical trials, such as sorafenib, sunitinib, everolimus, axitinib, gefitinib, imatinib, and motesanib, resulting in prolonged stable disease in patients with advanced MTC.[1] Despite the benefits of tyrosine kinase inhibitors, therapy has to be administered daily and continuously. As a result, adverse events are numerous and severe. Data on long-term toxicity and survival are insufficient, while significant short-term toxicity usually requires immediate dose reduction, and even complete withdrawal.[1] In addition, there are many issues on this therapy, regarding the dosage, mechanisms of resistance, benefit to overall survival and whether to terminate the treatment for patients with stable disease, or not.[1]

Treatment with *denosumab* (receptor activator of nuclear factor kappa-B ligand inhibitor) or *bisphosphonates* (zoledronic acid or pamidronate) is recommended by ATA for patients with painful bone metastases from thyroid cancer and for prevention or delay of other bone-related events.[1] On the contrary, the European Thyroid Association guidelines from 2012 do not recommend bisphosphonates in this setting due to insufficient data on this treatment in MTC patients.[120]

Patients with advanced MTC and symptoms caused by hormonally active metastases have to receive *additional symptoms-oriented therapy*. Diarrhea, caused by elevated serum Ct levels, should be initially treated with antimotility agents, such as loperamide, diphenoxylate/atropine, or codeine, with minimal side effects. Unlabeled somatostatin analogs were found to be useful in controlling severe diarrhea,[137] with better results if combined with interferon-alpha.[138] Local therapies, such as surgery for large tumor debulking or chemoembolization for large liver metastases, can decrease metastases burden and reduce the secretion of Ct, which consequently alleviates the severity of diarrhea. If Cushing's syndrome occurs, due to ectopic production of adrenocorticotropic hormone or corticotropin-releasing hormone, it can be treated medically, with aminoglutethimide, mifepristone, ketoconazole, mitotane, or metyrapone. In cases of Cushing's syndrome refractory to medical treatment, local therapies (tumor debulking or chemoembolization) and bilateral adrenalectomy can be useful.[1,139]

Based on the current results, combination of molecular targeted therapy agents and standard therapies, and symptoms-oriented therapy, appears as promising strategy for MTC treatment.

◇| REFERENCES

1. Wells SA Jr, Asa SL, Dralle H, Elisei R, Evans DB, Gage RF, et al.; American Thyroid Association Guidelines Task Force on Medullary Thyroid Carcinoma. Revised American Thyroid Association Guidelines for the Management of Medullary Thyroid Carcinoma. Thyroid. 2015;25(6):567-610.
2. Scollo C, Baudin E, Travagli JP, Caillou B, Bellon N, Leboulleux S, Schlumberger M. Rationale for central and bilateral lymph node dissection in sporadic and hereditary medullary thyroid cancer. J Clin Endocrinol Metab. 2003;88(5):2070-75.
3. Moley JF. Medullary thyroid carcinoma: management of lymph node metastases. J Natl Compr Canc Netw. 2010;8(5):549-56.
4. Bergholm U, Adami HO, Bergstrom R, Bäckdahl M, Akerström G. Long-term survival in sporadic and familial medullary thyroid carcinoma with special reference to clinical characteristics as prognostic factors. The Swedish MTC Study Group. Ann Med Interne (Paris). 1990;141:20-5.
5. Hundahl SA, Fleming ID, Fremgen AM, Menck HR. A National Cancer Data Base report on 53,856 cases of thyroid carcinoma treated in the US, 1985–1995. Cancer. 1998;83:2638-48.
6. Kebebew E, Ituarte PH, Siperstein AE, Duh QY, Clark OH. Medullary thyroid carcinoma: clinical characteristics, treatment, prognostic factors, and a comparison of staging systems. Cancer. 2000;88:1139-48.
7. Rendl G, Manzl M, Hitzl W, Sungler P, Pirich C. Long-term prognosis of medullary thyroid carcinoma. Clin Endocrinol (Oxf). 2008;69:497-505.
8. Perros P, Colley S, Boelaert K, Evans C, Evans RM, Gerrard GE, et al. British Thyroid Association Guidelines for the Management of Thyroid Cancer (3rd edition). Medullary thyroid cancer (chapter 17, pp. 69-79). Clin Endocr. 2014;81(Suppl. 1):1-122.
9. Machens A, Dralle H. Biomarker-based risk stratification for previously untreated medullary thyroid cancer. J Clin Endocrinol Metab. 2010;95:2655-63.
10. Machens A, Dralle H. Biological relevance of medullary thyroid microcarcinoma. J Clin Endocrinol Metab. 2012;97(5):1547-53.
11. Baber EC. Contributions to the minute anatomy of the thyroid gland of the dog. Phil Trans R Soc Lond. 1876;166:557-68.
12. Nonidez JF. The origin of the 'parafollicular' cell, a second epithelial component of the thyroid of the dog. Am J Anat. 1932;49:479-505.
13. Pearse AG. 5-Hydroxytryptophan uptake by dog thyroid 'C' cells, and its possible significance in polypeptide hormone production. Nature. 1966;211:598-600.
14. Pearse AG. The cytochemistry of the thyroid C cells and their relationship to calcitonin. Proc R Soc Lond B Biol Sci. 1966;164:478-87.
15. Nilsson M, Williams D. On the origin of cells and derivation of thyroid cancer: c cell story revisited. Eur Thyroid J. 2016;5(2):79-93.
16. Gauger PG, Delbridge LW, Thompson NW, Crummer P, Reeve TS. Incidence and importance of the tubercle of Zuckerkandl in thyroid surgery. Eur J Surg. 2001;167(4):249-4.
17. Fagman H, Andersson L, Nilsson M. The developing mouse thyroid: embryonic vessel contacts and parenchymal growth pattern during specification, budding, migration, and lobulation. Dev Dyn. 2006;235:444-55.
18. Kameda Y, Nishimaki T, Chisaka O, Iseki S, Sucov HM. Expression of the epithelial marker E-cadherin by thyroid C cells and their precursors during murine development. J Histochem Cytochem. 2007;55:1075-88.
19. Johansson E, Andersson L, Örnros J, et al. Revising the embryonic origin of thyroid C cells in mice and humans. Development. 2015;142(20):3519-28.
20. Pueblitz S, Weinberg AG, Albores-Saavedra J. Thyroid C cells in the DiGeorge anomaly: a quantitative study. Pediatr Pathol. 1993;13:463-73.
21. Yaday S, Singh I, Singh J, Aggarwal N. Medullary carcinoma in a lingual thyroid. Singapore Med J. 2008;49:251-3.
22. Vandernoot I, Sartelet H, Abu-Khudir R, Chanoine JP, Deladoey J. Evidence for calcitonin-producing cells in human lingual thyroids. J Clin Endocrinol Metab. 2012;97:951-6.
23. Dralle H, Musholt TJ, Schabram J, Steinmüller T, Frilling A, Simon D, et al.; German Societies of General and Visceral Surgery; Endocrinology; Nuclear Medicine; Pathology; Radiooncology; Oncological Hematology; and the German Thyroid Cancer Patient Support Organization Ohne Schilddrüse leben e.V. German Association of Endocrine Surgeons practice guideline for the surgical management of malignant thyroid tumors. Langenbecks Arch Surg. 2013;398(3):347-75.
24. Costante G, Durante C, Francis Z, Schlumberger M, Filetti S. Determination of calcitonin levels in C-cell disease: clinical interest and potential pitfalls. Nat Clin Pract Endocrinol Metab. 2009;5:35-44.
25. Walter MA, Meier C, Radimerski T, Iten F, Kränzlin M, Müller-Brand J, et al. Procalcitonin levels predict clinical course and progression free survival in patients with medullary thyroid cancer. Cancer. 2010;116:31-40.
26. Frank-Raue K, Machens A, Leidig-Bruckner G, Rondot S, Haag C, Schulze E, et al. Prevalence and clinical spectrum of nonsecretory medullary thyroid carcinoma in a series of 839 patients with sporadic medullary thyroid carcinoma. Thyroid. 2013;23(3):294-300.
27. Main C, Perrino MN, Colombo C, Cavedon E, Pennelli G, Ferrero S, et al. Refining calcium test for the diagnosis of medullary thyroid cancer: cutoffs, procedures, and safety. J Clin Endocrinol Metab. 2014;99:1656-64.

28. Trimboli P, Giovanella L, Crescenzi A, Romanelli F, Valabrega S, Spriano G, et al. Medullary thyroid cancer diagnosis: an appraisal. Head Neck. 2014;36:1216-33.

29. Toledo SP, Lourenco DM Jr, Santos MA, Tavares MR, Toledo RA, Correia-Deur JE. Hypercalcitoninemia is not pathognomonic of medullary thyroid carcinoma. Clinics (Sao Paulo). 2009;64: 699-706.

30. Basuyau JP, Mallet E, Leroy M, Brunelle P. Reference intervals for serum calcitonin in men, women, and children. Clin Chem. 2004;50:1828-30.

31. Guyetant S, Rousselet MC, Durigon M, Chappard D, Franc B, Guerin O, et al. Sex-related cell hyperplasia in the normal human thyroid: a quantitative autopsy study. J Clin Endocrinol Metab. 1997;82:42-7.

32. Elisei R, Pinchera A. Advances in the follow-up of differentiated or medullary thyroid cancer. Nat Rev Endocrinol 2012;8: 466-75.

33. Mendelsohn G, Wells SA Jr, Baylin SB. Relationship of tissue carcinoembryonic antigen and calcitonin to tumor virulence in medullary thyroid carcinoma. An immunohistochemical study in early, localized, and virulent disseminated stages of disease. Cancer. 1984;54:657-62.

34. Bockhorn M, Frilling A, Rewerk S, Liedke M, Dirsch O, Schmid KW, et al. Lack of elevated serum carcinoembryonic antigen and calcitonin in medullary thyroid carcinoma. Thyroid. 2004;14:468-70.

35. Dora JM, Canalli MH, Capp C, Punales MK, Vieira JG, Maia AL. Normal perioperative serum calcitonin levels in patients with advanced medullary thyroid carcinoma: case report and review of the literature. Thyroid. 2008;18:895-9.

36. Moo-Young TA, Traugott AL, Moley JF. Sporadic and familial medullary thyroid carcinoma: state of the art. Surg Clin North Am. 2009;89(5):1193-204.

37. Accardo G, Conzo G, Esposito D, Gambardella C, Mazzella M, Castaldo F, et al. Genetics of medullary thyroid cancer: an overview. Int J Surg. 2017;41 (Suppl 1):S2-S6.

38. Takahashi M, Ritz J, Cooper GM. Activation of a novel human transforming gene, RET, by DNA rearrangement. Cell. 1985;42:581-8.

39. Zordan P, Tavella S, Brizzolara A, Biticchi R, Ceccherini I, Garofalo S, et al. The immediate upstream sequence of the mouse Ret gene controls tissue-specific expression in transgenic mice. Int J Mol Med. 2006;18:601-8.

40. Santoro M, Carlomagno F. Central role of RET in thyroid cancer. Cold Spring Harb Perspect Biol. 2013;5(12):a009233.

41. Wells SA, Pacini F, Robinson BG, Santoro M. Multiple endocrine neoplasia type 2 and familial medullary thyroid carcinoma: an update. J Clin Endocrinol Metab. 2013;98(8):3149-64.

42. Marsh DJ, Learoyd DL, Andrew SD, Krishnan L, Pojer R, Richardson AL, et al. Somatic mutations in the RET proto-oncogene in sporadic medullary thyroid carcinoma. Clin Endocrinol (Oxf). 1996;44:249-57.

43. Boichard A, Croux L, Al Ghuzlan A, Broutin S, Dupuy C, Leboulleux S, et al. Somatic RAS mutations occur in a large proportion of sporadic RET-negative medullary thyroid carcinomas and extend to a previously unidentified exon. J Clin Endocrinol Metab. 2012;97:E2031-5.

44. Ciampi R, Mian C, Fugazzola L, Cosci B, Romei C, Barollo S, et al. Evidence of a low prevalence of RAS mutations in a large medullary thyroid cancer series. Thyroid. 2013;23:50-7.

45. Tuttle RM, Ball DW, Byrd D, Daniels GH. National Comprehensive Cancer Network. Medullary carcinoma—clinical practice guidelines in oncology. J Natl Compr Canc Netw. 2010;8(5):512-30.

46. Leboulleux S, Baudin E, Travagli JP, Schlumberger M. Medullary thyroid carcinoma. Clin Endocrinol. 2004;61:299-310.

47. Modigliani E, Cohen R, Campos JM, Conte-Devolx B, Maes B, Boneu A, et al.; The GETC Study Group (Groupe d'etude des tumeurs a calcitonine). Prognostic factors for survival and for biochemical cure in medullary thyroid carcinoma: results in 899 patients. Clin Endocrinol (Oxf). 1998;48:265-73.

48. Elisei R, Cosci B, Romei C, Bottici V, Renzini G, Molinaro E, et al. Prognostic significance of somatic RET oncogene mutations in sporadic medullary thyroid cancer: a 10-year follow-up study. J Clin Endocrinol Metab. 2008;93:682-7.

49. Smith DP, Houghton C, Ponder BA. Germline mutation of RET codon 883 in two cases of de novo MEN 2B. Oncogene. 1997;15:1213-7.

50. Melmed S, Polonsky KS, Larsen PR, Kronenberg HM. Williams Textbook of Endocrinology, 13th edition. Philadelphia, PA: Elsevier; 2016.

51. Imai T, Uchino S, Okamoto T, Suzuki S, Kosugi S, Kikumori T, et al.; MEN Consortium of Japan. High penetrance of pheochromocytoma in multiple endocrine neoplasia 2 caused by germ line RET codon 634 mutation in Japanese patients. Eur J Endocrinol. 2013;168:683-7.

52. Herfarth KK, Bartsch D, Doherty GM, Wells SA Jr, Lairmore TC. Surgical management of hyperparathyroidism in patients with multiple endocrine neoplasia type 2A. Surgery. 1996;120: 966-74.

53. Frank-Raue K, Rybicki LA, Erlic Z, Schweizer H, Winter A, Milos I, et al.; International RET Exon 10 Consortium. Risk profiles and penetrance estimations in multiple endocrine neoplasia type 2A caused by germline RET mutations located in exon 10. Hum Mutat. 2011;32:51-8.

54. Ceccherini I, Romei C, Barone V, Pacini F, Martino E, Loviselli A, et al. Identification of the Cys634/Tyr mutation of the RET proto-oncogene in a pedigree with multiple endocrine neoplasia type 2A and localized CLA. J Endocrinol Invest. 1994;17:201-4.

55. Verga U, Fugazzola L, Cambiaghi S, Pritelli C, Alessi E, Cortelazzi D, et al. Frequent association between MEN 2A and CLA. Clin Endocrinol (Oxf). 2003;59:156-61.

56. Decker RA, Peacock ML. Occurrence of MEN 2a in familial Hirschsprung's disease: a new indication for genetic testing of the RET proto-oncogene. J Pediatr Surg. 1998;33:207-14.

57. Kasprzak L, Nolet S, Gaboury L, Pavia C, Villabona C, Rivera-Fillat F, et al. Familial medullary thyroid carcinoma and prominent corneal nerves associated with the germline V804M and V778I mutations on the same allele of RET. J Med Genet. 2001;38:784-7.

58. Jasim S, Ying AK, Waguespack SG, Rich TA, Grubbs EG, Jimenez C, et al. Multiple endocrine neoplasia type 2B with a RET proto-oncogene A883F mutation displays a more indolent form of medullary thyroid carcinoma compared with a RET M918T mutation. Thyroid. 2011;21:189-92.

59. Kloos RT, Eng C, Evans DB, Francis GL, Gagel RF, Gharib H, et al.; American Thyroid Association Guidelines Task Force. Medullary Thyroid Cancer: Management guidelines of the American Thyroid Association. Thyroid. 2009;19: 565-612.

60. Machens A, Hauptmann S, Dralle H. Increased risk of lymph node metastasis in multifocal hereditary and sporadic medullary thyroid cancer. World J Surg. 2007;31:1960-5.

61. Kazaure HS, Roman SA, Sosa JA. Medullary thyroid microcarcinoma: a population-level analysis of 310 patients. Cancer. 2012;118:620-7.

62. Mitchell AL, Gandhi A, Scott-Coombes D, Perros P. Management of thyroid cancer: United Kingdom National Multidisciplinary Guidelines. J Laryngol Otol. 2016;130 (S2):S150-60.

63. Horvath E, Maylis S, Rossi R, Franco C, Niedmann JP, Castro A, et al. An ultrasonogram reporting system for thyroid nodules stratifying cancer risk for clinical management. J Clin Endocrinol Metab. 2009;94:1748-51.

64. Kim HJ. Updated guidelines on the preoperative staging of thyroid cancer. Ultrasonography. 2017;36(4):292-9.

65. Choi JS, Kim J, Kwak JY, Kim MJ, Chang HS, Kim EK. Preoperative staging of papillary thyroid carcinoma: comparison of ultrasound imaging and CT. Am J Roentgenol. 2009;193:871-8.

66. Roh JL, Park JY, Kim JM, Song CJ. Use of preoperative ultrasonography as guidance for neck dissection in patients with papillary thyroid carcinoma. J Surg Oncol. 2009;99:28-31.

67. Choi YJ, Lee JH, Baek JH. Ultrasound elastography for evaluation of cervical lymph nodes. Ultrasonography. 2015;34:157-64.

68. Paksoy N, Yazal K. Cervical lymphadenopathy associated with Hashimoto's thyroiditis: an analysis of 22 cases by fine needle aspiration cytology. Acta Cytol. 2009;53:491-6.

69. Choi JS, Chung WY, Kwak JY, Moon HJ, Kim MJ, Kim EK. Staging of papillary thyroid carcinoma with ultrasonography: performance in a large series. Ann Surg Oncol. 2011;18: 3572-8.

70. Choi JS, Lee HS, Kim EK, Moon HJ, Kwak JY. The influence of body mass index on the diagnostic performance of pre-operative staging ultrasound in papillary thyroid carcinoma. Clin Endocrinol (Oxf). 2015;83:550-5.

71. Loevner LA, Kaplan SL, Cunnane ME, Moonis G. Cross-sectional imaging of the thyroid gland. Neuroimaging Clin N Am. 2008;18:445-61.

72. Giraudet AL, Vanel D, Leboulleux S, Aupérin A, Dromain C, Chami L, et al. Imaging medullary thyroid carcinoma with persistent elevated calcitonin levels. J Clin Endocrinol Metab. 2007;92:4185-90.

73. Polyzos SA, Anastasilakis AD. A systematic review of cases reporting needle tract seeding following thyroid fine needle biopsy. World J Surg. 2010;34:844-51.

74. Trimboli P, Treglia, G, Guidobaldi L, Romanelli F, Nigri G, Valabrega S, et al. Detection rate of FNA cytology in medullary thyroid carcinoma: a meta-analysis. Clin Endocrinol (Oxf). 2015;82:280-5.

75. Papaparaskeva K, Nagel H, Droese M. Cytologic diagnosis of medullary carcinoma of the thyroid gland. Diagn Cytopathol. 2000;22:351-8.

76. Trimboli P, Cremonini N, Ceriani L, Saggiorato E, Guidobaldi L, Romanelli F, et al. Calcitonin measurement in aspiration needle washout fluids has higher sensitivity than cytology in detecting medullary thyroid cancer: a retrospective multicenter study. Clin Endocrinol. 2014;80:135-40.

77. Elisei R, Bottici V, Luchetti F, Di Coscio G, Romei C, Grasso L, et al. Impact of routine measurement of serum calcitonin on the diagnosis and outcome of medullary thyroid cancer: experience in 10,864 patients with nodular thyroid disorders. J Clin Endocrinol Metab. 2004;89:163-8.

78. The Japan Association of Endocrine Surgeons/The Japanese Society of Thyroid Surgery. Japanese clinical guidelines for treatment of thyroid tumors. Off J Jpn Assoc Endocrine Surg Jpn Soc Thyroid Surg. 2018; 35(3).

79. Faggiano A, Milone F, Ramundo V, Chiofalo MG, Ventre I, Giannattasio R, et al. A decrease of calcitonin serum concentrations less than 50 percent 30 minutes after thyroid surgery suggests incomplete C-cell tumor tissue removal. J Clin Endocrinol Metab. 2010;95(9):E32-6.

80. De Crea C, Raffaelli M, Milano V, Carrozza C, Zuppi C, Bellantone R, et al. Is intraoperative calcitonin monitoring useful to modulate the extension of neck dissection in patients with medullary thyroid carcinoma? World J Surg. 2014;38(3): 568-75.

81. Livhits MJ, Yeh MW. Calcitonin normalizes within 1 week after surgery in most patients with node-negative medullary thyroid cancer. Clin Thyroidol. 2019;31(4):162-4.

82. Machens A, Lorenz K, Dralle H. Time to calcitonin normalizaton after surgery for node-negative and node-positive medullary thyroid cancer. Br J Surg. 2019;106(4):412-8.

83. Sippel RS, Kunnimalaiyaan M, Chen H. Current management of medullary thyroid cancer. Oncologist. 2008;13(5): 539-47.

84. Eng C, Mulligan LM, Smith DP, Healey CS, Frilling A, Raue F, et al. Low frequency of germline mutations in the RET protooncogene in patients with apparently sporadic medullary thyroid carcinoma. Clin Endocrinol (Oxf). 1995;43:123-7.

85. Elisei R, Romei C, Cosci B, Agate L, Bottici V, Molinaro E, et al. RET genetic screening in patients with medullary thyroid cancer and their relatives: experience with 807 individuals at one center. J Clin Endocrinol Metab. 2007;92:4725-9.

86. Carlson KM, Bracamontes J, Jackson CE, Clark R, Lacroix A, Wells SA Jr, et al. Parent-of-origin effects in multiple endocrine neoplasia type 2B. Am J Hum Genet. 1994;55:1076-82.

87. Schuffenecker I, Ginet N, Goldgar D, Eng C, Chambe B, Boneu A, et al.; Prevalence and parental origin of de novo RET mutations in multiple endocrine neoplasia type 2A and familial medullary thyroid carcinoma. Le Groupe d'Etude des Tumeurs a Calcitonine. Am J Hum Genet. 1997;60:233-7.

88. Cerutti JM, Maciel RM. An unusual genotype-phenotype correlation in MEN 2 patients: should screening for RET double germline mutations be performed to avoid misleading diagnosis and treatment? Clin Endocrinol (Oxf). 2013;79: 591-2.

89. Farrag TY, Samlan RA, Lin FR, Tufano RP. The utility of evaluating true vocal fold motion before thyroid surgery. Laryngoscope. 2006;116:235-8.

90. Amin MB, Edge SB, Greene FL, Compton CC, Gershenwald JE, Brookland RL, et al. (Eds.); American Joint Committee on Cancer Thyroid. AJCC Cancer Staging Manual, 8th edition. New York: Springer; 2017.

91. Edge SB, Byrd DR, Compton CC, Fritz AG, Greene FL, Trotti A; American Joint Committee on Cancer Thyroid. AJCC Cancer Staging Manual, 7th edition. New York: Springer; 2010.

92. Dralle H, Damm I, Scheumann GFW, Kotzerke J, Kupsch E, Geerlings H, et al. Compartment-oriented microdissection of regional lymph nodes in medullary thyroid carcinoma. Surg Today. 1994;24:112-21.

93. Qubain SW, Nakano S, Baba M, Takao S, Aikouet T Distribution of lymph node micrometastasis in pN0 well-differentiated thyroid carcinoma. Surgery 2002;131:249-56.

94. Wittekind C, Greene FL, Henson DE, Hutter RVP, Sobin LH. TNM Supplement, 3rd edition. New York: Wiley-Liss; 2003. pp. 25-33.

95. Robbins KT, Shaha AR, Medina JE, Califano JA, Wolf GT, Ferlito A, et al. Consensus statement on the classification and

terminology of neck dissection. Arch Otolaryngol Head Neck Surg. 2008;134:536-8.

96. Villaret DB, Amdur RJ, Mazzaferri EL. Neck dissections to remove malignant lymph nodes. Essentials of Thyroid Cancer Management. New York: Springer Science & Business Media; 2005. pp. 147-53.

97. Jin LX, Moley JF. Surgery for lymph node metastases of medullary thyroid carcinoma: a review. Cancer. 2016;122(3):358-66.

98. Kelemen PR, Van Herle AJ, Giuliano AE. Sentinel lymphadenectomy in thyroid malignant neoplasms. Arch Surg. 1998;133:288-92.

99. Dzodic R, Markovic I, Inic M, Jokic N, Djurisic I, Zegarac M, et al. Sentinel lymph node biopsy may be used to support the decision to perform modified radical neck dissection in differentiated thyroid carcinoma. World J Surg 2006;30(5): 841-6. [Erratum in: World J Surg. 2006;30(5):918.]

100. Roh JL, Park CI. Sentinel lymph node biopsy as guidance for central neck dissection in patients with papillary thyroid carcinoma. Cancer. 2008;113:1527-31.

101. Balasubramanian SP, Harrison BJ. Systematic review and meta-analysis of sentinel node biopsy in thyroid cancer. Br J Surg. 2011;98:334-44.

102. Dzodic R, Buta M, Markovic I, Matovic M, Djurisic I, Milovanovic Z, et al. Surgical management of well-differentiated thyroid carcinoma in children and adolescents: 33 years of experience of a single institution in Serbia. Endocr J. 2014;61(11):1079-86.

103. Santrac N, Besic N, Buta M, Oruci M, Djurisic I, Pupic G, et al. Lymphatic drainage, regional metastases and surgical management of papillary thyroid carcinoma arising in pyramidal lobe—a single institution experience. Endocr J. 2014; 61(1):55-9.

104. Goran M, Pekmezovic T, Markovic I, Santrac N, Buta M, Gavrilovic D, et al. Lymph node metastases in clinically N0 patients with papillary thyroid microcarcinomas—a single institution experience. J BUON. 2017;22(1):224-31.

105. Grubbs EG, Evans DB. Role of lymph node dissection in primary surgery for thyroid cancer. J Natl Compr Canc Netw. 2007;5(6):623-30.

106. Dzodic R, Santrac N, Markovic I, Buta M, Goran M. Complications in thyroid surgery. In: Parameswaran R, Agarwal A (Eds). Evidence-based Endocrine Surgery. Singapore: Springer; 2018. pp. 187-99.

107. Skinner MA, Moley JA, Dilley WG, Owzar K, DeBenedetti MK, Wells SA. Prophylactic thyroidectomy in multiple endocrine neoplasia type 2A. N Engl J Med. 2005;353:1105-13.

108. Wells SA, Gunnells JC, Shelburne JD, Schneider AB, Sherwood LM. Transplantation of the parathyroid glands in man: clinical indications and results. Surgery. 1975;78:34-44.

109. Olson JA, DeBenedetti MK, Baumann DS, Wells SA. Parathyroid autotransplantation during thyroidectomy. Results of long-term follow-up. Ann Surg. 1996;223:472-78; discussion 478-80.

110. Lorente-Poch L, Sancho J, Muñoz JL, Gallego-Otaegui L, Martínez-Ruiz C, Sitges-Serra A. Failure of fragmented parathyroid gland autotransplantation to prevent permanent hypoparathyroidism after total thyroidectomy. Langenbecks Arch Surg. 2017;402(2):281-7.

111. Decker RA, Geiger JD, Cox CE, Mackovjak M, Sarkar M, Peacock ML. Prophylactic surgery for multiple endocrine neoplasia type IIa after genetic diagnosis: is parathyroid transplantation indicated? World J Surg. 1996;20:814-20; discussion 820-21.

112. Dralle H, Gimm O, Simon D, Frank-Raue K, Görtz G, Niederle B, et al. Prophylactic thyroidectomy in 75 children and adolescents with hereditary medullary thyroid carcinoma: German and Austrian experience. World J Surg. 1998;22:744-50; discussion 750-51.

113. Dzodic R, Santrac N. In situ preservation of parathyroid glands: advanced surgical tips for prevention of permanent hypoparathyroidism in thyroid surgery. J BUON. 2017;22(4): 853-55.

114. Asari R, Scheuba C, Kaczirek K, Niederle B. Estimated risk of pheochromocytoma recurrence after adrenal-sparing surgery in patients with multiple endocrine neoplasia type 2A. Arch Surg. 2006;141:1199-205.

115. Ito Y, Miyauchi A, Yabuta T, Fukushima M, Inoue H, Tomoda C, et al. Alternative surgical strategies and favorable outcomes in patients with medullary thyroid carcinoma in Japan: experience of a single institution. World J Surg. 2009;33(1):58-66.

116. Miyauchi A, Matsuzuka F, Hirai K, Yokozawa T, Kobayashi K, Ito Y, et al. Prospective trial of unilateral surgery for nonhereditary medullary thyroid carcinoma in patients without germline RET mutations. Word J Surg. 2002;26(8):1023-8.

117. Machens A, Dralle H. Prognostic impact of N staging in 715 medullary thyroid cancer patients: proposal for a revised staging system. Ann Surg. 2013;257:323-9.

118. Fialkowski E, DeBenedetti M, Moley J. Long-term outcome of reoperations for medullary thyroid carcinoma. World J Surg. 2008;32:754-65.

119. Machens A, Dralle H. Benefit-risk balance of reoperation for persistent medullary thyroid cancer. Ann Surg. 2013;257(4):751-7.

120. Schlumberger M, Basthold L, Dralle H, Jarzab B, Pacini F, Smit JWA. 2012 European thyroid association guidelines for metastatic medullary thyroid cancer. Eur Thyroid J. 2012;1:5-14.

121. Meijer JA, Bakker LE, Valk GD, de Herder WW, de Wilt JHW, Netea-Maier RT, et al. Radioactive iodine in the treatment of medullary thyroid carcinoma: a controlled multicenter study. Eur J Endocrinol. 2013;168:779-86.

122. Brierley J, Tsang R, Simpson WJ, Gospodarowicz M, Sutcliffe S, Panzarella T. Medullary thyroid cancer: analyses of survival and prognostic factors and the role of radiation therapy in local control. Thyroid. 1996;6:305-10.

123. Fife KM, Bower M, Harmer C. Medullary thyroid cancer: the role of radiotherapy in local control. Eur J Surg Oncol. 1996;22:588-91.

124. Martinez SR, Beal SH, Chen A, Chen SL, Schneider PD. Adjuvant external beam radiation for medullary thyroid carcinoma. J Surg Oncol. 2010;102:175-8.

125. Schwartz DL, Rana V, Shaw S, Yazbeck C, Ang K-K, Morrison WH, et al. Postoperative radiotherapy for advanced medullary thyroid cancer—local disease control in the modern era. Head Neck. 2008;30:883-8.

126. Call JA, Caudill JS, McIver B, Foote RL. A role for radiotherapy in the management of advanced medullary thyroid carcinoma: the Mayo Clinic experience. Rare Tumors 2013;5(3):e37.

127. Frassica DA. General principles of external beam radiation therapy for skeletal metastases. Clin Orthop Relat Res. 2003;415:S158–164.

128. Kim IY, Kondziolka D, Niranjan A, Flickinger JC, Lunsford LD. Gamma knife radiosurgery for metastatic brain tumors from thyroid cancer. J Neurooncol. 2009;93:355-9.

129. Santarpia L, El-Naggar AK, Sherman SI, Hymes SR, Gagel RF, Shaw S, et al. Four patients with cutaneous metastases from medullary thyroid cancer. Thyroid. 2008;18:901-5.

130. Iten F, Muller B, Schindler C, Rochlitz C, Oertli D, Mäcke HR, et al. Response to [90Yttrium-DOTA]-TOC treatment is associated with long-term survival benefit in metastasized medullary thyroid cancer: a phase II clinical trial. Clin Cancer Res. 2007;13(22 Pt 1):6696-702.

131. Maiza JC, Grunenwald S, Otal P, Vezzosi D, Bennet A, Caron P. Use of 131I-MIBG therapy in MIBG-positive metastatic medullary thyroid carcinoma. Thyroid. 2012;22:654-5.

132. Kraeber-Bodere F, Rousseau C, Bodet-Milin C, Ferrer L, Faivre-Chauvet A, Campion L, et al. Targeting, toxicity, and efficacy of 2-step, pretargeted radioimmunotherapy using a chimeric bispecific antibody and 131I-labeled bivalent hapten in a phase I optimization clinical trial. J Nucl Med. 2006;47(2): 247-55.

133. Wells SA Jr, Robinson BG, Gagel RF, Dralle H, Fagin JA, Santoro M, et al. Vandetanib in patients with locally advanced or metastatic medullary thyroid cancer: a randomized, double-blind phase III trial. J Clin Oncol. 2012;30(2):134-41. [Erratum in J Clin Oncol. 2013;31(24):3049.]

134. Elisei R, Schlumberger MJ, Muller SP, Schöffski P, Brose MS, Shah MH, et al. Cabozantinib in progressive medullary thyroid cancer. J Clin Oncol. 2013;31(29):3639-46.

135. Fox E, Widemann BC, Chuk MK, Marcus L, Aikin A, Whitcomb PO, et al. Vandetanib in children and adolescents with multiple endocrine neoplasia type 2B associated medullary thyroid carcinoma. Clin Cancer Res. 2013;19(15):4239-48.

136. Sherman SI, Cohen EEW, Schoffski P, Elisei R, Schlumberger M, Wirth LJ, et al. Efficacy of cabozantinib (Cabo) in medullary thyroid cancer (MTC) patients with RAS or RET mutations: results from a phase III study. J Clin Oncol. 2013;31(15 suppl):abstract 6000.

137. Vainas I, Koussis C, Pazaitou-Panayiotou K, Drimonitis A, Chrisoulidou A, Iakovou I, et al. Somatostatin receptor expression in vivo and response to somatostatin analog therapy with or without other antineoplastic treatments in advanced medullary thyroid carcinoma. J Exp Clin Cancer Res. 2004;23(4):549-59.

138. Lupoli G, Cascone E, Arlotta F, Vitale G, Celentano L, Salvatore M, et al. Treatment of advanced medullary thyroid carcinoma with a combination of recombinant interferon alpha-2b and octreotide. Cancer. 1996;78:1114-8.

139. Pozza C, Graziadio C, Giannetta E, Lenzi A, Isidori AM. Management strategies for aggressive Cushing's syndrome: from macroadenomas to ectopics. J Oncol. 2012:685213.

Poorly Differentiated Thyroid Carcinoma

Manohar H Martis, Elanthenral Sigamani, Deepak Abraham

INTRODUCTION

Thyroid malignancies have traditionally been classified based on cellular morphology and clinical behavior. At one end of the spectrum is the well-differentiated thyroid carcinoma (WDTC), with extremely good prognosis. At the other end of the spectrum is one of the most fatal malignancies known to mankind, anaplastic thyroid carcinoma (ATC).

With advancing medical knowledge and research, other aggressive variants of the well-differentiated thyroid were identified and subsequently added to the World Health Organization (WHO) classification of thyroid tumors. Researchers became increasingly aware of the existence of a unique group of tumors whose distinct morphologic appearance and biologic behavior lie between that of WDTC and ATC.

While it is possible that what Dr Langhans in Switzerland described as "Wuchernde Struma" (proliferating goiter) in 1907 due to its characteristic nesting pattern, may have been this particular tumor, it was Sakamoto et al. in 1983 and Carcangiu et al. in 1984 who first described it as poorly differentiated thyroid carcinoma (PDTC).[1-3] They classified it as a tumor with intermediate prognosis, positioning it between WDTC and ATC.

While there was universal agreement on the recognition of PDTC, pathologists differed on its histological definition. There were pathologists who based the diagnosis of PDTC purely on a solid, trabecular, and/or scirrhous growth pattern while others included an insular pattern with high mitotic rate and necrosis in a "peritheliomatous" pattern as necessary features for diagnosis. The definition of PDTC as a nonfollicular, nonpapillary, nonanaplastic, thyroglobulin-producing thyroid carcinomas was first included in the 2004 WHO classification of endocrine tumors. The proposed diagnostic criteria by WHO were heterogeneously applied by pathologists the world over, due to overlap with solid variant of PTC and solid/trabecular pattern of follicular thyroid carcinoma (FTC). The resulting confusion prompted expert pathologists to confer in Turin, Italy in 2006 and the "Turin proposal" was put forth to bring uniformity in the diagnosis of PDTC.

The clinical behavior of PDTC is much more aggressive than WDTC with higher rates of lymph nodal and distant metastasis at presentation. Recurrence rates are also higher when compared to WDTC. PDTC represents the main cause of morbidity and mortality from nonanaplastic follicular cell-derived thyroid cancer and is therefore clinically highly significant.

EPIDEMIOLOGY

Poorly differentiated thyroid carcinoma is a rare type of thyroid cancer, the incidence being between 2 and 15% of all thyroid malignancies.[4] The median age of presentation is 59 years.[5] The male to female ratio (1:1.16) is higher than WDTC (1:3).[6] From the available studies, Europe accounts for a higher incidence when compared to the United States.[7] An association with endemic goiter and PDTC has also been reported.[8]

CLINICAL PRESENTATION

Poorly differentiated thyroid carcinoma can occur de novo or as a result of progression from WDTC. The aggressiveness of PDTC is intermediate between that of WDTC and ATC.

Poorly differentiated thyroid carcinoma is known to be locally invasive. At the time of presentation, more than half of the patients have been found to have extrathyroidal disease.[8,9] Around 50–85% of the patients will present with regional lymph nodal metastasis, either clinically or imaging detected.[10,11] Distant metastasis has been reported to be present in up to 85% of the patients in some studies.[11]

Older age and male sex have been considered as adverse prognostic factors for WDTC.[6] This also holds good for PDTC. Age > 55 years at presentation and extrathyroidal extension have been documented as resulting in a significant reduced overall survival (OS).[12-14]

PATHOLOGY AND MOLECULAR ALTERATIONS

From the original description by Langhans as "Wuchernde Struma" in 1907 to the description as "Insular carcinoma" by Carcangiu et al. and the current classification as PDTC by WHO, PDTC has come a long way.[1,3]

Carcangiu et al. used the term "insular" in describing this tumor due to similarity in its appearance to insular type of carcinoid and pancreatic endocrine tumors.[3] Macroscopically, PDTC appears as a solid greyish-white tumor with multiple foci of necrosis. They are usually larger than 4 cm in size, display an invasive margin, and can appear as single or multiple nodules.

Microscopically, these tumors can have either insular, solid, trabecular, or a mixed pattern. Usually, it is the insular pattern **(Fig. 1A)** that predominates.[7] There are solid clusters of small and uniform tumor cells forming a variable number of microfollicles which may be separated by artifactual clefts. Other features which describe these tumors are increased mitosis, areas of necrosis **(Fig. 1C)** which may be in a peritheliomatous pattern (necrosis of cells away from a vessel), and capsular and vascular invasion **(Fig. 1B)**. These cells show typical dot positivity for thyroglobulin **(Fig. 2)** and nuclear positivity for thyroid transcription factor-1 (TTF-1), indicating their origin from thyroid cells. Immunohistochemistry (IHC) staining for calcitonin, chromogranin, and carcinoembryonic antigen is negative.

While PDTC may present as the only histological lesion most of the times, concomitant presence of WDTC and ATC has also been reported, as high as 59% in one study.[15] This finding lends further credibility to the hypothesis of dedifferentiation of WDTC to ATC with PDTC as the intermediate stage. However, the prognosis of the disease is determined by the PDTC component rather than the WDTC component.

Currently, the criteria as laid down by the "Turin proposal" in 2006 are used while making a histopathological diagnosis of PDTC.[16] They are as follows:

- Solid/trabecular/insular pattern of growth
- Absence of conventional nuclear features of papillary carcinoma
- *At least one of the following features*:
  - Convoluted nuclei and mitotic activity
  - ≥3/10 high power microscopic fields and tumor necrosis.

Convoluted nuclei have been defined as nuclei smaller and darker than those in papillary carcinoma, round and hyperchromatic with convolutions of the nuclear membrane ("raisin-like" contours).

A huge step forward in the management of thyroid carcinomas has been the identification of molecular markers responsible for the genesis and aggressiveness of the disease. Next-generation sequencing (NGS) techniques have been used to elucidate the molecular profile of PDTC. NGS also points to an intermediate position of PDTC as the mutation burden increases significantly from WDTC to ATC.

The two pathways implicated in the genetic alterations of follicular cells are either the mitogen-activated protein kinase (MAPK) pathway or the phosphatidylinositol 3-kinase (PI3K)/AKT pathway **(Fig. 3)**. The MAPK pathway is regulated by the

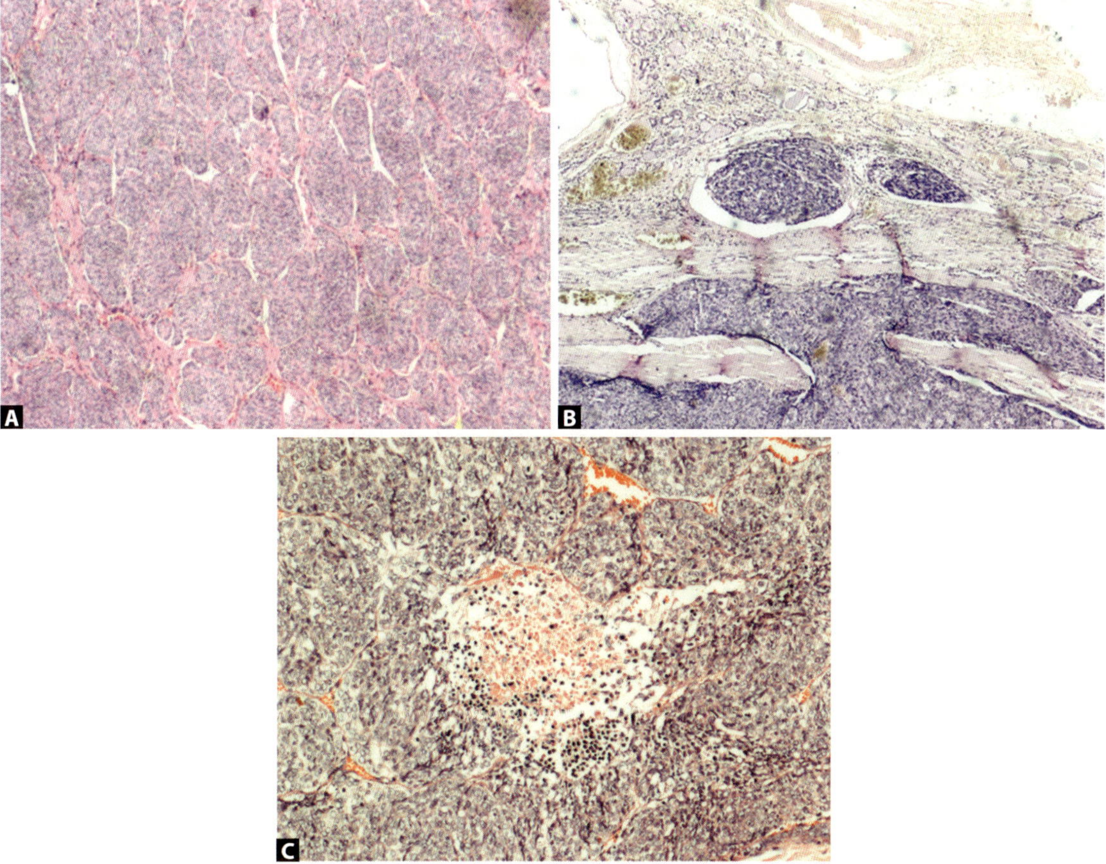

Figs. 1A to C: (A) Insular pattern (H&E at 50×); (B) Small lymphovascular invasion and capsular invasion (H&E at 100×); (C) Punctate necrosis (H&E at 10×).

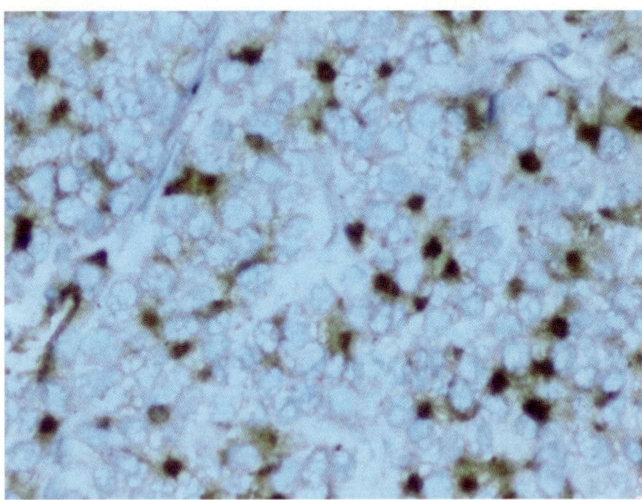

Fig. 2: Thyroglobulin cytoplasmic dot positivity (H&E at 400×).

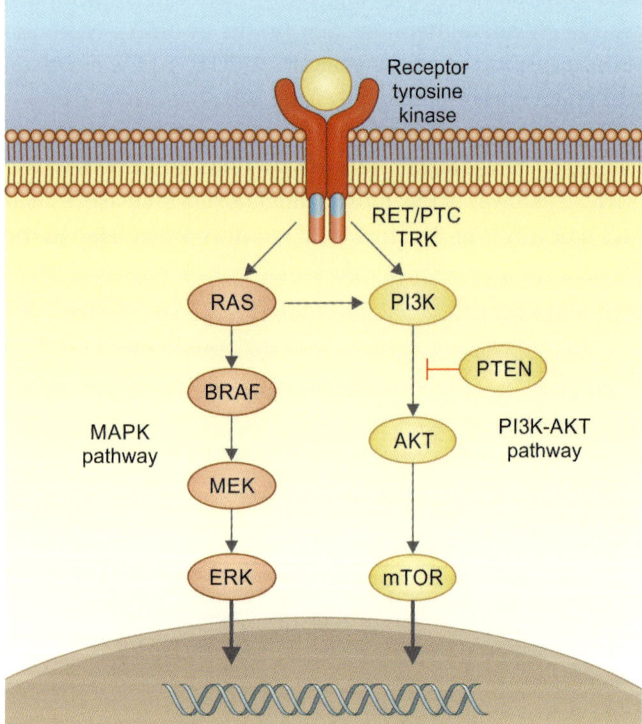

Fig. 3: Two pathways implicated in thyroid carcinogenesis are MAPK and PI3K-AKT.[19]
(PI3K: phosphatidylinositol 3-kinase; MAPK: mitogen-activated protein kinase; AKT: protein kinase B pathway; TRK: neurotrophin receptor signalling pathwa; ERK: extracellular signal-regulated kinase 1/2; mTOR: mammalian target of rapamycin)

RET, RAS, and *BRAF* genes. Point mutations in the *BRAF* and *RAS* genes or *RET/PTC* translocation can lead to unopposed activation of the MAPK pathway resulting in cellular proliferation and growth. The *BRAF* V600E mutation is seen in about 15% of PDTCs.[7] These are likely to arise from papillary thyroid cancers, as follicular cancers are unlikely to harbor the *BRAF* mutation. The *BRAF* gene is a marker of disease

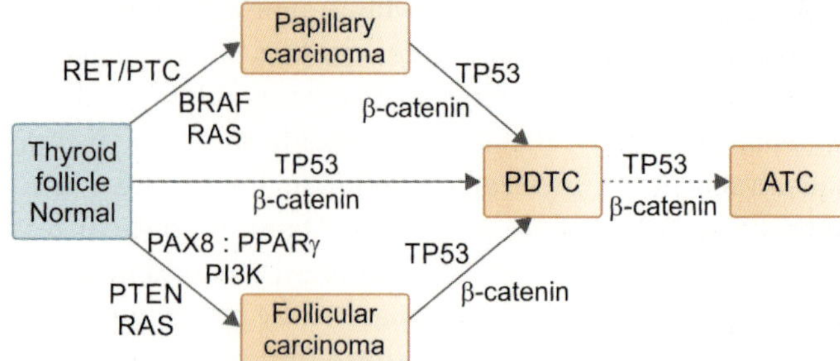

Flowchart 1: PDTC can arise de novo or from dedifferentiation of WDTC.[21]

(ATC: anaplastic thyroid carcinoma; PPAR: peroxisome proliferator-activated receptor; PDTC: poorly differentiated thyroid carcinoma; WDTC: well-differentiated thyroid carcinoma)

aggressiveness, tumor recurrence, lymph node or distant metastatic disease, and extrathyroidal extension.[17,18] *BRAF* mutations are also associated with a decreased capability to trap radioiodine and are more likely to be radioactive iodine (RAI) resistant.

RAS gene alterations are present in about 35% of patients with PDTCs. RAS can activate both the MAPK and the PI3K/AKT pathways. In PDTCs, oncogenic RAS activation is a prevalent genetic alteration and a marker of tumor dedifferentiation and adverse prognostic outcome.[8] However, many studies have reported that histological dedifferentiation is not necessarily driven by *BRAF* or *RAS* mutations individually, but rather represents the cooperation of multiple genetic alterations that likely stimulate dedifferentiation.[19,20]

The most frequently mutated tumor suppressor gene in PDTC is *p53* (about 28%; range, 17–38%).[7] These alterations are rarely associated with WDTCs. Studies indicate that unlike *BRAF* and *RAS, p53* mutations possess an exclusive function in triggering tumor dedifferentiation and evolution to PDTC and ATC.[7] Another tumor suppressor gene seen in both PDTC and ATC is the *ATM* gene.[8,9] The presence of this mutated gene in PDTC patients may indicate more aggressiveness as well as progression to ATC **(Flowchart 1)**.

Telomerase reverse transcriptase (TERT) promoter mutations represent the most common alterations in PDTC. They show a stepwise increase from PTC (9%) to PDTC (40%) and ATC (65–73%).[22] They are associated with increased aggressiveness and rates of mortality.[4]

The other mutations that have been recently reported are *EIF1AX, MED12,* and *RBM10* and may predict poor survival.[4]

Future research may help in developing targeted therapy toward these novel mutations and thus help in improving the prognosis in PDTC.

◇ DIAGNOSTIC WORKUP

The initial workup in PDTC is similar to that in any thyroid tumor and includes an ultrasound examination of the neck along with fine needle aspiration cytology (FNAC). Ultrasound helps in evaluation of the thyroid gland and the cervical lymph nodal basins.

Studies done on cytology in PDTC have found high cellularity, background of necrosis, low- to high-grade atypia, microfollicles, cytoplasmic vacuoles containing thyroglobulin, and nuclear inclusions.[7] While these features are not diagnostic of PDTC, they are definitely suggestive and should alert the clinician of the possibility of PDTC.

When PDTC is suspected, further evaluation should include a vocal cord assessment, given the high rate of extrathyroidal extension.

Suspicion of local invasion on history and clinical examination should also prompt the clinician to conduct a computed tomography (CT) scan of the neck, esophagoscopy, and bronchoscopy. If distant metastasis is suspected, then symptom-directed axial imaging with CT or magnetic resonance imaging (MRI) should be carried out.

TREATMENT

As PDTC is a rare tumor with paucity of prospective data and randomized control trials, it has not been possible to standardize its treatment. However, it is universally recognized by experts that surgery is the mainstay of treatment.

A total thyroidectomy with clearance of all gross disease offers the best possible chance of locoregional control in PDTC, reported in some studies to be as high as 81%.[9] Central and/or lateral neck dissection should be performed if there is clinical or radiological evidence of enlarged lymph nodes. If PDTC is suspected or diagnosed preoperatively, then the surgical plan should include a prophylactic central compartment neck dissection as per the recommendations of the American Thyroid Association, 2015 guidelines for differentiated thyroid cancers associated with an increased risk of metastasis and recurrence.[23]

The use of adjuvant treatment in PDTC is still controversial. Radioactive iodine (RAI) avidity of PDTC is variable, due to variation in tumor heterogeneity and existence of well and less well-differentiated tumor components.[12] Though some studies have demonstrated 80–85% uptake, they have failed to show statistical significance in 5-year survival rate. PDTC usually presents in the older age and at an advanced stage. Both these factors are associated with aggressive disease and loss of RAI avidity.

Similarly, external beam radiotherapy (EBRT) has not been proven to be beneficial in the OS. Most of the evidence for use of EBRT has been from retrospective studies and is therefore not entirely reliable. Patients who have unresectable disease, incomplete surgical excisions, and locoregional recurrences might benefit from EBRT.[7]

The use of chemotherapy in PDTC is still under investigation. While some studies have shown benefit in the form of nonoperable disease becoming operable, there has been no conclusive data to prove improvement in OS.[24]

Follow-up

Due to its propensity for recurrence, PDTC patients warrant a close surveillance. This can be achieved by serial monitoring of thyroglobulin. Serial RAI scans, ultrasound, and CT/MRI scans can help in detecting recurrences and metastasis earlier. Another important modality of detecting metastasis is fluorodeoxyglucose (FDG)-positron emission tomography (PET), since about 20% of thyroid metastasis may become RAI nonavid.[25]

OUTCOMES IN POORLY DIFFERENTIATED THYROID CARCINOMA

Poorly differentiated thyroid carcinoma is the most common cause for disease-specific death in fatal nonanaplastic follicular cell-derived thyroid carcinomas.

Poorly differentiated thyroid carcinoma has a 62–85% 5-year OS and a 66% 5-year DSS.[5,16] 5-year locoregional control rates up to 81% have been reported, if all gross disease is cleared at initial surgery. Locoregional disease is the cause of death in 18% of PDTC patients.[5] Distant control is achieved in only 59% patients at 5 years with the most common metastatic sites being lung and bone.[5] Distant disease also accounts for 85% of the deaths in PDTC.[5]

TARGETED THERAPY AND FUTURE PROSPECTS

The main challenge in the treatment of PDTC is tackling the distant spread since it does not respond to conventional therapy and is the leading cause for disease-specific death. Identification of the molecular makeup of PDTC in specific and thyroid cancer in general has led to research and identification of drugs specifically targeted toward these markers.

The US Food and Drug Administration (FDA) has approved the use of sorafenib and lenvatinib in the treatment of follicular cell-derived thyroid cancer, in cases of progressive, recurrent, or metastatic disease not responsive to RAI.[26] Both these drugs are multikinase inhibitors and inhibit tumor growth through antiangiogenic and antiproliferative mechanisms. Lenvatinib also targets fibroblast growth factor receptors (FGFRs). Two other drugs which have been approved for the treatment of ATC, dabrafenib (BRAF inhibitor) and tramctinib (MEK inhibitor), might also hold promise for PDTC given a similar aggressive nature as that of ATC.

Another area of research has been the restoration of RAI uptake, also known as redifferentiation, through inhibition of MAPK signaling. The drugs which are currently being studied for this mechanism are selumetinib (MEK inhibitor), dabrafenib (BRAF inhibitor), and panobinostat (histone deacetylase inhibitor). Studies have shown significant upregulation in the sodium/iodide symporter (NIS) transcripts with variable increase in RAI uptake.[27,28]

The usage of targeted therapy combined with the traditional chemotherapy/EBRT is also under investigation. Antiangiogenesis agents like the tyrosine kinase inhibitors (TKI), cabozantinib, and microtubule-depolymerizing agent combretastatin A-4 phosphate (CA4P) which blocks hypoxia-inducible factor 1-alpha (HIF1α) and vascular endothelial growth factor receptor (VEGFR) are believed to improve the resistance to chemotherapeutic agents.[29,30]

Besides these, molecules targeted against specific mutations in PDTC like TERT promoter and MED12 are also under current research and hold promise for the effective treatment of PDTC.[4]

◇| CONCLUSION

Poorly differentiated thyroid carcinoma is a rare malignancy of the thyroid. Over the years, it has carved its own place in the spectrum from WDTC to ATC. Dedicated study by clinicians and pathologists from Langhans to the those involved in the Turin proposal have provided us with a clearer understanding of its distinctive clinic-pathological and molecular picture. Surgery continues to be the best feasible option in curing PDTC while the role of RAI, chemotherapy, and EBRT is still controversial. Research into targeted molecular therapy will play a crucial role in the treatment of PDTC in the coming years.

◇| TAKE HOME MESSAGE

Poorly differentiated thyroid carcinoma is a rare thyroid malignancy whose pathological definition has reached a consensus after the Turin proposal. However, effective management still remains an enigma. Prompt and a complete surgery provides the maximum benefit, but this may not always be possible. More research into targeted therapy and its application is the way forward in the treatment of PDTC.

◇| REFERENCES

1. Langhans T. Über die epithelialen Formen der malignen Struma. Virchows Arch. 1907;189(1):69-152.
2. Sakamoto A, Kasai N, Sugano H. Poorly differentiated carcinoma of the thyroid. A clinicopathologic entity for a high-risk group of papillary and follicular carcinomas. Cancer. 1983;52(10):1849-55.
3. Carcangiu ML, Zampi G, Rosai J. Poorly differentiated ("insular") thyroid carcinoma. A reinterpretation of Langhans'" wuchernde Struma". Am J Surg Pathol. 1984;8(9):655-68.
4. Ibrahimpasic T, Ghossein R, Shah JP, Ganly I. Poorly differentiated carcinoma of the thyroid gland: current status and future prospects . Thyroid. 2019;29(3):311-21.
5. US Department of Health and Human Services. NIH. National Cancer Institute. Surveillance, Epidemiology, and End Results (SEER) Program. SEER Stat Fact Sheets: Colon and Rectum Cancer. [online] Available from https://seer.cancer.gov/statfacts/html/colorect.html [Last accessed June, 2021].
6. Shaha AR, Loree TR, Shah JP. Intermediate-risk group for differentiated carcinoma of thyroid. Surgery. 1994;116(6):1036-41.
7. Patel KN, Shaha AR. Poorly differentiated and anaplastic thyroid cancer. Cancer Control. 2006;13(2):119-28.
8. Nikiforov YEB, Paul W, Thompson LD (Eds). Diagnostic Pathology and Molecular Genetics of the Thyroid. Philadelphia: Lippincott Williams & Wilkins; 2009.
9. Ibrahimpasic T, Ghossein R, Carlson DL, Nixon I, Palmer FL, Shaha AR, et al. Outcomes in patients with poorly differentiated thyroid carcinoma. J Clin Endocrinol Metab. 2014;99(4):1245-52.
10. Sanders EM Jr, LiVolsi VA, Brierley J, Shin J, Randolph GW. An evidence-based review of poorly differentiated thyroid cancer. World J Surg. 2007;31(5):934-45.
11. Chao TC, Lin JD, Chen MF. Insular carcinoma: infrequent subtype of thyroid cancer with aggressive clinical course. World J Surg. 2004;28(4):393-6.
12. Hiltzik D, Carlson DL, Tuttle RM, Chuai S, Ishill N, Shaha A, et al. Poorly differentiated thyroid carcinomas defined on the basis of mitosis and necrosis: a clinicopathologic study of 58 patients. Cancer Interdiscip Int J Am Cancer Soc. 2006;106(6):1286-95.
13. de la Fouchardière C, Decaussin-Petrucci M, Berthiller J, Descotes F, Lopez J, Lifante JC, et al. Predictive factors of outcome in poorly differentiated thyroid carcinomas. Eur J Cancer. 2018;92:40-7.
14. Amin MB, Greene FL, Edge SB, Compton CC, Gershenwald JE, Brookland RK, et al. The Eighth Edition AJCC Cancer Staging Manual: Continuing to build a bridge from a population-based to a more "personalized" approach to cancer staging. CA Cancer J Clin. 2017;67(2):93-9.
15. Lam K, Lo C, Chan K, Wan K. Insular and anaplastic carcinoma of the thyroid: a 45-year comparative study at a single institution and a review of the significance of p53 and p21. Ann Surg. 2000;231(3):329-38.
16. Volante M, Collini P, Nikiforov YE, Sakamoto A, Kakudo K, Katoh R, et al. Poorly differentiated thyroid carcinoma: the Turin proposal for the use of uniform diagnostic criteria and an algorithmic diagnostic approach. Am J Surg Pathol. 2007;31(8):1256-64.
17. Xing M. BRAF V600E mutation and papillary thyroid cancer—in reply. JAMA. 2013;310(5):534-5.
18. Xing M, Alzahrani AS, Carson KA, Viola D, Elisei R, Bendlova B, et al. Association between BRAF V600E mutation and mortality in patients with papillary thyroid cancer. Jama. 2013;309(14):1493-501.
19. Nikiforov YE, Nikiforova MN. Molecular genetics and diagnosis of thyroid cancer. Nat Rev Endocrinol. 2011;7(10):569-80.
20. Nikiforov YE, Erickson LA, Nikiforova MN, Caudill CM, Lloyd RV. Solid variant of papillary thyroid carcinoma: incidence, clinical–pathologic characteristics, molecular analysis, and biologic behavior. Am J Surg Pathol. 2001;25(12):1478-84.
21. Hannallah J, Rose J, Guerrero MA. Comprehensive literature review: recent advances in diagnosing and managing patients with poorly differentiated thyroid carcinoma. Int J Endocrinol. 2013;2013:317487.

22. Agrawal N, Akbani R, Aksoy BA, Ally A, Arachchi H, Asa SL, et al. Integrated genomic characterization of papillary thyroid carcinoma. Cell. 2014;159(3):676-90.

23. Haugen BR, Alexander EK, Bible KC, Doherty GM, Mandel SJ, Nikiforov YE, et al. 2015 American Thyroid Association Management Guidelines for Adult Patients with Thyroid Nodules and Differentiated Thyroid Cancer: The American Thyroid Association Guidelines Task Force on Thyroid Nodules and Differentiated Thyroid Cancer. Thyroid. 2016;26(1): 1-133.

24. Auersperg M, Us-Krasovec M, Petric G, Pogacnik A, Besic N. Results of combined modality treatment in poorly differentiated and anaplastic thyroid carcinoma. Wien Klin Wochenschr. 1990;102(9):267-70.

25. Wang W, Macapinlac H, Larson SM, Yeh SD, Akhurst T, Finn RD, et al. [18F]-2-fluoro-2-deoxy-d-glucose positron emission tomography localizes residual thyroid cancer in patients with negative diagnostic 131I whole body scans and elevated serum thyroglobulin levels. J Clin Endocrinol Metab. 1999;84(7): 2291-302.

26. National Cancer Institute. Drugs Approved for Thyroid Cancer. [online] Available from https://www.cancer.gov/about-cancer/treatment/drugs/thyroid [Last accessed June, 2021].

27. Ho AL, Grewal RK, Leboeuf R, Sherman EJ, Pfister DG, Deandreis D, et al. Selumetinib-enhanced radioiodine uptake in advanced thyroid cancer. N Engl J Med. 2013;368(7):623-32.

28. Rothenberg SM, McFadden DG, Palmer EL, Daniels GH, Wirth LJ. Redifferentiation of iodine-refractory BRAF V600E-mutant metastatic papillary thyroid cancer with dabrafenib. Clin Cancer Res Off J Am Assoc Cancer Res. 2015;21(5):1028-35.

29. Viola D, Valerio L, Molinaro E, Agate L, Bottici V, Biagini A, et al. Treatment of advanced thyroid cancer with targeted therapies: ten years of experience. Endocr Relat Cancer. 2016;23(4): R185-205.

30. O'Reilly MS. Radiation combined with antiangiogenic and antivascular agents. Semin Radiat Oncol. 2006;16(1):45-50.

CHAPTER 17

Anaplastic Thyroid Carcinoma

Dhalapathy Sadacharan, Sabaretnam M, Siddhartha Chakravarthy N

INTRODUCTION

Anaplastic thyroid cancer (ATC) is an aggressive lethal thyroid cancer arising from the follicular epithelium and constitutes 1–2% of all thyroid cancers.[1] Thyroid cancer exhibits diverse presentation and prognosis, with well-differentiated thyroid cancer (WDTC) showing excellent prognosis whereas the ATC is the most lethal cancer and has the highest mortality among all thyroid cancers including all endocrine malignancies. It accounts for 20–50% of all deaths from thyroid cancer and causes death by suffocation.[2] The modality of treatment for any thyroid cancer is surgery, but in ATC upfront surgery is rarely feasible and it is a difficult thyroidectomy due to rapid local tumor invasion, end-of-life issues and plans for comfort care measures are integral part of initial disease management and planning. Majority of patients succumb to their disease within 6 months to a year as a result of local airway invasion or due to widespread systemic metastasis. Other modalities of treatment such as external beam radiotherapy (EBRT) and chemotherapy with multiple drugs when used as a single modality of treatment have shown poor outcomes. Therefore, the focus of the management of ATC has shifted to the understanding the genetic and molecular greater understanding of pathophysiology, new advances in treatment technologies, and the formulation and development of multiple innovative therapeutic clinical trials some of which have shown some promise.

The prevalence of ATC varies from 0.9 to 9.8%. An increased incidence is seen in areas with iodine deficiency where endemic goiters are prevalent. However, the incidence of WDTC is increasing due to revolution in imaging, primarily due to the rise in incidental papillary microcarcinomas of thyroid, the incidence of ATC seems most likely stable over the last few decades but mortality is still high. Suggested theories for this phenomenon include increased iodinization and improved management of WDTC.[3,4] ATC is a disease of the elderly, with a median age of diagnosis is 65 years and fewer than 10% are younger than 50 years of age. About 60–70% of tumors occur in women as with other thyroid disorders.[5]

ETIOPATHOGENESIS

Prior history of WDTC is seen only in 20% and coexisting differentiated thyroid cancer (DTC) is seen in 20–30% of patients. On further dedicated sectioning of the specimen the percentage may be higher, suggesting that a large proportion of ATCs reflect dedifferentiation of preexistent DTC into the more aggressive phenotype, and hence the aggressive behavior. The genomic events occurring in DTCs and ATCs suggest many overlapping alterations that are seen in conjunction with the DTC to poorly differentiated thyroid cancer (PDTC) to ATC transition, also indicate continuance of acquired alterations eventually leading to development of ATC. Landa et al. and Kunstman et al. published the first experience with a large cohort of ATCs and showed that they frequently carry all three BRAF, P53, and RAS mutations.[6,7]

Literature review conveys that nearly 80% of ATC arise in long-standing goiters, which suddenly increases in size.[2] ATC may arise through dedifferentiation from WDTC or de novo. Many molecular events have been described in the thyroid carcinogenesis and tumor progression. The primary events involve mitogen-activated protein kinase (MAPK) signaling pathway and phosphoinositide-3 kinase (PI3 K-AKT-mTOR) pathway. Late events in molecular pathway are commonly seen in ATC rather than the precursor WDTC include mutations in P53 tumor suppressor protein, 16p, catenin (cadherin-associated protein), beta 1, and PIK3CA.

Molecular and genetic alterations in ATC are extremely heterogeneous; next-generation molecular sequencing of the cancer should be performed to evaluate the presence of targetable mutations that might be treated either on clinical trial or through compassionate use program.[7-12]

- *BRAF*: Mutations in *BRAF* are present in 35% of ATC, encodes a protein called B-BRAF, a member of RAF kinases family of growth signal transduction protein kinases. This protein plays an important role in regulation of the MAPK/ERKs (extracellular signal-regulated kinases) signaling pathway, which affects cell division, differentiation, and secretion. *BRAF* mutations hinder the NIS (sodium/iodide symporter) gene expression and NIS membrane localization, consequently promoting dedifferentiation. BRAFV600E mutation increases the expression of vascular endothelial growth factor (VEGF) and hypoxia-inducible factor alpha.
- *RAS*: RAS family comprises H-RAS, K-RAS 4A, K-RAS 4B, N-RAS, and other homologous proteins. RAS protein

function is controlled by the guanosine triphosphate-guanosine diphosphate (GTP-GDP) cycle which regulate cell growth via MAPK and PI3K pathways. Mutation in RAS albeit important in diagnosis of follicular carcinoma of the thyroid and also it is seen in up to 60% of ATC.

- *RET/PTC*: Rearrangement of the *RET* gene, also known as RET/PTC rearrangement, is the most common genetic alteration identified in papillary thyroid carcinoma. RET/PTC3 rearrangements found in PTC also have dedifferentiation potential and can become ATC.
- *PIK3CA*: Mutation in PIK3CA functions is found in thyroid cancer progression. They promote the sequential progression of the thyroid adenomas to follicular carcinoma and ATC. These mutations have been found in up to 50% of ATC.
- *P53*: It is tumor suppressor gene whose activation induces apoptosis, cell cycle arrest, or senescence in response to the distinct stimuli, including DNA damage or aberrant oncogene activation. P53 mutation is found in up to 80% of ATC.
- *Telomerase reverse transcriptase (TERT)*: Mutation in TERT causes telomere lengthening which aids the thyroid cancer cells escape apoptosis and promote cell proliferation. These mutations are found in up to 50% of ATC.
- *HDAC*: BRAF mutation upregulates the HDAC and NIS silencing.
- *NOTCH 1 and HES 1*: Expression of Notch is decreased in ATC. This regulates cell proliferation and differentiation. HES 1 acts as a downstream effector of Notch 1 and plays an important function in thyrocyte proliferation and differentiation.
- *NF-KB*: This is linked to the member of transcription factors that is inactivated in the cytoplasm of resting cells including thyroid cells.
- *CTNNB1*: Mutations in this gene results in alteration of β-catenin phosphorylation which prevents its degradation, subsequently leads to Wnt signal activation. Reduction in membrane β-catenin leads to loss of tumor differentiation. Mutations in *CTNNB1* gene has been shown in 25–60% of ATC.
- *PTEN:* PI3K-AKT pathway activation occurs when PTEN is inactivated. They are reported in 10–20% of ATC.
- *Anaplastic lymphoma kinase (ALK):* Increased tyrosine kinase activity occurs in mutation of this protein. Mutation of ALK is shown in 11% of ATC.
- *Chromosomal aberrations:* Multiple chromosomal aberrations have been showed in ATC. Aurora kinase family is one such abnormality. Overexpression of Aurora A has been shown oncogenic potential.

◇ PATHOLOGY/HISTOLOGICAL SUBTYPES

Anaplastic thyroid cancer has various histologic types. Even though these histologic variants of ATC, they do not ultimately affect clinical management. ATCs are markedly invasive and WHO defines ATC as a highly malignant tumor wholly or partially composed of undifferentiated cells that retain features indicative of a follicular epithelial origin, on immunohistochemical or ultrastructural ground.

On gross examination of the specimen, ATC is composed of a white, fleshy tumor with extensive areas of necrosis and hemorrhage. Microscopically, they are composed of bizarre cells with marked cytological atypia and very high mitotic index. The variants of ATC include:[13–15]

- *Spindle variant*: It shows fascicular or storiform pattern of growth, indistinguishable from true sarcoma of thyroid. These tumors are generally well-vascularized resembling hemangiopericytoma-like pattern.
- *Pleomorphic giant cell variant*: Characterized by deep pleomorphism resembling osteoclasts like multinucleated giant cells with the connective tissue septae.
- *Squamoid variant*: Squamoid cells that are undifferentiated tumor appear epithelial with occasional focus of keratinization.
- Paucicellular variant
- Rhabdoid variant
- Carcinosarcoma variant

The spindle, pleomorphic giant cell, and squamoid variant are the more common variants. ATC may be comprised one of these variants or mixture of two or more variants. Immunohistochemistry can aid in differentiating these tumors from other neoplasms. Large numbers of these tumors are TTF1 and thyroglobulin negative and PAX8 positive.

◇ MANAGEMENT

Flowcharts 1 and **2** describe the management of ATC.

◇ CLINICAL PRESENTATION

Patients with ATC usually present with a rapidly enlarging mass in the neck with compressive symptoms. They can have hoarseness of voice, dysphagia, choking sensation, or pain

Flowchart 1: Initial management of anaplastic thyroid carcinoma.

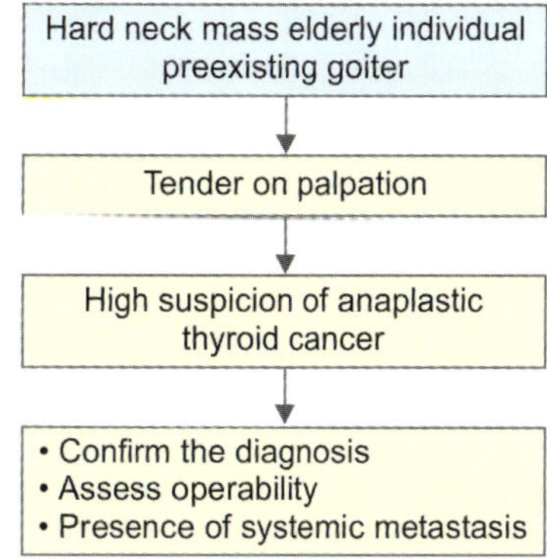

in the neck. On examination, these tumors are firm to hard usually restricted or fixed to the surrounding structures.

Cervical lymphadenopathy is present in 60% of the patients and most of them have distant metastasis either to the lung, bones, and brain. Infrequently ATC is diagnosed after thyroidectomy **(Figs. 1 to 4)**.

◇| DIAGNOSIS

The fine needle aspiration cytology (FNAC) is 95% sensitive in diagnosing ATC, but when it is inconclusive or the clinical suspicious is high, a core biopsy should be done under ultrasound guidance. The need for an urgent report has to be communicated to the pathologist. Whole body positron emission tomography-computed tomography (PET-CT)

Flowchart 2: Management of anaplastic thyroid carcinoma.

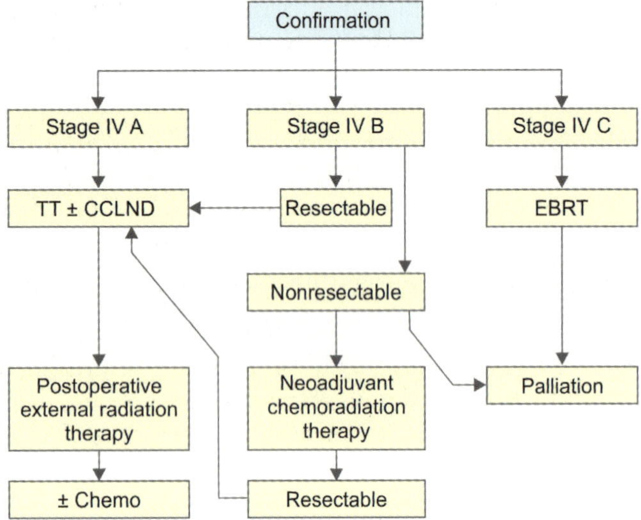

(CCLND: central compartment lymph nodes dissection; EBRT: external beam radiotherapy; TT: total thyroidectomy)

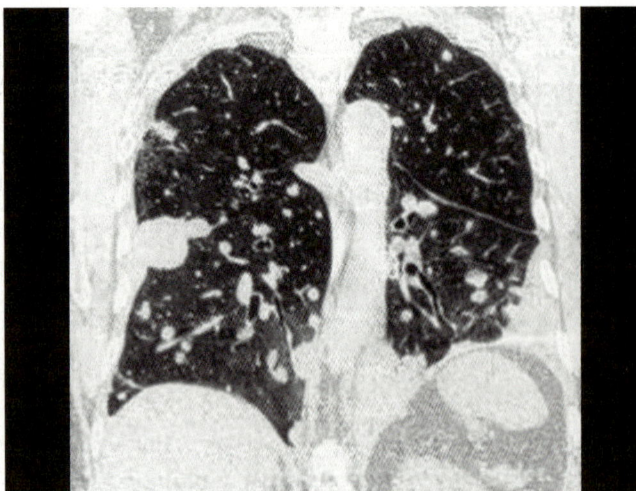

Fig. 1: Contrast-enhanced computed tomography of thorax of patient with anaplastic thyroid cancer with multiple lung metastasis.

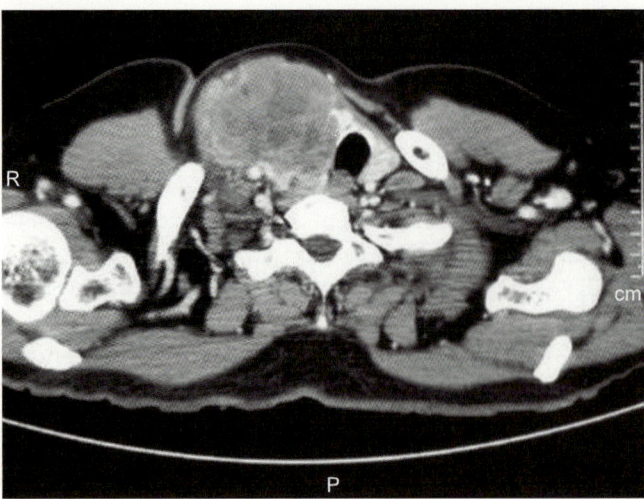

Fig. 2: Contrast-enhanced computed tomography of the neck with anaplastic thyroid cancer engulfing carotid artery and internal jugular vein.

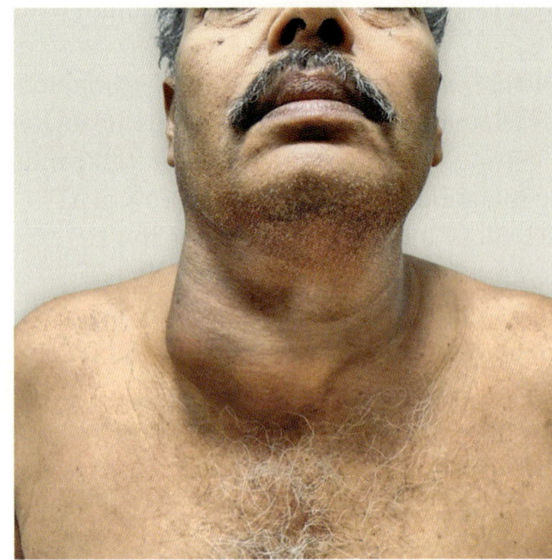

Fig. 3: Hard immobile swelling in the anterior aspect of the neck.

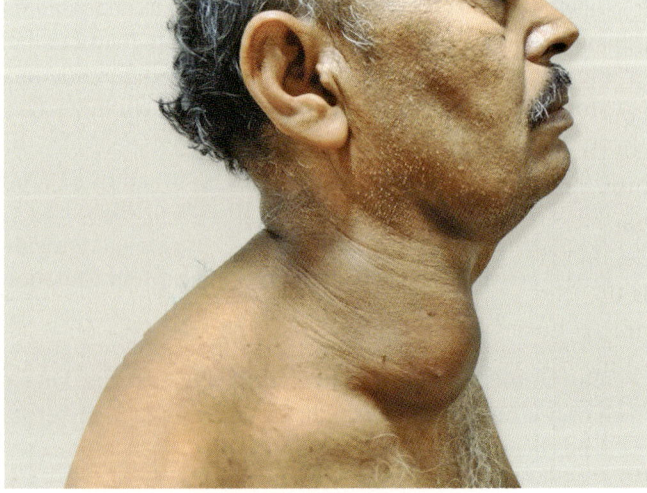

Fig. 4: Lateral aspect of the neck swelling which was immobile and tender.

Table 1: AJCC staging for ATC.

Stage	T	N	M
IV (A)	Intrathyroidal	No	M0
IV (B)	Gross extrathyroidal	Any N	M0
IV (C)	Any T	Any N	M1

(AJCC: American Joint Committee on Cancer; ATC: anaplastic thyroid cancer)

with contrast is done to check for local extent and systemic metastasis.

STAGING

All patients are classified as stage IV by American Joint Committee on Cancer (AJCC) **(Table 1)**.

TREATMENT

The rarity and aggressive behavior warrants a multidisciplinary approach and these patients are better managed in a tertiary care center. The comprehensive multidisciplinary team should include a surgeon, endocrinologist, medical oncologist, radiation oncologist, and a palliative specialist. The aggressive nature of the disease and the prognosis has to be discussed in detail with the patient and the family.

A combination of surgery followed by chemotherapy and radiation therapy might help in improving the long-term survival in selected patients, but in most the outcomes are poor. These tumors do not have NIS, hence there is no role of adjuvant radioactive iodine ablation.

SURGERY

It is important to discuss with a radiologist who has special interest in head and neck to assess the extent and resectability of the tumor. Preoperative nasolarnygopharyngoscopy is done to check the functionality of vocal cords. In locally advanced tumors, surgery should be avoided if the gross tumor cannot be excised. There is no role for surgery in patients with extensive systemic metastasis and tumor debulking is controversial. The extent of surgical resection is the best predictor for overall survival and remains the only chance for cure R0 resection is achieved in 20–30% of all planned surgery. The surgery consists of total thyroidectomy along with central and lateral compartment lymphadenectomy when involved. Prior planning is needed for laryngectomy, pharyngectomy, and other advanced procedures. It is essential to remove the gross tumor and keep the morbidity to a minimum.

AIRWAY MANAGEMENT

Sometimes few patients come to the emergency with stridor and surgeons are called to assess for tracheostomy. These patients typically have advanced and metastatic disease. ATC is aggressive and rapidly fungate through the incision site and grow inside the trachea. These factors have to be taken into consideration and better to avoid prophylactic tracheostomy.

Enteral Access

The need for percutaneous endoscopic gastrostomy (PEG) or gastrostomy has to be individualized depending on the extent of dysphagia.

External Beam Radiotherapy

Anaplastic thyroid carcinoma is a relatively radioresistant tumor, radiotherapy is either used as a part of definitive multimodality treatment or with palliative intent. As a part of definitive adjuvant therapy a total of 60 Gy is used and in palliative setting the doses are typically lower.

Cytotoxic Chemotherapy

Chemotherapy is used in combination with surgery and EBRT in stage IVA and IVB, but in metastatic disease (stage IVC) there is no survival advantage. The drugs used in retrospective analysis are doxorubicin, taxanes, and cisplatin. Tyrosine kinase receptors, sorafenib and pazopanib, have been used in clinical trials and have minimal effect on the tumor.

REFERENCES

1. Mao Y, Xing M. Recent incidences and differential trends of thyroid cancer in the USA. Endocr Relat Cancer. 2016;23(4): 313-22.
2. Lim H, Devesa SS, Sosa JA, Check D, Kitahara C. Trends in thyroid cancer incidence and mortality in the United States, 1974-2013. JAMA. 2017;317(13):1338-48.
3. Smallridge RC, Ain KB, Asa SL, Bible KC, Brierley JD, Burman KD, et al. American Thyroid Association Guidelines for

management of patients with anaplastic thyroid cancer. Thyroid. 2012;22(11):1104-39.

4. O'Neill JP, Shaha AR. Anaplastic thyroid cancer. Oral Oncol. 2013;49(7):702-6.

5. Ragazzi M, Ciarrocchi A, Sancisi V, Gandolfi G, Bisagni A, Piana S. Update on anaplastic thyroid carcinoma: morphological, molecular, and genetic features of the most aggressive thyroid cancer. Int J Endocrinol. 2014;2014:790834.

6. Landa I, Ibrahimpasic T, Boucai L, Sinha R, Knauf JA, Shah RH, et al. Genomic and transcriptomic hallmarks of poorly differentiated and anaplastic thyroid cancers. J Clin Invest. 2016;126(3):1052-66.

7. Kunstman JW, Juhlin CC, Goh G, Brown TC, Stenman A, Healy JM, et al. Characterization of the mutational landscape of anaplastic thyroid cancer via whole-exome sequencing. Hum Mol Genet. 2015;24(8):2318-29.

8. Viola D, Valerio L, Molinaro E, Agate L, Bottici V, Biagini A, et al. Treatment of advanced thyroid cancer with targeted therapies: ten years of experience. Endocr Relat Cancer. 2016;23(4): R185-205.

9. Papp S, Asa SL. When thyroid carcinoma goes bad: a morphological and molecular analysis. Head Neck Pathol. 2015;9(1):16-23.

10. Hsu K-T, Yu XM, Audhya AW, Jaume JC, Lloyd RV, Miyamoto S, et al. Novel approaches in anaplastic thyroid cancer therapy. Oncologist. 2014;19(11):1148-55.

11. Are C, Shaha AR. Anaplastic thyroid carcinoma: biology, pathogenesis, prognostic factors, and treatment approaches. Ann Surg Oncol. 2006;13(4):453-64.

12. Smith N, Nucera C. Personalized therapy in patients with anaplastic thyroid cancer: targeting genetic and epigenetic alterations. J Clin Endocrinol Metab. 2015;100(1): 35-42.

13. Feng G, Laskin WB, Chou PM, Lin X. Anaplastic thyroid carcinoma with rhabdoid features. Diagn Cytopathol. 2015;43(5): 416-20.

14. Lai ML, Faa G, Serra S, Senes G, Daniele GM, Boi F, et al. Rhabdoid tumor of the thyroid gland: a variant of anaplastic carcinoma. Arch Pathol Lab Med. 2005;129(3): e55-7.

15. Albores-Saavedra J, Sharma S. Poorly differentiated follicular thyroid carcinoma with rhabdoid phenotype: a clinicopathologic, immunohistochemical and electron microscopic study of two cases. Mod Pathol. 2001;14(2): 98-104.

Thyroidectomy

Anand Kumar Mishra, Kushagra Gaurav

◇| INTRODUCTION

In last 150 years, thyroid surgery has evolved from "Horrid Butchery" to a 100% safe operation especially when performed by experienced surgeons.[1-3] In last few decades, there have been technological breakthrough in gazettes and instrumentation, which have led to development of at one end more safe and fast surgery by conventional open technique like intraoperative nerve monitoring device, energy devices, and better intraoperative identification of parathyroid gland and at other end making possible endoscopic, remote access, and robotic thyroid surgery. There is also better understanding of the thyroid cancer etiology and its natural course. This all has led to the shift in the concept of surgery in thyroid from anatomical concept to embryological, subtotal to total excision of the gland.

In the present chapter, we discuss types of thyroid operations, surgical aspects of thyroidectomy with preoperative evaluation and preparation, operative management, postoperative care, and complications.

◇| TYPES OF THYROID OPERATIONS

Surgical procedures most commonly performed are:

- *Nodulectomy*: Excision or enucleation of nodule and leaving the rest lobe of the thyroid is nodulectomy. It is not a standard operation and should never be done.
- *Lobectomy*: It is the excision of an entire lobe of the thyroid gland.
- *Hemithyroidectomy*: It is the excision of lobe and isthmus. The trachea should be laid bare. Minimal surgery for a solitary thyroid nodule is lobectomy or hemithyroidectomy and indications are:
  - A solitary nodule that is "hot" or atypical on fine-needle aspiration biopsy (FNAB).
  - A dominant nodule in the context of a multinodular goiter (MNG) where only one lobe is significantly affected.
  - Differentiated thyroid cancer <1 cm.
- *Partial thyroidectomy*: Excision of undefined portion of thyroid gland is partial thyroidectomy. It is also not a standard operation.
- *Subtotal thyroidectomy*: Excision of the entire thyroid gland sparing 4–8 g on both sides in tracheoesophageal (t-o) gutter is subtotal thyroidectomy. This procedure was considered an operation of choice for hyperfunctioning goiter and euthyroid MNG. In other words, it can be defined as bilateral subtotal lobectomy and isthmusectomy.
- *Total thyroidectomy (TT)*: It is the complete removal of both the lobes as well as isthmus of the thyroid. It can be defined as hemithyroidectomy and lobectomy or bilateral lobectomy and isthmusectomy. Common indications of TT are:
  - All high-risk differentiated thyroid cancers size >4 cm or with gross extrathyroidal extension, clinically apparent metastatic lymph nodes or distant metastases, or thyroid cancer in a patient with prior radiation to head and neck or family history of differentiated thyroid cancer in a first-degree relative.[4]
  - Differentiat ed thyroid cancers size 1–4 cm without lymph nodes metastases or without gross evidence of extrathyroidal extension or clinical evidence of central or lateral compartment lymph node metastases depending on institutional protocol.
  - Medullary thyroid cancer and for those with a high-risk differentiated thyroid cancer. Differentiated thyroid cancer is defined by tumor ≥4 cm.
  - Hyperthyroidism due to Graves' disease when thyroid eye signs are present or medical management is unsuccessful or contraindicated.
  - Multinodular goiter where both lobes are significantly affected.
- *Near TT*: Excision of the entire thyroid gland sparing 1–2 g on both sides in t-o gutter or leaving the posterior capsule of the thyroid near Berry's ligament is near TT. The practice of near TT is to avoid the injury to recurrent nerves and superior parathyroid gland.

◇| INDICATIONS

The main indications for surgery in benign diseases of goiter can be remembered by 5Cs (**Table 1**).

◇| PREOPERATIVE PREPARATION

Thyroidectomy is an elective operation except certain situation of acute thyroiditis, compromised airway and stridor, or acute hemorrhage in a colloid nodule.

Table 1: Indications of thyroidectomy in benign cases.

Cosmesis	Solitary nodule, multinodular goiter, and large goiters
Control	Failure of medical treatment to control toxicity in hyperthyroidism or as definitive treatment of toxic goiters
Compression	Any symptom or signs suggestive of compression of airway and superior vena cava
Cancer	Fear of cancer and occult carcinoma, proven or suspected cancer on history, and examination or investigations (atypical, suspicious findings)
Come back	Recurrence of goiter

Hyperthyroidism and reoperative cases need certain additional preparation.

All patients undergoing thyroid surgery should undergo laryngeal examination to assess vocal cord function for occult recurrent laryngeal nerve (RLN) paresis and/or vocal cord paralysis. It is most commonly assessed by direct or indirect laryngoscopy. Other modalities are videostroboscopy (magnified, slow-motion view of vocal cords) and laryngeal ultrasound. Surgeon when examining the patient preoperatively should assess the thyromental distance, tracheal shifting, and neck length. If patient has short neck or gross tracheal deviation or short thyromental distance, then alert the anesthesia colleague about difficult intubation.

The American Thyroid Association and the American Head and Neck Society recommend preoperative vocal cord examination in special situations with high risk of having occult RLN paresis or vocal cord dysfunction,[5,6] however, voice change was observed only in one-third of patients with a vocal cord paralysis.[7] Special situations are:

- Preoperative hoarseness or voice changes
- History of prior neck or mediastinal surgery
- Invasive thyroid cancer or extrathyroidal extension posteriorly
- Bulky lymph nodes in central compartment or jugular chain.

Preoperative Management of Hyperthyroidism

The patient is made euthyroid with antithyroid medications.

- Clinically patient should be euthyroid. The sleeping pulse rate should be below 90 beats/min. Serum thyroid-stimulating hormone (TSH) may be suppressed in certain patients, so free thyroxine (T4) and total triiodothyronine (T3) should be in normal range.
- Continue preoperative antithyroid medications and/or beta-blockade till the morning of surgery.
- Start oral Lugol's solution [potassium iodide (SSKI)] 1 week prior to surgery as it blocks iodine uptake, secretion of thyroid hormone, makes the gland firm making handling of gland during operation easy, and decreases vascularity leading to reduced intraoperative bleeding.[8]

- Preoperative vitamin D and calcium supplementation are suggested to reduce the risk of symptomatic hypocalcemia postoperatively.[9]

Reoperative Thyroid Surgery

It is technically challenging as adhesions and scar tissues are present in the operative field. If it is being performed by different surgeons from the first surgery, it is not known what areas have been dissected during the previous surgery. Because of the above reasons, reoperative thyroid surgery can be associated with higher rates of complications such as RLN injury and hypoparathyroidism. Therefore, risks and benefits should be carefully weighed and discussed with the patient.

- Review of all operative and pathology reports from previous operations to determine the prior extent of disease and the visibility, location, and possible loss of parathyroid glands during the previous operations.
- Review of pathology slides from the previous surgeries may also be informative.
- *Imaging of thyroid*: Thyroid scan to see the residual mass and at least one anatomical imaging (high-resolution US, contrast-enhanced CT, or MRI).
- Completion thyroidectomy can be done in 7–10 days of the operation or after 6 weeks to allow the inflammation to subside. The timing of completion thyroidectomy after a partial thyroidectomy does not have any impact on complications; however, it should be done at high volume center or an experienced surgeon.

◇ SURGICAL ASPECTS OF THYROIDECTOMY

Antibiotics

It is a clean procedure performed in a well-vascularized area so infection rate is nil, however single dose of antibiotic prophylaxis is generally given and should be administered within 1 hour of incision. In patients at high risk for infection, poorly controlled diabetes and immunocompromised antibiotics are used as per the surgeon's protocol.

Venous Thromboembolism Prophylaxis

Mechanical methods of thromboprophylaxis (sequential compression devices) should be used and patients are ambulated in the evening of the surgery.

Anesthesia

Thyroidectomy is performed under general anesthesia with endotracheal intubation and the patient is placed in the thyroid position. It can be performed under local or regional anesthesia with cervical plexus block selectively provided that anatomy (nodule size) and pathology (benign, nontoxic) are favorable and patient is able to communicate with the operating room staff. It is safe to place an orogastric tube for identification of the esophagus in large goiters and malignancy.

Optional Equipment

Intraoperative nerve monitoring, intraoperative frozen section analysis, and vessel sealing devices are optional equipment to facilitate thyroid surgery. Intraoperative nerve monitoring technique and its use are discussed in other chapters of the book.

Positioning and Draping

The patient is placed in a supine position with the neck extended. An experienced anesthesiologist who is familiar with complex airway management can easily intubate the majority of patients even with large goiters with tracheal deviation. Fiber optic intubation may be necessary to safely secure airway in cases of marked tracheal deviation or compression. For intubation, "flex metallic or armored" endotracheal tubes are commonly used. They offer advantages of resistance to kinking and compression. Oral route of insertion is preferred to the nasal route which is done while performing transoral thyroidectomy.

The neck extension is achieved by placing a padded ring under the head of the patient and a rolled sheet under the shoulders or customized shoulder bags. Excessive neck extension during surgery can result in postoperative pain and hyperextension can lead to vertigo, headache, and postoperative nausea. The arms are kept by the side of the patient. The appropriate amount of extension is individually modified for each patient. It allows the thyroid to move both anteriorly and superiorly and thus making it more prominent. Usually 10–15° head elevation is done to allow gravitational drainage of the blood from the surgical site. The use of extension tubing provides an easy access to intravenous line. All patients and especially those with Graves' disease with ophthalmopathy should have their eyes covered with soft cotton pad **(Fig. 1)**.

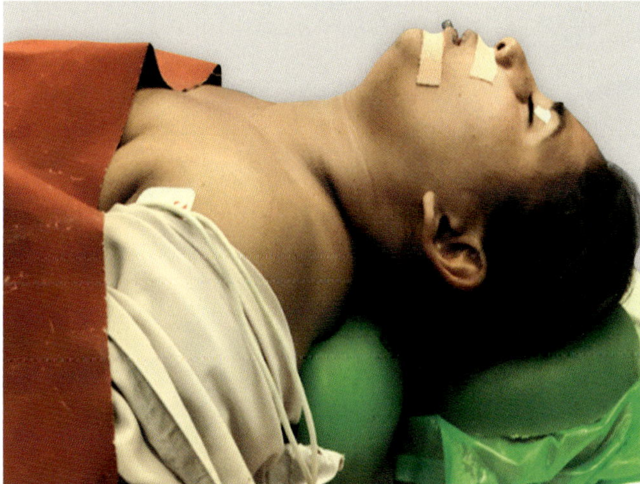

Fig. 1: Patient is positioned with hyperextended neck and with silicon head ring and silicon roll under neck and beneath shoulders (flexometallic endotracheal tube in situ).

In cases where intraoperative nerve monitoring is planned, the electromayographic [electromyography (EMG)] endotracheal tubes with neuromonitoring apparatus is used. These tubes are specialized in having electrodes near the cuff which come in contact with true vocal cords while intubation and, hence, record their electrical activity when recurrent nerve is stimulated by a probe. Long-acting muscle relaxants are avoided in such surgeries for correct documentation. Here one of the electrodes is placed in front of sternum area.

The patient is prepared with Savlon, spirit, and betadine scrub or as per institutional protocol from the chin to at least 4 cm below the clavicles and laterally to the trapezius, draped adequately so as to provide maximum exposure simultaneously avoiding unnecessary chances of breaking of sterility of operative area.

Incision and Skin Flaps

Neck incision (collar incision or Kocher's incision) is given about 2 cm above the suprasternal notch extending between medial edges of both sternocleidomastoid muscles. In short neck patients, it should be planned below cricoid cartilage and the length of the incision depends upon the thyroid nodule size. It should be symmetrical on both sides from midline and should be usually given in neck crease. If there are multiple neck creases, then the deepest should be chosen for the same. Incision length may vary as per goiter size and surgeon's preference often lengthened for large goiters, short neck, reoperative surgery, complicated cases, or patient is obese **(Fig. 2A)**. Incision with a knife is made through the skin, dermis, superficial cervical fascia, and the platysma. Some surgeons prefer to cut platysma by electrocautery **(Fig. 2B)**.

Raising Subplatysmal Flaps

Superior and inferior subplatysmal flaps are created, extending to the *thyroid cartilage and the sternal notch* for optimal exposure and laterally over sternocleidomastoid muscle. Technique of traction and countertraction (traction to flap, countertraction to thyroid gland) is used to open up this avascular plane. The anterior jugular veins will be deep to the superficial cervical fascia layer that may need to be ligated with either suture or the harmonic scalpel (Ethicon Endo-Surgery, Cincinnati, Ohio) or LigaSure (Covidien, Dublin, Ireland) if they interfere with exposure **(Figs. 3A and B)**. Smaller vessels may be cauterized, but use of cautery at skin edges is kept minimum, so as to avoid scar formation. The sternocleidomastoid muscles on both sides are mobilized.

Mobilization of the Gland

Strap muscles (sternothyroid and sternohyoid) are separated at midline raphe which is avascular and mobilized off the thyroid with sharp dissection **(Figs. 4A and B)**. Some surgeons prefer to divide the strap muscles transversally. It can be divided

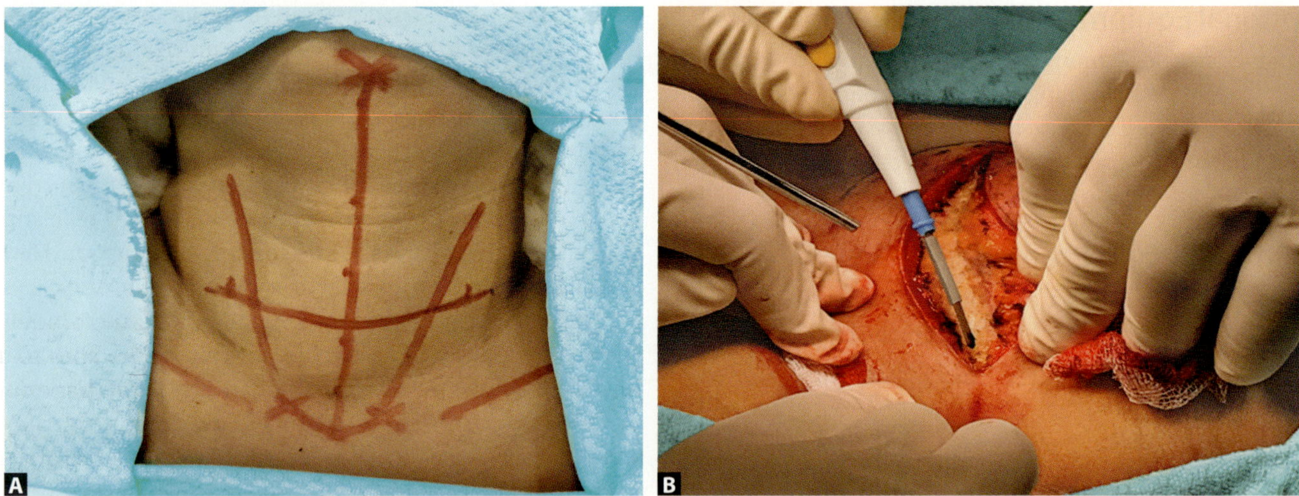

Figs. 2A and B: (A) Incision marked in natural neck crease with other surface markings; (B) After skin incision, platysma being cut with monopolar cautery.

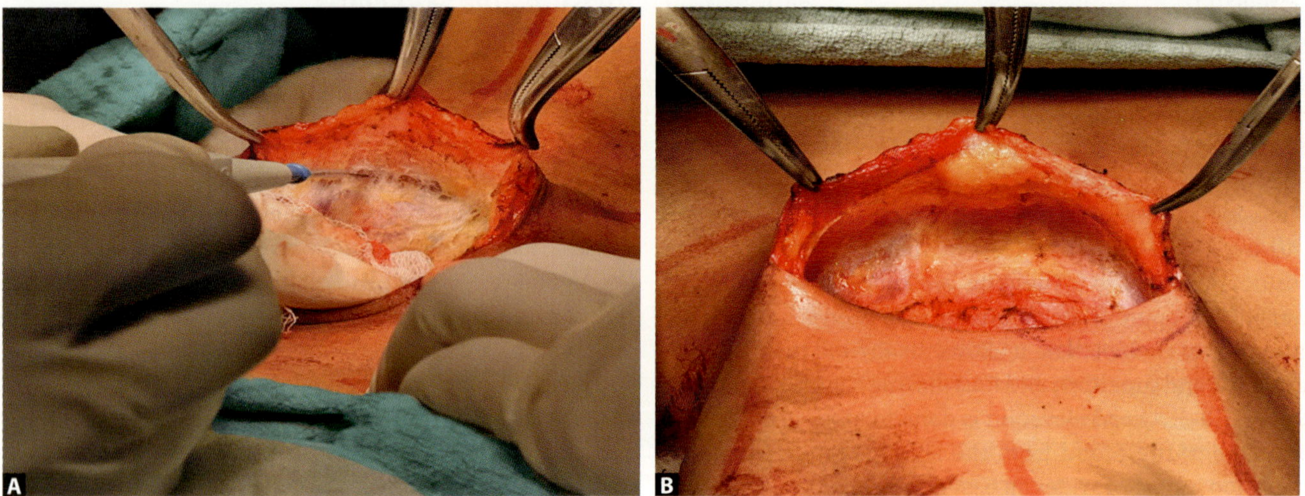

Figs. 3A and B: (A) Superior subplatysmal flap being raised; (B) Inferior subplatysmal flap raised till suprasternal notch.

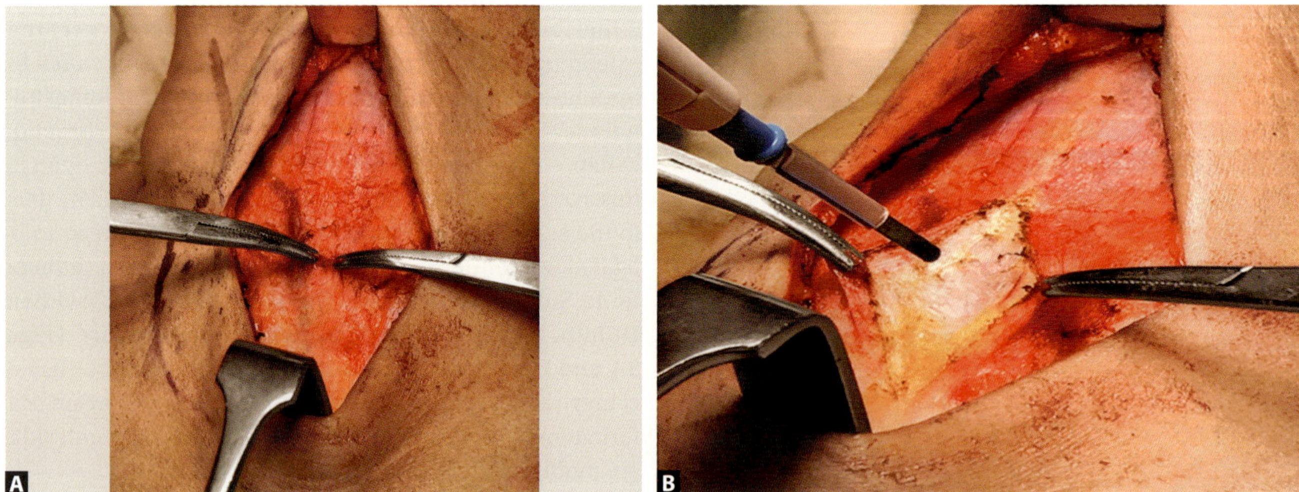

Figs. 4A and B: (A) Straps midline identified and held with two small hemostatic forceps before division; (B) Straps being divided in midline.

on both sides or on one side. The strap muscles are divided between hemostats with care not to damage the capsule of thyroid. Sometimes enlarged lymph nodes are visible in the midline prelaryngeal area (Delphian nodes) and it should be excised. If thyroid lobe is adherent or invades strap muscles, involved portion of the muscles should be resected en bloc with the tumor to maintain a negative margin. Few surgeons often advocate transverse division of sternothyroid muscle alone or along with sternohyoid muscle near the upper pole to increase exposure of the upper pole vessels.

Starting with the isthmus, one lobe of the thyroid gland is dissected from medial to lateral across the anterior capsule. When the lateral border of that lobe is reached, the middle thyroid vein should be identified and divided. Unless the middle thyroid veins which can be absent or one to multiple in numbers are tied and cut, the lobe cannot be rolled and delivered out of the tracheocarotid gutter. If middle thyroid veins are not tied and lobe is tried to deliver, there can be avulsion and hemorrhage. Further lobe is rolled lateral to medial to display its posterior capsule and the t-o groove. The flimsy attachment is separated by sharp or monopolar cautery.

Ligation of Superior Pedicle

Next is the dissection of superior thyroid pole to display the superior thyroid artery and the vein. Superior pole of the thyroid has superior thyroid artery, vein, and external branch of the superior laryngeal nerve (EBSLN). A medial thyroid space is created medial to the pole and lateral gutter is cleared off any tissue. Pole structures are identified and dissection is continued parallel to the superior thyroid vessels. The superior thyroid artery and veins are ligated individually after making adequate space and length to minimize the risk of injury to ESBLN.[10] Ligations can be done by silk sutures, clips, or by energy sources (bipolar, LigaSure, and harmonic scalpel) **(Fig. 5)**. In large sized glands, the anterior and the posterior branches of the superior thyroid artery may be ligated separately. Low ligation of the superior pole will ensure that ligation of the nerve is avoided. Care is taken to identify and preserve the EBSLN, but it is not mandatory to dissect and identify it in all cases. Usually just behind the superior pole when medial rotation is done, superior parathyroid gland can be identified in fat of pad. It is carefully dissected from thyroid capsule maintaining its blood supply and viability.

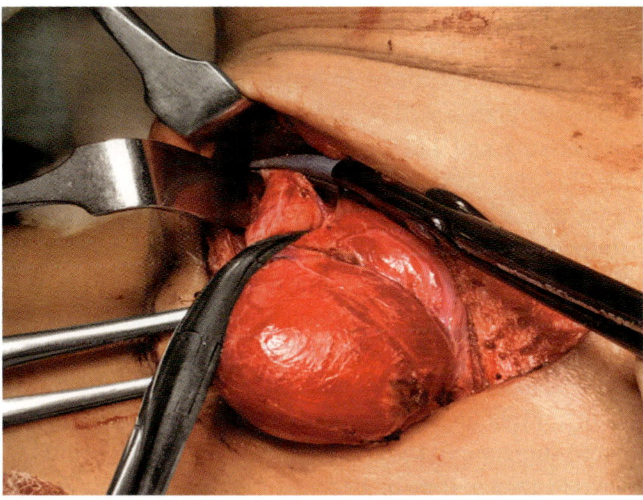

Fig. 5: Right superior pole vessels divided with LigaSure.

Recurrent Laryngeal Nerve and Parathyroid

For RLN, three structures need to be identified and defined: (1) trachea below isthmus and t-o groove, (2) inferior thyroid artery (ITA), and (3) landmark is entry point of RLN on lateral aspect of thyroid cartilage. The t-o groove can be identified by continuing the palpation of trachea laterally below isthmus. RLN runs in the t-o groove and in relation to ITA either below main trunk or between the branches of superficial to the trunk **(Fig. 6A)**. A mental mapping of the nerve can be done at this point and dissection within the fatty tissue of the t-o groove by fine Lahey's right angled forceps or hemostat is performed superior to the ITA. RLN runs most commonly posteriorly to ITA, but may lie in between or anterior to branches of ITA. Nerve stimulator probe is beneficial to aid in mapping the course of the RLN. Especially in this area, bipolar cautery and local pressure are used to control bleeding during dissection. RLN is identified as "pearly white tubular structure in t-o groove" with overlying "vasa nervosum" also called as "toothpaste sign". The RLN is then dissected both superiorly till insertion in trachea and inferiorly to the ITA. It is paramount that all branches of the RLN are saved as many times it has more than one. The use of nerve monitoring devices may improve the localization, detection, and viability of nerve branches.

In reoperative cases, RLN can be dissected and identified at the level of thoracic inlet where it is a single trunk (prior to branching) and this is typically below the last surgeon's scar.

Inferior parathyroid gland **(Fig. 6B)** most often lies anteromedial to RLN and over thyroid capsule. Capsular dissection refers to the tying all tertiary branches of ITA on the thyroid capsule. By capsular dissection, inferior parathyroid glands are gently dissected away from thyroid with the pedicle.

Ligation of Inferior Pedicle

The inferior pedicle contains the ITA trunk or its branches with RLN in relation to it. The vessels are skeletonized and tied individually close to the gland. ITA supplies 80% of the parathyroid glands, so it is prudent to tie all the branches of the thyroid capsule which is capsular dissection.

Removing Thyroid of Trachea

The posterior surface of thyroid gland now remains attached to the tracheal anterior surface and at oblique line of tracheal cartilage by condensation of pretracheal fascia which is also known as ligament of Berry. Ligament of Berry always has a vessel in its relation, so it should be tied or cut by bipolar or energy sources. If it is not properly burnt then after cutting, it retracts down and RLN is very close and can be damaged in spite of saving down. In fact, this is the most common area of RLN damage. Before removing thyroid off tracheal surface, entry of RLN must be ensured into cricothyroid region so as to avoid thermal damage to RLN by electrocautery. Isthmus should be separated from the anterior aspect of trachea

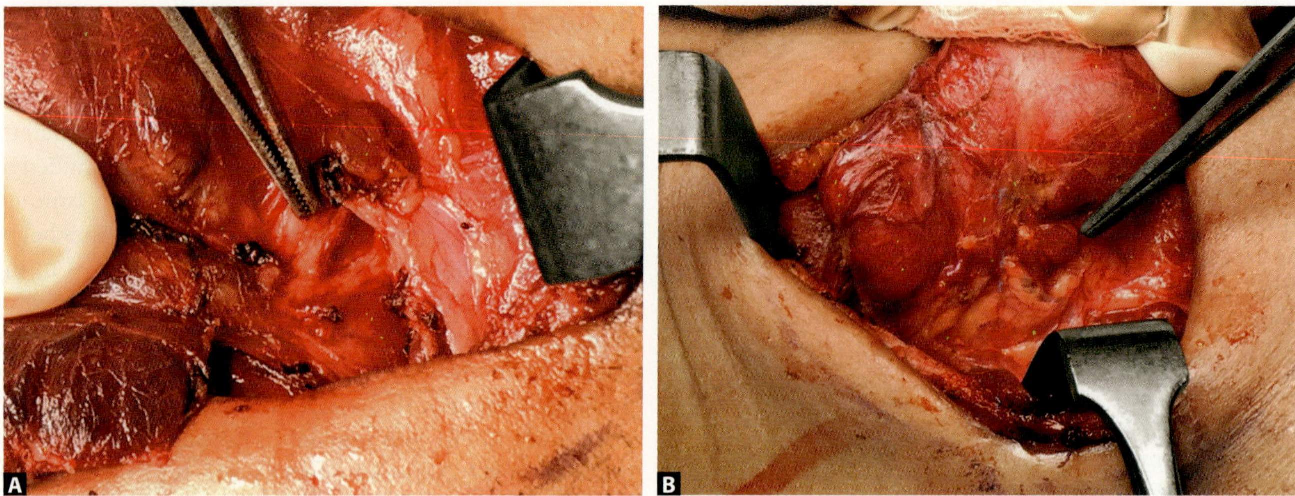

Figs. 6A and B: (A) Right recurrent laryngeal nerve in tracheoesophageal groove; (B) Right inferior parathyroid gland with feeder vessel.

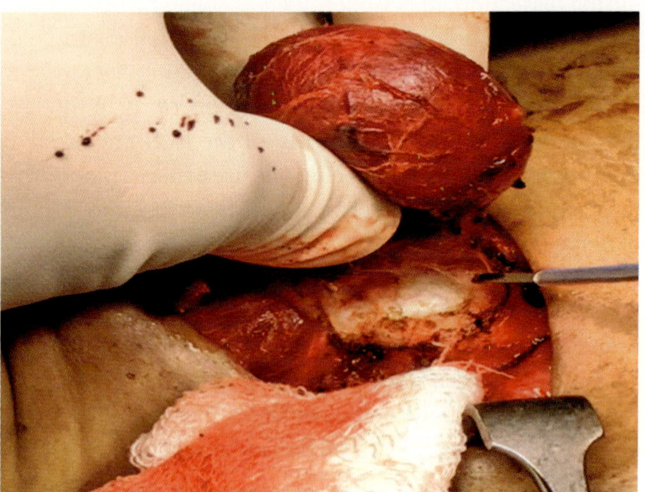

Fig. 7: Thyroid gland lifted off from tracheal surface.

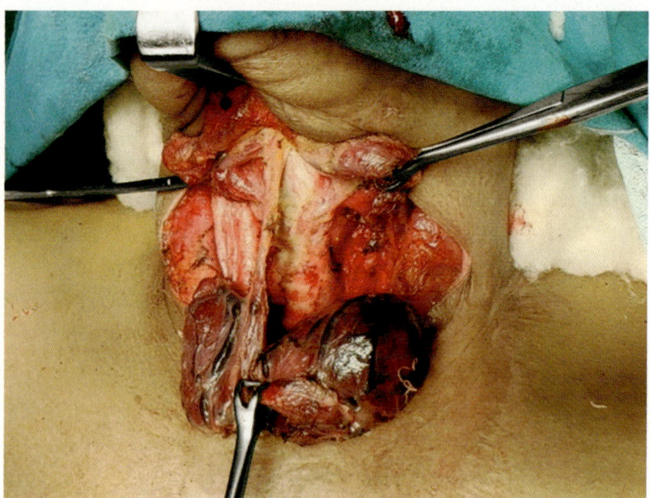

Fig. 8: Pyramidal lobe.

by monopolar cautery or blunt scissors and dissection is continued cephalad till pyramidal lobe and further up and the whole specimen is removed en bloc with the thyroid **(Fig. 7)**.

For hemithyroidectomy (lobectomy and isthmusectomy) operation, hemostat or Kelly clamp is applied across junction of isthmus to contralateral thyroid lobe and sharply divided. TT operation includes removal of both lobes, isthmus and pyramidal lobe **(Fig. 8)**. The stump is oversewn with a hemostatic absorbable suture. Alternatively, it can be divided by energy source or bipolar cautery. The specimen is then oriented and labeled for pathology. For TT, dissection is continued onto the contralateral lobe using gentle traction of the mobilized isthmus to help expose that lobe. All steps are repeated on contralateral side to complete the procedure. Central neck dissection or cervical thymectomy is performed after thyroidectomy and whole specimen is removed en bloc or separately after specimen has been removed. Thyroid specimen should be meticulously examined for any inadvertently excised parathyroid gland and if found gland should be autotransplanted immediately.

Closure

After the thyroid has been removed, wound is irrigated with saline and suctioned on gauze (to avoid damage to the parathyroid glands or RLN). Thyroid bed, strap muscle cut end and platysma, and skin flap are checked for hemostasis. At this time, the surgeon should check the colors of the parathyroid glands and if it is tan color, then a cut on the capsule of the parathyroid is given (knife cut test). Also newer technology such as indocyanine green fluorescence or near-infrared autofluorescence can help to identify the viability of parathyroid glands. Fresh bleeding from the cut denotes a viable gland. If there is no bleeding, it should be removed and transplanted. Parathyroid glands should always be saved with pedicle during thyroid surgery and removed only when grossly invaded by a thyroid malignancy or become severely ischemic during dissection. The removed glands are kept in ice and transplanted in well-vascularized sternocleidomastoid muscle after making a paste. Frozen section of a small portion of the gland should be performed before autotransplantation to ensure that tissue is of parathyroid origin in cases of obvious tumor involvement or a metastatic lymph node or a portion of the thyroid gland.

A meticulous hemostasis after saline wash and Valsalva testing before closure are two risk reduction strategies for avoiding postoperative bleeding **(Fig. 9)**. The anesthesiologist is requested for Valsalva maneuver (positive pressure ventilation). It will increase venous pressure in neck veins and will detect occult bleeders. Usage of drains after thyroidectomy is uncommon and totally depends upon the choice of operating surgeons; however, if drains are to be used, it should be suction drains only. Common indications for drain usage in thyroidectomy are thyroid bed with large dead space and/or extensive dissection.

The straps muscles are reapproximated with interrupted absorbable sutures in midline, leaving an opening of about 1–1.5 cm inferiorly to allow for blood or fluid to be evacuated to the subplatysmal plane, thereby minimizing the risk of tracheal compression by bleeding or seroma. So, midline closure is "noncontinuously" and leaving "weep holes" at lower end. The platysma is reapproximated with interrupted absorbable sutures. Skin is closed using a subcutaneous running closure **(Figs. 10A and B)**.

◇| POSTOPERATIVE CARE

After thyroid surgery, patients should be observed for pain, nausea, hypocalcemia, and hematoma.

◇| POSTOPERATIVE COMPLICATIONS

- *Hemorrhage*: In the postoperative period, hemorrhage is seen due to the slippage of the ligature on the superior thyroid artery, bleeding from the thyroid gland, or bleeding from the strap muscles. This may result in acute hematoma with respiratory distress. The skin sutures must be opened immediately and the patient should be wheeled into the operation theater for a re-exploration.
- *Respiratory distress*: Respiratory difficulty after thyroidectomy can be because of following reasons:
  - *Hemorrhage and hematoma*: It is seen from perioperative period to first 24 hours. The hemorrhage causes compression on airway or laryngeal edema.
  - Excessive wound edema causing pressure on the airway, larynx, and surrounding tissues.
  - Traumatic intubation
  - Recurrent or external branch of superior laryngeal nerve injury
  - Postoperative hypocalcemia
  - Tracheomalacia in long-standing large goiters[11]
  - Idiopathic.
- *Management*:
  - Use of ice packs on the neck after thyroidectomy. The ice pack may reduce wound edema.
  - Neck elevation and humidified oxygen support.

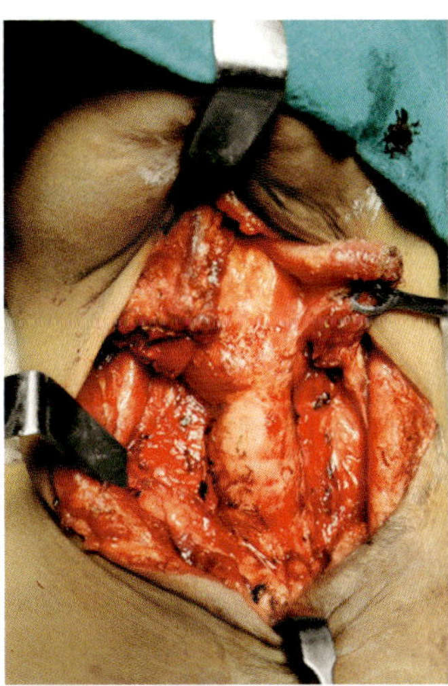

Fig. 9: Total thyroidectomy bed.

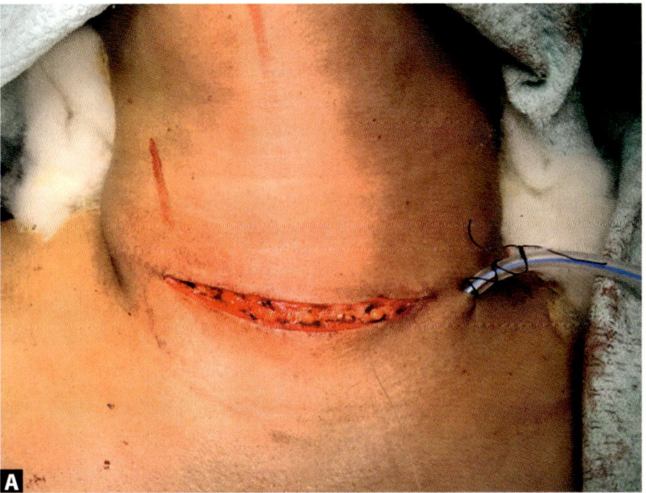

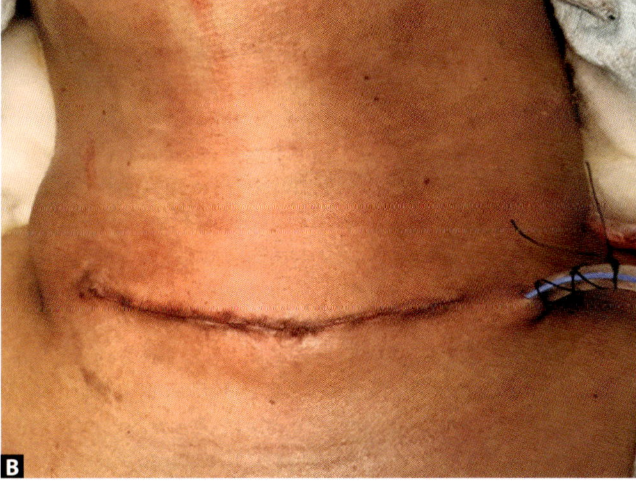

Figs. 10A and B: (A) Neck wound closed in layers—platysma closed with absorbable suture; (B) Incision after complete subcuticular closure and drain in situ.

- Endotracheal suction to remove subglottic mucus or sputum.
- Check clinical signs of hypocalcemia
- If major bleeding, then immediate surgical drainage.
- Patient can be intubated and observed. Tracheostomy is rarely required.

- *Hoarseness of voice*: Hoarseness which resolves spontaneously within 24–48 hours is typically due to vocal cord edema caused by endotracheal intubation. Persistent or severe hoarseness is caused by arytenoid dislocation or vocal cord dysfunction from a nerve injury. Hoarseness, uncontrolled coughing when talking, dyspnea (>24–48 hours) after surgery, or aspiration pneumonia should raise suspicion for possible vocal cord motion abnormalities. It results from injury to either the RLN or superior laryngeal nerve (more common). In unilateral RLN injury, the voice may be husky. Bilateral recurrent nerve injury is more serious as the vocal cords assume the midline position and lead to respiratory distress. This almost always requires a tracheostomy. Injury to the superior laryngeal nerve leads to an early fatigability during speaking.

- *Dysphagia*: Dysphagia is a frequent complaint after thyroidectomy. The etiology is uncertain but may be related to postoperative adhesions, decreased laryngeal elevation, cricothyroid trauma or inflammation, or nerve damage.

- *Parathyroid insufficiency*: Dissection often leads to disruption of the blood supply of the parathyroid glands and leads to transient hypocalcemia usually seen on the second or third postoperative day. Permanent hypocalcemia may follow inadvertent removal of all the parathyroids during TT. Patients in hypocalcemia present with circumoral tingling and carpopedal spasm. Intravenous bolus of calcium gluconate should be administered urgently (10 mL of 10% calcium gluconate) and the patient started on oral calcium and activated vitamin D.

- *Thyroid insufficiency*: Hypothyroidism is seen following unilateral or incomplete bilateral surgery (lobotomy or hemi or subtotal). A thyroid function test should be done when suspected or after 3 months once at least after unilateral surgery. Thyroid hormone supplementation requirement depends on both types of disease (benign vs. malignant disease) and extent of resection (unilateral or bilateral). After hemithyroidectomy, 15–30% patients require thyroid hormone supplementation because of various reasons. Risk factors for developing hypothyroidism after hemithyroidectomy are age, sex, preoperative TSH level >1.5 µIU/mL, lower free T4 levels, presence of antithyroid antibodies, autoimmune thyroiditis in the excised lobe, and volume of remnant thyroid lobe. Thyroid hormone requirements are usually calculated based on seven factors: (1) body weight, (2) age, (3) sex, (4) body mass index, (5) preoperative TSH, (6) iron supplementation, and (7) vitamin-mineral supplementation in patient after thyroidectomy. TT for benign disease is started on a daily dose of levothyroxine (LT4) at approximately dose of 1.6 µg/kg body weight after surgery. **Table 2** shows various schemes proposed in the literature for the estimation of LT4 requirements after thyroidectomy.[12-20] In malignancy, the thyroid hormone dose depends on thyroid cancer risk stratification whether low risk or high risk.

Total thyroidectomy for malignant disease planned for radioactive iodine (RAI) within 4 weeks of surgery may be discharged home without any thyroid hormone replacement. Thyroid hormone withdrawal makes hypothyroid, raises TSH level, which stimulates follicular cells for RAI uptake and improves efficacy. Alternatively, thyroid hormone may be started and recombinant human thyrotropin (rhTSH) can be used prior to RAI. Actual target of TSH suppression after RAI depends on the patient's age, stage, and aggressiveness of the cancer, however the starting dose is same (1.6 µg/kg body weight).

- *Thyrotoxic crisis (or thyroid storm)*: It is an uncommon but serious condition that may be seen in the postoperative period. This is usually seen in patients with Graves' disease and toxic MNG. In such patients, the antithyroid drugs should be continued postoperatively along with Lugol's iodine and beta-blockers. Hydrocortisone 100 mg can be given intravenously with correction of dehydration, heart failure, and control of hyperpyrexia.

- Wound problems—infection and keloid

- *Horner syndrome*: Horner syndrome is a neurologic syndrome caused by damage to the sympathetic pathway in the neck due to ischemic nerve damage, stretching of the cervical sympathetic chain by the retractor, or postoperative hematoma. The symptoms of Horner syndrome are miosis, ptosis, and anhidrosis. It is a very rare (0.2%) complication of thyroidectomy done along with a lateral neck dissection.

- *Chyle leak*: Chyle leaks or fistulas are caused by injury to thoracic duct usually during lateral neck dissection of left side but can occur with central neck dissection as well. Chyle leak is reported in 1.8–8.3% of thyroidectomies. Symptoms are excessive drains like milk, a bulging supraclavicular fossa, and induration or erythema of the skin. It can lead to severe fluid and electrolyte imbalances and even death if not treated properly. Low-output chyle leak (<500 mL/day) can be managed conservatively with fasting while high-output leaks require surgical ligation of the thoracic duct.[21]

- *Tracheal injury*: Tracheal necrosis secondary to excessive use of cautery on or around the trachea is a rare complication of thyroidectomy. The blood supply to the upper trachea is primarily from small branches of the inferior thyroid artery, which could be damaged during thyroid surgery. Tracheal necrosis can lead to air

Table 2: Methods in the literature for the estimation of LT4 requirements after thyroidectomy.

Author/location	Formula or scheme				
Cunningham JJ et al., 1984[12]	LT4 dose (µg/day) = 3.4 × LBM – 11				
	LBM (male) = (79.5 – 0.24 × weight – 0.15 × age) × weight/73.2				
	LBM (female) = (69.8 – 0.26 × weight – 0.12 × age) × weight/73.2				
Olubowale O et al., 2006[13]	LT4 dose (µg/day) = 100 if weight < 53 kg				
	= 125 if 53 ≤ weight ≤ 86 kg				
	= 150 if 86 < weight ≤ 108 kg				
	= 175 if weight > 108 kg				
Sukumar R et al., 2010[14]	Body surface area 2.04 µg/kg/day				
Mistry D et al., 2011[15]	LT4 dose (µg/day) = (0.943 × weight) + (–1.165 × age) + 125.8				
Ojomo KA et al., 2013[16]	LT4 dose (µg/day) = (–0.018 × BMI + 2.13) × weight				
Jin J et al., 2013[17]	LT4 dose (µg/day) = 1.5 × weight				
Di Donna V et al., 2014[18]	LT4 dose (µg/kg/day)	BMI	≤23	23–28	>28
		Age (years)			
		≤40	1.8	1.7	1.6
		>40–55	1.7	1.6	1.5
		>55	1.6	1.5	1.4
Elfenbein DM et al., 2016[19]	LT4 dose (µg/kg/day)	BMI	Male	Female	
		Age (years)			
		<21	2.1	1.8	
		22–26	1.9	1.7	
		27–32	1.7	1.6	
		33–40	1.5	1.4	
		>40	1.3	1.2	
Chen SS et al., 2019[20]	Poisson regression dosing scheme using Machine learning				

(BMI: body mass index; LBM: lean body mass; LT4: levothyroxine)

leak or subcutaneous emphysema and is potentially life-threatening. The treatment is neck re-exploration and tracheostomy.

- *Esophageal injury*: Esophageal and pharyngeal injury can occur with thyroid malignancy with extrathyroidal extension. The finding of extensive crepitus in the neck postoperatively should prompt immediate evaluation for a pharyngeal or esophageal perforation. For early identification, a nasogastric tube should be placed before starting the thyroidectomy in these cases.

◇ FOLLOW-UP

Follow-up after thyroidectomy is done within 2 weeks of surgery to:
- Evaluate the wound, any voice changes, subtle hypocalcemic symptoms, and overall recovery.
- Adjust doses of calcium/vitamin D supplementation in patients undergone TT.
- Review histopathology results.
- Plan and schedule multidisciplinary care for patients with thyroid cancer and RAI.

◇ THYROIDECTOMY TECHNIQUES: CURRENT TRENDS

Over recent years, with development of ultrasonic shears and small size endoscopes, it has allowed surgeons to perform thyroidectomies through much smaller incisions than using traditional techniques. Currently, there are two different approaches that are popular for minimal invasive thyroidectomy. First technique is "remote access thyroidectomy" often practiced in Japan, China, and Korea and involves making incisions away from the neck in hidden areas such as in the axillae, chest, or the areola of the breast—labeled as "axillary breast approach (ABA) or bilateral axillary breast approach (BABA)". Main advantage is that thyroidectomy is performed through a tunnel with endoscopic instruments up to neck thus avoiding neck incision. Other popular technique is Miccoli's "minimally invasive video-assisted thyroidectomy (MIVAT)" widely practiced in Europe and in US. A smaller incision is placed in conventional location in neck and a 5-mm 30º endoscope is introduced into the incision and thyroidectomy is performed guided by this endoscope.

A new technique gaining popularity these days is "transoral thyroidectomy"—where access to subplatysmal plane is through transvestibular space (between lip and gingiva) and thyroidectomy is performed with endoscopic instruments and hence leaving no scar in neck. Korean surgeons have popularized "robotic thyroidectomy" done using the da Vinci Surgical System [robotic arms, three-dimensional (3D) camera, and console] where 7–10 incisions are made unilaterally or in both axillae and the dissection progresses from the axilla to the neck with performance of a lobectomy or TT. Advantages are—better view and identification of critical structures, better dexterity, and no scar in neck.

◇| CONCLUSION

Thyroidectomy has evolved in the last 170-years from the time of Samuel Gross who described it as "Horrid Butchery" to the modern times when it has become a safe with a better understanding of surgical anatomy, the natural history of thyroid ailments, refinements in surgical techniques and use of modern adjuncts. Every surgeon practicing thyroidectomy should give paramount emphasis to understanding the anatomy of laryngeal nerves and parathyroid gland to prevent the two most dreaded complications of this operation and practice a safe thyroidectomy.

◇| REFERENCES

1. Rogers-Stevane J, Kauffman GL. A historical perspective on surgery of the thyroid and parathyroid glands. Otolaryngol Clin North Am. 2008;41:1059-67.
2. Adkisson CD, Howell GM, McCoy KL, Armstrong MJ, Kelley ML, Stang MT, et al. Surgeon volume and adequacy of thyroidectomy for differentiated thyroid cancer. Surgery. 2014;156:1453-59.
3. Adam MA, Thomas S, Youngwirth L, Hyslop T, Reed SD, Scheri RP, et al. Is there a minimum number of thyroidectomies a surgeon should perform to optimize patient outcomes? Ann Surg. 2017;265:402-7.
4. Haugen BR, Alexander EK, Bible KC, Doherty GM, Mandel SJ, Nikiforov YE, et al. 2015 American Thyroid Association Management Guidelines for Adult Patients with Thyroid Nodules and Differentiated Thyroid Cancer: The American Thyroid Association Guidelines Task Force on Thyroid Nodules and Differentiated Thyroid Cancer. Thyroid. 2016;26:1-133.
5. Sinclair CF, Bumpous JM, Haugen BR, Chala A, Meltzer D, Miller BS, et al. Laryngeal examination in thyroid and parathyroid surgery: An American Head and Neck Society consensus statement: AHNS Consensus Statement. Head Neck. 2016;38:811-9.
6. Steurer M, Passler C, Denk DM, Schneider B, Niederle B, Bigenzahn W. Advantages of recurrent laryngeal nerve identification in thyroidectomy and parathyroidectomy and the importance of preoperative and postoperative laryngoscopic examination in more than 1000 nerves at risk. Laryngoscope. 2002;112:124-33.
7. Cirocchi R, Arezzo A, D'Andrea V, Abraha I, Popivanov GI, Avenia N, et al. Intraoperative neuromonitoring versus visual nerve identification for prevention of recurrent laryngeal nerve injury in adults undergoing thyroid surgery. Cochrane Database Syst Rev. 2019;1:CD012483.
8. Erbil Y, Ozluk Y, Giriş M, Salmaslioglu A, Issever H, Barbaros U, et al. Effect of lugol solution on thyroid gland blood flow and microvessel density in the patients with Graves' disease. J Clin Endocrinol Metab. 2007;92:2182-9.
9. Oltmann SC, Brekke AV, Schneider DF, Schaefer SC, Chen H, Sippel RS, et al. Preventing postoperative hypocalcemia in patients with Graves disease: a prospective study. Ann Surg Oncol. 2015;22:952-8.
10. Mishra AK, Tamidari H, Singh N, Mishra SK, Agarwal A. External branch of superior laryngeal nerve in thyroid surgery: no more neglected nerve. Indian J Med Sci. 2007;61:3-8.
11. Agarwal A, Mishra AK, Gupta SK, Arshad F, Agarwal A, Tripathi M, et al. High incidence of tracheomalacia in longstanding goiters: experience from an endemic goiter region. World J Surg. 2007;31:832-7.
12. Cunningham JJ, Barzel US. Lean body mass is a predictor of the daily requirement for thyroid hormone in older men and women. J Am Geriatr Soc. 1984;32:204-7.
13. Olubowale O, Chadwick DR. Optimization of thyroxine replacement therapy after total or near-total thyroidectomy for benign thyroid disease. Br J Surg. 2006;93:57-60.
14. Sukumar R, Agarwal A, Gupta S, Mishra A, Agarwal G, Verma AK, et al. Prediction of LT4 replacement dose to achieve euthyroidism in subjects undergoing total thyroidectomy for benign thyroid disorders. World J Surg. 2010;34:527-31.
15. Mistry D, Atkin S, Atkinson H, Gunasekaran S, Sylvester D, Rigby AS, et al. Predicting thyroxine requirements following total thyroidectomy. Clin Endocrinol (Oxf). 2011;74:384-7.
16. Ojomo KA, Schneider DF, Reiher AE, Lai N, Schaefer S, Chen H, et al. Using body mass index to predict optimal thyroid dosing after thyroidectomy. J Am Coll Surg. 2013;216:454-60.
17. Jin J, Allemang MT, McHenry CR. Levothyroxine replacement dosage determination after thyroidectomy. Am J Surg. 2013;205:360-4.
18. Di Donna V, Santoro MG, de Waure C, Ricciato MP, Paragliola RM, Pontecorvi A, et al. A new strategy to estimate levothyroxine requirement after total thyroidectomy for benign thyroid disease. Thyroid. 2014;24:1759-64.
19. Elfenbein DM, Schaefer S, Shumway C, Chen H, Sippel RS, Schneider DF. Prospective intervention of a novel levothyroxine dosing protocol based on body mass index after thyroidectomy. J Am Coll Surg. 2016;222:83-8.
20. Chen SS, Zaborek NA, Doubleday AR, Schaefer SC, Long KL, Pitt SC, et al. Optimizing levothyroxine dose adjustment after thyroidectomy with a decision tree. J Surg Res. 2019;244:102-6.
21. Park I, Her N, Choe JH, Kim JS, Kim JH. Management of chyle leakage after thyroidectomy, cervical lymph node dissection, in patients with thyroid cancer. Head Neck. 2018;40:7-15.

CHAPTER 19

Surgery in Locally Advanced Thyroid Cancer

Gouri Pantvaidya, Karthik Rao, Anil D'Cruz

BACKGROUND

Papillary and follicular thyroid cancers are most commonly encountered differentiated thyroid cancers (DTC), encompassing >90% of all thyroid cancers.[1] Often, these tumors tend to be multifocal and have lymph node metastasis to central or lateral neck but are usually associated with good outcomes following optimal treatment. Around 10–25% of these tumors display aggressive behavior, characterized by local invasion, distant metastasis, treatment resistance, and increased mortality.[2-5] Although there is a lack of consensus in the definition of locally advanced thyroid cancers (LATC), thyroid cancers with tumor or nodal disease involving the recurrent laryngeal nerves (RLNs), aerodigestive tract, great vessels (internal jugular vein and internal carotid artery), and extensive soft-tissue involvement with or without multiple bulky bilateral nodal metastasis to central or lateral compartment encompass LATCs. The incidence of LATC is not accurate as tertiary referral centers that see larger number of malignancies have a higher incidence as compared to other centers. The incidence of early thyroid cancers is much higher in comparison with the LATC, probably attributable to the early detection and improved diagnostic modalities.[6] The age of tumor presentation, histology, size, presence of extrathyroid extension (ETE), and distant metastasis[7] must be considered to prognosticate the disease. From a surgical point of view, ETE is a critical factor. ETE determines the surgical planning, local recurrence, regional spread, and distant metastasis.[8,9] Certain pathological types such as tall cell, columnar cell, trabecular, insular, hobnail variants, and poorly differentiated thyroid carcinoma[10-14] have higher rates of ETE and distant metastasis. ETE occurs to the strap muscles, RLN, larynx, trachea, esophagus, and pharyngeal constrictors.[15] Lower extension of disease or metastatic nodes may lead to vascular involvement of the great vessels and extension to the mediastinum. The standard treatment for patients with locally aggressive thyroid cancer is en bloc surgical resection. Understanding local invasion and disease aggressiveness is crucial for adequate en block surgical resection and the need for postoperative adjuvant therapy in the form of radioactive iodine (RAI) and external beam radiation therapy (EBRT). This chapter explores the management of LATC involving the visceral and neural structures of central compartment.

ROUTES FOR VISCERAL INVASION BY THYROID CANCER

Extrathyroidal extension is related to increased frequency of both locoregional recurrence and disease-related death.[16] Instead of a true capsule, the thyroid gland has a pseudocapsule comprising an interrupted layer of fibroadipose tissue. The isthmic area is peculiar because of the proximity of thyroid parenchyma with subcutaneous fat and deep strap muscles.

In a large retrospective study by McCaffery et al.,[15] the pathways of spread of LATC into the laryngotracheal framework were described. There are four common routes of spread of thyroid cancer outside the capsule:

1. *Posteriorly*: Disease infiltration into the tracheoesophageal (TE) groove with involvement of the RLN.
2. *Superiorly*: Disease extension from the superior pole encircling or eroding the ala of thyroid cartilage and subsequent paraglottic space spread.
3. Tracheal infiltration by the adjacent disease or the metastatic central compartment nodes.
4. Cricotracheal infiltration due to central disease or metastatic nodes.

CLINICAL FEATURES

A sound clinical acumen is indispensable for preoperative recognition of LATC. This would allow for better planning of treatment strategies. Invasion into the visceral structures in the upper aerodigestive tract can have symptoms pointing to the structure involved **(Table 1)**. More commonly, the presenting symptom may be neck mass (98–100%), voice

Table 1: Clinical pointers for possible sites of involvement.[19,20]

Symptom	Possible site of involvement
Change in voice, voice weakness, hoarseness, and vocal fatigue	Recurrent laryngeal nerve
Change in voice, dyspnea, stridor, and hemoptysis	Laryngeal framework
Dyspnea and hemoptysis	Trachea
Odynophagia and dysphagia	Pharynx and esophagus
Neck pain and neck stiffness	Prevertebral facia and neck muscles

change (18–22%), swallowing discomfort (25%), hemoptysis (11–25%), or dyspnea (5–33%).[17,18] Several patients with a paralyzed vocal cord may not report abrupt voice changes due to the contralateral vocal cord's ability to gradually compensate for function loss.[19]

The data on the incidence of each subsite involvement was given by Thomas McCaffrey of Mayo Clinic in 1994.[15] In order of prevalence, the muscles (strap muscles and sternocleidomastoid muscle) 53%, laryngeal nerve 47%, trachea 37%, esophagus 21%, larynx 12%, and other sites (jugular vein, carotid artery, or prevertebral fascia) 30% were found to be involved.

A noticeable neck swelling on clinical examination has a low sensitivity to suggest an invasive cancer. A fixed thyroid nodule or nodal mass in the neck, or gross adhesion or involvement of the cervical skin may indicate advanced disease at the local level. The need for regular fiberoptic scopy to evaluate vocal cord functionality must be highlighted due to the lack of reliability in determining LATC just by the neck inspection and palpation. For LATC, on flexible scopy—vocal cord dysfunction, pooling of saliva, submucosal bulge, or change in vascular pattern or distinct intraluminal infiltration of the laryngotracheal complex should be thoroughly investigated. In summary, on clinical examination, patients who should be investigated for LATC are:

Patient with proven thyroid cancer presenting as:
- Extremes of age
- Symptoms of change in voice, dysphagia, dyspnea, or hemoptysis
- Fixed or restricted masses in the neck
- Multiple nodal masses
- Dilated neck and upper mediastinal veins
- Restricted/fixed vocal cords
- An intraluminal laryngotracheal bulge/mass

◇| DIAGNOSTIC INVESTIGATIONS

Preliminary evaluation of LATC is similar to evaluation of any thyroid nodule. Diagnostic modalities can be broadly categorized under two headings:
1. Routine investigations for evaluation of thyroid nodule
2. Investigations to assess the disease extent in a suspected case of LATC.

Routine Investigations for Evaluation of Thyroid Nodule

Ultrasonography

Fine-needle aspiration cytology (FNAC): FNAC is a reliable diagnostic modality to differentiate a benign from a malignant nodule. It, however, may not always be able to determine the poor histologic variants, which may point toward patients having an LATC. Upfront diagnosis of poorly differentiated thyroid malignancy, Hurthle cell neoplasm, and anaplastic

carcinoma thyroid should raise concerns of advanced disease and warrant further investigations.

The FNAC must be done under ultrasonography (USG) surveillance in cases with posteriorly located nodules and solid-cystic component in nodule. USG-guided FNAC is known to reduce the sampling error.[21,22]

Core needle biopsy (CNB): CNB is generally not the first method to obtain tissue specimen thyroid nodules. The tissue yield obtained is more from the CNB when compared to standard FNAC, this is more pronounced in individuals having sclerosis or calcification on sonography.[23,24] The CNB is indicated over conventional FNAC in cases with suspicion of lymphoma, medullary thyroid cancer, poorly differentiated cancers, anaplastic cancers, and in parathyroid lesions in concurrence with immunohistochemistry.[25,26]

Investigations to Assess the Disease Extent

Contrast-enhanced Computed Tomography

Contrast-enhanced computed tomography (CECT) is the most commonly performed imaging in patients with suspected LATC. CT for the evaluation of thyroid nodule is indicated in the presence of clinical signs and symptoms of ETE, lower mediastinum extension, and the presence of large metastatic lymph nodes.[27] The study by Ishigaki et al. has demonstrated the superior accuracy of CT over conventional sonography in identifying extrathyroidal extension.[28]

The CT scan characteristics of structures involved by thyroid cancer are as follows:
- *Recurrent laryngeal nerve invasion:* RLN is commonly found in fibrofatty tissue along with the TE groove, posterior to the lobe of the thyroid. The fibrofatty tissue and the RLN in the TE groove are not well visualized on the CT scan images due to the presence of an artefact caused by clavicles or by contrast content in the subclavian vein. In a study by Seo et al.,[29] they determined the following criteria for RLN involvement: When >25% of the tumor is in contact with posterior part of thyroid capsule along with fixed vocal cord on the side of nodule and loss of fatty tissue in the TE groove. The sensitivity and specificity of predicting RLN involvement were found to be 78.2% and 89.8%, respectively, when two-thirds criteria were fulfilled.
- *Tracheal invasion:* Invasion into the trachea can be determined by two criteria—the degree of encirclement[29] and depth of invasion[30]—deformity of the lumen, focal mucosal irregularity or thickening, and intraluminal mass.[31] In the study by Seo et al.,[29] if the tumor encircled >90° of tracheal circumference, the CT scan is sensitive in 68.1% and specific in 76.6% for prediction of tracheal involvement. If the degree of encirclement was >180°, the sensitivity dropped to 55% and specificity to 67%.

A seminal paper by Shin et al.[30] gave an overview into the degree of tracheal invasion by LATC. In his paper, he described four pathological stages of tracheal invasion based on the resected specimens.

- *Stage I*: Thyroid gland capsule is invaded and the disease is just in contact with the outer perichondrium of the trachea without invasion.
- *Stage II*: Outer tracheal cartilage invasion
- *Stage III*: Tracheal cartilage invasion and with invasion into the underlying tracheal lamina propria without mucosal invasion.
- *Stage IV*: A complete tracheal cartilage invasion with intraluminal disease, seen as ulceration or bulge.

The CECT validation of Shin's staging has not been performed, but radiologists should be encouraged to report tracheal involvement by thyroid cancers as per Shin's classification.[32-34] This will help the surgeon to plan the appropriate surgery preoperatively.

- *Esophageal invasion*: The esophageal wall is more difficult to evaluate than the trachea because it is usually not distended with air. CT scan is unable to detect invasion into the layers of the esophageal wall, especially the outer layer. The mean sensitivity, specificity, and accuracy of CT for esophageal invasion were found to be 28.6%, 96.2%, and 90.7% respectively, when the angle of tumor contact was >180° with the esophagus.[29]

Magnetic Resonance Imaging

The predictions of local invasion into RLN, laryngotracheal complex, and esophagus are comparable in both magnetic resonance imaging (MRI) and computed tomography (CT)[29,31,35,36] **(Table 2)**.

The presence or absence of tracheal invasion by LATC was diagnosed accurately (sensitivity 100%, specificity 84%, and accuracy of 90%) but prediction with MRI of the precise depth of tumor invasion to the trachea was unreliable.[31]

Takashima et al. investigated the diagnostic accuracy of MRI in predicting the RLN invasion with TE groove fat effacement as criteria, they found MRI to be 88% accurate (94% sensitivity, 82% specificity).

In a paper by Roychowdury,[37] the most suspicious finding for esophageal invasion is a focal T2 signal in the outer layer of the esophageal wall and other signs include esophageal wall thickening and effaced fat plane with the esophagus.

Positron Emission Tomography

Positron emission tomography (PET)-CT typically has limited sensitivity for use in DTCs. However, it may have a role to play in assessing extent of disease in dedifferentiated or poorly differentiated cancers.[38] The intensity of FDG (18-fluorodeoxyglucose) uptake is correlated with progressive dedifferentiation and a more aggressive tumor.[39]

Endoscopic Studies

Tracheobronchoscopy and esophagoscopy may provide additional information about the invasiveness of the disease and help the surgical planning. An endoscopic procedure can be used along with CT/MRI for the evaluation of submucosal bulges, altered mucosal vascularity, or intraluminal invasion. Additionally, endoscopy helps in determining the extent of intraluminal invasion and can also help to determine the surgical approach.

Endoscopic USG (EUS) is a procedure used in determining the size, depth of invasion, and presence of paratracheal and paraesophageal nodes in the esophageal cancers.[40] EUS was reported to be more sensitive in detecting esophageal invasion by thyroid cancer, especially in tumors involving lower and middle lobes, than esophagography, esophagoscopy, and MRI.[41,42] EUS examination of the thyroid gland has its limitations because it cannot visualize the upper lobes of the thyroid gland.[42]

There are several case reports where endobronchial USG (EBUS) has been utilized to determine the extent of tracheobronchial involvement and obtain the tissue sample by transluminal needle aspiration.[43,44] Although there are no studies which determine the use of EBUS in LATCs, it can have potential use in determining the submucosal disease, extent of involvement, free tracheal rings, and pretracheal and paratracheal nodes, this potential benefit can be extrapolated by the use of EBUS in tracheobronchial invasion in esophageal cancers.[45]

Balloon Test Occlusion

Conventional angiography with balloon occlusion procedures may be necessary in individual with extensive extrathyroidal extension and bulky nodes encasing the carotid arteries.

◇ SURGICAL TREATMENT

Preoperative Considerations

Inoperability, even with LATC, is very rare in patients with thyroid cancers, except in patients with anaplastic cancers where the disease invasion often precludes surgical treatment.

Table 2: Comparison between CT and MRI in determining the local invasion in LATC.[29,31,35,36]

Structure involved	CT scan			MRI scan		
	Sensitivity	Specificity	Accuracy	Sensitivity	Specificity	Accuracy
Trachea	59%	91%	83%	100%	84%	90%
RLN	29%	96%	91%	82%	94%	91%
Esophagus	78%	90%	86%	94%	82%	88%

(CT: computed tomography; LATC: locally advanced thyroid cancer; MRI: magnetic resonance imaging; RLN: recurrent laryngeal nerve)

Indications of Inoperability

- *Gross infiltration of great vessels*: If the tumor is encasing the carotid or great mediastinal vessels for 270° or more of its circumference, then the tumor may not be completely separable from the arteries.[46]
- *Prevertebral fascia involvement*: Infiltration of the disease into prevertebral tissues is difficult to determine preoperatively, a cross-sectional imaging is mandated to identify it and deems the disease unresectable. The involvement of the prevertebral fascia is also linked to a higher rates of retropharyngeal LN involvement, which results in poor prognosis.[47]
- *Mediastinal invasion*: Disease infiltrating into mediastinum and great vessels circumferentially is a relative contraindication for surgery.
- *Long-segment tracheal invasion*: The resection and reanastomosis/reconstruction of long-segment tracheal invasion (>5 cm) are often not possible and are associated with a high mortality rate.[48] Long-segment tracheal invasion may be a contraindication for surgery.

Once the patient is considered amenable to surgical resection, the following must be addressed:

- Patient counseling prior to surgery
- Functional assessment
- Anesthetic considerations
- Use of neuromonitoring

Preoperative Counseling

Surgical candidates must be systematically explained about the extent of surgery, removal of involved structures, reconstruction options, complications, and prolonged hospital stay. Patients also need to be counseled regarding chances of residual disease and the need for adjuvant treatment, hormone and calcium replacement, speech and swallowing issues.

Functional Assessment

It is critical to evaluate laryngotracheal, esophageal, and pulmonary functions prior to surgery.

Laryngotracheal function assessment: The three main functions of the laryngotracheal complex are: (1) phonation, (2) respiration, and (3) prevention of aspiration. Hoarseness caused because of preoperative vocal cord fixity should be documented by indirect laryngoscopy. The exact side of fixity should be noted with regard to disease extent so as to be able to save the contralateral recurrent laryngeal nerve during surgery. If the patient has stridor due to airway obstruction, a difficult airway should be anticipated. If patient has any clinical signs or symptoms of aspiration, a fiberoptic endoscopic evaluation of swallowing (FEES) may be performed to assess laryngeal function.

Anesthetic Considerations

Difficult intubation protocols must be followed in patients with LATC due to tumor infiltration into the upper aerodigestive tract. A thorough preanesthetic evaluation is necessary and discussion between operating surgeon and the anesthetist is needed for optimal patient management. In these scenarios, generally an awake fiberoptic nasotracheal intubation following topical anesthesia and laryngeal block is useful. A well-lubricated smaller lumen endotracheal tube can be used to pass beyond the laryngotracheal disease. Tracheostomy should be avoided as it leads to surgical site contamination and delays wound healing. If the tracheostomy is planned then the level of tracheostomy must be careful determined based on the endoscopic and CT/MRI reports to facilitate laryngotracheal resections when necessary.

Utility of Neuromonitoring

Intraoperative neuromonitoring (IONM) has been developed to confirm the location and function of the RLN based on electromyographic (EMG) integrity and is well accepted as an adjunct to visual identification of the RLN.[49-51] IONM can help the surgeon to identify the RLN in distorted anatomy, it can estimate the residual nerve function following surgery, it can provide pointers to decision-making when both the RLNs are at risk due to bilateral disease and the postoperative residual nerve potential might provide clues to possible postoperative complications.

However, the exact role of IONM has not been clearly defined and whether IONM can decrease the incidence of temporary or permanent RLN palsy, especially in thyroid cancers, is a matter of debate.

According to the findings of an Italian meta-analysis, IONM did not significantly decrease the rates of overall, transient, or permanent RLN palsy.[52] In a study by Si Yuan Wu et al., which investigated the routine use of IONM in patients undergoing thyroid cancer surgeries, they concluded that the routine use of IONM for thyroid cancer surgeries decreased the rate of RLN palsy over a period. No permanent RLN palsies occurred in nerves not invaded by tumor after routine IONM. Technetium-99m uptake and thyroglobulin levels also progressively decreased with the use of IONM.[53]

A recent Chinese meta-analysis, which evaluated the data from 1980 to 2017, consisting of 34 studies found a significant decrease in total injury, transient injury, and permanent injury with IONM in overall analysis. A subgroup analysis reported that IONM had prevented the complete, permanent, and transient RLN paralysis in total thyroidectomies. It also reduced the rate of complete and transient RLN injury in thyroidectomies for malignancies.[54]

Another systematic review and meta-analysis, which included 24 studies and 4 prospective randomized trials, had 3.15% overall RLN palsy, 1.82% transient palsy, and 0.67%

persistent RLN palsy in IONM and in control group, they were 4.37%, 2.58%, and 1.07%, respectively. There was a 40% reduction in temporary RLN palsy, which was statistically significant but there was no difference in permanent palsy rates.[54] However, most of these randomized trials and meta-analysis are done with a very heterogenous population largely consisting of benign diseases. The debate on whether IONM decreases incidence of RLN palsy in thyroid cancer patients undergoing surgery still remains. IONM can be a useful adjunct for surgery when dealing with locally advanced disease.

The indications (in order of priority) where IONM can be used are:

- Preexisting unilateral vocal cord palsy
- Revision or second surgery
- Gross ETE/extensive central compartment nodes
- Surgery for malignancy/large goiters

◇ MANAGEMENT OF RECURRENT LARYNGEAL NERVES

The fundamental principle of recurrent laryngeal nerve management in LATC is to have knowledge about its functional status, and surgical plan can be tailored accordingly **(Box 1)**. The nerve must be sacrificed only if there is a gross tumor infiltration into it.

Falk et al. and Nishida et al. studied the effect of RLN preservation versus resection in functionally intact nerves in LATC cases. They found that there was no differences in survival, if patients received adjuvant RAI therapy and there is no gross residual disease.[5,55]

A nonfunctioning RLN involved by tumor must be resected en bloc with the thyroid resection. If there is no evidence of tumor infiltrating into the RLN, then the nerve must be meticulously dissected to allow for recovery.[5,56]

If the RLN is resected for oncological purposes, then medialization thyroplasty must be performed in same sitting or in early postoperative period, mainly in elderly to prevent aspiration, poor voice, and ineffective cough. The wait-and-watch approach for vocal cord compensation can be followed in other low-risk cases.

Several studies have displayed the utility of IONM to prevent RLN injury in the revision surgeries[57,58] and for malignancies.[53,54,57-59]

◇ MANAGEMENT OF LARYNGOTRACHEAL INVASION

Laryngeal Invasion

Only 12% of patients with locally invasive thyroid cancers have laryngeal infiltration.[15] Surgical planning can be done based on the extent of infiltration.

- *Peeling or shave excision*: Peeling or shave excision to be considered, if the tumor is just abutting the outer perichondrium without involvement. No difference in survival when radical resection or shave procedures are done along with complete tumor resection.[15,60]
- *Partial laryngectomy*: McCaffery et al.[15] proposed that due to the laterality of the tumor even in cases with extensive laryngeal invasion, vertical laryngectomy can be performed. Up to 50% of the external laryngeal framework could be resected with internal laryngeal preservation as per Friedman et al.[61] Price et al. found that 30% of the cricoid can be resected without the need for composite reconstruction or a tracheostomy.[20]
- *Total laryngectomy*: It is indicated in varying degrees of airway obstruction, intraluminal bleed, intraluminal invasion, or loss of laryngeal function.[62-65] Ballantyne et al. demonstrated good control rates for LATC with gross laryngeal invasion[66] when treated with total laryngectomy. In comparison to the conservative laryngectomy surgeries, total laryngectomy was less morbid.[63] The placement of tracheoesophageal puncture (TEP) prosthesis may contribute to vocal rehabilitation for these patients.

Tracheal Invasion

Invasion of tracheal occurs in almost one-third of LATC cases, and is the third most common site of invasion.

In 1993, Shin and colleagues[30] defined the pathological staging system for the LATC with tracheal invasion based on the degree of tracheal infiltration.

Nishida et al.[5] studied 54 patients with Shin stage II and above who had airway resection (40 cases) or subtotal without airway resection. In the subtotal resection group, they reported a higher rate of recurrence (79% vs. 8%) and a shorter overall survival (1.5 years vs. 8.7 years). No difference in local and regional recurrence, distant metastasis, or overall survival was noted when Shin I patients underwent shave procedures versus LATC without involvement in trachea.[4,15,60,63] On the contrary, a few authors[61,67] suggested reduced local control rates and poor survival, when conservative procedures were performed for LATC with tracheal invasion; hence, some surgeons back a more radical approach even with shallow invasion to increase the disease-free survival.

Nonstandardized definitions of invasion, complete versus conservative procedures, different variants of DTC, and adjuvant treatment can explain the inconsistency.

- *Tracheal shaving*: Shin I tumors, with superficial tracheal invasion, can be amenable for shaving off procedures.
- *Window/sleeve resection*: It can be advocated in Shin II tumors, with lateral or anterior invasion of trachea.
- *Circumferential resection*: Shin III and IV tumors are amenable for circumferential resections.

Up to 5–6 cm of tracheal length can be excised and primary end-to-end anastomosis can be performed without the need for tracheal mobilization.[60] A supralaryngeal release with comprises separation of the thyrohyoid muscle, this leads to increase in length by 0.5 cm, and thyrohyoid membrane release produces 2.0 cm in length.[68] Grillo et al. have described stair-step tracheal incision to permit the lower tracheal part to jigsaw into the resected larynx.[69] Roughly 4% of primary cases and 15% of revision cases[70] have leaks at the site of anastomosis. Airway reconstruction provides no absolute benefit in scenarios with bilateral vocal cord paralysis.

Esophageal Invasion

Esophageal invasion typically occurs along with tracheal invasion, it also can occur when paratracheal or paraesophageal lymph nodes have extranodal extension.[71] It is usually considered a poor prognosis and correlates with significant reduction in overall survival.[5] In the series by McCaffrey et al., they noted that the tumor invades outside in, involving only the muscularis layer first and sparing the esophageal mucosa and submucosa.[15]

- *Cuff excision*: It can be considered in limited muscularis layer involvement without the involvement of submucosa or mucosa.[15] If the defect is through and through a complete tension less, multilayered, watertight closure is a must.
- *Segmental resection*: It can be performed if the tumor is extensively involving all three layers, appropriate reconstructive options should be considered, generally with free flaps.
- *Do nothing*: In inoperable patients with extensive esophageal involvement, stents can be used as a palliative measure to maintain the luminal patency.[72]

◁| ADJUVANT THERAPY

External Beam Radiation

The evidence for use of EBRT in LATC is from multiple retrospective studies[73-76] and it offers small benefits in improving the locoregional control in R1 resections with gross ETS and multiple nodes with PNE.[74] Intensity-modulated radiotherapy (IMRT) is preferred due to its low toxicity profile.[77] In cases with R2 resections, EBRT can be given but does not provide full local control of the disease.[20] It is important to balance the advantages versus the long-term side effects of EBRT in patient with thyroid cancers.

The benefit from EBRT has been highlighted in the latest ATA (American Thyroid Association) guidelines published in 2015. The recommendation 72 states to utilize EBRT as an adjuvant therapy following surgery with or without RAI ablation in LATCs of the aerodigestive tract.[78]

The ATA also recommends the use of EBRT in the treatment of spinal metastasis[79] and stereotactic radiotherapy in brain metastasis[80,81] (guidelines—C28 and C39).[78]

These recommendations have the following limitations:

- Evidence have been derived from nonrandomized trials, with multiple possible weaknesses raising apprehensions about internal validity or generalizing the findings.
- The studies have been retrospective, with heterogenous patient population, no clearly defined inclusion criteria and end points.
- The toxicity profile of radiation has not been highlighted in the studies.

Hence, the use of radiotherapy has not become a common clinical practice and standard of care, reflecting a lack of prospective data on toxicity and locoregional control in LATCs.

◁| CONCLUSION

Tremendous progress has been made in the treatment of LATC. Accurate patient identification and thorough clinical and radiological evaluation are necessary for proper treatment planning. Appropriate surgical management with adjuvant therapy, RAI with or without EBRT, remains the most effective course of treatment. IONM has helped in the intraoperative identification of recurrent laryngeal nerve in certain scenarios. Aggressive surgical treatment with en bloc removal of all gross tumor and possibly preserving vital structures when oncologically safe along with adjuvant therapy offers the best results. Incidence of locoregional and distant failure in this group of patients is high. Understanding tumor biology, such as poorly DTC and aggressive variants, is also important. Certain niche areas such as preoperative identification and predictors of these kind of tumors require more research.

◁| REFERENCES

1. Sherman SI. Thyroid carcinoma. Lancet Lond Engl. 2003;361(9356):501-11.
2. Britto E, Mbbs SS, Parikh DM, Rao RS. Laryngotracheal invasion by well-differentiated thyroid cancer: diagnosis and management. J Surg Oncol. 1990;44(1):25-31.
3. Djalilian M, Beahrs OH, Devine KD, Weiland LH, DeSanto LW. Intraluminal involvement of the larynx and trachea by thyroid cancer. Am J Surg. 1974;128(4):500-4.
4. Cody HS, Shah JP. Locally invasive, well-differentiated thyroid cancer. 22 years' experience at Memorial Sloan-Kettering Cancer Center. Am J Surg. 1981;142(4):480-3.
5. Nishida T, Nakao K, Hamaji M, Kamiike W, Kurozumi K, Matsuda H. Preservation of recurrent laryngeal nerve invaded by differentiated thyroid cancer. Ann Surg. 1997;226(1):85-91.

6. Davies L, Welch HG. Increasing incidence of thyroid cancer in the United States, 1973-2002. JAMA. 2006;295(18):2164-7.

7. Shah JP, Loree TR, Dharker D, Strong EW, Begg C, Vlamis V. Prognostic factors in differentiated carcinoma of the thyroid gland. Am J Surg. 1992;164(6):658-61.

8. Andersen PE, Kinsella J, Loree TR, Shaha AR, Shah JP. Differentiated carcinoma of the thyroid with extrathyroidal extension. Am J Surg. 1995;170(5):467-70.

9. Ito Y, Tomoda C, Uruno T, Takamura Y, Miya A, Kobayashi K, et al. Prognostic significance of extrathyroid extension of papillary thyroid carcinoma: massive but not minimal extension affects the relapse-free survival. World J Surg. 2006;30(5): 780-6.

10. Hawk WA, Hazard JB. The many appearances of papillary carcinoma of the thyroid. Cleve Clin Q. 1976;43(4):207-15.

11. Leung AK-C, Chow S-M, Law SCK. Clinical features and outcome of the tall cell variant of papillary thyroid carcinoma. Laryngoscope. 2008;118(1):32-8.

12. Wang X, Cheng W, Liu C, Li J. Tall cell variant of papillary thyroid carcinoma: current evidence on clinicopathologic features and molecular biology. Oncotarget. 2016;7(26):40792-9.

13. Ostrowski ML, Merino MJ. Tall cell variant of papillary thyroid carcinoma: a reassessment and immunohistochemical study with comparison to the usual type of papillary carcinoma of the thyroid. Am J Surg Pathol. 1996;20(8):964-74.

14. Falvo L, Catania A, Grilli P, Di Matteo FM, De Antoni E. Treatment of "locally advanced" well-differentiated thyroid carcinomas. Ann Ital Chir. 2004;75(1):17-21.

15. McCaffrey TV, Bergstralh EJ, Hay ID. Locally invasive papillary thyroid carcinoma: 1940-1990. Head Neck. 1994;16(2):165-72.

16. Kebebew E, Clark OH. Differentiated thyroid cancer: "complete" rational approach. World J Surg. 2000;24(8):942-51.

17. Segal K, Shpitzer T, Hazan A, Bachar G, Marshak G, Popovtzer A. Invasive well-differentiated thyroid carcinoma: effect of treatment modalities on outcome. Otolaryngol Head Neck Surg. 2006;134(5):819-22.

18. McCarty TM, Kuhn JA, Williams WL, Ellenhorn JD, O'Brien JC, Preskitt JT, et al. Surgical management of thyroid cancer invading the airway. Ann Surg Oncol. 1997;4(5):403-8.

19. Randolph GW, Kamani D. The importance of preoperative laryngoscopy in patients undergoing thyroidectomy: voice, vocal cord function, and the preoperative detection of invasive thyroid malignancy. Surgery. 2006;139(3):357-62.

20. Price DL, Wong RJ, Randolph GW. Invasive thyroid cancer: management of the trachea and esophagus. Otolaryngol Clin North Am. 2008;41(6):1155-68, ix-x.

21. Carmeci C, Jeffrey RB, McDougall IR, Nowels KW, Weigel RJ. Ultrasound-guided fine-needle aspiration biopsy of thyroid masses. Thyroid Off J Am Thyroid Assoc. 1998;8(4): 283-9.

22. Danese D, Sciacchitano S, Farsetti A, Andreoli M, Pontecorvi A. Diagnostic accuracy of conventional versus sonography-guided fine-needle aspiration biopsy of thyroid nodules. Thyroid Off J Am Thyroid Assoc. 1998;8(1):15-21.

23. Ha EJ, Baek JH, Lee JH, Song DE, Kim JK, Shong YK, et al. Sonographically suspicious thyroid nodules with initially benign cytologic results: the role of a core needle biopsy. Thyroid Off J Am Thyroid Assoc. 2013;23(6):703-8.

24. Ha EJ, Baek JH, Lee JH, Kim JK, Kim JK, Lim HK, et al. Core needle biopsy can minimise the non-diagnostic results and need for diagnostic surgery in patients with calcified thyroid nodules. Eur Radiol. 2014;24(6):1403-9.

25. Jung CK, Baek JH. Recent advances in core needle biopsy for thyroid nodules. Endocrinol Metab. 2017;32(4):407-12.

26. Ha EJ, Baek JH, Lee JH, Kim JK, Song DE, Kim WB, et al. Core needle biopsy could reduce diagnostic surgery in patients with anaplastic thyroid cancer or thyroid lymphoma. Eur Radiol. 2016;26(4):1031-6.

27. Weber AL, Randolph G, Aksoy FG. The thyroid and parathyroid glands. CT and MR imaging and correlation with pathology and clinical findings. Radiol Clin North Am. 2000;38(5): 1105-29.

28. Ishigaki S, Shimamoto K, Satake H, Sawaki A, Itoh S, Ikeda M, et al. Multi-slice CT of thyroid nodules: comparison with ultrasonography. Radiat Med. 2004;22(5):346-53.

29. Seo YL, Yoon DY, Lim KJ, Cha JH, Yun EJ, Choi CS, et al. Locally advanced thyroid cancer: can CT help in prediction of extrathyroidal invasion to adjacent structures? Am J Roentgenol. 2010;195(3):W240-4.

30. Shin DH, Mark EJ, Suen HC, Grillo HC. Pathologic staging of papillary carcinoma of the thyroid with airway invasion based on the anatomic manner of extension to the trachea: a clinicopathologic study based on 22 patients who underwent thyroidectomy and airway resection. Hum Pathol. 1993;24(8):866-70.

31. Wang J, Takashima S, Takayama F, Kawakami S, Saito A, Matsushita T, et al. Tracheal invasion by thyroid carcinoma. Am J Roentgenol. 2001;177(4):929-36.

32. Shimamoto K, Satake H, Sawaki A, Ishigaki T, Funahashi H, Imai T. Preoperative staging of thyroid papillary carcinoma with ultrasonography. Eur J Radiol. 1998;29(1):4-10.

33. Tomoda C, Uruno T, Takamura Y, Ito Y, Miya A, Kobayashi K, et al. Ultrasonography as a method of screening for tracheal invasion by papillary thyroid cancer. Surg Today. 2005;35(10):819-22.

34. Yamamura N, Fukushima S, Nakao K, Nakahara M, Kurozumi K, Imabun S, et al. Relation between ultrasonographic and histologic findings of tracheal invasion by differentiated thyroid cancer. World J Surg. 2002;26(8):1071-3.

35. Takashima S, Takayama F, Wang J, Kobayashi S, Kadoya M. Using MR imaging to predict invasion of the recurrent laryngeal nerve by thyroid carcinoma. AJR Am J Roentgenol. 2003;180(3):837-42.

36. Wang J, Takashima S, Matsushita T, Takayama F, Kobayashi T, Kadoya M. Esophageal invasion by thyroid carcinomas: prediction using magnetic resonance imaging. J Comput Assist Tomogr. 2003;27(1):18-25.

37. Roychowdhury S, Loevner LA, Yousem DM, Chalian A, Montone KT. MR imaging for predicting neoplastic invasion of the cervical esophagus. AJNR Am J Neuroradiol. 2000;21(9):1681-7.

38. Mirallié E, Guillan T, Bridji B, Resche I, Rousseau C, Ansquer C, et al. Therapeutic impact of 18FDG-PET/CT in the management of iodine-negative recurrence of differentiated thyroid carcinoma. Surgery. 2007;142(6):952-8; discussion 952-8.

39. Schlüter B, Bohuslavizki KH, Beyer W, Plotkin M, Buchert R, Clausen M. Impact of FDG PET on patients with differentiated thyroid cancer who present with elevated thyroglobulin and negative 131I scan. J Nucl Med. 2001;42(1):71-6.

40. Luo L, He L, Gao X, Huang XX, Shan HB, Luo GY, et al. Endoscopic ultrasound for preoperative esophageal squamous cell carcinoma: a meta-analysis. PLoS ONE. 2016;11(7):e0158373.

41. Ohshima A, Yamashita H, Noguchi S, Uchino S, Watanabe S, Toda M, et al. Usefulness of endoscopic ultrasonography (EUS) in diagnosing esophageal infiltration of thyroid cancer. J Endocrinol Invest. 2001;24(8):564-9.

42. Koike E, Yamashita H, Noguchi S, Ohshima A, Yamashita H, Watanabe S, et al. Endoscopic ultrasonography in patients with thyroid cancer: its usefulness and limitations for evaluating esophagopharyngeal invasion. Endoscopy. 2002;34(6):457-60.

43. Li P, Zheng W, Liu H, Zhang Z, Zhao L. Endobronchial ultrasound-guided transbronchial needle aspiration for thyroid cyst therapy: A case report. Exp Ther Med. 2017;13(5):1944-7.

44. Madan K, Mittal S, Hadda V, Jain D, Mohan A, Guleria R. Endobronchial ultrasound-guided transbronchial needle aspiration of thyroid: Report of two cases and systematic review of literature. Lung India Off Organ Indian Chest Soc. 2016;33(6):682-7.

45. Garrido T, Maluf-Filho F, Sallum RAA, Figueiredo VR, Jacomelli M, Tedde M. Endobronchial ultrasound application for diagnosis of tracheobronchial tree invasion by esophageal cancer. Clin Sao Paulo Braz. 2009;64(6):499-504.

46. Yousem DM, Hatabu H, Hurst RW, Seigerman HM, Montone KT, Weinstein GS, et al. Carotid artery invasion by head and neck masses: prediction with MR imaging. Radiology. 1995;195(3):715-720.

47. Yousem DM, Gad K, Tufano RP. Resectability issues with head and neck cancer. Am J Neuroradiol. 2006;27(10):2024-36.

48. Nagappan R, Parkin G, Wright CA, Walker CS, Vallance N, Buchanan D, et al. Adult long-segment tracheal stenosis attributable to complete tracheal rings masquerading as asthma. Crit Care Med. 2002;30(1):238-40.

49. Randolph GW, Dralle H, International Intraoperative Monitoring Study Group, Abdullah H, Barczynski M, Bellantone R, et al. Electrophysiologic recurrent laryngeal nerve monitoring during thyroid and parathyroid surgery: international standards guideline statement. Laryngoscope. 2011;121 Suppl 1:S1-16.

50. Dralle H, Sekulla C, Lorenz K, Brauckhoff M, Machens A, German IONM Study Group. Intraoperative monitoring of the recurrent laryngeal nerve in thyroid surgery. World J Surg. 2008;32(7):1358-66.

51. Hayward NJ, Grodski S, Yeung M, Johnson WR, Serpell J. Recurrent laryngeal nerve injury in thyroid surgery: a review. ANZ J Surg. 2013;83(1-2):15-21.

52. Pisanu A, Porceddu G, Podda M, Cois A, Uccheddu A. Systematic review with meta-analysis of studies comparing intraoperative neuromonitoring of recurrent laryngeal nerves versus visualization alone during thyroidectomy. J Surg Res. 2014;188(1):152-61.

53. Wu SY, Shen HY, Duh QY, Hsieh CB, Yu JC, Shih ML. Routine intraoperative neuromonitoring of the recurrent laryngeal nerve to facilitate complete resection and ensure safety in thyroid cancer surgery. Am Surg Atlanta. 2018;84(12):1882-8.

54. Bai B, Chen W. Protective effects of intraoperative nerve monitoring (IONM) for recurrent laryngeal nerve injury in thyroidectomy: meta-analysis. Sci Rep. 2018;8:1-8.

55. Falk SA, McCaffrey TV. Management of the recurrent laryngeal nerve in suspected and proven thyroid cancer. Otolaryngol Head Neck Surg. 1995;113(1):42-8.

56. Chiang FY, Wang LF, Huang YF, Lee KW, Kuo WR. Recurrent laryngeal nerve palsy after thyroidectomy with routine identification of the recurrent laryngeal nerve. Surgery. 2005;137(3):342-7.

57. Chan WF, Lang BHH, Lo CY. The role of intraoperative neuromonitoring of recurrent laryngeal nerve during thyroidectomy: a comparative study on 1000 nerves at risk. Surgery. 2006;140(6):866-72; discussion 872-873.

58. Dralle H, Sekulla C, Haerting J, Timmermann W, Neumann HJ, Kruse E, et al. Risk factors of paralysis and functional outcome after recurrent laryngeal nerve monitoring in thyroid surgery. Surgery. 2004;136(6):1310-22.

59. Shindo M, Chheda NN. Incidence of vocal cord paralysis with and without recurrent laryngeal nerve monitoring during thyroidectomy. Arch Otolaryngol Head Neck Surg. 2007;133(5):481-5.

60. Czaja JM, McCaffrey TV. The surgical management of laryngotracheal invasion by well-differentiated papillary thyroid carcinoma. Arch Otolaryngol Head Neck Surg. 1997;123(5):484-90.

61. Friedman M, Danielzadeh JA, Caldarelli DD. Treatment of patients with carcinoma of the thyroid invading the airway. Arch Otolaryngol Head Neck Surg. 1994;120(12):1377-81.

62. Breaux GP, Guillamondegui OM. Treatment of locally invasive carcinoma of the thyroid: how radical? Am J Surg. 1980;140(4):514-7.

63. Segal K, Abraham A, Levy R, Schindel J. Carcinomas of the thyroid gland invading larynx and trachea. Clin Otolaryngol Allied Sci. 1984;9(1):21-5.

64. Donnelly MJ, Timon CI, McShane DP. The role of total laryngectomy in the management of intraluminal upper airway invasion by well-differentiated thyroid carcinoma. Ear Nose Throat J. 1994;73(9):659-62.

65. Kim KH, Sung MW, Chang KH, Kang BS. Therapeutic dilemmas in the management of thyroid cancer with laryngotracheal involvement. Otolaryngol Head Neck Surg. 2000;122(5):763-7.

66. Ballantyne AJ. Resections of the upper aerodigestive tract for locally invasive thyroid cancer. Am J Surg. 1994;168(6):636-9.

67. Park CS, Suh KW, Min JS. Cartilage-shaving procedure for the control of tracheal cartilage invasion by thyroid carcinoma. Head Neck. 1993;15(4):289-91.

68. Dedo HH, Fishman NH. Laryngeal release and sleeve resection for tracheal stenosis. Ann Otol Rhinol Laryngol. 1969;78(2):285-96.

69. Grillo HC, Suen HC, Mathisen DJ, Wain JC. Resectional management of thyroid carcinoma invading the airway. Ann Thorac Surg. 1992;54(1):3-9; discussion 9-10.

70. Gaissert HA, Honings J, Grillo HC, Donahue DM, Wain JC, Wright CD, et al. Segmental laryngotracheal and tracheal resection for invasive thyroid carcinoma. Ann Thorac Surg. 2007;83(6):1952-9.

71. Fujimoto Y, Obara T, Ito Y, Kodama T, Yashiro T, Yamashita T, et al. Aggressive surgical approach for locally invasive papillary carcinoma of the thyroid in patients over forty-five years of age. Surgery. 1986;100(6):1098-107.

72. Ginsberg GG. Palliation of malignant esophageal dysphagia: would you like plastic or metal? Am J Gastroenterol. 2007;102(12):2678-9.

73. Tsang RW, Brierley JD, Simpson WJ, Panzarella T, Gospodarowicz MK, Sutcliffe SB. The effects of surgery, radioiodine, and external radiation therapy on the clinical outcome of patients with differentiated thyroid carcinoma. Cancer. 1998;82(2):375-88.

74. Farahati J, Reiners C, Stuschke M, Müller SP, Stüben G, Sauerwein W, et al. Differentiated thyroid cancer. Impact of adjuvant external radiotherapy in patients with perithyroidal tumor infiltration (stage pT4). Cancer. 1996;77(1):172-80.

75. O'Connell ME, A'Hern RP, Harmer CL. Results of external beam radiotherapy in differentiated thyroid carcinoma: a retrospective study from the Royal Marsden Hospital. Eur J Cancer Oxf Engl. 1994;30A(6):733-9.

76. Tubiana M, Haddad E, Schlumberger M, Hill C, Rougier P, Sarrazin D. External radiotherapy in thyroid cancers. Cancer. 1985;55(9 Suppl):2062-71.

77. Urbano TG, Clark CH, Hansen VN, Adams EJ, Miles EA, Mc Nair H, et al. Intensity modulated radiotherapy (IMRT) in locally advanced thyroid cancer: acute toxicity results of a phase I study. Radiother Oncol. 2007;85(1):58-63.

78. Haugen BR, Alexander EK, Bible KC, Doherty GM, Mandel SJ, Nikiforov YE, et al. 2015 American Thyroid Association management guidelines for adult patients with thyroid nodules and differentiated thyroid cancer: The American Thyroid Association Guidelines Task Force on Thyroid Nodules and Differentiated Thyroid Cancer. Thyroid. 2016;26(1):1-133.

79. Bernier MO, Leenhardt L, Hoang C, Aurengo A, Mary JY, Menegaux F, et al. Survival and therapeutic modalities in patients with bone metastases of differentiated thyroid carcinomas. J Clin Endocrinol Metab. 2001;86(4):1568-73.

80. Chiu AC, Delpassand ES, Sherman SI. Prognosis and treatment of brain metastases in thyroid carcinoma. J Clin Endocrinol Metab. 1997;82(11):3637-42.

81. McWilliams RR, Giannini C, Hay ID, Atkinson JL, Stafford SL, Buckner JC. Management of brain metastases from thyroid carcinoma: a study of 16 pathologically confirmed cases over 25 years. Cancer. 2003;98(2):356-62.

Newer Technology in Thyroid Surgery

Roma Pradhan, Amit Agarwal

INTRODUCTION

The history of thyroid surgery is the most fascinating for endocrine surgeons and endocrinologist dealing with thyroid disorders.

In 1600 BC, burnt sponge and seaweed were used by Chinese for treating goiters. Sushruta Samhita is probably the earliest written work which dealt with surgery (1500 BC). In 150 AD, Galen used an instrumental figure also referred to as "Spongia Usta" (burnt sponge) for the treatment of goiter. During the 12th century in Italy, hot irons and the setons were used through the enlarged gland as early surgical procedure. In 1791, during the French Revolution, Pierre-Joseph Desault performed the first partial thyroidectomy. However, the first total thyroidectomy (TT) was performed by Dupuytren in 1808; unfortunately, the patient died 36 hours after the surgery. In 19th century, thyroidectomy procedure carried a high mortality (40%) even in expert hands because of infection and hemorrhage. Therefore, the French and German Academy of Medicine banned thyroid surgery and across the Atlantic Samuel Gross also denounced thyroid surgery as "Horrid Butchery". The thyroidectomy procedure has evolved significantly over the past century with almost zero mortality now. This has been possible due to adoption of new technology which has made thyroidectomy very effective, very safe, and cosmetically less disfiguring. The areas in which new technology has made a difference are as follows:

- Use of surgeon-performed ultrasound (SPUS), thyroid imaging, reporting, and data system (TIRADS), and ultrasonography (USG)/elastography.
- New energy devices for achieving hemostasis
- Use of neuromonitoring to minimize the dreaded recurrent laryngeal nerve (RLN) palsy.
- Predicting and avoiding hypocalcemia
- Scarless in the neck thyroidectomy.

ELASTOGRAPHY AND THYROID IMAGING, REPORTING, AND DATA SYSTEM

Traditionally, a thyroid disorder or thyroid nodule is evaluated with thyroid-stimulating hormone (TSH), high frequency ultrasound, and cytology which are then followed by surgery or conservative management. The problem with this approach is that we get indeterminate cytology in 10–15% of patients and nondiagnostic results in 15%. Due to fear of malignancy, majority of patients with indeterminate nodules undergo a surgical procedure in practice but 80% turn out to be benign. Therefore, an area of continuous clinical interest is how to reduce unnecessary surgery in nodules with indeterminate cytology. One area was thyroid ultrasound where the system of TIRADS classification was first introduced by Horvath et al.[1] originating from the Breast Imaging, Reporting, and Data System (BIRADS).[2] We know that no single ultrasound feature of a nodule is sensitive or specific enough to confirm or rule out malignancy. Multiple studies report that combining the suspicious ultrasound features may better predict malignancy risk. It was considered that pattern recognition may be more precise for predicting whether a thyroid nodule is benign.

Thyroid imaging, reporting, and data system was based on 10 US patterns of thyroid nodules given by Horvath et al.[1] and they predicted the rate of malignancy according to the pattern. Due to its difficulty in use in clinical practice, other TIRADS classification systems have been also proposed.[3-6]

Thyroid imaging, reporting, and data system assessment is based on five high-risk characteristics of the nodule:

1. Hypoechogenicity
2. Irregular margins
3. Microcalcifications **(Figs. 1A and B)**
4. Taller than wide
5. Predominantly solid

The suspicious ultrasound features are classified and described in **Table 1**.[7]

The study by Maia et al.[8] showed high sensitivity and negative predictive value of Bethesda III nodules with a TIRADS score of 3/4a, which may suggest a conservative approach [follow-up and repeat US-fine-needle aspiration biopsy (FNAB)] is appropriate. In contrast, TIRADS scores 4b and 5 in combination with Bethesda III, IV, and V may suggest that proceeding directly to surgery is appropriate as such lesions have high incidence of malignancy.

Elastography

Palpation of the nodule is a clinical diagnostic method for thyroid evaluation as we know that the presence of a thyroid nodule which is hard in consistency is suggestive of increased

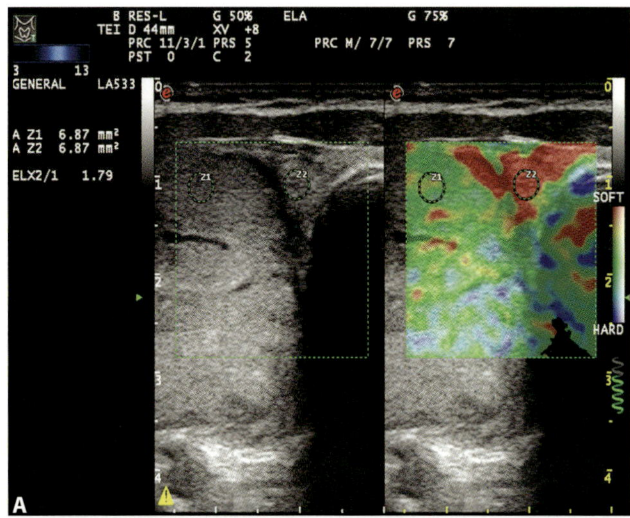

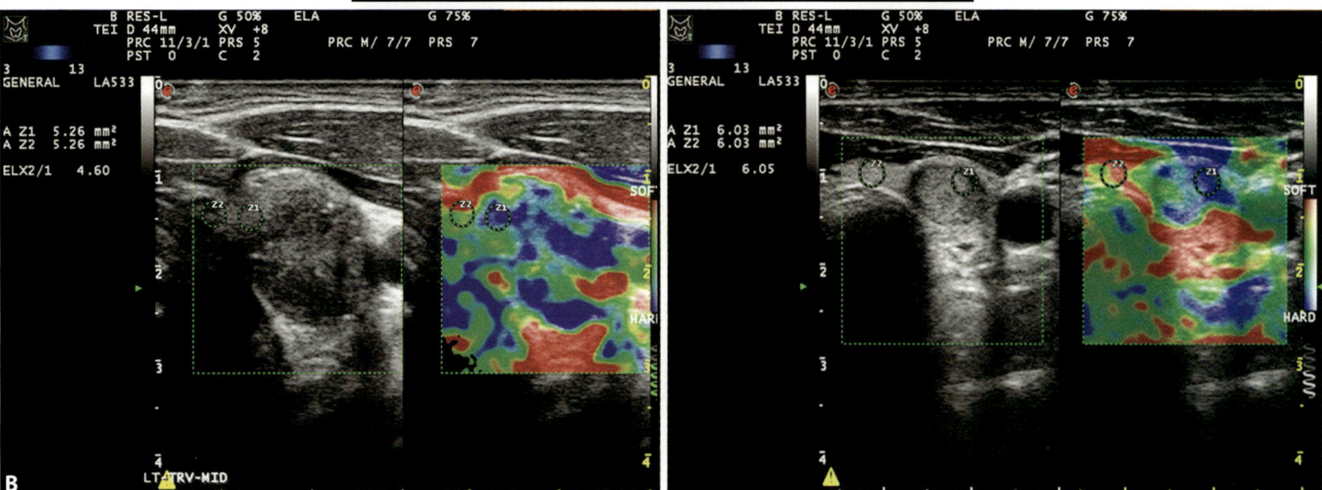

Figs. 1A and B: Elastography. (A) A 25-year-old man presented with STN measuring 5 × 4 cm with TIRADS score of 3 and FNAC of FLUS. Elastography revealed SR of 1.79% suggestive of benign lesion. HPE was benign thyroid lesion (follicular adenoma); (B) A 33-year-old man presented with MNG with USG showing multiple hypoechoic nodules with microcalcification in both lobes. Elastography revealed SR of 4.6 in left lobe nodule and 6.05 in right lobe nodule suggestive of malignant lesion. HPE turned out to be multifocal PTC.

(FLUS: follicular lesion of undetermined significance; FNAC: fine-needle aspiration cytology; HPE: histopathological examination; STN: solitary thyroid nodule; TIRADS: thyroid imaging, reporting, and data system; MNG: multinodular goiter; PTC: papillary thyroid carcinoma; USG: ultrasonography)

Table 1: Classification of suspicious ultrasound features.		
	Number of features	*Risk of malignancy*
Thyroid imaging, reporting, and data system 3 (TIRADS 3)	No suspicious features	0%
TIRADS 4a	One suspicious feature	4%
TIRADS 4b	Two suspicious features	12.5%
TIRADS 4c	Three or four suspicious features	62.2%
TIRADS 5	Five suspicious features	100%[1,7]

risk of malignancy. As this method is subjective, a more objective newer technique known as elastography to evaluate the stiffness of the lesion was developed. It is also known as "electronic palpation".

Ultrasound elastography was first used in thyroid by Lyshchik et al. in 2005.[9]

Principle of Elastography

Elastography depends on the degree of stiffness of the nodule when the nodule is subjected to external pressure. Malignant nodules have harder consistency or are less elastic than the benign ones.

There are two types of elastography:
1. *Strain elastography (SE):*
   - Strain elastography can be done with mechanical force (external or internal) or acoustic radiation force (ARF).
   - Relative displacement (strain) is greater in soft tissue as compared to stiff tissues.
   - Strain elastography tells us about the tissue elasticity through displacement which is induced by compression.

2. *Shear wave elastography (SWE)*: Shear wave elastography measures tissue elasticity by assessing the speed of transverse SWs.

Assessment strain elastography: Strain elastography indicates the stiffness in the tissues defined as the change in length during compression divided by the length before compression. The stress in SE is usually applied externally either by manual compression with the transducer or by acoustic radiation force impulse (ARFI) or an internal control such as carotid artery pulsations can be used. Stress with the transducer is applied by continuously and uniformly compressing and decompressing the skin of the patient a few millimeters at a time which is displayed as an elastogram which is calculated from the change in signals from before to after compression and the tissue stiffness is displayed in a spectrum of colors from red to green to blue, designating soft (high strain), intermediate (equal strain), and hard (no strain). Different machines display different color combinations. Besides this qualitative assessment of strain, semi-quantitative elastographic measurement can be done either by visual scoring system or by strain ratio. The cutoff value for strain ratio has been a matter of controversy and it can range from 1 to 5 in different studies.[10,11] Strain elastography can be performed as an extension to routine thyroid scanning and adds only 3–5 minutes to the examination time **(Fig. 2)**. The technique of SE can easily be mastered by novices after four to seven scans only. Briefly the method of SE is as follows: On pressing the elastography option, two boxes appear on screen, one for the B-mode ultrasound and another for elastography. Constant repetitive pressure is applied on nodule in perpendicular direction till

machine identified that the acquired image is appropriate for analysis by giving green signal. This image is then frozen on the screen and colorimetric score noted. After this, the measurement key on the keypad is pressed when two circles will pop-up on the screen. One circle is dragged and placed over normal thyroid tissue (Z1) and another on our targeted area (Z2). Machine automatically calculates the strain ratio (Z2/Z1).

Strain elastography using acoustic radiation force: ARFI imaging uses focused ultrasound beams to measure tissue deformity. Images are obtained before and after the application of force and displacement is measured. Strain changes are displayed on the screen as grayscale image. A lightshade indicates relatively soft tissue whereas a darker shade means relatively stiff tissue. Qualitative assessment is done by six-point scale devised by Xu et al.[12]

Shear wave elastography: The acoustic pulses from the probe target the nodule creating a SW traveling perpendicular to the conventional US waves. SWs are the transverse components of particle displacement that are rapidly attenuated by the tissue (1–10 m/s). This transverse component is measured as a numerical value corresponding to the shear wave speed (SWS). The elasticity index (EI) provides quantitative information about SWE (expressed in m/s) and the estimated tissue stiffness [expressed in kilopascals (kPa)].[13,14]

It relies on the degree of lesion stiffness. Malignant nodules have harder consistency or less elastic than benign ones due to the uncontrolled proliferation of cancer cells. The modulus of elasticity, also known as Young's modulus (in kPa), is calculated based on the SWE. The Young's modulus increases as the tissue becomes harder.[15,16]

In real clinical practice, elastography is usually performed with conventional high-resolution ultrasound and not as a standalone test. This is supported by the results of Trimboli et al.[17] who reported that the combination of these two modalities resulted in a high sensitivity (97%) and high negative predictive value (97%).

◇ HEMOSTASIS

Thyroid surgery involves meticulous dissection and removal of the thyroid gland which has one of the richest blood supplies. Therefore, hemostasis is of utmost importance. One of the major concerns following thyroid surgery is the risk of hematoma which can be life-threatening and the incidence of which is 0.3–3%.

Postoperatively drain is often used but presence or absence of drain does not have any influence on hematoma formation or bleeding.[18-21]

Two most commonly used techniques or methods for hemostasis are: (1) suture ligation and (2) electrocoagulation. The disadvantage of these techniques is the prolonged operating time, thermal damage to vital structures, and

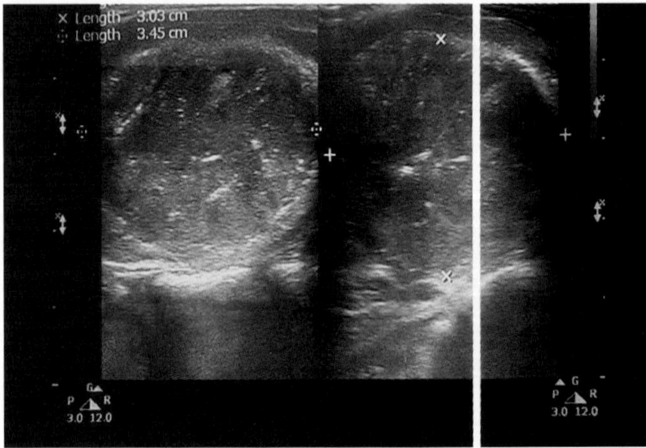

Fig. 2: TIRADS. A 26-year-old man presented with STN. USG revealed 3.3 × 3.0 × 3.5 cm well-defined solid isoechoic lesion wider than taller with punctate echogenic foci suggestive of microcalcification, replacing the left lobe. TIRADS 5, FNAC, and HPE revealed PTC.
(FNAC: fine-needle aspiration cytology; HPE: histopathological examination; PTC: papillary thyroid carcinoma; STN: solitary thyroid nodule; TIRADS 5: thyroid imaging, reporting, and data system 5; USG: ultrasonography)

possibility of granuloma formation. Evolutions in technology have allowed surgeons to achieve a better balance between hemostasis and preservation of important structures.

Newer devices include:
- Bipolar energy sealing system **(Fig. 3A)**
- Ultrasonic coagulation **(Fig. 3B)**.

Bipolar Energy Sealing System

It transfers radiofrequency energy to tissues through a bipolar device creating a coagulum by melting collagen and elastin. It can seal vessels up to 7 mm.

This has a unique design that prevents electrical power transmission and heat transfer thus avoiding thermal damage.[22] A significantly lower operation time for TT was seen in the study by Molnar et al. while using bipolar energy system.[22] In a randomized controlled trial comparing bipolar energy system with conventional thyroidectomy, a decrease in operative time and intraoperative bleeding was found compared to conventional technique.[23]

Ultrasonic Coagulation

It transfers frictional energy through vibrations at 55,000/s to tissues causing protein denaturation by rupture of hydrogen bonds. No electrical energy is transmitted to the patient.

With the use of ultrasonic coagulation, the duration of surgery can be shortened. This is due to the fact that tissue can be detached, coagulated, and dissected in a continuous operation without the need to change instruments which saves time. Lateral thermal spread is also less compared to monopolar cautery.

However, the evidence for showing the impact of these energy devises on postoperative complications is unclear. Some studies have reported lower rates of complications whereas others failed to demonstrate benefits over conventional hemostasis.[24-27]

Advantages of Energy Devices
- Minimal collateral damage for safe dissection near vital structure[28]
- Less smoke formation
- No neuromuscular stimulation
- No electrical energy to or through the patient (ultrasonic)
- Cuts, coagulates, grasps, and dissects by same instrument—no instrument exchanges
- Reliably seal and divide vessels.

◇| INTRAOPERATIVE NEUROMONITORING

The relationship of RLN with voice has a fascinating story which dates back as early as 6th century BC as written in Sushruta Samhita. Preservation of integrity of RLN seems to revolve around thyroid surgery.

Injury to the RLN is the most feared injury in thyroid surgery as compared to external branch of superior laryngeal nerve which supplies only the cricothyroid muscle, hence the damage of the nerve has varied effect on voice and is less troublesome except in singers and teachers.

Surgical Anatomy of Recurrent Laryngeal Nerve

The RLNs are derived from the sixth branchial arch and they originate from the tenth cranial nerves. Subsequently, the fifth and the distal portion of the sixth aortic arch regress on both the right and left sides and the two laryngeal nerves remain anchored to the structures that develop from the IV arch (i.e., the right subclavian artery and the aortic arch on the left side). When the heart descends into the thorax, these arteries take with them the nerves, which then assume their normal recurrent course.

Before the modern thyroid surgery developed, general surgeons never exposed the RLN for fear of damaging the RLN.

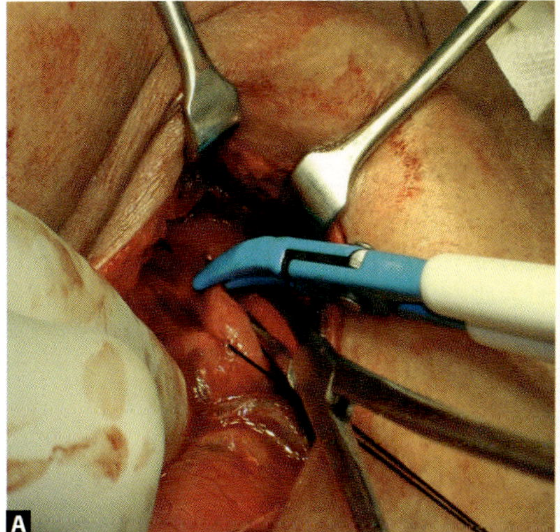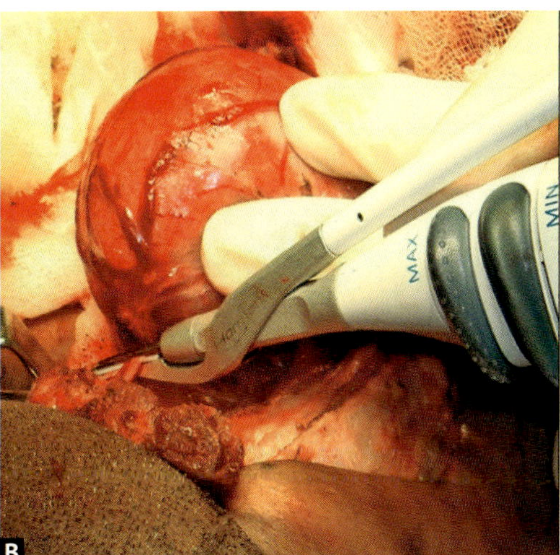

Figs. 3A and B: Sutureless thyroidectomy using energy devices. (A) Using bipolar energy sealing system for superior pedicle; (B) Using ultrasonic coagulation for superior pedicle.

However, modern thyroid surgery involved exposure and visualization of the entire course of RLN and this brought down the RLN damage rate to as low as 1–5%. But general surgeons and occasional thyroid surgeons continued to avoid exposure of the RLN perhaps because of lack of adequate training. Further, even for expert surgeons, certain challenging situations made exposure and identification of RLN very difficult. Head/neck surgeons have used electrophysiological monitoring routinely since long but it is only recently that thyroid surgeons started using intraoperative neuromonitoring (IONM).

Intraoperative neuromonitoring is considered a safe procedure to compliment the traditional method of visualizing the nerve which is considered the gold standard. It can also be used to prognosticate the postoperative nerve function, hence used as an adjunct tool for thyroid surgery.

There are two methods of neuromonitoring:
1. Intermittent
2. Continuous

Intermittent Neuromonitoring

The intermittent neuromonitoring in thyroid surgery for recognition of RLN was first done in Sweden way back in late 1960s.[29] All the 15 nerves investigated could be easily identified by it. Though its popularity and use is increasing still, it is considered as an adjunct in thyroid surgery and not a necessity. Visual identification of the nerve still remains the gold standard. The guidelines and literature suggest its importance in difficult cases like retrosternal goiter, toxic goiters, recurrent goiters, or recurrent thyroid cancer, however its use regularly in all cases is still debatable.

Equipment, technique, and operation course: Current neuromonitoring equipment is divided into audio only system or audio and visual waveform system. Audio only system is inferior as it provides less information regarding waveform, electromyography (EMG) response to nerve stimulation cannot be quantified, and absence of documentation of response.

Recording electrodes can be either needle based or endotracheal tube based. Use of needle electrodes may be traumatic leading to vocal cord or laryngeal hematoma, infection, deflation of cuff, or needle dislodgement. Endotracheal-based system records EMG data from vocal cord and does not require any additional equipment beyond endotracheal tubes.

The placement of endotracheal tube is the important step. Patient is induced with a short-acting intravenous neuroblocking agent. A larger size endotracheal tube is preferred as it snugly fits for good contact with vocal cords for better EMG signals. Baseline amplitude of 30–70 mV indicates proper positioning of the endotracheal tube.

Monitor settings need to be rechecked after proper positioning of the patient. The monitor should indicate an appropriate event threshold at 100 mV **(Figs. 4A and B)** and a stimulator probe should be set on a value of 1–2 mA.

To make sure proper functioning of the circuit, vagus stimulation should be done before dissection. The stimulator probe send signals at 4/s, hence the probe should be dragged over the tissue rather than just point touch.

Loss of signal: It is defined by EMG change from previous satisfactory EMG, very low or no response (<100 µV) with stimulation. Loss of signal (LOS) can be due to loss of nerve function or malfunctioning. Soon once the LOS occurs, the first thing to do is to see feel the laryngeal twitch. If it is present, then it is likely to be a recording side problem [endotracheal tube (ETT) malposition, ground electrodes detachment, interface box problems, or monitor/connections problems].

If with LOS, we have absent laryngeal twitch as well as absent strap muscle twitch, then the problem is from stimulating side (current problems, stimulator probe

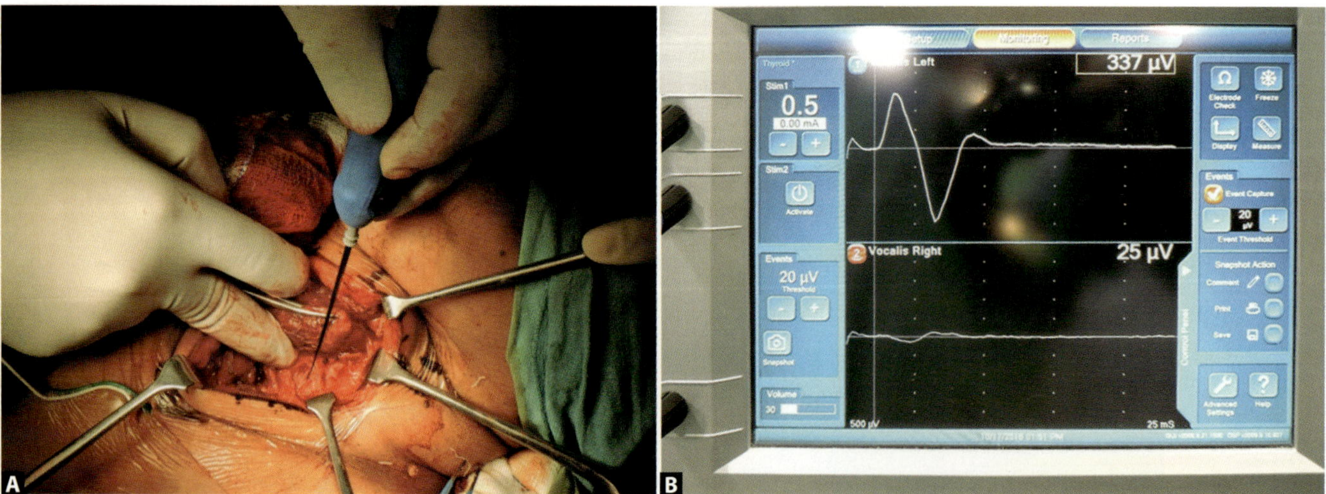

Figs. 4A and B: Intraoperative neuromonitoring. (A) Stimulating the recurrent laryngeal nerve with a voltage of 0.5 mA; (B) Electromyography response after stimulation; amplitude >100 µV is suggestive of functioning nerve.

problems, or neuromuscular blockade). If strap muscle twitch is present and signal is obtained after stimulating contralateral vagus nerve, then it indicates ipsilateral RLN injury.

Continuous Neuromonitoring

Continuous neuromonitoring is a step forward from intermittent neuromonitoring and helps us to react even before the injury is made. It tells us real-time status of the nerve function. It gives surgeons the opportunity to reverse the surgical maneuver which caused the EMG changes.

In continuous neuromonitoring, the endotracheal tube needs to be placed in same way as in intermittent monitoring. The addition in this is the automatic periodic stimulation (APS) electrode also called vagal electrode **(Figs. 5A and B)** that needs to be placed on the ipsilateral vagus nerve. This step in continuous neuromonitoring requires precision and experience.

Continuous intraoperative neuromonitoring technique and operation course: The initial stimulation is with 1 mA and 1 Hz and system calibration with highest amplitude is done which should preferably be ≥500 µV to guarantee a stable and reliable EMG signal.

After achieving the baseline, changes in amplitude and latency are displayed on a monitor timeline. It is possible to set an audio and visual alert when threshold values are exceeded to help the operating surgeon identify manipulations which may lead to nerve damage.

All continuous intraoperative neuromonitoring (CIONM) events are recorded and classified: Baseline amplitude reduction below 75%, 50%, and 25% or LOS as well as latency increase of 10%. Events with amplitudes <100 µV are counted as LOS regardless of the baseline amplitude.

After confirmation of LOS, the surgeons are expected to wait for 20 minutes to know if the affected nerve will recover fully or not and whether a staged surgery should be considered after the completion of one side.

The most common cause of RLN injury is due to traction of nerve especially at the area of ligament of Berry as suggested by Schneider[30] in their study and other authors subsequently.[31-33]

Dionigi et al. studied 281 injured nerves which were associated with postoperative vocal cord palsy (temporary or permanent) and identified intraoperatively by LOS found that only 14% of such injuries were identified intraoperatively emphasizing the importance of neural signal loss information and low sensitivity of visual inspection of the nerve.[34]

The most important controversy which hovers around neuromonitoring is its cost-effectiveness. The literature is varied with results of IONM use. Some meta-analysis has demonstrated IONM to reduce the overall and transient vocal cord palsy rates[35] whereas many others have failed to show that[36,37] cost-effectiveness of IONM was mentioned in few studies.[38,39] According to the study by Rocke et al.,[38] visual RLN identification was more cost-effective than using IONM. Further, IONM is cost-effective only if a surgeon can reduce palsy rate by 50.4% or more using IONM which is impossible to achieve. In fact, it is difficult to analyze the cost actually associated with IONM since it should also take into consideration the indirect costs associated with RLN palsy like rehabilitation cost and economic compensations for legal claims.

Although there is no consensus that IONM decreases RLN injury when compared to visual identification, it has many advantages:

- Intraoperative neuromonitoring may prevent bilateral RLN injury by allowing surgeons to stage the thyroidectomy when the signal is lost on the initial side, thus avoiding the need for tracheostomy.
- Intraoperative neuromonitoring can properly prognosticate postoperative function which is difficult to detect intra-operatively as most injured nerves appear intact.
- Intraoperative neuromonitoring can help detect anatomical variation and abnormal courses of the nerves which are at higher risk of injury if not detected.

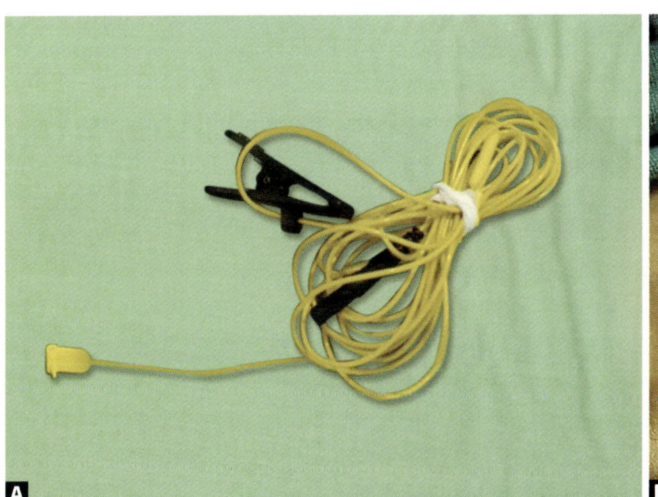
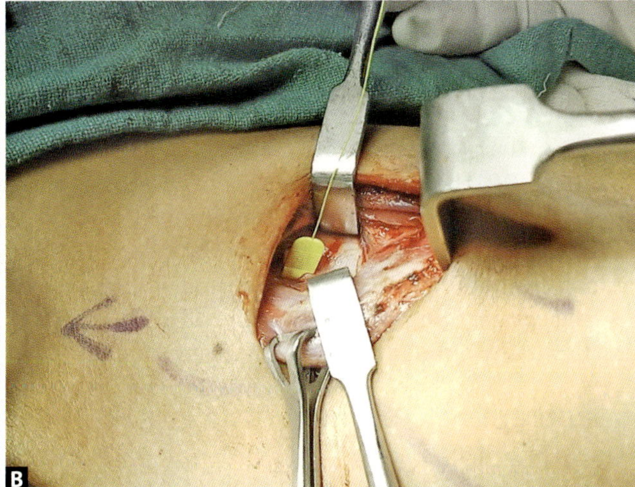

Figs. 5A and B: (A) Continuous intraoperative neuromonitoring. Vagal electrode is required for continuous neuromonitoring; (B) Placement of vagal electrode on the vagus nerve.

- *Especially beneficial in higher-risk patients which include*: Locally advanced thyroid cancer, patients with prior surgery and scarring, and patients with large goiters.
- Intraoperative neuromonitoring can prevent potential nerve injury by detecting signal changes indicating an adverse condition like suture compressing the nerve.
- Continuous intraoperative neuromonitoring is also able to detect the most proximal injuries which may be missed by intermittent monitoring.
- Several studies have suggested that low-volume thyroid surgeons may benefit from the use of neuromonitoring.

◇ PREDICTORS OF HYPOCALCEMIA

The reported incidence of transient hypocalcemia is 3–52% and that of permanent hypocalcemia is 0.4–13%.[40,41]

Various methods for diagnosing and managing postoperative hypocalcemia have been used. Postoperative hypocalcemia due to hypoparathyroidism is the most common complications after a TT. There are three methods of managing hypocalcemia. The most common approach used by surgeons is *supplementing* the calcium only if the patient develops signs and symptoms of hypocalcemia by monitoring the serum calcium but thus increasing the days of hospitalization. This method of managing hypocalcemia is still being used by many institutions worldwide because the nadir of hypocalcemia typically occurs within 48 hours after surgery. The *prophylactic or routine* use of postoperative oral calcium and/or vitamin D supplementation has been advocated by many surgeons to minimize the incidence of hypocalcemia and shorten hospital stay. More recently, the short half-life of the parathyroid hormone has led to increased interest in early postoperative *intact parathyroid hormone (IPTH)* as an early marker of hypocalcemia.[42] Various studies including a review[43] have evaluated the utility of postoperative IPTH measurement to predict postthyroidectomy hypocalcemia. Several studies have relied on the PTH to foresee hypocalcemia after TT using hemithyroidectomy procedure as control group,[44-46] but none could characterize an absolute PTH serum level or percentage hormone decline with 100% sensitivity and 100% specificity values. Some studies concluded that low perioperative PTH levels significantly correlate with the presence of postoperative hypocalcemia but cannot be used to predict it.[47]

Therefore, IPTH done early in the postoperative period has the potential to allow early discharge from the hospital without the need of the patient undergoing serial calcium monitoring.

Among the newer techniques, intraoperative parathyroid gland angiography during thyroidectomy can also be used to evaluate parathyroid gland perfusion and function.[48-50]

Intraoperative Detection of Parathyroid Gland

Detection of parathyroid gland presents greatest difficulty in cases such as TT, completion thyroidectomy (CT), central compartment lymph node dissection, and reoperative thyroid surgery. The incidence of inadvertent parathyroidectomy during thyroidectomy ranges from 8 to 19%, hence there is a need for an intraoperative technique to detect the parathyroid gland instantly and with high accuracy and more important to know if the in-situ parathyroid gland left is well-perfused or not. Laser Doppler flowmetry was initially tried for assessing parathyroid perfusion, but has not been widely practiced. Therefore, surgeons often have to rely on either visual inspection alone (i.e., by looking at the color changes) or the "knife" test as ways of estimating parathyroid perfusion and its viability. Indocyanine green (ICG) is an inert, water-soluble, nonradioactive, and nontoxic contrast agent approved by the US Food and Drug Administration since 1959. After intravenous injection, ICG is distributed throughout the intravascular space. When illuminated at 806 nm with a low-energy laser, these plasma-bound ICG molecules become fluorescent and this fluorescence is recorded by a device camera. Because the fluorescence intensity (FI) in a focused area is directly proportional to the perfusion in that area, the FI value of the in-situ gland measured on the ICG angiography (ICGA) **(Fig. 6)** may provide information regarding the perfusion and the extent of viability of the in-situ parathyroid gland. This technology has already been used in various other clinical scenarios like assessing perfusion of skin flaps, bowel anastomosis, and lower limbs. It is hypothesized that the FI in the in-situ gland may reflect not only the perfusion of the gland, but also parathyroid function and hence subsequent predictor of hypocalcemia. Given that parathyroid perfusion plays a vital role in normalizing early parathyroid function, perhaps patients with a greater FI value in their in-situ parathyroid glands have a lower chance of permanent hypocalcemia than those with a lower FI value.

In a recent randomized controlled trial[51] of 196 patients, a well-vascularized parathyroid gland could be identified in 146 patients (74.5%) and none of these patients presented with hypocalcemia. Therefore, calcium and/or PTH measurements may be omitted in patients with at least one

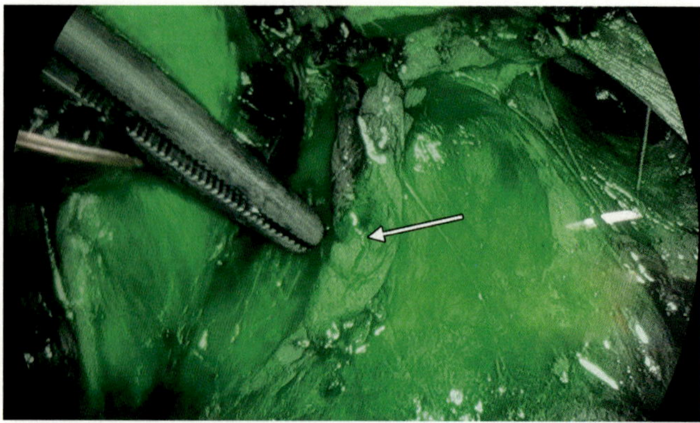

Fig. 6: Using indocyanine green dye to identify vascularized parathyroid gland.

well-perfused parathyroid gland as demonstrated by ICGA after thyroidectomy.

An issue which remains with ICGA is recognition or identification of parathyroid glands. Even an experienced thyroid surgeons might misinterpret other anatomical structures like fat or lymph node for a parathyroid gland. In experienced hands, the rate of correct identification of a structure as a parathyroid gland should exceed 95%[48] and hence a parathyroid biopsy is not necessary to confirm that the structure identified is indeed a parathyroid gland. In less experienced hands, a tool or procedure may be needed for detection of parathyroid glands. New studies on parathyroid gland autofluorescence[52,53] make use of a combination of autofluorescence first to identify the parathyroid glands which is then followed by ICGA to confirm about their vascularity.

◇ ENDOSCOPIC AND ROBOTIC-ASSISTED THYROIDECTOMY

The traditional thyroidectomy approach produces a long scar on the neck that is readily visible. Development of "alternative" approaches was driven by patient-centered efforts to improve the cosmetic impact of thyroid surgery. Novel approaches developed along two divergent avenues of innovation: (1) minimally invasive anterior cervical approaches and (2) remote access approaches **(Fig. 7)**. Chest/breast approaches included: Isolated anterior chest wall approach, bilateral transareolar approach, and unilateral transareolar approach. However, despite the lack of cervical scars, they involve incisions on the breast or anterior chest, more prone to hypertrophic scarring and may be an unappealing alternative to few patients. Also, these approaches may also be limited by a narrow operative field and restriction of movement by the rigid endoscopic equipment. Then came the axillary approach. The axillary approach is associated with improved cosmetic outcomes when compared to open surgery. However, it takes significantly longer to perform than a conventional open thyroidectomy. This approach is still subject to the constraints of carbon dioxide (CO_2)-assisted dissection—relatively narrow corridors, the need for rigid specialized endoscopic equipment, and the risks of CO_2-related morbidity. Then came the hybrid approaches which included: Axillobilateral breast approach (ABBA) and bilateral axillo-breast approach (BABA). These were designed to take advantage on the cosmetic benefit of the axillary approaches while providing additional anterior chest working ports without producing a transverse parasternal scar. Then came the transoral approach for thyroidectomy which was truly scarless.

Applying *robotic technology* to thyroidectomy was a step forward to minimally invasive thyroidectomy. Potential advantages included: More precise dissection, improved visualization, and hand tremor filtering system. Different techniques are:

- Two-incision (axillary and anterior chest)
- Bilateral axillary
- Bilateral areolar
- Single incision
- *Nonaxillary approach*:
  - Robotic facelift thyroidectomy (RFT)
  - Transoral

Robotic Transaxillary

Transaxillary approach was pioneered by Professor Chung and his team and they later published the largest series with 3,000 patients.[54] They selected patients with low body mass index (BMI) and small thyroid nodule with complication rates similar to open thyroidectomy.

The main disadvantage was of brachial plexus injury which decreased by placing the arm flexed at 90° position.

The meta-analysis published in 2014[55] summarized the comparison between robotic transaxillary, endoscopic transaxillary, and open thyroidectomy. Operative time was more in robotic as compared with open procedure, but with no difference in robotic and endoscopic thyroidectomy.

Transoral Robotic Thyroidectomy (Figs. 8A to E)

First described by Lee et al. in 2015 in four patients.[56] Though the procedure was successfully completed, three patients suffered mental nerve injury. Concern about the mental nerve injury did not escalate the acceptance of procedure until it was modified by Anuwong in 2016.[57] Anuwong positioned the lateral trocars toward the free edge of the lip to avoid excessive tension of the mental nerves. This helped in reducing the mental nerve paresthesia.

Advantages

- Avoidance of skin incision with invisible oral scar
- Less dissection required
- Equal access to both sides.

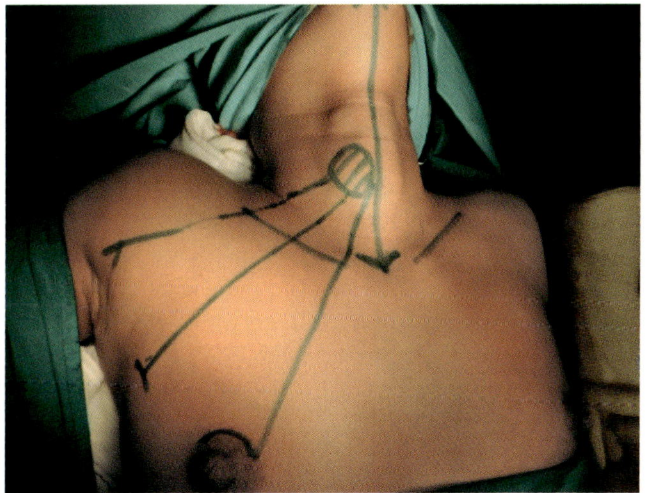

Fig. 7: Endoscopic thyroidectomy. Skin markings to show the area of dissection.

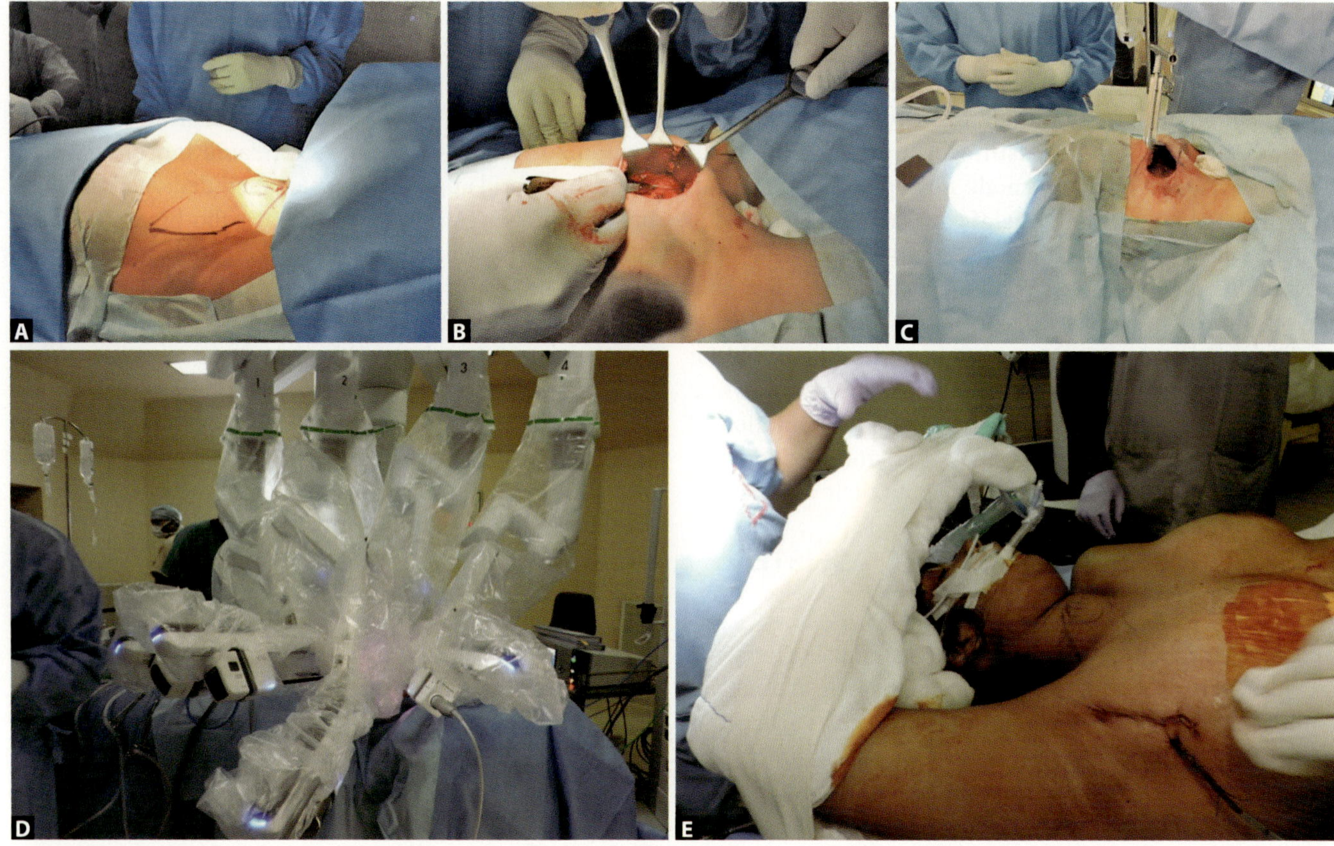

Figs. 8A to E: Robotic transaxillary thyroidectomy. (A) Marking of axillary incision; (B) Dissection of the skin flap to create access to thyroid; (C) Chung retractor in place; (D) Robot is docked on to the patient; (E) Axillary scar after robotic transaxillary thyroidectomy.

Disadvantages

- Introducing the oral infections into the neck requiring postoperative antibiotics.
- Increase length of stay due to dietary restriction (liquid then soft diet) in the first 24 hours and delayed drain removal on 3rd postoperative day.
- One of the biggest challenge was difficulty in dissection of the lateral borders of thyroid.[58]

Robotic Facelift Thyroidectomy

Advantages

- Reduced dissection area as compared with transaxillary approaches
- Easier to perform in obese patients
- No brachial plexus injury
- No paresthesia of the anterior chest unlike the transaxillary approach.

Disadvantages

- Transient hyperesthesia in the distribution of the greater auricular nerve
- Bilateral incisions are needed for TT procedure.

The da Vinci system (Intuitive Surgical Inc., USA) is the most common robotic system which offers a three-dimensional 10-times magnification with wristed robotic arms and 7° of freedom with tremor filtering system which enhances the safety of the procedure. However, important consideration regarding robotic-assisted thyroidectomy (RAT) is that there is a learning curve requiring at least 40 cases to master the technique and longer operative time. Comparing open and robotic thyroidectomy, there is no difference in surgical outcome; however, there was longer operative time (232 minutes vs. 109 minutes) in RAT.[59] Studies which objectively and subjectively analyzed found that there was no difference in complications.[60-62] In a systematic review and meta-analysis, studies again seem to confirm that both endoscopic and RAT are procedures that can be performed safely with good outcomes in appropriately selected patients.[63] The major drawback with robotic surgery is its cost. Cabot et al. mentioned that the costs of the robotic approach (transaxillary) are significantly more than that of conventional open thyroidectomy mainly due to expensive equipment and longer operative times.[39] However, there is a hope in future reduction of the cost of robotic surgery with increased medical equipment competition in this field.

CONCLUSION

Modern work-up of thyroid nodule now incorporates use of TIRADS and USG elastography along with molecular testing of thyroid aspirate. Various intraoperative adjuncts such as energy devices, use of Indo-cyanin green dye, using RLN/SLN neuromonitoring and IOPTH have made modern thyroid surgery almost bloodless and with minimal complications. Endoscopic and robotic approaches have made thyroid surgery cosmetically acceptable by either scarless surgery or by using remote incisions away from the neck. Also the treatment is now more personalized and tailored for individual patient. Sufficient data for application of endoscopic and robotic surgery in subset of thyroid patients is now available.

◇| REFERENCES

1. Horvath E, Majlis S, Rossi R, Franco C, Niedmann JP, Castro A, et al. An ultrasonogram reporting system for thyroid nodules stratifying cancer risk for clinical management. J Clin Endocrinol Metab. 2009;94:1748-51.
2. Vanel D. The American College of Radiology (ACR) Breast Imaging and Reporting Data System (BI-RADS): a step towards a universal radiological language? Eur J Radiol. 2007;61:183.
3. Park JY, Lee HJ, Jang HW, Kim HK, Yi JH, Lee W, et al. A proposal for a thyroid imaging reporting and data system for ultrasound features of thyroid carcinoma. Thyroid. 2009;19:1257-64.
4. Kwak JY, Jung I, Baek JH, Baek SM, Choi N, Choi YJ, et al. Image reporting and characterization system for ultrasound features of thyroid nodules: multicentric Korean retrospective study. Korean J Radiol. 2013;14:110-7.
5. Russ G, Royer B, Bigorgne C, Rouxel A, Bienvenu-Perrard M, Leenhardt L. Prospective evaluation of thyroid imaging reporting and data system on 4550 nodules with and without elastography. Eur J Endocrinol. 2013;168:649-55.
6. Na DG, Baek JH, Sung JY, Kim JH, Kim JK, Choi YJ, et al. Thyroid imaging reporting and data system risk stratification of thyroid nodules: categorization based on solidity and Echogenicity. Thyroid. 2016;26:562-72.
7. Kwak JY, Han KH, Yoon JH, Moon HJ, Son EJ, Park SH, et al. Thyroid imaging reporting and data system for US features of nodules: a step in establishing better stratification of cancer risk. Radiology. 2011;260:892-9.
8. Maia FF, Matos PS, Pavin EJ, Zantut-Wittmann DE. Thyroid imaging reporting and data system score combined with Bethesda system for malignancy risk stratification in thyroid nodules with indeterminate results on cytology. Clin Endocrinol (Oxf). 2015;82:439-44.
9. Lyshchik A, Higashi T, Asato R, Tanaka S, Ito J, Mai JJ, et al. Thyroid gland tumor diagnosis at US elastography. Radiology. 2005;237:202-11.
10. Ning CP, Jiang SQ, Zhang T, Sun LT, Liu YJ, Tian JW. The value of strain ratio in differential diagnosis of thyroid solid nodules. Eur J Radiol. 2012;81:286-91.
11. Xing P, Wu L, Zhang C, Li S, Liu C, Wu C. Differentiation of benign from malignant thyroid lesions: calculation of the strain ratio on thyroid sonoelastography. J Ultrasound Med. 2011;30:663-9.
12. Xu JM, Xu XH, Xu HX, Zhang YF, Zhang J, Guo LH, et al. Conventional US, US elasticity imaging, and acoustic radiation force impulse imaging for prediction of malignancy in thyroid nodules. Radiology. 2014;272:577-86.
13. Sebag F, Vaillant-Lombard J, Berbis J, Griset V, Henry JF, Petit P, et al. Shear wave elastography: a new ultrasound imaging mode for the differential diagnosis of benign and malignant thyroid nodules. J Clin Endocrinol Metab. 2010;95:5281-8.
14. Asteria C, Giovanardi A, Pizzocaro A, Cozzaglio L, Morabito A, Somalvico F, et al. US-elastography in the differential diagnosis of benign and malignant thyroid nodules. Thyroid. 2008;18:523-31.
15. Tanter M, Bercoff J, Athanasiou A, Deffieux T, Gennisson JL, Montaldo G, et al. Quantitative assessment of breast lesion viscoelasticity: initial clinical results using supersonic shear imaging. Ultrasound Med Biol. 2008;34:1373-86.
16. Bercoff J, Tanter M, Fink M. Supersonic shear imaging: a new technique for soft tissue elasticity mapping. IEEE Trans Ultrason Ferroelectr Freq Control. 2004;51:396-409.
17. Trimboli P, Guglielmi R, Monti S, Misischi I, Graziano F, Nasrollah N, et al. Ultrasound sensitivity for thyroid malignancy is increased by real-time elastography: a prospective multicenter study. J Clin Endocrinol Metab. 2012;97:4524-30.
18. Tübergen D, Moning E, Richter A, Lorenz D. Assessment of drain insertion in thyroid surgery? Zentralbl Chir. 2001;126:960-3.
19. Samraj K, Gurusamy KS. Wound drains following thyroid surgery. Cochrane Database Syst Rev. 2007;4:CD006099.
20. Memon ZA, Ahmed G, Khan SR, Khalid M, Sultan N. Postoperative use of drain in thyroid lobectomy—a randomized clinical trial conducted at Civil Hospital, Karachi, Pakistan. Thyroid Res. 2012;5:9.
21. Khanna J, Mohil RS, Chintamani, Bhatnagar D, Mittal MK, Sahoo M, et al. Is the routine drainage after surgery for thyroid necessary? A prospective randomized clinical study [ISRCTN63623153]. BMC Surg. 2005;5:11.
22. Molnar C, Voidazan S, Rad C, Neagoe V, Rosca C, Barna L. Total thyroidectomy with LigaSure Small Jaw versus conventional thyroidectomy: a clinical study. Chirurgia (Bucur). 2014;109:608-12.
23. Ramouz A, Rasihashemi SZ, Safaeiyan A, Hosseini M. Comparing postoperative complication of LigaSure Small Jaw instrument with clamp and tie method in thyroidectomy patients: a randomized controlled trial [IRCT2014010516077N1]. World J Surg Oncol. 2018;16:154.
24. Lombardi CP, Raffaelli M, Cicchetti A, Marchetti M, De Crea C, Di Bidino R, et al. The use of 'harmonic scalpel' versus 'knot tying' for conventional 'open' thyroidectomy: results of a prospective randomized study. Langenbecks Arch Surg. 2008;393:627-31.
25. Hallgrimsson P, Loven L, Westerdahl J, Bergenfelz A. Use of the harmonic scalpel versus conventional haemostatic techniques in patients with Grave disease undergoing total thyroidectomy: a prospective randomised controlled trial. Langenbecks Arch Surg. 2008;393:675-80.
26. Ecker T, Carvalho AL, Choe JH, Walosek G, Preuss KJ. Hemostasis in thyroid surgery: harmonic scalpel versus other techniques—a meta-analysis. Otolaryngol Head Neck Surg. 2010;143:17-25.
27. Miccoli P, Berti P, Dionigi G, D'Agostino J, Orlandini C, Donatini G. Randomized controlled trial of harmonic scalpel use during thyroidectomy. Arch Otolaryngol Head Neck Surg. 2006;132:1069-73.
28. Sutton PA, Awad S, Perkins AC, Lobo DN. Comparison of lateral thermal spread using monopolar and bipolar diathermy, the Harmonic Scalpel and the Ligasure. Br J Surg. 2010;97:428-33.
29. Flisberg K, Lindholm T. Electrical stimulation of the human recurrent laryngeal nerve during thyroid operation. Acta Otolaryngol Suppl. 1969;263:63-7.
30. Schneider R, Randolph G, Dionigi G, Barczyński M, Chiang FY, Triponez F, et al. Prospective study of vocal fold function after loss of the neuromonitoring signal in thyroid surgery: The International Neural Monitoring Study Group's POLT study. Laryngoscope. 2016;126:1260-6.

31. Phelan E, Schneider R, Lorenz K, Dralle H, Kamani D, Potenza A, et al. Continuous vagal IONM prevents recurrent laryngeal nerve paralysis by revealing initial EMG changes of impending neuropraxic injury: a prospective, multicenter study. Laryngoscope. 2014;124:1498-505.

32. Schneider R, Lamade W, Hermann M, Goretzki P, Timmermann W, Hauss J, et al. Continuous intraoperative neuromonitoring of the recurrent laryngeal nerve in thyroid surgery (CIONM): where are we now? An update to the European Symposium of Continuous Neuromonitoring in Thyroid Surgery. Zentralbl Chir. 2012;137:88-90.

33. Chiang FY, Lu IC, Kuo WR, Lee KW, Chang NC, Wu CW. The mechanism of recurrent laryngeal nerve injury during thyroid surgery—the application of intraoperative neuromonitoring. Surgery. 2008;143:743-9.

34. Dionigi G, Wu CW, Kim HY, Rausei S, Boni L, Chiang FY. Severity of recurrent laryngeal nerve injuries in thyroid surgery. World J Surg. 2016;40:1373-81.

35. Pisanu A, Porceddu G, Podda M, Cois A, Uccheddu A. Systematic review with meta-analysis of studies comparing intraoperative neuromonitoring of recurrent laryngeal nerves versus visualization alone during thyroidectomy. J Surg Res. 2014;188:152-61.

36. Higgins TS, Gupta R, Ketcham AS, Sataloff RT, Wadsworth JT, Sinacori JT, et al. Recurrent laryngeal nerve monitoring versus identification alone on post-thyroidectomy true vocal fold palsy: a meta-analysis. Laryngoscope. 2011;121:1009-17.

37. Rocke DJ, Goldstein DP, de Almeida JR. A Cost-Utility Analysis of recurrent laryngeal nerve monitoring in the setting of total thyroidectomy. JAMA Otolaryngol Head Neck Surg. 2016;142:1199-205.

38. Wang T, Kim HY, Wu CW, Rausei S, Sun H, Pergolizzi FP, et al. Analyzing cost-effectiveness of neural-monitoring in recurrent laryngeal nerve recovery course in thyroid surgery. Int J Surg. 2017;48:180-8.

39. Cabot JC, Lee CR, Brunaud L, Kleiman DA, Chung WY, Fahey TJ, et al. Robotic and endoscopic transaxillary thyroidectomies may be cost prohibitive when compared to standard cervical thyroidectomy: a cost analysis. Surgery. 2012;152:1016-24.

40. Vescan A, Witterick I, Freeman J. Parathyroid hormone as a predictor of hypocalcemia after thyroidectomy. Laryngoscope. 2005;115:2105-8.

41. Pisaniello D, Parmeggiani D, Piatto A, Avenia N, d'Ajello M, Monacelli M, et al. Which therapy to prevent post-thyroidectomy hypocalcemia? G Chir. 2005;26:357-61.

42. Lombardi CP, Raffaelli M, Princi P, Santini S, Boscherini M, De Crea C, et al. Early prediction of postthyroidectomy hypocalcemia by one single iPTH measurement. Surgery. 2004;136:1236-41.

43. Noordzij JP, Lee SL, Bernet VJ, Payne RJ, Cohen SM, McLeod IK, et al. Early prediction of hypocalcemia after thyroidectomy using parathyroid hormone: an analysis of pooled individual patient data from nine observational studies. J Am Coll Surg. 2007;205:748-54.

44. Alía P, Moreno P, Rigo R, Francos JM, Navarro MA. Postresection parathyroid hormone and parathyroid hormone decline accurately predict hypocalcemia after thyroidectomy. Am J Clin Pathol. 2007;127:592-7.

45. Di Fabio F, Casella C, Bugari G, Iacobello C, Salerni B. Identification of patients at low risk for thyroidectomy-related hypocalcemia by intraoperative quick PTH. World J Surg. 2006;30:1428-33.

46. Lo CY, Luk JM, Tam SC. Applicability of intraoperative parathyroid hormone assay during thyroidectomy. Ann Surg. 2002;236:564-9.

47. Ghaheri BA, Liebler SL, Andersen PE, Schuff KG, Samuels MH, Klein RF, et al. Perioperative parathyroid hormone levels in thyroid surgery. Laryngoscope. 2006;116:518-21.

48. Lang BH, Wong CK, Hung HT, Wong KP, Mak KL, Au KB. Indocyanine green fluorescence angiography for quantitative evaluation of in situ parathyroid gland perfusion and function after total thyroidectomy. Surgery. 2017;161:87-95.

49. Zaidi N, Bucak E, Yazici P, Soundararajan S, Okoh A, Yigitbas H, et al. The feasibility of indocyanine green fluorescence imaging for identifying and assessing the perfusion of parathyroid glands during total thyroidectomy. J Surg Oncol. 2016;113:775-8.

50. Vidal Fortuny J, Belfontali V, Sadowski SM, Karenovics W, Guigard S, Triponez F. Parathyroid gland angiography with indocyanine green fluorescence to predict parathyroid function after thyroid surgery. Br J Surg. 2016;103:537-43.

51. Vidal Fortuny J, Sadowski SM, Belfontali V, Guigard S, Poncet A, Ris F, et al. Randomized clinical trial of intraoperative parathyroid gland angiography with indocyanine green fluorescence predicting parathyroid function after thyroid surgery. Br J Surg. 2018;105:350-7.

52. De Leeuw F, Breuskin I, Abbaci M, Casiraghi O, Mirghani H, Ben Lakhdar A, et al. Intraoperative near-infrared imaging for parathyroid gland identification by autofluorescence: a feasibility study. World J Surg. 2016;40:2131-8.

53. McWade MA, Sanders ME, Broome JT, Solorzano CC, Mahadevan-Jansen A. Establishing the clinical utility of autofluorescence spectroscopy for parathyroid detection. Surgery. 2016;159:193-202.

54. Ban EJ, Yoo JY, Kim WW, Son HY, Park S, Lee SH, et al. Surgical complications after robotic thyroidectomy for thyroid carcinoma: a single center experience with 3,000 patients. Surg Endosc. 2014;28:2555-63.

55. Jackson NR, Yao L, Tufano RP, Kandil EH. Review safety of robotic thyroidectomy approaches: meta-analysis and systematic review. Head Neck. 2014;36:137-43.

56. Lee HY, You JY, Woo SU, Son GS, Lee JB, Bae JW, et al. Transoral periosteal thyroidectomy: cadaver to human. Surg Endosc. 2015;29:898-904.

57. Anuwong A, Ketwong K, Jitpratoom P, Sasanakietkul T, Duh QY. Safety and Outcomes of the Transoral Endoscopic Thyroidectomy Vestibular Approach. JAMA Surg. 2018;153:21-7.

58. Chang EHE, Kim HY, Koh YW, Chung WY. Review Overview of robotic thyroidectomy. Gland Surg. 2017;6:218-28.

59. Foley CS, Agcaoglu O, Siperstein AE, Berber E. Robotic transaxillary endocrine surgery: a comparison with conventional open technique. Surg Endosc. 2012;26:2259-66.

60. Lee J, Na KY, Kim RM, Oh Y, Lee JH, Lee J, et al. Postoperative functional voice changes after conventional open or robotic thyroidectomy: a prospective trial. Ann Surg Oncol. 2012;19:2963-70.

61. Lee J, Lee JH, Nah KY, Soh EY, Chung WY. Comparison of endoscopic and robotic thyroidectomy. Ann Surg Oncol. 2011;18:1439-46.

62. Yoo H, Chae BJ, Park HS, Kim H, Song BJ, Jung SS, et al. Comparison of surgical outcomes between endoscopic and robotic thyroidectomy. J Surg Oncol. 2012;105:705-8.

63. Lee S, Ryu HR, Park JH, Kim KH, Jeong JJ, Nam KH, et al. Excellence in robotic thyroid surgery: a comparative study of robot-assisted versus conventional endoscopic thyroidectomy in papillary thyroid microcarcinoma patients. Ann Surg. 2011;253:1060-6.

Neck Dissection in Differentiated Thyroid Cancer

Neeti Kapre, Madan Kapre

◇ INTRODUCTION

Thyroid cancers show a consistent rising trend in incidence over the past few decades. This has been in part attributed to improved diagnostic techniques. However, the survival outcomes have remained consistently promising. Differentiated thyroid cancers (DTCs) have superior outcomes compared to other head and neck cancers. Prognosis of nodal metastases in DTC is similarly much better than that in squamous cancers. However, appropriate management and successful outcomes require proper preoperative planning and sound surgical rationale.

◇ QUANTIFICATION OF THE PROBLEM

Reported prevalence of neck nodes in DTCs is approximately 50–80%, depending upon tumor factors, patient factors, and the imaging modality employed.[1-4] The first echelon for spread from DTC is the level VI or central compartment neck nodes. These may then subsequently metastasize to superior mediastinal (level VII) lymph nodes and lateral compartment (levels I–V, however levels II–IV are most commonly involved). Very rarely, there can be skip metastasis to level II lymph nodes in the absence of level VI nodes which is in fact the first echelon for DTCs. This phenomenon is generally seen with superior pole nodules.[5]

Although nodal disease does not impact significantly on survival, it does increase the risk of recurrence, especially when lymph node metastases are macroscopic. The impact of microscopic lymph node metastases on recurrence and survival is less clear.[6-10]

Following factors are prognosticators for increased risk of nodal metastases that are given in **Box 1**.[11-13]

◇ DIAGNOSIS

Preoperative neck ultrasonography for cervical lymph nodes is recommended for all patients undergoing thyroidectomy for malignant or suspicious for malignancy. US-guided fine-needle aspiration (FNA) of sonographically suspicious lymph nodes 8–10 mm in the smallest diameter should be performed to confirm malignancy if this would change management [Recommendation 33, American Thyroid Association (ATA) guidelines 2015].[14] There is adequate literature now to support

---

Box 1: Prognosticators of nodal metastasis.[11]

- Younger age[12]
- Male gender
- Extrathyroidal extension
- Aggressive pathological variants such as tall cell, columnar cell, and diffuse sclerosing or insular
- BRAF/TERT mutation positivity[13]

(TERT: telomerase reverse transcriptase ; BRAF: B-type RAF kinase)

---

the superiority of CT scan in nodal mapping.[15] Contrast-enhanced CT scan has incremental value over ultrasound in mapping central compartment nodes especially with thyroid gland in situ. It also delineates lateral compartment nodes and its relationship to vessels better. The myth regarding contraindication for use of iodinated contrast in thyroid cancer imaging is long broken now. Therefore, one need not shy away from using contrast-enhanced CT scans to provide more anatomical information on nodal metastasis preoperatively. Generally, presence of bulky nodal disease can also be associated with locally extensive disease and occasionally presence of distant metastasis also. Therefore, CT provides a good one time imaging opportunity to screen neck nodes, lung nodules, and mediastinal nodes along with precise information on local extension of disease into strap muscles or laryngotracheal framework MRI can be reserved for extensive vascular oroesophageal involvement.

There is no recommendation currently for positron emission tomography (PET) scan as an upfront imaging modality to assess nodal disease in thyroid cancers (Recommendation 33, ATA guidelines 2015).[14]

Thus, there are several advantages of CT scan such as:

- Improved nodal mapping especially in central compartment nodes.
- Detection of extrathyroidal extension including laryngotracheal involvement.
- Cross-sectional imaging of mediastinal nodes and lung nodules.
- Iodinated contrast no longer contraindicated.

Fine-needle aspiration cytology (FNAC) can be performed preoperatively to document metastatic nodal involvement. The addition of FNA-thyroglobulin (Tg) washout in the evaluation of suspicious cervical lymph nodes is appropriate in selected patients, but interpretation may be difficult in patients with an intact thyroid gland.[16] During surgery, frozen section provides a very reliable diagnostic tool. The authors have their own experience with crush imprint cytology as a surrogate to frozen section examination. This method of intraoperative pathology has accuracy of approximately 97%.

◇ SURGICAL MANAGEMENT OF CERVICAL NODAL METASTASES FROM DIFFERENTIATED THYROID CANCERS

Neck dissection for DTCs can be broadly classified into central compartment neck dissection (CCND) and lateral compartment neck dissection.

Central Compartment Neck Dissection

Performance of nodal clearance in the presence of documented central compartment nodes is therapeutic CCND whereas any nodal dissection done in the absence of clinico-radiologically proven disease is prophylactic CCND.

Therapeutic CCND is no longer a debatable issue (Recommendation 36, ATA guidelines 2015) and must be performed for:

- Clinically and radiologically manifest or pathologically proven central compartment nodal disease.
- Proven lateral compartment nodal diseases.

Prophylactic CCND on the other hand is a matter of great debate. Even in the presence of several meta-analysis, we still do not have consensus.[17-20]

Arguments in favor of prophylactic CCND are:

- No imaging or pathology examination is foolproof to detection of central compartment nodes preoperatively.[21]
- Intraoperative surgeon assessment is not reliable for decision-making.[22]
- Occult central compartment metastasis is seen up to 80%.
- Appropriate staging helps in better planning of adjuvant treatment.[23]
- Reoperation in central compartment has significantly higher incidence of recurrent laryngeal nerve (RLN) palsy and hypocalcemia.[24,25]

Arguments against prophylactic CCND are:

- Significantly higher rated of hypoparathyroidism, especially in lower volume centers.[26]
- No significant detriment to survival outcomes.[17,18]

The ATA consensus statement on CCND clearly defines anatomical boundaries, indications, and terminologies for surgical procedures.[27] Central compartment extends between the carotid arteries laterally on either side, superiorly from hyoid bone, and inferiorly up to the innominate artery. This includes the prelaryngeal (delphian), pretracheal, and paratracheal lymph nodes. Level VII lymph nodes are the superior mediastinal lymph nodes.

Each surgeon will have minimally differing philosophies on CCND surgery. Following surgical procedures are commonly practiced:

- *Central compartment exploration*:
  - Minimal dissection done to identify presence of central compartment nodes.
  - If there are no nodes seen, procedure is terminated and no further dissection is performed.
  - If nodes are identified, this is converted to a formal CCND clearance.
- *Central compartment sampling*:
  - Any clinically suspicious looking nodes are sent for intraoperative pathology assessment (frozen section or crush imprint cytology).
  - If the report is positive for metastatic nodes, formal CCND clearance is performed.
- *Central compartment nodal clearance*: This is generally more applicable for therapeutic CCND and it involves clearance of all lymph node and fibrofatty tissue from carotids on either side bilaterally and from hyoid to innominate artery in the vertical extent.

Some surgeons believe in performing *ipsilateral CCND* only in an attempt to preserve contralateral parathyroids and their vasculature. Ipsilateral CCND implies clearance of prelaryngeal, pretracheal, and paratracheal (between carotid and trachea) on the ipsilateral side, that is on the side of the primary thyroid tumor. Bilateral CCND implies clearance of all prelaryngeal, pretracheal, and bilateral paratracheal nodes.

Surgical Tips

Dissection in this area generally commences after the total thyroidectomy specimen has been separated off of the trachea and delivered out. However, a key initial tip during the ligating of the terminal branch of the inferior thyroid artery is to trace and identify vasculature of the inferior parathyroid gland. This can be marked or clipped with a Ligaclip to ease identification of the parathyroids with their supplying vessels during central compartment dissection. Some surgeons propose clearance of paratracheal nodes only medial to the RLN, i.e., between RLN and trachea. They believe that this results in lower hypoparathyroidism rates since majority of parathyroid blood supply comes laterally and yet ensures adequate oncological clearance since majority nodes are medial to RLN. The authors, however, believe in thorough ipsilateral CCND. It often helps if the operating surgeon stands at the head end of the table and an assistant applies gentle traction over the cricothyroid joint anteriorly. This allows the surgeon to work better along the RLN clearing all nodes on either sides of it **(Figs. 1A and B)**. One must also constantly bear in mind variations in the angulations of the nerve on either side. Being more angulated to the tracheoesophageal groove, the right RLN may be at more risk of injury. Caution must be exercised to keep the nerve attached to its fascial coverings and avoid handling to prevent neuropraxic damage. Microsurgical loops are preferred by

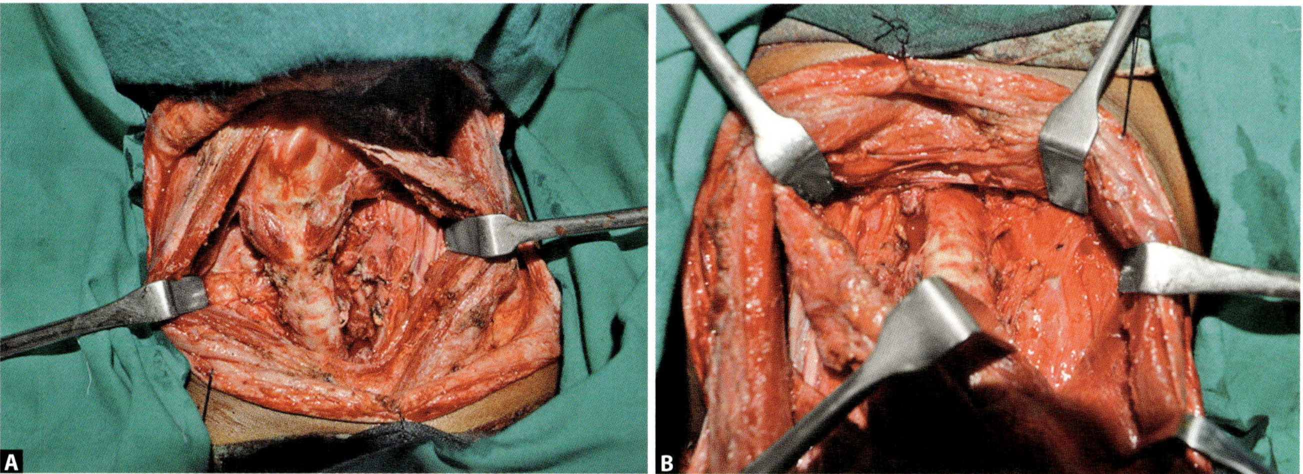

Figs. 1A and B: Completed central compartment neck dissection.

Flowchart 1: Algorithm for nodal disease severely engulfing or involving the recurrent laryngeal nerve (RLN).

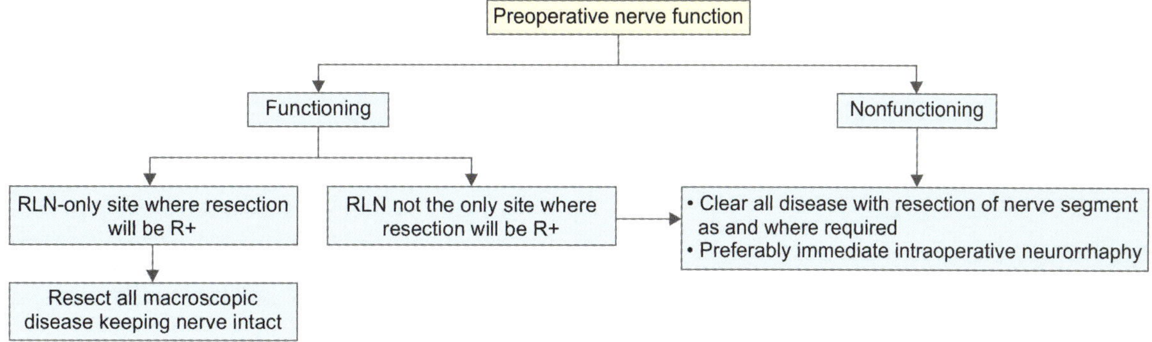

some surgeons for improved magnification allowing adequate clearance of disease and preservation of RLN and parathyroids with their vasculature. Use of intraoperative nerve monitoring during CCND is a useful adjunct for reducing chances of RLN injuries. This holds truer in the reoperative setting.

In case of nodal disease severely engulfing or involving the RLN, **Flowchart 1** may prove useful.

The rationale behind a neurorrhaphy is that published literature reports return of function in approximately 50% patients.[28] Also, it helps to maintain the bulk of the vocal cord muscles and therefore aids voice rehabilitation later on.

In case of an inadvertent parathyroidectomy along with CCND, autotransplantation of the concerned gland must be performed in the strap or the sternocleidomastoid (SCM) muscles. If at the end of procedure, the parathyroid gland appears dusky and a small nick with a scalpel or needle may help to relieve the hematoma. If the gland partially or completely regains its color, nothing further need be done. For a devascularized gland, however, autotransplantation may still yield a more successful outcome.

Lateral Compartment Neck Dissection

Indications for lateral neck dissection are:
- Extensive central compartment neck nodes
- Proven lateral compartment nodes.

There is no indication for performing prophylactic lateral compartment neck dissection (Recommendation 37, ATA guidelines 2015).[14]

Many philosophies for managing the lateral neck in DTC are presented in the literature including elective nodal sampling, US-directed compartment resections, and superselective nodal dissection, that is levels III–IV, leading to some controversy regarding when and how to manage the lateral neck in DTC.[29]

Berry picking or selective sampling and removal of nodes must be condemned. A selective neck dissection clearing all lymph nodes and fibrofatty tissue from levels II–IV should be practiced preserving SCM muscle, internal jugular vein, and the spinal accessory nerve. Sacrifice of any of these structures should be considered only in the presence of gross disease with obvious involvement of these nonlymphatic structures. Levels I and V should ideally be cleared only in the presence of obvious involvement by disease. Many surgeons follow the dictum of cleaning level V in case of level II nodal positivity. There has been much debate about clearance of level IIb in view of scant metastases at this nodal station and increased risk of traction injuries to the spinal accessory nerve during this dissection.[30] A thumb rule can be employed that level IIb clearance be mandatory in case of positive nodes at level IIa.

Table 1: Prognostic factors for nodal disease and risk of recurrence.

	Risk of recurrence—average (range)
Clinically N0, pN0	4% (0–9%)
Clinically N0, microscopic pN1	6% (4–11.5%)
Number of nodes ≤ 5	4% (3–8%)
Number of nodes > 5	19% (7–21%)
Nodes with extranodal extension	24% (15–32%)

PROGNOSTIC FACTORS

A very interesting study by Dr Randolph et al.[31] estimates chances of nodal recurrence in node-positive patients. Number of nodes, nodal dimensions, evidence of extranodal extension, and lymph node ratios are important prognostic factors. Small volume nodal disease, <five nodes, microscopic metastases, and without extranodal extension have lower chances of recurrence (approximately 5%) whereas patients with high volume nodal disease, >five nodes, >5 mm nodal diameter, and extranodal extension have a higher chances (approximately 20%) for nodal recurrence **(Table 1)**.

Reoperative Thyroid Surgery for Nodal Recurrence

Reoperative CCND has decidedly higher morbidity compared to lateral compartment neck dissection, hypoparathyroidism being the most dreaded one. Patient selection is a key factor. Such surgeries should ideally be undertaken at high volume centers by experienced surgeons. Precise localization studies including employment of intraoperative sonology if required is an important prerequisite. Intraoperative nerve monitoring and use of magnification are very useful adjuncts.

CONCLUSION

Differentiated thyroid cancers with nodal metastasis are an entirely surgical disease. Completeness of resection has always been one of the important prognostic factors in the various scoring systems. With the concept of dynamic risk stratification also being universally accepted, it is a surgeon's responsibility not to leave behind any structural disease. In the same vein, DTCs have very reasonable survival outcomes. Morbidity in the form of hypoparathyroidism remains the prime concern. It is this balance between adequate and safe surgery that the surgeon must always seek to achieve to improve results of thyroid surgery.

REFERENCES

1. Kim E, Park JS, Son KR, Kim JH, Jeon SJ, Na DG. Preoperative diagnosis of cervical metastatic lymph nodes in papillary thyroid carcinoma: comparison of ultrasound, computed tomography, and combined ultrasound with computed tomography. Thyroid. 2008;18:411-8.
2. Noguchi S, Noguchi A, Murakami N. Papillary carcinoma of the thyroid. I. Developing pattern of metastasis. Cancer. 1970;26:1053-60.
3. Stulak JM, Grant CS, Farley DR, Thompson GB, van Heerden JA, Hay ID, et al. Value of preoperative ultrasonography in the surgical management of initial and reoperative papillary thyroid cancer. Arch Surg. 2006;141:489-94.
4. Arturi F, Russo D, Giuffrida D, Ippolito A, Perrotti N, Vigneri R, et al. Early diagnosis by genetic analysis of differentiated thyroid cancer metastases in small lymph nodes. Endocrinol Metab. 1997;82:1638-41.
5. Lei J, Zhong J, Jiang K, Li Z, Gong R, Zhu J. Skip lateral lymph node metastasis leaping over the central neck compartment in papillary thyroid carcinoma. Oncotarget. 2017;8:27022-33.
6. Bardet S, Malville E, Rame JP, Babin E, Samama G, De Raucourt D, et al. Macroscopic lymph-node involvement and neck dissection predict lymph-node recurrence in papillary thyroid carcinoma. Eur J Endocrinol. 2008;158:551-60.
7. Lundgren CI, Hall P, Dickman PW, Zedenius J. Clinically significant prognostic factors for differentiated thyroid carcinoma: a population-based, nested case-control study. Cancer. 2006;106:524-31.
8. Podnos YD, Smith D, Wagman LD, Ellenhorn JD. The implication of lymph node metastasis on survival in patients with well-differentiated thyroid cancer. Am Surg. 2005;71:731-4.
9. Leboulleux S, Rubino C, Baudin E, Caillou B, Hartl DM, Bidart JM, et al. Prognostic factors for persistent or recurrent disease of papillary thyroid carcinoma with neck lymph node metastases and/or tumor extension beyond the thyroid capsule at initial diagnosis. Endocrinol Metab. 2005;90:5723-9.
10. Mazzaferri EL, Young RL. Papillary thyroid carcinoma: a 10 year follow-up report of the impact of therapy in 576 patients. Am J Med. 1981;70:511-8.
11. Stack BC, Ferris RL, Goldenberg D, Haymart M, Shaha A, Sheth S, et al. American Thyroid Association consensus review and statement regarding the anatomy, terminology, and rationale for lateral neck dissection in differentiated thyroid cancer. Thyroid. 2012;22:501-8.
12. Choi YJ, Yun JS, Kook SH, Jung EC, Park YL. Clinical and imaging assessment of cervical lymph node metastasis in papillary thyroid carcinomas. World J Surg. 2010;34:1494-9.
13. Xing M, Westra WH, Tufano RP, Cohen Y, Rosenbaum E, Rhoden KJ, et al. BRAF mutation predicts a poorer clinical prognosis for papillary thyroid cancer. J Clin Endocrinol Metab. 2005;90: 6373-9.
14. Cooper DS, Doherty GM, Haugen BR, Kloos RT, Lee SL, Mandel SJ, et al. Revised American Thyroid Association management guidelines for patients with thyroid nodules and differentiated thyroid cancer. Thyroid. 2009;19:1167-214.
15. Lesnik D, Cunnane ME, Zurakowski D, Acar GO, Ecevit C, Mace A, et al. Papillary thyroid carcinoma nodal surgery directed by a preoperative radiographic map utilizing CT scan and ultrasound in all primary and reoperative patients. Head Neck. 2014;36:191-202.
16. Salmaslıoğlu A, Erbil Y, Cıtlak G, Ersöz F, Sarı S, Olmez A, et al. Diagnostic value of thyroglobulin measurement in fine-needle aspiration biopsy for detecting metastatic lymph nodes in patients with papillary thyroid carcinoma. Langenbecks Arch Surg. 2011;396:77-81.
17. Zhao WJ, Luo H, Zhou YM, Dai WY, Zhu JQ. Evaluating the effectiveness of prophylactic central neck dissection with total thyroidectomy for cN0 papillary thyroid carcinoma: an updated meta-analysis. Eur J Surg Oncol. 2017;43:1989-2000.

18. Zhao W, You L, Hou X, Chen S, Ren X, Chen G, et al. The effect of prophylactic central neck dissection on locoregional recurrence in papillary thyroid cancer after total thyroidectomy: a systematic review and meta-analysis: pCND for the locoregional recurrence of papillary thyroid cancer. Ann Surg Oncol. 2017;24:2189-98.

19. Wang TS, Cheung K, Farrokhyar F, Roman SA, Sosa JA. A meta-analysis of the effect of prophylactic central compartment neck dissection on locoregional recurrence rates in patients with papillary thyroid cancer. Ann Surg Oncol. 2013;20:3477-83.

20. Zetoune T, Keutgen X, Buitrago D, Aldailami H, Shao H, Mazumdar M, et al. Prophylactic central neck dissection and local recurrence in papillary thyroid cancer: a meta-analysis. Ann Surg Oncol. 2010;17:3287-93.

21. Khokhar MT, Day KM, Sangal RB, Ahmedli NN, Pisharodi LR, Beland MD, et al. Preoperative high-resolution ultrasound for the assessment of malignant central compartment lymph nodes in papillary thyroid cancer. Thyroid. 2015;25:1351-4.

22. Scherl S, Mehra S, Clain J, Dos Reis LL, Persky M, Turk A, et al. The effect of surgeon experience on the detection of metastatic lymph nodes in the central compartment and the pathologic features of clinically unapparent metastatic lymph nodes: what are we missing when we don't perform a prophylactic dissection of central compartment lymph nodes in papillary thyroid cancer? Thyroid. 2014;24:1282-8.

23. Wang TS, Evans DB, Fareau GG, Carroll T, Yen TW. Effect of prophylactic central compartment neck dissection on serum thyroglobulin and recommendations for adjuvant radioactive iodine in patients with differentiated thyroid cancer. Ann Surg Oncol. 2012;19:4217-22.

24. Lang BH, Lee GC, Ng CP, Wong KP, Wan KY, Lo CY. Evaluating the morbidity and efficacy of reoperative surgery in the central compartment for persistent/recurrent papillary thyroid carcinoma. World J Surg. 2013;37:2853-9.

25. Tufano RP, Bishop J, Wu G. Reoperative central compartment dissection for patients with recurrent/persistent papillary thyroid cancer: efficacy, safety, and the association of the BRAF mutation. Laryngoscope. 2012;122:1634-40.

26. Sosa JA, Bowman HM, Tielsch JM, Powe NR, Gordon TA, Udelsman R. The importance of surgeon experience for clinical and economic outcomes from thyroidectomy. Ann Surg. 1998;228:320-30.

27. Carty SE, Cooper DS, Doherty GM, Duh QY, Kloos RT, Mandel SJ, et al. Consensus Statement on the Terminology and Classification of Central Neck Dissection for Thyroid Cancer. Thyroid. 2009;19:1153-8.

28. Nishida T, Nakao K, Hamaji M, Kamiike W, Kurozumi K, Matsuda H. Preservation of recurrent laryngeal nerve invaded by differentiated thyroid cancer. Ann Surg. 1997;226:85-91.

29. Roh JL, Kim JM, Park CI. Lateral cervical lymph node metastases from papillary thyroid carcinoma: pattern of nodal metastases and optimal strategy for neck dissection. Ann Surg Oncol. 2008;15:1177-82.

30. Farrag T, Lin F, Brownlee N, Kim M, Sheth S, Tufano RP. Is routine dissection of level II-B and V-A necessary in patients with papillary thyroid cancer undergoing lateral neck dissection for FNA-confirmed metastases in other levels. World J Surg. 2009;33:1680-3.

31. Randolph GW, Duh QY, Heller KS, LiVolsi VA, Mandel SJ, Steward DL, et al. The prognostic significance of nodal metastases from papillary thyroid carcinoma can be stratified based on the size and number of metastatic lymph nodes, as well as the presence of extranodal extension. Thyroid. 2012;22:1144-52.

CHAPTER 22

Principles of Neck Dissection in Medullary Thyroid Cancer

Aarathi Vijayashanker, Kushagra Gaurav, Akshay Anand, Abhinav Arun Sonkar

◇| INTRODUCTION

Unlike the more common differentiated thyroid carcinoma (DTC), medullary thyroid cancer or carcinoma (MTC) is an uncommon entity consisting for about 4–5% of all thyroid cancers. Parafollicular cells or C cells are the cells of origin of MTC.[1] MTC may be found in both hereditary and sporadic backgrounds. Although largely indolent in local growth, it can be invasive and metastatic, spreading most commonly to the locoregional group of lymph nodes (in neck and mediastinum), amplifying poor prognosis.[2] Because these parafollicular cells do not secrete the thyroid hormone, MTCs and their metastases do not typically concentrate radioactive iodine. Hence, MTCs are not amenable to hormonal manipulation or ablative therapy, leaving surgical clearance to be the only effective choice of curative therapy for residual/recurrent and nodal disease. For progressive or metastatic disease, in addition to re-resection, newer Food and Drug Administration (FDA)-approved targeted molecular therapies are becoming available. However, their long-term efficacy remains under scrutiny.

◇| C CELLS AND THEIR ORIGIN

First identified in dog thyroid by Baber in 1876, C cells initially were considered to have originated from the cephalic neural crest cells that supposedly invaded the branchial arches of the developing mammalian pharyngeal apparatus during early embryological development. These cells, of neuroectodermal origin, apparently migrate to diverse locations, including derivatives of the brachial arches such as the ultimobranchial glands, which are paired organs that arise from the foregut endoderm of future inferior pharynx (fourth pharyngeal pouch). During mammalian embryological development, the ultimobranchial glands coalesce with the embryonic thyroid, bringing C cell precursors to it and embedding them in its connective tissue. The C cells then spread into the thyroid, but mostly remain limited to the superolateral aspects of the thyroid, while the lower-third of the thyroid remains mostly devoid of C cells. However, this concept has been recently found to be faulty. Genetic lineage studies in mice have tilted the dispute of ancestry in favor of an endodermal origin of C cells in mammals.[3,4]

The C cells consist about 2–4% of the thyroid gland and produce calcitonin, important for calcium homeostasis. A rise of serum calcium concentration triggers C cells to release calcitonin, which in turn inhibit the osteoclast activity thereby reducing serum calcium levels. While important for calcium homeostasis, calcitonin from C cells is not indispensable to the human body. Post total thyroidectomy for various reasons, studies in humans have showed no change in bone mass or fracture rates, suggesting compensation from other sources. Thus, the exact physiological role of the hormone in humans remains to be elucidated. Thus, role of calcitonin in MTC is limited to its use and calibration as a biomarker of MTC disease and recurrence. The rarity of the tumor can be attributed partly to the minority of its progenitor cell population.[4,5]

◇| ETIOLOGY OF MTC

The development of MTC from C cells is believed through stepwise progression via C cell hyperplasia. Though yet to be elucidated in sporadic cases, such C cell hyperplasia arising before and giving rise to pathological MTC is more evident in hereditary cases. Identified to be a distinct tumor of the thyroid over 100 years ago, its origin from the C cell was not recognized until much later when immunohistochemical localization linked thyroidal calcitonin to the C cell.

The primary initiating event in tumorigenesis is somatic or germline mutations in the *RET* proto-oncogene. This gene is mapped on chromosome 10q11.2 and is responsible for encoding a single transmembrane protein of the receptor tyrosine kinase (RTK) family.[6] RET receptors are highly expressed in C cells as compared to most other cell types. Hence, their undue activation would be naturally leading to hyperplasia. While germline RET mutations are responsible for all hereditary MTC, up to 23–40% of sporadic tumors may also harbor somatic mutations in them.[7,8] Activation of *RAS* gene family members are alternate oncogenic pathways with mutations responsible in up to 43% of sporadic MTCs.[9] Other mutations may include members of RB1 and TP53 tumor suppressor pathways. While RAS mutations do not have a bearing on tumor biology, RB1 and TP53 mutations are known to cause aggressive disease. The autosomal dominant familial syndromes characterized by RET-mutated

MTCs, collectively known as multiple endocrine neoplasia type 2 (MEN 2), carry unique genotypic and phenotypic expression. The age of onset of disease, presence or absence of C cell hyperplasia, the tumor growth rate, and subsequent lymphatic and distant spread vary according to the causative mutation in the *RET* gene.[10] Therefore, knowledge of these mutations allows for stratification of patient into various risk groups—moderate, high, and highest risk groups—depending on risk of early development and progression of disease. Thus, it helps in identifying high-risk young children at an earlier age who have inherited these mutations and have high propensity to inherit the disease and curing them by "prophylactic" thyroidectomy (i.e., before the development of identifiable tumor) with or without central nodal dissection. Hence, reducing chances of morbidity and mortality due to disease spread.

MEN 2A presents with near total penetrance of bilateral and multifocal MTC in their patients. In addition, they also manifest with pheochromocytomas (50%), and primary hyperparathyroidism (25%). The most common mutation in MEN 2A is in *RET* 634. Other rare features include cutaneous lichen amyloidosis and Hirschsprung's disease. The natural course of MEN 2A depends on the codon mutation and commonly falls in the moderate (ATA-MOD) or high-risk (ATA-H) categories—mutation in MEN 2A is most commonly seen in codon 634 (up to 80%); others occurring in exons 10, 13, and 14—codons 609, 611, 618, and 620 (exon 10), codon 768 (exon 13), codon 804 (exon 14).

Meanwhile, MEN 2B is characterized by an early onset of disease at infancy or childhood. While also often having pheochromocytomas, and rarely hyperparathyroidism, they also show a variety of lesions such as ganglioneuromas of the gastrointestinal (GI) tract, neuromas in mucosal linings, megacolon, and characteristic marfanoid habitus. MEN 2B is characterized by most aggressive MTC disease—most frequently germline mutation is in codon 918 [exon 16, p.M918T (methionine to threonine)] 95%; second most common is in codon 883 (exon 15). These mutations pose the highest level of risk of aggressive MTC (ATA-highest). MTC in these cases usually develops during infancy and characterized by early lymph nodal metastases further disease spread.

Familial MTC is considered and classified as MEN 2A variant, with the least aggressive disease course. They only inherit MTC and no other endocrine tumor or any other lesion. The most common mutations in familial medullary thyroid cancer (FMTC) are detected in codons 620, 630, and 634.

◇| CLINICAL FEATURES OF MTC

True to their indolent nature, primary MTC may be locally invasive and may invade laryngotracheal complex, carotid arteries, internal jugular veins, recurrent laryngeal nerves (RLNs), and the esophagus. Hereditary variants are characterized by presence of bilateral C cell hyperplasia

ultimately leading to multiple foci of disease. When compared to the differentiated cancers of thyroid, propensity of lymph nodal spread is higher in MTC. Central compartment and mediastinal group of lymph nodes are commonly involved (85–98%). In about 50–75% cases ipsilateral cervical lymph nodes level I–V are involved **(Fig. 1)**. Contralateral or opposite side cervical nodes are seen in up to 15–20% of patients. Lymph node spread acts as an indirect prognostic indicator of disease. Higher the burden of primary tumor, greater is the locoregional lymph nodal burden and higher are the chances of distant spread. Though not uncommon, small subcentimetric MTC nodules present with distant metastasis; this scenario is more often observed in hereditary cases. Hematogenously spreads to the liver, lungs, bone, and other tissues.

Survival in MTC is influenced by multiple factors—age, disease stage, preoperative and postoperative calcitonin levels, and calcitonin doubling time (DT). A study quotes that the 10-year survival rate in those patients who did not achieve biochemical cure was reduced to 73% compared with 100% in patients who had achieved the same.[11] The fairly high survival rates of patients not achieving complete biochemical cure reconfirm the indolent nature and emphasize on utilizing therapeutic strategies that further enhances survival, including reoperation when feasible.

◇| PRINCIPLES OF TREATMENT OF MTC

Several unique features of MTC guide their treatment, making them different from the management of DTC. C cell origin results in no uptake/metabolism of iodine and hence radioiodine ablation and therapy remains essentially ineffective. Being parafollicular in origin, MTCs do not respond to thyroid-stimulating hormone (TSH) suppressive therapy as well, leaving surgery as the only possible curative option. Second, MTCs are multifocal and bilateral in over 90% of hereditary cases and 10–20% of sporadic cases with concomitant presence of diffuse C cell hyperplasia, making total thyroidectomy always the bare minimum surgical approach of choice over lobectomy or hemithyroidectomy. Third, occult or overt lymph nodal involvement is seen in approximately three-fourths of patients with clinical disease, correlating directly with serum calcitonin levels.[12] This makes central compartment neck dissection mandatory in all patients of primary MTC, increasing the morbidity of surgical therapy when compared to that for DTC. Finally, postoperative measurements of stimulated calcitonin and carcinoembryonic antigen (CEA) allow monitoring of persistent or recurrent disease.

It is recommended that all patients of histologically proven MTC should undergo genetic analysis to detect presence of germline RET mutation. If confirmed, pheochromocytomas and hyperparathyroidism should be screened for. Baseline serum calcitonin levels are documented. Regardless of high calcitonin levels, preoperative systemic imaging, primarily

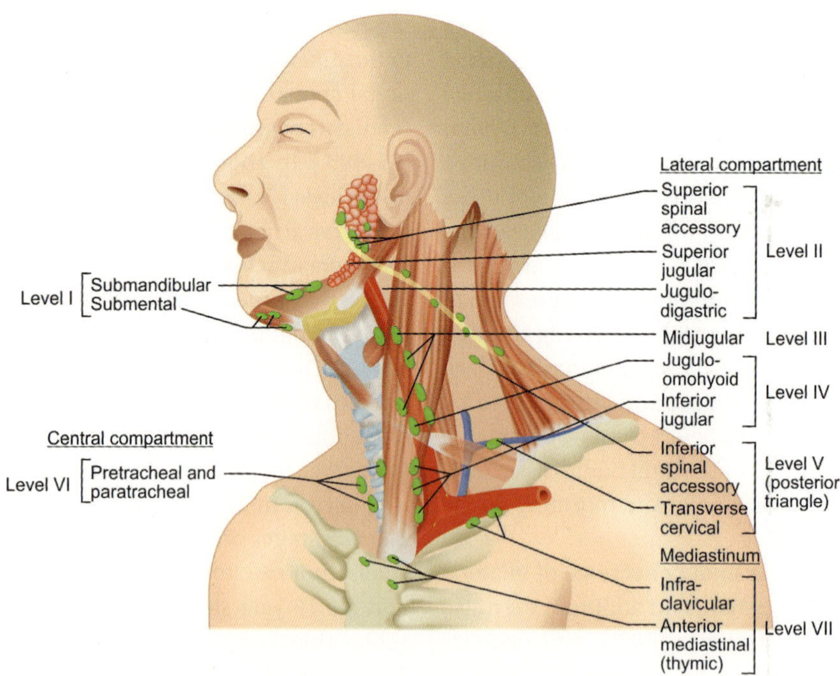

Fig. 1: Lymph node groups in the neck.
Source: Adapted from Fialkowski EA, Moley JF. Current approaches to medullary thyroid carcinoma, sporadic and familial. J Surg Oncol. 2006;94:737-47.

with contrast-enhanced chest computed tomography (CT) scan, axial magnetic resonance imaging (MRI) or CT of the abdomen, and bone scan, are indicated in case of extensive neck disease with or without signs and symptoms of metastases.[13,14]

EVALUATION OF CERVICAL LYMPH NODES

The management of lymph nodal metastases in MTC has seen a gradual evolution from the 1970s until now, from selective lymphadenectomy of grossly enlarged nodes to a more systematic lymphadenectomy of defined compartments according to the stage of tumor.[15,16] The extent of cervical lymph nodal dissection depends on the preoperative high frequency neck ultrasound, preoperative serum calcitonin levels as well as intraoperative examination of lymph nodal metastases. Intraoperative assessment of lymph nodes by surgeons, however useful, has an alarmingly low sensitivity (64%) and specificity (71%), missing more than one-third of the involved lymph nodes.[17] While the European societies often rely heavily on basal serum calcitonin levels for prediction of lymph nodal involvement, the Americans utilize preoperative ultrasound of the neck to map the same. Involved lymph nodes are usually multiple, hard nodes—abnormal in morphology with fatty hilum loss, and there may be certain areas of calcifications as well.[18,19]

The lymph nodal involvement depends moreover on two factors—the size of the primary tumor and its location. Elucidation of this pattern and their frequencies gain importance in the surgical plan, and hence all compartments should be deliberately addressed with utmost surgical

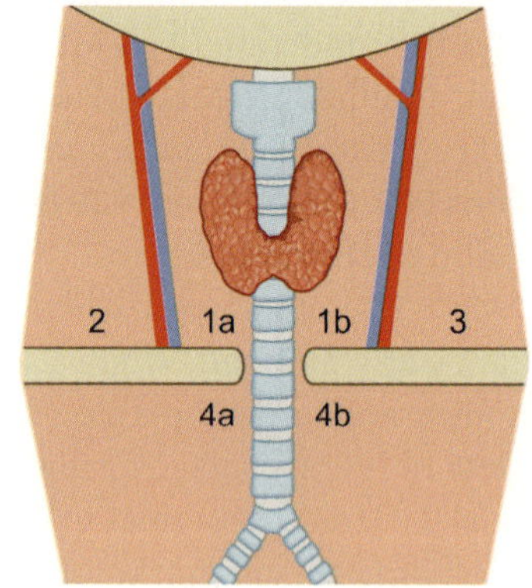

Fig. 2: Compartmental definition of the cervicomediastinal lymph nodal system.
Source: Adapted from Reference 15.

precision at the very first thyroidectomy surgery, given the increased rate of complications of redo neck surgery. In 1994, Henning Dralle et al. published a topographic definition of the anatomy of the cervicomediastinal compartments of lymph nodes for uniformity in accomplishment and analysis of the undertaken systematic lymphadenectomy. At this time, controversy regarding the ideal game plan for lymph nodes was ongoing. Nonetheless, this anatomic definition forms the basis of principles of lymphadenectomy even today **(Fig. 2)**.[15]

- *Compartment 1*: The cervicocentral lymph nodes, right and left paratracheal nodes, extend between the trachea in midline till the carotid sheath as lateral border in horizontal extent, and from the hyoid bone to the brachiocephalic vein in vertical extent (submandibular lymph nodes are included in this group).

Table 1: Compartmental hierarchy of locoregional lymph node involvement in 37 patients with recurrent node-positive sporadic medullary thyroid carcinoma.

Compartment involved	pT1 (n = 2)	pT2 (n = 23)	pT3 (n = 6)	pT4 (n = 6)	Total (n = 37)
Ipsilateral central neck (%)	100	70	50	75	70
Ipsilateral lateral neck (%)	100	71	60	60	66
Contralateral central neck (%)	100	32	50	100	48
Mediastinum (%)	50	29	25	83	39
Contralateral lateral neck (%)	0	27	33	50	30

Source: Adapted from Gimm O, Ukkat J, Dralle H. Determinative factors of biochemical cure after primary and reoperative surgery for sporadic medullary thyroid carcinoma. World J Surg. 1998;22:562-8.

- *Compartments 2 and 3*: The right and left cervicolateral lymph nodes between the carotid sheath and trapezius, from the subclavian vein up to the hypoglossal nerve, lymphatics around the fascicles of the cervical plexus.
- *Compartment 4*: Mediastinal lymph nodes on both sides of the trachea from the left brachiocephalic vein down to the tracheal bifurcation within the anterior and posterior part of the mediastinum.

Tumors located toward the upper pole of thyroid spread first to the upper and middle jugular group of nodes on same side, whereas tumors in the remaining gland metastasize initially to the level 6 and level 7 group of nodes. Also, tumors of the upper pole, involving the ipsilateral lateral compartment nodes, pre- and paratracheal group involvement may be absent in one-fourth of cases.[20] Apart from the location, the lateral cervical lymph nodal involvement on either side is also affected by central group of nodal involvement—higher the central group involved, higher is the lateral nodal involvement **(Table 1)**. While ipsilateral lymphatic spread is amenable to surgical cure in many patients, metastases to the contralateral lateral compartment usually herald incurable disease.[21]

The basal serum calcitonin levels (preoperative), although far from perfect, are a useful tool in determining the extent of lymph node metastases in MTC. Studies show that calcitonin levels correlate well with disease burden. Nodal involvement is commonly seen at levels 10–40 pg/mL. Levels >150 pg/mL almost always are associated with huge burden of locoregional disease and possible distant metastases and frequently with >1,000 pg/mL. Extensive distant metastasis in an incurable disease state is evident with levels >3,000 pg/mL.[19]

Carcinoembryonic antigen is nonspecific prognostic biomarker. Preoperative CEA levels are also helpful in risk stratification; normal levels suggest good prognosis disease with sufficiently good overall survival but levels >30 ng/mL are associated with highly likelihood of advanced incurable disease, hence a poorer prognosis.[22] Both serum calcitonin and CEA are recorded preoperatively and postoperatively at regular intervals—initially at 3–6 months and then annually. *Calcitonin and CEA DT*: The time, they need to double the serum concentration, is recorded in postoperative follow-up. Online calculators are available on internet for their calculation.

The curve of the DT signifies the rate of recurrence and poor prognosis in a recurrent disease.

◇ ROLE OF SENTINEL LYMPH NODE BIOPSY IN MTC

In the absence of central compartment nodes, in patients of subcentimetric, intrathyroidal MTCs with low serum calcitonin, there have been few studies indicating a possible future role of sentinel lymph node biopsy (SLNB) in identifying the jugulo-carotid group of lymph nodes. SLNB procedure is performed by injecting of 1% methylene blue dye (0.2–0.5 mL) subcapsularly. After total thyroidectomy and central neck dissection, blue-stained *"Sentinel"* lateral cervical lymph nodes (level II/III) on either side are sent are frozen section evaluation. If SLNB report comes out to be benign, additional lymph nodal sampling is done for more accurate results. If SLNB report comes out to be malignant, a single-setting modified radical neck dissection is done. More studies with larger sample sizes and higher evidence are however needed to validate the true usefulness of this procedure.[23]

Central Compartment Dissection

In patients with histologically proven MTC, total thyroidectomy along with lymph nodal dissection of the central compartment (level VI) is the most apt surgical approach of choice in view of frequent multicentricity and occult nodes. In the absence of palpable nodes in the central compartment, en bloc microdissection (using magnifying glasses) of central compartment for staging purpose of even tumors of size 10 mm or less (pT1) may show metastasis in as high as 33% of them.[24] Some authors advocate avoid addressing level VI prophylactically in the absence of enlarged nodes when the serum calcitonin levels are <20 pg/mL.[19] However, the Task Force of American Thyroid Association published their recommendations in 2015 and did not support this practice unanimously.[13] A stepwise, compartment-based dissection of neck nodes can improve survival rates and decrease recurrence rates. A berry picking approach to lymph node removal has long been discouraged. The thyroidectomy technique follows the principles of oncological clearance, including central compartment dissection as well. The standard procedure includes a collar incision in front of the neck, elevating superior and inferior preplatysmal flaps. Incising the midline linea, retracting strap muscles laterally, exposes the thyroid gland. The strap muscles may need to be excised only in T4 cancers or reoperative operations. The lobe on the tumor side is mobilized first, and the middle thyroid vein ligated and divided. The RLN needs to be carefully identified in tracheoesophageal groove, while using adjuncts like intraoperative nerve monitoring for preservation. The pedicles are controlled one after the other, in inferior to superior fashion, as the gland and lymphatics are reflected from the underlying cartilages till the midline. The contralateral dissection is done similarly, by lateral to medial approach. Ultimately, thyroid lobes, lymph nodal tissue, and all fibrofatty tissue are removed. This will extirpate prelaryngeal, pretracheal, and unilateral or bilateral paratracheal lymph nodes. All the parathyroids are identified and preserved. Some surgeons believe that leaving the parathyroids in place may compromise the adequacy of lymph node clearance while also risking devascularizing the glands. In that case, the parathyroid glands are retrieved from neck and kept in ice cold saline, confirmed by parathyroid hormone (PTH) aspirate or frozen section analysis and then autotransplanted into the muscle (sternocleidomastoid/brachioradialis).[10,13,25]

Lateral Compartment Dissection

As previously mentioned, regionally involved lymph nodes in MTC are managed exclusively with surgical extirpation since they are NOT radioactive iodine-avid. The volume of disease in the central compartment lymph nodes can often help in predicting lateral compartment metastasis. The ground work for this prediction was laid by a retrospective analysis of compartment-oriented lymphadenectomy for MTC that showed that is approximately 10% chances of lymph nodal involvement in lateral compartment (same side) in the absence of involved central nodes.[21] A modified radical neck dissection should be performed in meticulous manner dissecting out all lymph nodal tissue from level I–V in all cases with clinical/sonological evidence of enlarged pathological lymph nodes I lateral compartment, locally advanced disease and based on calcitonin levels. Prophylactic ipsilateral lateral neck dissection is done if there is evidence of central lymph node involvement (preoperative or intraoperative), while prophylactic contralateral dissection is advised in the presence of similarly enlarged ipsilateral lateral nodes or serum calcitonin levels above 200 pg/mL. The standard incision includes a U-shaped collar incision, and when required, a Y-shaped median extension onto manubrium sterni for median sternotomy. In case of lateral compartment involvement, it is cleared first, followed by en bloc central compartment dissection. After raising adequate subplatysmal flaps, the flaps are retracted and fixed on both sides. The carotid sheath is accessed from the medial aspect of the sternocleidomastoid muscle. The sheath is bared from the carotid bifurcation cranially, to the level of venous angle (subclavian-internal jugular venous junction) inferiorly. Similarly, the lateral compartment of lymphatics along the internal jugular vein is prepared from caudal to cranial fashion. The level V lymph nodes along with all fibrofatty tissues are removed, preserving the cervical plexus and the spinal accessory nerve. If anterior mediastinal nodes are involved, the suprabrachiocephalic and infrabrachiocephalic nodes are dissected en bloc with the mediastinal and cervical thymus via the transsternal approach before central neck dissection.[26,27]

HEREDITARY MTC AND LYMPH NODAL METASTASES

While the goal of surgery in primary MTC is complete removal of tumor, in hereditary MTC syndromes, the goal is resection before malignant transformation. Children with MEN 2A fall within the category of moderate or high risk depending on the harbored mutation. Central compartment dissection can be safely avoided in such cases where basal calcitonin is not raised. Only total thyroidectomy will suffice to their surgical treatment. This obviously also reduces injury chances to RLN and parathyroid. In case of enlarged lymph nodes or raised calcitonin levels, central compartment dissection is recommended. Those at moderate risk should be annually examined starting at 5 years of age—for occurrence of any suspicious thyroid nodules and/or cervical lymphadenopathy along with neck imaging by high resolution ultrasound, and measurement of annual serum calcitonin levels, and undergo surgery in early childhood or young adulthood. It is recommended that children of high-risk category should be operated at or before 5 years of age. MEN 2B patients harboring *RET* M918T mutations belonging to the highest risk category, the MTC is highly aggressive, often established at birth and therefore, thyroidectomy with central compartment dissection is recommended within the period of infancy, even as early as in the first 6 months of life. Central compartment dissection may be avoided in cases with normal calcitonin levels and in the absence of suspicious lymph nodes. The parathyroid glands should be identified and handled with utmost care to be left in situ. In cases of inadvertent parathyroidectomy, gland should be autotransplanted or cryopreserved for future if hypoparathyroidism occurs. All efforts should be made to avoid such events because hypoparathyroidism in a child can be disastrous.[13]

IDENTIFICATION AND MANAGEMENT OF RECURRENT MTC

Unduly raised calcitonin levels after primary surgery hint toward residual or recurrent disease, most commonly occurring due to residual central compartment lymph nodes.

Postsurgery calcitonin and CEA levels should be checked at 3 months initially and further repeat measurement should be after every 6 months for 1 year, and then annually thereafter in cases if values are found to be normal or near normal. Though debatable but many authors support the fact that calcitonin levels reach normalcy with 3 months of period. Serum CEA takes longer and is hence less preferred as a predictor.[28] Levels below 150 pg/mL warrant a fresh neck ultrasound and examination, while levels above 150 pg/mL warrants workup for distant metastases.[28,29] For patients with nonmetastatic, persistent biochemical or locoregional disease, Tisell introduced his technique of microdissection involving a meticulous clearance of all lymphatics and fat of the central and lateral compartment.[30] MTC is an indolent tumor, and many patients may present with biochemical evidence of persistently raised calcitonin despite all possible surgical clearance and with no evidence of disease on imaging, such patients are grouped under an entity—"Persistent hypercalcitoninemia." These patients continue to fare well with remarkable 5- and 10-year survival rates of 90% and 86%, respectively.[31] Palliative debulking of tumor is only indicated in certain scenarios—with tracheal compression features, metastatic disease with intractable pain, and systemic symptoms of flushing and diarrhea. While resurgery in experienced hands can lead to biochemical cure in over 33% of patients, the procedure bears the disadvantage of significantly increased morbidity and chances of complications, such as chyle fistula, RLN injury, and permanent hypoparathyroidism.[32] For such reoperative cases, preoperative imaging in form of CT scan or MRI is must. Other intraoperative adjuncts like intraoperative neuromonitoring, surgical loupes, harmonic or vessels sealer as advanced generation bipolar energy devices in reoperation increase precision and accuracy of surgery thereby complications are minimized in experienced hands. In children, these reoperative surgeries could be lead to permanent hypoparathyroidism as there is difficulty in identifying parathyroids—due to the small size of the parathyroids and absence of surrounding fat. A lateral approach (instead of the traditional, midline access through the center of strap muscles) through opening the lateral space between the straps and carotids to reach thyroid bed provides less chances of injury as this is usually a naive plane with minimal fibrous scar tissue and surgically at ease to address; important structures like RLN and parathyroids lie in tracheoesophageal groove quite far from point of entry—theoretically, this decreases their injury.[33]

ROLE OF RADIOTHERAPY

No level 1 evidences are available at the moment that validates the benefit of adjuvant radiotherapy following thyroidectomy in MTC. Since long-term survival is good in patients of MTC,

a valid end point in most patients can also be locoregional disease control. Although radiotherapy may not have any advantages in terms of overall survival, studies have shown that they may have a role in reducing locoregional recurrence-free survival in given postoperatively (86% vs. 52%).[34] Progressive disease in the neck can significantly impact the quality of life of patients. Since radiotherapy will make redo surgery more difficult, patient choice is of utmost importance. After weighing the potential benefits of this therapy against the risks of acute and chronic toxicities of external beam radiotherapy, postoperative doses ranging from 60 to 66 Gy to the thyroid bed over a span of 6 weeks can be given to patients who are having high risk of recurrence and are poor candidates of reoperative surgery with multiple comorbidities. In case of gross residual disease, 70 Gy or more may be used. Intensity modulated radiotherapy (IMRT) may allow for dose escalations. Depending on necessity, one or both of the lateral compartments may be encompassed in the filed.[13]

ROLE OF TARGETED THERAPY FOR LOCOREGIONAL DISEASE

While predominantly used for systemic control of symptomatic metastases and secretory symptoms, targeted therapy also has locoregional benefits. It may be used in conditions where resurgery and radiotherapy are not viable treatment options or have been exhausted. The primarily used families of drugs are tyrosine kinase inhibitors (TKIs) and monoclonal antibodies (mAbs). TKIs, cabozantinib and vandetanib, are FDA-approved, first-line TKIs of choice. Vandetanib and cabozantinib provide progression-free survivals of 30.5 and 11.2 months, respectively. The main limitation of these modes of management is that after a variable period of treatment, the cancer cells develop resistance. Studies on new and reliable molecular therapies are underway.[13,35]

CONCLUSION

Medullary thyroid cancer is a unique tumor of thyroid with a definite surgical role in its management in each clinical setting, beginning with prophylactic surgery in RET mutation carriers, through curative surgery for early tumors, re-explorative surgery in locally advanced, recurrent or persistent disease, to palliative debulking in metastatic, symptomatic disease. The tumor's predilection to affect lymph nodes is its defining characteristic. Adequate primary surgery of the tumor and lymph nodes is the mainstay of treatment. Eradication of involved lymph nodes along with the primary tumor confers disease control and long-term survival. Therefore, an excellent knowledge of the surgical anatomy of thyroid and its lymph nodal drainage system is necessary. One must also need to know the concepts of both sporadic and hereditary domains of disease.

◇| REFERENCES

1. Hundahl SA, Fleming ID, Fremgen AM, Menck HR. A National Cancer Data Base report on 53,856 cases of thyroid carcinoma treated in the US, 1985–1995. Cancer. 1998;83(12):2638-48.
2. Machens A, Hauptmann S, Dralle H. Increased risk of lymph node metastasis in multifocal hereditary and sporadic medullary thyroid cancer. World J Surg. 2007;31(10):1960-5.
3. Cote GJ, Grubbs EG, Hofmann M-C. Thyroid C-cell biology and oncogenic transformation. Recent Results Cancer Res. 2015;204:1-39.
4. Nilsson M, Williams D. On the origin of cells and derivation of thyroid cancer: C cell story revisited. Eur Thyroid J. 2016;5(2): 79-93.
5. Felsenfeld AJ, Levine BS. Calcitonin, the forgotten hormone: does it deserve to be forgotten? Clin Kidney J. 2015;8(2):180-7.
6. Santoro M, Carlomagno F, Romano A, Bottaro DP, Dathan NA, Grieco M, et al. Activation of RET as a dominant transforming gene by germline mutations of MEN2A and MEN2B. Science. 1995;267(5196):381-3.
7. Eng C, Mulligan LM, Smith DP, Healey CS, Frilling A, Raue F, et al. Mutation of the RET protooncogene in sporadic medullary thyroid carcinoma. Genes Chromosomes Cancer. 1995;12(3):209-12.
8. Romei C, Ciampi R, Casella F, Tacito A, Torregrossa L, Ugolini C, et al. RET mutation heterogeneity in primary advanced medullary thyroid cancers and their metastases. Oncotarget. 2018;9(11):9875-84.
9. Moura MM, Cavaco BM, Leite V. RAS proto-oncogene in medullary thyroid carcinoma. Endocr Relat Cancer. 2015;22(5):R235-52.
10. Jin LX, Moley JF. Surgery for lymph node metastases of medullary thyroid carcinoma: a review. Cancer. 2016;122(3):358-66.
11. Rendl G, Manzl M, Hitzl W, Sungler P, Pirich C. Long-term prognosis of medullary thyroid carcinoma. Clin Endocrinol (Oxf). 2008;69(3):497-505.
12. Dralle H. Lymph node dissection and medullary thyroid carcinoma. Br J Surg. 2002;89(9):1073-5.
13. Wells SA, Asa SL, Dralle H, Elisei R, Evans DB, Gagel RF, et al. Revised American Thyroid Association Guidelines for the Management of Medullary Thyroid Carcinoma. Thyroid. 2015;25(6):567-610.
14. Giraudet AL, Vanel D, Leboulleux S, Aupérin A, Dromain C, Chami L, et al. Imaging medullary thyroid carcinoma with persistent elevated calcitonin levels. J Clin Endocrinol Metab. 2007;92(11):4185-90.
15. Dralle H, Damm I, Wilhelm Scheumann GF, Kotzerke J, Kupsch E, Geerlings H, et al. Compartment-oriented microdissection of regional lymph nodes in medullary thyroid carcinoma. Surg Today. 1994;24(2):112-21.
16. Fleming JB, Lee JE, Bouvet M, Schultz PN, Sherman SI, Sellin RV, et al. Surgical strategy for the treatment of medullary thyroid carcinoma. Ann Surg. 1999;230(5):697-707.
17. Moley JF, DeBenedetti MK. Patterns of nodal metastases in palpable medullary thyroid carcinoma: recommendations for extent of node dissection. Ann Surg. 1999;229(6):880-7; discussion 887-8.
18. Daniels GH. Screening for medullary thyroid carcinoma with serum calcitonin measurements in patients with thyroid nodules in the United States and Canada. Thyroid. 2011;21(11):1199-207.
19. Machens A, Dralle H. Biomarker-based risk stratification for previously untreated medullary thyroid cancer. J Clin Endocrinol Metab. 2010;95(6):2655-63.
20. Dralle H, Machens A. Surgical management of the lateral neck compartment for metastatic thyroid cancer. Curr Opin Oncol. 2013;25(1):20-6.
21. Machens A, Hauptmann S, Dralle H. Prediction of lateral lymph node metastases in medullary thyroid cancer. Br J Surg. 2008;95(5):586-91.
22. Machens A, Ukkat J, Hauptmann S, Dralle H. Abnormal carcinoembryonic antigen levels and medullary thyroid cancer progression: a multivariate analysis. Arch Surg. 2007;142(3):289-93.
23. Dzodic R, Santrac N, Goran M, Buta M, Djurisic I, Pupic G, et al. Sentinel lymph node biopsy in medullary thyroid microcarcinomas after methylene blue dye mapping: a pilot study. J Clin Oncol. 2016;34(15_suppl):e17549-e17549.
24. Niccoli P, Wion-Barbot N, Caron P, Henry JF, de Micco C, Saint Andre JP, et al. Interest of routine measurement of serum calcitonin: study in a large series of thyroidectomized patients. The French Medullary Study Group. J Clin Endocrinol Metab. 1997;82(2):338-41.
25. Machens A, Dralle H. Surgical treatment of medullary thyroid cancer. Recent Results Cancer Res. 2015;204:187-205.
26. Machens A, Holzhausen H-J, Dralle H. Prediction of mediastinal lymph node metastasis in medullary thyroid carcinoma. Br J Surg. 2004;91(6):709-12.
27. Zhang TT, Qu N, Hu JQ, Shi RL, Wen D, Sun GH, et al. Mediastinal lymph node metastases in thyroid cancer: characteristics, predictive factors, and prognosis. Int J Endocrinol. 2017;2017:1868165.
28. Elisei R, Pinchera A. Advances in the follow-up of differentiated or medullary thyroid cancer. Nat Rev Endocrinol. 2012;8(8):466-75.
29. Pellegriti G, Leboulleux S, Baudin E, Bellon N, Scollo C, Travagli JP, et al. Long-term outcome of medullary thyroid carcinoma in patients with normal postoperative medical imaging. Br J Cancer. 2003;88(10):1537-42.
30. Tisell LE, Hansson G, Jansson S, Salander H. Reoperation in the treatment of asymptomatic metastasizing medullary thyroid carcinoma. Surgery. 1986;99(1):60-6.
31. van Heerden JA, Grant CS, Gharib H, Hay ID, Ilstrup DM. Long-term course of patients with persistent hypercalcitoninemia after apparent curative primary surgery for medullary thyroid carcinoma. Ann Surg. 1990;212(4):395-400.
32. Moley JF, Wells SA, Dilley WG, Tisell LE. Reoperation for recurrent or persistent medullary thyroid cancer. Surgery. 1993;114(6):1090-5; discussion 1095-6.
33. Singaporewalla RM, Tan BC, Rao AD. The lateral "backdoor" approach to open thyroid surgery: A comparative study. Asian J Surg. 2018;41(4):384-8.
34. Brierley J, Tsang R, Simpson WJ, Gospodarowicz M, Sutcliffe S, Panzarella T. Medullary thyroid cancer: analyses of survival and prognostic factors and the role of radiation therapy in local control. Thyroid. 1996;6(4):305-10.
35. Viola D, Valerio L, Molinaro E, Agate L, Bottici V, Biagini A, et al. Treatment of advanced thyroid cancer with targeted therapies: ten years of experience. Endocr Relat Cancer. 2016;23(4): R185-205.

Complications of Thyroidectomy

Gyan Chand, Sudhi Agarwal

INTRODUCTION

Thyroid surgery is being practiced since ages, but it was associated with high morbidity and mortality. It was considered so morbid during ancient time that it was once banned in many countries. However, with the availability of safe anesthesia, antisepsis, and homeostasis, the thyroid surgery evolved as a major reform. Due to his major contribution in reducing the surgical complications of thyroid surgeries, Theodor Kocher (1841–1917) was awarded the Nobel Prize in medicine in 1909; in fact, he was the first surgeon to receive the prestigious award. He reported in his important article in thyroid surgery in 1878 that improvement in the surgical technique reduces the mortality to practically nil; however, the morbidity from thyroidectomy is still a concern. Meticulous attention to surgical technique is required to balance between the adequacies of resection to avoid recurrences against the risk of complications. Most complications of thyroidectomy can be avoided by the detailed anatomy and the careful surgical dissection.[1-3]

The adequate experience in thyroid surgery and future collaboration with thyroid physicians will improve the quality of care and also provide confidence to deal with any legal issues. The extent of thyroid surgery must be evaluated carefully to determine benefit versus morbidity from thyroidectomy.[4]

COMPLICATIONS VERSUS NATURAL SEQUEL

Complication is an unexpected adverse result caused by thyroidectomy. Before proceeding further in details of complications, it is prudent to emphasize that there may be certain sequel, maybe of temporary or permanent in nature, which are the (1) natural results of thyroidectomy such as hypothyroidism or (2) result of the disease itself for which the thyroidectomy was performed such as tracheomalacia, which may be recognized during or after surgery.

In this chapter, we will discuss the complications as unfavorable and unintended outcome of thyroidectomy.

The post-thyroidectomy complications rate may vary in various studies. The rate of complications depends on the expertise of the surgeon, the meticulous technique used, the extent and type of goiter, and the extent of thyroidectomy.[5-8]

Hypothyroidism

Following thyroidectomy, hypothyroidism is expected as a natural sequel either immediately following total thyroidectomy or delayed, in less than total thyroidectomy. Postoperative hypothyroidism is the reasonable price for the patient to pay to avoid recurrent hyperthyroidism and cancer.

The complications of thyroidectomy may be divided into:
- *General complications:* Independent of surgical technique, e.g., circulatory, respiratory, and urinary
- *Specific complications*: Directly related to surgical technique, such as:
  - *Nerve palsy*: Laryngeal nerves (external branch of superior and recurrent)
  - Hypoparathyroidism and hypocalcemia
  - Hemorrhage
  - Injury to neighboring structures such as aerodigestive tracts, chyle leak, and pleural injury
  - Wound-related complications
- *Other complications*: Tracheomalacia, hyperthyroid crisis, and complications related to remote access thyroid surgery.

Nerve Injury

Recurrent Laryngeal Nerve Injury

The right recurrent laryngeal nerve (RLN) is a small branch of the right vagus nerve, which ascends along the tracheoesophageal groove after looping around the subclavian artery and runs an oblique course in the neck which makes it more prone to injury in the neck. The left RLN arises from the left vagus nerve at the level of arch of aorta and loops around it and then ascends along the tracheoesophageal groove, leading to longer course and making it more prone to injury than the right one.[9,10]

In 0.05% of cases, the right nerve is nonrecurrent (i.e., it arises high up in neck from vagus and enters directly into larynx without coursing back), and in unsuspected cases, it is highly prone to injury.[11,12]

Mechanisms of injury to the RLN include extensive handling and dissection along nerve, thermal insult, traction injury, crush injury, misplaced ligature, complete or partial transection, and compromised blood supply.

Injury to RLN leads to the paralysis of all the intrinsic laryngeal muscles sparing cricothyroid muscle.

Presentation:[13,14] The most important cause of postoperative hoarseness is RLN injury. Depending upon the duration of injury, the paralysis may be temporary or permanent. When the trauma is minimal, the nerve goes into neuropraxia and resumes function after a certain duration, usually within 6 months. However, when the injury is significant, the nerve may be permanently paralyzed.

- *Unilateral RLN injury*: Unilateral RLN injury paralyzes all the intrinsic laryngeal muscles leaving the cricothyroid muscle, which fixes the vocal folds in the median or paramedian position, and it does not move laterally while the patient phonates or takes a deep breath. Majority of the unilateral RLN injury usually pass undetected clinically; however, in some patients, there may be minor hoarseness without difficulty in breathing or aspiration. With the gradual compensation of healthy cord by crossing the midline and approximating the paralyzed cord, there will be improvement in voice quality over time, precluding any specific treatment.
- *Bilateral RLN injury*: Following bilateral RLN injury, all the intrinsic laryngeal muscles become paralyzed and the unopposed action of the bilateral cricothyroid muscles leads to both vocal folds fixed in the median or paramedian position. The fixed vocal cords in the paramedian position cause inadequate airway and are clinically presented as dysphonia or stridor, which becomes worst during exertion or during the attack of acute laryngitis. The voice is usually good in this situation.

Bilateral RLN palsy is very rare. More commonly, such situations are often seen in cases with already paralyzed RLN due to malignant infiltration or post-hemithyroidectomy of the contralateral lobe.

If bilateral RLN injury is unnoticed during surgery, the vocal folds go into cadaveric position and the patient expresses difficulty in breathing, requiring even tracheostomy either temporary or permanent depending upon the pattern of recovery. The possibility of bilateral RLN palsy is high in the patients undergoing reoperative thyroid surgery, malignant goiter, central compartment, lymph nodes dissection, and preoperatively diagnosed unilateral RLN palsy.

Requiring immediate reintubation due to falling saturation, or repeated failure to extubate a patient, highly suggests the possibility of bilateral RLN palsy. If the surgical team is sure about the integrity of RLN during the surgery, it is justifiable to treat the patient with systemic steroids and assisted endotracheal ventilation for few days. After weaning off the ventilator gradually, the patient is extubated in the operating room. The flexible fiberoptic is used to evaluate the larynx. No further intervention is done, if an adequate airway with functioning cords is demonstrated; otherwise, an elective tracheostomy is done to facilitate the discharge and domiciliary care of the patient. The patient is followed up for at least 6 months for spontaneous recovery.

In cases with no recovery, the patient has two options: (1) He may opt for permanent tracheostomy with speaking valves, which relieves their stridor and gives reasonably good voice, with disadvantage of tracheostomy hole in the neck or (2) he may opt for surgical lateralization of the cord with compromised quality of voice without a hole in the neck.

Evaluation: Various mechanisms may lead to postoperative hoarseness. If it occurs in the first 2–5 postoperative days, it is most likely caused by edema in the operative field.

Preoperative direct or indirect laryngoscopy must be performed in all patients with a voice change, with proven malignancy or with history of neck surgery in the past. Postoperative laryngoscopy may not be performed routinely but reserved for patients with vocal cord dysfunction, seen at the time of extubation and in patients with voice change after thyroid surgery. When vocal cord dysfunction continues for 1 year, it is most likely permanent. However, in cases with nerve re-anastomosis, the functional recovery is still possible in 1–2 years.

The functionality of vocal fold can be assessed by laryngoscopy (indirect or direct) and laryngeal electromyography (EMG). Laryngoscopy helps in demonstrating the range of mobility of the vocal cords, while laryngeal EMG helps in demonstrating the power of laryngeal muscle which helps in differentiating between the neural and extraneural factors of muscle dysfunction. The follow-up studies may give information concerning the recovery and prognosis of the patient.[15]

Prevention: The following strategies can reduce the risk of injury. The first and the foremost is the visual identification of the nerve and its extralaryngeal course. Visual identification of nerve and its extralaryngeal course, dissecting it medially and gradually separating it away from thyroid. The second method is the intraoperative electrical nerve stimulation of the nerve in addition to the visual identification to characterize the position, functionality and possibly the trajectory of RLN by observing the contractions of the cricopharyngeus muscles. The third is the uninterrupted monitoring of the laryngeal EMG activity through the electrodes placed against the posterior cricoarytenoid muscles. It reveals the changes in mechanical activities due to manipulation of the RLN during dissection.

The latter two techniques are costlier and require special instruments which may not be available at every center. They may be relatively more useful in recurrent, reoperative, and advanced malignancy cases. To conclude, the importance of the detailed anatomical knowledge and its application cannot be surpassed.[16]

Treatment: The RLN injury, if detected during the surgery, then assess the proximity of the cut ends. If the two cut ends are approximated without any tension, the end-to-end primary anastomosis must be performed. If there is loss of length, then primary neurorrhaphy may be performed by using either phrenic nerve, ansa cervicalis, or preganglionic sympathetic neurons. The animal models demonstrated good results of these neurorrhaphy; however, the results are not as impressive in humans, because of the nonselective reinnervation of abductor and adductor muscles, resulting in synkinesis.

If the nerve palsy is detected in the postoperative period, it is recommended to defer any corrective procedures before 6 months following surgery, which help to recover the reversible injury as much as possible.

Medialization (preferred) and reinnervation procedures are the available surgical options for the patients with permanent unilateral vocal cord paralysis.

In medialization, with the help of either injection laryngoplasty or laryngeal framework surgery, the impaired vocal fold is medialized to improve the contact of affected vocal fold with the contralateral normal mobile fold.

In type I thyroplasty, which is a commonly done procedure, an implant is placed at the level of the true vocal cords through a window to push the vocal fold medially. These implants are made of different materials including absorbable or not absorbable. The silicon or polytetrafluoroethylene (PTFE) are permanent implants whereas the gelatin sponge provides temporary treatment as it reabsorbs over time.

The vocal cord loses its contact with the contralateral healthy cord due to atrophy following denervation leading to voice weakness. The various reinnervation procedures help to conserve or reinstate tone of the intrinsic laryngeal musculature, which helps to maintain and improve the voice quality.[17,18]

In bilateral vocal cord paralysis, the main issue is compromised airway. Thus, the first step must be to ensure patent airway and respiration, preferably with endotracheal intubation as an initial treatment. In suspicious cases, the neck can be re-explored to ensure there is no reversible cause of nerve dysfunction such as misplaced ligature. In patients with good preservation of RLN, a trial of extubation can be attempted after few days, preferably in operation theater with full preparedness for emergency tracheostomy, if extubation fails. Supportive treatment such as intravenous steroids, neurotropics, and head elevation may help to reduce the edema. Few centers consider a second trial of extubation before emergency tracheostomy.

In most of the cases with intact nerves, the recovery occurs within 6 months following surgery and the tracheostomy is decannulated. But in cases with no recovery, the patient has to opt between the permanent tracheostomy with speaking valves or the lateralization procedures. The principal goal of lateralization procedures such as cordotomy and arytenoidectomy is to improve the airway patency but at the cost of the quality of the voice.[19]

External Branch of Superior Laryngeal Nerve[13,20]

Superior laryngeal nerve (SLN) is the branch of the vagus (inferior ganglion), which travels down behind the internal carotid artery and divides into external and internal branches at the level of the greater cornua of the hyoid bone. The internal branch enters the larynx high up and therefore is usually not at risk of injury during thyroidectomy. It provides sensory innervations to the larynx and hypopharynx. The external branch is positioned cranial to the dissection area of superior pole of thyroid juxtaposition to the superior thyroid artery. It curves medially above the superior pole of the thyroid lobe to provide motor function to the cricothyroid muscle, which helps in elongation of the ipsilateral vocal cord and creates a high-pitched sound. In singers and professional vocal, the injury to the external branch of superior laryngeal nerve (EBSLN) is a serious problem, although for some patients, symptoms are minimal and are often overlooked.

Two aspects of its anatomy are important determinants of the risk of being injured during dissection of the superior pole of thyroid:

1. The level at which it traverses the superior thyroid vessels at the superior pole of thyroid. The more near the thyroid, the more chances of injury.
2. Whether it runs superficial to or is covered with the inferior constrictor of the pharynx. More superficial are more prone for injury.

To summarize, all the muscles of the larynx except cricothyroid are supplied by RLN except cricothyroid, which receives its blood supply from the EBSLN. Above the vocal folds, the sensory innervations is by the internal laryngeal nerve and below the vocal folds is by the RLN.

Presentation

- *Unilateral EBSLN injury*: The unilateral EBSLN palsy causes paralysis of the ipsilateral cricothyroid muscle and the anesthesia of the larynx above the cord. Clinically, the voice becomes weak and the pitch cannot be raised. Unilateral supralaryngeal anesthesia may go unnoticed or may cause occasional aspiration or reflex coughing or swallowing.

  Though the EBSLN injury is difficult to describe clinically and the patient may notice mild hoarseness, reflex cough, weak vocal stamina, or loss of high pitch, the impact on the vocal professionals such as the singers and teachers is very high and may impose a threat on their career.
- *Bilateral EBSLN injury*: In bilateral paralysis of EBSLN injury, both cricothyroid muscles are paralyzed along with the anesthesia to the supralaryngeal mucosa. Clinically, presence of both paralysis and anesthesia causes reflex coughing, especially during deglutition, with voice weakness and huskiness. Cuffed tracheostomy with feeding esophageal tube may be required in some cases with repeated aspirations. Alternatively, by epiglottopexy (reversible procedure), patients can close the inlet to protect the lungs from repeated aspiration.

Evaluation: On laryngeal examination, due to the rotation of the anterior commissure to the healthy side, the glottis becomes a skew in position and the affected cord is shortened and wavy with loss of tension. This loss of tension may lead to the paralyzed cord, becomes floppy, and sags down during inhalation and bulges during exhalation.

Prevention: Most of the time, EBSLN is neglected compared to the RLN. It is considered prudent to ligate the superior thyroid pedicle close to the upper pole of thyroid rather than identifying and preserving it; therefore, most of the injuries went unnoticed.

Though supervising of the SLN by electrophysiologic study is reported, its use is not routinely advised.

Sometimes, cricothyroid muscle injury can compromise the muscle function and present as insult to the external branch of the SLN, even when the nerve is conserved.[20]

Treatment: No specific therapy is recommended for nerve recovery; however, speech therapy can be used for voice improvement.[20]

Combined Paralysis of RLN and EBSLN[21]

The innervations from the contralateral nerve to the interarytenoid spare it from the paralysis during unilateral combined RLN and EBSLN injury; rest other intrinsic muscles become paralyzed. On examination, the vocal cord will present in cadaveric position (3.5 mm from the midline). The glottis becomes incompetent, because the healthy cord will not be able to approximate with paralyzed cord and that leads to hoarseness of voice, repeated aspiration, and ineffective cough. The management includes speech therapy, medialize procedure of cords by Teflon paste injection, implantation of muscle or cartilage, type 1 thyroplasty, or arthrodesis of cricoarytenoid joints.

In bilateral paralysis, since all the intrinsic muscles of both the sides are paralyzed, both vocal cords lie in the cadaveric position along with total anesthesia of the larynx. Clinically, the patient may present with aphonia, ineffective cough, and bronchopneumonia due to recurrent aspirations.

The condition with bilateral RLN and EBSLN nerve palsies is extremely rare but may be a possibility in surgeries requiring extended thyroid resections such as malignancy and high thyroid altering the cervical anatomy, in cases where the nerve is not identified and in reoperative cases.

Hypoparathyroidism[22,23]

Another clinically important complication of thyroid surgery is post-thyroidectomy hypoparathyroidism. The parathyroid hormone (PTH) is an essential hormone to control the serum calcium homeostasis in human body, which is secreted by parathyroid glands.

Majority have four parathyroid glands, two on either side. Each gland normally weighs 30–40 mg. Anatomical studies have demonstrated that 80–85% of the superior parathyroid and 90–95% of the inferior parathyroid arteries originate from the inferior thyroid arteries. The truncal ligation of the inferior thyroid arteries may therefore significantly jeopardize the parathyroid vascularity and function. However, due to partial supply by the superior thyroid vessels and the development of the collaterals from the tracheal and esophageal vessels, the overall parathyroid functions may remain intact.

The upper parathyroid glands emerge embryologically from the fourth pharyngeal pouch. They come down only slightly during the embryologic development. It is usually found close to the posterior surface of the middle part of the thyroid lobe, just anterolateral to the RLN at the level of Berry's ligaments and thus easiest to preserve during thyroidectomy. The inferior parathyroid glands arise from the third pharyngeal pouch, along with the thymus. They have a wide range of distribution since they travel far in embryologic life, from just below the mandible to the anterior mediastinum. These glands usually present on the posterolateral surface of the inferior pole of the thyroid lobes and are almost always anterior to the RLN and are more vulnerable for injury.

The PTH regulates calcium metabolism in the body. It increases the serum calcium by resorption of bone, reabsorption from kidney, and activation of vitamin D.

Injury to the parathyroid glands during surgery either by direct trauma of gland or by their vascularity or inadvertent excision may lead to hypoparathyroidism and consequently hypocalcemia. This hypocalcemia can be temporary or permanent depending upon the extent and severity of injury.

Other proposed causes of post-thyroidectomy transient hypocalcemia include reversible ischemia of the parathyroid glands, the release of an acute-phase reactant protein known to suppress PTH production (endothelin-1), the release of calcitonin, and hungry bone syndrome.

Presentation

Acute hypocalcemia: Sudden decrease in serum calcium causes neuromuscular instability, paresthesia, and numbness of the fingertips and perioral area. The neuromuscular rigidity can be elicited by provocation tests such as *Chvostek's sign* or *Trousseau's sign.*

Chvostek's sign is the twitching of the ipsilateral facial muscles (perioral, nasal, and eyes muscles) by tapping over the ipsilateral cranial nerve VII at the ear.

Though helpful, it is neither sensitive nor specific for hypocalcemia since it is absent in 30% of patients with the hypocalcemia and is present in 10–15% of normocalcemic patients.

Trousseau's sign of latent tetany is a carpopedal spasm induced by inflation of the blood pressure cuff around the arm. It is more sensitive and specific than Chvostek's sign, present in 94% of hypocalcemic patients and only observed in 1% of normocalcemic patients.

Laboratory Evaluation

- Serum calcium (<8.5 mg/dL); critical (<6 mg/dL)
- Ionized calcium levels < 3.8 mg/dL; critical <3.2 mg/dL

Chronic Permanent Hypocalcemia

Depending upon the duration of hypoparathyroidism, in cases with partial injury, the function may recover after sometime (6 months) and the hypoparathyroidism will be temporary; however, if the damage is complete and not recoverable (>12 months), the hypoparathyroidism will be permanent. Such patients have high serum phosphate levels. Despite frequent testing and adjustments for the therapy, fatigue, paresthesia, and irritability are common. Cataracts have been reported in 70–80% of permanent hypoparathyroidism cases despite laboratory evidence of normocalcemia.

Patients with hypocalcemia may initially complain of generalized body tingling and paresthesia, which may start from circumoral or fingertip paresthesias and rigidity. In severe cases, it may present with psychiatric changes, tetany, carpopedal spasm, laryngeal spasm, seizures, QT prolongation on ECG, and cardiac arrest.

Evaluation

The effective method of evaluation of parathyroid function is to consider ionized calcium levels in the postoperative period.

- Serum calcium (<8.5 mg/dL); critical (<6 mg/dL)
- Ionized calcium levels < 3.8 mg/dL; critical <3.2 mg/dL
  Alternatively, the postoperative PTH level in normal range may predict normocalcemia after thyroid surgery. Identification of low PTH levels indicates patients at risk of hypocalcemia which can be managed with prompt calcium replacement therapy, which helps to facilitate safe and early discharge from hospital.

Hypocalcemia with normal PTH levels may present in patients with renal failure, hypomagnesemia, and some medications. The management is unchanged regardless of the etiology. In cases with permanent deficiency, biochemical re-evaluation can be done 6 months after surgery to check the revival of the parathyroid glands' function.

Prevention

The most important way to protect a parathyroid during surgery is to identify it with its color, shape, and position and gently separate it from the thyroid capsule, preserving its blood supply. The key of dissection during surgery is to ligate the vessels as close to the thyroid capsule as feasible.

For the better identification of the PTGs and their vascularity, magnifying glasses (×2.5) are helpful. Meticulous dissection avoiding cautery or extensive dissection near the PTGs is an important factor. When the parathyroid cannot be safely separated from the thyroid capsule, it has been advised to remove it and autotransplanted in the sternocleidomastoid muscle or in the brachioradialis muscle of the nondominant arm.

Recognition of the parathyroid during surgery is of great importance. The following features are very helpful such as:

- The position
- Mobility independent of thyroid gland
- Brownish color
- Smooth, finely granular surface
- Presence of vascular pedicle
- Easy bleeding on manipulation
- The presence of small fatty hood

Management Protocol

Different institutes follow different management protocols based on their clinical experiences. However, the most commonly followed are as follows:

- Initiation of 3 g of elemental calcium PO per day as soon as the patient starts orally, unless there are specific contraindications to oral calcium.
- Check ionized calcium q8 hourly postoperative.
- If two consecutive calcium values are within the normal range or increasing, discontinue checking calcium and patient is tapered off calcium supplementation gradually over weeks.
- If serum calcium is decreasing, increase oral calcium to 4 g elemental calcium per day. If this stabilizes the calcium, arrangements for the above tapered regimen begin at 1 g/week. Check and correct abnormal serum magnesium. The patient should have calcium checked every week after discharge.
- If serum calcium continues to decrease <3.8 mg/dL and the patient becomes symptomatic, add 0.5 µg of 1,25 DOH vitamin D per day. The first dose is to be given immediately. If there is a continued decrease in calcium or symptoms increase, increase the dose to 0.5 BD and consult the endocrinologist involved.
- For patients who are severely symptomatic with serum ionized calcium <3.8 mg/dL, IV calcium may be administered.
- 1 amp of calcium gluconate (10 mL of calcium gluconate 10% contains 1 g of calcium gluconate in 500 mL D5W). This infusion will eventually stop the symptoms.
  - Recheck the calcium after administration.
  - Check magnesium levels and correct if needed.
  - Maximize oral 1,25 DOH vitamin D and oral calcium in consultation with the endocrinologist.

Important points regarding IV calcium administration:

- *Avoid rapid IV infusion*: It may lead to GI side effects such as nausea, vomiting, calcium taste, local thrombophlebitis, cardiotoxicity, hypotension, tingling sensation, and flushing
- Extravasations during injection cause irritation.
- Subcutaneous or intramuscular administration is contraindicated, as it may cause severe injection site necrosis and sloughing.

- If overdose—stop the infusion immediately and if required, rehydrate with normal saline infusion
- Caution in dialysis patient and those with kidney disease
- Serum calcium/ionized calcium must be closely monitored.

Other Complications

Thyrotoxic Storm[24]

An unusual complication of thyroid surgery is thyrotoxic storm. It occurs due to outpouring of the stored hormone from the thyroid gland during surgical manipulation in patients with uncontrolled hyperthyroidism such as Graves' disease. If neglected, thyrotoxic storm may be potentially lethal.

Clinical presentation: During surgery under general anesthesia, the patient may present with tachycardia, hyperthermia, or delayed weaning. Patients without anesthesia may present with tachycardia, palpitation, anxiety, restlessness, and increased body temperature. The patient may have complaints of nausea, tremors, cardiac arrhythmia, and altered mental function. If untreated, the patient may progress to unconsciousness.

Prevention: The key factor for the prevention is to make every hyperthyroid patient as euthyroid as possible before surgery depending upon the time available and the severity of the symptoms. Drug treatment must be directed to decrease the synthesis [methimazole, propylthiouracil (PTU), and iodine] and peripheral conversion pathways (propylthiouracil, β-blockers, and steroids) of thyroid hormone.

In adequately prepared patients, the morbidity and mortality related to thyroid storm rates are less.

Intraoperative management: As soon as the thyrotoxic crises are diagnosed, stop the manipulation. Target on the synthetic and peripheral pathways with the help of sodium iodine, intravenous β-blockers, steroids, and PTU which also help to control the sympathetic activities. Manage hyperthermia with cooling blankets. Oxygen support and IV fluids are given as the demand increases during these crises.

Postoperative management: Since the half-life of circulating T4 is 7–8 days, even after removal of thyroid, the thyrotoxic symptoms are not relieved immediately. By the time the thyroid hormone levels decrease, the patient is given supportive care which is gradually weaned over the weeks after surgery.

Surgical Site Infection and Seroma

During 1800s, infection was the major cause of death from thyroid surgery. With the advances in medical science, presently, the overall infection rate is less than 1–2% of all thyroid surgery. If recognized and treated early, it is unlikely to have any mortality due to infection. *It is usually caused by gram-positive cocci. These are considered clean cases where antibiotics prophylaxis is recommended only in patients with cardiovascular disorders and in immunocompromised patients.*

Presentation: The clinical manifestation of post-thyroidectomy infection is either superficial cellulitis or deep abscess. Superficial cellulitis is clearly visible with features of acute inflammation such as warmth, erythema, and tenderness around the incision with or without wound discharge. A deep neck abscess may not be clinically visible; however, it can be suspected in post-thyroidectomy patients with fever, pain, leukocytosis, and tachycardia.

Evaluation: Laboratory investigation includes complete blood counts and pus aspirate or swab for bacterial culture and sensitivity. Contrast-enhanced computed tomography (CECT) neck may be helpful to find out the extent of the problem and is especially useful for the deep abscesses. Esophageal perforation must be ruled out in cases with deep abscess. Delay in prompt treatment may lead to devastating mediastinitis.

Prevention: The most important point for preventing postoperative infection is respecting the surgical planes and the use of aseptic surgical technique. Recommendation is against the excessive use of the antibiotics in thyroid surgery.

Treatment: Drain any drainable abscess and send the pus for bacterial culture and sensitivity. Start with broad-spectrum antibiotics and escalate or deescalate the antibiotic spectrum according to the culture and sensitivity reports as soon as made available.

Percutaneous aspiration and compression usually relieve the clinically evident seroma.

Edema

Postoperative mild edema is usual; however, major disturbance of the lymphatic flow, caused by bilateral lymphadenectomy in cases with extensive thyroidectomy, may lead to laryngotracheal edema causing respiratory compromise. Endotracheal intubation or anaphylactoid reaction may also cause the pharyngolaryngeal edema.

Management: Head elevation, steroid therapy, oxygen support, and occasional temporary re-intubation help in tiding the crisis.

Hemorrhage

The incidence of symptomatic bleeding requiring intervention is 0.1–1.5%. Thyroid is a highly vascular structure. The postoperative bleeding can be manifested as tachycardia, cervical pain, swelling and pressure, soakage and increased drain discharge, respiratory distress, and dysphagia.

The key to prevent this situation is to carefully recognize the anatomic detail and meticulous homeostasis during surgery. If still uncertain, Valsalva maneuver is of great help.

By elevating the intrapulmonary pressure, it helps in the identification of at-risk bleeding vessels.

Routine use of suction drains does not prevent postoperative bleeding; however, they are useful in early detection and decompression.

Management: Once recognized, the hematoma must be evacuated. Even emergency bed side stitch opening and hematoma evacuation are warranted in cases with significant respiratory distress, with consideration for endotracheal intubation, if required. Tracheostomy either in emergency or due to persisting airway obstruction after hematoma evacuation is rarely required.

Malposition

Brachial plexus injury, though rare, is a possibility on the operating table when the patient is malpositioned. Bilateral adducted and secured arms avoid nerve injury. Similarly, avoiding hyperextension of neck prevents cervical pain, nausea, and headache in the postoperative period.

Rare Neural, Visceral, and Vascular Complications

Cervical sympathetic trunk injury (1:5,000 cases) may occur while dissecting in prespinal areas like for retroesophageal goiter.

Damage to the phrenic nerve leads to ipsilateral hemidiaphragmatic elevation; dropping of shoulder due to spinal accessory nerve injury and limited movements of shoulder and arm due to muscle atrophy are rare but can occur during dissection for thyroid cancer.

Dissection of the retrosternal goiter or mediastinal lymphadenectomy may lead to *pneumothorax or subclavian vessels injury.*

Clinically significant pneumothorax requires air evacuation via percutaneous needle insertion or thoracic drain placement.

Arteriovenous (AV) fistula of the superior thyroid vessels may occur. Individual ligation of superior thyroid vessels may help to prevent this phenomenon. This will also prevent injury to the EBSLN.

The carotid artery injury is very rare; however, excessive lateral retraction of the carotid sheath containing an atherosclerosed artery during mobilization of an enlarged gland may injure the vessel wall or damage the blood flow to the brain.

Injury to the Lymphatic

Patients with thyroid cancers requiring lymph nodes dissection are prone to injury to the thoracic duct on the left side and lymphatic duct on the right side. Care should be taken to identify and ligate the major lymphatic duct with nonabsorbable sutures peroperatively. However, if detected in the postoperative period (frank milky fluid from drain), conservative management by continuous drainage, external compression, and low-fat and high-protein diet with or without addition of somatostatin is effective in most of the cases. The surgical ligation of the fistula must be considered, in cases with persistent high leak.

Injury to Esophagus

Though rare, it may be encountered in patients with altered anatomy due to huge goiters, locally advanced thyroid cancer, and difficult localization of RLN. If detected peroperative, primary suturing with absorbable sutures, Ryle's tube insertion, and total parenteral nutrition (TPN) are helpful. If detected in the postoperative period as an esophagocutaneous fistula, wound care and insertion of feeding Ryle's tube are helpful which serve the purpose of giving rest to the wounded area while maintaining low-cost, high-value nutrition to the patient.

Injury to Trachea

Though rare in experienced hands, this injury usually occurs while separating the thyroid off the anterolateral tracheal surface. The risk increases further with the presence of tracheomalacia, tracheal infiltration, or adhesion. It can be avoided by using the low thermal cautery very meticulously and clearing the plane with continuous suction. If injury is detected peroperatively, primary closure of the defect with buttressing with strap or sternocleidomastoid muscle flap with external compression suffices in most of the cases. In the postoperative period, undetected tracheal injuries manifest as the surgical emphysema and respiratory distress. Percutaneous drainage of surgical emphysema with local compression eventually subsides this complication.

◇ CONCLUSION

The surgeon plays a very vital role in the practice of thyroid surgery. A clear understanding of not only the thyroid and its diseases, anatomy, embryology, and surgical pathology but also the molecular biology is very prudent. Still, the common disorders presented to a surgeon are the nodular goiters, thyroid cancer, and thyrotoxicosis. Dedicated surgeons enjoy their surgeries and they make efforts to practice it at the highest level to achieve the best outcome. Achieving this level requires a sound training system. The postoperative complications are infrequent in the hands of the experienced thyroid surgeon and are best avoided by a meticulous surgical technique. Successful outcome depends on the timely recognition and immediate management of complications.

◇ REFERENCES

1. Sarkar S, Banerjee S, Sarkar R, Sikder B. A review on the history of 'Thyroid Surgery'. Indian J Surg. 2016;78(1):32-6.
2. Dorairajan N, Pradeep PV. Vignette thyroid surgery: a glimpse into its history. Int Surg. 2013;98(1):70-5.
3. Hannan SA. The magnificent seven: a history of modern thyroid surgery. Int J Surg. 2006;4(3):187-91.

4. Zbären P, Shah JP, Randolph GW, Silver CE, Olsen KD, Shaha AR et al. Thyroid surgery: whose domain is it? Adv Ther. 2019;36(10):2541-6.

5. Caulley L, Jhonson-Obaseki S, Luo L, Javidnia H. Risk factors for postoperative complications in total thyroidectomy: a retrospective, risk-adjusted analysis from the National Surgical Quality Improvement Program. Medicine (Baltimore). 2017;96(5):e5752.

6. Bhattacharyya N, Fried MP. Assessment of the morbidity and complications of total thyroidectomy. JAMA. 2002;128(4): 389-92.

7. Christou N, Mathonnet M. Complications after total thyroidectomy. J Visc Surg. 2013;150(4):249-56.

8. Chand G, Agarwal S, Mishra A, Agarwal G, Verma AK, Mishra SK et al. The impact of uniform capsular dissection technique of total thyroidectomy on postoperative complications: an experience of more than 1000 total thyroidectomies from an endocrine surgery training centre in North India. Indian J Endocrinol Metab. 2018;22(3):362-7.

9. Myssiore D. Recurrent laryngeal nerve paralysis: anatomy and etiology. Otolaryngol Clin North Am. 2004;37(1):25-44.

10. Shindo ML, Wu JC, Park EE. Surgical anatomy of the recurrent laryngeal nerve revisited. Otolaryngol Head Neck Surg. 2005;133(4):514-9.

11. Defechereux T, Alexandre J, Albert V, Bonnet P, Hamoir E, Meurisse M. The inferior non-recurrent laryngeal nerve: a major surgical risk during thyroidectomy. Acta Chir Belg. 2000;100(2):62-7.

12. Abboud B, Aouad R. Non-recurrent inferior laryngeal nerve in thyroid surgery: Report of three cases and review of the literature. J Laryngol Otol. 2004;118(2):139-42.

13. Pradeep PV, Jayashree B, Harshita SS. A closer look at laryngeal nerves during thyroid surgery: a descriptive study of 584 nerves. Anat Res Int. 2012;1-6. Article ID 490390

14. Vachha B, Cunnen MB, Mallur P, Moonis G. Losing your voice: Etiologies and imaging features of vocal fold paralysis. J Clin Imaging Sci. 2013;3(1):1-8.

15. Parnes SM, Satya-Murti S. Predictive value of laryngeal electromyography in patients with vocal cord paralysis of neurogenic origin. Laryngoscope. 1985;95(11):1323-6.

16. Shen C, Xiang M, Wu H, Ma Y, Li Chen, Cheng L. Routine exposure of recurrent laryngeal nerve in thyroid surgery can prevent nerve injury. Neural Regen Res. 2013;8(17):1568-75.

17. Lahey FH. Hoover WB. Injuries to the recurrent laryngeal nerve in thyroid operations. Their management and avoidance. Ann Surg. 1938;108(4):545-62.

18. Hartl DM, Tivagli J-P, Leboulleux S, Baudin E, Brasnu DF, Schlumberger M. Current concepts in the management of unilateral recurrent laryngeal nerve paralysis after thyroid surgery. J Clin Endocrinol Metab. 2005;90(5): 3084-8.

19. Dispenza F, Dispenza C, Marchese D, Kulamarva G Saraniti C. Treatment of bilateral vocal cord paralysis following permanent recurrent laryngeal nerve injury. Am J Otolaryngol. 2012;33(3):285-8.

20. Orestes ML, Chhetri DK. Superior laryngeal nerve injury: Effects, clinical findings, prognosis, and management option. Curr Opin Otolaryngol Head Neck Surg. 2014;22(6):439-43.

21. Dhingra PL. Diseases of Ear, Nose and Throat, 7th edn. Elsevier, 2017.

22. Clark OH. Textbook of Endocrine Surgery, 2nd edn. Elsevier, 2005.

23. Stack BC, Bimston DN, Bodenner DL, Brett EM, Dralle H, Orloff LA, et al. American Association of Clinical Endocrinologists and American College of Endocrinology Disease State Clinical Review: Postoperative hypoparathyroidism—definitions and management. Endocr Pract. 2015; 21(6):674-85.

24. Carroll R, Matfin G. Endocrine and metabolic emergencies: thyroid storm. Ther Adv Endocrinol Metab. 2010;1(3):139-45.

Alok Thakar, R Chandra Shekar Reddy, Harsha Yadav CT

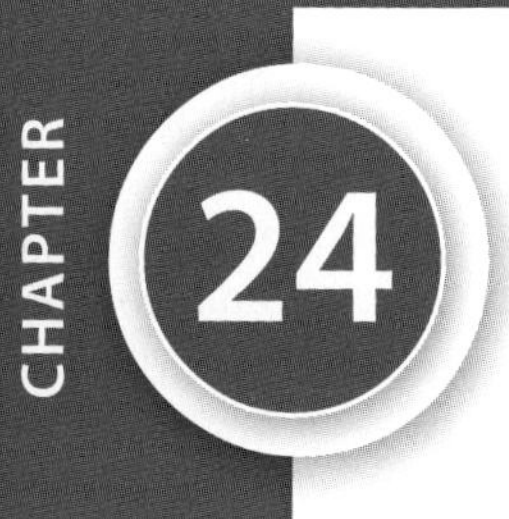

Voice Changes Following Thyroidectomy

CHAPTER 24

INTRODUCTION

The most frequent voice changes after thyroidectomy are consequent to injury to the recurrent laryngeal nerve (RLN) or the superior laryngeal nerve (SLN). Mild degrees of voice change may also occur because of injury to the strap muscles or their innervation, and similarly injury to cricothyroid muscle and laryngeal framework, or injury consequent to the act of intubation. These are, however, generally minor and will not be discussed further in this chapter.

In simplistic terms, the larynx may be considered an organ with two antagonistic functions—one of a conduit for breathing, which requires an open glottis with abducted vocal folds, and the other functions of voicing and of aspiration-free swallow, which require a closed glottis with adducted vocal folds. These functions are well undertaken with intact laryngeal nerves and muscles but are alternately affected with vocal cord paralysis. Bilateral RLN paralysis causes predominantly respiratory difficulty and inspiratory stridor but a relatively good voice. Unilateral RLN paralysis causes, however, predominantly voice problems as the paralyzed vocal fold does not approximate fully well with the contralateral mobile cord. Other less frequent affectations are a poorly effective cough and some aspiration with liquids, but the airway is not compromised.[1]

RELEVANT ANATOMY AND PHYSIOLOGY

Each hemilarynx is primarily innervated by the ipsilateral two laryngeal branches from the vagus trunk, i.e., the SLN and the RLN. Identification of the nerve is the key to its preservation during surgery. This necessitates thorough understanding of the course of the laryngeal nerves and variations.

Superior Laryngeal Nerve

The SLN arises from nodose ganglion of the vagus. It begins posteriorly and then runs medial to the internal carotid artery and divides into an internal (sensory and autonomous) and external branch (motor). The internal laryngeal branch pierces the thyrohyoid membrane, enters the larynx along with the superior laryngeal artery, and subsequently divides into upper and lower branches.[2] The external branch runs medially on the lateral surface of the larynx overlying the inferior pharyngeal constrictor muscle and deep to the straps to supply only the cricothyroid muscle.[2] Contraction of the cricothyroid muscle distracts the cricoid and thyroid cartilages in the plane of the vocal fold and so causes a tensioning and stretching of the vocal fold. The stretch and tensioning also lead to a mild adduction of the vocal fold.

The external branch of the superior laryngeal nerve (EBSLN) is particularly at risk during thyroidectomy at the time of ligation of superior thyroid pedicle. The course of EBSLN is variable,[2-4] and there may also be variations between the two sides in 535 cases.[3] Cernea's classification of EBSLN types as stated below is the most popular and is based on its relation to superior thyroid pedicle:[3]

- *Type 1 (60%)*: Nerve crossing the superior thyroid vessels 1 or more cm above a horizontal plane passing the upper border of the superior thyroid pole
- *Type 2a (17%)*: Nerve crossing <1 cm above the plane
- *Type 2b (20%)*: Nerve crossing below the plane of the upper border of superior thyroid pole

Kierner's new classification defines a type 4 EBSLN based on Cernea's classification as a nerve descending dorsal to the artery and only crossing the branch of the superior thyroid artery immediately above the upper pole of the gland. This was noted in 14% of cadavers and is another anatomic configuration at high risk for injury during thyroidectomy.[4]

Friedman's classification[2] highlights importance of identification of EBSLN at the site of insertion into the cricothyroid muscle, i.e., the inferior constrictor–cricothyroid junction. This may be helpful, especially in cases where the nerve was not identified in relation to superior thyroid pedicle.

Recurrent Laryngeal Nerve

The RLN is given off lower down from the vagus, which hooks around the subclavian artery on the right and the arch of aorta on the left and ascends in tracheoesophageal groove to enter larynx through posterior aspect larynx at cricoarytenoid joint.

In 20–65% cases, the RLN branches into an anterior and posterior division before entering into the larynx.[5-7] As per recent investigations, the anterior is believed to be motor and posterior branch mainly sensory.[5] Failing to identify this will lead to misinterpretation of a thicker posterior branch to be the main trunk and inadvertent injury to the anterior branch.[5]

The RLN supplies all the intrinsic muscles of the larynx except the cricothyroid and is responsible for both vocal cord abduction and adduction.[1] Abductor motor units contain more muscle fibers but there are four times as many adductor nerve fibers as abductor (4:1). As a result, the adductor motor units greatly outnumber the abductors.[8]

In case of laryngeal denervation, a spontaneous re-innervation process can be observed as soon as 2 months after denervation.[9] Regeneration is most remarkable in RLN but also likely to be synkinetic.[1] The difference in the number of motor units (4:1) favors reinnervation of adductor muscle fibers. Reinnervation may, therefore, lead to progressive predominance of adductor function over abductor and a shift of the paralyzed cord from a lateral to a more medial position.[8]

The incidence of EBSLN injury varies from 0 to 58% globally, depending on the experience of surgeon. Paralysis of EBSLN nerve leads to loss of motor innervations to cricothyroid. Ipsilateral vocal fold becoming lax and sagging can lead to a lesser degree of weak and breathy voice or it may manifest only as an inability to raise the pitch of the voice when the vocal fold needs to be tightened.[10] Objectively, EBSLN injury is evaluated by laryngeal electromyography (EMG) and videostroboscopy. Due to loss of tension on the vocal cord, videostroboscopy shows bowing and inferior displacement of the vocal cord and rotation of the posterior glottis toward the paralytic side suggestive of EBSLN palsy.[11]

The RLN injury in thyroid surgeries is 1–2% when performed by experienced neck surgeons.[12] Although the incidence of RLN injury may be less than that of EBSLN, the voice disability following RLN injury is far more pronounced and easily identified on endoscopy as compared to subtle symptomatology of EBSLN injury. The incidence of RLN injury has been found to be higher during re-explorations, Graves' disease, and thyroid carcinoma procedures.[13,14] Ipsilateral injury to the RLN leads to an immobile vocal fold, which generally settles in a paramedian position about 1.5 mm from the midline. This results in the true vocal folds not opposing when speaking and therefore a weak and breathy voice whereas bilateral RLN injury leads to bilateral vocal cords in paramedian position resulting in dyspnea and often life-threatening glottal obstruction.[15,16]

Injury to RLN and SLN motor branches may be permanent or transient. Transient paralysis occurs due to manipulation or stretch of the nerve. Such an injury may subsequently recover with return of function.

◇| ASSESSMENT

The most important parameter to discern in a patient with a laryngeal paralysis is whether it is permanent or transient. This can be discerned by going through the exact nature of injury during the operation and the surgeon's impression. It is always fruitful to speak to the surgeon who has undertaken the operation regarding whether the nerve was identified or not and if it was injured.

A careful videolaryngoscopy is necessary. Recording the same can allow for a better initial evaluation and provide a baseline to judge subsequent improvement (or lack of it) over time. The laryngoscopy should be assessed for features of EBSLN and RLN paralysis as listed above. Further assessment is of the degree and pattern of the glottic gap, the laxity of the vocal fold, and the degree of paralysis (partial or complete).

Laryngoscopy also assesses the compensatory mechanisms used by the patient for voicing. These may include excessive strain or squeezing of the contralateral laryngeal muscles, or excessive tension in the cricothyroid muscle so as to attempt glottic approximation and so make voice. Alternately, some patients may switch to a rough supraglottic voicing by approximating the false vocal folds.

Voice disability may be assessed by the vocal handicap index (VHI) or the abridged VHI-10. VHI-10 is a reliable and validated self-assessment tool that measures voice quality and its effect on quality of life.[17] A set of 10 preset questions are asked, with responses ranging from 0 to 4. Total score ranging from 0 to 40 implies nil to maximal handicap. The maximum phonation time (MPT) and S/Z ratio are simple, quick, and reliable measures of glottic efficiency and are affected in patients with glottic gap/glottic insufficiency consequent to unilateral vocal fold paralysis. MPT is undertaken by asking the patient to sustain a vowel in a single breath after maximal inspiration.[18] MPT values expected are 25–35 seconds in males and 15–25 seconds in females, and a score <10 is considered pathological.[19] The S/Z ratio looks at the ratio of the MPTs while voicing the |s| (voiceless phonation) and the |z| (voiced phonation) and approximates to 1 in normal individuals. It is increased to >1.4 (95% CI) in patients with glottic insufficiency consequent to unilateral vocal fold paralysis.[20]

In ambiguous situations, if a vocal fold paralysis is noted as partial (paresis), then that indicates to an anatomically intact nerve and predicates toward a good chance of spontaneous recovery.

A complete paralysis, however, may be consequent to muscle stretch or manipulation or possibly nerve section and it is difficult to predicate clinically on the chances of recovery. A laryngeal EMG, if available, can inform in this situation with regard to the extent of denervation. The laryngeal EMG can demonstrate electrical activity in the muscle initiated by attempted vocalization, and even if no muscle activity is clinically discernible, this indicates to residual innervation. In the setting of recent paralysis, vocalization-induced electrical activity would suggest to a reasonable chance of recovery and opting for a conservative nonsurgical option. If nerve injury is noted as complete due to denervation of the muscle, then this predicates to a less favorable prognosis for spontaneous recovery.

Surgical intervention by thyroplasty violates the paraglottic space with the laryngeal muscles and is traditionally not undertaken till it is certain that further recovery is not anticipated. In a situation, wherein it is indiscernible as to whether the injury is permanent or transient, it has traditionally been considered to wait for 6–9 months for spontaneous recovery.

Even in patients with no recovery, there can be spontaneous improvement in voice because of compensation from the contralateral vocal fold, which may cross over the midline and meet the contralateral paralyzed cord to bring about improvement in voice.

◇ TREATMENT OPTIONS

The treatment options available can broadly be divided into:
- Conservative watchful waiting with voice therapy to strengthen compensation
- Temporary measures such as vocal fold injection so as to cause vocal fold medialization and thus improve voice
- More permanent surgical measures such as laryngeal framework surgery (thyroplasty) to medialize and tauten the vocal folds
- Reinnervation procedures

The choice between treatments depends on a multifactorial assessment evaluating the anticipated chances for spontaneous recovery, the degree of voice and swallow dysfunction, and also the patient's specific voice needs. An initial period of voice therapy is, however, invariable and also aids the response to injection laryngoplasty and surgical procedures **(Fig. 1)**.

Voice Therapy

The main aim of voice therapy is to improve glottal closure while simultaneously reducing compensatory hyperfunctional behaviors such as supraglottic compression (lateral and anteroposterior). This is aided by an appropriate assessment and laryngeal examination by the otolaryngologist and an objective assessment of the degree of voice dysfunction by the speech pathologist.

Therapy is best undertaken under the supervision of a speech therapist so that unintentional strain patterns are not erroneously learnt in. Therapy works on the contralateral normally functional muscles and aims to improve intrinsic laryngeal muscle strength and agility. At the very basic, the therapy involves relaxed voicing/humming with forced glottic closure by standing and forcefully pushing one's hands against a wall. Additional exercises for breathing control are undertaken. Further specific details are beyond the scope of this chapter and the reader may refer to a comprehensive review by Miller.[21]

In a study of 41 patients with RLN lesions (22 male and 19 female), Heuer et al. found that 64% of males and 68% of females did not elect to have surgery after voice therapy.[22] This is because partial spontaneous recovery and also contralateral compensation as encouraged by voice therapy can limit voice disability in a large proportion of patients with mild and isolated dysfunction of the RLN. More severe dysfunction with significant breathiness or glottic incompetence would, however, require additional vocal fold medialization by injection laryngoplasty or thyroplasty. Patients with poor glottic competence and aspiration and a poorly effective cough would also require a surgical procedure for appropriate improvement.

Voice therapy is also an inalienable adjunct to injection or surgical medialization as it helps to develop a good and relaxed vocal technique and to avoid and treat developing strain patterns.

Injection Laryngoplasty

In this procedure, a material is injected into the paralyzed vocal fold so as to add bulk to it and to medialize the edge of the vocal fold. The injection is usually positioned in the paraglottic space and was traditionally undertaken under general anesthesia through a rigid laryngoscope. With the recent advances in technology and improved videolaryngoscopes, it is now generally undertaken under local anesthetic as an office-based procedure and has therefore gained popularity. An additional advantage of undertaking the procedure under local anesthesia is that one may have an immediate feedback on the vocal outcome.

Autologous fat has the advantage of being cheap and easily available but is variably absorbed over time. It is usually obtained from the periumbilical region, centrifuged, and injected into the paralyzed vocal cord paraglottic space. Its chief disadvantage is its viscosity making it difficult to inject and so limiting its applicability for office-based injections.

A host of easy-to-inject materials used for injection laryngoplasty is now available which is biocompatible and cause minimal inflammation. These include calcium hydroxyapatite (Radiesse Voice), carboxymethylcellulose

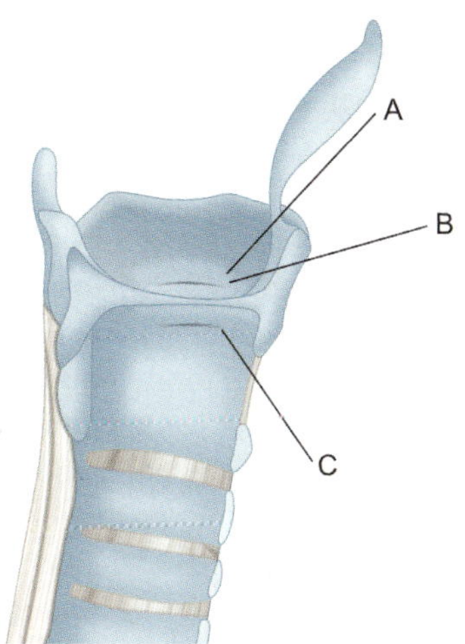

Fig. 1: Percutaneous approaches to injection laryngoplasty. A—suprathyroid through epiglottis, B—transthyroid through thyroid cartilage, and C—transcricothyroid.

(Radiesse voice gel), hyaluronic acid (Restylane), collagen, micronized acellular dermal matrix (Cymetra), and Gelfoam. Older materials, such as Teflon, are no longer used because of subsequent immunogenic reaction leading to granuloma formation.[23] The amount injected varies from 1.5 to 3 mL depending on the degree of glottic insufficiency.[24] It is usual to aim for slight overcorrection.

Various routes of injection may be used for office injection under local anesthetic. They are currently all undertaken under visual guidance with a flexible fiberoptic laryngoscope. The following injection routes are usual:

- *Transoral*: This can be done using a long, curved injection needle guided by flexible nasopharyngoscopy.
- Percutaneous anterior superior approach through the thyroid notch. The needle is entered into the supraglottis midline at the petiole of the epiglottis and is then directed inferiorly onto the superior surface of the vocal fold.
- Percutaneous transthyroid where injection is through the ala of the thyroid cartilage at the level of vocal fold.
- Percutaneous transcricothyroid injection where the injection needle is inserted through the cricothyroid membrane anteriorly and directed upward and laterally into the vocal fold.

We personally prefer the percutaneous approaches to the transoral approach and have maximal experience with the cricothyroid approach.

The medialization of vocal fold injection is, however, transient and the injected material typically resorbs in a period of 3–18 months depending on the material used. It is therefore ideally suited to be undertaken in the initial phase of the paralysis when there is yet uncertainty re the expectation of recovery and a more definitive thyroplasty procedure is therefore not appropriate.

Laryngeal Framework Surgery/Thyroplasty

The ideal treatment for glottic incompetence due to RLN injury should be to position the vocal fold in its original phonatory position, similar to the opposite vocal fold. Although injection laryngoplasty can improve voice outcomes and glottal competence in the initial phases, it is a short-term option. Laryngeal framework surgery is a better option for long-term and sustained improvement.

Most of the laryngeal framework surgery is based on thyroplasty techniques by Isshiki et al.[25] Of these techniques, type 1 thyroplasty is the most commonly used technique used for medialization of the vocal fold. This involves creating a window through the thyroid cartilage at the level of the vocal fold and inserting a wedge-shaped carved silastic block. Other implant materials used include Gor-Tex and prefabricated implants of hydroxyapatite and titanium.

Occasionally, vocal fold medialization needs to be supplemented with additional medialization of the arytenoid. Arytenoid adduction was described by Isshiki et al. to correct the position of the arytenoid cartilage after RLN injury.[26] The arytenoid tends to get displaced anteriorly, inferiorly, and laterally on the cricoid facet, which results in a shortened and lateralized vocal fold. In this procedure, the posterior border of the thyroid lamina on the affected side is released and its posterior edge partly removed to gain access to the muscular process of the arytenoid cartilage. A suture is then placed through the muscular process and anchored forward by passing it through the thyroid lamina anteriorly. Two ends are tied outside the thyroid lamina to simulate the action of the lateral cricoarytenoid muscle (LCA). This provides medial rotation of the vocal process of arytenoid.

Ipsilateral cricothyroid approximation (ipsilateral type IV thyroplasty) is a procedure described to correct the residual flaccidity and loss of tension in the vocal fold. Two sutures are passed anteriorly to approximate the thyroid and cricoid cartilages anteriorly, and this approximation leads to stretching and tensioning of the ipsilateral vocal fold. Physiologically, it simulates the action of the cricothyroid muscle and is therefore best applied to any residual deficits following a SLN palsy or a combined paralysis of the SLN and RLN.[27] In our experience, it may also be usefully combined with a type I medialization laryngoplasty with some cord atrophy, wherein stretching and tensioning the vocal fold provide additional improvement over medialization alone.

Thyroplasty Type I (Surgical Procedure)

A flexible nasopharyngoscopic laryngeal examination is undertaken prior to confirm the side of immobility, the degree of glottic gap that needs correction, any loss of vocal fold tension and tone and sagging in the vertical plane, arytenoid position and posterior glottis closure, and function of the opposite vocal fold.

The first step at surgery, if using a silastic implant, is to precut the implant as per specifications required (**Figs. 2A and B**). The silastic implant thickness is configured as per the desired medialization. The author's practice is to have the implant thickness 2–3 mm greater than the glottic gap to allow for some compression of tissues on inserting the implant.

The operation is best performed with the patient being awake under monitored local anesthesia with or without additional sedation. Awake surgery helps to optimize voice results as it allows voice assessments in real time. The patient is placed supine in reverse Trendelenburg position with a shoulder bag placed for neck extension. Some surgeons prefer to insert a flexible laryngoscope and fix it in position for a continuous view of larynx during the surgery. This allows real-time visual assessment of the correction.

The skin crease overlying the ipsilateral cricothyroid region is usually used for incision and injected with 2% lignocaine with 1:200,000 epinephrine. This can be mixed with a solution of bupivacaine 0.5% and 1:100,000 epinephrine

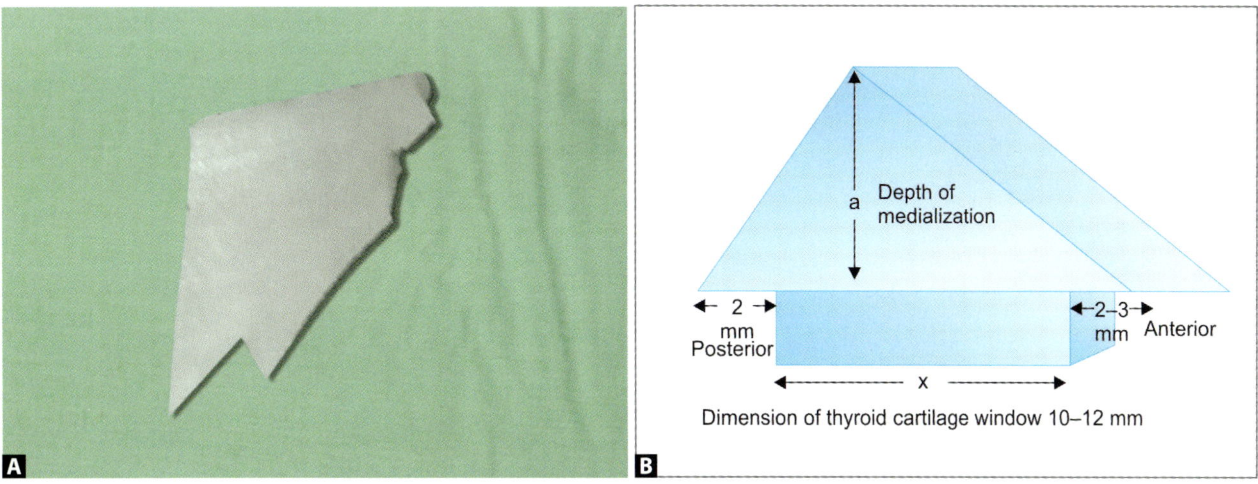

Figs. 2A and B: (A) Silastic implant; (B) Measurements of implant.

for a longer effect. The patient is then prepared and draped from nose above to clavicle below. Unless contraindicated, dexamethasone injection is administered in anticipation of laryngeal edema due to surgical manipulation.

Skin incision is given over the skin crease over the cricothyroid membrane. Subplatysmal flaps are elevated, the midline raphe is dissected, and strap muscles are retracted to expose the thyroid cartilage. The transversely horizontal window for the implant is planned with its superior margin at the level of the vocal fold, which lies approximately midway between the superior and the inferior notch of the thyroid cartilage. The external perichondrium of the thyroid cartilage is incised along with the midline and the ipsilateral superior border and a perichondrial flap elevated. A rectangular window is created approximately 5–7 mm posterior to the midline of thyroid cartilage and 3–4 mm above the inferior border of thyroid cartilage **(Fig. 3)**. In older individuals with calcified cartilage, this may require a drill.

The inner perichondrium may be preserved or incised. In the author's practice with a silastic implant, the inner perichondrium is sought to be preserved and it is raised along the peripheral rim of the window to allow for its medial displacement and so create a sizeable pocket. The silastic implant is then positioned in the extraperiosteal pocket **(Figs. 4A to D)**. With the prefabricated implants (Montgomery implant-hydroxyapatite; TVPMI implant-titanium), it is usual to incise the inner perichondrium and place the implant in the paraglottic space. Care should be taken to avoid surgical dissection further medially as this can exacerbate local edema and may also increase chances of implant extrusion.

Proper placement of implant can be assessed subjectively by checking the patient's voice as well as by looking at the flexible nasolaryngoscope monitor. Intraoperative assessment may however overestimate the improvement due to the impact of superimposed tissue edema. The implant is then secured in place by nonabsorbable sutures. The outer perichondrium is

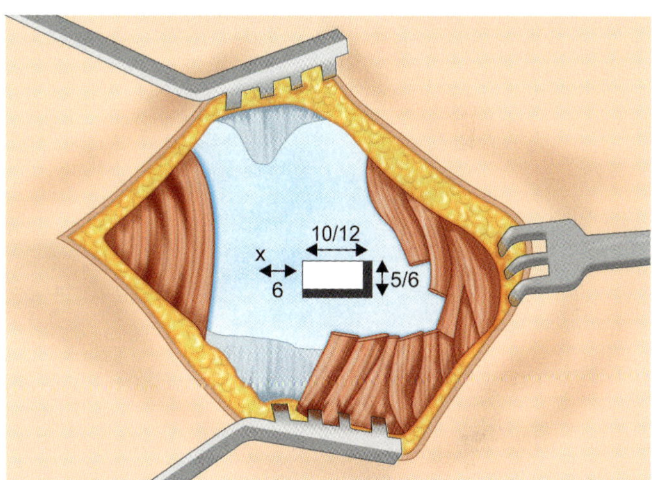

Fig. 3: Making a thyroid cartilage window on left side (exposed after retracting and dividing the strap muscles). x—midpoint of the height of the thyroid cartilage, suggestive of the level of vocal folds. Window to be around 6 mm lateral to midline, 10–12 mm long, and 5–6 mm in height. A minimum of 3 mm of cartilage should be present below the level of thyroplasty window.

repositioned and tacked with sutures, and the wound is closed in layers. A drain may be placed.

Reinnervation Procedures

Medialization thyroplasty, though a very effective procedure, is noted as suboptimal in cases with complete RLN denervation or section as the laryngeal muscles undergo denervation atrophy with reduced bulk and tone. Reinnervation has the potential to restore muscle tone and is therefore emerging as an alternate option for unilateral vocal fold paralysis. Reinnervation is usually "non-selective" with restoration of neural impulses to the adductors and abductors. Its impact is mainly in restoring muscle tone, and restoration of controlled voluntary vocal fold mobility is unusual.[28] Reports have occasionally combined it with a type I medialization thyroplasty.

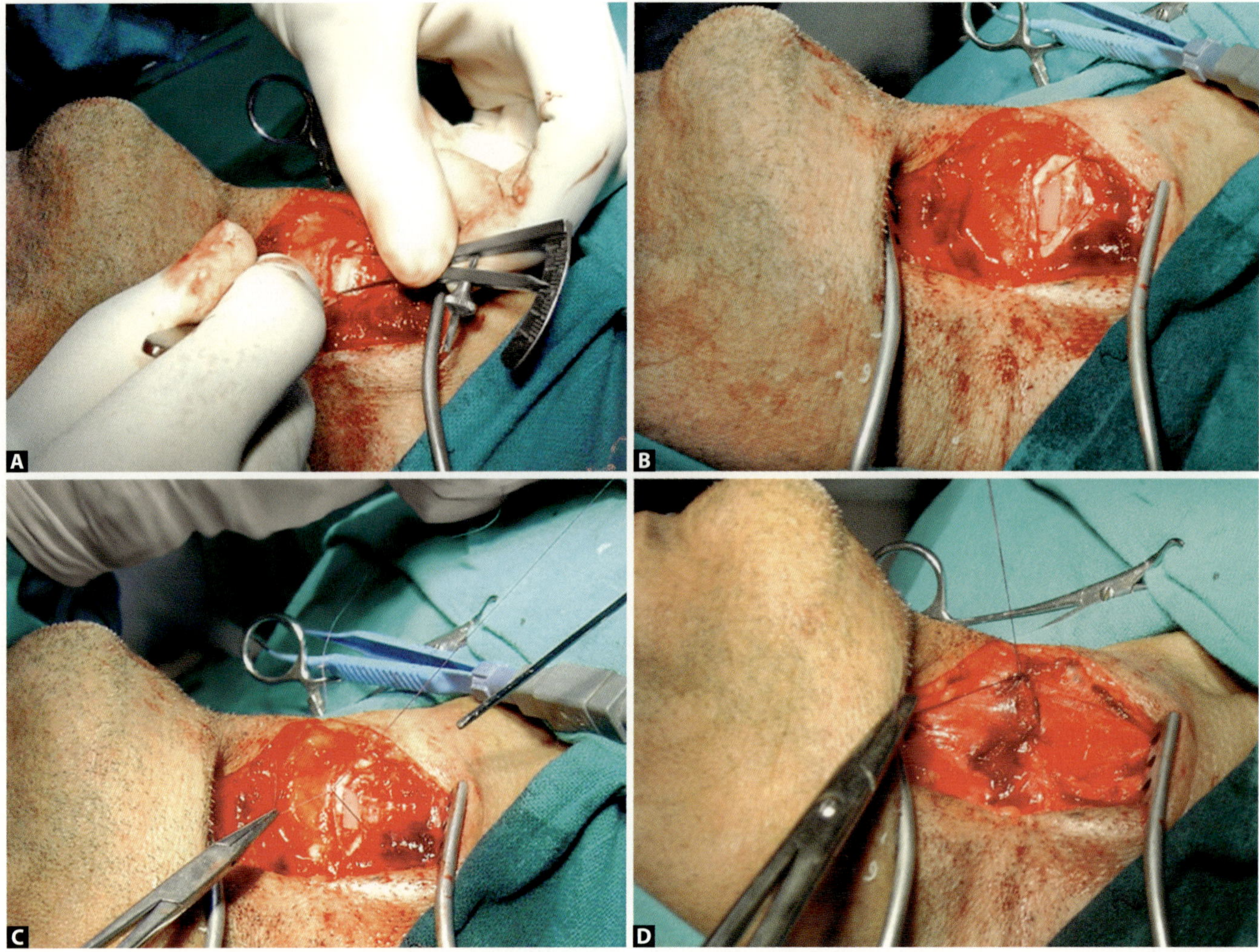

Figs. 4A to D: (A) Measurements for thyroplasty window; (B) Prosthesis in place; (C) External perichondrium sutured; (D) Strap muscles sutured.

The currently applicable laryngeal reinnervation options for unilateral laryngeal paralysis include:

- Neural anastomosis of the cut edges of a divided RLN. Direct end-to-end anastomosis, however, is difficult to achieve as the nerve edges tend to retract away, and a nerve graft is usually required.
- *Nerve transfer to the distal RLN (ansa cervicalis to RLN):*
  - *Ansa cervicalis*: RLN transfer was reported by Frazier and colleagues in 1924 in an attempt to restore vocal fold mobility.[29] The ansa cervicalis nerve supplies the pretracheal strap muscles which contract with voluntary phonation and is therefore an appropriate nerve to rennervate the laryngeal adductors. Anatomically, its abundant length enables an easy mobilization and tension-free transfer for anastomosis to the distal stump of the RLN. The minimal morbidity with the sacrifice of innervation to the strap muscles has made it the preferred donor nerve for vocal fold renervation.[30]

Surgical Technique

The procedure is done under general anesthesia. The RLN is identified in the tracheoesophageal groove and dissected till its entry into the larynx to ensure its integrity. The ansa cervicalis is found at the lateral border of the thyrohyoid muscle at the level of omohyoid muscle and is transected at its point of entry into the muscle. It is gently mobilized and positioned alongside the distal end of the RLN. The anastomosis is undertaken with 9-0 or 10-0 nylon and may be further supplemented with fibrin glue.

Return of laryngeal muscle tone and some movement can be anticipated no sooner than 4–6 months. The surgery may therefore be supplemented with a vocal fold injection as a temporary procedure to improve the voice in the interim.

Reinnervation appears to provide adequate tone to stabilize and position the vocal fold and arytenoid appropriately. Consistent and reliable voice improvement at rates of 90–95% has been reported.[31-33]

◇| REFERENCES

1. Finck C. Laryngeal dysfunction after thyroid surgery: diagnosis, evaluation and treatment. Acta Chirurgica Belgica. 2006;106(4):378-87.
2. Friedman M, LoSavio P, Ibrahim H. Superior laryngeal nerve identification and preservation in thyroidectomy. Arch Otolaryngol Head Neck Surg. 2002;128(3):296-303.
3. Cernea CR, Ferraz AR, Nishio S, Dutra Jr A, Hojaij FC, Dos Santos LR. Surgical anatomy of the external branch of the superior laryngeal nerve. Head Neck. 1992;14(5):380-3.
4. Kierner AC, Aigner M, Burian M. The external branch of superior laryngeal nerve: its topographical anatomy as related to surgery of the neck. Arch Otolaryngol Head Neck Surg. 1998;124:301-3.
5. Chandrasekhar SS, Randolph GW, Seidman MD, Rosenfeld RM, Angelos P, Barkmeier-Kraemer J, et al. Clinical practice guideline: improving voice outcomes after thyroid surgery. Otolaryngol Head Neck Surg. 2013;148(6_suppl):S1-37.
6. Serpell JW, Yeung MJ, Grodski S. The motor fibers of the recurrent laryngeal nerve are located in the anterior extralaryngeal branch. Ann Surg. 2009;249(4):648-52.
7. Beneragama T, Serpell JW. Extralaryngeal bifurcation of the recurrent laryngeal nerve: a common variation. ANZ J Surg. 2006;76(10):928-31.
8. Woodson GE. Configuration of the glottis in laryngeal paralysis. II: animal experiments. Laryngoscope. 1993;103:1235-41.
9. Hirano M, Nozoe I, Shin T, Maeyama T. Electromyography for laryngeal paralysis. In: Hirano M, Kirchner J, Bless D (Eds). Neurolaryngology: Recent Advances. Boston: College Hill Press; 1987. pp. 232-43.
10. Teitelbaum B, Wenig B. Superior laryngeal nerve injury from thyroid surgery. Head Neck. 1995;17:36-40.
11. Aluffi P, Policarpo M, Cherovac C, Olina M, Dosdegani R, Pia F. Post-thyroidectomy superior laryngeal nerve injury. Eur Arch Otorhinolaryngol. 2001;258(9):451-4.
12. Zakaria HM, Al Awad NA, Al Kreedes AS, Al-Mulhim AM, Al-Sharway MA, Hadi MA, et al. Recurrent laryngeal nerve injury in thyroid surgery. Oman Med J. 2011;26(1):34-8.
13. Hisham AN, Lukman MR. Recurrent laryngeal nerve in thyroid surgery: a critical appraisal. ANZ J Surg. 2002;72(12):887-9.
14. Kasemsuwaran L, Nubthuenetr SJ. Recurrent laryngeal nerve paresis: a complication of thyroidectomy. Otorhinolaryngology. 1997;26:365-7.
15. Jatzko GR, Lisborg PH, Müller MG, Wette VM. Recurrent nerve palsy after thyroid operations: principal nerve identification and a literature review. Surgery. 1994;115(2):139-44.
16. Fewins J, Simpson CB, Miller FR. Complications of thyroid and parathyroid surgery. Otolaryngol Clin North Am. 2003;36(1):189-206, x.
17. Lifante JC, McGill J, Murry T, Aviv JE, Inabnet III WB. A prospective, randomized trial of nerve monitoring of the external branch of the superior laryngeal nerve during thyroidectomy under local/regional anesthesia and IV sedation. Surgery. 2009;146(6):1167-73.
18. Neiman GS, Edeson B. Procedural aspects of eliciting maximum phonation time. Folia Phoniatr. 1981;33:285-93.
19. Boone DR. The Voice and Voice Therapy, 1st edition. Englewood Cliffs, NJ: Prentice-Hall; 1971. p. 169.
20. Eckel FC, Boone DR. The s/z ratio as an indicator of laryngeal pathology. J Speech Hear Disord. 1981;46(2):147-9.
21. Miller S. Voice therapy for vocal fold paralysis. Otolaryngol Clin North Am. 2004;37(1):105-19.
22. Heuer RJ, Sataloff RT, Emerich K, Rulnick R, Baroody M, Spiegel JR, et al. Unilateral recurrent laryngeal nerve paralysis: The importance of "preoperative" voice therapy. J Voice. 1997;11(1):88-94.
23. Salinas JB, Chhetri DK. Injection laryngoplasty: techniques and choices of fillers. Curr Otorhinolaryngol Rep. 2014;2(2):131-6.
24. Khadivi E, Akbarian M, Khazaeni K, Salehi M. Outcomes of autologous fat injection laryngoplasty in unilateral vocal cord paralysis. Iran J Otorhinolaryngol. 2016;28(86):215-9.
25. Isshiki N, Morita H, Okamura H, Hiramoto M. Thyroplasty as a new phonosurgical technique. Acta Otolaryngol. 1974;78:451-7.
26. Isshiki N, Tanabe M, Sawada M. Arytenoid adduction for unilateral vocal cord paralysis. Arch Otolaryngol. 1978;104:555-8.
27. Thakar A, Sikka K, Verma R, Preetam C. Cricothyroid approximation for voice and swallowing rehabilitation of high vagal paralysis secondary to skull base neoplasms. Eur Arch Otorhinolaryngol. 2011;268(11):1611-6.
28. Fancello V, Nouraei SR, Heathcote KJ. Role of reinnervation in the management of recurrent laryngeal nerve injury: current state and advances. Curr Opin Otolaryngol Head Neck Surg. 2017;25(6):480-5.
29. Frazier CH. Anastomosis of the recurrent laryngeal nerve with the descendens noni. JAMA. 1924;83:1637-41.
30. Paniello RC, West SE. Laryngeal adductory pressure as a measure of post-reinnervation synkinesis. Ann Otol Rhinol Laryngol. 2000;109(5):447-51.
31. Crumley RL. Nerve transfer technique as it relates to phonatory surgery. In: Cummings CW, Fredrickson JM, Harker LA, Krause CJ, Schuller DE, Smith RA (Eds). Otolaryngology-head and neck surgery: update II. St. Louis: Mosby-Year Book; 1990. pp. 100-6.
32. Miyauchi A, Matsusaka K, Kawaguchi H, Nakamoto K, Maeda M. Ansa-recurrent nerve anastomosis for vocal cord paralysis due to mediastinal lesions. Ann Thorac Surg. 1994;57(4):1020-1.
33. Wang W, Chen D, Chen S, Li D, Li M, Xia S, et al. Laryngeal reinnervation using ansa cervicalis for thyroid surgery-related unilateral vocal fold paralysis: a long-term outcome analysis of 237 cases. PLoS One. 2011;6(4):e19128.

Genetic Landscape and Molecular Mechanisms in Thyroid Cancer

Nelson George, Amit Agarwal

INTRODUCTION

In the past two decades, the molecular mechanisms and molecular alterations in thyroid cancer have been unraveled, largely due to the next-generation sequencing (NGS) platform. What was a mere hypothesis for many years, there is now clear evidence for a step-wise tumorigenesis in follicular-derived thyroid cancers. The genetic landscape and the mechanisms can be understood through the following sections:

- Molecular alterations in thyroid cancer
- Epigenetic alterations in thyroid cancer
- Pathways involved in tumor genesis
- *Early molecular events*:
  - *Genetic alterations in early thyroid tumorigenesis*:
    - *Gene mutations: BRAF and RAS*
    - *Gene translocations*: *RET*/papillary thyroid carcinoma (*PTC*), *PAX8/PPAR-gamma*, *NTRK*, *AKAP9/BRAF*
  - *Genetic pathways:* Mitogen-activated protein kinase (*MAPK*)/*PIK3-AKT*
- *Late molecular events*:
  - *Genetic alterations in late progression of tumor:* TP53, TERT, EIF1AX, phosphatase and tensin homolog (PTEN), RCAN 1-4, PIK3CA (amplification)
  - *Genetic pathways:* WNT/BETA-Catenin, PIK3-AKT, nuclear factor kappa B (NF-κβ), hypoxia-inducible factor-α (HIF-α), and thyroid-stimulating hormone receptor (TSHR) pathway
- Downregulation of iodine-metabolizing genes
- Genotype–phenotype correlation
- Translational utility of molecular/genetic alterations

MOLECULAR ALTERATIONS IN THYROID CANCER

These can be divided into three types:

1. *Genetic alterations*: These include various mutations of genes such as *BRAF, RAS, PTEN, TP53*, β-catenin (*CTNNB1*), *TERT*.
2. *Gene amplification and copy number gains*
3. *Gene translocations/rearrangements*: This includes RET/PTC rearrangement and PAX8–PPGAMMAG fusions.

BRAF Mutations

The most common genetic mutation in thyroid cancer, particularly PTC, is the *BRAF* mutation, which results from the T1799A transverse point mutation in exon 15 and causes a V600E amino acid change in BRAF protein resulting in constitutive and oncogenic activation of mutated BRAF kinase, which in turn causes two events: (1) Aberrant activation of MAPK cascade, which renders the thyroid cells susceptible to transforming growth factor-β (TGF-β) induced epithelial mesenchymal transition, and (2) *BRAF* mutation increases the production of cancer-promoting molecules such as extracellular matrix proteins, thrmobospondin-1, vascular endothelial growth factor (VEGF), metalloproteinase-3 (MMP3), c-Met, and platelet-derived growth factor (PDGF).[1-3] It has also been hypothesized that once PTC has been initiated by *BRAFV600E* mutation, secondary genetic alterations drive the tumorigenesis.[4] Alternatively, it has been suggested that *BRAF* mutations could be a secondary genetic event in PTC rather than a primary initiating event.[5] A third hypothesis proposes that *BRAF* mutation not only initiates tumorigenesis, but is also required to maintain and promote progression of PTC.[6,7] The average prevalence of BRAF mutation is 44% which reaches up to 70% in Asian countries.[8,9]

Thus, three features of *BRAF* mutation: (1) Its exclusive occurrence (that it is sufficient on its own to drive PTC tumorigenesis) in PTC or PTC-derived anaplastic thyroid cancer (ATC); (2) Its specificity as it does not occur in follicular thyroid carcinoma (FTC), and (3) Its high prevalence in PTC—make it the prime oncogenic driver of PTC.

The *BRAF* mutation is not only pathognomonic of PTC; the meta-analysis by Kim et al. in 2002[10] confirmed that it also correlates with high-risk clinicopathological features and poor clinical outcome. Despite some conflicting studies, most studies from widespread diverse geographical areas across the globe have demonstrated a significant correlation of *BRAF* mutation with one or more high-risk features of PTC such as LNM, ETE, DM, and RAIR.[11-13] It has been proposed that silencing of major tumor suppressor genes in a CIMP-like manner may play an important role in BRAF-promoted progression of PTC.[14] *BRAF* mutation causes aberrant methylation of several important tumor suppressor genes such as *TIMP3, DAPK, SLC5A8*, and

RARBETA2.[15-17] Methylation-mediated silencing of *TIMP3* gene may play a unique role in *BRAF* mutation-promoted invasiveness.[18]

RAS Mutations

The second-most prevalent mutation in thyroid cancer is another point mutation, the *RAS* mutation. In normal thyroid follicular cells, the intrinsic GTPases of *RAS* hydrolyze GTP to inactivate RAS. However, *RAS* mutations result in loss of its GTPase activity, thus rendering *RAS* in a permanently constitutively active GTP-bound state which then preferentially activates the PI3K-AKT pathway resulting in thyroid tumorigenesis.[19] There are three isoforms of *RAS*: HRAS, KRAS, and NRAS, and NRAS is predominantly mutated in thyroid tumors, mostly involving codons 12, 13, and 61. *RAS* mutations are commonly detected in follicular adenoma, and this suggests that *RAS* may play an exclusive role in early follicular thyroid cell tumorigenesis. However, additional genetic alterations other than *RAS* mutation are apparently required to promote transformation of follicular thyroid adenoma (FTA) into thyroid cancer, particularly the PTEN deletions.[20]

PTEN

Specifically, *PTEN* inhibits PI3K-AKT pathway promoting PIP3 dephosphorylation. The study on Cowden's syndrome, a congenital disease characterized by germline mutations of PTEN, provided the first evidence that *PTEN* deletion shows a strong predisposition to FTA and FTC.[21] Mutations or deletions of the tumor suppressor gene *PTEN* activate the PI3K-AKT pathway and are the genetic basis for follicular thyroid cell tumorigenesis in Cowden's syndrome.[22] Mutations of *PIK3CA*, which encodes the p110α catalytic subunit of *PI3K*, are also common in thyroid cancer, particularly FTC, poorly differentiated thyroid cancer (PDTC), and ATC.

There is an interesting co-occurrence with *BRAFV600E* in the undifferentiated tumors.[23]

TP53

It is well documented that thyroid carcinoma initiation and progression occur through the gradual accumulation of multiple genetic alterations. One of the pivotal molecular alterations discriminating ATCs from well-differentiated thyroid carcinomas (WDTCs) is the inactivation of the *p53* tumor suppressor gene. *p53* mutations are common in undifferentiated thyroid tumors (50–80% in ATCs).[24,25] However, several findings indicate that alterations in the *p53* sequence may also play a role in the early stages of thyroid carcinogenesis. Indeed, *p53* mutations were recently found in up to 40% of PTCs and in 22% of oncocytic FTCs. Usually, *p53* point mutations are located in the region between exons 5 and 8. DNA-damaging agents activate *p53*, leading to its binding of specific DNA responsive elements that transcriptionally regulate selected target genes. In thyroid cancer cells, *p53* tumor suppressor activity is inhibited by three different mechanisms hindering *p53* transcriptional activity, protein stability, and downstream signaling.

Beta-catenin (CTNNB1)

Mutations in β-catenin have been identified in the most aggressive forms of thyroid cancer, such as poorly differentiated and anaplastic carcinomas, and they act via activation of the WNT-β signaling pathway. Interestingly, it has been shown that mutations in β-catenin have a role to play even in initiation of some thyroid cancers, particularly those associated with *RAS* mutations. *RAS*, particularly HRAS signals through PI3K/AKT to stabilize β-catenin via two mechanisms—GSK3b inhibition and direct β-catenin phosphorylation at Ser552–PI3K/AKT-mediated β-catenin activation protects cells from senescence and increases cell proliferation, epithelial–mesenchymal transition (EMT), and cell invasion.

TERT

It was as early as 2013, when two point mutations, C228T and C250T, on *TERT* gene promoter were detected in thyroid carcinoma.[26,27] The *TERT* gene encodes the reverse transcriptase subunit of the telomerase complex, the specialized DNA polymerase that elongates the telomere portion of chromosomes adding repeated sequences. Its expression and activity are usually absent/low in normal cells whereas it is strongly increased in cancer cells[28] including aggressive thyroid cancers[29] with a lower prevalence in PTCs (~10%) compared to PDTCs (40%) and ATCs (~70%). It has been shown that *TERT* promoter mutations have higher prevalence in FTCs and aggressive *BRAFV600E*-positive PTCs while no *TERT* mutation was found in benign thyroid lesions; *TERT* mutation correlated with a worse clinical outcome in patients with DTCs,[30] and coexistence of *TERT* mutation with *BRAFV600E* results in more aggressive PTC.

RET–PTC

RET is a proto-oncogene encoding an RTK. *RET–PTC* occurs due to genetic recombination between the 3′ tyrosine kinase portion of RET and the 5′ portion of a partner gene.[31] There are more than 10 types of *RET–PTC* translocation; the most common types are *RET–PTC1* and *RET–PTC3*.[32] The rearrangement results in ligand-independent dimerization and constitutive tyrosine kinase activity of RET, which causes activation of both MAPK and PI3K-AKT pathways.[33] *RET–PTC* then activates the dual pathways by recruiting signaling adaptors to phosphorylated Tyr1062 on the intracellular domain of the *RET* fusion protein 60. Because of the fact that *RET-PTC* activates the PI3-AKT pathway, *RET-PTC* mutations are also seen in follicular thyroid adenomas.

AKAP9/BRAF

The prevalence of this fusion protein in sporadic PTC is very low and can be considered a rare event.[34]

PAX8/PPARγ

This gene rearrangement (somatic translocation) in thyroid cancer results from the fusion between the paired box 8 (*PAX8*) and peroxisome proliferator-activated receptor gamma (*PPARγ*) (*PAX8/PPARγ*). *PAX8* is an essential transcription factor for thyroid gland development[35] and in the mature organ, it is responsible for thyroid-specific gene expression.[36] On the other hand, PPARγ, a nuclear hormone receptor, has no known physiological role in the thyroid but is well described as a promoter of anti-inflammatory phenotype in macrophage and as a master regulator of adipogenesis. The *PAX8–PPARγ* gene is another prominent recombinant oncogene in thyroid cancer, occurring in up to 60% of FTC and FVPTC. *PAX8–PPARγ* also occurs in FTA, but its prevalence is low in benign thyroid tumors. PTC detection of *PAX8/PPARγ* is strongly associated with follicular features; tumors are encapsulated and likely have an indolent clinical course.[37] In thyroid cells, *PAX8/PPARγ* expression can induce activation of the WNT/TCF pathway, causing an increase of invasiveness and aggressiveness features, such as anchorage-independent growth.

Epigenetic Alterations

Like in other human cancers, aberrant gene methylation is also commonly seen in thyroid cancer.[14] This results in silencing of a gene. In thyroid cancers, *BRAFV600E* mutation results in hypermethylation of tumor suppressor genes such as *TIMP3*, *SLC5A8*, *DAPK1*, and *RARB*.[16] The hypermethylation of these genes results in alteration of several metabolic and cellular functions. Even RAS mutations, via activation of the PIK3-AKT pathway, result in silencing of *PTEN* gene, which also causes alteration of cellular and metabolic functions of thyroid follicular cells.[38]

Pathways Involved in Tumor Genesis

Aberrant signaling of two major pathways results in tumori-genesis in thyroid cancer:

1. *MAPK signaling pathway*: This pathway plays a central role in initiation of thyroid tumorigenesis particularly PTC.
   - *The driver mutations* of this pathway are— *BRAF*, *RAS*, and *ALK* mutations; PET/PTC rearrangement
   - *Secondary molecular alterations:* Hypermethylation and upregulation of oncogenic proteins such as chemokines, VEGFA, MET, NF-κβ, MMP, and HIF-α, TGF-β
   - *Oncogenic mechanism*: Cell proliferation, growth, migration, tumor angiogenesis, invasion, and metastases
2. *PIK3-AKT pathway*: It has a fundamental role in thyroid cancer progression, especially FTC. The driver mutation of this pathway is RAS. Invasion and metastatic ability of FTC are promoted by the PIK3-AKT pathway (especially AKT1 isoform).[39] Further, the fact that the aberrant signaling of the PIK3-AKT pathway is far more prevalent in FTC than its precursor FA supports the hypothesis that aberrant activation of PIK3-AKT signaling promotes conversion of FA to FTC by conferring tumor cell invasiveness.

Early and Late Molecular Events

Early molecular events occur in the MAPK pathway and are seen in PTC, FTC, and Hurthle cell carcinoma (HCC). Late molecular events are seen in PIK3-AKT pathway and are seen in PDTC and ATC.

Early Molecular Events

Constitutive activation of the MAPK signaling pathway plays a central role in initiation of thyroid cancer. The successive cascade of downstream events in this pathway leads to altered cell proliferation and differentiation. Interestingly, the genetic alterations in the MAPK pathway are mutually exclusive of the alterations in the PIK3-AKT pathway (i.e., the alterations in each of these pathways are not dependent on each other). Genetic alterations in this pathway are highly prevalent and seen in as much as 80% of all PTCs.[40]

Late Molecular Events

In the process of de-differentiation, two important events occur late in thyroid tumor genesis:

1. *Progressive accumulation of genetic alteration*: Aggressive thyroid cancers such as radioiodine refractory PTC (RAIR), PDTC, and ATC are characterized by the accumulation of genetic alterations which otherwise are mutually exclusive in well-differentiated cancers.[41] Thus, mutation of *NRAS*, *PIK3CA*, and *PTEN* as well as amplification of *PIK3CA* progressively increases in frequency from FTA to FTC and then to PDTC and ATC.[42-44] Similarly, these aggressive PTCs also show coexistence of *BRAF/RAS* mutations along with *RET/PTC* rearrangement. This gives support to the hypothesis that aggressive thyroid cancers result from amplification of the oncogenic process brought on by the synergistic co-operation of multiple accumulated genetic alterations.
2. *Co-operation of MAPK and PIK3-AKT pathways*: Genetic alterations that cause aberrant signaling of the MAPK pathway cause tumorigenesis toward PTC while activation of the PIK3-AKT pathway results in FTC. However, in PDTC and ATC, additional or secondary genetic alterations such as mutation in *TP53* and *CTNNB1* can cause dual activation of both pathways resulting in tumor progression of PTC and FTC toward PDTC and ATC.

Downregulation of Iodine-metabolizing Genes

Five iodine-metabolizing genes are involved in the iodine-metabolizing system of the thyroid cell. These are *NIS*, *SLC26A4* (Pendrin), *TPO*, *TSHR*, and *TG*. Expression of these genes is impaired or lost (silencing) in thyroid cancer, especially those cancers that harbor *BRAF* mutation, and the methylation of these genes are proposed to be the mechanism responsible for silencing of these genes.[45,46] *BRAF* mutation not only results in downregulation of these genes through the MEK-ERK pathway; it also directly affects the targeting of the gene to the cell membrane, particularly that of NIS. NIS is thus rendered nonfunctional because it has been established that targeting to and retention of NIS in the plasma membrane rather than cytoplasm are essential for NIS to be fully functional.[47]

Activation of the PIK3-AKT pathway by RAS/RET-PTC has also been shown to downregulate the iodide-handling machinery in thyroid cancer cells.[48] Thus, even though the three oncoproteins (BRAF, RAS, and RET/PTC) work together along a single cascade (MAPK), they are also mutually exclusive (independent) and are able to trigger different specific signals. The implication of this finding is that therapies that target inhibition of MEK-ERK pathway may not be able to redifferentiate RAIR tumors to express NIS in the basolateral membrane and therefore specific BRAF/RAS/RET-PTC inhibitors will be required to induce radioactive iodine (RAI) uptake.

Genotype–Phenotype Correlation

There is a strong correlation between histology of thyroid cancer, including various variants and the underlying genotype **(Table 1)**.

◇ GENETIC LANDSCAPE OF VARIOUS THYROID CANCERS

Papillary Thyroid Carcinoma

It has a relatively low mutational burden and a stable genome exhibiting only a few copy number alterations. The Cancer Genome Atlas (TGCA) study of 500 PTCs[49] confirmed that PTC is characterized by a few dominant, largely mutually exclusive oncogenic somatic mutations which manifest either as a single nucleotide substitution, or as small insertions and deletions, or as fusions. These involve a small set of genes whose protein products are typically members of MAPK and PI3K/PTEN/AKT/mechanistic target of rapamycin (mTOR) signaling pathways. Common genetic alteration in conventional PTC is the T1799A transverse point mutation in exon 15 of *BRAFV600E* (60%), which causes a V600E amino acid change in BRAF protein residues, RAS (15%), gene fusions of RET/PTC (6%), BRAF, NRTK1/3 and ALK (<5%), and TP53 (<5%). Based on gene-expression profiles, PTC can be divided into two distinct types—BRAF-like PTC and RAS-like PTC. BRAF-like PTCs are characterized by activation of the MAPK signaling pathway activated by *BRAFV600E* mutations as well as RET/PTC and NTRK1/3 fusions; RAS-like PTCs are characterized by HRAS, EIEAX, and BRAF K601E point mutations and PPARγ fusions, which activate both MAPK and PI3K/AKT signaling pathways. All these mutations are exclusive of each other even though the two groups and pathways are correlated.

Impact of TERT Promoter Mutations in PTC

In 2014, Xing et al.[50] were the first to prove the role of synergistic effect of coexisting *TERT* promoter mutations and *BRAFV600E* in PTC in aggressive behavior and poor clinical outcome of PTC.

There is a strong genotype–phenotype correlation in the variants of PTC:

- Tall cell variant shows strong *BRAFV600E* mutation and strong MAPK output and is prone to de-differentiation.
- FVPTC has a RAS-dominant (30%) mutational profile but also exhibits *BRAF* mutation in 15%.[51]
- Noninvasive follicular thyroid neoplasm with papillary-like nuclear features (NIFTP) is dominated by *RAS* mutations and absent *BRAF* mutations.[52]
- *Pediatric* PTC shows a higher incidence of RET/PTC and BRAF fusions.

Follicular Thyroid Carcinoma

Mutations of *RAS* and rearrangements of PPAR-γ (e.g., PAX8-PPAR-γ translocation) are common in follicular thyroid cancer. The prevalence of RAS and PAX8-PPARγ varies considerably between studies. *RAS* mutations are found in up to 40–50% of FTC and 20–40% of FA; PAX8-PPARγ fusions are found in 30–40% of FTC and a smaller percentage of FA (2–13%).[53] RAS and PAX8-PPARγ are mutually exclusive. RAS is an activator of both the mitogen-activated protein kinase and PI3K-AKT pathways. *RAS* (NRAS, HRAS, and less KRAS) mutations are also seen frequently in follicular adenomas and it is hypothesized that additional genetic alterations are required to transform an adenoma into follicular thyroid cancer, for example, deletions of the tumor suppressor gene *PTEN* or mutations of *PIK3CA*.[54,55]

Table 1: Genotype–Phenotype correlation.

Genotype	Phenotype	(%) prevalence
BRAFV600E	TCV	89
	CVPTC	67
RAS	FVPTC	38
	NIFTP	40
PAX8-PPARg	FTC	45
	FVPTC	38
RET/PTC1	CVPTC	06
TERT	ATC	70
	HCC	
	PDTC	40
TP53	ATC	65
	PDTC	40

(ATC: anaplastic thyroid cancer; CVPTC: classical variant of papillary thyroid carcinoma; FTC: follicular thyroid carcinoma; FVPTC: follicular variant of papillary thyroid carcinoma; PDTC: poorly differentiated thyroid cancer; NIFTP: noninvasive follicular thyroid neoplasm with papillary-like nuclear features; PAX8: paired box 8; PPARγ: peroxisome proliferator-activated receptor gamma)

Hurthle Cell Carcinoma

The genetic landscape of HCC is different from the one in FTC and PTC. HCC is distinct from other cancers, as it shows two unique features: extensive mitochondrial DNA mutation in complex 1 of electron transport chain[56] as well as the whole chromosome losses. These genetic alterations lead to decreased oxidative phosphorylation, enhanced aerobic glycolysis, and oxidative stress as well as the overactivation of the PI3K/AKT/mTOR and RAS/RAF/MEK/ERK signaling pathways. Moreover, high-risk HTC is characterized by a significant mutation burden and aneuploidy, which may result in the enhanced immunogenicity of the tumor and consequently a better response to immunotherapy. These tumors also exhibit a distinct gene expression profile; RAS point mutations and PAX8-PPARγ fusions are much less common than in FTC.[57]

Poorly Differentiated Thyroid Cancer

The study by Landa et al.[58] using the MSK-IMPACT NGS platform has been the largest and the most comprehensive published study on PDTC to date. It examined the largest PDTC cohort of 84 patients. NGS showed molecular level evidence for the intermediate position of PDTC; mutation burden increased significantly from PTC toward PDTC[59] and ATC (median number of mutations: 1, 2, and 6, respectively).

The *BRAFV600E* and *RAS* mutations remain the mutually exclusive main driver mutations in PDTC, occurring in 33 and 45% of PDTCs, respectively. Interestingly, in PDTC, the BRAF/RAS signatures are closely correlated with the histologic phenotypes and dictate distinct metastatic patterns—those with *RAS*-mutated PDTC tend to metastasize to distant sites while *BRAF*-mutated PDTC tends to spread to lymph node (LN) only.[60] *TERT* mutations represent the most common molecular alteration in PDTC with a step-wise increase from PTC (9%) to PDTC (40%) and ATC (65–73%). *TERT* mutations tend to co-occur with RAS and *BRAF* mutations, and this has a synergistic effect on the aggressiveness of PDTC.[61] *TP53* mutations, although highly prevalent in ATCs, were relatively rare in PDTCs (73% vs. 8%).[62] Another tumor suppressor gene *ATM* is also mutated in PDTC and has a similar frequency (8%) to ATC (9%). The higher frequency of RAS family mutations compared with *BRAF* mutations suggests that more PDTCs may be related to FTC or follicular variant of PTC than classical type PTC. The low percentage of *BRAF* mutations found in PDTC compared with ATC could indicate that when BRAF-mutant PTCs progress, they progress straight to ATC or progress quickly through a poorly differentiated state. Finally, the paucity of RET/PTC and PAX8/PPARγ rearrangements and ALK fusions in PDTCs (14%) suggest that well-differentiated tumors harboring these alterations may be less predisposed to de-differentiation.[62]

◇| ANAPLASTIC THYROID CANCER

Anaplastic thyroid cancers harbor a higher number of mutations than PDTCs and PTCs. There is a high prevalence of *TERT* mutations (75%), followed by *TP53* (70%) followed by *BRAF* (45%) and *RAS* (24%). Mutations of genes encoding members of the PI3K/AKT/mTOR pathway were seen more frequently in ATCs than PDTCs (39% vs. 11%). Besides *PIK3CA* and *PTEN*, mutations of *PIK3C2G*, *PIK3CG*, *PIK3C3*, *PIK3R1*, *PIK3R2*, *AKT3*, *TSC1*, *TSC2*, and *mTOR* were also present. Genes encoding components of the SWI/SNF chromatin remodeling complex were mutated in 36% of ATCs and 6% of PDTCs. Mutations of genes encoding members of the WNT signaling pathway—i.e., CTNNB1 (β-catenin), *AXIN1*, and *APC*—have previously been reported as genetic hallmarks of ATCs.[63] Due to their accumulation in ATC, PI3K/AKT/ mTOR pathway mutations, TERT promoter mutations, TP53 mutations, mutations in SWI/SNF complexes, and HMTs may represent key genetic events distinguishing ATC and PDTC. It has been observed that in ATCs, there is a much lower expression of vascular endothelial growth factor receptors 1, 2, and 3; fibroblast growth factor receptors 1, 2, 3, and 4; and platelet-derived growth factor receptor-α, RET, and KIT.[64] Thus, generally, inhibitors of growth factors and their receptors appear to have a very limited effect on the survival of ATC patients. Similarly, rearrangements such as RET/PTC and ALK are rare in ATC. Studies on ATCs have found *PIK3CA* mutations/copy number gains to be overlapping with the presence of *BRAF* or *RAS* mutations, or increased *p53* expression,[65] suggesting that PIK3CA alterations often cooperate with other oncogenic events in ATC. Thus, in ATC, both genetic instability and clonal heterogeneity are responsible for genetic heterogeneity of ATC. TP53 damage in a differentiated carcinoma is likely a key factor of de-differentiation and major chromosomal instability leading to ATC.

The poor prognosis and the inefficiency of conventional and targeted therapies in ATC may be explained by the fact that besides oncogenic mutations, there are other mechanisms such as abnormalities in gene expression, alterations in miRNAs, and epigenetic modifications that interact with mutations in onco-genes and tumor suppressors to result in such a virulent tumor.

Translational Utility of Molecular/Genetic Alterations

This information can be utilized in three ways:
1. For enhancing the diagnostic utility of conventional cytology
2. For systemic therapy for advanced DTC, PDTC, and ATC
3. For prognostication

Enhancing the Diagnostic Utility of Conventional Cytology

Gene expression is being used to assist in the diagnostic evaluation of Bethesda category 3, 4, 5, and thyroid nodules as a "rule-in test." 7-gene mutation panel including BRAF, RAS, RET/PTC, and PAX8-PPARG has been used in aspirates as a "rule-out test" to improve the diagnostic accuracy of conventional cytology in indeterminate nodules.

Therapeutic Utility

Targeted therapy has been developed against aggressive thyroid cancers and includes:

- Tyrosine kinase inhibitors (TKIs)
- Therapies targeting gene fusions
- mTOR inhibitors
- Re-differentiating agents
- Immunomodulators

Tyrosine kinase inhibitors: Novel, small-molecule protein-kinase inhibitors have been proven to be effective against many components of MAPK and PI3K-AKT pathways, which are the therapeutic targets. Both selective kinase inhibitors and multikinases have been developed since it is known that simultaneously inhibiting the MAPK and PI3K-AKT pathways can result in better response. Five drugs or drug combinations have been approved by the Food and Drug Administration (FDA):

1. *Vandetanib*: It has been approved only for treatment of advanced and progressive and/or symptomatic medullary thyroid cancer (MTC). However, efficacy of vandetanib in advanced RAIR differentiated thyroid cancer (DTC) has been studied in a randomized double-blinded trial, which showed enhanced PFS in vandetanib group (11.1 months vs. 5.9 months).[66]
2. *Cabozantinib*: It has also been approved only for MTC and again its utility in advanced DTC has been studied in two trials.[67]
3. Sorafenib
4. Lenvatinib
5. Dabrafenib and trametinib

Limitations of TKIs: Two major limitations are: (1) adverse effects which result either in de-escalation of dose or in stoppage of drug; and (2) development of tumor resistance leading to transient response.

Neoadjuvant therapy with TKIs: There are anecdotal case reports of use of TKI inhibitors in a neoadjuvant setting with the goal of shrinking the tumor and making it amenable to surgical resection. Most TKIs can be used in neoadjuvant setting but since they all are VEGF inhibitors, they can lead to poor wound healing and fistula formation and need to be discontinued at least 2 weeks prior to surgery. On the other hand, selective BRAF, RET, NTRK inhibitors can be used in the neoadjuvant setting without the risk of poor would healing as they have little or no angiogenic properties and they need not be discontinued prior to surgery.

Therapies targeting gene fusions: Several drugs aimed at targeting *NTRK* and *AKL* gene fusions have been tested, and some of them have been approved by the FDA. Larotrectinib is a highly selective inhibitor of tropomyosin receptor kinase (TRKA, TRKB, and TRKC) which has been approved by the FDA for the treatment of solid tumors with NTRK fusion.[68] The objective response rate in phase I and II clinical trials was high (80%) with 63% of patients with NTRK-positive tumors experiencing partial response and 13% complete response. Entrectinib is also a selective inhibitor of TRKA, TRKB, and TRKC that also inhibits ALK and ROS1 tyrosine kinases. In August 2019, it received FDA approval for the treatment of TRK-positive solid tumors, based on results of phase 1 and 2 clinical trials documenting an objective response rate of 57%, a partial response in 50%, and a complete response in only 7%.[69] One of the major advantages of this drug is that it penetrates the blood–brain barrier making it feasible to target brain metastases of the solid tumors.

mTOR inhibitors: Everolimus is a serine–threonine kinase inhibitor of mTOR. It is FDA approved for the treatment of renal cell carcinoma. Everolimus has been studied in several trials for the treatment of thyroid cancer. All trials required disease progression for trial entry.[70]

Re-differentiating agents: RAIR DTC results from decreased NIS expression due to *BRAF* mutation. BRAF and MEK inhibitors have been used to restore RAI uptake in these aggressive DTC enabling treatment with RAI resulting in increased PFS. The two commonly used agents are selumetinib (75 mg/day) and the selective BRAF inhibitor dabrafenib (150 mg twice a day).[71]

Immunotherapy for DTC: Another emerging potential therapeutic target is the immune landscape of the thyroid cancer. The two important immune checkpoints, such as pro-grammed cell death protein 1 (PD1) and its ligand-PDL-1, as well as cytotoxic T-lymphocyte-associated protein 4 (CTLA-4) inhibitors, exhibit antitumor effects by changing the inter-action between the immune system cells and tumor cells.[72] The expression of PDL1 was studied in one meta-analysis by Aghajani et al.,[73] which concluded that the expression of PDL1 in thyroid cancer was associated with tumor recurrence and poor survival. However, DTC is a poorly immunogenic cancer due to a low mutation burden and therefore it has shown relatively poor response to immunotherapy with checkpoint inhibitors.[74] On the other hand, response of these therapies may be more in de-differentiated tumors, such as PDTC and ATC, as they are characterized by high mutation burden and higher likelihood of introducing immunogenicity.[75]

◇ CLINICAL PEARLS

- There is step-wise tumorigenesis in follicular-derived thyroid cancers
- The most common genetic mutation in thyroid cancer, particularly PTC, is the T1799A transverse point mutation in exon 15 of *BRAFV600E*, which causes a V600E amino acid change in BRAF protein.

- Genetic landscape of thyroid cancer includes mutations such as *BRAF, RAS, PTEN, TP53*, β-catenin (*CTNNB1*), *TERT*; gene rearrangements/fusions such as RET/PTC and PAX8-PPGAMMAG; and epigenetic alterations such as hypermethylation of tumor suppressor genes such as *TIMP3, SLC5A8, DAPK1*, and *RARB*.
- The two major signaling pathways are the MAPK pathway (major drivers are BRAF and RAS) and the PI3K-AKT (main driver mutation is RAS).
- Early molecular events occur in the MAPK pathway and seen in PTC, FTC, and HCC. Late molecular events are seen in PIK3-AKT pathway and are seen in PDTC and ATC.
- *BRAF* works through MAPK pathway to downregulate the five iodine-metabolizing genes and also directly preventing the targeting of *NIS* gene to the cell membrane making it nonfunctional.
- Three unique features of *BRAF* mutation make it the prime oncogenic driver of PTC: (1) Its exclusive occurrence (that it is sufficient on its own to drive PTC tumorigenesis) in PTC or PTC-derived ATC, (2) Its specificity as it does not occur in FTC, and (3) Its high prevalence in PTC.
- There is a strong correlation between histology of thyroid cancer, including various variants, and the underlying genotype.
- *BRAF* mutation also correlates with high-risk clinicopathological features and poor clinical outcome.
- *RAS* mutations may have a role in early follicular thyroid cell tumorigenesis. However, additional genetic alterations other than RAS mutation are apparently required to transform FTA into thyroid cancer, particularly the pTEN deletions.
- PTC has a relatively low mutational burden and a stable genome.
- HCC shows two unique features: (1) Extensive mitochondrial DNA mutation in complex 1 of electron transport chain and (2) Whole chromosome losses.
- *BRAFV600E* and *RAS* mutations remain the mutually exclusive main driver mutations in PDTC, occurring in 33% and 45% of PDTCs, respectively.
- Those with RAS-mutated PDTC tend to metastasize to distant sites while BRAF-mutated PDTC tends to spread to LN only.
- *TERT* mutations represent the most common molecular alteration in PDTC.
- ATCs harbor a higher number of mutations than PDTCs and PTCs. There is a high prevalence of *TERT* mutations (75%), followed by TP53 (70%) followed by *BRAF* (45%) and *RAS* (24%).

◇ REFERENCES

1. Knauf JA, Sartor MA, Medvedovic M, Lundsmith E, Ryder M, Salzano M, et al. Progression of BRAF-induced thyroid cancer is associated with epithelial-mesenchymal transition requiring concomitant MAP kinase and TGF-β signaling. Oncogene. 2011;30:3153-62.

2. Nucera C, Porrello A, Antonello ZA, Mekel M, Nehs MA, Giordano TJ, et al. B-Raf(V600E) and thrombospondin-1 promote thyroid cancer progression. Proc Natl Acad Sci USA. 2010;107:10649-54.

3. Wang Y, Ji M, Wang W, Miao Z, Hou P, Chen X, et al. Association of the T1799A BRAF mutation with tumor extrathyroidal invasion, higher peripheral platelet counts, and over-expression of platelet-derived growth factor-B in papillary thyroid cancer. Endocr Relat Cancer. 2008;15:183-90.

4. Xing M. BRAFV600E mutation and papillary thyroid cancer: chicken or egg? J Clin Endocrinol Metab. 2012;97:2295-8.

5. Vasko V, Hu S, Wu G, Xing JC, Larin A, Savchenko V, et al. High prevalence and possible de novo formation of BRAF mutation in metastasized papillary thyroid cancer in lymph nodes. J Clin Endocrinol Metab. 2005;90:5265-9.

6. Salvatore G, Falco V, Salerno P, Nappi T, Pepe S, Troncone G, et al. BRAF is a therapeutic target in aggressive thyroid carcinoma. Clin Cancer Res. 2006;12:1623-9.

7. Liu D, Liu Z, Condouris S, Xing M. BRAFV600E maintains proliferation, transformation, and tumorigenicity of BRAF-mutant papillary thyroid cancer cells. J Clin Endocrinol Metab. 2007;92:2264-71.

8. Xing M. BRAF mutation in thyroid cancer. Endocr Relat Cancer. 2005;12:245-62.

9. George N, Agarwal A, Kumari N, Agarwal S, Krisnani N, Gupta SK. Mutational profile of papillary thyroid carcinoma in an endemic goiter region of north India. Indian J Endocrinol Metab. 2018;22(4):505-10.

10. Kim TH, Park YJ, Lim JA, Ahn HY, Lee EK, Lee YJ, et al. The association of the BRAF(V600E) mutation with prognostic factors and poor clinical outcome in papillary thyroid cancer: a meta-analysis. This is a large meta-analysis on the relationship of BRAF mutation with clinicopathological behaviours of PTC. Cancer. 2012;118:1764-73.

11. Namba H, Nakashima M, Hayashi T, Hayashida N, Maeda S, Rogounovitch TI, et al. Clinical implication of hotspot BRAF mutation, V599E, in papillary thyroid cancers. J Clin Endocrinol Metab. 2003;88:4393-7. .

12. Adeniran AJ, Zhu Z, Gandhi M, Steward DL, Fidler JP, Giordano TJ, et al. Correlation between genetic alterations and microscopic features, clinical manifestations, and prognostic characteristics of thyroid papillary carcinomas. Am J Surg Pathol. 2006;30:216-22.

13. Riesco-Eizaguirre G, Gutierrez-Martinez P, Garcia-Cabezas MA, Nistal M, Santisteban P. The oncogene BRAF V600E is associated with a high risk of recurrence and less differentiated papillary thyroid carcinoma due to the impairment of Na_/I_ targeting to the membrane. Endocr Relat Cancer. 2006;13:257-69.

14. Xing M. Gene methylation in thyroid tumorigenesis. Endocrinology. 2007;148:948-53.

15. Hoque MO, Rosenbaum E, Westra WH, Xing M, Ladenson P, Zeiger MA, et al. Quantitative assessment of promoter methylation profiles in thyroid neoplasms. J Clin Endocrinol Metab. 2005;90:4011-8.

16. Hu S, Liu DX, Tufano RP, Carson KA, Rosenbaum E, Cohen Y, et al. Association of aberrant methylation of tumor suppressor genes with tumor aggressiveness and *BRAF* mutation in papillary thyroid cancer. Int J Cancer. 2006;119:2322-9.

17. Porra V, Ferraro-Peyret C, Durand C, Selmi-Ruby S, Giroud H, Berger-Dutrieux N, et al. Silencing of the tumor suppressor gene *SLC5A8* is associated with BRAF mutations in classical papillary thyroid carcinomas. J Clin Endocrinol Metab. 2005;90:3028-35.

18. Anand-Apte B, Bao L, Smith R, Iwata K, Olsen BR, Zetter B, et al. A review of tissue inhibitor of metalloproteinases-3 (TIMP- 3) and experimental analysis of its effect on primary tumor growth. Biochem Cell Biol. 1996;74:853-62.

19. Liu Z, Hou P, Ji M, Guan H, Studeman K, Jensen K, et al. Highly prevalent genetic alterations in receptor tyrosine kinases and phosphatidylinositol 3-kinase/akt and mitogen-activated protein kinase pathways in anaplastic and follicular thyroid cancers. J Clin Endocrinol Metab. 2008;93:3106-16.

20. Miller KA, Yeager N, Baker K, Liao XH, Refetoff S, Di Cristofano A. Oncogenic Kras requires simultaneous PI3K signaling to induce ERK activation and transform thyroid epithelial cells in vivo. Cancer Res. 2009;69:3689-94.

21. Liaw D, Marsh DJ, Li J, Dahia PL, Wang SI, Zheng Z, et al. Germline mutations of the *PTEN* gene in Cowden disease: an inherited breast and thyroid cancer syndrome. Nat Genet. 1997;16:64-7.

22. Dahia PLM, Marsh DJ, Zheng Z, Zedenius J, Komminoth P, Frisk T, et al. Somatic deletions and mutations in the Cowden disease gene, PTEN, in sporadic thyroid tumors. Cancer Res. 1997;57:4710-3.

23. Burke JE, Perisic O, Masson GR, Vadas O, Williams RL. Oncogenic mutations mimic and enhance dynamic events in the natural activation of phosphoinositide 3-kinase p110α (PIK3CA). Proc Natl Acad Sci USA. 2012;109:15259-64.

24. Cancer Genome Atlas Research Network. Integrated genomic characterization of papillary thyroid carcinoma. Cell. 2014; 159:676-90.

25. Farid NR. P53 mutations in thyroid carcinoma: Tidings from an old foe. J. Endocrinol. Investig. 2001;24:536-45.

26. Landa I, Ganly I, Chan TA, Mitsutake N, Matsuse M, Ibrahimpasic T, et al. Frequent somatic TERT promoter mutations in thyroid cancer: higher prevalence in advanced forms of the disease. J Clin Endocrinol Metab. 2013;98: E1562-6.

27. Liu X, Bishop J, Shan Y, Pai S, Liu D, Murugan AK, et al. Highly prevalent TERT promoter mutations in aggressive thyroid cancers. Endocr Relat Cancer. 2013;20:603-10.

28. Meyerson M, Counter CM, Eaton EN, Ellisen LW, Steiner P, Caddle SD, et al. hEST2, the putative human telomerase catalytic subunit gene, is up-regulated in tumor cells and during immortalization. Cell. 1997;90:785-95.

29. Brousset P, Chaouche N, Leprat F, Branet-Brousset F, Trouette H, Zenou RC, et al. Telomerase activity in human thyroid carcinomas originating from the follicular cells. J Clin Endocrinol Metab. 1997;82:4214-6.

30. Melo M, da Rocha AG, Vinagre J, Batista R, Peixoto J, Tavares C, et al. TERT promoter mutations are a major indicator of poor outcome in differentiated thyroid carcinomas. J Clin Endocrinol Metab. 2014;99:E754-765.

31. Ciampi R, Nikiforov YE. RET/PTC rearrangements and BRAF mutations in thyroid tumorigenesis. Endocrinology. 2007;148:936-41.

32. Santoro M, Melillo RM, Fusco A. RET/PTC activation in papillary thyroid carcinoma: European Journal of Endocrinology Prize Lecture. Eur J Endocrinol. 2006;155.645-53.

33. Castellone MD, De Falco V, Rao DM, Bellelli R, Muthu M, Basolo F, et al. The β-catenin axis integrates multiple signals downstream from RET/papillary thyroid carcinoma leading to cell proliferation. Cancer Res. 2009;69:1867-76.

34. Lee JH, Lee ES, Kim YS, Won NH, Chae YS. BRAF mutation and AKAP9 expression in sporadic papillary thyroid carcinomas. Pathology (Phila). 2006;38:201-4.

35. Macchia PE, Lapi P, Krude H, Pirro MT, Missero C, Chiovato L, et al. PAX8 mutations associated with congenital hypothyroidism caused by thyroid dysgenesis. Nat Genet. 1998;19:83-6.

36. Pasca di Magliano M, Di Lauro R, Zannini M. Pax8 has a key role in thyroid cell differentiation. Proc Natl Acad Sci USA. 2000;97:13144-9.

37. Armstrong MJ, Yang H, Yip L, Ohori MP, McCoy KL, Stang MT, et al. PAX8/PPARγ rearrangement in thyroid nodules predicts follicular-pattern carcinomas, in particular the encapsulated follicular variant of papillary carcinoma. Thyroid. 2014;24: 1369-74.

38. Hou P, Ji M, Xing M. Association of PTEN gene methylation with genetic alterations in the phosphatidylinositol 3-kinase/AKT signaling pathway in thyroid tumors. Cancer. 2008;113:2440-7.

39. Vasko V, Saji M, Hardy E, Kruhlak M, Larin A, Savchenko V, et al. Akt activation and localisation correlate with tumour invasion and oncogene expression in thyroid cancer. J Med Genet. 2004;41:161-70.

40. Gao J, Aksoy BA, Dogrusoz U, Dresdner G, Gross B, Sumer SO, et al. Integrative analysis of complex cancer genomics and clinical profiles using the cBioPortal. Sci Signal. 2013;6(269):l1.

41. Kimura ET, Nikiforova MN, Zhu Z, Knauf JA, Nikiforov YE, Fagin JA. High prevalence of BRAF mutations in thyroid cancer: genetic evidence for constitutive activation of the RET/PTC-RAS-BRAF signaling pathway in papillary thyroid carcinoma. Cancer Res. 2003;63:1454-7.

42. Wang Y, Hou P, Yu H, Wang W, Ji M, Zhao S, et al. High prevalence and mutual exclusivity of genetic alterations in the phosphatidylinositol-3-kinase/akt pathway in thyroid tumors. J Clin Endocrinol Metab. 2007;92:2387-90.

43. Santarpia L, El Naggar AK, Cote GJ, Myers JN, Sherman SI. Phosphatidylinositol 3-kinase/akt and ras/raf-mitogen-activated protein kinase pathway mutations in anaplastic thyroid cancer. J Clin Endocrinol Metab. 2008;93:278-84.

44. Hou P, Liu D, Shan Y, Hu S, Studeman K, Condouris S, et al. Genetic alterations and their relationship in the phosphati-dylinositol 3-kinase/Akt pathway in thyroid cancer. Clin Cancer Res. 2007;13:1161-70.

45. Ringel MD, Anderson J, Souza SL, Burch HB, Tambascia M, Shriver CD, et al. Expression of the sodium iodide symporter and thyroglobulin genes. Mod Pathol. 2001;14(4):289-96.

46. Liu D, Hu S, Hou P, Jiang D, Condouris S, Xing M. Suppression of BRAF/MEK/MAP kinase pathway restores expression of iodide-metabolizing genes in thyroid cells expressing the V600E BRAF mutant. Clin Cancer Res. 2007;13:1341-9.

47. Dohan O, Baloch Z, Banrevi Z, Livolsi V, Carrasco N. Rapid communication: predominant intracellular overexpression of the Na(+)/I(x) symporter (NIS) in a large sampling of thyroid cancer cases. J Clin Endocrinol Metab. 2001;86:2697-700.

48. de Souza EC, Padrón AS, Braga WMO, de Andrade BM, Vaisman M, Nasciutti LE, et al. MTOR downregulates iodide uptake in thyrocytes. J Endocrinol. 2010;206:113-20.

49. Agrawal N, Akbani R, Aksoy BA, Ally A, Arachchi H. Integrated genomic characterization of papillary thyroid carcinoma. Cell. 2014;159:676-90.

50. Xing M, Liu R, Liu X, Murugan AK, Zhu G, Zeiger MA, et al. BRAF V600E and TERT promoter mutations cooperatively identify the most aggressive papillary thyroid cancer with highest recurrence. J Clin Oncol. 2014;32:2718-26.

51. Yoo SK, Lee S, Kim SJ, Jee HG, Kim BA, Cho H, et al. Comprehensive analysis of the transcriptional and mutational landscape of follicular and papillary thyroid cancers. PLoS Genet. 2016;12:e1006239.

52. George N, Agarwal A, Kumari N, Agarwal S, Krisnani N, Gupta SK. Molecular profiling of follicular variant of papillary thyroid cancer reveals low-risk noninvasive follicular thyroid neoplasm with papillary-like nuclear features: a paradigm shift to reduce aggressive treatment of indolent tumors. Indian J Endocrinol Metab. 2018;22(3):339-46.

53. Nikiforov YE. Molecular diagnostics of thyroid tumors. Arch Pathol Lab Med. 2011;135:569-77.

54. Sponziello M, Lavarone E, Pegolo E, Di Loreto C, Puppin C, Russo MA, et al. Molecular differences between human thyroid follicular adenoma and carcinoma revealed by analysis of a murine model of thyroid cancer. Endocrinology. 2013;154:3043-53.

55. Xing M. Molecular pathogenesis and mechanisms of thyroid cancer. Nat Rev Cancer. 2013;13:184-99.

56. Gasparre G, Porcelli AM, Bonora E, Pennisi LF, Toller M, Iommarini L, et al. Disruptive mitochondrial DNA mutations in complex I subunits are markers of oncocytic phenotype in thyroid tumors. Proc Natl Acad Sci USA. 2007;104:9001-6.

57. Ganly I, Ricarte Filho J, Eng S, Ghossein R, Morris LG, Liang Y, et al. Genomic dissection of Hürthle cell carcinoma reveals a unique class of thyroid malignancy. J Clin Endocrinol Metab. 2013;98:E962-72.

58. Landa I, Ibrahimpasic T, Boucai L, Sinha R, Knauf JA, Shah RH, et al. Genomic and transcriptomic hallmarks of poorly differentiated and anaplastic thyroid cancers. J Clin Invest. 2016;126:1052-66.

59. Cheng DT, Mitchell TN, Zehir A, Shah RH, Benayed R, Syed A, et al. Memorial sloan kettering-integrated mutation profiling of actionable cancer targets (MSK-IMPACT): a hybridization capture-based next-generation sequencing clinical assay for solid tumor molecular oncology. J Mol Diagn. 2015;17: 251-64.

60. Jeon M, Chun SM, Kim D, Kwon H, Jang EK, Kim TY, et al. Genomic alterations of anaplastic thyroid carcinoma detected by targeted massive parallel sequencing in a BRAFV600E mutation-prevalent area. Thyroid. 2016;26(5):683-90.

61. Caillou B, Talbot M, Weyemi U, Pioche-Durieu C, Al Ghuzlan A, Bidart AM, et al. Tumor-associated macrophages (TAMs) form an interconnected cellular supportive network in anaplastic thyroid carcinoma. PLoS One. 2011;6(7):e22567.

62. Takeuchi Y, Daa T, Kashima K, Yokoyama S, Nakayama I, Noguchi S. Mutations of p53 in thyroid carcinoma with an insular component. Thyroid. 1999;9(4):377-81.

63. Garcia-Rostan G, Tallini G, Herrero A, D'Aquila TG, Carcangiu ML, Rimm DL. Frequent mutation and nuclear localization of beta-catenin in anaplastic thyroid carcinoma. Cancer Res. 1999;59(8):1811-5.

64. Kasaian K, Wiseman SM, Walker BA, Schein JE, Zhao Y, Hirst M, et al. The genomic and transcriptomic landscape of anaplastic thyroid cancer: implications for therapy. BMC Cancer. 2015;15:984.

65. Abubaker J, Jehan Z, Bavi P, Sultana M, Al-Harbi S, Ibrahim M, et al. Clinicopathological analysis of papillary thyroid cancer with PIK3CA alterations in a Middle Eastern population. J Clin Endocrinol Metab. 2008;93:611-8.

66. Leboulleux S, Bastholt L, Krause T, de la Fouchardiere C, Tennvall J, Awada A, et al. Vandetanib in locally advanced or metastatic differentiated thyroid cancer: a randomised, double-blind, phase 2 trial. Lancet Oncol. 2012;13(9):897-905.

67. Cabanillas ME, de Souza JA, Geyer S, Wirth LJ, Menefee ME, Liu SV, et al. Cabozantinib as salvage therapy for patients with tyrosine kinase inhibitor-refractory differentiated thyroid cancer: results of a multicenter phase II International Thyroid Oncology Group trial. J Clin Oncol. 2017;35(29):3315-21.

68. Drilon A, Laetsch TW, Kummar S, DuBois SG, Lassen UN, Demetri GD, et al. Efficacy of larotrectinib in TRK fusion-positive cancers in adults and children. N Engl J Med. 2018;378(8):731-9.

69. Demetri GD, Paz-Ares L, Farago AF, Liu SV, Chawla SP, Tosi D, et al. Efficacy and safety of entrectinib in patients with NTRK fusion-positive (NTRK-fp) tumors: pooled analysis of STARTRK-2, STARTRK-1 and ALKA-372-001 [abstract]. Ann Oncol. 2018;29(Suppl 8):VIII713.

70. Hanna GJ, Busaidy NL, Chau NG, Wirth LJ, Barletta JA, Calles A, et al. Genomic correlates of response to everolimus in aggressive radioiodine-refractory thyroid cancer: a phase II study. Clin Cancer Res. 2018;24(7):1546-53.

71. Ho AL, Grewal RK, Leboeuf R, Sherman EJ, Pfister DG, Deandreis D, et al. Selumetinib-enhanced radioiodine uptake in advanced thyroid cancer. N Engl J Med. 2013;368(7):623-32.

72. Fu G, Polyakova O, MacMillan C, Ralhan R, Walfish PG. Programmed death-ligand 1 expression distinguishes invasive encapsulated follicular variant of papillary thyroid carcinoma from noninvasive follicular thyroid neoplasm with papillary-like nuclear features. EBioMedicine. 2017;18:50-5.

73. Aghajani M, Graham S, McCaerty C, Shaheed CA, Roberts T, DeSouza P, et al. Clinicopathologic and prognostic significance of programmed cell death ligand 1 expression in patients with non-medullary thyroid cancer: a systematic review and meta-analysis. Thyroid. 2018;28:349-61.

74. Lawrence MS, Stojanov P, Polak P, Kryukov GV, Cibulskis K, Sivachenko A, et al. Mutational heterogeneity in cancer and the search for new cancer-associated genes. Nature. 2013;499: 214-8.

75. Gopal RK, Kubler K, Calvo SE, Polak P, Livitz D, Rosebrock D, et al. Widespread chromosomal losses and mitochondrial DNA alterations as genetic drivers in Hurthle cell carcinoma. Cancer Cell. 2018;34:242-255.e5.

Primary Hyperparathyroidism

Julie A Miller, Edwina C Moore

INTRODUCTION

Primary hyperparathyroidism (PHPT) is the most common cause of hypercalcemia, particularly in postmenopausal females.[1,2] It is caused by autonomous production of parathyroid hormone (PTH) by one or more parathyroid glands.[3,4] The understanding of PHPT has evolved significantly over the past 40 years and as a consequence, the clinical presentation has changed to such a degree that there are now three recognized phenotypes.[4]

RELEVANT ANATOMY

The parathyroid glands are endodermal in origin and develop from the third (lower) and fourth (upper) pharyngeal pouches.[5,6] Most people have four parathyroid glands.[7] They are located in the central neck, "para," or next to the thyroid but are distinct endocrine organs. The upper glands are usually behind the upper two-thirds of the thyroid, while the lower parathyroid glands can have a more variable location due to a longer migration from their embryological origin.[7]

Usually, the upper and lower glands are symmetrical.[8] The recurrent laryngeal nerve (RLN) is the most important landmark in delineating the superior gland from the inferior gland. If a coronal plane is made along the path of the RLN, the superior gland lies posterior and the inferior anterior to this plane.[9] Therefore, a gland located on the vertebral body in the upper mediastinum would be a prolapsed upper parathyroid, rather than a lower parathyroid, due to its posterior position **(Fig. 1)**.

About 10% of patients have supernumerary glands or fewer than the standard four glands.[7,8] Ectopic parathyroid glands are not uncommon. Ectopic upper glands can be located in the carotid sheath **(Figs. 2A and B)**, retroesophageal and retropharyngeal spaces, or are rarely intrathyroidal **(Fig. 3)**. Ectopic lower glands can also be located within the thyroid, i.e., thymus, carotid sheath and superior mediastinum.[8,9,11-13] The most commonly missed parathyroid gland is an upper gland in its usual anatomical location.

A normal parathyroid gland is about the size and color of a lentil (30–50 mg, tan). It may be difficult to identify by standard imaging techniques (preoperatively) or to differentiate from fat or lymphoid tissue (at operation). By contrast, an abnormal parathyroid gland can be quite variable: enlarged,

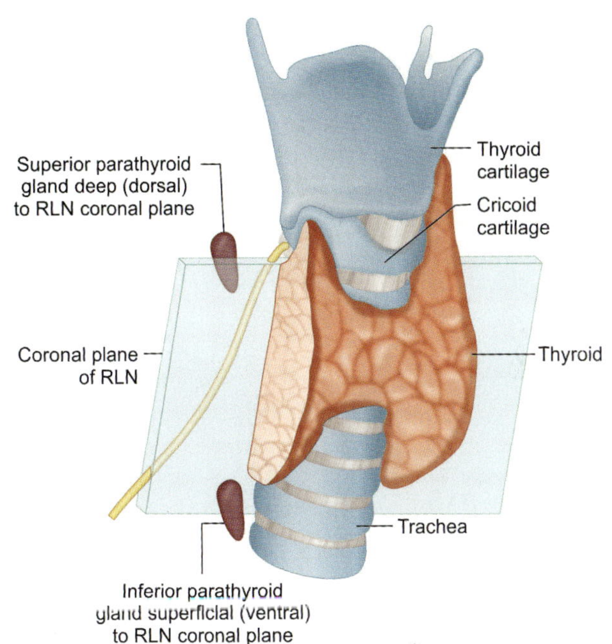

Fig. 1: The superior PTG is often just posterior and deep to the RLN, just prior to the RLN entry point into the larynx.[10] (PTG: parathyroid gland; RLN: recurrent laryngeal nerve)

firm, bilobed, and deep red in color. Both upper and lower parathyroid glands are predominantly supplied by the inferior thyroid artery.[12]

In most cases (70%), PHPT is caused by a single adenoma. Double adenomas occur less often (15%) and are typically bilateral upper adenomas.[1,4,15-17] In multigland disease, all four glands are abnormal (hyperplastic) and this is more common in familial cases of hyperparathyroidism, secondary or tertiary HPT.[4]

DEFINITIONS

The diagnosis of PHPT is made biochemically. It is characterized by hypercalcemia and *inappropriately* elevated PTH or inappropriately normal (nonsuppressed) PTH **(Table 1)**.[3,4] In determining hypercalcemia, it is important to correct the serum calcium for albumin, as this is the major calcium-binding protein.

Corrected calcium = Serum calcium + 0.8 ×
(4 – Serum albumin)

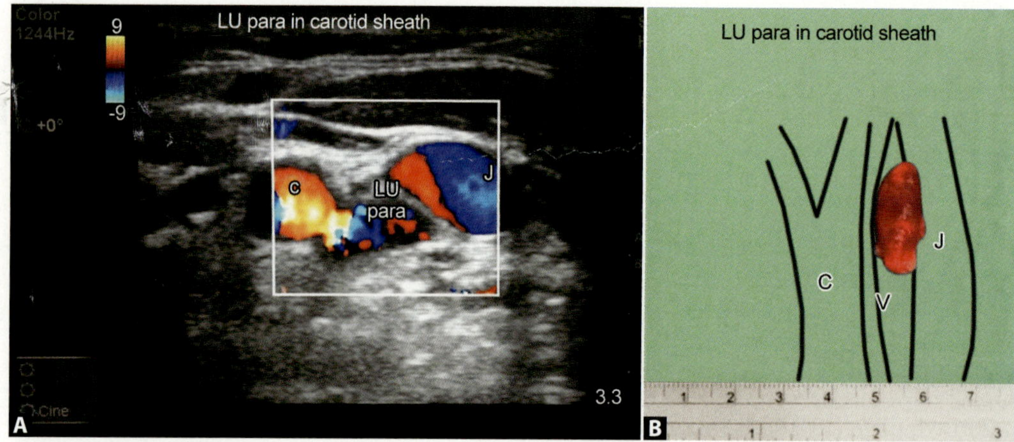

Figs. 2A and B: Ectopic left upper parathyroid gland (PTG) within the left carotid sheath. Seen on preoperative surgeon performed ultrasound (US) and confirmed at operation (C: carotid artery; V: vagus nerve; J: internal jugular vein).

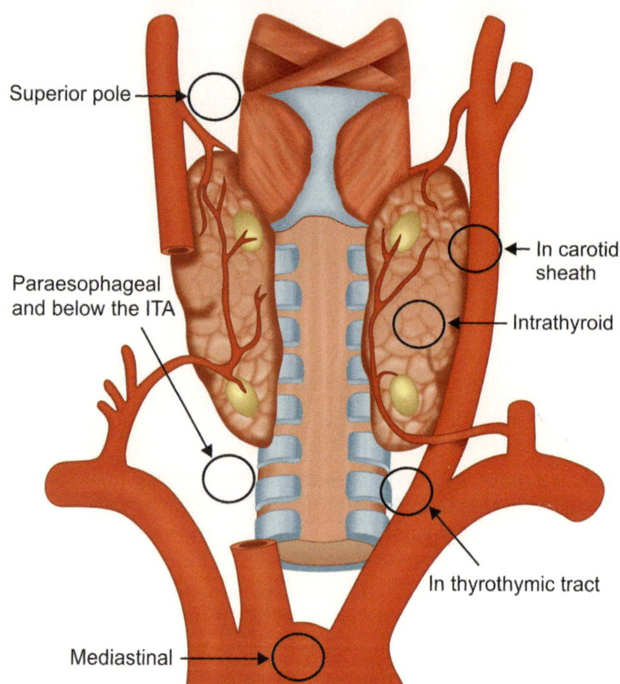

Fig. 3: Location of ectopic and ectopic parathyroid glands from behind, in relation the inferior thyroid artery (ITA).[14]

Box 1: Differential diagnosis of increased PTH.

- Primary hyperparathyroidism
- Vitamin D deficiency
- Renal failure
- Malabsorption syndromes
- *Medications*:
  - Thiazides
  - Lithium
  - Denosumab
- Malignancy-associated PTHrP*
- Ectopic PTH (malignant secretion of PTH by nonparathyroid cancer)†

*Most modern immunoassays can differentiate between true PTH and PTHrP.
†Very uncommon. More likely that a patient has two pathologies concurrently: malignancy and PHPT.
(PHPT: primary hyperparathyroidism; PTH: parathyroid hormone; PTHrP: parathyroid hormone-related protein)

Typically, the PTH is elevated in the setting of elevated serum calcium (classic PHPT). Elevated serum calcium in the setting of inappropriately normal PTH is still classified as PHPT and referred to as normohormonal PHPT. In both scenarios, the elevated or normal PTH is inappropriate for the hypercalcemic state. A third subtype, whereby the calcium is normal but the PTH is elevated (normocalcemic PTH), is increasingly recognized.[18,19] It is necessary to exclude all causes of secondary hyperparathyroidism before making a diagnosis of normocalcemic PTH. Common causes of secondary HPT include vitamin D insufficiency, poor dietary calcium intake, and renal impairment **(Box 1)**.

The typical reference range for PTH is 10–62 pg/mL but is influenced by the ambient 25-hydroxyvitamin D levels.[1,4] It has also been observed that patients with PHPT with vitamin D deficiency seem to have a more severe disease presentation than those without.[20] If a patient has a mildly elevated PTH and is vitamin D deficient, a practical strategy would be to replace vitamin D to a target of >75 nmol/L and then recheck biochemistry after 3–6 months of replacement therapy. Younger patients tend to demonstrate values lower than the common reference ranges.[1]

Table 1: Differential diagnosis of hypercalcemia.

Increased bone resorption	• Hyperparathyroidism (all types) • Thyrotoxicosis
Increased calcium absorption	• Chronic renal failure • Hypervitaminosis • Milk-alkali syndrome
Malignancy	Primary bone tumors, e.g., multiple myeloma or bony metastases from other primary tumors, e.g., breast, prostate hypercalcemia of malignancy PTHrP
Miscellaneous	• Familial hypercalcemic hypocalciuria (FHH)[27] • Medications, e.g., lithium and thiazides • Adrenal insufficiency • Rhabdomyolysis • Theophylline toxicity

(PTHrP: parathyroid hormone-related protein)

Table 2: Biochemical profiles of primary HPT.

	Serum calcium	PTH	ALP	25-hydroxyvitamin D	1,25-hydroxyvitamin D	Urine calcium
Classical	↑	↑	Mildly increased	Low normal	High normal	Normal or ↑
Normohormonal	↑	Normal	Mildly increased	Low normal	High normal	↑
Normocalcemic	Normal	↑	Mildly increased	Low normal	High normal	Normal

In evaluating a patient for potential PHPT, it is also important to eliminate interfering substances and medications prior to biochemical testing **(Table 2)**. Biotin is often self-administered for hair loss and can spuriously lower PTH with certain immunoassays.[21] In addition, patients taking lithium or thiazide diuretics can appear to have classic PHPT (high calcium and high PTH) but on ceasing these medications, these parameters can normalize.[22,23]

Persistent PHPT is defined as ongoing hypercalcemia within 6 months following surgery, with no period of normocalcemia.[3,4,25]

Recurrent PHPT is defined by recurrence of hypercalcemia after a normocalcemic interval, at more than 6 months after parathyroidectomy.[4,25,26]

Secondary hyperparathyroidism is a physiological reactive hyperparathyroidism. It occurs with vitamin D deficiency, renal impairment, or malabsorption syndromes whereby parathyroid tissue is chronically stimulated by low serum calcium. The biochemical profile is high PTH, normal calcium, usually in the lower half of the normal range and often evidence of renal impairment.

Tertiary hyperparathyroidism evolves from secondary hyperparathyroidism when the original stimulus is removed, for example after a renal transplant.[4] Serum calcium levels are corrected but parathyroid tissue behaves autonomously and continues to produce and secrete excess PTH. The biochemical profile shows a trend from low calcium/high PTH to normal calcium/normal PTH to corrected calcium/recurrently elevated PTH. The point at which the biochemistry normalizes corresponds to the timing of renal transplantation.

◇ OTHER LABORATORY ABNORMALITIES

Phosphate

Phosphate levels are often low normal in patients with mild PHPT. Hypophosphatemia occurs in severe PHPT because of increased excretion after proximal tubule reabsorption.

1,25-Dihydroxyvitamin D

Parathyroid hormone acts to convert 25-hydroxyvitamin D to 1,25-dihydroxyvitamin D; therefore in PHPT, it is common to see low normal 25-D and high normal 1,25-D.

Magnesium

Magnesium excretion tends to be slightly increased in PHPT and a few patients have mild hypomagnesemia. If identified, levels should be replete.

Hemoglobin

Severe PHPT is sometimes associated with a normocytic, normochromic anemia and is presumably related to reversible bone marrow fibrosis.[24]

Acid–base Balance

Metabolic acidosis is unusual in patients with PHPT unless they have underlying renal disease or significantly high PTH levels. PTH decreases proximal tubule bicarbonate absorption, which is counteracted by increased alkali liberation from osteoclastic activity in bone.

Ionized Calcium

This is needed to establish a diagnosis of normocalcemic hyperparathyroidism.[18,19,25] If ionized calcium is high, then patient has classical PHPT.

◇ INCIDENCE

Primary hyperparathyroidism is a common endocrine disorder. The incidence of PHPT is approximately 1% of the general population and increases with age.[25,28] It is more common in women, with a male-to-female ratio of 1:3–4.[1] The prevalence in postmenopausal women is up to 5% of the population.[29] PHPT in younger patients (<35 years)[30] may be associated with a hereditary syndrome (in which case multigland disease is more common). Prevalence varies by race and geographical location and is in part related to active screening protocols. PHPT is more common in Western European and North American countries, where screening is routine.[31] Overall, the incidence and prevalence of PHPT have been increasing, due to increased awareness and recognition of the disease. However, the disorder remains vastly underdiagnosed due to a large proportion of asymptomatic patients or patients with vague, nonspecific symptoms.[32]

◇ CLASSIFICATION

Primary hyperparathyroidism can be classified in several ways—biochemically, clinically, pathologically, and by etiology.

It should be noted that there is no recognized relationship between degree of biochemical derangement and pathology; however, patients with higher calcium values are often more symptomatic.[33]

Biochemical Subtypes

- Classical
- Normohormonal
- Normocalcemic

Clinical Subtypes

- Overt hypercalcemia with symptoms or end-organ involvement
- Mild and asymptomatic hypercalcemia
- Elevated PTH with persistently normal, albumin corrected, and ionized calcium

Etiological Subtypes

- Sporadic (>90%)—no family history
- Genetic (<10%)—limited to parathyroid glands or affecting multiple endocrine organs, e.g., MEN1, familial isolated pHPT, and MEN2A.[34-37]

Pathological Subtypes

- Single adenoma (hypercellular)—70% **(Fig. 4)**
- Double adenoma (hypercellular)—15%
- Multigland disease (four gland hyperplasia)—15% **(Fig. 5)**
- Parathyroid carcinoma: This is extremely rare (<1% of cases of PHPT). Red flags may be a palpable mass, younger age, or higher than anticipated serum values (calcium >14 mg/dL and PTH >500 pg/mL). At operation, the field may be densely scarred, and planes of dissection are difficult to establish. Parathyroid cancer is rarely associated with genetic syndromes, e.g., Jaw tumor syndrome.[38,39]

PATHOPHYSIOLOGY

Primary hyperparathyroidism is caused by abnormal and unregulated secretion of PTH from one or more parathyroid glands. It is usually a sporadic disease, with no family history. PTH has multiple physiologic actions, the outline of which is shown in **Flowchart 1**.

Modifiable risk factors associated with PHPT include chronically low dietary intake of calcium, certain medications (such as lithium or thiazide diuretics), obesity, hypertension, and reduced physical activity. External beam radiation is a nonmodifiable risk factor, with a very long lag period up to 20 years.[40,41] There is also a weak association with radioiodine ablation which is more significant in elderly patients.[42] Thiazide diuretics reduce urinary calcium and can cause mild hypercalcemia. They are not a direct cause of PHPT but can mask underlying disease (which is obvious once the medication is ceased). Lithium increases serum and ionized calcium levels and causes a persistent defect in calcium-PTH regulation.[1,3]

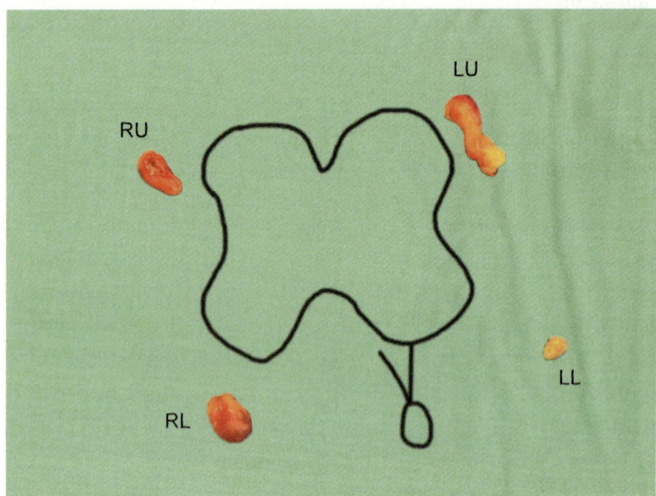

Fig. 5: In four-gland hyperplasia, all of the parathyroid tissues are abnormal. (RU = right upper PTG, RL = right lower PTG, LU = left upper PTG, LL = left lower PTG)

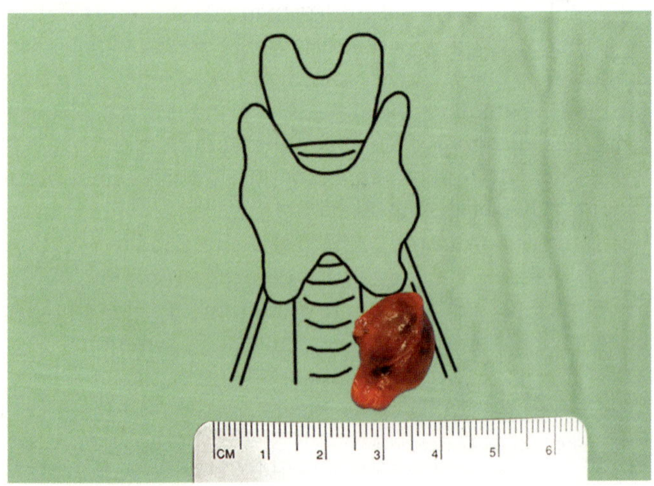

Fig. 4: A single enlarged left lower parathyroid adenoma.

Flowchart 1: Schematic algorithm of physiological properties of PTH.

(PTG: parathyroid glands; PTH: parathyroid hormone; 25(OH)D$_3$ = 25-hydroxycholecalciferol; 1,25(OH)$_2$D$_3$ = 1,25-dihydroxycholecalciferol)

◇| CLINICAL EVALUATION

Evaluation of a patient with suspected PHPT begins with history and examination.

Symptoms of hypercalcemia have low sensitivity and specificity for PHPT. In countries with higher healthcare accessibility, most patients (80%) are found to have PHPT on routine biochemical testing but careful questioning often elicits symptoms of which the patient may be unaware.[1,4,25] It is also important to ascertain for evidence of end-organ damage **(Table 3)**.

By contrast, in countries where biochemical testing is not a part of standard healthcare, classic presentations that mirror the famous axiom "stones, moans, bones, and groans" are more relevant.

There are few signs associated with PHPT, and a detailed neck examination is often unrevealing. Patients with severe disease may have evidence of band keratopathy (along the exposed cornea), but this finding is only seen with a slit lamp.

Many endocrine surgeons utilize cervical ultrasound (US) as part of their clinical examination, in an attempt to localize abnormal parathyroid glands before surgery and concurrently assess for coexistent thyroid disease.[1,25]

◇| INVESTIGATIONS

Recommendations for the evaluation of a patient with suspected PHPT are given in **Table 4**. While very rare, it is prudent to consider familial hypercalcemic hypocalciuria (FHH) within the differential diagnosis, especially in younger patients and males who are outside the most common demographic, or prior to re-exploration in patients with failed surgery. Patients with FHH may have a history of elevated serum calcium since childhood and a family history of unsuccessful parathyroid surgery. FHH is usually differentiated from PHPT based on urinary calcium creatinine clearance ratio (CCCR). However, some patients with PHPT will also have a low CCCR.[43] The gold standard is genetic testing for mutations within the *calcium-sensing receptor (CASR)* gene.[35]

Localization Studies

Localization studies are performed as part of preoperative planning but are not part of the diagnostic algorithm.[25] Negative localizing studies do not contradict the initial biochemical diagnosis. Preoperative parathyroid localization

Table 3: Symptoms and end-organ effects of hypercalcemia.	
Renal	• Hypercalciuria • Nephrolithiasis "stones"—common • Nephrocalcinosis "diffuse calcification of renal parenchyma" • Reduced renal function • Polyuria • Polydipsia
Skeletal	• Reduced bone density (cortical > cancellous)* • Bone and joint pains • Fragility fractures • Skeletal deformities "osteitis fibrosa cystica" (salt and pepper degranulation of the skull, distal tapering of the clavicles and phalanges, bone cysts, Brown tumors) **(Fig. 6)**
Neurocognitive	• Fatigue • Anxiety • Poor concentration • Irritable mood • Memory loss • Cognitive decline • Altered mental status • Poor sleep
Cardiovascular	• Arrythmias • Hypertension • Left ventricular hypertrophy • Valvular calcification
Gastrointestinal	• Abdominal pain "moans" • Reduced appetite • Reflux • Peptic ulcer disease • Constipation • Vague abdominal pain "gut atony" • Pancreatitis • Vomiting
Neuromuscular	Proximal muscle weakness

*Bone density loss seen in postmenopausal women with estrogen deficiency is the reverse (cancellous > cortical). Three points should be assessed in bone densitometry—distal radius, hip, and spine.

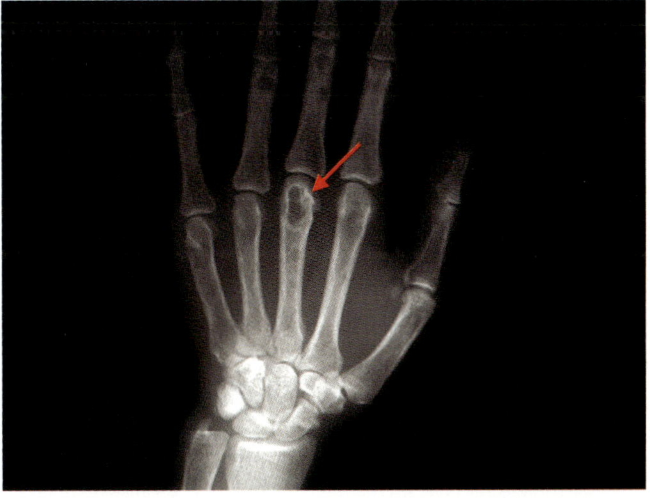

Fig. 6: Brown tumor in primary hyperparathyroidism.

Table 4: Initial investigations for a patient with suspected PHPT.	
Blood tests	Serum calcium, PTH, phosphate, ALP, GFR, 25-hydroxyvitamin D, eGFR
Urine (24-hour collection)	Calcium and creatinine*
Imaging	DEXA (including hip, lumbar spine, and distal one-third of radius)

*If urinary calcium >400 mg/day, consider urinary stone risk profiling.
(ALP: alkaline phosphatase; GFR: glomerular filtration rate; PHPT: primary hyperparathyroidism; PTH: parathyroid hormone)

should be performed only following biochemical confirmation of disease and confirmed suitability for surgery.[25,44,45] Imaging studies are unnecessary to make the diagnosis of PHPT and can cause confusion with false-positive and false-negative results. The aim of localization is to select patients who might be suitable for focused parathyroid surgery, to identify ectopic parathyroid glands (outside of the central neck) and to minimize surgical dissection and thereby the risk of complications.

Ultrasound and sestamibi scintigraphy or parathyroid four-dimensional computed tomography (4DCT) are the most common modalities for localization, and the choice of study depends on local expertise. Additional studies such as selective venous sampling may be used in re-operative cases.

Ultrasound

High-resolution US is highly sensitive and noninvasive and is the preferred imaging modality in PHPT.[46] It can also assess for concurrent thyroid disease.[47] A normal parathyroid gland cannot be reliably visualized; however, an abnormal parathyroid gland will appear enlarged, ovoid, hypoechoic, and vascular. US is operator dependent and limited by the patient's body habitus. Inferior parathyroid adenomas are easier to identify, as they are more superficial. Deep superior adenomas, especially in the retroesophageal or prevertebral space, or inferior adenomas in the upper mediastinum, are difficult to visualize on ultrasound. A large goiter also makes parathyroid identification more challenging, as does autoimmune thyroiditis, which often produces reactive adenopathy in level VI.

Sestamibi Scintigraphy

Technetium-99m methoxyisobutylisonitrite (99m-Tc sestamibi) is the dominate isotope in parathyroid scintigraphy **(Fig. 7)**. It was initially used for cardiac scintigraphy during which it was noted to concentrate in parathyroid glands which are rich in mitochondria.[48] The radiolabeled isotope is administered intravenously to the patient, uptaken by both the thyroid and the parathyroid glands but retained for longer by the oxyphilic cells within parathyroid tissue. A series of images (dual phase) are taken over 2 hours or more. Parathyroid adenomas demonstrate increased uptake and persistence of activity compared with normal thyroid **(Fig. 7)**. Unfortunately, false negatives are not uncommon (12–25%) and in particular are associated with small or superior glands, adenomas with scant oxyphil cells or hyperplasia, and in the presence of thyroid nodules.[49-51] False positives can be seen with thyroid adenomas or thyroid cancer. Scintigraphy alone does not provide clear anatomical detail.

Dual isotope scintigraphy and subtraction scanning can be used to enhance parathyroid identification. A thyroid-specific isotope such as 123 I-sodium iodine is used in addition to the technetium-99m and the thyroid images are digitally subtracted from the parathyroid images.

Sestamibi SPECT (single-photon emission computed tomography) and SPECT-CT: This is a sestamibi scan that provides higher resolution with three-dimensional imaging compared with planar scintigraphy.[52] A low-dose CT can be added to create a hybrid SPECT/CT. Sestamibi SPECT can potentially identify ectopic parathyroids outside the central neck.

Four-dimensional Computed Tomography

Four-dimensional computed tomography relies on the rapid uptake and washout of contrast by parathyroid adenomas in a multiphase contrast CT, and in some centers, it has replaced sestamibi as the initial imaging of choice. The protocol involves a pre-contrast scan, arterial phase, venous phase, and delayed phase **(Figs. 8A to C)**. The main disadvantages are cost and that it typically requires a much larger radiation dose than other localizing studies.[53,54]

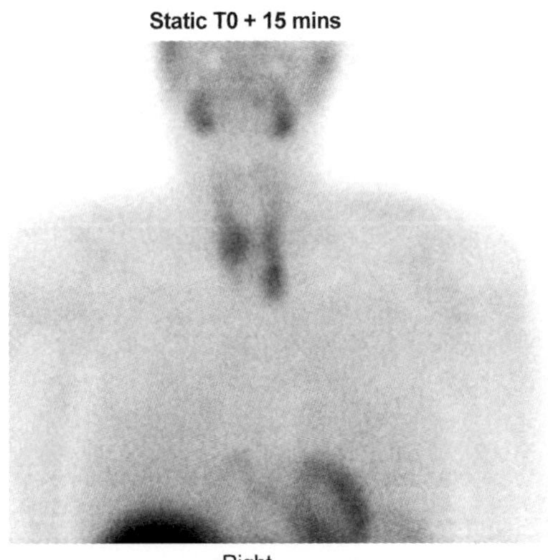

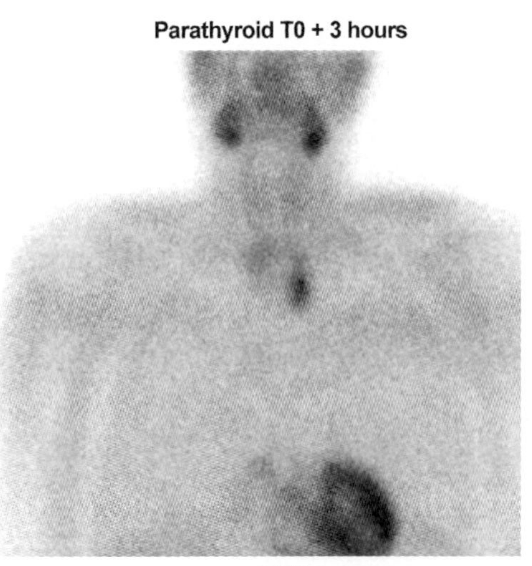

Fig. 7: Retention of isotope in the left lower region is suspicious for a left lower parathyroid adenoma.

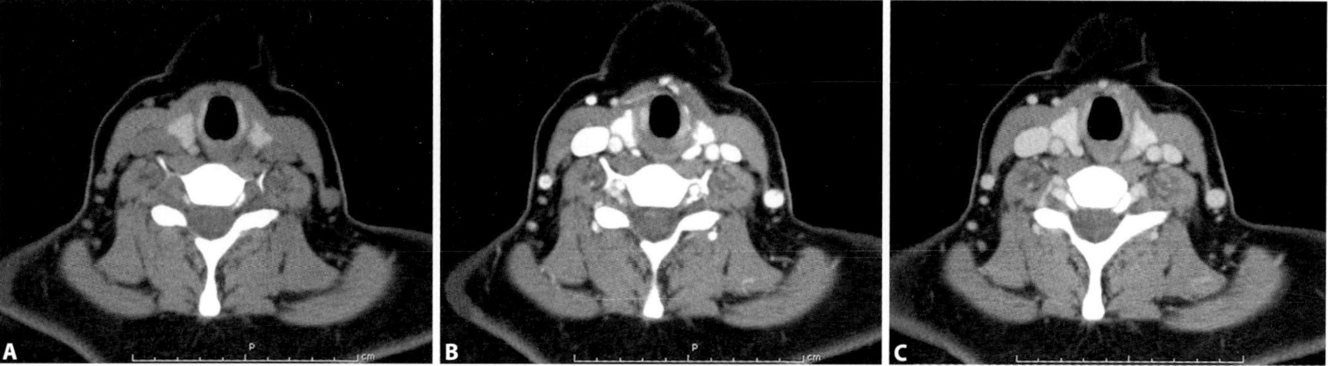

Figs. 8A to C: Four-dimensional computed tomography (4DCT) showing LU parathyroid adenoma in noncontrast, arterial, and venous phases.

It is possible to reduce the effective radiation dose by eliminating the delayed phase and by decreasing the length of the remaining phases to levels associated with SPECT-CT, although this may limit spatial resolution and needs further investigation.[55]

Selective Venous Sampling

This is an invasive procedure that requires a high level of skill by an interventional radiologist and patient cooperation. It is usually reserved for complicated reoperative cases when all other localization studies have been negative. Samples are drawn via a femoral catheter from representative cervical drainage sites (inferior, middle, superior thyroid, thymic, and vertebral veins) and compared with peripheral veins to identify a PTH gradient of 1.5–2-fold between sites.[56]

Other

Magnetic resonance imaging is rarely used for parathyroid imaging.[25,45] Recently, newer positron emission tomography (PET) tracers, e.g., 18F-fluorocholine, have been gaining attention for detection of parathyroid adenomas. Compared with nuclear imaging, they have improved sensitivity, resulting in the detection of smaller adenomas and reduced scanning time (due to the rapid kinetics of choline within the highly metabolically active parathyroid cell).[57] However, large prospective validation studies are required to evaluate the usefulness of F18-choline PET/CT and compare them with other more established imaging modalities.[58]

Different centers utilize different imaging modalities in different combinations based on local expertise.[59,60] Just like with surgery, the success of imaging is often dependent on the experience and expertise of those protocolling and interpreting the images. Therefore, parathyroid imaging should ideally be performed in a high-volume center. Nonlocalizing (negative) studies do not preclude surgery, especially for patients with classic disease.

Intraoperative Localization

There are several intraoperative adjuncts that can assist with parathyroid localization. These are especially important in reoperative cases. Some examples are intraoperative PTH measurement (with a rapid throughput assay), bilateral venous sampling, intraoperative ultrasound, and autofluorescence, but are beyond the scope of this chapter.[61-63]

◇| MANAGEMENT

Surgery for PHPT is the only course of treatment that offers definitive cure and is recommended for all patients with symptomatic disease. It is important to screen carefully for symptoms, as many patients attribute symptoms such as fatigue and bodily aches and pains to their age or their stress levels or anything but their hypercalcemia.

For asymptomatic patients, there are guidelines that help to determine the need for surgery.[26] These are:

- Hypercalcemia >1 mg/dL above normal
- Fragility fracture
- Renal stones
- Hypercalciuria (>400 mg/day)
- T-score <2.5 (and should be considered for those with osteopenia)
- Age <50 years
- Creatinine clearance <60 mL/min

The surgical criteria published by the American Association of Endocrine Surgeons (AAES) also consider neurocognitive symptoms and other nontraditional symptoms such as muscle weakness and abnormal sleep patterns when offering surgical intervention to patients.[25] Some authors recommend surgery for *all patients* with asymptomatic disease and reasonable life expectancy, and there is increasing evidence that these patients benefit from fracture risk reduction.[64,65] Currently, it is uncertain whether the same benefits of parathyroidectomy apply to patients with normocalcemic PHPT.[30]

Surgical Treatment

The operation performed for PHPT has varied over the past few decades.[66-69] Traditionally, a complete exploration of all glands was performed. With increasing use of localization studies and rapid immunoassay for PTH measurement, many surgeons have moved toward a minimally invasive parathyroidectomy (MIP), whereby only a preoperatively identified abnormal gland is targeted and removed.[69-73] By contrast, others continue to advocate routine four-gland exploration via a bilateral neck exploration (BNE), as the sensitivity and specificity of localization studies are approximately 70% and up to 30% of patients have more than one abnormal gland.[74]

Both techniques are effective for the treatment of PHPT.[75,76] The safety profile of MIP appears superior to BNE (lower rate of hypocalcemia and RLN injury) but there is conflicting evidence, some of which show a slightly lower success rate with MIP due to the risk of undiagnosed multigland disease,[72] but other large studies showing equivalent efficacy with MIP.[59]

Overall, the morbidity associated with parathyroid surgery is very low (approximately 1%). Recognized complications include RLN injury, hypocalcemia, postoperative bleeding, and very rarely infection. Operative mortality is exceptionally low. The risk of failed parathyroidectomy (i.e., persistent hyperparathyroidism) is approximately 2%.[77]

Advocates of MIP argue that subsequent exploration of the contralateral side in the event of recurrence can be performed with minimal morbidity and that a vast majority of patients (>85–90%) experience a long-term cure with unilateral exploration. In addition, some glands may appear slightly enlarged but are not overactive. Therefore, in patients with concordant imaging studies, bilateral exploration exposes the patient to increased risk with questionable benefit. Advocates of routine bilateral exploration continue to argue that the only effective way to determine whether a gland is abnormal is to examine it and that complication rates for re-operative surgery are still higher than for the initial operation.

There is good evidence of a strong volume–outcome relationship with parathyroid surgery. Therefore, the most important aspect of parathyroid surgery is locating a well-trained, high-volume parathyroid surgeon who understands the intracacies of the disease and operative strategies.[25,26] Even following a successful operation, biochemical cure may not be immediately apparent and PTH may continue to fluctuate for several months.[69] Parathyroidectomy leads to an improvement in skeletal strength, in reverse order of demineralization, meaning that the patients with the worst disease preoperatively have the greatest improvement. For patients with a history of renal stones, recurrent nephrolithiasis after successful parathyroid surgery is extremely unlikely.[78]

Operative Technique

The patient's skin creases are marked prior to induction of anesthesia, preferably with the patient sitting upright. The patient is positioned supine with their neck extended using a shoulder roll, head ring and arms tucked (being mindful of pressure areas). We use a lower body warmed air blanket and calf compressors. Local anesthetic is administered in bilateral superficial cervical plexus blocks and local wound infiltration. We routinely perform a cervical ultrasound at this point in order to visualize the parathyroid adenoma and to choose the most appropriate incision placement **(Figs. 9A and B)**.

The patient is then prepped and draped. Prophylactic antibiotics are not indicated in primary neck surgery, although may be considered for patients with increased risk factors or in re-operative cases. A midline or lateral approach may be chosen depending on the patient's anatomy and the location of the parathyroid adenoma.

A 3-cm incision is made through the chosen skin crease with a 15-blade scalpel and continued through the subcutaneous fat. Larger incisions may be required for a patient with obesity, a large goiter, or fixed neck flexion. Meticulous

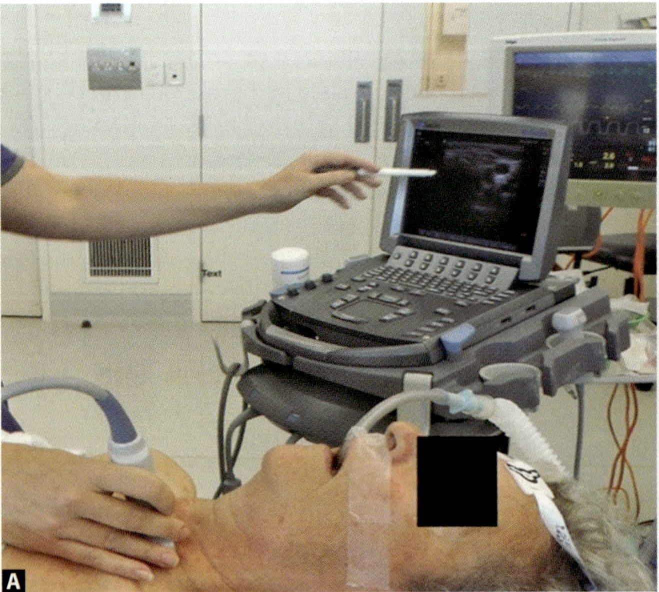
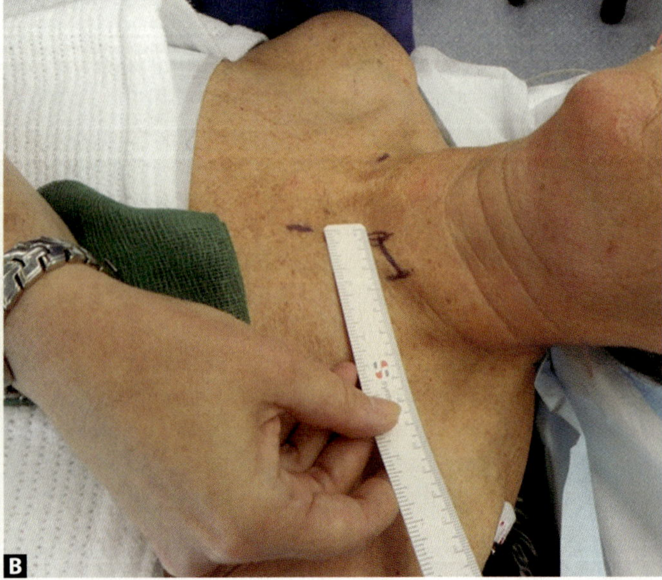

Figs. 9A and B: An on-table ultrasound is performed after the patient is anesthetized. The precise location of the incision is determined using the natural skin creases (which were marked in advance with the patient in an upright position).

hemostasis is important at all steps of the operation. Even the smallest amount of bleeding can stain the tissues and make identification of PTGs more difficult. The platysma is divided and small subplatysmal flaps are raised with cautery on a low setting, being mindful to avoid the anterior jugular veins. Spring retractors are used to retract the skin edges. For a midline approach (ideal for lower parathyroid glands or bilateral parathyroid exploration), the midline is identified, and the median raphe is divided. Then the strap muscles are separated, subtly undermined and retracted laterally. The lateral approach is ideal for focused parathyroidectomy for a well-localized superior adenoma. The incision is placed laterally and after raising of a subplatysmal flap, the sternocleidomastoid is mobilized and retracted laterally and the strap muscles are retracted medially in order to enter the deep cervical space. The thyroid is mobilized from its surrounding soft-tissue attachments and retracted to expose a superior parathyroid adenoma. When using the lateral approach, the RLN is typically medial to the parathyroid adenoma.

When localization studies have failed, it is important to have a systematic approach to dissection.

Finding an Upper Gland

The upper PTG is usually located posterior to the RLN, at the junction of the upper two-thirds and lower one-third of the thyroid. It is typically located on the superoposterior aspect of the tubercle of Zuckerkandl, just posterior to the coronal plane of the RLN. The most commonly missed PTG is the upper gland in its usual anatomical location. Not infrequently all that is required to find a hidden upper gland is to medially rotate the thyroid further, which reveals it hiding on the posterior surface of the gland. Ectopic upper parathyroid glands may be found in the retroesophageal (or prevertebral space), sometimes prolapsed into the posterior mediastinum.

Finding a Lower Gland

The lower PTG has a more variable location but tends to be more anterior, in association with the lower pole of thyroid, sometimes under the thyroid capsule. It may be necessary to examine the thyrothymic ligament or perform a cervical thymectomy, if the lower gland cannot be located. This is achieved with gentle traction on the thymus arising from the lower pole, "like pulling worms out of the ground." In case of a missing parathyroid, the carotid sheath should also be examined and is best incised longitudinally.

Four-gland Hyperplasia

Approximately 10–15% of parathyroid disease is caused by multigland disease, either multiple adenomata or four-gland hyperplasia, whereby all the PTGs are equally abnormal. In cases of hyperplasia, the surgeon attempts to leave just enough parathyroid tissue to maintain normal calcium homeostasis but to avoid permanent hypoparathyroidism.

Depending on the size of the glands, a patient may undergo a 3 or 3.5 gland resection. Typically, the smallest and least abnormally looking PTG is selected to be the remnant and if this is a lower gland, that is ideal (as it is more superficial, putting the RLN at decreased risk during reoperative surgery). The remnant gland should be selected only after all of the PTGs have been identified. However, it should be fashioned (with a large clip, placed across the distal portion which is then removed) before the other more abnormal PTGs are removed. This technique enables viability of the remnant to be checked before there is no longer an alternative. A remnant is usually 30–40 mg or about the size of a normal PTG.

Intraoperative Confirmation

An abnormal parathyroid gland looks different to its normal counterpart. It is often enlarged, slightly firmer than normal parathyroid tissue, and darker tan or brown in color compared with the peanut-butter color of normal parathyroid tissue. Parathyroid glands also have a characteristic "bobbling" movement when manipulated, sliding within the surrounding fat. It can be difficult to differentiate a suppressed PTG from the surrounding fat or lymphoid tissue, or a nodular thyroid rest. Lymph nodes are more typically pinkish white, while thyroid rests are more reddish brown. Experienced parathyroid surgeons are often confident in identifying parathyroid tissue based on its appearance. In cases of uncertainty, several intraoperative adjuncts are available [frozen section, technetium Tc99, PRH monitoring, intraoperative parathyroid hormone (IoPTH),[61] indocyanine green (ICG), autofluorescnce[79]] but are beyond the scope of this chapter.

Other Adjuncts

Bilateral internal jugular vein (IJV) sampling can be utilized to assess PTH when none of the glands can be found. Care must be taken so that the blood is drawn from a site, which is appropriately distal to include the outflow from the whole neck. If the PTH levels are significantly greater on one side, it suggests that the missing gland can be found on that side at an ectopic location. If the right and left PTH levels drawn centrally are the same as peripheral levels, it is reasonable to assume that the ectopic gland is not in the neck (and probably in the chest). At this point, the operation should be terminated, new imaging obtained, and a thoracic surgeon consulted (for video-assisted thoracoscopic surgery).

Intraoperative ultrasound can be used to assess for a potential intrathyroidal PTG (or the preoperative imaging can be re-reviewed). Ideally, any candidate lesions would have been identified in the preoperative US. By filling the central neck with normal saline, the ultrasonic waves are conducted with relative ease. However, in the absence of any potential targets on imaging, blind lobectomy is not typically recommended.

One of the most important lessons in parathyroid surgery is that if a pathological gland cannot be identified following a systematic search, it is prudent to seek help from a more experienced surgeon, if available, rather than to continue with an increasingly frustrating operation. In addition, normal parathyroid glands should not be excised.

Meticulous and anatomical dissection is used to protect and preserve the RLNs. Vocal cord palsy is a serious but uncommon complication of parathyroid surgery.

At the end of the procedure, hemostasis is checked. The strap muscles are reapproximated and the platysma is closed with an absorbable suture. For a lateral approach, the straps do not need reapproximation. Closing the platysma does not have a functional advantage but achieves a better cosmetic result. The skin is closed, and the wound dressed according to the preference of the surgeon. Firm and direct pressure may be applied to the wound and the surrounding soft tissues, until the patient is extubated **(Fig. 10)**.

Postoperative Care

Most patients have relatively little pain after parathyroid surgery and opioid analgesia is often not required. The most common complaint is actually a sore throat for which a local anesthetic spray or warm or cold soft foods can be helpful. Patients are prescribed paracetamol and NSAID, plus a small dose of narcotics, if requested. Vitamin D repletion in the perioperative period ensures efficient absorption of dietary calcium, and if the patient does not have adequate dietary calcium intake, calcium supplementation may be recommended. There are no dietary restrictions after surgery. Patients are encouraged to mobilize freely and therefore it is not necessary to prescribe deep venous thrombosis (DVT) prophylaxis. Serum PTH is sent from recovery and serum calcium is checked on the first postoperative day.

Follow-up

In our practice, patients are discharged home the day after surgery, although many centers safely perform day case parathyroidectomy. We review patients 2 weeks after surgery to remove the dressing, check if wound healing is satisfactory, review pathology, and assess the voice quality. We recommend a serum calcium at 6 months and thereafter annually. Recent studies have identified that long-term recurrence (>3 years) is significantly higher than anticipated for reasons that are incompletely understood.[80] Improvements in bone densitometry can be seen in 6–12 months and is most apparent for patients with worse premorbid disease. Improvement in quality of life and nonspecific symptoms is often observed and seems to be more noticeable in younger patients.[81,82]

Nonsurgical Treatment

Some patients are not suitable for surgery due to medical comorbidities, personal preference, or failing to meet acceptable criteria. In these situations, surveillance with repeated annual testing is reasonable **(Table 5)**. However, the long-term natural history of patients who do not undergo surgery is ultimately disease progression.[64,83]

Alendronate, a bisphosphonate, may be used to improve bone density but will not alter serum calcium levels and therefore will not improve symptoms related to hypercalcemia.[64] Cinacalcet hydrochloride is a calcimimetic agent and may be used for symptomatic hypercalcemia. Cinacalcet partially reduces PTH synthesis, by interfering with calcium-sensing receptors to increase the calcium signal to the parathyroid cell; however, it has no effect on bone mineral density (BMD).[84] These medications are commonly used as combination therapy for patients who are nonsurgical candidates.

Patients with hypercalcemia secondary to PHPT should not restrict their dietary calcium intake. Low-dietary calcium can become a further stimulus for already abnormal parathyroid tissue to synthesize and secrete more PTH, thus exacerbating the problem. Dietary intake of calcium should mirror normal guidelines, even for patients with PHPT.

Management Algorithm

- Confirm the diagnosis (typically two sets of blood tests)
- Assess for end-organ damage
- Assess suitability for surgery
- Preoperative localization
- Surgery
- Surveillance

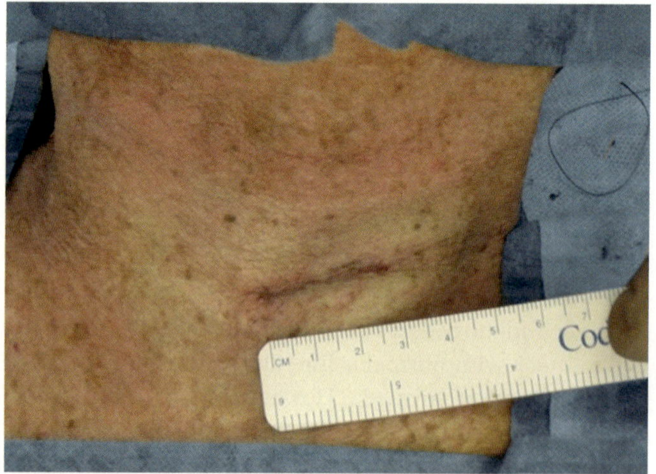

Fig. 10: A small lateral incision (for a superior minimally invasive para-thyroidectomy) is closed with an absorbable suture.

Table 5: Guidelines for medical monitoring in nonsurgical candidates.

Serum calcium	Annually
DEXA (three sites: hip, spine and forearm)	1–2 years
eGFR	Annually

(DEXA: dual-energy X-ray absorptiometry; eGFR: estimated glomerular filtration rate)

◇ CLINICAL PEARLS

- PHPT is a common endocrine disorder that is under-diagnosed and under-treated.
- Symptoms can be subtle and non-specific, or occasionally absent.
- In regions with lower healthcare accessibility, PHPT is less commonly diagnosed, and more advanced disease is encountered.
- Typical symptoms include bodily aches and pains, fatigue, "brain fog," irritable mood, reflux, constipation, polyuria, poor sleep quality, and increased risk of kidney stones.
- If untreated, PHPT often results in accelerated bone loss and increased fracture risk.
- Most cases are caused by a single adenoma, but up to 20-30% of patients have multigland disease.
- Consider familial disease in patients <35 years.
- Localization studies have no role in the diagnosis PHPT. However, once the diagnosis has been made, localization studies are useful for operative planning. Negative imaging does not influence the diagnosis or indication for surgery.
- Surgery is the only option for definitive cure and, in experienced hands, is associated with 98% success and a very low risk of complications.
- Diagnosis of PHPT is made biochemically.
- Localization studies have no role in the initial evaluation of a patient with suspected PHPT and may be confusing.
- In areas of routine health screening, PHPT is a common and usually asymptomatic disease.
- In areas where screening is not performed routinely, PHPT is uncommon and often symptomatic.
- Consider familial disease in patients <40 years.
- Surgery is the only option for definitive cure and, in experienced hands, is associated with 98% lifelong success.

◇ REFERENCES

1. Machado NN, Wilhelm SM. Diagnosis and evaluation of primary hyperparathyroidism. Surg Clin North Am. 2019;99(4):649-66.
2. Press DM, Siperstein AE, Berber E, Shin JJ, Metzger R, Monteiro R, et al. The prevalence of undiagnosed and unrecognized primary hyperparathyroidism: a population-based analysis from the electronic medical record. Surg (United States). 2013;154(6):1232-8.
3. Bilezikian JP, Bandeira L, Khan A, Cusano NE. Hyperparathyroidism. Lancet (London, England). 2018;391(10116):168-78.
4. O'Connor C, Levine JA, Hahr A. Primary hyperparathyroidism. In: Camacho P (Ed). Metabolic Bone Diseases. Springer, Cham. 2019;103(6):15-25.
5. Larsen WJ, Sherman LS, Potter SS SW. Human Embryology, 3rd edition. New York: Churchill Livingstone; 2001.
6. Fancy T, Gallagher D, Hornig JD. Surgical anatomy of the thyroid and parathyroid glands. Otolaryngol Clin North Am. 2010;43(2):221-7, vii.
7. Sadler TW LJ. Langman's Medical Embryology, 10th edition. Philadelphia: Lippincott Williams and Wilkins; 2006.
8. Akerstrom G, Malmaeus J, Bergstrom R. Surgical anatomy of human parathyroid glands. Surgery. 1984;95(1):14-21.
9. Alveryd A. Parathyroid glands in thyroid surgery. I. Anatomy of parathyroid glands. II. Postoperative hypoparathyroidism: identification and autotransplantation of parathyroid glands. Acta Chir Scand. 1968;389:1-120.
10. Genden EM, Varvares MA. Head and neck cancer: An evidence-based team approach. Ann R Coll Surg Engl. 2010;92(8):718.
11. Wang C. The anatomic basis of parathyroid surgery. Ann Surg. 1976;183(3):271-5.
12. Mohebati A, Shaha AR. Anatomy of thyroid and parathyroid glands and neurovascular relations. Clin Anat. 2012;25(1):19-31.
13. Wang C. Hyperfunctioning intrathyroid parathyroid gland: a potential cause of failure in parathyroid surgery. JR Soc Med. 1981;74(1):49-52.
14. Jason DS, Balentine CJ. Intraoperative decision making in parathyroid surgery. Surg Clin North Am. 2019;99(4):681-91.
15. Bartsch D, Nies C, Hasse C, Willuhn J, Rothmund M. Clinical and surgical aspects of double adenoma in patients with primary hyperparathyroidism. Br J Surg. 1995;82(7):926-9.
16. Ruda JM, Hollenbeak CS, Stack BC. A systematic review of the diagnosis and treatment of primary hyperparathyroidism from 1995 to 2003. Otolaryngol Head Neck Surg. 2005;132(3):359-72.
17. Tezelman S, Shen W, Shaver JK, Siperstein AE, Duh QY, Klein H. Double parathyroid adenomas: clinical and biochemical characteristics before and after parathyroidectomy. Ann Surg. 1993;218(3):300-7; discussion 307-9.
18. Silverberg SJ, Bilezikian JP. "Incipient" primary hyperparathyroidism: a "forme fruste" of an old disease. J Clin Endocrinol Metab. 2003;88(11):5348-52.
19. Cusano NE, Silverberg SJ, Bilezikian JP. Normocalcemic primary hyperparathyroidism. J Clin Densitom. 2013;16(1):33-9.
20. Silverberg SJ. Vitamin D deficiency and primary hyperparathyroidism. J Bone Miner Res. 2007;22 (Suppl 2):V100-4.
21. Piketty ML, Prie D, Sedel F, Bernard D, Hercend C, Chanson P, et al. High-dose biotin therapy leading to false biochemical endocrine profiles: Validation of a simple method to overcome biotin interference. Clin Chem Lab Med. 2017;55(6):817-25.
22. Griebeler ML, Kearns AE, Ryu E, Thapa P, Hathcock MS, Melton LJ 3rd, et al. Thiazide-associated hypercalcemia: Incidence and association with primary hyperparathyroidism over two decades. J Clin Endocrinol Metab. 2016;101(3):1166-73.
23. Szalat A, Mazeh H, Freund HR. Lithium-associated hyperparathyroidism: Report of four cases and review of the literature. Eur J Endocrinol. 2009;160(2):317-23.
24. Boxer M, Ellman L, Geller R, Wang CA. Anemia in primary hyperparathyroidism. Arch Intern Med. 1977;137(5):588-93.
25. Wilhelm SM, Wang TS, Ruan DT, Lee JA, Asa SL, Duh QY, et al. The American Association of Endocrine Surgeons Guidelines for Definitive Management of Primary Hyperparathyroidism. JAMA Surg. 2016;151(10):959-68.
26. Bilezikian JP, Brandi ML, Eastell R, Silverberg SJ, Udelsman R, Marcocci C, et al. Guidelines for the management of asymptomatic primary hyperparathyroidism: Summary statement from the fourth international workshop. J Clin Endocrinol Metab. 2014;99(10):3561-9.
27. Christensen SE, Nissen PH, Vestergaard P, Mosekilde L. Familial hypocalciuric hypercalcaemia: a review. Curr Opin Endocrinol Diabetes Obes. 2011;18(6):359-70.
28. Griebeler ML, Kearns AE, Ryu E, Hathcock MA, Melton LJ, Wermers RA. Secular trends in the incidence of primary hyperparathyroidism over five decades (1965–2010). Bone. 2015;73:1-7.

29. Rao SD. Epidemiology of parathyroid disorders. Best Pract Res Clin Endocrinol Metab. 2018;32(6):773-80.

30. Milat F, Ramchand S, Herath M, Gundara J, Harper S, Farrell S, et al. Primary hyperparathyroidism in Adults (Part I). Assessment and Medical Management: Position Statement of the Endocrine Society of Australia, Australian and New Zealand Endocrine Surgeons, and the Australian and New Zealand Bone and Mineral Society. Clinical Endocrinology. 2021. DOI: 10.1111/ cen.14659.

31. Yeh MW, Ituarte PHG, Zhou HC, Nishimoto S, Liu ILA, Harari A, et al. Incidence and prevalence of primary hyperparathyroidism in a racially mixed population. J Clin Endocrinol Metab. 2013;98(3):1122-9.

32. Dombrowsky A, Borg B, Xie R, Kirklin JK, Chen H, Balentine CJ. Why is hyperparathyroidism underdiagnosed and undertreated in older adults? Clin Med Insights Endocrinol Diabetes. 2018;11:1179551418815916.

33. Wallace LB, Parikh RT, Ross LV, Mazzaglia PJ, Foley C, Shin JJ, et al. The phenotype of primary hyperparathyroidism with normal parathyroid hormone levels: How low can parathyroid hormone go? Surgery. 2011;150(6):1102-12.

34. Agarwal SK, Kester MB, Debelenko LV, Heppner C, Emmert-Buck MR, Skarulis MC, et al. Germline mutations of the *MEN1* gene in familial multiple endocrine neoplasia type 1 and related states. Hum Mol Genet. 1997;6(7):1169-75.

35. Marini F, Cianferotti L, Giusti F, Brandi ML. Molecular genetics in primary hyperparathyroidism: the role of genetic tests in differential diagnosis, disease prevention strategy, and therapeutic planning: a 2017 update. Clin Cases Miner Bone Metab. 2017;14(1):60-70.

36. Lee M, Pellegata NS. Multiple endocrine neoplasia type 4. Front Horm Res. 2013;41:63-78.

37. Marx SJ, Simonds WF, Agarwal SK, Burns AL, Weinstein LS, Cochran C, et al. Hyperparathyroidism in hereditary syndromes: special expressions and special managements. J Bone Miner Res. 2002;17 Suppl 2:N37-43.

38. Mohebati A, Shaha A, Shah J. Parathyroid carcinoma: challenges in diagnosis and treatment. Hematol Oncol Clin North Am. 2012;26(6):1221-38.

39. Duan K, Mete Ö. Parathyroid carcinoma: diagnosis and clinical implications. Turk Patoloji Derg. 2015;31:80-97.

40. Schneider AB, Gierlowski TC, Shore-Freedman E, Stovall M, Ron E, Lubin J. Dose-response relationships for radiation-induced hyperparathyroidism. J Clin Endocrinol Metab. 1995;80(1):254-7.

41. Fujiwara S, Sposto R, Ezaki H, Akiba S, Neriishi K, Kodama K, et al. Hyperparathyroidism among atomic bomb survivors in Hiroshima. Radiat Res. 1992;130(3):372-8.

42. Colaço SM, Si M, Reiff E, Clark OH. Hyperparathyroidism after radioactive iodine therapy. Am J Surg. 2007;194(3):323-7.

43. Moore EC, Berber E, Jin J, Krishnamurthy V, Shin J, Siperstein A. Calcium-creatinine clearance ratio is not helpful in differentiating primary hyperparathyroidism from familial hypercalcemic hypocalciuria: a study of 1,000 patients. Endocr Pract. 2018;24(11). Online ahead of print.

44. Clark OH. Presidential address: "Asymptomatic" primary hyperparathyroidism: is parathyroidectomy indicated? Surgery. 1994;116(6):947-53.

45. Zafereo M, Yu J, Angelos P, Brumund K, Chuang HH, Goldenberg D, et al. American Head and Neck Society Endocrine Surgery Section update on parathyroid imaging for surgical candidates with primary hyperparathyroidism. Head Neck. 2019;41(7):2398-409.

46. Haber RS, Kim CK, Inabnet WB. Ultrasonography for preoperative localization of enlarged parathyroid glands in primary hyperparathyroidism: comparison with (99m) technetium sestamibi scintigraphy. Clin Endocrinol (Oxf). 2002;57(2):241-9.

47. Bentrem DJ, Angelos P, Talamonti MS, Nayar R. Is preoperative investigation of the thyroid justified in patients undergoing parathyroidectomy for hyperparathyroidism? Thyroid. 2002;12(12):1109-12.

48. Palestro CJ, Tomas MB, Tronco GG. Radionuclide imaging of the parathyroid glands. Semin Nucl Med. 2005;35(4):266-76.

49. Stephen AE, Roth SI, Fardo DW, Finkelstein DM, Randolph GW, Gaz RD, et al. Predictors of an accurate preoperative sestamibi scan for single-gland parathyroid adenomas. Arch Surg. 2007;142(4):381-6.

50. Civelek AC, Ozalp E, Donovan P, Udelsman R. Prospective evaluation of delayed technetium-99m sestamibi SPECT scintigraphy for preoperative localization of primary hyperparathyroidism. Surgery. 2002;131(2):149-57.

51. Berber E, Parikh RT, Ballem N, Garner CN, Milas M, Siperstein AE. Factors contributing to negative parathyroid localization: an analysis of 1000 patients. Surgery. 2008;144(1):74-9.

52. Lavely WC, Goetze S, Friedman KP, Leal JP, Zhang Z, Garret-Mayer E, et al. Comparison of SPECT/CT, SPECT, and planar imaging with single- and dual-phase 99mTc-sestamibi parathyroid scintigraphy. J Nucl Med. 2007;48(7):1084-9.

53. Mahajan A, Starker LF, Ghita M, Udelsman R, Brink JA, Carling T. Parathyroid four-dimensional computed tomography: evaluation of radiation dose exposure during preoperative localization of parathyroid tumors in primary hyperparathyroidism. World J Surg. 2012;36(6):1335-9.

54. Day KM, Elsayed M, Beland MD, Monchik JM. The utility of 4-dimensional computed tomography for preoperative localization of primary hyperparathyroidism in patients not localized by sestamibi or ultrasonography. Surg (United States). 2015;157(3):534-9.

55. Czarnecki CA, Einsiedel PF, Phal PM, Miller JA, Lichtenstein M, Stella DL. Dynamic CT for parathyroid adenoma detection: how does radiation dose compare with nuclear medicine? Am J Roentgenol. 2018;210(5):1118-22.

56. Lebastchi AH, Aruny JE, Donovan PI, Quinn CE, Callender GG, Carling T, et al. Real-time super selective venous sampling in remedial parathyroid surgery. J Am Coll Surg. 2015;220(6):994-1000.

57. Prabhu M, Damle NA. Fluorocholine PET Imaging of parathyroid disease. Indian J Endocrinol Metab. 2018;22(4):535-41.

58. Taywade SK, Damle NA, Behera A, Devasenathipathy K, Bal C, Tripathi M, et al. Comparison of 18F-Fluorocholine positron emission tomography/computed tomography and four-dimensional computed tomography in the preoperative localization of parathyroid adenomas-initial results. Indian J Endocrinol Metab. 2017;21(3):399-403.

59. Norlén O, Glover A, Zaidi N, Aniss A, Sywak M, Sidhu S, et al. The weight of the resected gland predicts rate of success after image-guided focused parathyroidectomy. World J Surg. 2015;39(8):1922-7.

60. Yeung M. Parathyroidectomy without the utilisation of iPTH: the gold standard is still a good operation—how understanding the anatomy and a simple US can help. World J Surg. 2020;44(2):622-4.

61. Patel KN, Caso R. Intraoperative parathyroid hormone monitoring. optimal utilization. Surg Oncol Clin N Am. 2016;25(1):91-101.

62. Moore EC, Rudin A, Alameh A, Berber E. Near-infrared imaging in re-operative parathyroid surgery: first description of autofluorescence from cryopreserved parathyroid glands. Gland Surg. 2019;8(3):283-6.

63. Moore EC, Berber E. Fluorescence techniques in adrenal surgery. Gland Surg. 2019;8:S22-S27.

64. Yeh MW, Zhou H, Adams AL, Ituarte PHG, Li N, Liu ILA, et al. The relationship of parathyroidectomy and bisphosphonates with fracture risk in primary hyperparathyroidism: an observational study. Ann Intern Med. 2016;164(11): 715-23.

65. Zanocco KA, Wu JX, Yeh MW. Parathyroidectomy for asymptomatic primary hyperparathyroidism: A revised cost-effectiveness analysis incorporating fracture risk reduction. Surg (United States). 2017;161(1):16-24.

66. Jinih M, O'Connell E, O'Leary DP, Liew A, Redmond HP. Focused versus bilateral parathyroid exploration for primary hyperparathyroidism: a systematic review and meta-analysis. Ann Surg Oncol. 2017;24(7):1924-34.

67. Schneider DF, Mazeh H, Chen H, Sippel RS. Predictors of recurrence in primary hyperparathyroidism: an analysis of 1386 cases. Ann Surg. 2014;259(3):563-8.

68. Hodin R, Angelos P, Carty S, Chen H, Clark O, Doherty G, et al. No need to abandon unilateral parathyroid surgery. J Am Coll Surg. 2012;215(2):297.

69. Siperstein A, Berber E, Barbosa GF, Tsinberg M, Greene AB, Mitchell J, et al. Predicting the success of limited exploration for primary hyperparathyroidism using ultrasound, sestamibi, and intraoperative parathyroid hormone: analysis of 1158 cases. Ann Surg. 2008;248(3):420-8.

70. Noureldine SI, Gooi Z, Tufano RP. Minimally invasive parathyroid surgery. Gland Surg. 2015;4(5):410-9.

71. Chen H, Sokoll LJ, Udelsman R. Outpatient minimally invasive parathyroidectomy: a combination of sestamibi-SPECT localization, cervical block anesthesia, and intraoperative parathyroid hormone assay. Surgery. 1999;126(6):1016-22.

72. Norman J, Chheda H, Farrell C. Minimally invasive parathyroidectomy for primary hyperparathyroidism: decreasing operative time and potential complications while improving cosmetic results. Am Surg. 1998;64(5):391-5; discussion 395-6.

73. Lowney JK, Weber B, Johnson S, Doherty GM. Minimal incision parathyroidectomy: cure, cosmesis, and cost. World J Surg. 2000;24:1442-5.

74. Norman J, Lopez J, Politz D. Abandoning unilateral parathyroidectomy: why we reversed our position after 15,000 parathyroid operations. J Am Coll Surg. 2012;214(3):260-9.

75. Singh Ospina NM, Rodriguez-Gutierrez R, Maraka S, de Ycaza AEE, Jasim S, Castaneda-Guarderas A, et al. Outcomes of parathyroidectomy in patients with primary hyperparathyroidism: a systematic review and meta-analysis. World J Surg. 2016;40(10):2359-77.

76 Miller JA, Gundara J, Harper S, Herath M, Ramchand SK, Farrell S, et al. Primary hyperparathyroidism in adults (Part II) surgical management and postoperative follow-up: Position statement of the Endocrine Society of Australia, The Australian & New Zealand Endocrine Surgeons, and The Australian & New Zealand Bone and Mineral Society. Clin Endocrinol (Oxf). 2021. doi: 10.1111/cen.14650.

77. Zheng F, Zhou H, Li N, Haigh PI, Adams AL, Yeh MW. Skeletal effects of failed parathyroidectomy. Surg (United States). 2018;163(1):17-21.

78. Silverberg SJ, Shane E, Jacobs TP, Siris E, Bilezikian JP. A 10-year prospective study of primary hyperparathyroidism with or without parathyroid surgery. N Engl J Med. 1999;341(17): 1249-55.

79. Kose E, Rudin AV, Kahramangil B, Moore E, Aydin H, Donmez M, et al. Autofluorescence imaging of parathyroid glands: an assessment of potential indications. Surg (United States). 2020;167(1):173-9.

80. Mallick R, Nicholson KJ, Yip L, Carty SE, McCoy KL. Factors associated with late recurrence after parathyroidectomy for primary hyperparathyroidism. Surgery. 2020;167(1):160-5.

81. Blanchard C, Mathonnet M, Sebag F, Caillard C, Hamy A, Volteau C, et al. Surgery for "asymptomatic" mild primary hyperparathyroidism improves some clinical symptoms postoperatively. Eur J Endocrinol. 2013;169(5): 665-72.

82. Blanchard C, Mathonnet M, Sebag F, Caillard C, Kubis K, Drui D, et al. Quality of life is modestly improved in older patients with mild primary hyperparathyroidism postoperatively: results of a prospective multicenter study. Ann Surg Oncol. 2014;21(11):3534-40.

83. Rubin MR, Bilezikian JP, McMahon DJ, Jacobs T, Shane E, Siris E, et al. The natural history of primary hyperparathyroidism with or without parathyroid surgery after 15 years. J Clin Endocrinol Metab. 2008;93(9):3462-70.

84. Peacock M, Bilezikian JP, Klassen PS, Guo MD, Turner SA, Shoback D. Cinacalcet hydrochloride maintains long-term normocalcemia in patients with primary hyperparathyroidism. J Clin Endocrinol Metab. 2005;90(1):135-41.

Parathyroid Surgery

Roma Pradhan

◇ INTRODUCTION

An inappropriately high parathyroid hormone (PTH) level for a particular calcium level is considered as hyperparathyroidism (HPT). It occurs in three forms **(Table 1)**:

1. *Primary hyperparathyroidism (PHPT)*: It is a biochemical syndrome characterized by inappropriately high PTH due to increased secretion of PTH from either one or more parathyroid glands (PTGs). In outpatients, it is the most frequent cause of hypercalcemia. About 10% are familial and are inherited as autosomal dominant disease [three common familial HPTs are familial isolated HPT (FIHPT), multiple endocrine neoplasia type 1 (MEN1)/multiple endocrine neoplasia type 2a (MEN2a), or HPT-jaw tumor (HPT-JT) syndrome].
2. Secondary hyperparathyroidism
3. Tertiary hyperparathyroidism

◇ PRIMARY HYPERPARATHYROIDISM

Primary hyperparathyroidism is not an uncommon disorder. PHPT in the western world is still a disease of postmenopausal women[1] whereas in our country, it is symptomatic at presentation. The most common cause of PHPT is enlargement of single gland, which is found in 80–85% of patients, followed by hyperplasia (enlargement of all glands) in 15–20% and carcinoma in <1%. The management also evolved with first parathyroidectomy performed by Mandl[2] in 1924 in which an attempt was made to visualize all the four PTGs and with excision of a single enlarged gland. As the clinical presentation of PHPT evolved from severe symptomatic to asymptomatic disease, the surgical approach also evolved from visualization of all the four glands (bilateral neck exploration) to focused approach (visualization and removal of single gland) with advancement in various preoperative investigations along with operative adjuncts.

◇ INDICATIONS OF PARATHYROID SURGERY

Primary Hyperparathyroidism

It has been clearly documented that the only curable treatment for PHPT is parathyroidectomy. A study of natural history of PHPT has revealed that 25–30% of patients of PHPT who are medically followed up show progression of disease and meet criteria for surgery.[3-5] Considerations in favor of early parathyroidectomy in asymptomatic patients include minimization of cardiovascular (CV) risk, prevention of continued progressive bone loss, prevention of progression of renal dysfunction, and alleviation of neurocognitive symptoms of PHPT and improving quality of life. Surgical intervention is needed in all patients of symptomatic PHPT. The patient can have classical symptoms of psychic moans, abdominal groans, renal stones, and painful bone. The other symptoms include:

- Polydipsia and polyuria
- Nephrolithiasis or nephrocalcinosis
- Hypercalciuria (24-hour urine calcium level >400 mg/dL)
- Impaired renal function [glomerular filtration rate (GFR) <60 mL/min]
- Osteoporosis (bone density score <−2.5)
- Fragility fracture or vertebral compression fracture
- Pancreatitis
- Peptic ulcer disease or gastroesophageal reflux disease (GERD)
- Neurocognitive dysfunction or neuropsychiatric symptoms

Table 1: Forms of hyperparathyroidism and their causes and treatment.

Type	Cause	Treatment
Primary HPT	Unregulated overproduction of parathyroid hormone resulting in high calcium in the presence of normal renal function and normal levels of vitamin D due to adenoma, hyperplasia, or carcinoma	*Surgery*: Open/minimal access parathyroidectomy
Secondary HPT	Excessive production of parathyroid hormone secondary to a chronic abnormal stimulus such as chronic renal failure and vitamin D deficiency and malabsorption syndromes	Medical management + Surgery
Tertiary HPT	Autonomous hypersecretion of parathyroid hormone causing hypercalcemia often seen in chronic secondary hyperparathyroidism (prolonged compensatory stimulation)	Medical management + Surgery total parathyroidectomy with autotransplantation, surgery

(HPT: hyperparathyroidism)

Table 2: Guidelines for surgery in asymptomatic primary hyperparathyroidism.[6]

	1990	2002	2008	2013
Serum calcium (>Upper limit of normal)	1–1.6 mg/dL	1.0 mg/dL	1.0 mg/dL	1.0 mg/dL
Skeletal	BMD by DXA:Z score < −2.0	BMD by DXA:T score <−2.0 at any site	• BMD by DXA:T score < −2.0 at any site • Previous fragility fracture	• BMD by DXA:T score <−2.0 at lumbar spine, total hip, femoral neck, or distal radius • Vertebral fracture by X-ray, CT, MRI, or VFA
Renal	• eGFR reduced by >30% from expected • 24-hour urine for calcium >400 mg/day	• eGFR reduced by >30% from expected • 24-hour urine for calcium >400 mg/day	• eGFR <60 cc/min • 24-hour urine for calcium not recommended	• Creatinine clearance <60 cc/min • 24-hour urine for calcium >400 mg/day • Presence of nephrolithiasis or nephrocalcinosis by X-ray, ultrasound or CT
Age in years	<50	<50	<50	<50

(BMD: bone mineral density; DXA: dual-energy X-ray absorptiometry; eGFR: estimated glomerular filtration rate; VFA: vertebral fracture assessment)

The indications for surgery in *asymptomatic PHPT* are summarized in **Table 2**.

PARATHYROID SURGERY FOR PRIMARY HYPERPARATHYROIDISM

In parathyroid surgery, the following need to be discussed:
- General principles of parathyroid surgery
- Preoperative preparation
- Imaging studies
- Surgical approach or exposure
- Extent of parathyroidectomy
- Novel approaches
- Postoperative considerations
- Outcome
- Special situations

General Principles of Parathyroid Surgery

The following general principles in parathyroid surgery should be followed for a successful outcome:
- Maintaining a bloodless field
- Meticulous dissection
- *Identification of all four PTGs in a bilateral exploration*: Inferior PTGs are typically identified within 1 cm circle around intersection of inferior thyroid artery and recurrent laryngeal nerve (RLN). Superior PTGs are typically located near the entry of RLN into larynx at the cricothyroid joint.
- *Attention to embryological migration*: While exploring, the extent of embryological migration of PTGs, especially the inferior glands, should be kept in mind. If inferior PTG is not identified, then ectopic sites lie thymus, carotid sheath and possibility of an undescended inferior parathyroid gland (PTG) should be kept in mind. If superior PTG is not located, then ectopic sites such as retropharyngeal/retroesophageal site and intrathyroidal site should be explored.

- RLN identification with or without use of intraoperative neuromonitoring (IONM) is very important to avoid injury to RLN.
- Avoid direct handling or holding of the PTA so as to avoid rupture of capsule, which later results in parathyromatosis. One of the methods to avoid rupture of capsule is to use sponge on stick for blunt dissection of the PTA from the surrounding structures.
- Never remove a normal PTG.
- Biopsy of one or more normal glands should be avoided as it may lead to an increased incidence of hypocalcemia.

PREOPERATIVE PREPARATION

- Careful history and physical examination to establish whether the patient is symptomatic/minimally symptomatic/asymptomatic.
- All medications should be inquired, especially with respect to intake of lithium and thiazide diuretics.
- Any family history suggestive of familial endocrine predisposition syndromes should be documented.
- Although a palpable parathyroid adenoma should raise a suspicion of parathyroid carcinoma, in developing countries such as ours, a palpable benign PTA is not uncommon. Whatever the etiology, a palpable PTA should alert to the possibility of profound postoperative hypocalcemia.
- Preoperative vocal cord evaluation by indirect laryngoscopy (IDL)
- It is also incumbent upon the endocrine surgeon to reconfirm the biochemical diagnosis of PHPT by reviewing the reports of serum calcium, phosphorus, PTH, vitamin D, serum creatinine, 24-hour urinary calcium, bone mineral density (BMD), echocardiography, etc.

Imaging Studies

These are necessary if a decision for minimally invasive parathyroidectomy (MIP) has been taken. It is emphasized that the imaging studies do not play any role in making the diagnosis of PHPT. Preoperative localization studies allow the surgeon to establish/predict whether a patient is likely to have a single gland disease (which allows to plan an MIP) or multiglandular disease (in which case a bilateral exploration is preferred). Though there are a number of imaging studies, the preference of choosing the studies varies from center to center. But typically, a commonly used protocol is to do an ultrasonography (USG) and myocardial perfusion imaging (MIBI) scan. If both are concordant, then MIP is planned. If the studies are negative or discordant, then one can either proceed directly to bilateral exploration or do a 4D-CT scan.

Surgical Approach or Exposure

The traditional and gold standard approach was bilateral neck exploration for all situations, whether the gland was localized or nonlocalized.

However, over the years, it was thought that in keeping with the concept of minimally invasive surgery, surgeons developed two other approaches:
1. Unilateral approach where only the side of the localized gland was explored.
2. Focused approach where only the offending gland was explored and removed.

Focused Parathyroidectomy

Focused or limited parathyroidectomy can be performed by either small incision right over the offending gland **(Fig. 1)** or a conventional Kocher incision. Focused parathyroidectomy (FP) is attempted preferably after we have a concordant imaging on preoperative evaluation.

Focused parathyroidectomy is a procedure, which utilizes preferably a small incision (<2 cm), minimal dissection, and removal of the single enlarged gland without making any effort to either find or visualize the other normal gland on that side. Briefly, the procedure involves making a small incision **(Fig. 1)**, either central or oblique, then dilating the space with

index finger **(Fig. 2)**, and dissecting the space between the strap muscles and the sternocleidomastoid muscle (SCM). Once the adenoma is visualized, it is bluntly dissected out from the surrounding tissues keeping in mind not to damage its capsule. This can be facilitated using a small peanut taking care to keep hugging the adenoma **(Fig. 3)** during dissection to avoid injury to the RLN.

Many randomized controlled trials (RCTs) have compared MIP and bilateral exploration.[7-10]

Minimally invasive parathyroidectomy has been found to be associated with many advantages.

Advantages of FP:
- Minimally invasive
- Less analgesic requirement
- Allows for outpatient surgery
- Enables surgery under local anesthesia
- Provides excellent cosmesis
- Cure rates > 98%
- Less postoperative hypocalcemia

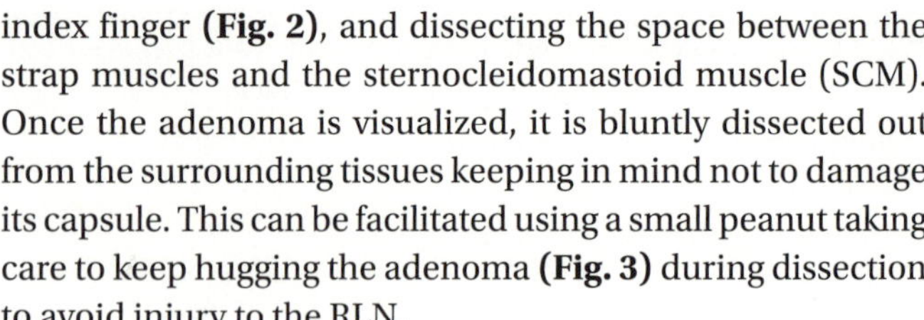

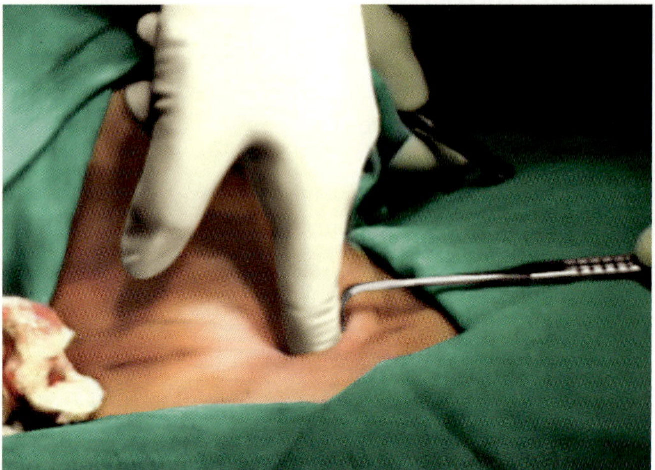

Fig. 2: Dilatation of the space.

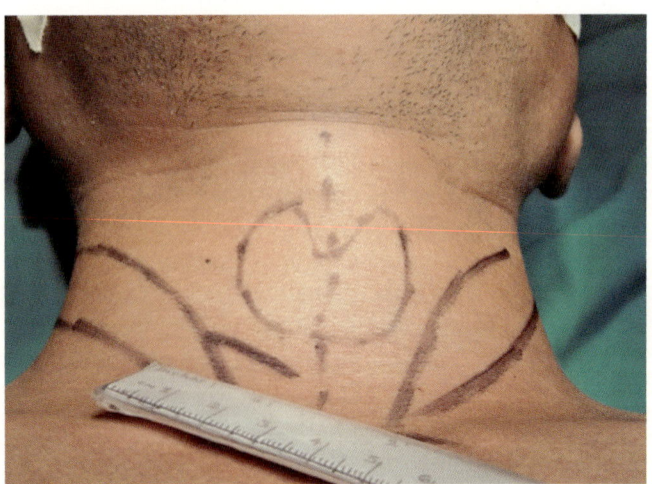

Fig. 1: Mini incision marked over the adenoma localized by ultrasound in the operating room.

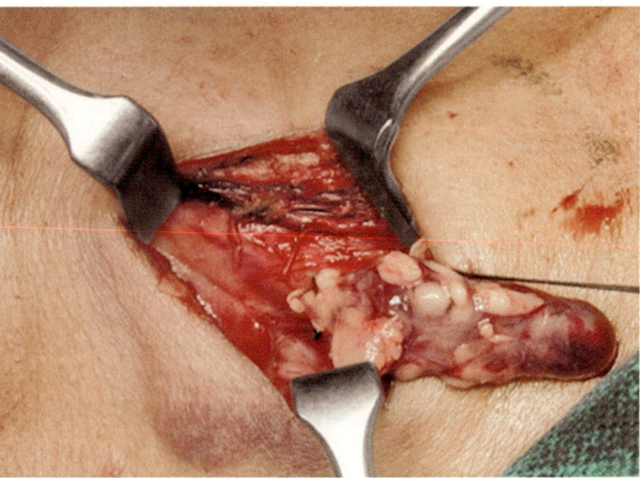

Fig. 3: Adenoma excised.

Bilateral Neck Exploration

Even after FP being the surgical procedure of choice by majority of endocrine surgeons, bilateral neck exploration is still considered the gold standard and is the procedure of choice in certain situations:

Absolute indications:
- MEN1
- Negative preoperative localization studies
- Inadequate fall of intraoperative PTH

Relative indications:
- Isolated familial PHPT
- MEN2 syndrome
- History of lithium therapy or treatment
- History of head and neck irradiation
- Discordant preoperative localization studies

These are some general principles which one should keep in mind during bilateral neck exploration—we need to find at least four PTGs, do not resect normal PTGs, and remember the dictum "every parathyroid you see should be thought of as last parathyroid." Biopsy should be done sparingly in normal-appearing parathyroids and to confirm all tissues on frozen section biopsy.

Extent of Parathyroidectomy

Single Adenoma

When a single adenoma is there, we need to excise only that enlarged gland which may or may not be sent for frozen section confirmation. However, frozen section enables us to know only about the tissue of origin and not the pathology (adenoma or hyperplasia). Routine biopsy of all normal PTGs is strictly discouraged. Intraoperative PTH monitoring is usually preferred as an adjunct. If intraoperative PTH monitoring during MIP shows no fall in PTH hormone and suggests the presence of residual hypersecreting parathyroid tissue, then a decision to explore the other glands showed be made (bilateral neck exploration).

Double Adenomas

Finding of a macroscopically abnormal PTG during FP does not preclude the absence of other abnormal PTGs such as double adenoma or multiglandular disease (MGD). Hence, intraoperative PTH monitoring is especially useful in such circumstances which tell us the probable presence of another hyperfunctioning gland. In the literature, double adenomas have been found in 2–15% of patients undergoing parathyroid surgery;[11-16] however, some investigators suggest it to be asymmetrical hyperplasia.[17] Various studies which have shown normalization and maintenance of hypocalcemia after excision of double adenoma[16] point toward the existence of double adenoma and not merely missed cases of hyperplasia. We had three cases of double adenoma out of 246 parathyroid specimens.[18]

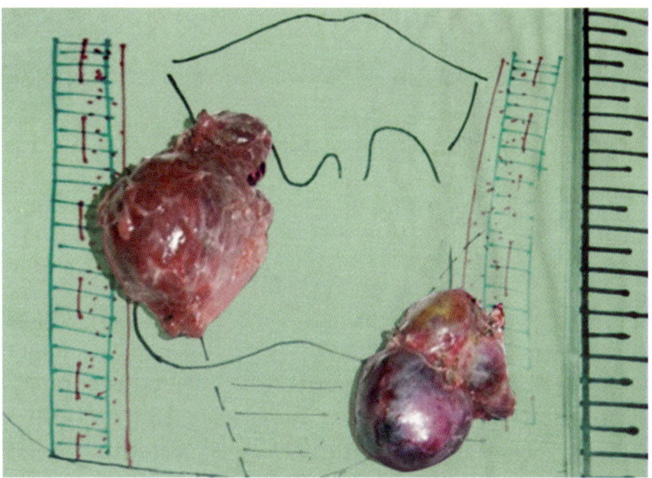

Fig. 4: Double adenoma.

In case of double adenoma **(Fig. 4)**, we remove the two enlarged parathyroid lesions and also identify the other two normal glands. Unlike in case of single adenoma where we avoid biopsy of normal glands, here we must biopsy one of the normal glands in order to rule out hyperplasia.

Sporadic Hyperplasia/Sporadic Multiglandular Disease

Sporadic MGD has been reported in literature in 7–33% of patients with PHPT.[11,18-24]

Diagnosis of sporadic hyperplasia is usually made in the following situations such as:
- Negative preoperative localization
- Discordant preoperative localization
- No curative fall of intraoperative parathyroid hormone (IOPTH) following excision of one or two glands
- Intraoperative finding of more than one gland enlargement

In such a scenario of sporadic MGD, treatment options ranged from 3 gland excision, 31/2 or total with or without autotransplantation. All these three procedures differ in their recurrence/persistence and complication rates:
- Therefore, we need to individualize treatment.
- However, thymectomy should never be done as a part of procedure for sporadic MGD.

◁ NOVEL APPROACHES

In quest for a cosmetically acceptable incision or still better a scarless operation, novel approaches have been developed which include:
- Video-assisted endoscopic parathyroidectomy—through a small 1.5-cm central cervical incision
- Endoscopic transaxillary or axillo-breast approaches which do not leave a cervical scar.
- Robotic transaxillary or axillo-breast approach
- Natural orifice transoral approach which does not leave a skin incision.

◇| POSTOPERATIVE CONSIDERATIONS

Three major complications that may occur after parathyroid surgery include:

1. *Hematoma*: This life-threatening complication may occur with or without respiratory obstruction and has to be managed emergently either at bedside or in the operation theater.

2. Profound hypocalcemia resulting either from hungry bone syndrome, especially in patients with severe bone disease or large adenomas, or due to hypoparathyroidism resulting from ischemia to the normal PTGs in bilateral exploration.

   The term *"hungry bone syndrome (HBS)"* has been coined to the rapid, profound, and prolonged (longer than 4th day postoperatively) hypocalcemia, which happens following parathyroidectomy for severe HPT, followed by normal or elevated PTH levels. In patients with preoperative accelerated bone turnover, successful parathyroidectomy curbs osteoclastic resorption, leading to a decrease in the activation frequency of new remodeling sites and to a reduction in remodeling space leading to a consequent gain in bone mass. Increase in bone uptake also results in hypophosphatemia and hypomagnesemia in HBS. Severe hypocalcemia (serum calcium concentration <2.1 mmol/L) may manifest as neuromuscular irritability, carpopedal spasms, perioral paresthesia, tingling extremities, Chvostek sign, and Trousseau sign. Patients can also develop generalized convulsions, which can lead to pathological fractures and ultimately, if uncorrected, to coma and even death. Congestive heart failure, which is reversible after normalization of serum calcium concentration, has also been reported. The treatment of HBS is aimed primarily at replenishing the depleted skeletal calcium stores. The amount of calcium supplementation required to treat the severe hypocalcemia can vary between 6 and 12 g/day along with adequate doses of active metabolites of vitamin D (calcitriol) or alfacalcidol (2–4 mg/day) Replenishment of magnesium stores is required which is given intravenously as magnesium chloride or sulfate or orally as magnesium sulfate.

3. *RLN palsy*: Temporary/permanent

◇| OUTCOMES

In symptomatic patients, "immediate improvement" (>50% of patients reporting improvement by postoperative week 1) may be seen for fatigue and bone pains, whereas the majority of symptoms will show peak improvement at 6 weeks ("delayed improvement"). "Continuous improvements" were those which show progressive improvement up to 6 months postoperatively (polydipsia, headaches, and nausea/vomiting). There is significant improvement in BMD and this improvement is maximum in the first 2 years. There

is vigorous but disorderly remineralization in brown tumors which heal within a median period of 3 months but persistent vitamin D deficiency after operation delays bone recovery. Therefore, vitamin D stores should be replenished in the follow-up. Recovery from renal disease is gradual and may never occur in some patient while in others, it may progress to end-stage renal disease (ESRD). Patients recover fully from pancreatitis and they are unlikely to experience any further attack of acute pancreatitis.

◇| SPECIAL SITUATIONS

Parathyroid Carcinoma

Management of parathyroid carcinoma is challenging for the following reasons:

- Parathyroid carcinoma is difficult to differentiate from benign PHPT based on just biochemical values, although serum calcium and intact PTH levels are usually elevated more in patients with parathyroid carcinoma.

- *It may appear as an intraoperative surprise*: In the operating room, a supposedly benign PTA may typically appear as a gray or white, firm mass that is densely adherent to the thyroid and other surrounding structures. In such a case, an intraoperative diagnosis of parathyroid carcinoma is made and en bloc resection of the ipsilateral thyroid lobe and overlying strap muscles is performed.

- The histopathological diagnosis (both under- and over-reporting) is common and one may have to resort to immunohistochemical markers such as parafibromin, Galecti-3, and PGP9.5[17,25] (**Fig. 5**).

- Even after a complete clearance of all tissues on the side of parathyroid carcinoma including the lymph nodes (LNs), there is a very high rate of local recurrence and distant relapse (>60%).

Hypercalcemic Crisis

Hypercalcemic crisis is an uncommon complication of PHPT in which patients usually have accelerated hypercalcemia [serum ≥14 mg/dL (≥3.5 mmol/L)] along with rapid deterioration of central nervous system, cardiac, gastrointestinal, and renal functions as well as life-threatening cardiac arrhythmias when severe hyperparathyroid-induced hypercalcemic crisis (HIHC) is not treated promptly.[26] Prompt diagnosis and aggressive measures to reduce serum calcium levels help in reducing morbidity and mortality and these measures include rapid intravascular volume expansion with isotonic saline solution and diuretics such as frusemide to induce calciuresis, with or without bisphosphonates followed by semiurgent or expeditious parathyroidectomy. Although no strong data exist, surgery may be performed when the serum calcium levels have been lowered to at least 14 mg/dL.[27]

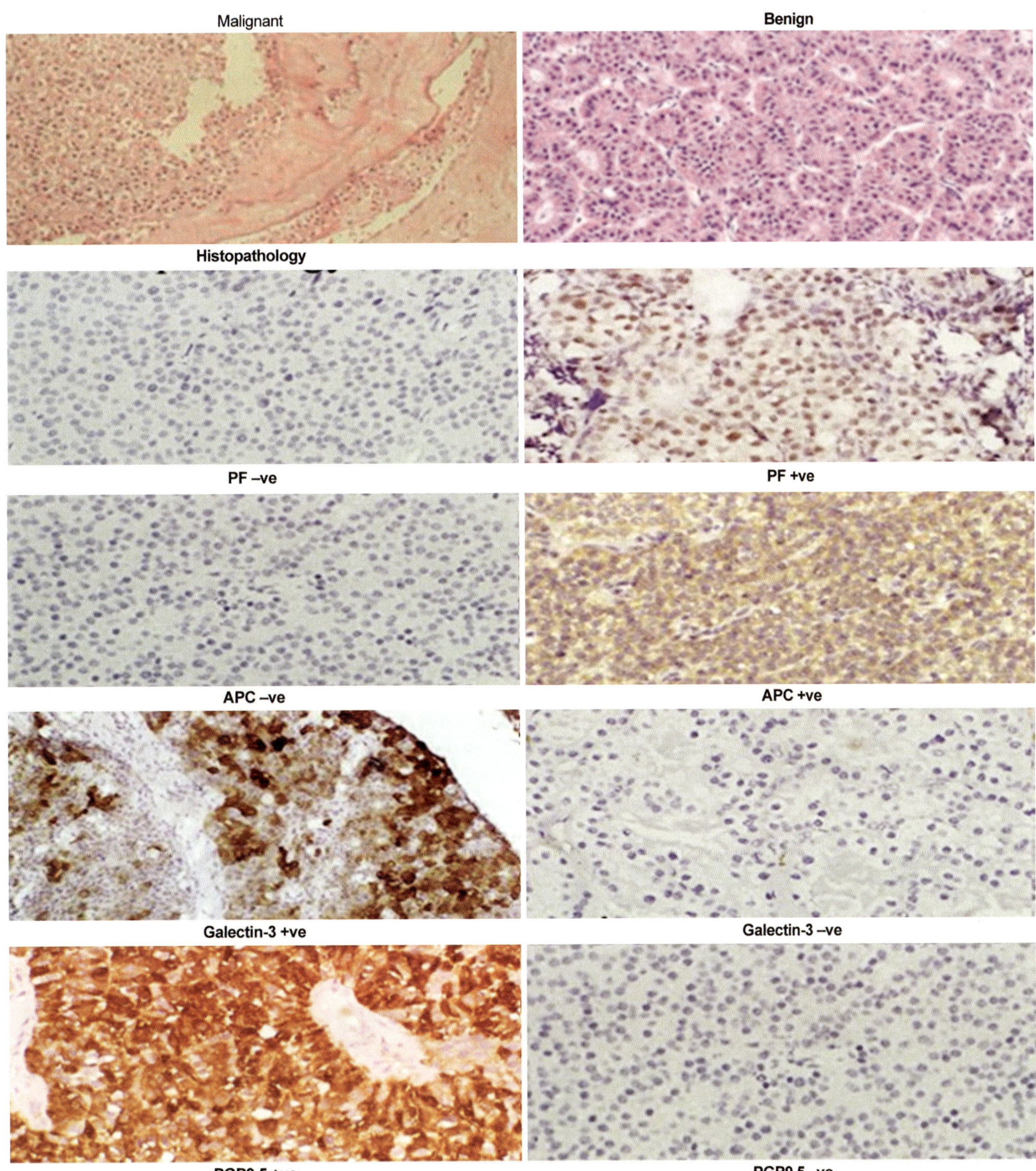

Fig. 5: Immunohistochemistry in benign and malignancy parathyroid lesions.

Familial Hyperparathyroidism

Familial HPT includes MEN1, MEN2a, HPT-JT, and FIHPT. All these comprise 2–5% of PHPT cases.

- MEN1: Multiple Endocrine Neoplasia 1
- MEN2a: Multiple Endocrine Neoplasia 2a
- FIHPT: Familial Isolated Hyperparathyrodism
- HPT-JT: Hyperparathyrodism Jaw Tumor

Multiple Endocrine Neoplasia Type 1 PHPT

Multiple endocrine neoplasia type 1 PHPT is characterized by earlier onset in 2nd or 3rd decade of life as compared to sporadic PHPT, which is more common after the 5th decade of life.[28,29] MEN1 is an autosomal-dominant disorder caused by mutation in tumor suppressor gene *Menin*. PHPT occurs in 90% of patients of MEN1 and usually the initial clinical manifestation.

Primary HPT in MEN1 is characterized by multiglandular hyperplasia which is usually asymmetrical and asynchronous. The main modality of treatment in MEN1 PHPT is surgery. HPT in MEN1 is monoclonal or oligoclonal, which causes the parathyroid tissue susceptible to enlargement after the second somatic mutation.[30] Supernumerary glands are found in 20% of MEN1 patients.[31]

Considering the multiglandular nature of the disease, routine preoperative investigations such as cervical USG, sestamibi scan, or newer modalities such as 4D-CT or MRI are not very helpful before the first surgery but nonetheless they may be useful in knowing about the location of any ectopic glands. However, preoperative investigations are mandatory in a reoperative setting.

The choice of surgery for PHPT in MEN1 is debatable between two options—total parathyroidectomy and subtotal parathyroidectomy. Both the procedures differ in their recurrence/persistence and complication rates **(Table 3)**.

The three goals of surgery are to:
1. Maintain normal calcium levels (eucalcemia) for the longest time possible
2. Avoid iatrogenic surgical hypocalcemia and other operative complications
3. Facilitate future surgery for recurrent disease

Transcervical thymectomy should be performed at the initial operation because of two reasons: there is approximately 15% chance of finding parathyroid in thymus and due to occurrence of thymic carcinoids which is part of MEN1 pathology.

Total parathyrodiectomy with autotransplantation and subtotal parathyroidectomy, both have their pros and cons.

Total parathyroidectomy with AT which is an extensive surgery still poses some risk of recurrence with a high rate of permanent hypoparathyroidism or hypocalcemia and RLN damage. The less extensive surgery of subtotal parathyroidectomy, on the other hand, has high rates of recurrence leading to more reoperations and further increase in rates of complications. Any procedure less than subtotal parathyroidectomy tends to have the highest rate of both recurrent and persistent PHPT. **Table 3** shows a comparison of surgical procedures of recent studies in MEN1 PHPT patients. Most surgeons prefer 3½ parathyroidectomy but with cervical thymectomy and removal of any supernumerary glands.

Multiple Endocrine Neoplasia Type 2a

MEN type 2a is a familial disorder characterized by medullary thyroid cancer and pheochromocytoma caused by RET gene mutation. It is known as MEN2a when associated with PHPT and MEN2b when associated with neuromas and gastrointestinal tumors. PHPT in MEN2a is usually mild, asymmetrical, and can be detected as enlargement of PTG during thyroid surgery for MTC,[40] as it is rarely the first manifestation of MEN2a.

Indications for surgery in MEN2a PHPT are the same as in sporadic PHPT or MEN1 PHPT patients. The operative approach most commonly followed for PHPT in MEN2a is removal of only affected or enlarged glands.

Majority of times, PHPT in MEN2a presents after the initial surgery has already been performed for MTC; hence, parathyroid surgery is usually done in reoperative settings.

Table 3: Comparison of surgical procedures of recent studies in MEN1 PHPT patients.						
Study	*Surgery*	*Number of patients*	*Permanent hypocalcemia*	*Persistent PHPT*	*Recurrent PHPT*	*Follow-up*
Salmeron, 2010[32]	SPTX	69	3 (4%)		9 (13%)	75 (9–300)
Waldmann, 2010[33]	<SPTX	13	0	3 (23%)	6 (46%)	84 (36–180)
	SPTX	11	5 (45%)	0	2 (18%)	118 (32–132)
	TPTX	23	5 (22%)	1 (4%)	1 (4%)	84 (4–204)
Schreinemaker, 2011[34]	<SPTX	29	2 (7%)	9 (31%)	17 (59%)	99 (44–162)
	SPTX	17	4 (24%)	1 (7%)	11 (65%)	144 (71–207)
	TPTX	6	4 (67%)	1 (17%)		16 (4–201)
Pieterman, 2012[35]	<SPTX	17	4 (24%)	9 (53%)	9 (53%)	Overall 51 (21–78)
	SPTX	23	9 (39%)	4 (17%)	4 (17%)	
	TPTX	32	21 (66%)	6 (19%)	6 (19%)	
Versnick, 2013[36]	<SPTX	6				19
	SPTX	10	4 (40%)		3 (30%)	106
	TPTX	10	6 (60%)		3 (30%)	133
Lairmore, 2014[37]	SPTX	17	2 (12%)	1 (6%)	4 (24%)	7.5 ± 5.7
	PTPX	15	1 (7%)		2 (13%)	7.5 ± 5.7
Frysten, 2015[38]	<SPTX	31	2 (7%)	7 (23%)		247
	SPTX	30	5 (16%)	2 (7%)		155
	TPTX	8	6 (75%)	1 (13%)		234
Marini, 2018[39]	PPTX	35	0		14	
	SPTX	17	0		2	
	TPTX	37	5			

Due to reoperative settings, detailed operative notes should be identified, if the previous surgery happened in another institute. The patient should preferably undergo thorough preoperative investigations with high-resolution ultrasound of neck and MIBI scan with or without 4D CT in order to localize the offending gland. If the previous surgery included autograft in the forearm, the upper extremities should also be included in the sestamibi scan.

If the offended gland or glands are localized on preoperative imaging, then FP can be performed with intraoperative PTH monitoring. If the PTH falls >50%, then we can conclude surgery without further exploration.

Hyperparathyroidism-jaw Tumor

Hyperparathyroidism-jaw tumor syndrome is a rare disease, which is caused by mutation in the tumor suppressor gene *CDC73*. It is associated with higher frequency of parathyroid carcinoma with frequency of up to 38%.[41]

Compared with MEN1-related hyperparathyroidism, the HTP-JT syndrome has a more aggressive course: the patients tend to present with severe hypercalcemia or even hypercalcemic crisis.

Pathologically, PHPT in HPT-JT syndrome is more often one- or two-gland involvement (adenoma or double adenoma) that may or may not present synchronously.[42] This is in contrast with MEN1 in which usually all the glands are involved. The other unique feature of parathyroid neoplasia in HPT-JT syndrome is the high incidence of cystic change in resected glands, also called familial cystic parathyroid adenomatosis.[43] The cystic change in parathyroid neoplasia associated with HPT-JT syndrome can range from numerous follicle-like or crypt-like glandular dilatations to large cysts, which distort the overall parathyroid architecture, all of which are lined by parathyroid cells. Parathyroid carcinoma has been reportedly associated with HPT-JT syndrome in many cases. However, the diagnosis of parathyroid carcinoma is extremely difficult and relies upon the evidence of metastatic disease or demise of the patient caused by persistent locally aggressive disease.

Hence, patients with benign adenomas harboring *HRPT2* mutations should be kept on lifelong follow-up as few studies provide correlation between *HRPT2* mutation and sporadic carcinoma.[44]

CONCLUSION

Modern-day parathyroid surgery requires:
- Understanding of the disease process
- Adequate preoperative work-up
- Accurate preoperative localization
- Tailoring the extent and approach of parathyroid surgery
- Adhering to the principles of parathyroid surgery, especially the algorithm for exploring the ectopic sites
- Judiciously utilizing the intraoperative adjuncts such as IOPTH, IONM, and Indocyanine green (ICG) dye

- Situations such as parathyroid carcinoma and hypercalcemic crisis are especially challenging to the endocrine surgeon.
- Vigilant postoperative monitoring, especially for life-threatening complications such as severe hypocalcemia.

CLINICAL PEARLS

- Diagnosis of HPT is biochemical.
- In any patient, it is imperative to establish the form of HPT—PHPT/SHPT/THPT as the imaging studies and extent of surgery differ.
- MIP is a modern approach to parathyroid surgery and as compared to four-gland exploration, it offers equivalent cure along with many advantages.
- A concordant USG and MIBI with IOPTH results in >95% cure rate.
- One should be careful about the possibility of HBS postoperatively.
- Familial HPT requires four-gland exploration except if a single gland is localized in MEN2a.
- *Extent of surgery*: PHPT: single-gland excision, SHPT: 3½ gland parathyroidectomy, MEN1: subtotal parathyroidectomy with thymectomy, and MEN2a: single gland excision

REFERENCES

1. Silverberg SJ, Walker MD, Bilezikian JP. Asymptomatic primary hyperparathyroidism. J Clin Densitom. 2013;16(1):14-21.
2. Mandl F. Therapeutischer versuch bein einem falle von ostitis fibrosa generalisata mittels exstirpation eines epithelk orperchen tumors. Zentralbl Chir. 1926;5:260.
3. Purnell DA, Smith LH, Scholz DA, Elveback LR, Arnaud CD. Primary hyperparathyroidism: a prospective clinical study. Am J Med. 1971;50:670-8.
4. Scholz DA, Purnell DC. Asymptomatic primary hyperpara-thyroidism: 10-year prospective study. Mayo Clin Proc. 1981;56:473-8.
5. Silverberg SJ, Shane E, Jacobs TP, Siris E, Bilezikian JP. A 10-year prospective study of primary hyperparathyroidism with or without parathyroid surgery. N Engl J Med. 1999;341:1249-55.
6. Bilezikian JP, Brandi ML, Eastell R, Silverberg SJ, Udelsman R, Marcocci C, et al. Guidelines for the management of asymptomatic primary hyperparathyroidism: summary statement from the Fourth International Workshop. J Clin Endocrinol Metab. 2014;99(10):3561-9.
7. Slepavicius A, Beisa V, Janusonis V, Strupas K. Focused versus conventional parathyroidectomy for primary hyperparathyroidism: a prospective, randomized, blinded trial. Langenbecks Arch Surg. 2008;393:659-66.
8. Miccoli P, Berti P, Materazzi G, Ambrosini CE, Fregoli L, Donatini G. Endoscopic bilateral neck exploration versus quick intraoperative parathormone assay (qPTHa) during endoscopic parathyroidectomy: a prospective randomized trial. Surg Endosc. 2008;22:398-400.
9. Aarum S, Nordenstrom J, Reihner E, Zedenius J, Jacobsson H, Danielsson R, et al. Operation for primary hyperparathyroidism: the new versus the old order. A randomized controlled trial of preoperative localisation. Scand J Surg. 2007;96:26-30.

10. Sozio A, Schietroma M, Franchi L, Mazzotta C, Cappelli S, Amicucci G. Parathyroidectomy: bilateral exploration of the neck versus minimally invasive radioguided treatment. Minerva Chir. 2005;60:83-9.

11. Attie JN, Bock G, Auguste LJ. Multiple parathyroid adenomas: report of thirty-three cases. Surgery. 1990;108(6):1014-19.

12. Bergson EJ, Heller KS. The clinical significance and anatomic distribution of parathyroid double adenomas. J Am Coll Surg. 2004;198(2):185-9.

13. Tezelman S, Shen W, Shaver JK, Siperstein AE, Duh QY, Klein H, et al. Double parathyroid adenomas: clinical and biochemical characteristics before and after parathyroidectomy. Ann Surg. 1993;218(3):300-7.

14. Milas M, Wagner K, Easley KA, Siperstein A, Weber CJ. Double adenomas re-visited: nonuniform distribution favors enlarged superior parathyroids (fourth pouch disease). Surgery. 2003;134(6):995-1004.

15. Kandil E, Alabbas HH, Bansal A, Islam T, Tufaro AP, Tufano RP. Intraoperative parathyroid hormone assay in patients with primary hyperparathyroidism and double adenoma. Arch Otolaryngol Head Neck Surg. 2009;135(12):1206-8.

16. Ghandur-Mnaymneh L, Kimura N. The parathyroid adenoma: a histopathologic definition with a study of 172 cases of primary hyperparathyroidism. Am J Pathol. 1984;115(1):70-83.

17. Kumari N, Chaudhary N, Pradhan R, Agarwal A, Krishnani N. Role of histological criteria and immunohistochemical markers in predicting risk of malignancy in parathyroid neoplasms. Endocr Pathol. 2016;27(2):87-96.

18. Alhefdhi A, Schneider DF, Sippel R, Chen H. Recurrent and persistence primary hyperparathyroidism occurs more frequently in patients with double adenomas. J Surg Res. 2014;190:198-202.

19. Vandenbulcke O, Delaere P, Vander Poorten V, Debruyne F. Incidence of multiglandular disease in sporadic primary hyperparathyroidism. B-ENT. 2014;10:1-6.

20. Mazeh H, Chen H, Leverson G, Sippel RS. Creation of a "Wisconsin index" nomogram to predict the likelihood of additional hyperfunctioning parathyroid glands during parathyroidectomy. Ann Surg. 2013;257:138-41.

21. Chneider DF, Burke JF, Ojomo KA, Clark N, Mazeh H, Sippel RS, et al. Multigland disease and slower decline in intraoperative PTH characterize mild primary hyperparathyroidism. Ann Surg Oncol. 2013;20:4205-11.

22. Hughes DT, Miller BS, Doherty GM, Gauger PG. Intraoperative parathyroid hormone monitoring in patients with recognized multiglandular primary hyperparathyroidism. World J Surg. 2011;35:336-41.

23. Cayo AK, Sippel RS, Schaefer S, Chen H. Utility of intra-operative PTH for primary hyperparathyroidism due to multigland disease. Ann Surg Oncol. 2009;16:3450-4.

24. Szabo E, Lundgren E, Juhlin C, Ljunghall S, Akerström G, Rastad J. Double parathyroid adenoma, a clinically nondistinct entity of primary hyperparathyroidism. World J Surg. 1998;22:708-13.

25. Agarwal A, Pradhan R, Kumari N, Krishnani N, Shukla P, Gupta SK, et al. Molecular characteristics of large parathyroid adenomas. World J Surg. 2016;40(3):607-14.

26. Singh DN, Gupta SK, Kumari N, Krishnani N, Chand G, Mishra A, et al. Primary hyperparathyroidism presenting as hypercalcemic crisis: Twenty-year experience. Indian J Endocrinol Metab. 2015;19(1):100-5.

27. Starker LF, Bjorklund P, Theoharis C, Long WD 3rd, Carling T, Udelsman R. Clinical and histopathological characteristics of hyperparathyroidism-induced hypercalcemic crisis. World J Surg. 2011;35:331-5.

28. Giusti F, Cavalli L, Cavalli T, Brandi ML. Hereditary hyperparathyroidism syndromes. J Clin Densitom. 2013;16:69-74.

29. Romero Arenas MA, Morris LF, Rich TA, Cote GJ, Grubbs EG, Waguespack SG, et al. Preoperative multiple endocrine neoplasia type 1 diagnosis improves the surgical outcomes of pediatric patients with primary hyperparathyroidism. J Pediatr Surg. 2014;49(4):546-50.

30. Carling T. Molecular pathology of parathyroid tumors. Trends Endocrinol Metab. 2001;12(2):53-8.

31. Hellman P, Skogseid B, Oberg K, Juhlin C, Akerstrom G, Rastad J. Primary and reoperative parathyroid operations in hyperparathyroidism of multiple endocrine neoplasia type 1. Surgery. 1998;124:993-9.

32. Salmeron MD, Gonzalez JM, Sancho Insenser J, Goday A, Perez NM, Zambudio AR, et al. Causes and treatment of recurrent hyperparathyroidism after subtotal parathyroid-ectomy in the presence of multiple endocrine neoplasia 1. World J Surg. 2010;34(6):1325-31.

33. Waldmann J, López CL, Langer P, Rothmund M, Bartsch DK. Surgery for multiple endocrine neoplasia type 1-associated primary hyperparathyroidism. Br J Surg. 2010;97(10): 1528-34.

34. Schreinemakers JM, Pieterman CR, Scholten A, Vriens MR, Valk GD, Rinkes IH. The optimal surgical treatment for primary hyperparathyroidism in MEN1 patients: a systematic review. World J Surg. 2011;35(9):1993-2005.

35. Pieterman CR, van Hulsteijn LT, den Heijer M, van der Luijt RB, Bonenkamp JJ, Hermus AR, et al. Primary hyperparathyroidism in MEN1 patients: a cohort study with long-term follow-up on preferred surgical procedure and the relation with genotype. Dutch MEN1 Study Group. Ann Surg. 2012;255(6):1171-8.

36. Versnick M, Popadich A, Sidhu S, Sywak M, Robinson B, Delbridge L. Minimally invasive parathyroidectomy pro-vides a conservative surgical option for multiple endocrine neoplasia type 1; primary hyperparathyroidism. Surgery. 2013;154(1):101-5.

37. Lairmore TC, Govednik CM, Quinn CE, Sigmond BR, Lee CY, Jupiter DC. A randomized, prospective trial of operative treatments for hyperparathyroidism in patients with multiple endocrine neoplasia type 1. Surgery. 2014;156(6):1326-34.

38. Fyrsten E, Norlén O, Hessman O, Stalberg P, Hellman P. Long-term surveillance of treated hyperparathyroidism for multiple endocrine neoplasia type 1: recurrence or hypoparathyroidism? World J Surg. 2016;40:615-21.

39. Marini F, Giusti F, Brandi ML. Multiple endocrine neoplasia type 1: extensive analysis of a large database of Florentine patients. Orphanet J Rare Dis. 2018;13:205.

40. Romei C, Pardi E, Cetani F, Elisei R. Genetic and clinical features of multiple endocrine neoplasia types 1 and 2. J Oncol. 2012;2012:705036.

41. Mehta A, Patel D, Rosenberg A, Boufraqech M, Ellis RJ, Nilubol N, et al. Hyperparathyroidism-jaw tumor syndrome: results of operative management. Surgery. 2014;156:1315-24.

42. Jackson CE, Norum RA, Boyd SB, Talpos GB, Wilson SD, Taggart RT, et al. Hereditary hyperparathyroidism and multiple ossifying jaw fibromas: a clinically and genetically distinct syndrome. Surgery. 1990;108:1006-12.

43. Mallette LE, Malini S, Rappaport MP, Kirkland JL. Familial cystic parathyroid adenomatosis. Ann Intern Med. 1987;107:54-60.

44. Cetani F, Pardi E, Borsari S, Viacava P, Dipollina G, Cianferotti L, et al. Genetic analyses of the *HRPT*2 gene in primary hyperparathyroidism: germline and somatic mutations in familial and sporadic parathyroid tumors. J Clin Endocrinol Metab. 2004;89:5583-91.

CHAPTER 28

Secondary and Tertiary Hyperparathyroidism: An Endocrine and Renal Perspective

Manju Chandran, Jiunn Wong

◇ INTRODUCTION

The parathyroid gland(s) play a pivotal role in bone mineral homeostasis through its secretion of parathyroid hormone (PTH). PTH increases calcium efflux from the bone, increases tubular reabsorption of calcium and phosphate excretion in the kidneys, and, by stimulating the renal production of 1,25-dihydroxyvitamin D [(1,25(OH)$_2$D], increases gastrointestinal absorption of calcium.

It is important to distinguish between a primary disorder of the parathyroid glands in which there is dysregulated and excessive production of PTH [as in the case of primary hyperparathyroidism (PHPT)] and situations in which the parathyroid gland responds secondarily to a stimulus such as malabsorption or renal failure and reacts by increasing PTH secretion. These latter forms of hyperparathyroidism are collectively known as secondary hyperparathyroidism (SHP; **Box 1**).

Tertiary hyperparathyroidism refers to the hypercalcemic state in which, after long-standing SHP, the stimulated parathyroid glands assume a quasi-autonomous role akin to that seen in PHPT. The differentiation of tertiary from PHPT is usually made possible since in the former, a clearly identifiable long-standing disorder such as malabsorption or renal failure is present predating the onset of hypercalcemia **(Table 1)**.

Though SHP and its eventual progression to tertiary hyperparathyroidism have many causes as outlined in **Box 1**, this review will focus on and will highlight recent research related to the pathogenic, clinical, and therapeutic aspects of these conditions in the setting of chronic kidney disease (CKD).

Secondary hyperparathyroidism is a frequent complication of CKD. The SHP associated with CKD is characterized by a complicated, multifaceted, and as yet incompletely understood pathophysiology. Renal replacement therapy has turned this once terminal illness to a chronic one. It is estimated that 30–50% of stage-5 CKD patients have intact parathyroid hormone (iPTH) levels of >300 pg/mL.[1] As the kidneys fail, gross derangements in fluid and solute clearance occur. Initially an adaptive response that over time becomes maladaptive, it leads to the clinical syndrome loosely termed chronic kidney disease-metabolic bone disorder (CKD-MBD).[2] CKD-MBD is defined as a systemic disorder of mineral and bone metabolism due to CKD, manifested by either one or a combination of the following:

- Abnormalities of calcium, phosphorus, PTH, or vitamin D metabolism
- Abnormalities in bone turnovers, mineralization, volume, linear growth, or strength
- Vascular or other soft-tissue calcification

◇ PATHOPHYSIOLOGY

The pathophysiology of CKD-MBD is complex and not fully understood **(Flowchart 1)**. The kidneys are complex

---

Box 1: Causes of secondary hyperparathyroidism.

- Chronic kidney disease
- Decreased calcium intake

Decreased absorption of calcium:
- Vitamin D deficiency
- Bariatric surgery
- Celiac disease
- Pancreatic diseases with fat malabsorption

Renal calcium losses:
- Idiopathic hypercalciuria
- Loop diuretics

Secondary to phosphate replacement therapy in conditions such as X-linked hypophosphatemia, autosomal-dominant hypophosphatemia, and tumor-induced osteomalacia.

Table 1: Biochemical differentiation between primary, secondary, and tertiary hyperparathyroidism.

Biochemical parameter	Primary hyperparathyroidism	Secondary hyperparathyroidism	Tertiary hyperparathyroidism
Calcium	↑	↓	↑
Phosphate	↓	↑*	↑
iPTH	↑	↑	↑

* Secondary hyperparathyroidism in patients with normal renal function (unlike as in those with CKD) is usually associated with low levels of phosphate given the inhibitory effect of PTH on sodium–phosphate co-transporters in the renal tubules.
(CKD: chronic kidney disease; iPTH: intact parathyroid hormone)

Flowchart 1: Schematic representation of the current understanding regarding the pathophysiology of secondary hyperparathyroidism.

↑ PTH

↓ Calcium

↓ 25 D　　↓ 1, 25 D

↓ 1 α-hydroxylase　　Urinary phosphate excretion　　Normal serum phosphate

↑ FGF-23

↑ Phosphate

? PTH / ? Phosphate / ? Calcium　　Normal phosphate intake

↓ eGFR

↓ Phosphate excretion

Kidney disease

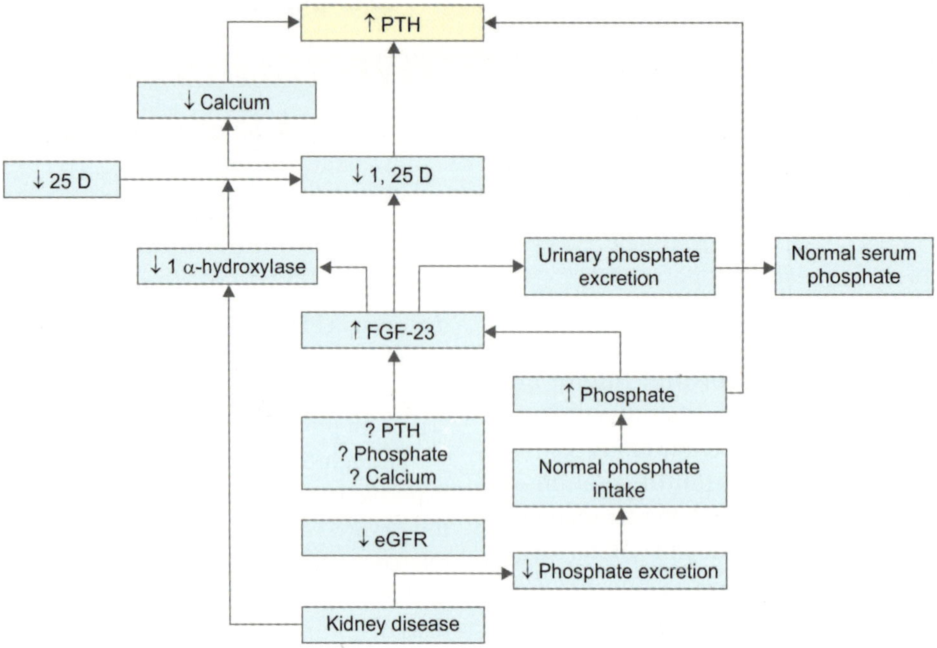

organs that have multiple functions. They regulate fluid and electrolyte balance in the body, generating urine of different volumes and solute make-up to maintain mineral homeostasis. In addition, they regulate blood pressure via the renin–angiotensin system. Peritubular interstitial cells in the kidney regulate erythropoietin production and the proximal tubules of the kidney express the enzyme 1α-hydroxylase that converts 25-hydroxyvitamin D to 1,25(OH)$_2$D, the biologically active form of the molecule.

The parathyroid glands play a closely integrated role with the kidneys in maintaining bone mineral homeostasis. The secretion of PTH is closely regulated by extracellular ionized calcium through the calcium-sensing receptor (CaSR) on parathyroid cells.[3] PTH synthesis and secretion are also influenced by 1,25(OH)$_2$D, which by binding to vitamin D receptor (VDR) in parathyroid tissue inhibits PTH mRNA synthesis.[4] Inorganic phosphate (Pi) may also act as an important regulator of PTH, although the exact sensing mechanism through which it does this still remains to be elucidated. In addition, the relatively recently identified and characterized fibroblastic growth factor-23 (FGF-23), an osteocyte, and an osteoblast-derived phosphaturic hormone[5] have been shown to decrease PTH synthesis and secretion[6] by acting on the parathyroid glands through its receptor Klotho-FGF.[7,8]

Secondary hyperparathyroidism develops early in the course of CKD and is characterized by persistently elevated levels of PTH and parathyroid hyperplasia.[9] It has long been considered that the failure of the kidney to excrete serum phosphate with resultant hyperphosphatemia is the key driver of SHP in CKD patients.[10] The formation of calcium–phosphate salts with a reduction in serum ionized

calcium,[11] the inhibitory effect of Pi on the enzyme CYP27B1 [25(OH)D-1-alpha hydroxylase] that is involved in the conversion of 25-hydroxyvitamin D to 1,25(OH)$_2$ vitamin D in the proximal renal tubular cell,[12] and the decreased viable renal mass[13,14] in chronic renal insufficiency with resultant lesser 1-α-hydroxylase activity all are believed to result in hypocalcemia and to initiate the cascade of events that lead to dysregulation of PTH in SHP. However, these postulations do not explain the clinical observation that serum 1,25(OH)$_2$D begins to decline even in early kidney disease before overt hyperphosphatemia develops. It has been noted that hyperparathyroidism develops early in chronic renal failure at a time when plasma calcium and phosphorous are within normal limits. As creatinine clearance decreases <80 mL/m, there is a significant decrease in plasma calcitriol and a slow and progressive significant increment in plasma PTH.[15]

The identification and characterization of FGF-23 in the last decade have provided important clues toward understanding the early phases in the pathogenesis of SHP.[16,17] This 22.5-kDa protein is encoded by the *FGF-23* gene located on chromosome 12 and is secreted mainly by osteocytes and osteoblasts. Its synthesis and release are mainly stimulated by 1,25 D and also by Pi, PTH, and calcium by as yet incompletely defined mechanisms, though it is thought that PTH induces FGF-23 transcription through activation of the orphan receptor Nurr1 and through activation of PKA and Wnt signaling in bones, thereby constituting a bone-parathyroid-endocrine loop[18-20] FGF-23 together with its coreceptor, the membrane-bound α-Klotho, functions to increase phosphate excretion in the urine through downregulation of sodium–phosphate cotransporters and inhibits 1,25-hydroxy vitamin D synthesis in the kidney by inhibiting 1-α hydroxylase and stimulates 24-hydroxylase and thereby the catabolism of active vitamin sterols.[21] This subsequently leads to hypocalcemia and stimulation of the parathyroid gland **(Fig. 1)**. A soluble and circulating form of α-Klotho produced mainly by the kidney may also have additional autonomous (i.e., independent of FGF-23) phosphaturic and anticalciuric effects.[22] A progressive renal reduction in production of both membrane-bound and circulating α-Klotho, increasing levels of FGF-23 secondary to its reduced renal clearance and due to Pi retention, and resistance to the phosphaturic effect of FGF-23 due to deficiency of α-Klotho characterize the progression of CKD.

Fibroblast growth factor-23 is the initial marker to be elevated as CKD progresses. This initial appropriate physiological response maintains phosphate balance by increasing phosphate excretion.[23] As the FGF-23 level increases, a trade-off occurs between maintaining normophosphatemia versus 1,25-hydroxyvitamin D deficiency with the latter progressing relentlessly and causing elevated PTH levels.[24] The phosphate level will start to rise only as CKD progresses and the adaptive compensation by FGF-23 becomes inadequate. At this advanced stage, hyperphosphatemia, continued decreased $1,25(OH)_2D$, and hypocalcemia all contribute to further increase in PTH mRNA levels and PTH synthesis. Persistently increased PTH synthesis in CKD results in parathyroid cell proliferation with resultant initial diffuse hyperplasia and then ultimately nodular hyperplasia. It has recently been shown that microRNA (miRNA) dysregulation within the parathyroid glands may also play a role in the development of SHP in rodents as well as humans.[25] This may constitute a CaSR-independent mechanism for hypocalcemia to stimulate PTH secretion. However, whether specific miRNAs can be utilized or targeted for therapeutic intervention in SHP needs to be studied further.

Though conflicting data also exists,[26] it appears that FGF-23 may also act directly on the parathyroid gland to suppress PTH secretion through the Klotho-FGFR1 complex.[27] In patients with advanced SHP, the parathyroid expression of the Klotho-FGFR1 complex is downregulated.[28] This likely contributes to the resistance to the inhibitory effect of FGF-23 on PTH secretion in progressive and advanced SHP.

As parathyroid hyperplasia progresses, both CaSR and VDR on the parathyroid glands become downregulated and reduced expression of these receptors has been observed in the most severe forms of SHP.[29-33] However, whether this reduced expression of VDR on parathyroid cells really plays a prominent causal role in SHP development is unclear, since knocking out VDR in parathyroid cells only while maintaining the intestinal VDR was not found to be associated with any major change in PTH secretion in mice in one study[20] suggesting that perhaps the reduction of receptors on the parathyroid cells may just be a consequence of the histological changes that characterize the most severe stages of secondary

and tertiary hyperparathyroidism rather than playing a causal role in their development and/or progression.

Recently, it has been suggested that the production of $1,25(OH)_2D$ by oxyphil cells in the parathyroid glands might inhibit PTH secretion through autocrine/paracrine pathways.[34] These cells characterized by abundant mitochondria that are the site of $1,25(OH)_2$ D synthesis are almost completely absent in normal parathyroid glands but consistently increased in SHP. In the most advanced stages of secondary and tertiary hyperparathyroidism, this inhibitory mechanism might fail with consequent hypersecretion of PTH, increased bone resorption, and hypercalcemia. Oxyphil cells in addition to expressing CYP27B1 (1-alpha hydroxylase) also show higher levels of CaSR. This increases the sensitivity of these cells to calcium as well as calcimimetics.[35] The increase in the number of these cells during the course of SHP may represent an attempt to counteract the latter's progression to tertiary hyperparathyroidism, which is characterized by reduced expression of CaSR in parathyroid glands[31] with a decreased response of PTH to the inhibitory effect of calcium.

The size of the parathyroid glands progressively increases as SHP due to any cause worsens and gland size is positively correlated with serum PTH levels **(Fig. 1)**. The cellular etiology of tertiary hyperparathyroidism is unknown, but it is postulated to be due to a monoclonal expansion of parathyroid cells in which the set point of the CaSRs has been altered such that semiautonomous secretion of PTH occurs despite high serum calcium levels. Monoclonal chief cell growth results in the formation of nodules. Nodular glands have less VDRs and CaSRs[29-33] compared to diffusely hyperplastic glands and this as mentioned earlier exacerbates parathyroid gland resistance to calcitriol and calcium. Even postrenal transplantation, though phosphate and $1,25(OH)_2D$ homeostasis may have normalized, if the tissue mass has increased significantly enough to function autonomously, PTH levels and serum calcium levels may not return to normal.

◇| CLINICAL FEATURES

Skeletal Manifestations

Parathyroid hormone binds to the PTH/PTHrP receptor on osteoblasts and thus by indirectly stimulating osteoclastic activity, it leads to a high turnover bone disease. The most common and clinically relevant skeletal manifestation in CKD is the increased bone fragility and susceptibility to fractures that have been reported to be—two to four times more frequent when compared to age- and gender-matched normal populations. This increased risk is associated with an increased risk of mortality[36] and an association between PTH levels and fracture risk has been observed, with intact PTH levels >900 pg/mL shown to be independently associated with an increased risk of incident fractures in the Dialysis Outcomes and Practice Patterns Study (DOPPS).[37] It has to be remembered, however that the bone fragility

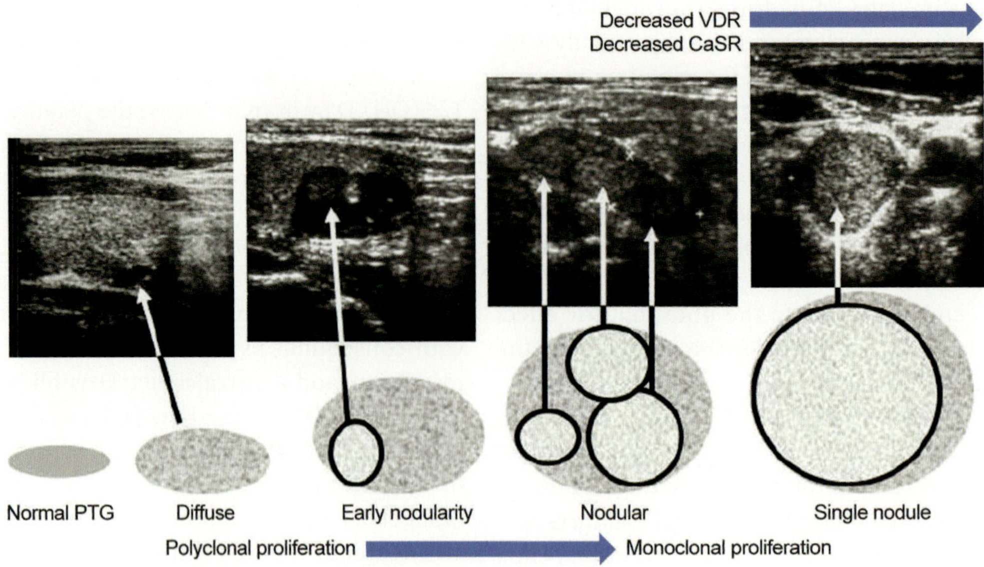

Fig. 1: The stages in the evolution of secondary and teritory hyperparathyroidism.
Source: Modified from Ultrasonographic evaluation of parathyroid hyperplasia in dialysis patients. February 2006—The Scientific World Journal 6:1599-608. DOI:10.1100/tsw.2006.273 Via License: CC By 3.0 *https: creativecommons.org/licenses/by/3.0/* (VDR: vitamin D receptor; CaSR: calcium sensing receptor)

in CKD may have several causes other than SHP, such as metabolic acidosis, anemia, hypogonadism, inflammation, β_2 microglobulin-associated amyloidosis, vitamin D deficiency, and bone formation inhibition secondary to Wnt inhibition in osteocytes, to name a few.

Extraskeletal Manifestations

Elevated PTH levels may be associated with an increased sympathetic drive and endothelial stress, and it has long been recognized that SHP might play a causal role in the development of vascular calcifications, ischemic cardiovascular events, and cardiac failure.[38] Other metabolic changes associated with CKD such as dyslipidemia, impaired insulin sensitivity or secretion, and hyperphosphatemia may also contribute to these vascular changes. Elevated PTH levels have been found to be independently associated with anemia, which is a hallmark of CKD and severe SHP is associated with a resistance to erythropoietin therapy in CKD.[39]

It should be borne-in-mind that despite the associations noted between the different extraskeletal manifestations noted above and SHP, no clear causal relationship has been established neither has it been shown that correction of elevated PTH levels can result in a complete remission of these clinical conditions.

FGF-23-mediated Manifestations

Recent studies have identified diverse adverse effects of FGF-23 on various organs in a Klotho-independent manner.[40] Causal roles for FGF-23 in the development of left ventricular hypertrophy (LVH),[41] renal anemia,[42] and immune dysfunction[43] have been suggested. Since PTH is one of the main drivers of FGF-23,[19] it is possible that this latter molecule may be the link between SHP and these clinical manifestations. The relative importance of and possible interactions between PTH and FGF-23 in the pathogenesis of these adverse events should be studied in greater detail.

◇ CLINICAL EVALUATION

The diagnoses of secondary and tertiary hyperparathyroidism are purely biochemical. Accurate measurement of PTH is therefore essential in the management of this condition. PTH is a hormone of 84 amino acids. Retention of various PTH fragments can occur in CKD. Over the last few decades, three generations of PTH assays have been developed that measure different parts of the molecule **(Fig. 2)**. PTH exerts its classical biological effects on the bone and kidney through its first 34 amino acids (N terminal). The first radioimmunoassay for PTH was developed in 1963 by generating a single polyclonal antibody against epitopes in the carboxy terminal (C terminal) end of the PTH molecule.[44] The first-generation assays had poor specificity as the antibodies used mainly targeted the nonbioactive portion of the PTH molecule, the C-terminal which is retained in CKD. The second-generation assays that were developed to overcome this problem use two sets of antibodies: (1) Capture antibodies against epitopes located within the C-terminal; and (2) Detection antibodies directed to amino acid sequences 12–20 within the amino terminal end.[45] This assay is currently the most widely used and is called iPTH assay, as it is assumed that it captures intact PTH 1–84. However, the detection antibodies have been found to cross-react with PTH 7–84 fragments that also tend to accumulate in patients with CKD due to insufficient renal clearance.[46,47]

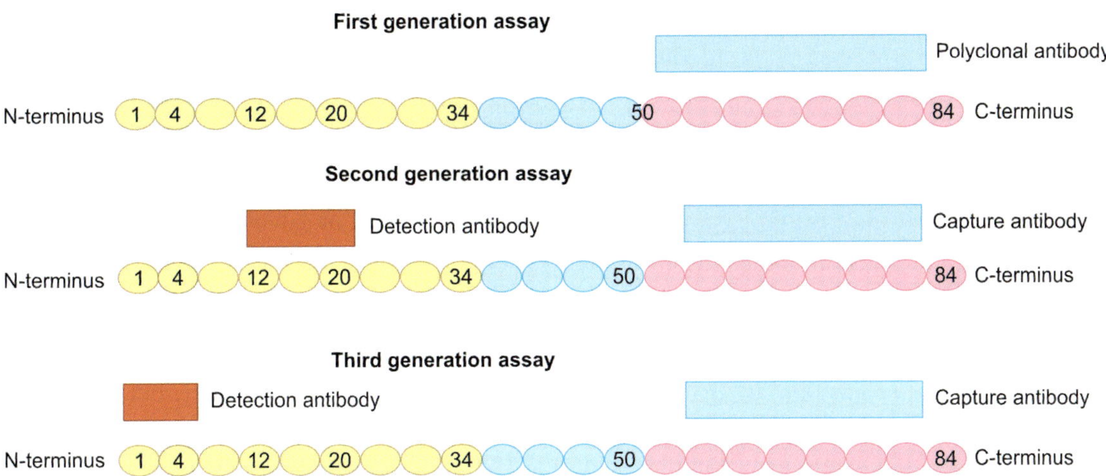

Fig. 2: Schematic representation of the 3 generation of PTH assays.

It has also become apparent that high concentrations of 7–84 PTH and some other C-terminal PTH fragments may oppose the biochemical and bone-metabolic effects of 1–84 PTH, aggravating the potential undesirable clinical consequences of overestimating 1–84 PTH concentrations in renal failure patients,[48,49] i.e., the physician might mistakenly assume the erroneously high PTH reading as the correct value and may institute further PTH-lowering therapies with disastrous consequences. To overcome these shortcomings, third-generation PTH assays such as the whole PTH assay and the Bio-Intact PTH assay have been developed.[50] Though the capture antibody used in the third-generation assay is the same as that used in the second-generation assay, the detection antibody used in the former is directed toward the first four amino acids. These assays do not thus recognize 7–84 PTH and are therefore considered more specific to 1–84 PTH than second-generation assays. Two automated third-generation PTH assays are now available.[51] However, there is little evidence to show that they provide any better clinical information than the second-generation assays with regard to the diagnosis of CKD-MBD[52] and, therefore, have not been adopted for use in current guidelines for management of SHP. In general, PTH levels measured with second-generation assays are higher than those obtained with third-generation ones. The ratio of whole (biointact)/iPTH levels has been noted to be between 0.6 and 0.7 in dialysis patients,[53] though exceptions to this rule have been reported in patients with severe SHP with a new molecular form of PTH with an intact N-terminus[54,55] that can be detected by third-generation PTH assays but not by second-generation ones identified in these patients. In these patients, thus PTH levels measured with third-generation assays are paradoxically higher than those with second-generation ones. Existing clinical data suggests that an overproduction of N-PTH may be associated with rapid progression of SHP and that NPTH has significant bioactivity.[56,57]

The Kidney Disease Improving Global Outcomes (KDIGO) guidelines recommend target iPTH levels of 2–9 times of the upper limit of normal for the given assay to noninvasively monitor bone status in dialysis patients. iPTH values above the target suggest high bone turnover bone disease with a specificity of 86% and values below the target values suggest low bone turnover with a sensitivity of 66%. The latest update to the CKD-MBD guideline published by the KDIGO in 2017 suggests that in patients with CKD G3a–G5D, treatment for CKD-MBD should be based on serial assessments of phosphate, calcium, and PTH levels, considered together and not absolute values of any of these parameters.[58]

◇ **TREATMENT OPTIONS**

A paradigm shift has occurred in the approach to the treatment of secondary and tertiary hyperparathyroidism in CKD with the understanding that the alterations in calcium and phosphate metabolism in CKD do not only cause renal osteodystrophy and bone abnormalities but also are linked to increased risk of cardiovascular disease and all-cause mortality potentially mediated through vascular calcification.[59]

The complex pathophysiology of secondary and tertiary hyperparathyroidism makes it necessary that their treatment should be multipronged. The three main targets are thus phosphate, 1,25-vitamin D, and PTH.

Controlling Phosphate Levels

The management of hyperphosphatemia has formed the cornerstone of therapy for SHP for decades. Dietary phosphate restriction and treatment with oral phosphate binders can decrease PTH levels up to stage 3 and 4 CKD.[60] The reduction of protein intake (particularly protein of animal origin) has been the basis of dietary prescriptions in CKD for the last several years. However, such a diet is difficult to maintain, and such dietary restrictions should be counterbalanced by the awareness that they may be associated with an increased risk of malnutrition in CKD patients. Nevertheless, all attempts should be made to have a diet that contains more vegetable than animal proteins to avoid processed foods, etc. Most often, as CKD progresses and hyperphosphatemia ensues, dietary phosphate restriction alone is not helpful and phosphate binding medications are needed. An ever-increasing number of phosphate binders have been developed over the last few decades. They can be broadly grouped into calcium-based and noncalcium-based agents. All these agents are more or less equally effective in the control of phosphate levels and SHP. However, the debate on whether calcium-based Pi binders are associated with a higher risk for vascular calcifications and consequently for cardiovascular mortality continues.[61] Tenapanor, a new agent, that inhibits the intestinal absorption of phosphate through the inhibition of intestinal sodium/hydrogen exchanger isoform 3 has recently been shown to effectively reduce phosphate in patients who are on maintenance dialysis.[61] This opens up a potential new therapeutic option in controlling serum phosphate in patients with CKD. Phosphate is also removed during dialysis. Hence, it is vital that dialysis dose is adequate to optimize phosphate control. This can be achieved by adjusting dialysis time as well as blood flow settings during dialysis. It has been shown that patients who are on long/frequent dialysis have much better control of phosphate than their counterparts who are on conventional dialysis.[61]

Vitamin D Analogs

Treatment with vitamin D receptor activators (VDRAs) has long been a very important therapeutic strategy in the management of SHP. Calcitriol, the first synthetic VDRA, decreases serum PTH levels[62] in CKD and has also been shown to reduce bone turnover and to thus ameliorate osteitis fibrosa in dialysis patients,[63] though their effect on risk of fractures in CKD has not been adequately studied. The inhibitory effect on PTH synthesis is mediated through binding of calcitriol to its specific receptor (VDR) and subsequent regulation of gene transcription and inhibition of PTH mRNA synthesis. This is important to know because in advanced SHP, with nodular hyperplasia of the parathyroid glands, there is decreased expression of CaSR and VDRs in the parathyroid gland[32,33] and in such a situation, VDRAs are not as effective in suppressing PTH secretion.[64] The downside of calcitriol therapy is that through its effect on enhancing intestinal calcium absorption, there is increased risk of hypercalcemia, which limits its clinical utility. The newer selective VDRAs such as paricalcitol (19-nor-1,25-dihydroxyvitamin D2) and maxacalcitol (22-oxa-1,25-dihydroxyvitamin D3) may be preferable in this regard because they have more modest effects on serum calcium levels, though it has to be noted that these agents can also cause hypercalcemia.

Although it has long been known that vitamin D deficiency is common in CKD patients, the common belief has been that the need for its correction is not as stringent in this clinical setting provided that active vitamin D is administered.

However, the administration of native vitamin D may have other pluripotent benefits and it has also been demonstrated that early use of native vitamin D esters is effective in lowering PTH levels at least in the early stages of SHP.[65]

Calcimimetics

The introduction of calcimimetics, agents that mimic the action of calcium on tissues by allosteric activation of the CaSR, has significantly mitigated the need for high doses of activated vitamin D and the risk of hypercalcemia in SHP. These agents "mimic" calcium at the parathyroid receptor and increase the sensitivity of CaSRs on the parathyroid gland. As a result, the receptor "thinks" there is sufficient calcium, leading to reduced PTH secretion. Currently, the only oral calcimimetic approved by the Food and Drug Administration (FDA) is cinacalcet. Cinacalcet effectively reduces PTH levels and serum calcium levels in patients with SHP.[66] Notably, cinacalcet is effective even in patients with marked parathyroid hyperplasia,[67] thus making it an acceptable alternative to parathyroidectomy for the treatment of severe SHP. The advent of these medications and the practice of renal physicians to initiate it early in the course of mild-to-moderate SHP are claimed to be the reason for the marked reduction in parathyroidectomy rates in countries such as Japan.[68] Appropriate and timely dose increases in cinacalcet are required to achieve effective control of SHP. However, this is accompanied by gastrointestinal adverse effects such as nausea and vomiting. The introduction of a new intravenous calcimimetic, Etelcalcetide, offers a therapeutic alternative to oral cinacalcet.[69] Etelcalcetide has a longer half-life than cinacalcet and can be administered intravenously every other day at the end of dialysis treatment, thus overcoming the problem of compliance with a daily oral regimen. Etelcalcetide has been shown to markedly decrease PTH levels in patients on hemodialysis with moderate-to-severe SHP and may be superior to cinacalcet in this regard,[70] though further studies are needed to assess clinical outcomes as well as long-term efficacy and safety of this agent.

The effects of PTH lowering with cinacalcet on bone turnover and bone histology in patients with CKD and evidence of high-turnover bone disease have been studied in the Bone Histomorphometry Assessment for Dialysis patients with Secondary Hyperparathyroidism of End-Stage Renal Disease (BONAFIDE) study.[71] This study has demonstrated that long-term treatment with cinacalcet lowers biochemical markers of high bone turnover and improves bone histology in this setting. In the Evaluation of Cinacalcet Hydrochloride therapy to Lower Cardiovascular Events (EVOLVE) trial, a randomized controlled trial to assess the effects of cinacalcet on clinical outcomes, though no significant effect of cinacalcet in the primary intention to treat analysis was seen, a significant reduction in the risk of fracture in the cinacalcet group was found when differences in baseline characteristics, multiple fractures, and/or events prompting discontinuation of study drug were taken into account.[72] The results of the EVOLVE trial also suggested a beneficial effect of cinacalcet with regard to reduction in the risk of death or cardiovascular outcomes, though it has to be noted that this again was not in the primary unadjusted intention to treat analysis but in the log-sensing analysis.[73] It also has to be noted that in the EVOLVE trial, no apparent clinical advantage on long-term clinical outcomes for the use of cinacalcet as compared with traditional therapy for the control of SHP was proven.[73]

Parathyroidectomy

Despite the availability of newer vitamin D analogs and calcimimetics, parathyroidectomy continues to be a necessity in certain patient groups. Prolonged parathyroid stimulation leads initially to diffuse polyclonal hyperplasia followed by monoclonal nodular hyperplasia. At this stage when hypercalcemia and hyperphosphatemia that are recalcitrant to medical therapy develop, parathyroidectomy may be the only viable option. It is estimated that parathyroidectomy is required in about 15% of patients after 10 years and in 38% of patients after 20 years of ongoing dialysis therapy.[74] Successful surgical treatment results in a dramatic reduction in PTH levels and improvement of clinical symptoms such as bone pain and itching. Parathyroidectomy is also associated with better patient survival[75-77] and reduced risk of fractures[78] in patients with severe SHP.

A description of the surgical techniques for parathyroidectomy is beyond the scope of this chapter and we leave that to our surgical colleagues to elaborate. There is no one technique that has proven to be superior and the choice of surgical technique, namely subtotal parathyroidectomy versus total parathyroidectomy with autotransplantation, ultimately depends on operator experience and expertise and has to be individualized to the patient. However, parathyroidectomy is not without its risk. The most commonly seen and most feared is the phenomenon of Hungry Bone Syndrome[79] characterized by severe hypocalcemia postparathyroidectomy. The abrupt withdrawal of very high and sustained levels of PTH following parathyroidectomy turns off osteoclast activity and bone resorption in the remodeling space. However, osteoblast activity and new bone formation continue, which lead to the influx of calcium, phosphate, and magnesium into bone resulting in their abrupt drops in the serum. This condition remains poorly defined, and the prevalence of this condition has been reported to range from 8 to 87% following parathyroidectomy for SHP.[80] The other concern is the occurrence of adynamic bone disease and hypoparathyroidism postparathyroidectomy. This is less well described in the literature. Hypoparathyroidism typically is reported following surgery for PHPT and there is no study that reports the incidence or prevalence of this condition in patients who undergo parathyroidectomy for SHP. Low turnover bone disease, however, has been reported to occur postparathyroidectomy and has been associated with worsening of vascular calcification in hemodialysis patients.[81-83]

Chemical Ablation of Parathyroid Gland

Percutaneous fine-needle ethanol injection of the parathyroid gland was first reported in 1985 in 12 patients with SHP.[84] These included patients who had developed recurrence of parathyroid tumors after previous subtotal surgery, had high surgical risk, or who had refused surgery. In 2003, the Japanese Society of Parathyroid Intervention published its guideline for selective percutaneous ethanol injection therapy of the parathyroid glands in chronic dialysis patients in which it recommended that enlarged parathyroid glands with nodular hyperplasia could be "selectively" destroyed by ethanol injection and other glands with diffuse hyperplasia could be then managed by medical therapy.[85]

Percutaneous injection using the vitamin D analog— calcitriol instead of alcohol has also been described.[86] The rationale behind this approach is to introduce a high level of vitamin D around the parathyroid gland without the systemic complications that could potentially be caused by its systemic administration.

These local approaches could be considered in patients who refuse surgery or are not candidates for surgery although long-term control of SHP is unlikely to be obtained.

PERSISTENT HYPERPARATHYROIDISM AFTER KIDNEY TRANSPLANTATION

Though successful kidney transplantation reverses most bone and mineral abnormalities associated with CKD, hyperparathyroidism might persist in some allograft recipients. It is most likely to be present in patients with advanced SHP with nodular hyperplasia of the parathyroid glands before transplant. It is the most common cause of hypercalcemia[87] in renal transplant patients and may result in poor graft outcomes and progression of vascular calcification.[88] Surgical parathyroidectomy should be considered in kidney transplant patients with persistent hyperparathyroidism, especially when it is associated with severe hypercalcemia. Cinacalcet appears to be a promising therapeutic option for patients with persistent hypercalcemia post-transplantation at least as a bridging agent before parathyroidectomy.[89-91]

CONCLUSION

Our knowledge of the pathophysiology of secondary and tertiary hyperparathyroidism has vastly improved during the past few years. They may be caused by various conditions; however, that associated with CKD has been the one most studied and yet remains incompletely defined. The clinical consequences of these disorders of the parathyroid gland are not limited to the musculoskeletal system but are multifold and systemic. It is however difficult to define clearly whether there is a causal relationship between the elevated levels of PTH seen in these disorders and the protean clinical manifestations or whether they simply are associations in a complex clinical setting. The number of available therapeutic options for the management of secondary and tertiary hyperparathyroidism has increased significantly and control of PTH and phosphate and calcium levels can be successfully achieved in most cases with these medications. However, convincing benefits on major clinical outcomes such as prevention of fractures, cardiovascular events, or survival have not been demonstrated so far and a significant percentage of patients still need parathyroidectomy—the approach to which should be undertaken on an individualized basis.

◇| REFERENCES

1. Hedgeman E, Lipworth L, Lowe K, Saran R, Do T, Fryzek J, et al. International burden of chronic kidney disease and secondary hyperparathyroidism: a systematic review of the literature and available data. Int J Nephrol. 2015;2015:184321.

2. Kidney Disease: Improving Global Outcomes (KDIGO) CKD-MBD Work Group. KDIGO clinical practice guideline for the diagnosis, evaluation, prevention, and treatment of chronic kidney disease-mineral and bone disorder (CKD-MBD). Kidney Int Suppl. 2009;(113):S1-130.

3. Brown EM, Pollak M, Seidman CE, Seidman JG, Chou YH, Riccardi D, et al. Calcium-ion-sensing cell-surface receptors. N Engl J Med. 1995;333(4):234-40.

4. Dusso AS, Brown AJ, Slatopolsky E. Vitamin D. Am J Physiol Renal Physiol. 2005;289(1):F8-28.

5. Quarles LD. Endocrine functions of bone in mineral metabolism regulation. J Clin Invest. 2008;118(12):3820-8.

6. Galitzer H, Ben-Dov I, Lavi-Moshayoff V, Naveh-Many T, Silver J. Fibroblast growth factor 23 acts on the parathyroid to decrease parathyroid hormone secretion. Curr Opin Nephrol Hypertens. 2008;17(4):363-7.

7. Urakawa I, Yamazaki Y, Shimada T, Iijima K, Hasegawa H, Okawa K, et al. Klotho converts canonical FGF receptor into a specific receptor for FGF-23. Nature. 2006;444(7120):770-4.

8. Kurosu H, Ogawa Y, Miyoshi M, Yamamoto M, Nandi A, Rosenblatt KP, et al. Regulation of fibroblast growth factor-23 signaling by Klotho. J Biol Chem. 2006;281(10):6120-3.

9. Drüeke TB. Cell biology of parathyroid gland hyperplasia in chronic renal failure. J Am Soc Nephrol. 2000;11(6):1141-52.

10. Slatopolsky E, Caglar S, Pennell JP, Taggart DD, Canterbury JM, Reiss E, et al. On the pathogenesis of hyperparathyroidism in chronic experimental renal insufficiency in the dog. J Clin Invest. 1971;50(3):492-9.

11. Brown EM. Extracellular Ca²⁺ sensing, regulation of parathyroid cell function, and role of Ca²⁺ and other ions as extracellular (first) messengers. Physiol Rev. 1991;71(2): 371-411.

12. Tanaka Y, Deluca HF. The control of 25-hydroxyvitamin D metabolism by inorganic phosphorus. Arch Biochem Biophys. 1973;154(2):566-74.

13. Llach F. Secondary hyperparathyroidism in renal failure: the trade-off hypothesis revisited. Am J Kidney Dis. 1995;25(5):663-79.

14. Slatopolsky E, Delmez JA. Pathogenesis of secondary hyperparathyroidism. Nephrol Dial Transplant. 1996;11 (Suppl 3): 130-5.

15. Martinez I, Saracho R, Montenegro J, Llach F. The importance of dietary calcium and phosphorous in the secondary hyperparathyroidism of patients with early renal failure. Am J Kidney Dis. 1997;29(4):496-502.

16. Elias RM, Dalboni MA, Coelho ACE, Moysés RMA. CKD-MBD: from the pathogenesis to the identification and development of potential novel therapeutic targets. Curr Osteoporos Rep. 2018;16(6):693-702.

17. Gutiérrez OM. Fibroblast growth factor 23 and disordered vitamin D metabolism in chronic kidney disease: updating the "trade-off" hypothesis. Clin J Am Soc Nephrol. 2010;5(9): 1710-6.

18. Fukagawa M, Nii-Kono T, Kazama JJ. Role of fibroblast growth factor 23 in health and in chronic kidney disease. Curr Opin Nephrol Hypertens. 2005;14(4):325-9.

19. Lavi-Moshayoff V, Wasserman G, Meir T, Silver J, Naveh-Many T. PTH increases FGF-23 gene expression and mediates the high-FGF-23 levels of experimental kidney failure: a bone parathyroid feedback loop. Am J Physiol Renal Physiol. 2010;299(4): F882-9.

20. Meir T, Durlacher K, Pan Z, Amir G, Richards WG, Silver J, et al. Parathyroid hormone activates the orphan nuclear receptor Nurr1 to induce FGF-23 transcription. Kidney Int. 2014;86(6):1106-15.

21. Shimada T, Hasegawa H, Yamazaki Y, Muto T, Hino R, Takeuchi Y, et al. FGF-23 is a potent regulator of vitamin D metabolism and phosphate homeostasis. J Bone Miner Res. 2004;19(3): 429-35.

22. Kuro-O M. The Klotho proteins in health and disease. Nat Rev Nephrol. 2019;15(1):27-44.

23. Shigematsu T, Kazama JJ, Yamashita T, Fukumoto S, Hosoya T, Gejyo F, et al. Possible involvement of circulating fibroblast growth factor 23 in the development of secondary hyperparathyroidism associated with renal insufficiency. Am J Kidney Dis. 2004;44(2):250-6.

24. Gutierrez O, Isakova T, Rhee E, Shah A, Holmes J, Collerone G, et al. Fibroblast growth factor-23 mitigates hyperphosphatemia but accentuates calcitriol deficiency in chronic kidney disease. J Am Soc Nephrol. 2005;16(7):2205-15.

25. Shilo V, Mor-Yosef Levi I, Abel R, Mihailović A, Wasserman G, Naveh-Many T, et al. Let-7 and MicroRNA-148 regulate parathyroid hormone levels in secondary hyperparathyroidism. J Am Soc Nephrol 2017;28(8):2353-63.

26. Kawakami K, Takeshita A, Furushima K, Miyajima M, Hatamura I, Kuro-O M, et al. Persistent fibroblast growth factor 23 signalling in the parathyroid glands for secondary hyperparathyroidism in mice with chronic kidney disease. Sci Rep. 2017;7:40534.

27. Krajisnik T, Björklund P, Marsell R, Ljunggren O, Akerström G, Jonsson KB, et al. Fibroblast growth factor-23 regulates parathyroid hormone and 1alpha-hydroxylase expression in cultured bovine parathyroid cells. J Endocrinol. 2007;195(1): 125-31.

28. Krajisnik T, Olauson H, Mirza MAI, Hellman P, Akerström G, Westin G, et al. Parathyroid Klotho and FGF-receptor 1 expression decline with renal function in hyperparathyroid patients with chronic kidney disease and kidney transplant recipients. Kidney Int. 2010;78(10):1024-32.

29. Tokumoto M, Tsuruya K, Fukuda K, Kanai H, Kuroki S, Hirakata H, et al. Reduced p21, p27 and vitamin D receptor in the nodular hyperplasia in patients with advanced secondary hyperparathyroidism. Kidney Int. 2002;62(4):1196-207.

30. Yano S, Sugimoto T, Tsukamoto T, Chihara K, Kobayashi A, Kitazawa S, et al. Association of decreased calcium-sensing receptor expression with proliferation of parathyroid cells in secondary hyperparathyroidism. Kidney Int. 2000;58(5): 1980-6.

31. Gogusev J, Duchambon P, Hory B, Giovannini M, Goureau Y, Sarfati E, et al. Depressed expression of calcium receptor in parathyroid gland tissue of patients with hyperparathyroidism. Kidney Int. 1997;51(1):328-36.

32. Kifor O, Moore FD, Wang P, Goldstein M, Vassilev P, Kifor I, et al. Reduced immunostaining for the extracellular Ca^{2+}-sensing receptor in primary and uremic secondary hyperparathyroidism. J Clin Endocrinol Metab. 1996;81(4):1598-606.

33. Fukuda N, Tanaka H, Tominaga Y, Fukagawa M, Kurokawa K, Seino Y, et al. Decreased 1,25-dihydroxyvitamin D3 receptor density is associated with a more severe form of parathyroid hyperplasia in chronic uremic patients. J Clin Invest. 1993;92(3):1436-43.

34. Ritter CS, Haughey BH, Miller B, Brown AJ. Differential gene expression by oxyphil and chief cells of human parathyroid glands. J Clin Endocrinol Metab. 2012;97(8):E1499-505.

35. Ritter C, Miller B, Coyne DW, Gupta D, Zheng S, Brown AJ, et al. Paricalcitol and cinacalcet have disparate actions on parathyroid oxyphil cell content in patients with chronic kidney disease. Kidney Int. 2017;92(5):1217-22.

36. Tentori F, McCullough K, Kilpatrick RD, Bradbury BD, Robinson BM, Kerr PG, et al. High rates of death and hospitalization follow bone fracture among hemodialysis patients. Kidney Int. 2014;85(1):166-73.

37. Jadoul M, Albert JM, Akiba T, Akizawa T, Arab L, Bragg-Gresham JL, et al. Incidence and risk factors for hip or other bone fractures among hemodialysis patients in the Dialysis Outcomes and Practice Patterns Study. Kidney Int. 2006;70(7):1358-66.

38. Kestenbaum B, Katz R, de Boer I, Hoofnagle A, Sarnak MJ, Shlipak MG, et al. Vitamin D, parathyroid hormone, and cardiovascular events among older adults. J Am Coll Cardiol. 2011;58(14):1433-41.

39. Tanaka M, Komaba H, Fukagawa M. Emerging association between parathyroid hormone and anemia in hemodialysis patients. Ther Apher Dial. 2018;22(3):242-5.

40. Komaba H, Fukagawa M. The role of FGF-23 in CKD—with or without Klotho. Nat Rev Nephrol. 2012;8(8):484-90.

41. Faul C, Amaral AP, Oskouei B, Hu MC, Sloan A, Isakova T, et al. FGF-23 induces left ventricular hypertrophy. J Clin Invest. 2011;121(11):4393-408.

42. Coe LM, Madathil SV, Casu C, Lanske B, Rivella S, Sitara D, et al. FGF-23 is a negative regulator of prenatal and postnatal erythropoiesis. J Biol Chem. 2014;289(14):9795-810.

43. Rossaint J, Oehmichen J, Van Aken H, Reuter S, Pavenstädt HJ, Meersch M, et al. FGF-23 signaling impairs neutrophil recruitment and host defense during CKD. J Clin Invest. 2016;126(3):962-74.

44. Berson SA, Yalow RS, Aurbach GD, Potts JT. Immunoassay of bovine and human parathyroid hormone. Proc Natl Acad Sci USA. 1963;49(5):613-7.

45. Nussbaum SR, Zahradnik RJ, Lavigne JR, Brennan GL, Nozawa-Ung K, Kim LY, et al. Highly sensitive two-site immunoradiometric assay of parathyrin, and its clinical utility in evaluating patients with hypercalcemia. Clin Chem. 1987;33(8):1364-7.

46. Brossard JH, Cloutier M, Roy L, Lepage R, Gascon-Barré M, D'Amour P, et al. Accumulation of a non-(1-84) molecular form of parathyroid hormone (PTH) detected by intact PTH assay in renal failure: importance in the interpretation of PTH values. J Clin Endocrinol Metab. 1996;81(11):3923-9.

47. D'Amour P. Circulating PTH molecular forms: what we know and what we don't. Kidney Int Suppl. 2006;(102):S29-S33.

48. Nguyen-Yamamoto L, Rousseau L, Brossard JH, Lepage R, D'Amour P. Synthetic carboxyl-terminal fragments of parathyroid hormone (PTH) decrease ionized calcium concentration in rats by acting on a receptor different from the PTH/PTH-related peptide receptor. Endocrinology. 2001;142(4):1386-92.

49. Divieti P, John MR, Jüppner H, Bringhurst FR. Human PTH-(7-84) inhibits bone resorption in vitro via actions independent of the type 1 PTH/PTHrP receptor. Endocrinology. 2002;143(1):171-6.

50. Joly D, Drueke TB, Alberti C, Houillier P, Lawson-Body E, Martin KJ, et al. Variation in serum and plasma PTH levels in second-generation assays in hemodialysis patients: a cross-sectional study. Am J Kidney Dis. 2008;51(6):987-95.

51. Cavalier E, Delanaye P, Lukas P, Carlisi A, Gadisseur R, Souberbielle JC, et al. Standardization of DiaSorin and Roche automated third generation PTH assays with an International Standard: impact on clinical populations. Clin Chem Lab Med. 2014;52(8):1137-41.

52. Lehmann G, Stein G, Hüller M, Schemer R, Ramakrishnan K, Goodman WG, et al. Specific measurement of PTH (1-84) in various forms of renal osteodystrophy (ROD) as assessed by bone histomorphometry. Kidney Int. 2005;68(3):1206-14.

53. Nakanishi S, Kazama JJ, Shigematsu T, Iwasaki Y, Cantor TL, Kurosawa T, et al. Comparison of intact PTH assay and whole PTH assay in long-term dialysis patients. Am J Kidney Dis. 2001;38(4 Suppl 1):S172-4.

54. Arakawa T, D'Amour P, Rousseau L, Brossard JH, Sakai M, Kasumoto H, et al. Overproduction and secretion of a novel amino-terminal form of parathyroid hormone from a severe type of parathyroid hyperplasia in uremia. Clin J Am Soc Nephrol. 2006,1(3).525-31.

55. Tanaka M, Itoh K, Matsushita K, Fujii H, Fukagawa M. Normalization of reversed bio-intact-PTH(1-84)/intact-PTH ratio after parathyroidectomy in a patient with severe secondary hyperparathyroidism. Clin Nephrol. 2005;64(1):69-72.

56. Tanaka M, Komaba H, Itoh K, Matsushita K, Matsushita K, Hamada Y, et al. The whole-PTH/intact-PTH ratio is a useful predictor of severity of secondary hyperparathyroidism. NDT Plus. 2008;1(Suppl 3):iii59-iii62.

57. Komaba H, Takeda Y, Shin J, Tanaka R, Kakuta T, Tominaga Y, et al. Reversed whole PTH/intact PTH ratio as an indicator of marked parathyroid enlargement: five case studies and a literature review. NDT Plus. 2008;1(Suppl 3):iii54-iii58.

58. Kidney Disease: Improving Global Outcomes (KDIGO) CKD-MBD Update Work Group. KDIGO 2017 Clinical Practice Guideline update for the diagnosis, evaluation, prevention, and treatment of chronic kidney disease-mineral and bone disorder (CKD-MBD). Kidney Int Suppl. 2017;7(1):1-59.

59. Palmer SC, Hayen A, Macaskill P, Pellegrini F, Craig JC, Elder GJ, et al. Serum levels of phosphorus, parathyroid hormone, and calcium and risks of death and cardiovascular disease in individuals with chronic kidney disease: a systematic review and meta-analysis. JAMA. 2011;305(11):1119-27.

60. Sprague SM, Abboud H, Qiu P, Dauphin M, Zhang P, Finn W, et al. Lanthanum carbonate reduces phosphorus burden in patients with CKD stages 3 and 4: a randomized trial. Clin J Am Soc Nephrol. 2009;4(1):178-85.

61. Palmer SC, Gardner S, Tonelli M, Mavridis D, Johnson DW, Craig JC, et al. Phosphate-binding agents in adults with CKD: a network meta-analysis of randomized trials. Am J Kidney Dis. 2016;68(5):691-702.

62. Palmer SC, McGregor DO, Craig JC, Elder G, Macaskill P, Strippoli GF, et al. Vitamin D compounds for people with chronic kidney disease requiring dialysis. Cochrane Database Syst Rev. 2009;(4):CD005633.

63. Andress DL, Norris KC, Coburn JW, Slatopolsky EA, Sherrard DJ. Intravenous calcitriol in the treatment of refractory osteitis fibrosa of chronic renal failure. N Engl J Med. 1989;321(5):274-9.

64. Okuno S, Ishimura E, Kitatani K, Chou H, Nagasue K, Maekawa K, et al. Relationship between parathyroid gland size and responsiveness to maxacalcitol therapy in patients with secondary hyperparathyroidism. Nephrol Dial Transplant. 2003;18(12):2613-21.

65. Miskulin DC, Majchrzak K, Tighiouart H, Muther RS, Kapoian T, Johnson DS, et al. Ergocalciferol supplementation in hemodialysis patients with vitamin D deficiency: a randomized clinical trial. J Am Soc Nephrol. 2016;27(6):1801-10.

66. Block GA, Martin KJ, de Francisco ALM, Turner SA, Avram MM, Suranyi MG, et al. Cinacalcet for secondary hyperparathyroidism in patients receiving hemodialysis. N Engl J Med. 2004;350(15):1516-25.

67. Komaba H, Nakanishi S, Fujimori A, Tanaka M, Shin J, Shibuya K, et al. Cinacalcet effectively reduces parathyroid hormone secretion and gland volume regardless of pretreatment gland size in patients with secondary hyperparathyroidism. Clin J Am Soc Nephrol. 2010;5(12):2305-14.

68. Tentori F, Wang M, Bieber BA, Karaboyas A, Li Y, Jacobson SH, et al. Recent changes in therapeutic approaches and association with outcomes among patients with secondary hyperparathyroidism on chronic hemodialysis: the DOPPS study. Clin J Am Soc Nephrol. 2015;10(1):98-109.

69. Martin KJ, Bell G, Pickthorn K, Huang S, Vick A, Hodsman P, et al. Velcalcetide (AMG 416), a novel peptide agonist of the calcium-sensing receptor, reduces serum parathyroid hormone and FGF-23 levels in healthy male subjects. Nephrol Dial Transplant. 2014;29(2):385-92.

70. Block GA, Bushinsky DA, Cheng S, Cunningham J, Dehmel B, Drueke TB, et al. Effect of etelcalcetide vs cinacalcet on serum parathyroid hormone in patients receiving hemodialysis with secondary hyperparathyroidism: a randomized clinical trial. JAMA. 2017;317(2):156-64.

71. Behets GJ, Spasovski G, Sterling LR, Goodman WG, Spiegel DM, De Broe ME, et al. Bone histomorphometry before and after long-term treatment with cinacalcet in dialysis patients with secondary hyperparathyroidism. Kidney Int. 2015;87(4):846-56.

72. Moe SM, Abdalla S, Chertow GM, Parfrey PS, Block GA, Correa-Rotter R, et al. Effects of cinacalcet on fracture events in patients receiving hemodialysis: the EVOLVE trial. J Am Soc Nephrol. 2015;26(6):1466-75.

73. EVOLVE Trial Investigators, Chertow GM, Block GA, Correa-Rotter R, Drüeke TB, Floege J, et al. Effect of cinacalcet on cardiovascular disease in patients undergoing dialysis. N Engl J Med. 2012;367(26):2482-94.

74. Lau WL, Obi Y, Kalantar-Zadeh K. Parathyroidectomy in the management of secondary hyperparathyroidism. Clin J Am Soc Nephrol. 2018;13(6):952-61.

75. Kestenbaum B, Andress DL, Schwartz SM, Gillen DL, Seliger SL, Jadav PR, et al. Survival following parathyroidectomy among United States dialysis patients. Kidney Int. 2004;66(5):2010-6.

76. Costa-Hong V, Jorgetti V, Gowdak LHW, Moyses RMA, Krieger EM, De Lima JJG, et al. Parathyroidectomy reduces cardiovascular events and mortality in renal hyperparathyroidism. Surgery. 2007;142(5):699-703.

77. Trombetti A, Stoermann C, Robert JH, Herrmann FR, Pennisi P, Martin PY, et al. Survival after parathyroidectomy in patients with end-stage renal disease and severe hyperparathyroidism. World J Surg. 2007;31(5):1014-21.

78. Rudser KD, de Boer IH, Dooley A, Young B, Kestenbaum B. Fracture risk after parathyroidectomy among chronic hemodialysis patients. J Am Soc Nephrol. 2007;18(8):2401-7.

79. Jain N, Reilly RF. Hungry bone syndrome. Curr Opin Nephrol Hypertens. 2017;26(4):250-5.

80. Witteveen JE, van Thiel S, Romijn JA, Hamdy NAT. Hungry bone syndrome: still a challenge in the post-operative management of primary hyperparathyroidism: a systematic review of the literature. Eur J Endocrinol. 2013;168(3):R45-R53.

81. Yajima A, Ogawa Y, Ikehara A, Tominaga T, Inou T, Otsubo O, et al. Development of low-turnover bone diseases after parathyroidectomy and autotransplantation. Int J Urol. 2001;8(8):S76-9.

82. Chan HWH, Chu KH, Fung SKS, Tang HL, Lee W, Cheuk A, et al. Prospective study on dialysis patients after total parathyroidectomy without autoimplant. Nephrology (Carlton). 2010;15(4):441-7.

83. Hernandes FR, Canziani MEF, Barreto FC, Santos RO, Moreira VDM, Rochitte CE, et al. The shift from high to low turnover bone disease after parathyroidectomy is associated with the progression of vascular calcification in hemodialysis patients: a 12-month follow-up study. PloS One. 2017;12(4):e0174811.

84. Giangrande A, Castiglioni A, Solbiati L, Allaria P. Ultrasound-guided percutaneous fine-needle ethanol injection into parathyroid glands in secondary hyperparathyroidism. Nephrol Dial Transplant. 1992;7(5):412-21.

85. Fukagawa M, Kitaoka M, Tominaga Y, Akizawa T, Kakuta T, Onoda N, et al. Guidelines for percutaneous ethanol injection therapy of the parathyroid glands in chronic dialysis patients. Nephrol Dial Transplant. 2003;18(Suppl 3):iii31-iii33.

86. Nakanishi S, Yano S, Nomura R, Tsukamoto T, Shimizu Y, Shin J, et al. Efficacy of direct injection of calcitriol into the parathyroid glands in uraemic patients with moderate to severe secondary hyperparathyroidism. Nephrol Dial Transplant. 2003;18 (Suppl 3):iii47-iii49.

87. Gwinner W, Suppa S, Mengel M, Hoy L, Kreipe HH, Haller H, et al. Early calcification of renal allografts detected by protocol biopsies: causes and clinical implications. Am J Transplant. 2005;5(8):1934-41.

88. Hernández D, Rufino M, Bartolomei S, González-Rinne A, Lorenzo V, Cobo M, et al. Clinical impact of preexisting vascular calcifications on mortality after renal transplantation. Kidney Int. 2005;67(5):2015-20.

89. Zavvos V, Fyssa L, Papasotiriou M, Papachristou E, Ntrinias T, Savvidaki E, et al. Long-term use of cinacalcet in kidney transplant recipients with hypercalcemic secondary hyperparathyroidism: a single-center prospective study. Exp Clin Transplant. 2018;16(3):287-93.

90. Ważna-Jabłońska E, Gałązka Z, Durlik M. Treatment of persistent hypercalcemia and hyperparathyroidism with cinacalcet after successful kidney transplantation. Transplant Proc. 2016;48(5):1623-5.

91. Dulfer RR, Koh EY, van der Plas WY, Engelsman AF, van Dijkum EJMN, Pol RA, et al. Parathyroidectomy versus cinacalcet for tertiary hyperparathyroidism: a retrospective analysis. Langenbeck's Arch Surg. 2019;404(1):71-9.

Parathyroid Carcinoma

Sai Krishna Vittal, Sai Vishnupriya Vittal, V Sucharitha, Sivapatham Vittal

INTRODUCTION

Parathyroid carcinoma (PC) is a rare cause of primary hyperparathyroidism (PHPT) (0.5–5%). This entity was first described by Fritz D'Quervain in 1904. Subsequently, the first functioning PC was described by Sainton and Millet in 1933. Since that time, less than a thousand cases have been reported in the literature, with them being either case reports or retrospective studies. This disease is an enigma and there are challenges in diagnosis, management, and adjuvant treatment. The treating surgeon should have a high index of suspicion based on clinical findings and investigations, which is the key to preoperative diagnosis. However, most cases are diagnosed intraoperatively or are a histological surprise postoperatively. Since the disease is rare, there are limited large-scale studies leading to controversies regarding management, staging, and follow-up.

INCIDENCE

Parathyroid carcinoma is one of the rare cancers with a prevalence of 0.005% of all cancers. The incidence of PC varies from country to country ranging from 1% of all PHPT patients in USA to about 5% in Japan, Italy, and India. Survival after diagnosis of this cancer ranges from 1 month to 20 years or more. In contrast to PHPT due to benign causes which demonstrates a strong female preponderance, PC appears to have no gender predominance. The 5- and 10-year survival rates for PC have been estimated between 78–85% and 49–70%, respectively.[1] Disease recurrence is common occurring from 33 to 78% in different series and may manifest within 3 years from the initial intervention. Metastases to lymph nodes are rare and most patients succumb to profound hypercalcemia than due to tumor burden of metastatic disease.

ETIOLOGY AND PATHOGENESIS

The etiology is still not fully understood. Till date, there have been no predisposing factors identified. However, few cases of PC occurring in patients previously treated with radiation therapy have been described. The predisposing factors include secondary and tertiary hyperparathyroidism associated with end-stage renal disease. PC may occur sporadically or may be part of a familial syndrome. The genetic syndromes associated with PC include multiple endocrine neoplasia type 1 (MEN1), MEN2a, hyperparathyroidism-jaw tumor syndrome, and isolated familial hyperparathyroidism. The origin of PC has been a matter of debate; however, there is recent evidence that indicates that PC may originate de novo rather than progression from adenoma to carcinoma sequence.

MOLECULAR BIOLOGY

Germline mutations in *HRPT2* gene (also known as *CDC73*), a tumor suppressor gene, play a fundamental role in the molecular pathogenesis of PC. The incidence of *HRPT2* mutations in PC, however, is variable (15–100%). An important point is that only very rarely (<1%) these mutations are found in benign parathyroid disease.[2,3] Hence, it is advisable and a good practice for all PC patients to be considered for this germline testing. The *HRPT2* gene is a tumor suppressor gene, which codes for a protein parafibromin. Parafibromin functions involve the regulation of gene expression and inhibition of cell proliferation. Immunohistochemistry can be used to identify parafibromin expression and hence it could be used to identify patients with *HRPT2* mutations. Other genetic markers include cyclin D1, Rb, BRCA2 and p53, which exhibit abnormal expressions in some parathyroid cancers.

PRESENTATION

The distinction between PHPT due to benign and malignant cause can be difficult. There are, however, few manifestations which should arouse suspicion of PC in a patient with PHPT.

- PHPT due to PC is rarely asymptomatic. Most patients of PC are functional and present with simultaneous manifestations of skeletal disease and renal disease. The skeletal manifestations which are seen include severe bone pain, osteopenia in cortical bone, osteitis fibrosis cystica **(Fig. 1)**, and pathological fractures following trivial trauma. The renal features include decreased glomerular filtration rate (GFR), nephrolithiasis, and nephrocalcinosis. Simultaneous skeletal and renal disease are seen in >50% of cases of PC.
- About 7–12% of patients of PC present with hypercalcemic crisis or parathyrotoxicosis which is a less common initial manifestation of benign PHPT.

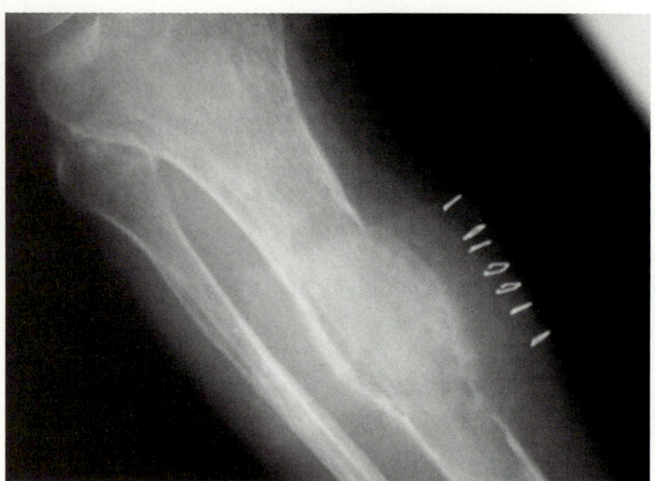

Fig. 1: X-ray showing severe bone disease in tibia and fibula.
Source: Reproduced with kind Permission from Indian Journal of Surgery

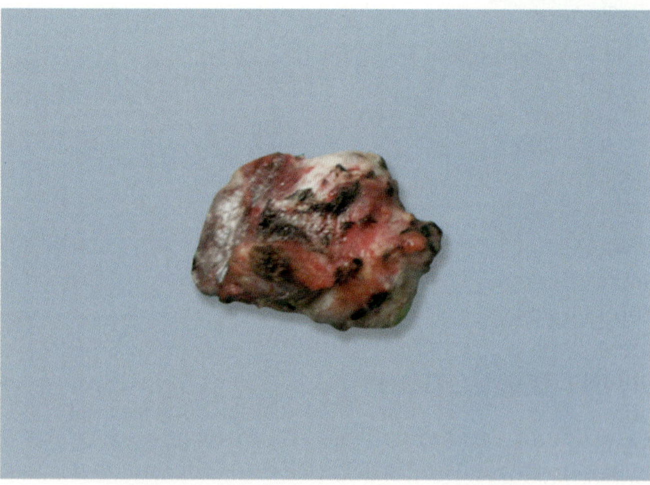

Fig. 2: Gross specimen of parathyroid carcinoma.

- Clinical examination may reveal a palpable neck mass in 40–70% of patients, which should alert the clinician about the possibility of PC.
- Other suspicious factors are when a patient with PHPT presents with recurrent laryngeal nerve palsy (especially if the patient has no previous history of neck surgery)
- About 15–30% of patients may present with regional lymph nodal involvement and about 30% may present with distant metastatic lesions, especially in the lungs, liver, and bone.
- Biochemically, the degree of hypercalcemia is marked in PC then in benign PHPT.[4] Serum calcium levels are 2–4 mg/dL more than normal levels unlike benign PHPT where the calcium levels are 1–2 mg/dL more than the reference range. Many patients have serum calcium level >14 mg/dL.
- Serum PTH is markedly elevated up to 5–10 times the upper limit of normal.[5]
- Alkaline phosphatase levels are higher in patients with PC than in benign PHPT with the exception being patients with osteitis fibrosa cystica in developing countries who may also have high alkaline phosphatase levels.

Although the distinction between PC and benign PHPT can be difficult, especially in the developing countries where patients with benign PHPT present with severe disease, it is a good practice to consider PC as a differential diagnosis in cases of severe hypercalcemia which would enable early diagnosis resulting in more complete resection and good prognosis on follow-up.

◇ IMAGING

In PHPT, once biochemically proven, localization tests are required to locate the abnormal parathyroid gland/s. The most commonly used localization tests are ultrasound scan neck and sestamibi scan preferably with single-photon emission computed tomography (SPECT). It is difficult to differentiate between benign PHPT and PC using sestamibi scan. Ultrasound scan of the neck cannot diagnose PC; however, there are certain sonological features which would arouse suspicion of PC. The ultrasound features include lobulation, hypoechogenicity, and large parathyroid gland with irregular borders.[6] Other features suggestive of malignancy include infiltration into surrounding structures, suspicious calcification, suspicious vascularity, and presence of thick and broad capsule. When PC is suspected preoperatively, it would be a good practice to do a cross-sectional imaging such as contrast-enhanced computed tomography (CECT) of neck or magnetic resonance imaging of neck to detect local infiltration which may guide surgical management.

◇ CYTOLOGY

Needle aspiration should be avoided in case PC is suspected because of an increased risk of tumor seeding along the needle tract.

◇ PATHOLOGY

On gross examination, PC is a hard, lobulated mass which is tan to grayish white in color with or without adherence to the surrounding structures **(Fig. 2)**. The adenoma is usually soft, red, or brownish in color and shows no sign of local infiltration. However, in a large number of cases, it may be difficult to differentiate between adenoma and carcinoma intraoperatively and the final diagnosis made only after histopathology. Grossly, the tumors are large (>3 cm) and majority weigh between 2 and 10 g.

So, the diagnosis of PC is a challenge for the pathologist and still remains a dilemma. Frozen section done intraoperatively is not reliable in differentiating benign adenoma from PC.

The histological criteria for diagnosis of PC were first described by Shantz and Castleman, which are as follows:

- Trabecular pattern of arrangement
- Thick and broad fibrous bands **(Fig. 3)**
- Presence of excess mitotic figures
- Invasion of capsule and blood vessel **(Figs. 4 and 5)**

However, the clinical outcomes diagnosed on these criteria showed that a large number do not clinically progress and the number of reported cases with proven lymph node involvement and metastatic spread outside the neck is very small suggesting that these criteria may overdiagnose the condition. Moreover, McKeown , et al.[7] indicated that cellular pleomorphism and atypia are not very reliable indicators of malignancy. Ronald DeLellis[8] postulated that although fibrosis and mitotic activity are common in carcinomas, these features are not specific only for malignancy. The diagnosis of carcinoma should be restricted to tumors that show invasion of blood vessels, perineural spaces, soft tissues, thyroid gland, or other adjacent structures or to tumors with documented metastases.

Immunohistochemistry staining may assist in the differentiation of PC from adenoma. The most commonly used marker is parafibromin, which is encoded by the *HRPT2* gene.

When this *HRPT2* gene is mutated, a loss of parafibromin expression and loss of staining are seen, making it a highly specific test for PC. Additional markers for the diagnosis of malignancy in parathyroid tumors include increased expression of galectin-3 and protein gene product (PGP) 9.5 and the loss of the adenomatous polyposis coli (APC) gene product. However, use of these markers requires additional studies.

◇| STAGING

In 2017, the American Joint Committee on Cancer (AJCC) guidelines recognized that sufficient data on tumor characteristics and prognosis for PC was not available.

The AJCC has proposed and defined specific variables to be recorded prospectively in order to develop a formal staging system, which will be useful in future. The proposed registry variables for PC included the age at initial diagnosis, gender, race, size of primary tumor, location of tumor, presence of invasion into the surrounding structures, distant metastatic disease, number of lymph nodes removed, number of positive lymph nodes, highest preoperative calcium reading, highest preoperative PTH, presence of lymphovascular invasion, histological grade (high grade or low grade), weight of tumor, mitotic rate, and time to recurrence.

The tumor, node, metastasis (TNM) definitions for PC currently followed are as follows:
- *Primary tumor*:
    - Tis—atypical parathyroid neoplasm
    - T1—tumor localized to the parathyroid gland with extension limited to soft tissue
    - T2—tumor invades the thyroid gland (direct invasion)
    - T3—tumor invades surrounding structures—recurrent laryngeal nerve, esophagus, trachea, and skeletal muscle
    - T4—tumor invades major blood vessels or spine

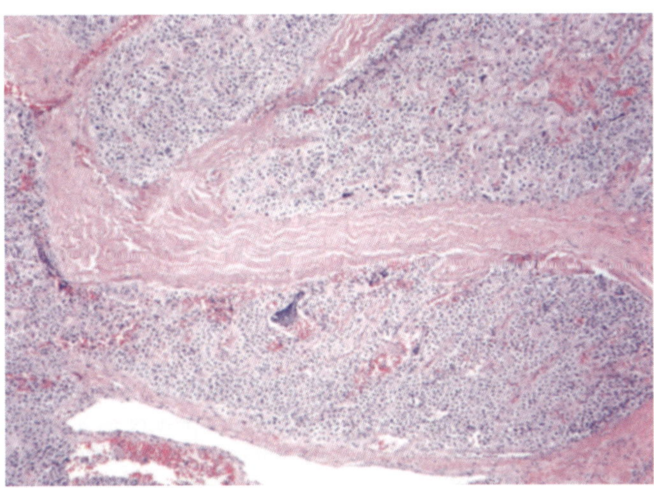

Fig. 3: Thick fibrous bands in parathyroid carcinoma.

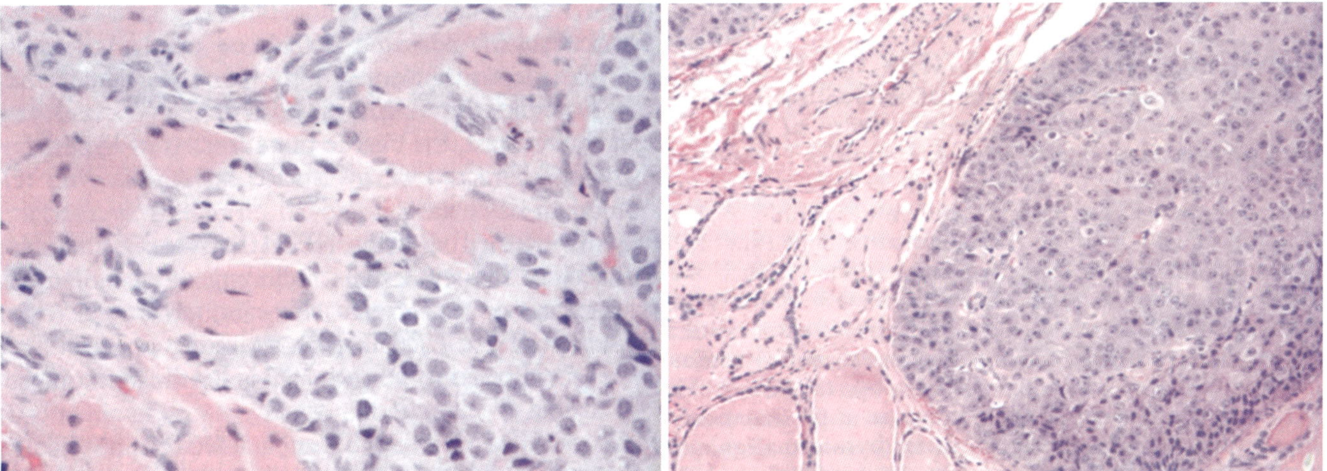

Fig. 4: Vascular invasion in parathyroid carcinoma seen in low-power field.

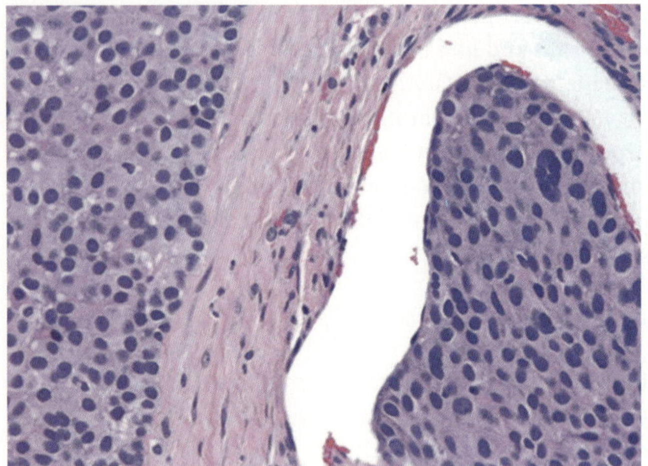

Fig. 5: Vascular invasion in parathyroid carcinoma seen in high-power field.

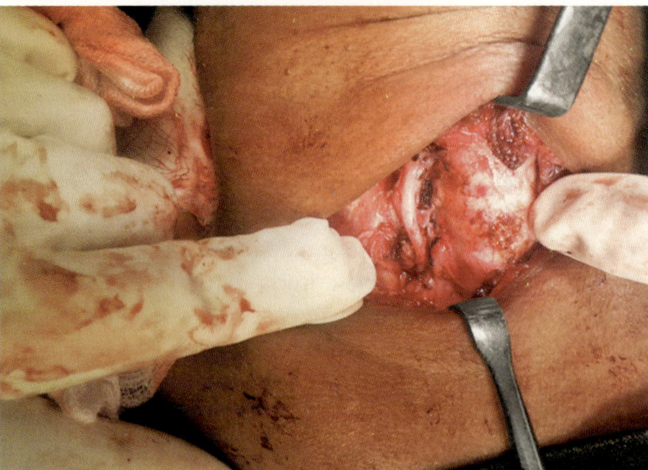

Fig. 6: Intraoperative photograph after en bloc resection of parathyroid carcinoma with intact recurrent laryngeal nerve.

- *Regional lymph nodes*:
  - N0—no lymph node metastasis present
  - N1a—presence of lymph nodes in central compartment of neck
  - N1b—presence of lymph nodes in lateral compartment of neck
- *Distant metastasis*:
  - M0—no distant metastasis present
  - M1—distant metastasis

◇| MANAGEMENT

Surgery

Surgery is the mainstay of treatment and the only curative treatment in the management of PC. The recognition of this disease during the initial neck exploration followed by en bloc resection offers the best chance of cure **(Fig. 6)**.

En bloc resection includes removal of the tumor along with removal of the ipsilateral thyroid lobe, removal of contiguous lymph nodes, and any suspicious or adherent components of the ipsilateral central neck compartment. During surgery, it is important to prevent the rupture of parathyroid capsule to prevent tumor seedling which may increase the likelihood of recurrence of disease.

The recurrent laryngeal nerve is preserved, if not involved by tumor. If the tumor involves a functioning recurrent laryngeal nerve then effort must be made to preserve the nerve unless it is circumferentially involved.

Most studies recommend ipsilateral central compartment lymph nodal clearance as part of the en bloc resection.[9,10] Modified neck dissection is done only if the lateral compartment lymph nodes are involved.

The main issue of controversy is the appropriate surgical management in a patient with postoperative pathological diagnosis of PC who was not suspected to have PC preoperatively or intraoperatively. Does the patient warrant re-exploration and en bloc resection or can the patient be observed? There is no concrete evidence to support one way or the other. Some surgeons advocate close observation of serum calcium and PTH levels for evidence of recurrence and utilizing en bloc resection as a reserve in the event of recurrence.

Adjuvant Treatment

Parathyroid carcinoma is primarily a radioresistant tumor. However, postoperative radiotherapy has been beneficial in terms of local control and reduced recurrence rate in few studies.[11] It has been mainly used in high-risk patients with local recurrence (incomplete excision), multifocal recurrence, or soft tissue deposits in patients with recurrent disease.

No chemotherapeutic regimen has been found to be useful in PC.[12]

Medical Management

Hypercalcemic crisis or parathyrotoxicosis is a medical emergency and associated with functioning PCs. Surgical intervention is contraindicated until the hypercalcemia is brought under control. Patient is initially managed with aggressive fluid resuscitation with isotonic saline and once adequate urine output is assured, loop diuretic such as furosemide is given to promote calcium diuresis. Patients with renal failure may require hemodialysis. Agents that inhibit bone resorption such as bisphosphonates (pamidronate and zoledronate) and salmon calcitonin are used to control hypercalcemia. For patients not responding, calcimimetics can be used. Cinacalcet which is a long-acting calcimimetic drug that binds to calcium-sensing receptors and decreases PTH secretion has been used **(Box 1)**.

◇| RECURRENT CARCINOMA

Recurrence of PC occurs in 40–60% patients, of which majority recur 2–5 years after the initial surgery. Recurrence is generally biochemically picked up with high calcium and PTH levels. Most of the recurrences are locoregional probably due to

Box 1: Medical management of hypercalcemic crisis.

- Fluid resuscitation
- Loop diuretic, e.g., furosemide
- Bisphosphonates, e.g., pamidronate, zoledronate
- Calcitonin
- Calcimimetic, e.g., cinacalcet
- Hemodialysis in renal failure

inadequate resection or intraoperative tumor spillage. Distant metastasis is usually to the lungs, followed by bones and liver.

Hypercalcemia is the cause of morbidity and mortality in recurrent PC. The management of recurrence is primarily surgical since surgical intervention results in significant lowering of calcium levels. For isolated recurrence in the neck, re-exploration and resection of tumor and its contiguous structures with regional lymphatics are ideal. Resection of isolated metastatic lesions is recommended to lower calcium levels and to improve patient survival.

PROGNOSIS

Parathyroid carcinoma is a progressive disease with variable outcome. The Surveillance, Epidemiology, and End Results (SEER) database reports 5-year survival of 86% and 10-year survival of 49%. The important factor affecting prognosis is the completeness of tumor resection in the initial intervention. Recurrence of PC ranges from 40 to 60% and usually occurs within 2–5 years after the initial surgical intervention. Most patients with PC usually die due to hypercalcemia rather than due to tumor spread.

CONCLUSION

Parathyroid carcinoma is a rare endocrine malignancy, which often presents with severe hypercalcemia and diagnosis can be difficult. A high index of suspicion is essential to diagnose it preoperatively or intraoperatively. Surgery is the main modality of treatment. The initial recognition with en bloc resection offers the best chance of cure. Postoperative radiotherapy is generally not effective, except in few selected cases. Patients with PC ultimately succumb to refractory hypercalcemia. Due to the rarity of this disease, patients should be managed by a multidisciplinary team in dedicated centers.

CLINICAL PEARLS

- PC is a rare malignancy accounting for 0.5–5% of all cases of PHPT.
- Germline mutations of *HRPT2* gene play a key role in the molecular pathogenesis of PC.
- PC presents with hypercalcemia. It is not uncommon for patients to present with hypercalcemic crisis.
- Differentiation between parathyroid adenoma and carcinoma can be difficult for surgeons and pathologists and a high index of suspicion is necessary.

- Fine-needle aspiration cytology (FNAC) should be avoided in a suspected case of PC due to the risk of parathyromatosis.
- Histological diagnosis can sometimes be difficult and complementary immunohistochemical markers such as parafibromin, PGP9.5, and galectin-3 may be required.
- Surgical intervention is the mainstay. The initial en bloc resection offers the best chance of cure.
- Postoperative radiotherapy may be useful in selected cases.
- Principles of medical management of severe hypercalcemia include aggressive fluid resuscitation, loop diuretic, bisphosphonates, calcitonin, and calcimimetic.
- The SEER database reports 5-year survival of 86% and 10-year survival of 49%.

REFERENCES

1. Cetani F, Pardi E, Marcocci C. Parathyroid carcinoma. Front Horm Res. 2019;51:63-76.
2. Li Y, Zhang J, Adikaram PR, Welch J, Guan B, Weinstein LS, Chen H, Simonds WF. Genotype of CDC73 germline mutation determines risk of parathyroid cancer. Endocr Relat Cancer. 2020;27(9):483-94.
3. Cetani F, Pardi E, Borsari S, Viacava P, Dipollina G, Cianferotti L, Ambrogini E, Gazzerro E, Colussi G, Berti P, Miccoli P, Pinchera A, Marcocci C. Genetic analyses of the *HRPT2* gene in primary hyperparathyroidism: germline and somatic mutations in familial and sporadic parathyroid tumors. J Clin Endocrinol Metab. 2004;89(11):5583-91.
4. Wei CH, Harari A. Parathyroid carcinoma: update and guidelines for management. Curr Treat Options Oncol. 2012;13(1):11-23.
5. Harari A, Waring A, Fernandez-Ranvier G, Hwang J, Suh I, Mitmaker E, Shen W, Gosnell J, Duh QY, Clark O. Parathyroid carcinoma: a 43-year outcome and survival analysis. J Clin Endocrinol Metab. 2011;96(12):3679-86.
6. Sidhu PS, Talat N, Patel P, Mulholland NJ, Schulte KM. Ultrasound features of malignancy in the preoperative diagnosis of parathyroid cancer: a retrospective analysis of parathyroid tumours larger than 15 mm. Eur Radiol. 2011;21(9):1865-73.
7. McKeown PP, McGarity WC, Sewell CW. Carcinoma of the parathyroid gland: is it overdiagnosed? A report of three cases. Am J Surg. 1984;147(2):292-8.
8. DeLellis RA. Parathyroid tumors and related disorders. Mod Pathol. 2011;24 (Suppl 2):S78-93
9. Villar-del-Moral J, Jiménez-García A, Salvador-Egea P, Martos-Martínez JM, Nuño-Vázquez-Garza JM, Serradilla-Martín M, Gómez-Palacios A, Moreno-Llorente P, Ortega-Serrano J, de la Quintana-Basarrate A. Prognostic factors and staging systems in parathyroid cancer: a multicenter cohort study. Surgery. 2014;156(5):1132-44.
10. Talat N, Schulte KM. Clinical presentation, staging and long-term evolution of parathyroid cancer. Ann Surg Oncol. 2010;17(8):2156-74.
11. Chow E, Tsang RW, Brierley JD, Filice S. Parathyroid carcinoma: the Princess Margaret Hospital experience. Int J Radiat Oncol Biol Phys. 1998;41(3):569-72.
12. Bukowski RM, Sheeler L, Cunningham J, Esselstyn C. Successful combination chemotherapy for metastatic parathyroid carcinoma. Arch Intern Med. 1984;144(2):399-400.

Jnaneshwari Jayaram, Chitresh Kumar

◇ INTRODUCTION

The term incidentaloma was coined by Geelhoed and Druy in 1982. They recognized that with the advent of improved resolution of radiological techniques, clinicians were facing an unfamiliar dilemma of early diagnosis of an asymptomatic adrenal mass.[1] In recent times, the further technological advancements and easy availability of ultrasonography (USG), computed tomography (CT) scan, magnetic resonance imaging (MRI), and positron emission tomography (PET) led to even more frequent detection of unexpected lesions in the adrenals.[2]

◇ DEFINITION

Adrenal incidentaloma (AI) is defined as clinically inapparent adrenal mass discovered inadvertently during radiological imaging done for the symptoms not related to adrenal conditions.

In 2002, the National Institute of Health coined the term as "clinically inapparent adrenal mass."[3] The terms adrenaloma or clinically "inapparent adrenal mass" or the "incidentaloma" are interchangeably used.[4]

In the annual meeting held at the American Association of Endocrine Surgeons, when Prinz presented his first nine cases of AI, he said, "Does detection of these anatomic abnormalities offer hope for early diagnosis and treatment of adrenal tumors so that the complications from the hormone producing tumors can be lessened and the dismal prognosis of malignant tumors can be improved? Or does CT merely bring up to clinical attention adrenal enlargements that do not pose a threat to the patient's overall health?"[5] After so many advancements in the imaging, hormonal evaluation, and treatment, this dilemma is still persisting.

◇ EPIDEMIOLOGY

The prevalence depends on the data source (autopsy, radiology, and surgery) or group of patient population as said by Black et al.[6] The prevalence of any disease increases with enhanced ability of the observer to detect abnormalities.[6] In a large autopsy series conducted by Kokko et al. and Hedeland et al., the prevalence of AIs was found between 1.05 and 8.7%.[7,8] At the Mayo Clinic, in a study done by Herrera et al., 61,054 patients underwent CT scanning over a period of 5 years. Out of them, 2,066 (3.4%) patients were found to have an adrenal abnormality.[9] Recent studies have also reported a frequency of AIs about 4.2–7.3%.[10] So, in the era of modern imaging modalities such as high-resolution USG, CT, and MRI, we anticipate the incidence of AIs to remain around 5%.

◇ DEMOGRAPHIC CHARACTERISTICS

A large retrospective autopsy study by Kobayashi et al. demonstrated that the prevalence of AIs increases with age. Around 25% of AIs are found in <50 years and 75% identified in patients >50 years.[11] Other autopsy and radiology series also demonstrated that the occurrence of AIs increases with age, showing a peak incidence in the 5th to 7th decades.[12,13] AIs are less common in <30 years of age group. If present, it should be evaluated for functional status of the adenomas and also evaluated for malignancy and familial syndromes.[14,15] AIs are more commonly found in females as per autopsy studies.

Malignant Potential

Various large clinical studies have also investigated the various characteristics of AIs. Many studies have found that the mean diameter of AI discovered by a CT scan is 30 mm ranging from 8 to 230 mm.[16] As many studies were retrospective, they had their limitations. However, all the studies consistently reported a higher incidence of adrenocortical carcinoma in masses >4 cm in size.[17] The risk of malignancy increases from 6 to 25% as size increases from 4 to 6 cm. There is higher incidence of malignancy in adrenal tumors secreting, steroid precursors such as dehydroepiandrosterone sulfate (DHEAS), sex steroids, or multiple hormones.

Laterality

There is development in the techniques of CT protocols, which has led to detection rate of adrenal masses equally on both sides.[18] However, study done by Ahn et al. suggested higher prevalence of left-sided adrenal tumor detection on imaging.[19] This reflects a detection bias as radiologists can easily visualize left-side compared to right-side lesions. This was concluded by Sangwaiya et al. that detection bias may result in under-recognition of small (<30 mm) right-sided lesions and also bilateral disease.[20]

◇| PATHOLOGICAL DIAGNOSIS

Adrenal incidentalomas can be functioning or nonfunctioning, with nonfunctioning benign being the most common cause comprising 80% of AI cases.[21] The benign conditions are cysts, ganglioneuroma, myelolipoma, and hematoma. Kim's study reported functional adrenal tumors of 41.3%. Among the hormone-producing tumors, pheochromocytoma (PCC) is the most frequently encountered with average incidence of 6.2% (range: 2.1–20.0%), which may have normal laboratory values followed by subclinical Cushing's syndrome (SCS) average of 8.1% (3–11.3%) and rarely hyperaldosteronism with an average of 3.9% (1.5–10%), malignant tumors (adrenal cortical carcinoma and adrenal metastases) averaged 2.6% (range: 0.7–15.0%).[22-24] According to a study by Terzo et al., the prevalence of PCC is 1.5–23.0%, adrenocortical carcinoma is 1.2–12% **(Table 1)**.[24] It cannot be underestimated that adrenal gland is a site of metastasis for a variety of cancers from the lung, breast, kidney, melanoma, and lymphoma.

◇| DIAGNOSTIC APPROACH

Although the AIs are rarely associated with life-threatening disorders, the question of whether an incidentally detected adrenal lesion is malignant or producing hormones needs to be addressed. Therefore, a detailed medical history and a careful clinical examination are a must before evaluating the imaging characteristics and biochemical parameters.

Clinical Evaluation

According to definition, AIs should not have any signs or symptoms related to adrenal diseases before the radiological detection of the adrenal lesion. The physicians who are not familiar with endocrine diseases may overlook mild signs of hormone excess and start clinical evaluation of adrenal function after the incidental discovery of an adrenal mass.

Table 1: Frequency of the different types of adrenal incidentaloma.[25]

Type	Average %	Range %
Clinical studies		
Adenoma:	80	33–96
• Nonfunctioning	75	71–84
• Cortisol secreting	12	1.0–29
• Aldosterone secreting	2.5	1.6–3.3
Pheochromocytoma	7.0	1.5–14
Carcinoma	8.0	1.2–11
Metastasis	5.0	0–18
Surgical studies		
Adenoma:	55	49–69
• Nonfunctioning	69	52–75
• Cortisol secreting	10	1.0–15
• Aldosterone secreting	6.0	2.0–7.0
Pheochromocytoma	10	11–23
Carcinoma	11	1.2–12
Metastasis	7.0	0–21
Myelolipoma	8.0	7–15
Cysts	5.0	4–22
Ganglioneuroma	4.0	0–8

In this scenario, these cases should not be labeled as AIs and highlight the need for detailed and careful clinical history and examination. History and clinical examination of a patient found to have AIs should be aimed at subclinical Cushing's syndrome and PCC in normotensive patients. In hypertensive patients/patients having hypokalemia, the aldosterone-secreting tumor should be ruled out.

To suspect Cushing's syndrome, enquiry to be made about substantial weight gain, centripetal obesity, easy bruisability, difficulty in get up from sitting position, development of hypertension, diabetes, fatigue, or rarely virilization. History of bone fractures is also to be enquired (because of osteoporosis). On examination, round facies, buffalo hump, thinned skin, purple striae, hirsutism, hypertension, proximal muscle weakness, and central obesity to be looked specifically. To suspect PCC, history should include the presence of sudden or severe headache, palpitation, heavy sweating, anxiety attacks, and weight loss. On examination, hypertension, tachycardia, arrhythmias, low BMI, wet and warm skin, tremors, and hyperreflexia may be found. To suspect aldosteronoma, history of muscle cramps, weakness, fatigue, headache, excessive thirst, and frequent need to urinate should be sought. On examination, hypertension, pedal edema, and fluid overload to be carefully looked upon.

To suspect metastasis to adrenal gland, history of recent weight loss, fever, smoking, and previous malignancy (lung, breast, kidney, melanoma, and lymphoma) to be enquired. A thorough systemic examination is a must to look for primary malignancy.

Biochemical Evaluation

As per the American Association of Clinical Endocrinology (AACE) guidelines, AI detection should prompt for biochemical evaluation unless it is confirmatory of myelolipoma.[26] Adrenal myelolipomas are of low CT attenuation on noncontrast (–10 to –20) and also contain fat; hence, diagnosis is straightforward.[27] Along with functionality of the tumor, tumor characterization into benign or primary malignancy or metastatic should be done which leads us for further investigation and treatment.

- 1-mg overnight dexamethasone suppression test (ONDST) or/and late-night salivary cortisol
- Plasma-free metanephrines, normetanephrine levels, and 24-hour total urinary metanephrines and fractionated catecholamines.
- Plasma aldosterone concentration (PAC) (ng/dL) to plasma renin activity (PRA) (ng/mL/h) (spironolactone and mineral corticoid receptor blockers should be stopped).
- Testing for sex hormones is indicated when the patient has obvious signs.

Cushing's Syndrome

Screening for Cushing's syndrome is important as it is the most common pathology found in AI. 1-mg overnight dexamethasone suppression test is enough for screening and can be done on outpatient basis. There is a disagreement about reference range and its sensitivity and specificity.[26,28] A value <1.8 µg/dL is considered normal. A value of 5 µg/dL or more suggests asymptomatic hypercortisolism. Values between 1.8 and 5 µg/dL needs additional investigations.[24] When the values of basal serum cortisol are at 1.8 µg/dL (50 nmol/L), sensitivity of DST is >95% and specificity is 70–80%. When the baseline is at 5 µg/dL (138 nmol/L), specificity is >95% but sensitivity decreases **(Table 2)**.[24] More accurate diagnosis can be obtained by finding a low or suppressed adrenocorticotropic hormone (ACTH) level.[29] A second abnormal test result of hypothalamic-pituitary-adrenal (HPA) axis function, such as a 48-hour low-dose dexamethasone test and plasma cortisol, measured at 9 AM on day 0 and again 48 hours later, after administration of dexamethasone 0.5 mg every 6 hours for 48 hours, may be needed to establish the diagnosis of SCS **(Flowchart 1)**.[14] Certain drugs (e.g., phenytoin and rifampicin) may increase the metabolic clearance rate of dexamethasone, leading to false-positive results.

Late-night salivary cortisol is the earliest and most sensitive marker of hypercortisolism. The diagnostic accuracy of a single midnight salivary cortisol level has been established in several studies: a cortisol value >2.0 ng/mL (5.5 nmol/L) has a 100% sensitivity and a 96% specificity for diagnosis of Cushing's syndrome.[30-32]

24-hour urinary free cortisol (UFC) levels are unaffected by the factors that influence corticosteroid-binding globulins. UFC elevation above four times the normal value is diagnostic of Cushing's syndrome.[33] When it is up to threefold elevated, it can be associated with pseudo-Cushing's syndrome seen in chronic anxiety, depression, alcoholism, and obesity. In this situation, a confirmatory test is required.[30]

Adrenal Incidentaloma with Autonomous Cortisol Secretion

Clinical features of Cushing's syndrome are well known. Many a time, there can be a situation wherein the patient has

Table 2: Steps of hypercortisolism evaluation by different guidelines.

	NIH (2002)[3]	AACE/AAES (2009)[26]	IACE (2011)[24]	ESE/ENSAT (2016)[25]
Terminology				
	SCS	ACS	SCS	ACS
Primary screening test				
ONDST	Recommended cut-off >5 µg/dL—possible SCS	Recommended cut-off >5 µg/dL	Recommended cut-off <1.8 µg/dL exclude >5 µg/dL consider 1.8–5 µg/dL = intermediate	Recommended cut-off >5 µg/dL—possible SCS
Secondary screening test				
24-h UFC	Not mentioned	Not recommended	Yes	Yes
Late-night serum cortisol	Not mentioned	Not mentioned	Yes	Yes
Late-night salivary cortisol	Not mentioned	Not recommended	Not recommended	Yes

(AACE: American Association of Clinical Endocrinologists; AAES: American Association of Endocrine Surgeons; ACS: autonomous cortisol secretion; ESE: European Society of Endocrinology; ENSAT: European Network for the Study of Adrenal Tumors; IACE: Italian Association of Clinical Endocrinologists; NIH: National Institutes of Health; SCS: subclinical Cushing's syndrome)

Flowchart 1: Algorithm for hormonal evaluation of hypercortisolism in adrenal incidentaloma.

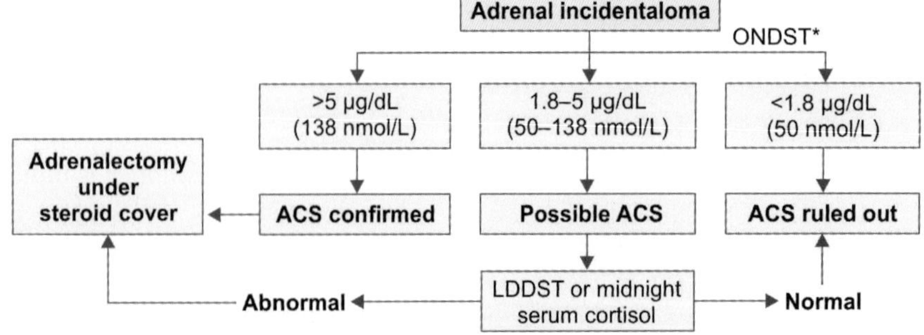

*24 hour urinary free cortisol or late night salivary cortisol can also be used in place of ONDST
(ACS: autonomous cortisol suppression; LDDST: low-dose dexamethasone suppression test; ONDST: overnight dexamethasone suppression test)

Flowchart 2: Algorithm for hormonal evaluation of pheochromocytoma in adrenal incidentaloma.

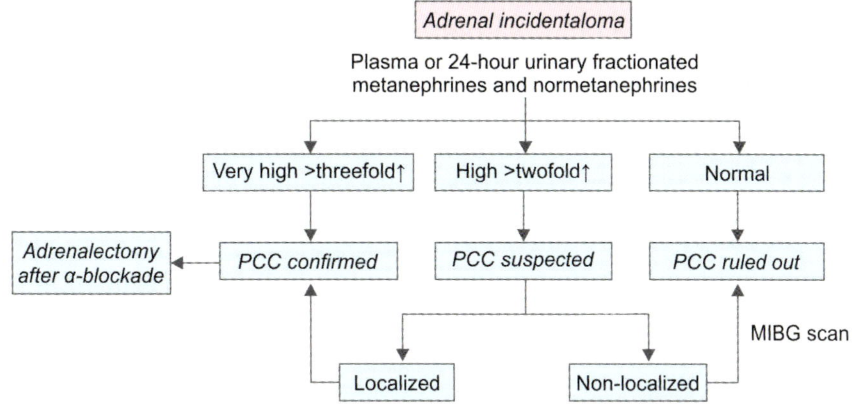

(MIBG: metaiodobenzylguanidine; PCC: pheochromocytoma)

ACTH-independent cortisol secretion without overt clinical features attributing to excessive secretion of cortisol termed autonomous cortisol secretion (ACS), which makes diagnostic challenging.

Autonomous cortisol secretion is defined as alteration of HPA axis characterized by ACTH-independent cortisol excess often without clinical signs and symptoms of overt Cushing's syndrome. Other names used are SCS (as per NIH), subclinical hypercortisolism, and preclinical Cushing's syndrome, which cause confusion. As proposed by the European Society of Endocrinology (ESE)/European Network for the Study of Adrenal Tumors (ENSAT), the ACS term is used.[25]

Even though there are no florid signs, ACS in AI patients has been seen to be associated with hypertension, insulin resistance, type 2 diabetes mellitus, obesity, metabolic syndrome, and increased mortality.[34] In a study by Vassilatou, ACS has emerged as the most common functional abnormality in patients with AI with up to 20%.[35]

Pheochromocytoma

Pheochromocytomas secrete norepinephrine, epinephrine, and rarely dopamine (can have hypotension). Earlier urinary vanillylmandelic acid (VMA), catecholamines, and unfractionated metanephrines were used to confirm the PCC. Nowadays, either 24-hour urinary fractionated metanephrines or plasma fractionated metanephrines are recommended to confirm the diagnosis. To ensure adequacy of the collection, we should measure creatinine in all collections of urine. The collection container should be dark and acidified and should be kept cold to avoid degradation of the catecholamines. Optimally, collect urine during or immediately after a crisis.

Although dopamine is a major catecholamine, measurement of dopamine levels in 24-hour urine is not useful, because most urinary dopamine is derived from renal extraction. A 24-hour urine total metanephrine >1,800 µg in the clinical setting is diagnostic of PCC. A fractionated plasma-free metanephrine level may be measured in a standard venipuncture sample, drawn about 15–20 minutes after

Flowchart 3: Algorithm for hormonal evaluation of hyperaldosteronism in adrenal incidentaloma.

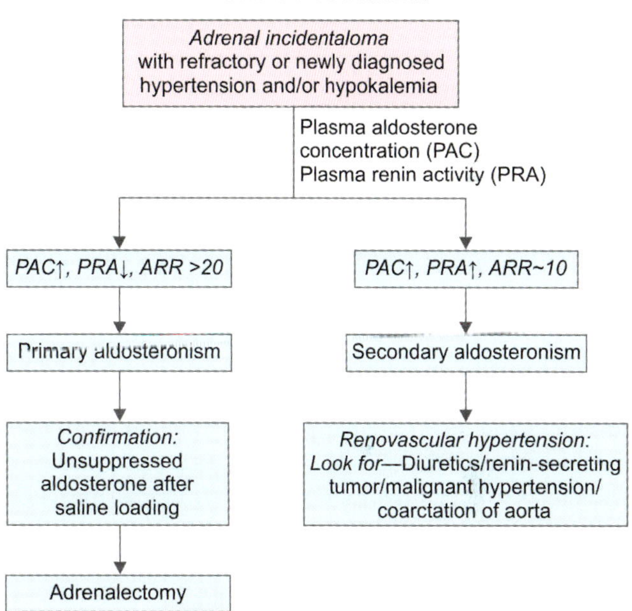

(ARR: aldosterone-to-renin ratio; PRA: plasma renin activity; PAC: plasma aldosterone concentration)

intravenous catheter insertion in supine position. A plasma metanephrine level exceeding three to four times normal is diagnostic with sensitivity ranging from 77 to 97% and specificity from 69 to 98%. The measurement of plasma-free metanephrines and normetanephrines, which have sensitivity (97–100%) and specificity (85–89%), appears to be the initial screening test for PCC **(Flowchart 2)**.[36]

Aldosteronoma

The universal accepted screening modality for aldosteronism is determining the ratio of PAC (ng/dL) to PRA (ng/mL).[37] At the Mayo Clinic, investigators found that the aldosterone-to-renin ratio (ARR) > 20 along with PAC >15 ng/dL was highly sensitive **(Flowchart 3)**.[38] Weinberger et al. found that ARR of >30 along with PAC >20 ng/dL had a sensitivity of 90% and a specificity of 91%.[39]

Drugs which interfere with values such as spironolactone and eplerenone (mineralocorticoid receptor blocker) should be stopped for 4–6 weeks. Thiazide diuretics, calcium channel blockers (dihydropyridines), angiotensin-converting enzyme (ACE) inhibitors, and angiotensin receptor blockers (ARBs) can actually improve the diagnostic discriminatory power of the ARR; in contrast, β-adrenergic blocking agents and clonidine suppress PRA and thus may cause false-positive results. The ARR is most sensitive when blood samples are collected in the morning, after patients have been out of bed for at least 2 hours and have been seated for 5–15 minutes.

Imaging

According to definition, AI is imaging-detected adrenal lesion in patients who do not have any symptoms related to adrenal pathology. AI can be detected by any abdominal imaging, but most commonly AI is being detected either by USG or by noncontrast CT abdomen because these are the frequently advised abdominal imaging.

Any adrenal lesion measuring >1 cm in short axis needs further characterization to determine if the lesion is benign or malignant at the time of initial diagnosis. The evaluation is emphasized more because of tumor size correlation with risk of adrenocortical cancer. It is a well-known fact that tumors <4 cm have 2% risk, tumors with 4.1–6 cm harbor 6% risk, and tumors >6 cm have 25% risk of being malignant.[3]

Normal adrenal glands have distinctive shape equate to a lambda or Y, V, and inverted T shape on CT (axial) or MRI. Adrenal gland has three parts, namely medial limb, body, and lateral limb. The limbs are thin with a normal maximum diameter of 6 mm for right adrenal and left adrenal measuring 8 mm.[40] Apart from a definitive lesion, thickened adrenal limbs (>10 mm) are considered abnormal as well. The various imaging modalities are described as follows.

Ultrasonography of Abdomen

Ultrasonography can detect adrenal lesions measuring >2 cm in size. The main drawback of USG is that it is operator dependent and any lesion detected by USG needs further anatomical characterization. Therefore, USG has no place in imaging of AI.

Computed Tomography

The unenhanced (noncontrast) CT scan is the first step of anatomical characterization mainly used for measuring Hounsfield units (HUs). The HU measurement is a method of quantifying the X-ray absorption of the body tissues when compared with water. The HU assessment is more valid for homogeneous lesions as in heterogeneous lesions, HUs are variable in different areas of the same lesion. The HU of water is taken as zero; the air has a low attenuation value (–600 to –1,000 HU) as does fat (–100 HU). Adrenal lesions with bulk macroscopic fat are myelolipoma (–90 to –120 HU). These tumors do not require further evaluation as myelolipomas are nonfunctional tumors. In any patient, without a history of extra-adrenal malignancy, HU ≤10 on an unenhanced CT is expected to be lipid-rich adenoma.[41]

Among the benign adrenal adenomas, 30% do not contain large amount of lipid and hence its attenuation value will be >10 which is called lipid-poor adenoma. These lesions cannot be safely characterized on noncontrast CT scan because of overlapping density with PCCs and malignant lesions.[42] A meta-analysis done by Boland et al. reported that a threshold of 10 HU in unenhanced CT resulted in diagnosing adrenal adenoma with sensitivity of 71% and specificity of 98%.[41] Once the lesion shows HU >10, the adrenal protocol needs to be followed to characterize the lesion in terms of size, homogeneity, borders, relation to other structures, and most importantly kinetics (washout) study.

A dedicated triple-phased adrenal protocol is mandatory to characterize the lesions. The first phase is unenhanced, second phase is early enhanced 1-min postcontrast, and the third phase is delayed enhanced 10–15-min postcontrast scan. The main intention of following this protocol is to differentiate between lipid-poor adenoma and malignant lesion depending on washout kinetics. The percentage of washout in delayed images is helpful in characterizing a lesion. Adenomas, including the lipid-poor adenomas, have rapid loss of attenuation soon after enhancement with intravenous contrast material, i.e., washout decreases more quickly in adenomas compared to malignant lesions in delayed images.[43]

Absolute percentage washout (APW) is calculated using the following formula:

$$(Enhanced\ HU - 15\text{-}min\ delayed\ HU) / (Enhanced\ HU - Unenhanced\ HU) \times 100\%$$

Relative percentage washout (RPW) is used when unenhanced CT value is not available, and the enhanced values are compared with 15-minutre delayed scans, by using the following formula:

$$(Enhanced\ HU - 15\text{-}min\ delayed\ HU)/(Enhanced\ HU) \times 100\%$$

If the APW is >60% or RPW is >40% after 15 minutes from contrast administration, this is indicative of adenoma, with sensitivity and specificity of 88% and 96% at the APW and sensitivity and specificity of 83% and 93% at the RPW, respectively.[44]

On broad terms, benign adrenal lesions, on immediate contrast enhancement, show up to 80–90 HU, and >50% on delayed scan (**Figs. 1A and B**), whereas metastatic lesions, carcinomas, and PCC show lesser washout. PCC shows enhancement to >100 HU, which distinguishes from adenomas.[27]

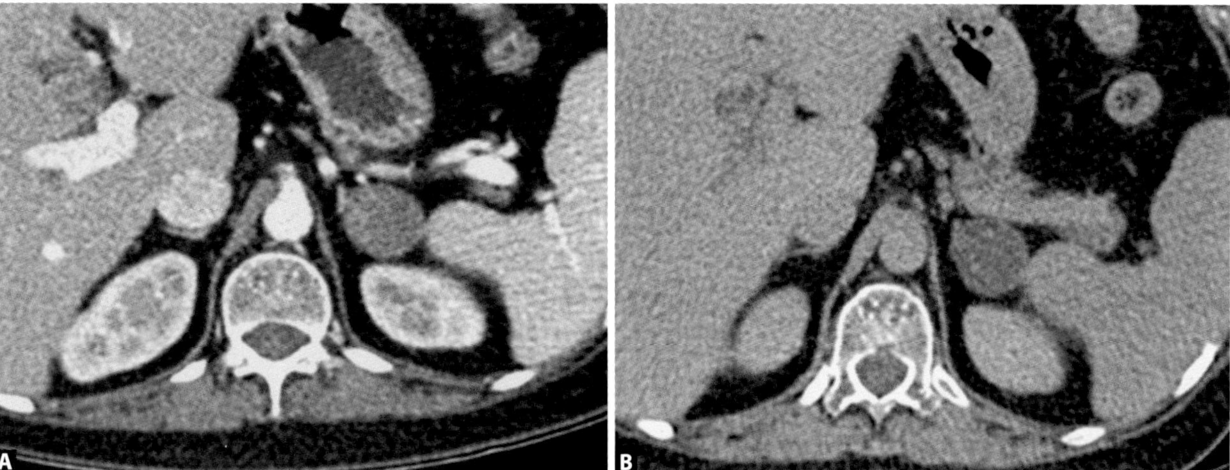

Figs. 1A and B: (A) A left-sided adrenal incidentaloma—postcontrast 1-minute CT image showing enlarged enhancing left adrenal gland (circle) with HU = 50; (B) Postcontrast 15-minute CT image showing relative washout of 80% with HU = 10.

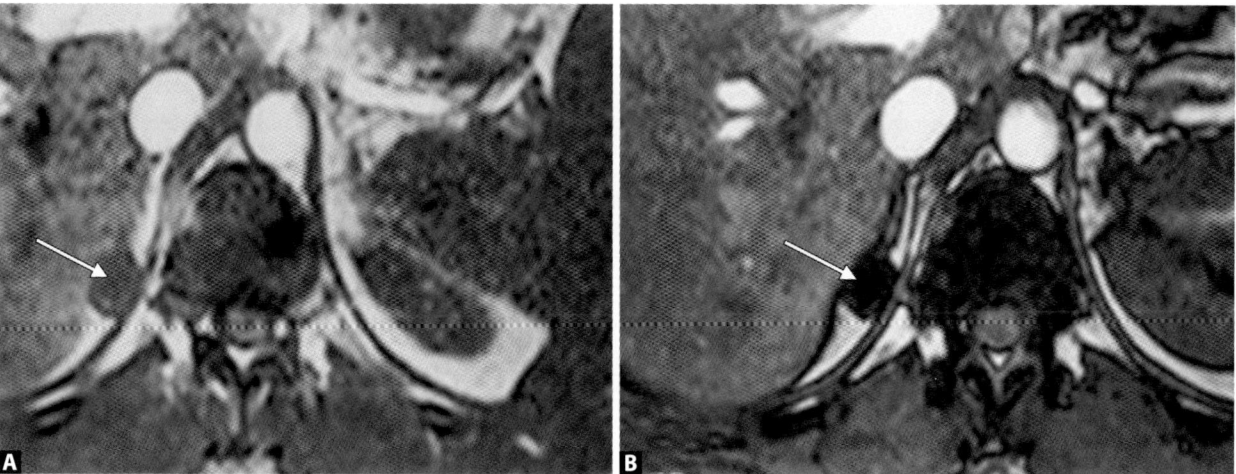

Figs. 2A and B: (A) MRI of a right adrenal incidentaloma (arrow) on T1-weighted image; (B) Loss of signal on out-of-phase compared to in-phase imaging favoring fat-rich adenoma.
Source: Dr Devasenathipathy K, Additional Professor, Department of Radiodiagnosis, AIIMS, New Delhi, India.

Dual-energy CT

Dual-energy CT is nowadays being investigated for clinical use; it can provide additional specific data about attenuation properties of different materials at different energies. It can be useful when the detection of AI on single-phase contrast-enhanced CT is typically performed 60–90 seconds after contrast administration that is when the HU value of benign and doubtful lesions overlaps.[45] Virtual noncontrast CT data set can be derived from the routinely acquired variable energy single-phase contrast-enhanced CT.[46]

Magnetic Resonance Imaging

The recent guidelines suggest that MRI imaging should be used primarily as a problem-solving tool. It can be used in patient's situation where CT cannot be used like in pregnancy, children, and patients allergic to iodinated contrast.[27] The best MRI technique to differentiate benign from malignant adrenal masses is chemical shift. The first use of chemical shift MRI was described in 1992 by Platzek et al.[47] The most characteristic feature of adrenal adenoma is the presence of intracellular lipid. Within the magnetic fields, protons in water and fat vibrate at slightly different frequencies. That means water and fat protons oscillate in and out of phase with respect to one another and we can get separate images for oscillating water and fat protons by selecting appropriate sequencing parameters. Adrenal adenomas with a high fat content lose signal intensity on out-of-phase images compared with in-phase images **(Figs. 2A and B)**, whereas malignant lesions, PCCs, and adrenal adenomas with low fat content remain unchanged.

Semelka et al. identified adrenal adenoma on chemical shift MRI with sensitivity of 78% and specificity reaching 87%. They used adrenal signal intensity index threshold value of >16.5%.[48] Adenomas have typical homogeneous enhancement on immediate contrast-enhanced images. Adrenocortical carcinomas are most of the time large at the time of diagnosis,

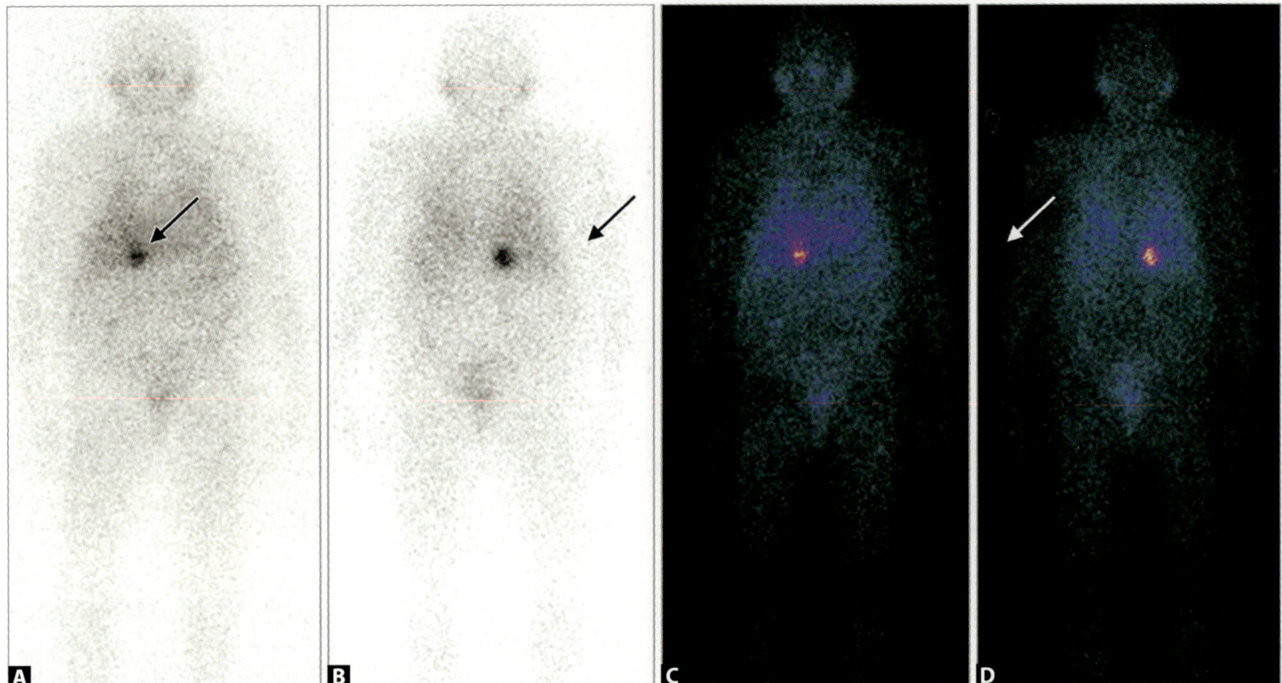

Figs. 3A to D: ^{131}I-mIBG scan showing focal area of increased tracer uptake is seen in right suprarenal region (arrow). (A) Anterior image; (B) Posterior image, SPECT images also confirming a structural lesion in right suprarenal region; (C) Anterior image; (D) Posterior image. (SPECT: single-photon emission computed tomography)
Source: Dr Nishikant A Damle, Associate Professor, Department of Nuclear Medicine, AIIMS, New Delhi, India.

tend to show higher signal intensity on T2-weighted images, and are heterogeneous on both T1-weighted and T2-weighted images due to the presence of necrosis/internal hemorrhage. PCCs are hyperintense on T2-weighted images and with gadolinium contrast, they show rapid enhancement referred to as the light bulb sign.

Functional Imaging

Iodine-labeled metaiodobenzylguanidine (MIBG), a guanethidine analog, has been used for functional imaging of tumors arising from the adrenal medulla for over 30 years **(Figs. 3A to D)**.[49] The ^{123}I-MIBG has significant limitations, including a 2-day imaging protocol and the need for thyroid blockade with potassium iodide prior to tracer injection. Other PET tracers including dopamine analogs such as 18F-fluorodopamine and 18F-fluorodihydroxyphenylalanine (DOPA) which image norepinephrine (noradrenaline) may be useful. Recently, ^{68}Ga-labeled (1,4,7,10-tetraazacyclododecane-1,4,7,10-tetraacetic acid)-1-NaI[3]-octreotide (DOTA-NOC) is being increasingly used as a functional imaging to evaluate AI **(Figs. 4A to C)**.

[18]Fluorodeoxyglucose (FDG)-PET is not recommended until there is a high suspicion of malignancy or negative DOTA-NOC scan. Normal adrenal glands do exhibit mild FDG uptake but equal or less than the liver uptake with maximum standardized uptake values (max SUV) ranging between 0.95 and 2.46.[50] Sometimes, CT and MRI scans will not be able to definitively characterize adrenal nodules, due to either heterogeneous density making HU measurements unreliable and also difficulty in evaluating lipid poor adenomas—termed indeterminate nodules.[51] In these situations, FDG-PET has a promising role in distinguishing benign from malignant adrenal masses, which can be either adrenocortical cancer or metastatic with sensitivity of 74–100% and specificity of 66–100% in the population of patients with and without past history of cancer.[52-56] When adrenal max SUV cutoff of 3.1 used by Metser et al., FDG PET/CT had a sensitivity of 98.5% and a specificity of 92% for differentiating adenomas (lipid rich/poor) from malignant.[57]

Adrenal Metastasis

Due to its rich sinusoidal blood supply, the adrenal gland is a common site for metastasis.[58] There is usually bilateral involvement in cases of adrenal metastasis. Melanoma, breast, lung, colon, lymphoma, kidney, thyroid, esophagus, pancreas, and stomach cancers are the malignancies that commonly metastasize to the adrenals.[59] Small metastases might appear homogeneous on CECT or MRI, but large metastases tend to have regions of heterogeneous appearance due to necrosis, hemorrhage, or both, though calcification is rare.

Other causes of bilateral adrenal enlargement are lymphoma, ectopic ACTH-induced macrohyperplasia, tuberculosis, histoplasmosis, blastomycosis, and other granulomatous diseases affecting the adrenals that usually have bilateral involvement but are often asymmetrical. Fine-needle aspiration cytology (FNAC) or biopsy is needed to

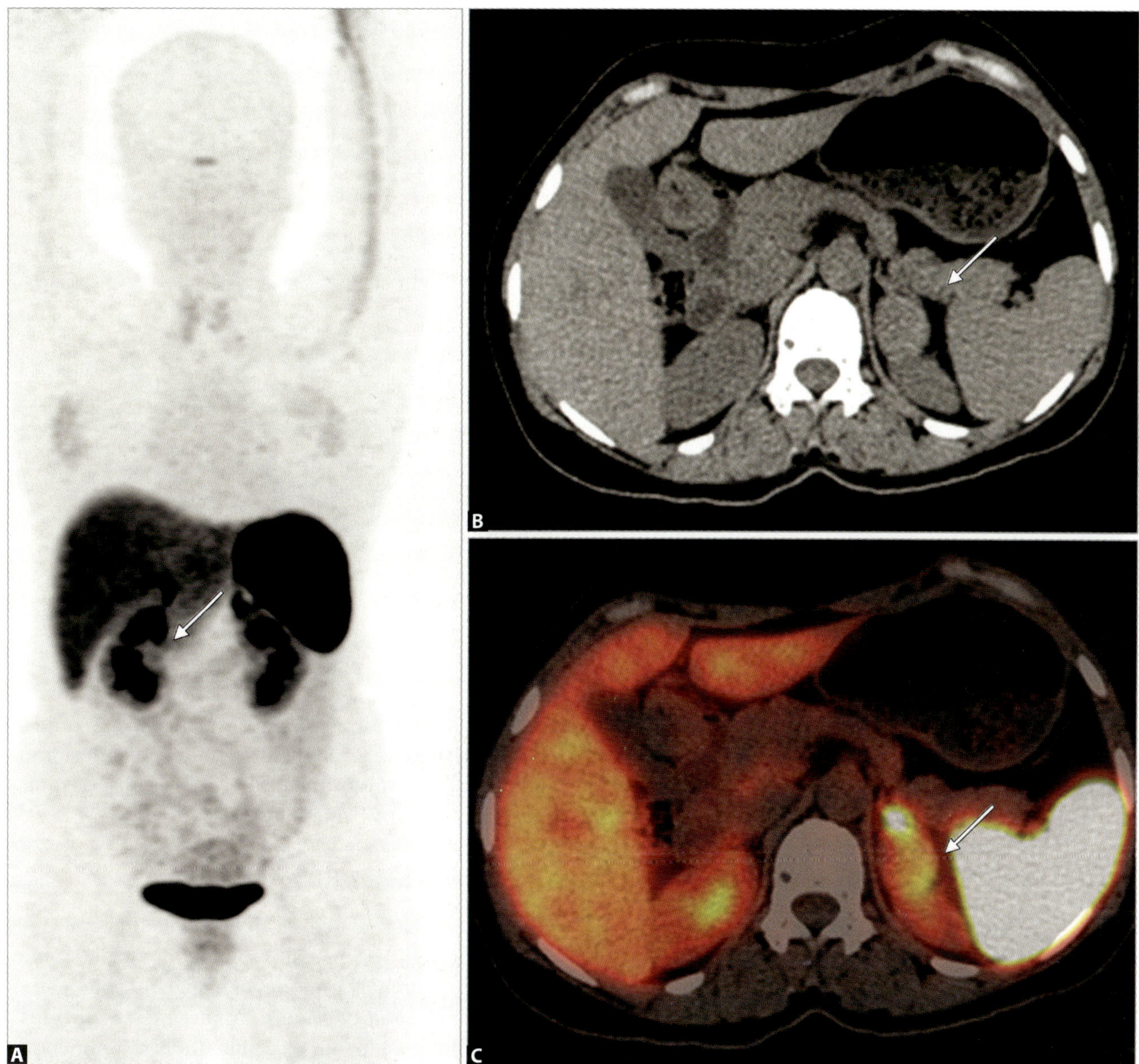

Figs. 4A to C: (A) ^{68}Ga-DOTANOC positron emission tomography (PET)/computed tomography (CT) unfused coronal view; (B) Axial non-contrast CT (HU = 10); (C) Axial fused PET/CT images. A well-defined rounded soft-tissue density mass is seen in the left adrenal (arrow), arising from its medial limb with increased radiotracer uptake (indicating SSTR expression) (white arrows).
Source: Dr Nishikant A Damle, Associate Professor, Department of Nuclear Medicine, AIIMS, New Delhi, India.

confirm the diagnosis and identify the responsible organism. In case of metastasis or cancer, biopsy should be avoided for AIs due to risk of seeding of adrenal cancer, and adverse hemodynamic changes when performed in an undiagnosed PCC.

TREATMENT OF ADRENAL INCIDENTALOMA

The appropriateness of surgical intervention should be guided by the likelihood of malignancy, the presence and degree of hormone excess, age, general health, and patient's preference. Surgery is not usually indicated in patients with an asymptomatic, nonfunctioning unilateral adrenal mass (<4 cm) and obvious benign features on imaging studies **(Flowchart 4)**. These patients should be kept under surveillance and repeat imaging should be done after 6–12 months **(Table 3)**. Rapid increase in size (>20% or >1 cm in a year), development of malignant features, or functionality is the indication for surgery. All the functional AIs should undergo laparoscopic or retroperitoneoscopic adrenalectomy. Large (>7 cm) benign and malignant AIs should undergo open surgery. The HPA axis is suppressed in case of hypercortisolism and after removal of Cushing's adenoma, the other hypofunctional adrenal may not produce the physiological amount of corticosteroids and

Table 3: Recommendations for follow-up of adrenal incidentaloma.

Guidelines	Image follow-up period	Hormone test follow-up period
NIH consensus statement, 2002[3]	Two CTs, at least 6 months apart, if there is no change in size, there is no basis for further follow-up	• 1 mg DST • Plasma-free metanephrine • K+ and renin/aldosterone ratio (when accompanied by high blood pressure) • Every year for 4 years
Young, NEJM, 2007[38]	Repeat imaging at 6, 12, and 24 months	• 1 mg DST • Plasma-free metanephrine • K+ and renin/aldosterone ratio (when accompanied by high blood pressure) • Every year for 5 years
AACE/AAES guidelines, 2009[26]	• Imaging at 3–6 months, then annually for 1–2 years • Repeat imaging at 6, 12, and 24 months	
IACE, 2011[24]	Imaging at 3–6 months for size >2 cm and density >10 HU	The panel agrees that the value of periodic hormonal screening is uncertain but, if felt necessary, the 1 mg DST may serve the purpose
ESE/ESNAT clinical practice guidelines, 2016[25]	Repeat imaging at every 6–12 months	Not recommended unless new clinical signs of endocrine activity appear or there is worsening of comorbidities (e.g., hypertension and type 2 diabetes)

(AACE: American Association of Clinical Endocrinologists; AAES: American Association of Endocrine Surgeons; ACS: autonomous cortisol secretion; CT: computed tomography; DST: dexamethasone suppression test; ESE: European Society of Endocrinology; ENSAT: European Network for the Study of Adrenal Tumors; IACE: Italian Association of Clinical Endocrinologists; NEJM: New England Journal of Medicine, NIH: National Institutes of Health; SCS: subclinical Cushing's syndrome)

the patient may land up in adrenal insufficiency. To avoid this life-threatening situation, all AIs with hypercortisolism should be operated under steroid cover. The need of steroid replacement has to be confirmed 1–2 months after surgery with appropriate testing. If postsurgical adrenal insufficiency is confirmed, steroid replacement could be subsequently tapered guided by clinical data and re-evaluation of the HPA axis every 3–6 months. It is pertinent to say that adrenal insufficiency may last for many months. All the PCCs should be operated after adequate preoperative α blockade to avoid perioperative hypertensive crisis. In case of bilateral adrenal tumors adrenal insufficiency, infection and metastasis should be ruled out before any kind of intervention.

NATURAL HISTORY OF ADRENAL INCIDENTALOMAS

Since AIs do not represent a single clinical entity, their natural history varies depending on the underlying etiology. Primary malignant adrenal tumors typically display rapid growth (>2 cm/year) and a poor outcome with an overall 5-year survival <50%. PCCs grow slowly and are mostly benign, but if untreated, these are potentially lethal displaying high cardiovascular mortality and morbidity.

A recent meta-analysis of 32 studies including 2,690 patients with nonfunctioning AIs and adrenal tumors associated with ACS provided important insights into the natural history of such tumors that help in solving controversy and informing practice. Only 4.7% of AIs grew by 10 mm or more over a mean follow-up. Similarly, inapparent autonomous cortisol

and catecholamine excess were developed in 5.2% and 0.4% patients, respectively. More importantly hyperaldosteronism and malignant transformation were never observed till the end of follow-up of 49 months.[60]

CLINICAL PEARLS

- All patients found to have an AI should undergo clinical, biochemical, and imaging examinations to determine an excess of adrenal hormones or malignant potential.
- An ONDST and plasma or urinary metanephrines are recommended for all AIs while ARR is recommended in presence of hypertension and hypokalemia.
- Until proven otherwise, AIs of size <4 cm and HU <10 are benign.
- All functional and >4-cm AI should be surgically removed.
- Washout CT, MRI, and FDG-PET may be recommended in case of indeterminate adrenal nodules (size ≤ 4 cm, heterogeneous, irregular, and HU > 10).
- Nonfunctional ≤ 4 cm AI should be followed up with yearly hormonal and imaging evaluation till 5 years.
- Laparoscopic or retroperitoneoscopic adrenalectomy is the preferred surgical approach.
- Steroid administration is needed before and after adrenalectomy for cortisol-producing adrenal adenomas until the hypothalamus-pituitary-adrenal axis has recovered.
- To prevent perioperative cardiovascular complications, 7–14 days of preoperative α-blocker therapy is recommended to all patients with PCC.

Flowchart 4: Algorithm on the management of patients with adrenal incidentalomas.

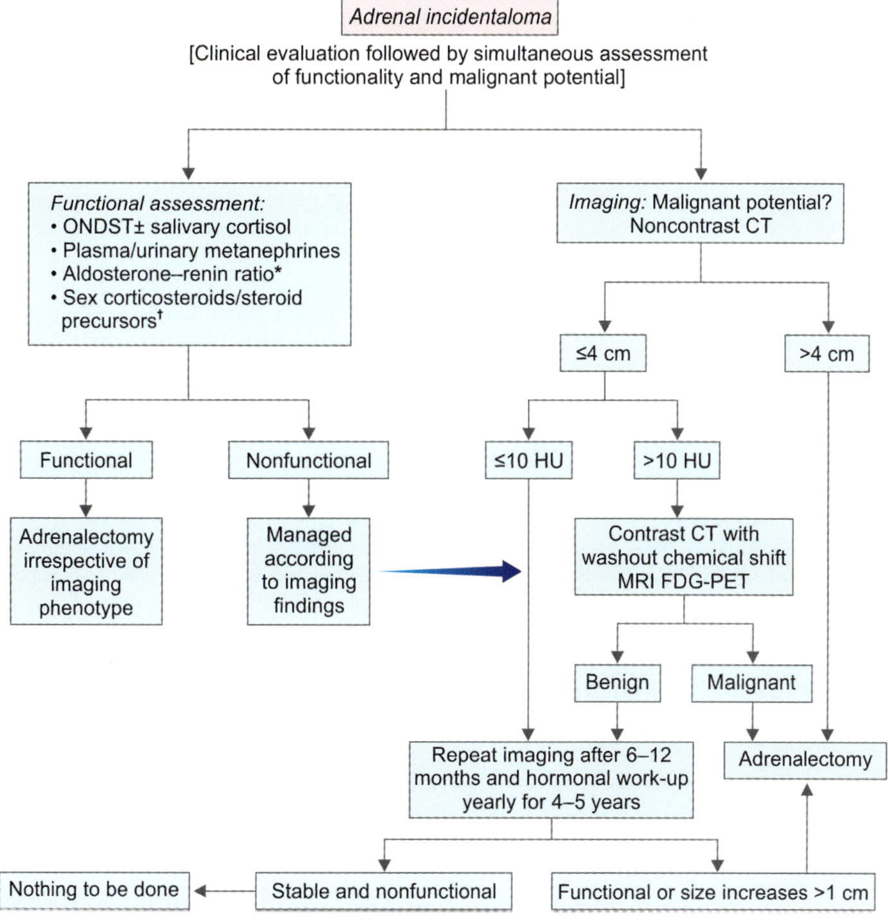

*Indicated in case of concomitant hypertension and/or hypokalemia.
†Indicated in case of clinical or radiological suspicion of adrenal carcinoma.
(CT: computed tomography; FDG-PET: fluorodeoxyglucose-positron emission tomography; MRI: magnetic resonance imaging)

◇| REFERENCES

1. Geelhoed GW, Druy EM. Management of the adrenal "incidentaloma". Surgery. 1982;92(5):866-74.
2. Vassiliadi DA, Tsagarakis S. Endocrine incidentalomas: challenges imposed by incidentally discovered lesions. Nat Rev Endocrinol. 2011;7(11):668-80.
3. National Institutes of Health. NIH State-of-the-science Statement on Management of the Clinically Inapparent Adrenal Mass ("incidentaloma"). NIH Consens State Sci Statements. 2002;19(2):1-25.
4. Shen WT. "Operating on Shadows" The discovery and naming of adrenal "incidentaloma". In: Zeiger MA, Shen WT, Felger EA (Eds). The Supreme Triumph of the Surgeon's Art: a narrative History of Endocrine Surgery. San Francisco, CA: University of California Medical Humanities Press; 2013.
5. Prinz RA, Brooks MH, Churchill R, Graner JL, Lawrence AM, Paloyan E, et al. Incidental asymptomatic adrenal masses detected by computed tomographic scanning. Is operation required? JAMA. 1982;248(6):701-4.
6. Black WC, Welch HG. Advances in diagnostic imaging and overestimations of disease prevalence and the benefits of therapy. N Engl J Med. 1993;328(17):1237-43.
7. Kokko JP, Brown TC, Berman MM. Adrenal adenoma and hypertension. Lancet. 1967;1(7488):468-70.
8. Hedeland H, Ostberg G, Hökfelt B. On the prevalence of adrenocortical adenomas in an autopsy material in relation to hypertension and diabetes. Acta Med Scand. 1968;184(3):211-4.
9. Herrera MF, Grant CS, van Heerden JA, Sheedy PF, Ilstrup DM. Incidentally discovered adrenal tumors: an institutional perspective. Surgery. 1991;110:1014-21.
10. Reimondo G, Castellano E, Grosso M, Priotto R, Puglisi S, Pia A, et al. Adrenal incidentalomas are tied to increased risk of diabetes: findings from a prospective study. J Clin Endocrinol Metab. 2020;105(4):dgz284.
11. Kobayashi S, Iwase H, Matsuo K, Fukuoka H, Ito Y, Masaoka A. Primary adrenocortical tumors in autopsy records: a survey of "Cumulative Reports in Japan" from 1973 to 1984. Jpn J Surg. 1991;21:494-8.
12. Caplan RH, Strutt PJ, Wickus GG. Subclinical hormone secretion by incidentally discovered adrenal masses. Arch Surg. 1994;129(3):291-6.
13. Goh Z, Phillips I, Hunt PJ, Soule S, Cawood TJ. Characteristics of adrenal incidentalomas in a New Zealand centre. Intern Med J. 2018;48(2):173-8.
14. Mantero F, Terzolo M, Arnaldi G, Osella G, Masini AM, Alì A, et al. A survey on adrenal incidentaloma in Italy. Study Group on Adrenal Tumors of the Italian Society of Endocrinology. 2000;85(2):637-44.

15. Comlekci A, Yener S, Ertilav S, Secil M, Akinci B, Demir T, et al. Adrenal incidentaloma, clinical, metabolic, follow-up aspects: single centre experience. Endocrine. 2010;37(1):40-6.

16. Song JH, Chaudhry FS, Mayo-Smith WW. The incidental adrenal mass on CT: prevalence of adrenal disease in 1,049 consecutive adrenal masses in patients with no known malignancy. Am J Roentgenol. 2008;190(5):1163-8.

17. Kasperlik-Załuska AA, Otto M, Cichocki A, Rosłonowska E, Słowińska-Srzednicka J, Jeske W, et al. Incidentally discovered adrenal tumors: a lesson from observation of 1,444 patients. Horm Metab Res. 2008;40(5):338-41.

18. Foti G, Malleo G, Faccioli N, Guerriero A, Furlani L, Carbognin G. Characterization of adrenal lesions using MDCT wash-out parameters: diagnostic accuracy of several combinations of intermediate and delayed phases. Radiol Med. 2018;123(11): 833-40.

19. Ahn SH, Kim JH, Baek SH, Kim H, Cho YY, Suh S, et al. Characteristics of adrenal incidentalomas in a large, prospective computed tomography-based multicenter study: the COAR study in Korea. Yonsei Med J. 2018;59(4):501-10.

20. Sangwaiya MJ, Boland GW, Cronin CG, Blake MA, Halpern EF, Hahn PF. Incidental adrenal lesions: accuracy of characterization with contrast-enhanced washout multidetector CT—10-minute delayed imaging protocol revisited in a large patient cohort. Radiology. 2010;256:504-10.

21. Hammarstedt L, Muth A, Wangberg B, Björneld L, Sigurjónsdóttir HA, Götherström G, et al. Adrenal lesion frequency: a prospective, cross sectional CT study in a defined region, including systematic reevaluation. Acta Radiol. 2010;51:1149-56.

22. Kim HY, Kim SG, Lee KW, Seo JA, Kim NH, Choi KM, et al. Clinical study of adrenal incidentaloma in Korea. Korean J Intern Med. 2005;20:303-9.

23. Kebebew E, Siperstein AE, Clark OH, Duh QY. Results of laparoscopic adrenalectomy for suspected and unsuspected malignant adrenal neoplasms. Arch Surg. 2002;137(8): 948-53.

24. Terzolo M, Stigliano A, Chiodini I, Loli P, Furlani L, Arnaldi G, et al. AME position statement on adrenal incidentaloma. Eur J Endocrinol. 2011;164:851-70.

25. Fassnacht M, Arlt W, Bancos I, Dralle H, Newell-Price J, Sahdev A, et al. Management of adrenal incidentalomas: European Society of Endocrinology clinical practice guideline in collaboration with the European Network for the Study of Adrenal Tumors. Eur J Endocrinol. 2016;175(2):G1-G34.

26. Zeiger MA, Thompson GB, Duh QY, Hamrahian AH, Angelos P, Elaraj D, et al. The American Association of Clinical Endocrinologists and American Association of Endocrine Surgeons medical guidelines for the management of adrenal incidentalomas. Endocr Pract. 2009;15(5):1-20.

27. Caoili EM, Korobkin M, Francis IR, Cohan RH, Platt JF, Dunnick NR, et al. Adrenal masses: characterization with combined unenhanced and delayed enhanced CT. Radiology. 2002;222:629-33.

28. Nieman LK. Approach to the patient with an adrenal incidentaloma. J Clin Endocrinol Metab. 2010;95:4106-13.

29. Mansmann G, Lau J, Balk E, Rothberg M, Miyachi Y, Bornstein SR. The clinically inapparent adrenal mass: update in diagnosis and management. Endocr Rev. 2004;25:309-40.

30. Findling JW, Raff H. Newer diagnostic techniques and problems in Cushing's disease. Endocrinol Metab Clin North Am. 1999;28:191-210.

31. Findling JW, Raff H. Diagnosis and differential diagnosis of Cushing's syndrome. Endocrinol Metab Clin North Am. 2001;30:729-47.

32. Findling JW, Raff H. Cushing's syndrome: important issues in diagnosis and management. J Clin Endocrinol Metab. 2006;91:3746-53.

33. Arnaldi G, Angeli A, Atkinson AB, Bertagna X, Cavagnini F, Chrousos GP, et al. Diagnosis and complications of Cushing's syndrome: a consensus statement. J Clin Endocrinol Metab. 2003;88:5593-602.

34. Giordano R, Marinazzo E, Berardelli R, Picu A, Maccario M, Ghigo E, et al. Long-term morphological, hormonal, and clinical follow-up in a single unit on 118 patients with adrenal incidentalomas. Eur J Endocrinol. 2010;162(4):779-85.

35. Vassilatou E, Vryonidou A, Michalopoulou S, Manolis J, Caratzas J, Phenekos C, et al. Hormonal activity of adrenal incidentalomas: results from a long-term follow-up study. Clin Endocrinol (Oxf). 2009;70(5):674-9.

36. Lenders JW, Pacak K, Walther MM, Linehan WM, Mannelli M, Friberg P, et al. Biochemical diagnosis of pheochromocytoma: which test is best? JAMA. 2002;287:1427-34.

37. Montori VM, Young WF Jr. Use of plasma aldosterone concentration-to-plasma renin activity ratio as a screening test for primary aldosteronism: a systematic review of the literature. Endocrinol Metab Clin North Am. 2002;31:619-32.

38. Young WF Jr. Management approaches to adrenal incidentalomas: a view from Rochester, Minnesota. Endocrinol Metab Clin North Am. 2000;29:159-85.

39. Weinberger MH, Fineberg NS. The diagnosis of primary aldosteronism and separation of two major subtypes. Arch Intern Med. 1993;153:2125-9.

40. Vincent JM, Morrison ID, Armstrong P, Reznek RH. The size of normal adrenal glands on computed tomography. Clin Radiol. 1994;49:453-5.

41. Boland GW, Lee MJ, Gazelle GS, Halpern EF, McNicholas MM, Mueller PR. Characterization of adrenal masses using unenhanced CT: an analysis of the CT literature. Am J Roentgenol. 1998;171(1):201-4.

42. Pena CS, Boland GW, Hahn PF, Lee MJ, Mueller PR. Characterization of indeterminate (lipidpoor) adrenal masses: use of washout characteristics at contrast-enhanced CT. Radiology. 2000;217(3):798-802.

43. Blake MA, Kalra MK, Sweeney AT, Lucey BC, Maher MM, Sahani DV, et al. Distinguishing benign from malignant adrenal masses: multidetector row CT protocol with 10-minute delay. Radiology. 2006;238:578-5.

44. Johnson PT, Horton KM, Fishman EK. Adrenal mass imaging with multidetector CT: pathologic conditions, pearls, and pitfalls. Radiographics. 2009;29(5):1333-51.

45. Patel J, Davenport MS, Cohan RH, Caoili EM. Can established CT attenuation and washout criteria for adrenal adenoma accurately exclude pheochromocytoma? AJR Am J Roentgenol. 2013;201(1):122-7.

46. Marin D, Boll DT, Mileto A, Nelson RC. State-of-the-art: dual-energy CT of the abdomen. Radiology. 2014;271(2): 327-42.

47. Platzek I, Sieron D, Plodeck V, Borkowetz A, Laniado M, Hoffmann RT. Chemical shift imaging for evaluation of adrenal masses: a systematic review and meta-analysis. Eur Radiol. 2019;29(2):806-17.

48. Semelka RC, Shoenut JP, Lawrence PH, Greenberg HM, Maycher B, Madden TP, et al. Evaluation of adrenal masses with gadolinium enhancement and fat-suppressed MR imaging. J Magn Reson Imaging. 1993;3:337-43.

49. Avram AM, Fig LM, Gross MD. Adrenal gland scintigraphy. Semin Nucl Med. 2006;36(3):212-27.

50. Bagheri B, Maurer AH, Cone L, Doss M, Adler L. Characterization of the normal adrenal gland with 18F-FDG PET/CT. J Nucl Med. 2004;45:1340-3.

51. Sundin A, Imaging of adrenal masses with emphasis on adrenocortical tumors. Theranostics. 2012:2;516-22.

52. Erasmus JJ, Patz Jr EF, McAdams HP, Murray JG, Herndon J, Coleman RE, et al. Evaluation of adrenal masses in patients with bronchogenic carcinoma using 18F-fluorodeoxyglucose positron emission tomography. Am J Roentgenol. 1997;168:1357-60.

53. Gupta NC, Graeber GM, Tamim WJ, Rogers JS, Irisari L, Bishop HA. Clinical utility of PET-FDG imaging in differentiation of benign from malignant adrenal masses in lung cancer. Clin Lung Cancer. 2001;3:59-64.

54. Kumar R, Xiu Y, Yu JQ, Takalkar A, El-Haddad G, Potenta S, et al. 18F-FDG PET in evaluation of adrenal lesions in patients with lung cancer. J Nucl Med. 2004;45:2058-62.

55. Sung YM, Lee KS, Kim BT, Choi JY, Chung MJ, Shim YM, et al. (18)F-FDG PET versus (18)F-FDG PET/CT for adrenal gland lesion characterization: a comparison of diagnostic efficacy in lung cancer patients. Korean J Radiol. 2008;9:19-28.

56. Brady MJ, Thomas J, Wong TJ, Franklin KM, Ho LM, Paulson EK. Adrenal nodules at FDG PET/CT in patients known to have or suspected of having lung cancer: a proposal for an efficient diagnostic algorithm. Radiology. 2009;250:523-30.

57. Metser U, Miller E, Lerman H, Lievshitz G, Avital S, Sapir E. 18F-FDG PET/CT in the evaluation of adrenal masses. J Nucl Med. 2006;47:32-7.

58. Osella G, Terzolo M, Borretta G, Magro G, Ali A, Piovesan A, et al. Endocrine evaluation of incidentally discovered adrenal masses (incidentalomas). J Clin Endocrinol Metab. 1994;79:1532-9.

59. Abrams HL, Spiro R, Goldstein N. Metastases in carcinoma: analysis of 1000 autopsied cases. Cancer. 1950;3:74-85.

60. Elhassan YS, Alahdab F, Prete A, Delivanis DA, Khanna A, Prokop L, et al. Natural history of adrenal incidentalomas with and without mild autonomous cortisol excess: a systematic review and meta-analysis. Ann Intern Med. 2019;171(2):107-16.

CHAPTER 31

Primary Hyperaldosteronism

Farheen Khan, Dileep Ramesh Hoysal, Sushohbhan Pradhan, Yuvraj Devgan, Sarah Idrees, Arjun Raja A, Amit Agarwal

"I plan to make a scientific report to you about a clinical syndrome, the investigation of which has been most exciting to Me."

–Dr Jerome W Conn
(At meeting of Central Society for Clinical Research, Chicago, Illinois, October 29, 1954)

◇ INTRODUCTION

Primary hyperaldosteronism (PHA) is the most frequent cause of secondary hypertension (HTN). It is characterized by inappropriately elevated aldosterone in setting of low plasma renin.[1] Initially, the predicted prevalence rate of PHA was reported as 0.5–1% of all hypertensive patients. However, it has now been proven that in approximately 10–20% of all patients with HTN, PHA is the underlying cause.[1]

◇ ETIOPATHOGENESIS

Normal Physiology

In order to understand the pathophysiology of PHA, one needs to revisit the normal physiology of aldosterone and its regulators. The renin–angiotensin system (RAS) is the primary regulator of aldosterone production. In states of volume depletion or decreased renal perfusion (e.g., renal artery stenosis), the juxtaglomerular apparatus cells in kidney release renin. Upon activation, renin cleaves angiotensinogen to angiotensin I in the liver, which is, in turn, converted to angiotensin II by angiotensin-converting enzyme (ACE) found in lungs. Binding of angiotensin II on its receptors on the zona glomerulosa in adrenal cortex causes depolarization of cell membrane potential, increased intracellular calcium, and, through these, induction of enzymatic machinery to synthesize aldosterone–aldosterone synthase[2] **(Flowchart 1)**. Aldosterone thus produced binds to its receptors in the distal nephrons and helps in sodium retention, in exchange for potassium, and volume expansion. The renin–angiotensin–aldosterone system (RAAS) is highly sensitive to dietary sodium intake. High plasma potassium also stimulates aldosterone production by potentiating angiotensin II. Adrenocorticotropic hormone (ACTH) transiently stimulates aldosterone synthesis as well[2] **(Fig. 1)**. The net effect of this entire physiology is that renin and aldosterone normally rise and fall in parallel.

◇ PATHOPHYSIOLOGY OF PRIMARY HYPERALDOSTERONISM

The hallmark of primary aldosteronism is autonomous secretion of aldosterone from adrenal glands, independent

Flowchart 1: Components of the renin–angiotensin system.

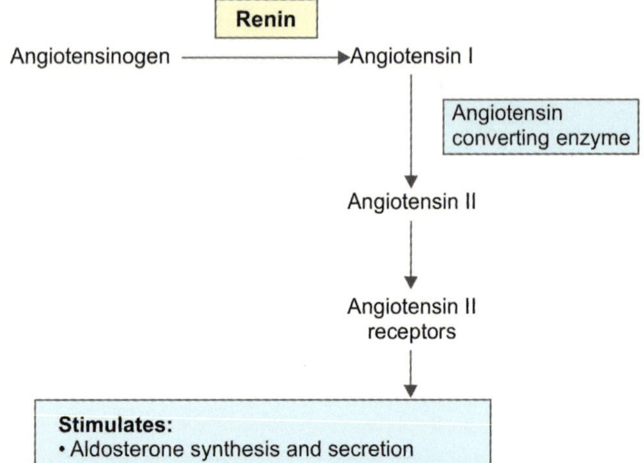

of its primary regulators: angiotensin II, hyperkalemia, and ACTH. Excess aldosterone causes suppression of renin and angiotensin II. Since angiotensin II is an important mediator of proximal nephron sodium reabsorption, suppression of angiotensin II results in greater sodium delivery to the distal nephron, thereby amplifying the aldosterone-driven sodium reabsorption and volume expansion as well as potassium and acid excretion. Thus, excess aldosterone has the following effects on normal physiology:

- Mineralocorticoid-induced expansion of plasma and extracellular fluid
- Increased total peripheral vascular resistance
- Sodium retention, increased excretion of potassium and hydrogen ions
- Release of norepinephrine and epinephrine from adrenal medulla

All these lead to HTN, hypokalemia, and metabolic alkalosis.[3] Patients with PHA are at an increased risk of myocardial infarction, atrial fibrillation, stroke, and renal damage, all attributable to the deleterious effects of excess aldosterone. Further aldosterone promotes cardiac and vascular fibrosis and tissue damage independent of blood pressure levels by augmenting expression of several collagen genes [transforming growth factor-β (TGF-β), plasminogen activator inhibitor (PAI)][4] **(Flowchart 2)**.

However, of particular note is the observation made in the Primary Aldosteronism Prevalence in Italy (PAPY) study, wherein >50% of patients with PHA were not found to be hypokalemic indicating that one of the classical signs of PHA is absent in majority of the cases. Hence, hypokalemia is not a "sine quo non" for searching a PHA.[4]

◇ CAUSES OF PRIMARY HYPERALDOSTERONISM

The causes of PHA can be simply classified as given in **Table 1**.[4]

All the above-mentioned conditions are caused due to excess/autonomous aldosterone production due to either somatic or germline mutations.

The mutations in PHA lead to abnormalities in the ion channels or pumps involved in mineralocorticoid signaling. The primary end-point of all mutations is increased intracellular calcium causing induction of CYP11B2 aldosterone synthase and subsequent autonomous aldosterone secretion. The underlying mechanisms leading to the activation of intracellular calcium signaling are, however, different and are discussed in **Table 2**.[5]

Development of Aldosterone-producing Adenoma[5]

Among surgically curable causes of PHA, aldosterone-producing adenoma (APA) is the most frequent cause.[6] Two hypotheses have been given for its development:

1. *Aldosterone-producing cell cluster (APCC) model*: APA-driven genes lead to formation of APCCs, which subsequently turn into APCC-to-APA translational lesions and ultimately APA development. This hypothesis is supported by the evidence that a subgroup of APCC has a similar metabolic profile to that of APA lesions.

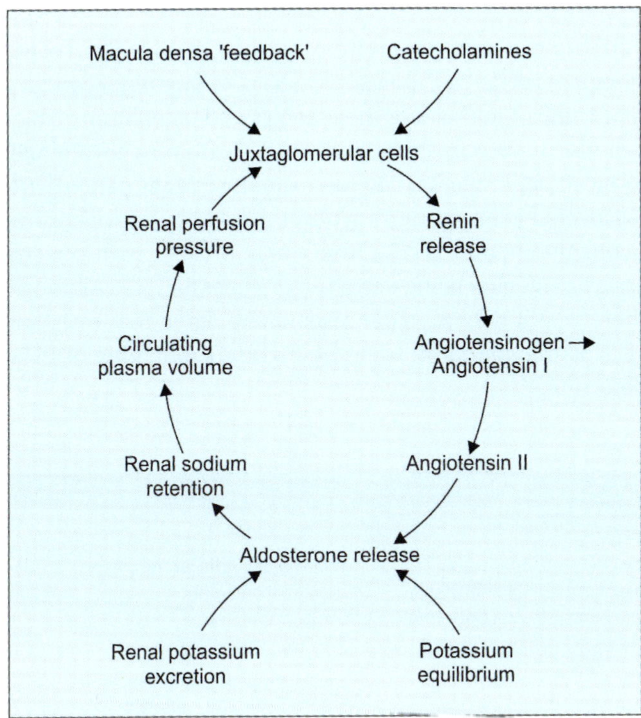

Fig. 1: Feedback loop of the Renin—Angiotensin—Aldosterone system. Aldosterone production is determined by each loop.

Flowchart 2: Sequence of events leading to increased risk of cardiovascular morbidities in PHA.

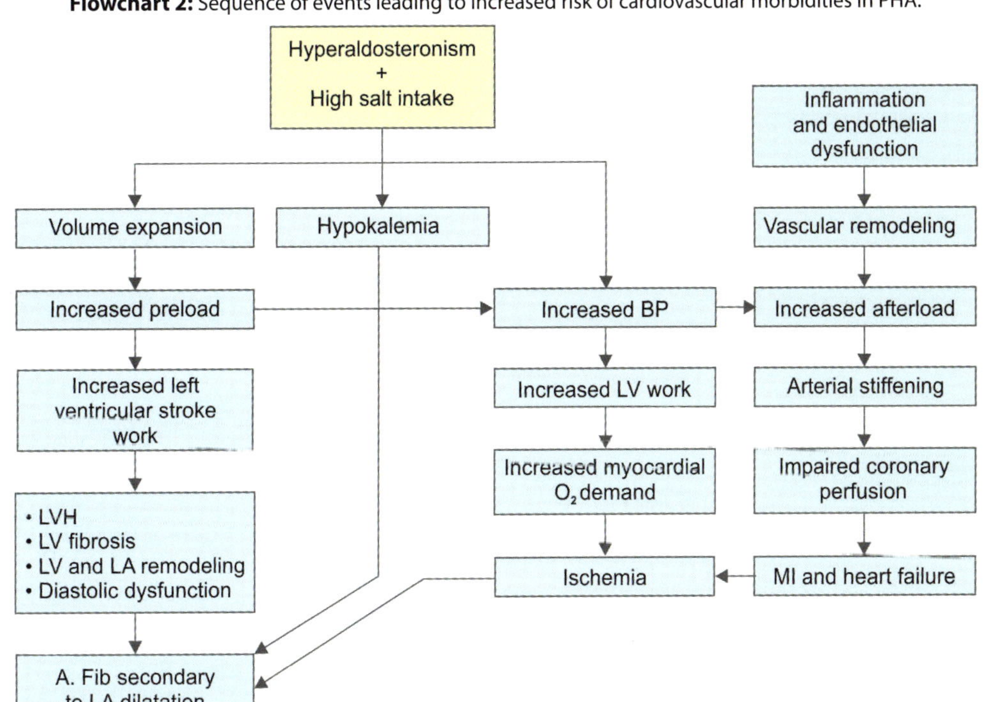

2. *Two-hit model*: Two consecutive events leading to abnormal proliferation create a prolific environment for occurrence of somatic mutations in APA-driver genes. Adrenal cortex remodeling or zona glomerulosa hyperplasia due to first-hit mutations may escalate into activation of Wnt-B catenin signaling (second hit) in the entire adrenal cortex and thus APA formation.

Improved understanding of the mechanisms leading to PHA has led to improved diagnostics and treatment strategies for PHA and shall be discussed subsequently.

CLINICAL PRESENTATION

Patients are asymptomatic often but may present with symptoms of fatigue, muscle weakness, cramping (secondary to wasting of potassium), headaches, and palpitations. They can also have polydipsia and polyuria from hypokalemia-induced nephrogenic diabetes insipidus.[1] Many patients are discovered to have Conn's syndrome as a result of persisting hypokalemia and HTN. Others may present with serious arrhythmias after being started on diuretics for HTN. Although there is still debate, most researchers agree that resistant HTN is the condition with the highest probability of PHA detection.[2,3]

Table 1: Classification of primary hyperaldosteronism based on management by surgery.

Curable by surgery	Not curable by surgery
Aldosterone-producing adenoma (unilateral or bilateral)	Bilateral adrenal hyperplasia
Primary micronodular unilateral adrenocortical hyperplasia	Unilateral aldosterone-producing adenoma or bilateral adrenal hyperplasia (aldosterone-producing cell clusters)
Ovary aldosterone-producing tumor	Familial hyperaldosteronism type I–V
Aldosterone-producing adenoma or bilateral adrenal hyperplasia with concomitant pheochromocytoma	
Aldosterone-producing teratoma	

Table 2: Underlying mechanisms leading to the activation of intracellular calcium signaling.

Germline mutations	Underlying abnormality	Disease developed
CYP11B1–CYP11B2 chimeric gene: *CYP11B1* encodes for cortisol production in zona fasciculata whereas *CYP11B2* encodes for aldosterone production in zona glomerulosa	Fusion of CYP11B1 with CYP11B2 leads to ectopic expression of CYP11B2 throughout the adrenal cortex (instead of only zona glomerulosa). Excess aldosterone synthesis with inappropriate regulation by ACTH	• Familial hyperaldosteronism type I • Autosomal dominant • Young-onset HTN
CLCN2 mutation—chloride channel	Sustained chloride efflux from cell causes stimulation of calcium signaling and thus induction of aldosterone synthase (CYP11B2)	• Familial hyperaldosteronism type II • >2 family members affected
KCNJ5 mutation—potassium channel	This gene codes for G-protein for potassium channel GIRK4. Loss of selectivity for potassium causes depolarization and calcium influx	• Familial hyperaldosteronism type III • Severe early onset HTN
CACNA1H	Affects T-type voltage-dependent calcium channel	Familial hyperaldosteronism type IV
CACNA1D	Affects voltage-dependent L-type calcium channel subunit	• PASNA—Primary hyperaldosteronism (PHA) • Seizures • Neurological abnormalities
Somatic mutations		
• *Aldosterone-producing adenoma (APA):*		
KCNJ5	Loss of potassium channel selectivity	Most frequent mutation found in APA, >40%
CACNA1D	Affects voltage-dependent L-type calcium-channel subunit	Most frequent mutation in African–Americans with APA
ATPases *ATP1A1* *ATP2B3*	Mutation in Na–K ATPase causing loss of pump activity and decreased affinity for potassium	
CTNNB1		In 2–5% of APAs
PRKACA	Mutation involving sarcoplasmic reticulum calcium channel	
• *Micronodular adrenal glands with APA*	Different micronodules within the same gland may have different mutations	
• *Aldosterone-producing cell clusters (APCC): Groups of aldosterone expressing cells found in normal adrenal glands*	*CACNA1D, ATP1A1*, and *KCNJ5* mutations involved	Precursor to APA

(ACTH: adrenocorticotropic hormone; APA: aldosterone-producing adenoma; HTN: hypertension)

Periodic paralysis as a presentation of PHA is commonly reported among the oriental races. In a series of 50 patients with PHA from Taiwan, 42% presented with periodic paralysis, although all 50 had hypokalemia.[7]

Physical Findings

- Hypertension
- Abdominal distension
- Ileus associated with hypokalemia
- Hypertension-associated bruits, altered mental status, and retinopathy

Primary hyperaldosteronism is now known to be the most common cause of secondary HTN, with a prevalence of 20% among patients with resistant HTN,[4,5] 10% in those with severe HTN [systolic blood pressure (SBP) $\geq$ 180 mm Hg, diastolic blood pressure $\geq$110 mm Hg],[6,7] and 6% in those with otherwise uncomplicated HTN.

The prevalence of target organ damage to the heart and kidney is increased in patients with PHA compared to those with essential HTN.[8-10] Long-standing undiagnosed PHA frequently leads to chronic kidney disease.[8,9] In a recent meta-analysis of 31 studies, including 3,838 patients with PHA and 9,284 patients with essential HTN, patients with APA and IHA had an increased risk of stroke [odds ratio (OR) 2.58], coronary artery disease (OR 1.77), atrial fibrillation (OR 3.52), and heart failure (OR 2.05).[10] In addition, the diagnosis of PHA increased the risk of diabetes (OR 1.33), metabolic syndrome (OR 1.53), and left ventricular (LV) hypertrophy (OR 2.29).[10] Thus, the cardiovascular toxicity in PHA extends beyond HTN; there is an aldosterone-specific toxicity.

The hypokalemia occurs in only 30–40% of cases of primary aldosteronism. Clinical manifestations resulting from hypokalemia in Conn's syndrome are most often moderate and potentially reversible.

Patients suffer rarely from neuromuscular symptoms, including mild muscle weakness, uncontrolled contractions, and paresthesias. In rare cases, hypokalemia caused by PHA may be profound enough to induce rhabdomyolysis. Involvement of respiratory muscles or cardiac arrhythmia due to hypokalemia can result in life-threatening consequences.[3]

Other rare presentations include neurological complications presenting with seizure and coma metabolic myopathy with rhabdomyolysis, potentially due to severe hypokalemia,[12] presenting with subarachnoid hemorrhage complicated by severe HTN. It is important to note that Conn's syndrome is not associated with edema because of spontaneous natriuresis.[17]

◇ EVALUATION OF HYPERALDOSTERONISM

Primary aldosteronism now is considered the most common form of secondary HTN, and the most common cause of potentially correctable HTN.

Initially thought to have a prevalence of 1% in hypertensive patients, with increased screening, it is now thought to affect 7–12% of patients with HTN.

Although primary aldosteronism is still a considerable diagnostic challenge, recognizing the condition is critical because primary aldosteronism-associated HTN can often be optimally controlled with the proper surgical or medical intervention.

Indications of screening for hyperaldosteronism:
- Finding of hypokalemia and HTN (spontaneous or diuretic induced)
- Treatment-resistant HTN (three hypertensive drugs and poor control)
- Severe HTN [patients with Joint National Commission stage 2 (>160–179/100–109 mm Hg), stage 3 (>180/110 mm Hg)]
- Hypertension and incidental adrenal mass
- Onset of HTN at a young age
- Hypertension and a family history of early onset HTN or cerebrovascular accident at a young age (<40 years)
- Workup for secondary HTN evaluation (i.e., when testing for renovascular disease and pheochromocytoma)
- Hypertensive first-degree relatives of patients with PHA

The diagnosis is generally three-tiered, involving an initial screening, a confirmation of the diagnosis, and a determination of the specific subtype of primary aldosteronism. However, according to studies by Zarnegar et al., the combination of plasma aldosterone concentration (PAC)/plasma renin activity (PRA) ratio and computed tomography (CT) imaging (if adrenal tumor >1 cm) alone is highly sensitive for the diagnosis of hyperaldosteronism, and confirmatory subtype tests are necessary only if any of those tests are equivocal.

Screening (First-Tier) Tests

Serum Potassium and Bicarbonate Levels

- Hypokalemia (serum potassium level <3.6 mEq/L) has a sensitivity of 75–80% while the patient is on a normal sodium diet.[6]
- Mild metabolic alkalosis (serum bicarbonate level >31 mEq/L) and inappropriate kaliuresis (urinary potassium excretion >30 mmol/day)

Sodium and Magnesium Levels

Mild serum hypernatremia in the 143–147 mEq/L range and mild hypomagnesemia from renal magnesium wasting are other associated biochemical findings in established primary aldosteronism.

Plasma Aldosterone Concentration/Plasma Renin Activity Ratio[11]

Because the random plasma aldosterone/PRA ratio is fairly constant over many physiologic conditions, it can be used for screening. This is the most frequently used test and considered the standard screening test for determining PHA biochemically.

This ratio should be measured in the morning (8–10 am) and may be performed while the patient is taking most anti-hypertensive medications and without postural stimulation.

Medication interference: The plasma aldosterone/PRA ratio should not be calculated when the patient is taking medications that can interfere with this measurement.[19] Spironolactone, an aldosterone receptor antagonist and high-dose amiloride, should be stopped for 6 weeks prior to testing. Eplerenone, another aldosterone receptor antagonist, can also interfere with testing and should be stopped for at least 2 weeks before testing.

Alpha-blockers, such as doxazosin, do not interfere with the plasma aldosterone concentration/PRA ratio. Beta-blockers and calcium-channel blockers do not affect the diagnostic accuracy of the ratio in most cases.[2]

However, if renin remains suppressed despite these medications, the renin, aldosterone, and aldosterone-to-renin ratio (ARR) remain valid and interpretable, and, therefore, testing while on these medications is reasonable **(Table 3)**.

Primary hyperaldosteronism should be suspected if:
- The PAC is elevated and the PRA is suppressed.

Secondary hyperaldosteronism (i.e., renal artery stenosis) should be suspected if:
- Both PAC and PRA are increased

Alternate sources of mineralocorticoid receptor (MR) agonism (i.e., hypercortisolism) should be suspected if:
- Both PAC and PRA are suppressed

Lack of uniformity in diagnostic protocols and assay methods for ARR measurement has been associated with substantial variability in cut-off values used by different groups ranging from 20 to 100.

Based on various studies, an ARR of >20–40 with a minimum aldosterone value of 15 ng/dL is recommended when testing is performed in the morning on a seated ambulatory patient.

Some authors argue that having a minimum aldosterone value requirement would exclude 15–20% of patients with PHA.

The minimum aldosterone level is recommended to ensure that patients with low-renin HTN are excluded to avoid falsely elevated ARR.

An ARR of at least 35 has been shown to have a sensitivity of 100% and specificity of 92.3% for the diagnosis of PHA.

Confirmatory (Second-Tier) Tests

There are certain instances in practice where confirmatory testing is not always performed. An example of this would be in a patient with spontaneous hypokalemia who has undetectable plasma renin with PAC >20 ng/dL (550 pmol/L). This is most likely PHA, and confirmatory testing is not necessary.

Table 3: Effects of antihypertensive drugs on the renin–angiotensin system.

Medication class	Plasma renin activity	Aldosterone levels
Diuretics (hydrochlorthiazide, furesemide)	Decreased	Increased
Angiotensin receptor blockers	Increased	Decreased
Beta-blockers (metoprolol, labetolol, propranolol)	Decreased	Decreased
Alpha-blockers (prazosin, doxazosin, terazosin)	No effect	No effect
Vasodilators (minoxidil, SNP)	No effect	No effect
Calcium-channel blockers	Increased or no effect	Decreased
ACE-I	Increased	Decreased

(ACE: angiotensin-converting enzyme)

Confirmatory tests are based on the concept that aldosterone is secreted in an unregulated fashion in primary aldosteronism and, therefore, cannot be suppressed by usual physiologic regulatory inputs. In a similar fashion, the PRA is chronically and tonically suppressed and cannot be stimulated.

The four main recommended confirmatory tests are as follows:

1. *Oral sodium loading test*: Patients are instructed to consume an approximately 4–6 g sodium diet for 3–4 days (with or without sodium chloride tablets). Additional potassium supplementation is also commonly required due to an increase in kaliuresis. On the final day of the diet, a 24-hour urine specimen is collected. A 24-hour urine aldosterone excretion of >10–12 µg in the setting of 24-hour urine sodium excretion of >200 mEq is diagnostic of PHA. This test is not recommended in patients with severe uncontrolled HTN, renal insufficiency, cardiac arrhythmia, or severe hypokalemia.

2. *Intravenous salt loading test*: The patient stays in a recumbent position/sitting an hour before and during the infusion of 2 L of 0.9% saline over 4 hours in the morning. Renin, aldosterone, cortisol, and potassium are drawn at time 0 and after 4 hours. Blood pressure and heart rate are monitored throughout the test. A postinfusion aldosterone <5 ng/dL (140 pmol/L) makes PHA less likely and levels >10 ng/dL (280 nmol/L) makes PHA more likely. Values between 5 and 10 ng/dL are intermediate. This test is also contraindicated in patients with severe uncontrolled HTN, renal insufficiency, cardiac arrhythmia, or severe hypokalemia.

3. *Fludrocortisone suppression test*: Patients receive fludrocortisone 0.1 mg every 6 hours for 4 days together with sodium and potassium supplementation. On day 4, serum cortisol is measured at 7 am, while serum aldosterone (S-Aldo), PRA, and cortisol are measured at 10 am with the patient in a seated position. A S-Aldo >6 ng/dL with a

PRA <1.0 ng/mL/h and a 10 am serum cortisol less than the 7 am value is diagnostic of primary aldosteronism.

4. *Captopril challenge test*: Individuals are given 25–50 mg of captopril after sitting or standing for at least 1 hour. S-Aldo and PRA are measured at time zero and at 1 and 2 hours after captopril administration, with the patient remaining seated during this period. S-Aldo will be suppressed in normal individuals; however, in primary aldosteronism, aldosterone will remain elevated and PRA will remain suppressed. Many different diagnostic thresholds have been proposed. A less than 30% suppression of aldosterone from baseline while PRA remains suppressed confirms primary aldosteronism.

Determination of Primary Aldosteronism Subtype (Third-Tier) Tests

Once the diagnosis of primary aldosteronism has been confirmed by a first- or second-tier test, the next step is to determine the subtype of primary aldosteronism and to identify surgically curable disease. For practical purposes, this means distinguishing between an adrenal adenoma and idiopathic adrenal hyperplasia (IAH).

Postural Stimulation Test

With upright posture, a rise in plasma aldosterone occurs in cases of IAH but not in aldosterone-producing adrenocortical adenoma/APA (Conn's syndrome).

Aldosteronomas are associated with an anomalous decrease in the aldosterone level with upright posture, in contrast to patients with IAH, in whom a RAS-mediated increase in aldosterone level occurs with upright posture.

Similarly, a S-Aldo level surge occurs in patients with renin-responsive adenomas (RRAs), low-renin essential HTN, and very rare cases of unilateral adrenal hyperplasia (the latter presenting with features intermediate between IAH and aldosterone-producing adrenal adenoma, occasionally designated as "intermediate aldosteronism").[10]

When abdominal CT and magnetic resonance imaging (MRI) scans are combined with postural stimulation, the positive-predictive value (PPV) of an abnormal postural test in predicting surgically correctable primary aldosteronism due to a single adenoma is 98%.

The standard postural test protocol involves obtaining baseline values for S-Aldo and PRA levels, as well as these levels 2 hours after the patient has assumed an erect posture. S-Aldo levels typically rise in this setting at least 50% above baseline in healthy persons, in persons with essential HTN, and in the subgroup of patients with primary aldosteronism who have either IAH or RRAs.

Among patients with aldosteronomas (APAs), S-Aldo levels typically do not rise or paradoxically fall to this level. The sensitivity and specificity of this test in the differential diagnosis of the main causes of primary aldosteronism have been reported to be as high as 80–85%.

Furosemide (Lasix) Stimulation Test

This test is often combined with the upright posture test. A typical test involves the oral administration of 40 mg of furosemide the night before as well as the morning of the test. On the morning of the test, after the furosemide dose has been administered, the patient remains upright 2–3 hours; then, S-Aldo and PRA levels are assayed.

Normally, furosemide stimulates PRA within 4 hours because of natriuresis and so produces an increase in the aldosterone level of at least 50% from the baseline in healthy individuals. Failure to do so is suggestive of PH.

Diurnal Rhythm of Aldosterone

The circadian rhythm of aldosterone secretion in healthy individuals parallels that of cortisol and is corticotropin dependent. The lowest values are observed around 11:30 pm to midnight, and the highest values occur early in the morning around 7:30–8:00 am (assuming a normal sleep–wake cycle). While this is preserved in patients with aldosteronomas, it is typically lost in patients with IAH.

Elevated levels of 18-OH corticosterone and/or 18-OH cortisol in plasma and urine may be found in some patients with aldosteronomas but are uncommon in IAH.

Localization

It should be kept in mind that reliance on cross-sectional imaging to determine laterality is not widely recommended and can be misleading.

CT Scanning

The initial radiologic investigation in the workup of primary aldosteronism is high-resolution, thin-sliced (2–2.5 mm) adrenal CT scanning with contrast **(Fig. 2)**.

Aldosteronomas tend to be small, in contrast to cortisol-producing adrenocortical adenomas; only aldosteronomas that are at least 1 cm in diameter can be detected reliably and consistently.

The overall sensitivity of high-resolution, thin-slice adrenal CT scanning is >90%, but the picture is complicated by the many false-positive findings associated with incidentalomas, which are reported in some series to be found in up to 10–15% of the general population (their prevalence increases with age).

Moreover, high-resolution CT studies can actually be detrimental, because these scans often detect the hyperplasia accompanying adenomas and may result in a tendency to overdiagnose IAH. Similarly, because long-term adrenal hyperplasia is associated with pseudonodule and nodule formation, this radiographic picture may often be confused with the diagnosis of autonomous adenomas.

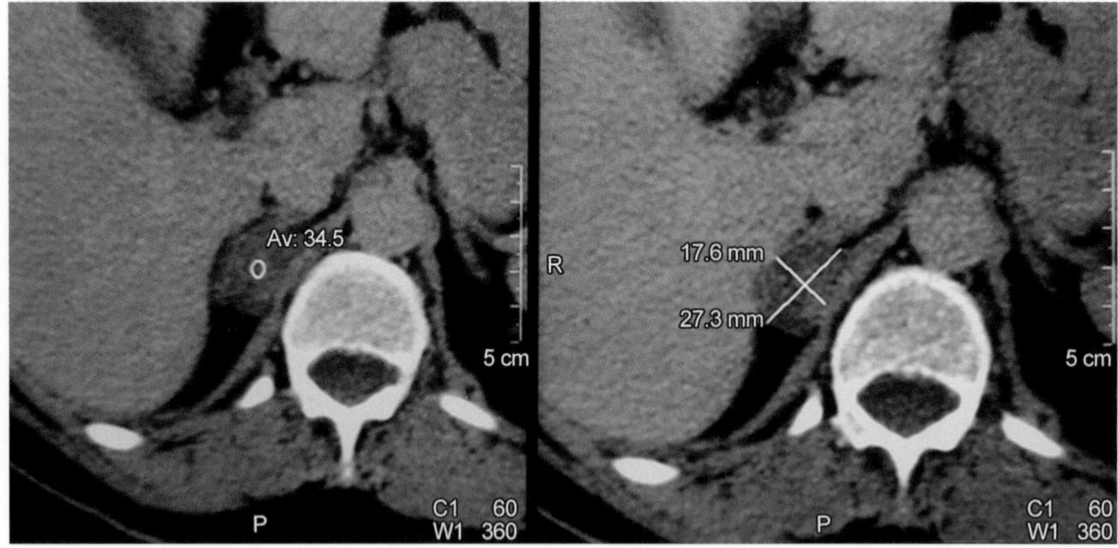

Fig. 2: Contrast-enhanced computed tomography (CECT) showing Conn's adenoma of right adrenal gland.

Some investigators suggest that when a solitary, unilateral macroadenoma (>1 cm) is detected with a suppressed opposite adrenal gland on a CT scan in a young patient (<35) in the setting of unequivocal aldosteronism, adrenal vein sampling (AVS) is not required and unilateral adrenalectomy is indicated.

However, because of the age-dependent risk that a solitary, unilateral adrenal macroadenoma may be a nonfunctioning adenoma, some experts believe that AVS[6] should be performed in patients >40 years.

Selective Adrenal Venous Sampling

Because this procedure is highly dependent on the availability of technically proficient interventional radiologists, it cannot (and should not) be performed universally, despite the fact that it is the criterion standard for the confirmation of lateralizable aldosterone excess.

Indications

- Indeed, adrenal venous sampling may be performed selectively only when preoperative imaging cannot definitively lateralize a presumed unilateral aldosteronoma.
- Adrenal venous sampling probably has its greatest utility when adrenal imaging findings are completely normal despite biochemical evidence for primary aldosteronism.
- Settings in which bilateral adrenal pathology is present on imaging and the biochemistry suggest the presence of a functional aldosteronoma.
- To resolve the exact etiology in cases of primary aldosteronism in which discordance exists between the biochemical findings and the radiologic findings with regard to whether the primary aldosteronism is due to IAH or an aldosteronoma

Technique

The adrenal veins are catheterized via a percutaneous femoral venous approach. The right and left venous catheters should be placed in the ipsilateral adrenal veins to prevent errors in handling the samples (Cannulation of the right adrenal vein is technically difficult because of the short length of this vessel. The left adrenal vein is longer, allowing for more stable catheter placement).

At baseline and following corticotropin stimulation (preferably by continuous infusion at 50 µg/hour for the duration of the sampling study), blood samples are obtained simultaneously from both adrenal veins and from the inferior vena cava, and the samples are assayed for aldosterone and cortisol.

In order to document the placement of the catheters within the adrenal veins, an adrenal-to-vena cava cortisol ratio (post corticotropin) is calculated; it should be >5–10.

Diagnosis

The accuracy of the test exceeds 95% when the procedure is technically successful. If autonomous, unilateral secretion of aldosterone is present on either side, the ratio of aldosterone concentrations between the right and left adrenal veins generally exceeds 10:1. False-positive results can occur when renal artery stenosis is present; hence, renal artery stenosis needs to be thoroughly excluded, especially before a highly invasive test is performed.

Most patients with a unilateral source of aldosterone have adrenal-to-adrenal aldosterone-to-cortisol ratios of >4. Ratios of <3 suggest hyperplasia, and values of 3–4 are considered indeterminate results.

Risks

Adrenal venous sampling is not without risks. Adrenal and iliac venous thrombosis, adrenal hemorrhage, adrenal insufficiency, or even major venous hemorrhage due to transmural tears and catheter dislocations are among the potential complications.

◇| MANAGEMENT OF CONN'S SYNDROME[12]

The overall treatment plan in patients with Conn's syndrome is to prevent the adverse outcomes associated with excess aldosterone such as HTN, hypokalemia, renal toxicity, and cardiovascular damage.

Subtypes of PHA:
- Bilateral idiopathic hyperaldosteronism or IAH 60–70%
- Unilateral APAs 30–40%
- Unilateral hyperplasia or primary adrenal hyperplasia (PAH) approximately 3%

Treatment goals:
- The overall treatment plan in patients with primary aldosteronism is to prevent the morbidity and mortality associated with HTN, hypokalemia, renal toxicity, and cardiovascular damage. Excessive secretion of aldosterone is associated with an increased risk of cardiovascular events (which are independent of hypokalemia), including an increase in LV mass measurements, stroke, myocardial infarction, heart failure, and atrial fibrillation.
- So, the goals of therapy for PHA due to either unilateral or bilateral adrenal disease include:
  - Reversal of the adverse cardiovascular effects of hyper-aldosteronism
  - Normalization of the serum potassium in patients with hypokalemia
  - Normalization of the blood pressure

Type of Therapy

Determination of the correct subtype diagnosis is essential since the treatment of PHA is based upon the cause. Once the correct subtype diagnosis is confirmed, the plan of management includes the following:
- For patients with unilateral disease, laparoscopic adrenalectomy is advised.
- For patients with bilateral idiopathic hyperaldosteronism, medical therapy is advised.

Medical Therapy

This involves restriction of intense dietary sodium intake (<50 mmol/day) and use of MRs. Lifelong MR antagonist therapy is recommended for patients with bilateral primary aldosteronism and in rare situations of unilateral primary aldosteronism patients who are unable to or unwilling to undergo surgical adrenalectomy. The two most common MR antagonists are spironolactone and eplerenone. Though spironolactone has approximately double the potency of eplerenone, it carries with it a risk for gynecomastia in men which may necessitate discontinuation of drug.

MR antagonists reduce HTN and improve potassium levels by decreasing epithelial sodium channel (ENaC)-mediated sodium reabsorption and consequent volume expansion and decrease potassium and hydrogen ion excretion. However, despite treatment with MR antagonists, patients with primary aldosteronism had a two-fold higher risk for developing myocardial infarction, heart failure hospitalization, stroke, atrial fibrillation, and chronic kidney disease compared with patients with essential HTN, despite similar blood pressure control.

Surgical Therapy

Surgical therapy in the form of unilateral laparoscopic adrenalectomy is indicated in the following situations:
- *Unilateral adenoma*: In this situation, it is curative.
- *Unilateral hyperplasia*: It can be curative.
- *Bilateral hyperplasia*: In cases of bilateral primary aldosteronism, where the disease is difficult to control with maximal doses of MR or where MR antagonist dosing is limited by side effects such as gynecomastia or hyperkalemia (e.g., in patients with coexisting chronic kidney disease), unilateral surgical adrenalectomy could reduce the amount of autonomous aldosterone secretion which can then become amenable to medical treatment.

Laparoscopic adrenalectomy (Fig. 3): Unilateral adrenalectomy shows a marked reduction in aldosterone secretion and correction of hypokalemia in almost all patients. HTN is improved in all and is cured in approximately 35–60% of patients. Laparoscopic adrenalectomy is preferred over open adrenalectomy because it is associated with shorter hospital stays and fewer complication **(Fig. 4)**. Resection of the entire adrenal gland is preferred over partial adrenalectomy.

Preoperative optimization: Preoperatively, HTN should be controlled, and hypokalemia should be corrected with potassium supplementation or a MR antagonist.

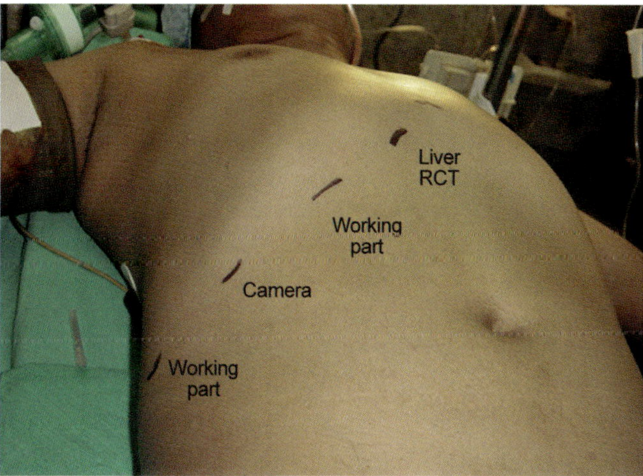

Fig. 3: Port positions in right laparoscopic adrenalectomy for Conn's adenoma.

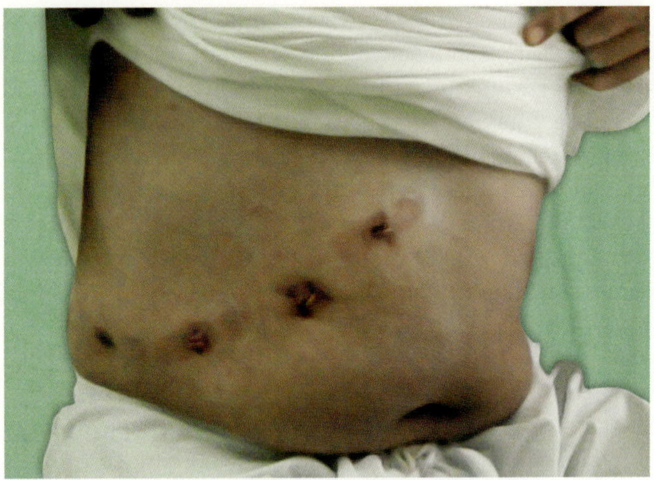

Fig. 4: Postoperative view of laparoscopic scars.

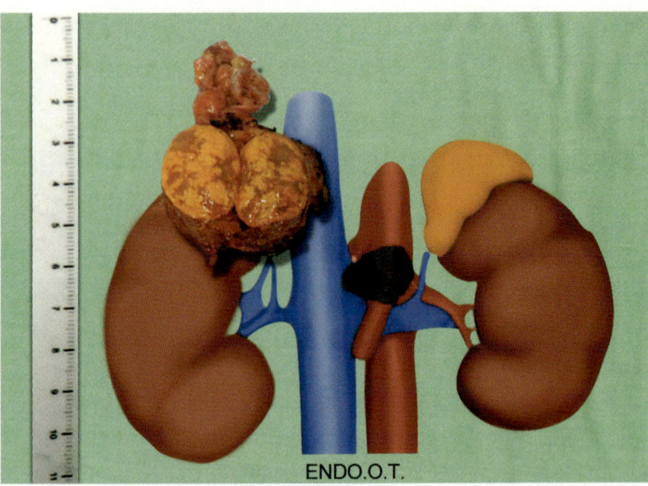

Fig. 5: Gross specimen of right adrenalectomy showing bright yellow Conn's adenoma.

Postoperative issues:[13] Plasma aldosterone is measured day after surgery to assess for cure. An undetectable plasma aldosterone concentration confirms correct preoperative subtype assignment and long-term cure. However, if the postoperative plasma aldosterone concentration is >5 ng/dL, the patient should be followed closely by monitoring daily home blood pressure measurements and weekly serum potassium concentrations. Re-evaluation for persistent hyperaldosteronism is indicated in those patients with either persistent hypokalemia or lack of blood pressure improvement postoperatively. Potassium supplements and mineralocorticoid receptor antagonists should be discontinued in all patients, and, if possible, antihypertensive therapy should be decreased. When patients are treated with multiple antihypertensive agents prior to surgery, postoperatively either discontinue or decrease the doses of those drugs that may predispose to hyperkalemia [e.g., ACE inhibitors and angiotensin II receptor blockers (ARBs)] and, if needed for blood pressure control, continue those that are potassium neutral (e.g., calcium-channel blockers). Postoperatively, patients should be monitored closely for hyperkalemia, which may result from transient hypoaldosteronism due to chronic suppression of renal renin release and contralateral adrenal gland aldosterone secretion. Serum potassium should be measured during the hospitalization and, subsequently as an outpatient, once weekly for 4 weeks. Serum creatinine should be followed serially in patients who had renal insufficiency preoperatively. Primary aldosteronism has been associated with renal toxicity and improvement of HTN corrects renal hyperfiltration and may unmask the pre-existing renal damage. The preferred intravenous fluid after surgery is isotonic saline without potassium (unless the patient is still hypokalemic), and a sodium-rich diet should be considered before and after discharge.[17]

Pathology: Grossly Conn's adenoma appear bright yellow **(Fig. 5)**. Microscopic appearance is of a nodule composed of cells with foamy cytoplasm and round nuclei.

◇ OUTCOMES[14,15]

Hypertension

Though HTN is cured in some patients, a small degree of HTN persists in as many as 40–65% of cases.

A number of factors help to identify patients who have more chances of resolution after adrenalectomy, which are:

- Shorter duration of HTN
- Lack of family history of HTN
- Preoperative use of two or fewer antihypertensive agents
- Younger age
- Higher preoperative ratio of plasma aldosterone concentration to PRA
- Higher urine aldosterone level

Persistent HTN may be related to underlying primary HTN and/or the development of nephrosclerosis after a prolonged period of uncontrolled HTN.

Hypokalemia

Hypokalemia resolves in almost 100% cases. The immediate postoperative plasma aldosterone concentration should be low. In maximum cases, aldosterone secretion from the remaining adrenal gland recovers over a couple of weeks as renal renin release recovers from chronic suppression. If preoperative hypokalemia was present, it resolves in a matter of days. The concern in the first several weeks after surgery is for hyporeninemic hypoaldosteronism and resultant hyperkalemia. Patients who have recurrent hypokalemia at any point following surgery should undergo formal re-evaluation.

Left Ventricular Mass

Though it is suggested that adrenalectomy is more effective than medical therapy for reduction of LV mass, a meta-analysis of four studies including 355 patients reported that while adrenalectomy was more effective than medical therapy for blood pressure reduction, both treatments had a similar effect on LV mass change.[16]

Quality of Life

The quality of life is low in patients with unilateral disease (APAs or unilateral hyperplasia) when compared with healthy individuals but improves to normal within 3–12 months of unilateral adrenalectomy. The improvement appears to be constant at 6 months. The quality of life is also improved by medical therapy but not to the level found in the general population.

◇| PROGNOSIS AND FOLLOW-UP

Hypokalemia and HTN related to PHA contribute to the morbidity and mortality. Chronic HTN can lead to complications such as myocardial infarction, cerebrovascular disease, and congestive heart failure. Cardiac exposure to chronic aldosteronism in itself irrespective of elevated blood pressure is associated with increased risk for cardiac injury—ischemic, hypertrophic, and fibrotic injury. Evidence shows that patients with primary aldosteronism are more likely to develop LV hypertrophy, stroke, and acute coronary syndromes than patients with similar degrees of HTN from other causes. Prevalence of cardiovascular disease is approximately 9.4% in patients with primary aldosteronism when compared to patients with essential HTN. The risk factors for cardiovascular disease in primary aldosteronism were found to include hypokalemia, unilateral primary aldosteronism, and plasma aldosterone levels at or above 125 pg/mL. HTN related to PHA also contributes to a spectrum of complications secondary to HTN such as nephropathy causing chronic renal failure and retinopathy.

Surgical removal of a unilateral source of aldosterone overproduction results in resolution of hypokalemia in 98–100% of patients and biochemical cure by normalization of aldosterone levels, in similar patient percentages. Only one-third of patients report complete resolution of HTN after adrenalectomy, while the majority of patients (75–98%) will see improvement in HTN with a reduction in the number of required antihypertensive agents.

The earlier the diagnosis is made, the better is the outcome in terms of cardiovascular damage, cardiorenal, and cerebrovascular events. In 2008, a study by Zarnegar et al.[17] proposed the aldosteronoma resolution score. In clinical practice, this score system uses four items to predict the likelihood of complete resolution of HTN after adrenalectomy.

This scoring system is an easy tool to advise patients of their probable outcomes before proceeding to surgery. Complete resolution of HTN postoperatively was achieved in 80% of patients with a score of four or five and in only 13.7% of patients with a score of zero or one. However, even without complete resolution, 98% of patients with a score of five have normalization of potassium and over 95% have improved blood pressure control. However, despite the scoring system, absence of vascular remodeling and/or renal chronic kidney disease is the strongest predictor of cure of HTN.

Studies show that negative end-organ effect of hyperaldosteronism is slowed down and sometimes even reversed 1-year postadrenalectomy. Cardiovascular risks in patients with PHA become equal to patients with essential HTN postadrenalectomy for APA. There is also reversal of ventricular hypertrophy, septal thickening, and myocardial fibrosis. Renal function shows improvement, with resolution of microalbuminuria and no difference in long-term progression of renal dysfunction from those with essential HTN.

In patients with Conn's adenoma who have undergone unilateral adrenalectomy, regular follow-up visits are advised. Adrenalectomy-induced correction of the hyperfiltration caused by hyperaldosteronism and hyperkalemia require monitoring and follow-up postoperatively. Follow-up visits with biochemical retesting are necessary, at least in the first 6 months.

◇| CLINICAL PEARLS

- Conn's syndrome should be suspected in a hypertensive patient who is having resistant hypertension with hypokalemia.
- In Asian countries spontaneous, periodic but reversible motor paralysis is a common presentation of primary hyperaldosteronism.
- Confirmatory tests are essential to differentiate the Conn's adenoma requiring surgery, from the bilateral idiopathic primary hyperaldosteronism which is a medical disease.
- Patients of Conn's syndrome who show a enlarged unilateral gland with suppressed contralateral adrenal gland on adrenal protocol CECT do not require adrenal venous sampling to confirm the laterality.
- A composite tumor (Conn's adenoma with Cushing's adenoma) should be suspected if the adenoma is more than 2 cm, suppressed ONDST, positive saline loading test)
- All patients of biochemically proven Conn's adenoma should be offered surgery because it reduces cardiovascular risk and resulting mortality in these patients.
- All patients of Conn's adenoma can be treated by laparoscopic or robotic approach.
- Postoperatively patients should be monitored closely for hyperkalemia, which may result from transient hypoaldosteronism.

◇| REFERENCES

1. Bobanga I, Bénay C, Krishnamurthy VD. Primary hyperaldosteronism (Conn's syndrome). In: Docimo Jr S, Pauli E (Eds). Clinical Algorithms in General Surgery. Cham: Springer; 2019.

2. Melmed, Shlomo, Williams RH. Williams Textbook of Endocrinology, 13th edition. Philadelphia: Elsevier/Saunders; 2016.

3. Jameson J. Harrison's Endocrinology, 4th edition. China: McGraw-Hill Education; 2016. pp. 119-23.

4. Rossi GP. Primary hyperaldosteronism. JACC. 2019;74(22): 2799-811.

5. Zennaro MC, Boulkroun S, Fernandes-Rosa FL. Pathogenesis and treatment of primary aldosteronism. Nat Rev Endocrinol. 2020;16(10):578-89.

6. Bernini G, Galetta F, Franzoni F, Bardini M, Taurino C, Bernardini M, et al. Arterial stiffness, intima-media thickness and carotid artery fibrosis in patients with primary aldosteronism. J Hypertens. 2008;26(12):2399-405.

7. Ma JT, Wang C, Lam KS, Yeung RT, Chan FL, Boey J, et al. Fifty cases of primary hyperaldosteronism in Hong Kong Chinese with a high frequency of periodic paralysis: evaluation of techniques for tumour localisation.QJ Med. 1986;61(235):1021-37.

8. Young WF, Primary aldosteronism: renaissance of a syndrome. Clin Endocrinol (Oxf). 2007;66(5):607.

9. Ohno Y, Sone M, Inagaki N, Yamasaki T, Ogawa O, Takeda Y, et al. Prevalence of cardiovascular disease and its risk factors in primary aldosteronism: a multicenter study in Japan. Hypertension. 2018;71(3):530-7.

10. Monticone S, D'Ascenzo F, Moretti C, Williams TA, Veglio F, Gaita F, et al. Cardiovascular events and target organ damage in primary aldosteronism compared with essential hypertension: a systematic review and meta-analysis. Lancet Diabetes Endocrinol. 2018;6(1):41.

11. Hundemer GL, Vaidya A. Primary aldosteronism diagnosis and management: a clinical approach. Endocrinol Metab Clin North Am. 2019;48(4):681-700.

12. Lee FT, Elaraj D. Evaluation and management of primary hyperaldosteronism. Surg Clin N Am. 2019;99:731-45.

13. Kim RM, Lee J, Soh EY. Predictors of resolution of hypertension after adrenalectomy in patients with aldosterone-producing adenoma. J Korean Med Sci. 2010;25(7):1041-4.

14. Quillo AR, Grant CS, Thompson GB, Farley DR, Richards ML, Young WF. Primary aldosteronism: results of adrenalectomy for nonsingle adenoma. J Am Coll Surg. 2011;213(1):106-12; discussion 12-3.

15. Proye CA, Mulliez EA, Carnaille BM, Lecomte-Houcke M, Decoulx M, Wémeau JL, et al. Essential hypertension: first reason for persistent hypertension after unilateral adrenalectomy for primary aldosteronism? Surgery. 1998;124:1128-33.

16. Marzano L, Colussi G, Sechi LA, Catena C. Adrenalectomy is comparable with medical treatment for reduction of left ventricular mass in primary aldosteronism: meta-analysis of long-term studies. Am J Hypertens. 2015;28(3):312-8.

17. Zarnegar R, Young WF Jr, Lee J, Sweet MP, Kebebew E, Farley DR, et al. The aldosteronoma resolution score: predicting complete resolution of hypertension after adrenalectomy for aldosteronoma. Ann Surg. 2008;247(3):511-8.

Adrenal Surgery and Cushing's Syndrome

MJ Paul, Aravindan Nair

INTRODUCTION

The evolution of adrenal surgery encompasses the medical developments in anatomy, physiology, genetics, imaging, and surgery. Scientific progress has helped physicians and surgeons to develop a degree of mastery over the mysterious behavior of tumors of this fascinating gland.

ANATOMICAL DISCOVERY

The adrenal glands were first described and illustrated in 1552 on copper plates by Bartholomaeus Eustachius, the Roman anatomist, who named them the "glandulae renibus incumbents" meaning "glands lying on the kidneys." Many others described additional features of black content and ducts until Riolan of Paris in 1629 introduced the term "capsulae suprarenales." The cortex and medulla were recognized only in the 19th century. The cortex was found to be of mesodermal origin and the medulla resembled nerve elements; it stained yellow or brown with potassium bichromate earning the term "pheochrome." Fragments of aberrant adrenal tissue were recognized in up to 90% of people and termed "paraganglia."[1,2]

FUNCTIONAL ELUCIDATION

Gulliver suggested in 1840 that they "poured a special matter into the blood." Thomas Addison reported 11 cases of debility and peculiar skin color in connection with a diseased condition of the suprarenal capsules including tuberculosis, metastatic cancer, and atrophy at autopsy. Armand Trousseau observed a similar finding in Paris and proposed the name "Addison's disease." Spurred by the report, the physiologist Brown Sequard in Paris performed animal experiments with adrenalectomy and suggested they were essential to life. In 1893, Oliver and Schafer in London prepared an extract of the suprarenals that produced a dramatic rise in blood pressure, constriction of the arterioles, and a forcible contraction of the heart when injected intravenously in dogs; the active principle was isolated later in 1897—"epinephrine" the term used in the American continent. The purified product was termed "adrenaline" in 1901 in Britain and was the first hormone to be discovered. A long search for cortical hormones moved from cortin (cortical extracts) in the 1930s to the first synthesized steroid deoxycorticosterone by Kendall

and Reichstein in 1937 before it was realized in 1940 that the cortex produced several hormones, two of which were essential to life—the glucocorticoid and mineralocorticoid.[3] By 1948, a few grams of cortisone produced spectacular results in rheumatoid arthritis and earned Kendall, Hench, and Reichstein a Nobel Prize in 1950. A simpler method of cortisone production emerged to meet the subsequent demand and changed the face of medicine forever. The potent mineralocorticoid was isolated and synthesized by Tait and co-workers in 1955 and named aldosterone, and further work resulted in the discovery of sex steroids. Synthetic steroids prednisolone, dexamethasone, and fludrocortisone were available for use by 1956.[1,2,4]

REPORTS OF ADRENAL TUMORS

Tumors and their syndromes were described only from late 19th century such as ganglioneuroma by Loretz in 1870, "medullary adenoma with chromaffin reaction" by Manasse in 1896, carcinoma of adrenal cortex with hirsutism and sexual precocity by Bulloch and Sequeira in 1905, paraganglioma by Alezais and Peyron in 1908, neuroblastoma by Wright in 1910, and pheochromocytoma by Pick in 1912. It was later in 1954 following the discovery of aldosterone that Jerome Conn described the syndrome of primary hyperaldosteronism.[1,2]

IMAGING OF ADRENAL TUMORS

In the 1930s, X-rays were used regularly to locate hyper-functioning adrenal masses that were suspected clinically. Plain radiographs and pyelograms suggested the presence of tumors till tomography became available. Lumbar retroperitoneal insufflation of gas was used to delineate the edge of adrenal tumors first in Europe in 1920. Early complications were reported, but the technique was improved using CO_2 and presacral insufflation with simultaneous pyelography remaining the best imaging technique for a period even up to the 1970s. Selective sampling of caval blood was used first in 1955 for catecholamines and later for steroids; phlebography was attempted but led to infarctions of the adrenal and was given up shortly. Aortography by the lumbar route to outline vascular tumors was used in the 1930s; selective angiography was used by the 1960s and refined later by subtraction images. All these invasive techniques required skill and experience, liable to cause bleeding, hypertensive crises, and rarely death.

Noninvasive imaging was introduced in the 1970s with scintigraphy of the adrenal cortex developed in 1970 when analogs of cholesterol were labeled with 131-I and concentrated by hyperplastic cortical tissue; they were not taken up by malignant or nonfunctioning tumors. Ultrasonography was applied to adrenal lesions in 1973 and was adopted widely because of the lack of ionizing radiation. Computed tomography was introduced in 1975 and adopted slowly because of the cost but became the best imaging modality. By the 1980s, radiologists were deluged with CT scans performed with low clinical suspicion producing many unsuspected adrenal tumors that we now label "adrenal incidentalomas." The CT density of <20 HU is a guide to the lipid-rich adenoma, which is the typical cortisol-producing lesion of the adrenal. Large tumors with enhancing solid periphery, necrotic areas, calcifications, and unclear planes raise the suspicion of carcinoma.

The modern imaging armamentarium includes magnetic resonance imaging (MRI) with T1/T2 weighting, gadolinium enhancement, and chemical shift characteristics to diagnose adenomas not typical on CT scan. The other large advancement was made in nuclear imaging techniques, especially with metaiodobenzylguanidine (MIBG tagged to 131-I) for functioning adrenal medullary tumors and positron emission tomography to fuse functional characteristics with structural detail of CT scanning.

◇| SURGICAL ANATOMY AND PHYSIOLOGY

The adrenal gland is composed of a cortex and medulla, each having a different embryological origin. The cortex is of mesodermal origin, arising from the coelomic epithelium in the 5th week of gestation and the medulla is of neurectodermal origin, arising from the neural crest at around the same time. The adrenal glands are situated atop the kidneys on their superomedial aspect lateral to the diaphragmatic crura. Each measures $50 \times 30 \times 10$ mm^3 and weighs 4–5 gm. The right adrenal gland is triangular and the left is crescentic. This dark golden yellow gland has a defined capsule and is supplied by multiple small branches from the inferior phrenic, renal artery, and direct branches from the aorta. These arterioles form a rich subcapsular plexus supplying the parenchyma— the venous drainage mainly via a single large adrenal vein. The right adrenal vein is short and drains directly into the inferior cava; the left adrenal vein drains into the left renal vein. The lymphatic vessels drain into the para-aortic, paracaval, and perirenal lymph nodes.

The cortex has three zones—glomerulosa, fasciculata, and reticularis (GFR)—from superficial to deep. The cortex constitutes 85% of the whole gland. Plasma cholesterol is the major source of substrate used for steroid synthesis.

Aldosterone produced by the zona glomerulosa is regulated by the renin–angiotensin system and potassium and sodium ion concentrations in the blood. Increased aldosterone production causes sodium retention, potassium loss, and increase in plasma volume. Adrenocorticotropic hormone (ACTH) has only a permissive role in aldosterone production. The zonae fasciculata and reticularis produce the glucocorticoids and the sex steroids. Production of cortisol is regulated through the hypothalamic–pituitary–adrenal axis. Synthesis of cortisol is normally completely regulated by ACTH. Glucocorticoid hormones are responsible for glycogen metabolism, peripheral glucose utilization, lipid metabolism, cells of the immune system, bone soft tissue, and mineral metabolism. In addition, they play a vital role in fluid, electrolyte homeostasis, and the nervous system. Dehydroepiandrosterone (DHEAS) and androstenedione are the prohormones of androgens that are produced in the adrenal cortex.

Like all endocrine glands, the adrenal gland can present with features of hypo- or hyperfunction.

Primary adrenal cortical deficiency is a medically treated condition, commonly known as Addison's disease, and is a result of disease process which destroys the adrenal cortex.[4] The more common causes include autoimmune adrenalitis, granulomatous diseases (tuberculosis, histoplasmosis, and sarcoidosis), metastatic deposits, or bilateral adrenal hemorrhage (due to coagulopathy or sepsis). Secondary deficiency is usually caused by pituitary hypofunction leading to decreased ACTH production most often caused by exogenous steroid therapy—surgical or radioablation. When corticotropin-releasing hormone (CRH) production from the hypothalamus is affected by brain tumors, irradiation, or sarcoidosis, the condition is referred to as tertiary adrenal insufficiency.

◇| CUSHING'S SYNDROME

Harvey Cushing's report in 1932 of a pituitary basophilic adenoma presenting with central obesity, cutaneous striae, osteoporosis, hypertensions, diabetes, and hirsutism first drew attention to this condition.[5] Cortisol is the adrenal glucocorticoid hormone that can be produced in response to ACTH stimulation from pituitary or elsewhere—autonomously from the adrenal. The most common cause of the syndrome seen in clinical practice is the secondary effect of exogenous steroid administration. The endogenous or primary causes of Cushing's syndrome may be classified thus as **(Flowchart 1)**:

- *ACTH-dependent causes:*
  - Pituitary-dependent Cushing's disease (up to 70%) **(Fig. 1)**
  - *Ectopic ACTH-producing tumors:*
    - Thymic and bronchial carcinoid tumors—indolent surgically correctible
    - Medullary carcinoma thyroid, pancreatic neuro-endocrine tumor (NET), and pheochromocytoma

Flowchart 1: Surgical management of endogenous Cushing's syndrome.

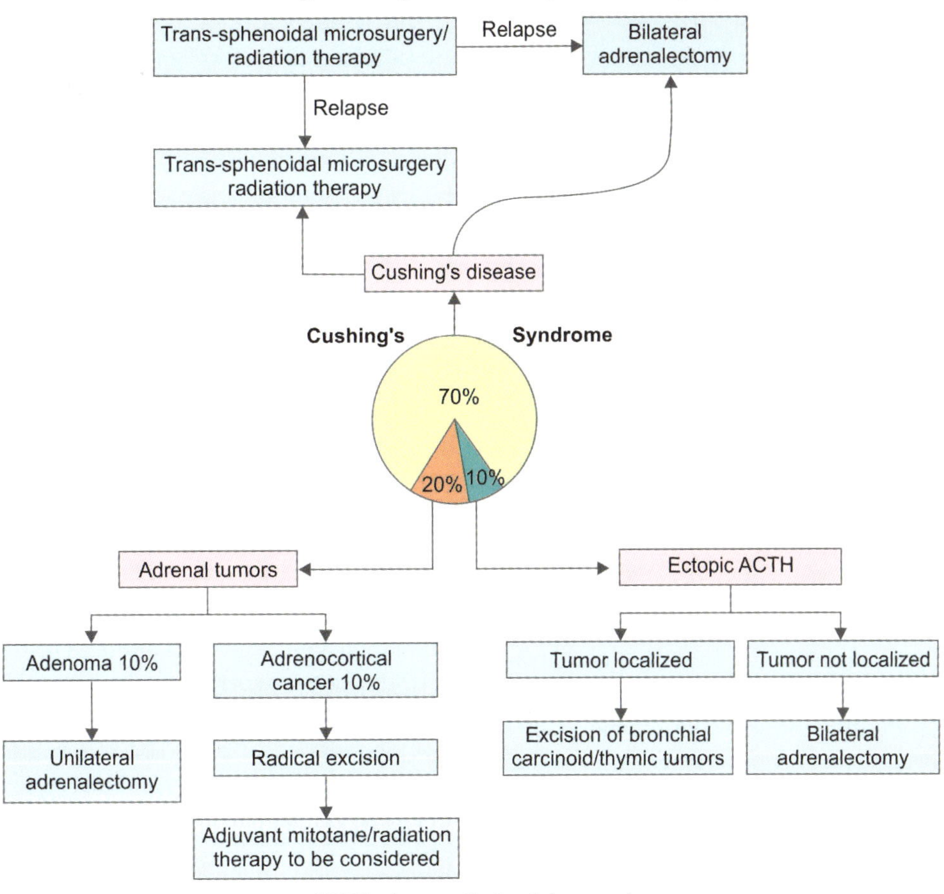

(ACTH: adrenocorticotropic hormone)

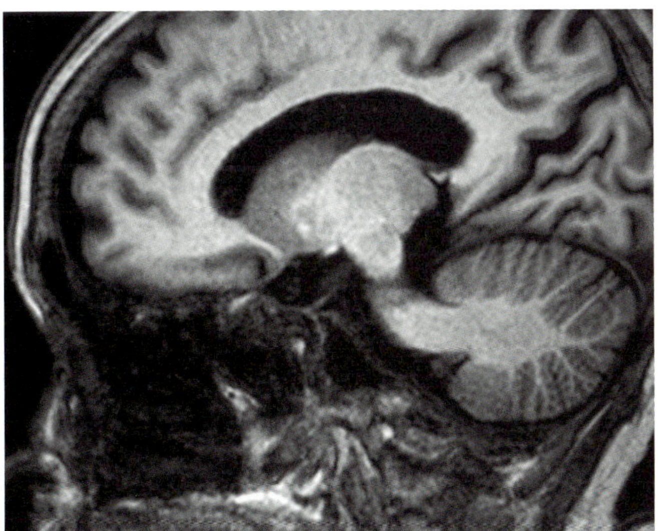

Fig. 1: Pituitary tumor secreting adrenocorticotropic hormone (ACTH).

- Highly malignant small cell carcinomas of the lung, though numerically more common, produce very high levels of ACTH and cortisol with rapid deterioration and atypical presentations such as pigmentation.
- *ACTH-independent causes*:
  - Adrenal adenoma and carcinoma **(Fig. 2)**

- Primary pigmented nodular adrenal hyperplasia (nodules are small 2–4 mm and pigmented); may occur as part of Carney's complex (occurring with mesenchymal tumors, skin spotty pigmentation, breast, testicular and pituitary tumors)
- *McCune–Albright syndrome*: Sexual precocity and growth hormone (GH) excess with Cushing's in some cases.
- *ACTH independent macronodular hyperplasia (AIMAH)*: Nonpigmented nodules >5 mm may attain much larger sizes.

Clinical Features

These include *in order of frequency of occurrence*—weight gain causing truncal or generalized obesity with moon face, buffalo hump, cutaneous striae, facial plethora, hypertension, menstrual disturbances, hirsutism, psychiatric disturbances, proximal muscle weakness, acne, headache, easy bruising, fractures, and loss of scalp hair. Males may manifest a lack of libido and gynecomastia. Many of these are not specific to Cushing's syndrome, and the more specific clinical features have been given *a higher discriminatory index* including easy bruising, muscle weakness, facial plethora, hypertension, hirsutism, menstrual irregularity, and truncal obesity.[6,7]

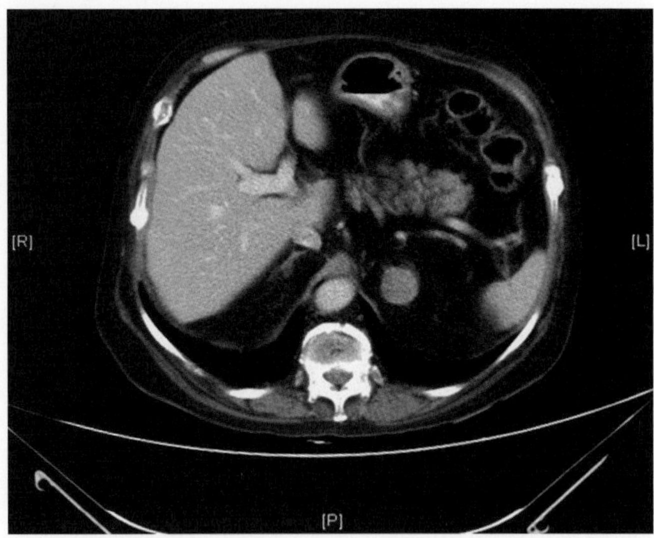

Fig. 2: Left adrenal adenoma with cortisol hypersecretion.

Initially, one should exclude exogenous intake of steroids by a detailed history and physical inspection of medication where necessary. Rarely, factitious ingestion and physiologic hypercortisolism may be the problem. Testing is recommended in multiple progressive clinical features, features unusual for age, unexplained severe manifestations, or workup of an adrenal incidentaloma to exclude subclinical Cushing's syndrome.

Diagnosis

- *The first step in diagnosis is to confirm hypercortisolism through laboratory diagnosis*: The baseline plasma cortisol level is elevated with a loss of the normal diurnal variation but is not sufficient for a diagnosis (normal range is 5–20 µg/dL with a lower evening value). Guidelines recommend using one of three screening tests in low clinical suspicion—elevated 24-hour urinary free cortisol (UFC) (threefold upper limit of normal, normal <100 µg/24 hour), elevated late-night salivary cortisol (>1.6 ng/mL), and nonsuppressed overnight 1 mg dexamethasone suppression test (>1.8 ug/dL). At least two values are required of urinary and salivary tests to confirm hypercortisolism.[8]
- *The next step is to identify the cause of hypercortisolism*: To differentiate between ACTH-dependent hyperplasia and a primary adenoma, the low-/high-dose dexamethasone suppression tests are helpful. Here, dexamethasone is given in 0.5 mg/2 mg doses every 6 hours and a plasma cortisol is done after 48 hours. In a patient with hyperplasia, since it is ACTH dependent, the cortisol will be <1% of the basal value, whereas in a tumor, there will be no suppression. Additionally, measurement of plasma ACTH will be in the low normal range (10–60 pg/mL) in adrenal tumors, around 80–200 pg/mL in pituitary tumors, and >200 pg/mL in ectopic ACTH tumor syndromes. In ectopic ACTH syndrome also, there will be no suppression of the cortisol level. In patients with adrenocortical carcinoma, there will be high levels of urinary 17 ketosteroids (>20 mg/24 hours). Serum DHEAS, which is produced solely by the adrenal and a marker of androgen secretion, may be elevated in adrenocortical neoplasms (>700 ng/dL). In patients with pituitary adenoma when suppression tests are not conclusive, bilateral selective inferior petrosal vein sampling following CRH stimulation will show a 50% increase in ACTH as compared to the basal and peripheral values.[9,10]

Imaging

Magnetic resonance imaging is preferable for pituitary imaging and for ectopic sites such as the bronchus and pancreas. CT and MRI will give the anatomical details of the adrenal mass. CT scan is the standard for adrenal imaging, and a solid homogeneous mass with density <20 HU confirms an adenoma. Necrosis and irregular borders raise suspicion of adrenocortical cancer. MRI may be added when indicated to confirm doubtful features on the CT scan or when there is hyperplasia. Chemical shift MRI shows a loss of signal in lipid-rich adenomas when the CT is not clearly in the adenoma density <20 HU. Iodocholesterol scintigraphy is not easily available but can be used to show a hot spot in an adenoma/carcinoma or bilateral uptake in hyperplasia.

Treatment

It is essential to reduce mortality and associated comorbidities of Cushing's syndrome. An effective treatment strategy first includes the normalization of cortisol levels and its effects. It also includes the adequate control of associated hypertension and diabetes. A detailed clinical assessment for other sites of infection and appropriate treatment is required. Surgical resection of the underlying tumor(s) is generally the first-line approach. The choice of second-line treatments, including medication, bilateral adrenalectomy, and radiation therapy, must be individualized to each patient and can be guided by standard published guidelines.[11]

- *Pituitary-dependent Cushing's syndrome:* If both transsphenoidal microsurgery and irradiation for residual/recurrent disease fail, then bilateral adrenalectomy can be done to control hypercortisolism. In patients who have bilateral adrenalectomy for hyperplasia, Nelson's syndrome is a complication seen in up to 20%, characterized by cutaneous hyperpigmentation and expanding intrasellar neoplasm. This can be treated with pituitary irradiation/surgical debulking.

  Drugs such as ketoconazole (antifungal), metyrapone, and mitotane (derivative of DDT) have been tried successfully as a temporary or palliative therapy to control hypercortisolism.[11]
- *Adrenal adenomas* can be treated by a unilateral adrenalectomy.

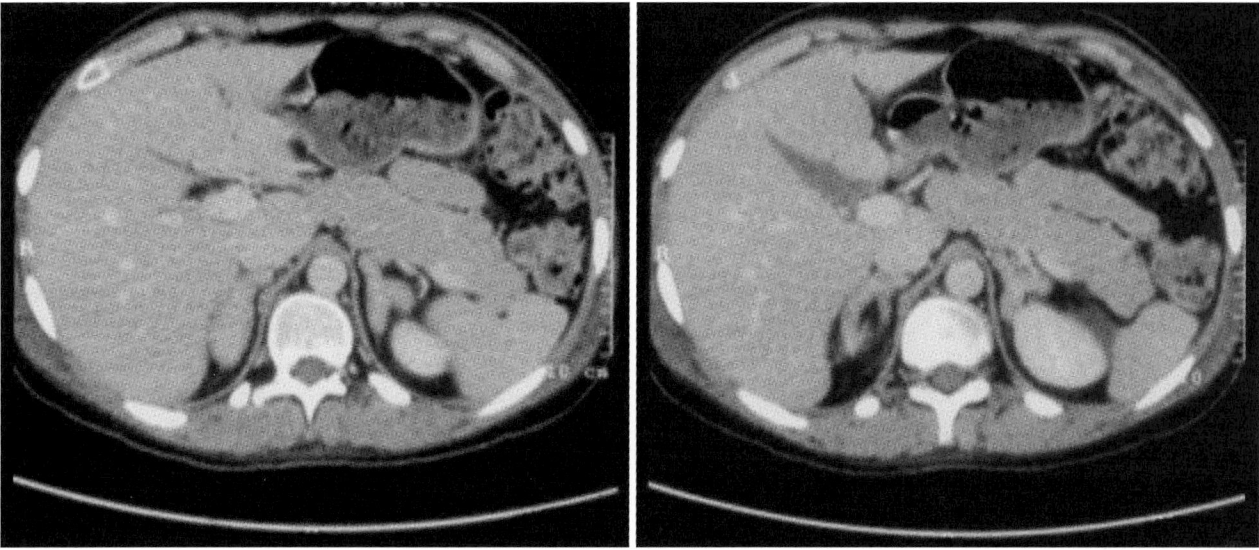

Fig. 3: Bilateral adrenal hyperplasia in ectopic Cushing's syndrome.

- *Macronodular adrenal hyperplasia* may be treated by bilateral adrenalectomy for clinically overt disease associated with significant enlarged glands bilaterally or unilateral adrenalectomy in selected cases with asymmetric involvement. Medical therapy is being explored **(Fig. 3)**.
- *Adrenal cortical carcinomas* are rare tumors. They may be functioning or nonfunctioning. Presentation can be as a mass, as an overt clinical syndrome, or as an incidentaloma. Assessment is made for function by checking serum potassium, plasma aldosterone, and plasma cortisol. These neoplasms have a grim prognosis. Early detection and surgical resection offer the only chance of cure. Radiotherapy and chemotherapy (platinum based) are not very effective. *Staging according to McFarlane modified by Sullivan*:
  - *Stage I*: <5 cm with no nodes or metastases
  - *Stage II*: >5 cm with local invasion/nodes
  - *Stage III*: Any size with metastases

  The survival is limited to 20% at 2 years from this lethal tumor, most patients developing metastatic disease. Adjuvant therapy includes local radiation, which has no proven benefit, and mitotane, which has been shown to prolong survival.
- *Ectopic ACTH-producing tumors*, typically in the lung and thymus, are removed when localized. Other sites are pancreatic NET and thyroid medullary cancer. In these patients, the key is to reduce adrenal corticosteroid and mitotane can be tried. Bilateral adrenalectomy is recommended only for patients in whom medications fail to control corticosteroid synthesis.

Surgical Approach

Multiple options are available to the surgeon approaching Cushing's syndrome and a familiarity with the development of techniques can be useful.

Traditional open adrenalectomy: Thornton, having trained under Joseph Lister and Spencer Wells, was well versed with the antiseptic technique and surgical hemostasis and reported the first known case of adrenalectomy in 1889.[12] He used the T-shaped subcostal incision of cholecystectomy advocated by Langenbuch and removed a large tumor along with the kidney; the patient developed an abscess, which fortuitously discharged via the bronchus saving the deteriorating patient. Other surgeons employed horizontal or vertical paramedian incisions and encountered difficulty with capsular rupture and hemorrhage from the vena cava. Open surgery of the adrenal was approached for long in the same way as the kidney tumors. Three main approaches emerged in the early 20th century and surgeons chose different approaches depending on the patient and tumor characteristics.[13]

1. The anterior bilateral subcostal incision with later modifications and extensions (rooftop/tri-radiate) was suitable for a wide subcostal angle, but a midline approach extendable by a right-angle incision was better for a narrow costal angle. The benefit was the ability to explore the whole abdomen and both adrenals, especially because localization was not possible in the early 20th century.[14]

A lateral retroperitoneal approach through an eleventh or twelfth rib bed incision allowed one adrenal to be examined thoroughly and a tumor to be removed. The patient was turned over at surgery to permit assessment of the opposite gland; this approach was difficult in Cushing's syndrome and required a staged procedure with two operations. Borstal of London pioneered a long intercostal incision in the tenth interspace, which was deepened via the pleural cavity and through diaphragm to approach larger adrenal tumors with excellent access. Temporary pneumothorax caused problems in the early days but could be managed later with the use of positive-pressure ventilation. The thoracoabdominal incision still

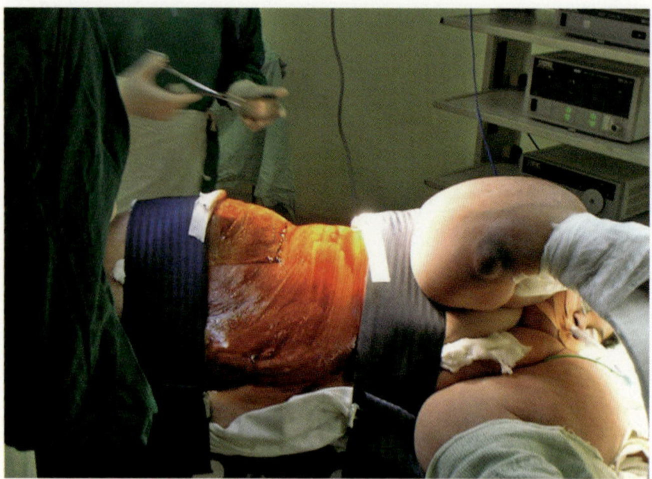

Fig. 4: Laparoscopic approach helps in access for bilateral adrenalectomy in a case of extreme obesity due to delayed presentation of Cushing's disease after failed pituitary surgery.

remains a useful approach when ease of access is paramount for large tumors with liver or cardiovascular involvement though the postoperative morbidity is higher. However, the extended subcostal incision into the xiphisternum and use of a fixed iron retractor with mobilization of the liver are the current most commonly used approaches for large/invasive adrenal tumors, avoiding the painful recovery of the thoracic incision.

2. The posterior approach with the patient supine as described by Young with or without 11th/12th rib excision allowed both adrenals to be examined in the same position but only small tumors could be removed, this being a useful approach for Cushing's syndrome, now largely abandoned for the laparoscopic approaches **(Fig. 4)**.

The open approach is still needed for large or malignant invasive tumors. The special situation when adrenocortical cancer invades is the adrenal vein must be handled carefully planning the access with appropriate help from urology or cardiac surgery colleagues where required. The removal of a tumor thrombus from the inferior vena cava (IVC) can be straightforward but can sometimes extend all the way to the right atrium and trans-diaphragmatic access and even cardiac bypass with a cardiac surgical team may be needed as standby.

Advances in minimally invasive surgery: Laparoscopic adrenalectomy was introduced by Gagner in 1992 and is now widely used as the procedure of choice in most adrenal pathologies.[15] Mirroring the varied open approaches, multiple endoscopic approaches have been described. Though no randomized trials are available to compare the laparoscopic with the open technique, multiple reports from around the world demonstrate the well-known benefits of improved cosmesis and shorter recovery time.[16,17] Functional cure and oncological safety have also been demonstrated and relative cost-effectiveness is an added benefit.

The controversies that persist include the following:

- Is there a maximum size that is deemed safe for the laparoscopic approach? Authors have suggested 6–8 cm as a guide, which will vary according to tumor characteristics and surgical expertise.[16,17]

- Is it safe to use the laparoscopic approach in the resection of a proven or potentially malignant lesion? There is no controversy when the lesion is large and frankly invasive on imaging. However, several reports of safe resection of smaller malignant tumors, which have well-defined planes, have been published. Laparoscopy can be advantageous in careful dissection of planes because of the magnified view though surgeons must be careful with capsular rupture during retraction and removal of larger tumors.

- Is it justified to lower the threshold size for resection of incidentaloma from 4 to 3 cm because of the ease of excision laparoscopically? The risk of malignancy is spectrum and even 3-cm lesions do have a small risk of being malignant. So, clinical judgment is required to make an appropriate decision in each case.

- When should surgery be indicated for subclinical Cushing's syndrome? When there is biochemical cortisol excess without classic clinical features, several authors have recommended surgical excision of an adenoma to mitigate the metabolic effects. However, clear benefits remain hard to prove.

- The choice of endoscopic technique is another matter of surgeon preference—*lateral transperitoneal adrenalectomy (LTA)* or *posterior retroperitoneoscopic adrenalectomy (PRA)*? A meta-analysis of the literature shows only minor differences in patient outcomes between the techniques.[16,17] Each surgeon has to choose according to his skill and the characteristics of the patient and tumor. Single-access endoscopic procedures are a further development. *Robot-assisted laparoscopic adrenalectomy* is being used to reduce the difficulty of advanced laparoscopic techniques, which requires a high level of skill and experience; the high cost of the equipment and disposables as well as no improvement in disease outcomes over laparoscopy remains an impediment to widespread adoption. However, this appears to be the future of minimally invasive surgery once the barriers are overcome.[16,17]

Bilateral adrenalectomy can be done via the transperitoneal route that requires changing the patient position to access the opposite gland or recently described CoBRA *(Combined Bilateral Retroperitoneoscopic Adrenalectomy)* procedure simultaneously via the posterior retroperitoneoscopic approach, an advancement over the staged procedure. Reports from India show encouraging results.[18-20] *Natural orifice surgery* is a new concept with reports of transvaginal excision of adrenal tumors trialed on cadaver and porcine models.[21]

Perioperative Precautions

Patients with Cushing's syndrome are at a higher risk for local wound complications because of weakened tissues and compromised healing, respiratory complications, deep vein thrombosis (DVT), and pulmonary embolism. The major dictums of surgical management include careful technique, prophylactic antibiotic cover, respiratory physiotherapy, DVT prophylaxis, and awareness that complications may not give overt symptoms in view of the cortisol excess state.[22]

Postoperative stress prophylaxis with corticosteroid supplementation tapered over 3–6 months with careful monitoring and addition of mineralocorticoid when required can be managed in partnership with medical colleagues. Special advice is needed for patients' post bilateral adrenalectomy, and a multidisciplinary approach will go a long way in providing the best care.

◇ CLINICAL PEARLS

- Cushing's syndrome is mostly exogenous in a general clinic setting; one should assess carefully for steroid use before pursuing endogenous causes.
- Pituitary tumors causing Cushing's disease are the most common endogenous cause at 70%. Surgical treatment and radiation have a small failure rate worldwide and some need bilateral adrenalectomy.
- Ectopic ACTH tumours should be considered in cases with significantly high biochemical values and rapid clinical deterioration usually without classic weight gain.
- Timely medical treatment to control hypercortisolism and treat associated infections are life-saving.
- Close cooperation with a skilled colleagues endocrinologist. Radiology, biochemistry and pathology team is paramount in successful management.

◇ REFERENCES

1. Welbourne RB. The History of Endocrine Surgery. Westport: Praeger; 1990.
2. Schumacker HB. The early history of the adrenal glands. Bull Hist Med. 1936;4:39-56.
3. Kendall EC. Cortisone. New York, NY: Charles Scribner's Sons; 1971.
4. Addison T. On the constitutional and local effects of disease of the suprarenal capsules. London: Samuel Highley; 1855.
5. Cushing H. The basophil adenomas of the pituitary and their clinical manifestations (pituitary basophilism). Bull Johns Hopkins Hosp. 1932;50:137-95.
6. Ross EJ, Linch DC. Cushing's syndrome—killing disease: discriminatory value of signs and symptoms aiding early diagnosis. Lancet. 1982;2:646 9.
7. Newell-Price J, Bertagna X, Grossman AB, Nieman LK. Cushing's syndrome. Lancet. 2006;367;1605-17.
8. Arnaldi G, Angeli A, Atkinson AB, Bertagna X, Cavagnini F, Chrousos GP, et al. Diagnosis and complications of Cushing's syndrome: a consensus statement. J Clin Endocrinol Metab. 2003;88:5593-602.
9. Findling JW, Raff H. Screening and diagnosis of Cushing's syndrome. Endocrinol Metab Clin North America. 2005;34:385-402.
10. Oldfield EH, Doppmann JL, Niemann LK, Chrousos GP, Miller DL, Katz DA, et al. Petrosal sinus sampling with and without corticotropin-releasing hormone for the differential diagnosis of Cushing's syndrome. N Engl J Med. 1991;325:897-905.
11. Lynette BLK, Biller BMK, Findling JW, Murad MH, Newell-Price J, Savage MO, et al. Treatment of Cushing's syndrome: an Endocrine Society Clinical Practice Guideline. J Clin Endocrinol Metab. 2015;100(8):2807-31.
12. Thornton JK. Abdominal nephrectomy for large sarcoma of the left suprarenal capsule: recovery. Trans Clin Soc London. 1890;23:150-3.
13. Iacobone M, Citton M, Scarpa M, Viel G, Boscaro M, Nitti D. Systematic review of surgical treatment of subclinical Cushing's syndrome. Br J Surg. 2015;102(4):318-3.
14. Young HH. Technique for simultaneous exposure and operation on the adrenals. Surg Gynecol Obstet. 1936;63:179-88.
15. Gagner M, Lacroix A, Bolté E. Laparoscopic adrenalectomy in Cushing's syndrome and pheochromocytoma. N Engl J Med. 1992;327:1003-12.
16. Walz MK, Alesina PF, Wenger FA, Deligiannis A, Szuczik E, Petersenn S, et al. Posterior retroperitoneoscopic adrenalectomy—results of 560 procedures in 520 patients. Surgery. 2006;140(6):943-8.
17. Lee CR, Walz MK, Park S, Park JH, Jeong JS, Lee SH, et al. A comparative study of the transperitoneal and posterior retroperitoneal approaches for laparoscopic adrenalectomy for adrenal tumors. Ann Surg Oncol. 2012;19(8):2629-34.
18. Raffaelli M, Brunaud L, De Crea C, Hoche G, Oragano L, Bresler L, et al Synchronous bilateral adrenalectomy for Cushing's syndrome: laparoscopic versus posterior retroperitoneoscopic versus robotic approach. World J Surg. 2014;38(3):709-17.
19. Prajapati OP, Verma AK, Mishra A, Agarwal G, Agarwal A, Mishra SK. Bilateral adrenalectomy for Cushing's syndrome: pros and cons. Indian J Endocrinol Metab. 2015;19(6):834-40.
20. Tiyadatah BN, Kalavampara SV, Sukumar S, Mathew G, Pooleri GK, Prasanna AT, et al. Bilateral simultaneous laparoscopic adrenalectomy in Cushing's syndrome: safe, effective and curative. J Endourol. 2012;26(2):157-63.
21. Perretta S, Allemann P, Asakuma M, Dallemagne B, Marescaux J. Adrenalectomy using natural orifice transluminal endoscopic surgery (NOTES: a transvaginal retroperitoneal approach. J Surg Endosc. 2009;23(6):1390.
22. Schreiner F, Anand G, Beuschlein F. Perioperative management of endocrine active adrenal tumours. Exp Clin Endocrinol Diabetes. 2019;127(2-03):137-46.

CHAPTER 33

Pheochromocytoma

Deependra Narayan Singh, Amit Agarwal

INTRODUCTION

Pheochromocytomas and paragangliomas (PGs) are neuro-endocrine tumors arising from chromaffin cells of the adrenal medulla (80%) or extra-adrenal paraganglia (20%) and produce catecholamines.

- *Head and neck PGs*: Non-catecholamine producing
- *Abdominal PGs*: Catecholamine producing

Pheochromocytoma derives its name from phaios (dusky), chroma (color), and cytoma (tumor). The term "pheochromocytoma" was coined by Pick in 1912. Fränkel was the first to report a pheochromocytoma during autopsy in 1886. In 1926, there were two successful operations of a pheochromocytoma first reported by Cesar Roux in Lausanne, Switzerland, and later by CH Mayo in the United States. A notable researcher in this area was the 1970 Nobel Prize laureate, Ulf Svante von Euler at the Karolinska Institute, who was recognized for his discoveries of prostaglandin in 1935, piperidine in 1942, and norepinephrine in 1946.

ETIOLOGY

Pheochromocytoma is a rare tumor with an overall prevalence of 1–2 per 100,000 in western literature and is the cause of secondary hypertension in 0.1–0.6% of hypertensive patients. Presently as much as 30% of incidentally discovered adrenal masses on anatomical imaging turn out be pheochromocytoma. It does not have a sex or side predilection. Sporadic phaeochromocytomas present in the fourth decade, whereas hereditary forms present a decade earlier. Pheochromocytoma was initially labeled as a "10% tumor," but recent evidence suggests that it is more likely to be a 0% tumor:

- 20% are extra-adrenal.
- 20% are multifocal.
- 20% are malignant.
- 20% are bilateral.
- 2 × 20% (40%) are familial.
- 20% occur in children.

RISK FACTORS

- *Multiple endocrine neoplasia (MEN) syndrome types 2A and B*: Even if unilateral at presentation, 50% will develop contralateral tumors.

- *Von Hippel–Lindau (VHL) disease*: The prevalence is 10–20%.
- *Succinate dehydrogenase (SDH) subunit B, C, and D gene mutations*: These germline mutations predispose to pheochromocytomas and have a predilection for head and neck PGs. Malignancy rate is high in such patients.
- *Neurofibromatosis type 1 (NF1)*: 1–5% of patients with pheochromocytomas have been found to have NF1.

FAMILIAL AND HEREDITARY PHEOCHROMOCYTOMAS

Approximately 40% of pheochromocytoma and paraganglio-mas (PPGLs) are hereditary. Two striking features of PPGLs need to be remembered which make genetic testing mandatory: one is its high penetrance because it is caused by a single driver germline mutation and hence has a clear family history. The second striking characteristic of PPGLs is their *genetic heterogeneity*-mutated genes that can be grouped in two clusters: cluster 1—hypoxia-related signals and cluster 2—increased kinase signaling **(Figs. 1 and 2)**. Newer susceptibility genes are being discovered every year, and presently 18 genes have been implicated in familial cases.

Cluster 1 genes include *VHL, RET, SDH, IDF, FH, HIF2A,* and *IOMA*, while the mutations of rearranged during trans-fection protooncogene (*RET*), *myc-associated factor X* (MAX), transmembrane protein 127 (TMEM127), neurofibromin 1 (NF1), and kinesin family member1B β (KIF1Bβ) are the cluster 2 genes **(Table 1)**.

In MEN2, pheochromocytomas have certain features which differ from pheochromocytomas in VHL disease **(Table 2)**.

EXTRA-ADRENAL PHEOCHROMOCYTOMAS

Twenty percent of catecholamine-producing tumors can be extra-adrenal and their incidence is still higher in children, where it accounts for 30%.

Similarly, the incidence of multicentricity and malignancy is higher in them as compared to adrenal pheochromocytoma (36% vs. 10%).

The most common locations of extra-adrenal pheochromo-cytomas are renal hilum and organ of Zuckerkandl at the

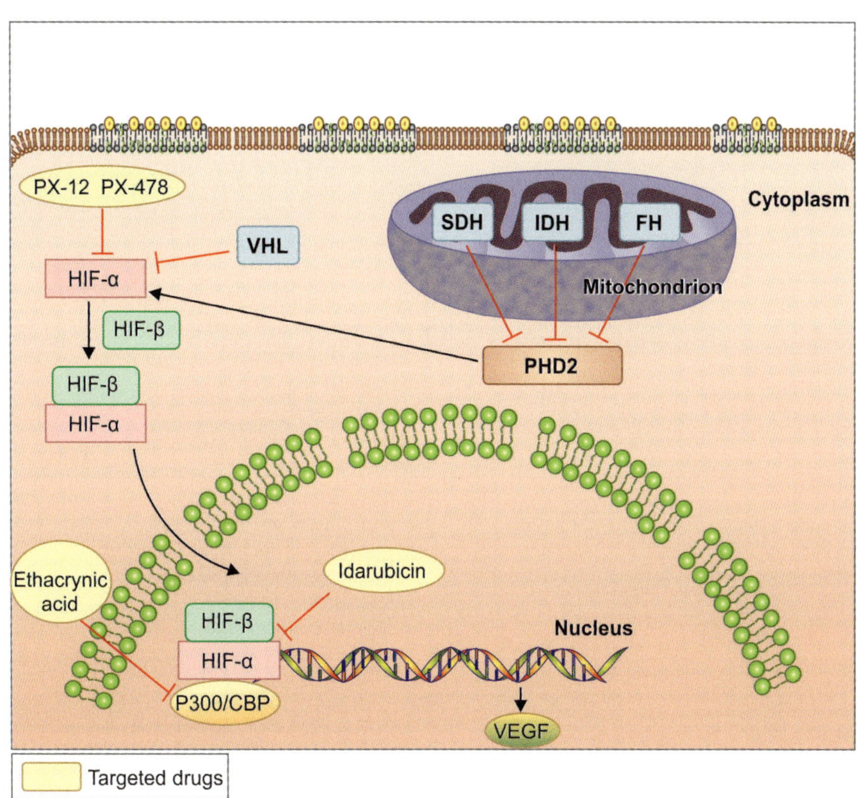

Fig. 1: The hypoxia-related signal pathway, cluster 1 genes, and their potential molecular-targeted medicines.
(FH: fumarate hydratase; HIF: hypoxia-inducible factor; IDH: isocitrate dehydrogenase; PHD2: prolyl hydroxylase domain protein 2; SDH: succinate dehydrogenase; VEGF: vascular endothelial growth factor; VHL: von Hippel–Lindau)

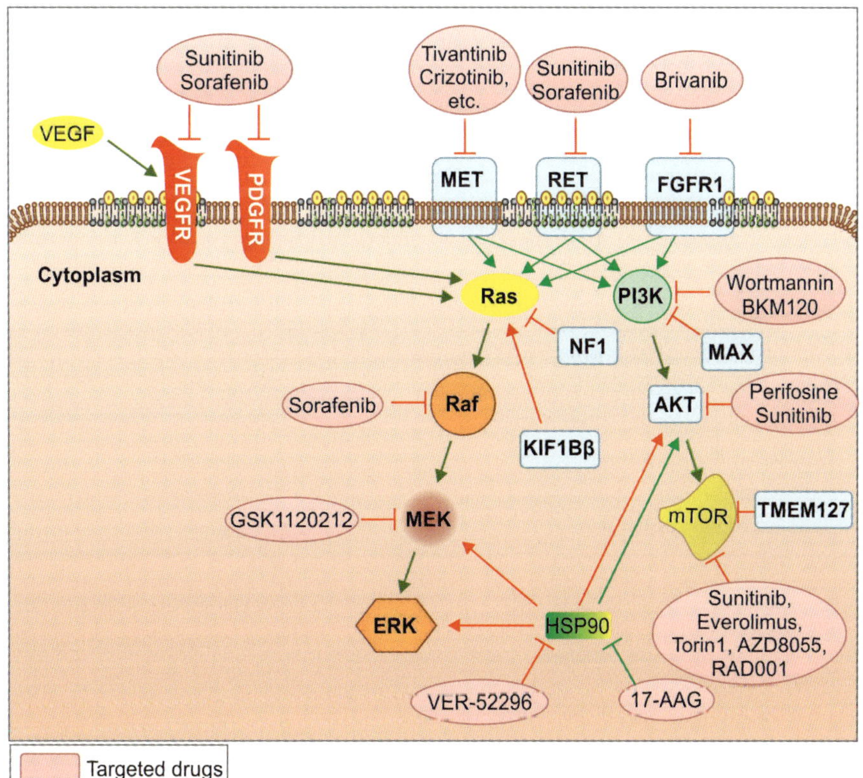

Fig. 2: Increased kinase signal pathways and cluster 2 genes.
(ERK: extracellular regulated protein kinases; FGFR1: fibroblast growth factor receptor 1; HSP: heat shock protein; KIF1Bβ: kinesin family member1B β; MAX: myc-associated factor X; MET: *MET* proto-oncogene; mTOR: mammalian target of rapamycin; MEK,MAPK/ERK kinase; NF1: neurofibromin 1; PDGF: platelet-derived growth factors receptor; PI3K: phosphatidylinositol 3-kinase; RET: rearranged during transfection protooncogene; TMEM127: transmembrane protein 127; VEGF: vascular endothelial growth factor; VEGFR: vascular endothelial growth factor receptor)

Table 1: Genetic syndromes associated with pheochromocytoma.

Syndrome	Gene affected	Components
MEN2A (Sipple's syndrome)	Germline mis-sense mutations in extracellular *cysteine* codons of *RET*	• Medullary carcinoma of thyroid • Pheochromocytoma • Hyperparathyroidism *Cutaneous lichen amyloidosis* (variant)
MEN2B	Germline mis-sense mutation in *tyrosine kinase* domain of *RET*	• Medullary carcinoma of the thyroid • Pheochromocytoma *Mucosal neuroma* *Marfanoid habitus* *Ganglioneuromas of the gastrointestinal tract*
Neurofibromatosis (von Recklinghausen's disease) type I **(Fig. 3)**	*NF1* gene	• Multiple freckling • Cafe-au-lait spots • Axillary freckling • Multiple neurofibromas on skin and mucosa • Pheochromocytoma
Von Hippel–Lindau disease	*VHL* gene	*Type 1 (no pheochromocytoma):* • Renal-cell cysts and carcinomas • Retinal and CNS hemangioblastomas • Pancreatic neoplasms and cysts • Endolymphatic sac tumors • Epididymal cystadenomas *Type 2 (with pheochromocytoma)* **(Fig. 4)**: *2A:* • Retinal and CNS hemangioblastomas • Pheochromocytomas • Endolymphatic sac tumors • Epididymal cystadenomas *2B:* • Renal-cell cysts and carcinomas • Retinal and CNS hemangioblastomas • Pancreatic neoplasms and cysts • Pheochromocytomas • Endolymphatic sac tumors • Epididymal cystadenomas *2C*: Pheochromocytomas only
Familial paraganglioma (PG) syndrome	Germline mutations of *SDHD* and *SDHC* genes	• Head and neck tumors (carotid-body tumors; vagal, jugular, and tympanic paragangliomas) • Pheochromocytomas • Abdominal or thoracic paragangliomas (or both)

(CNS: central nervous system; MEN: multiple endocrine neoplasia)

Table 2: Differentiating features betweeen MEN2A and VHL.

Characteristics	MEN2A	VHL disease
Bilaterality	Bilateral in 30–50%	50%
Hyperplasia	Associated with hyperplasia in 25%	No hyperplasia
Multicentricity	Usually, multicentric	Not multicentric
Extra-adrenal	They are rarely extra-adrenal	Extra-adrenal pheochromocytoma is rare
Malignancy	<5%	<2%
Biochemistry	Epinephrine secretion	Norepinephrine secretion
Blood pressure	Sustained HTN	Normotensive/paroxysmal HTN
Histopathology	Tumor capsule is thin	Tumor capsule is thick

(HTN: hypertension; MEN: multiple endocrine neoplasia; VHL: Von Hippel–Lindau)

origin of the inferior mesenteric artery. 85% of these extra-adrenal tumors are located below the diaphragm **(Figs. 5A to C)**.

Extra-adrenal pheochromocytoma locations are listed in **Box 1** in a decreasing order of frequency.

Pathophysiology and Symptomatology

High levels of epinephrine are suggestive of pheochromocytoma of adrenal origin because pheochromocytomas secrete predominantly norepinephrine, which is converted to

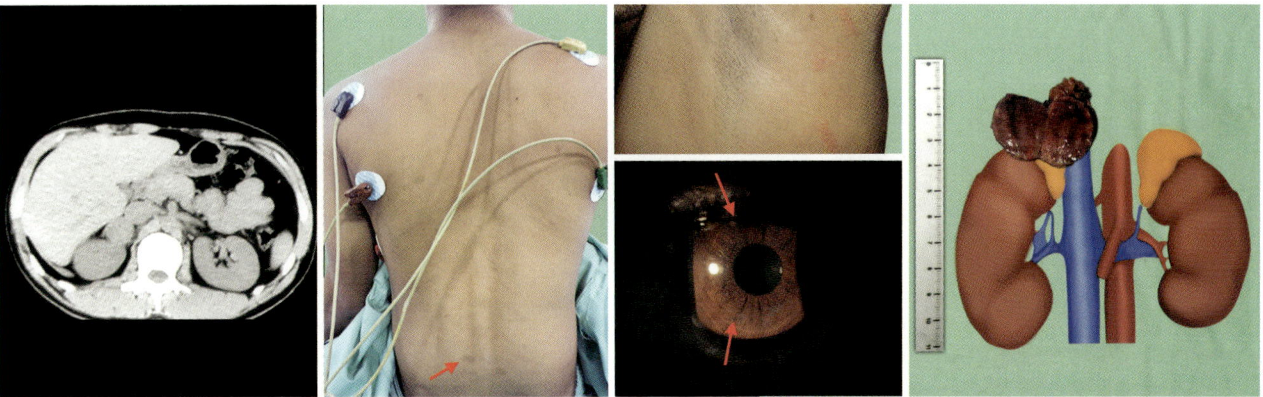

Fig. 3: *Familial Pheochromocytoma (NF-1):* A 26-year-old man presented with a right adrenal mass with elevated NMN. Found to be having multiple Cafe-au-lait patches over neck and trunk (3 of them >15 mm in diameter). Along with bilateral axillary freckling (1–3 mm); slit-lamp examination revealed more than 2 Lisch nodules (≥2 mm), thus fulfilling 3 criteria to make a clinical diagnosis of NF-1. Underwent laparoscopic adrenalectomy.

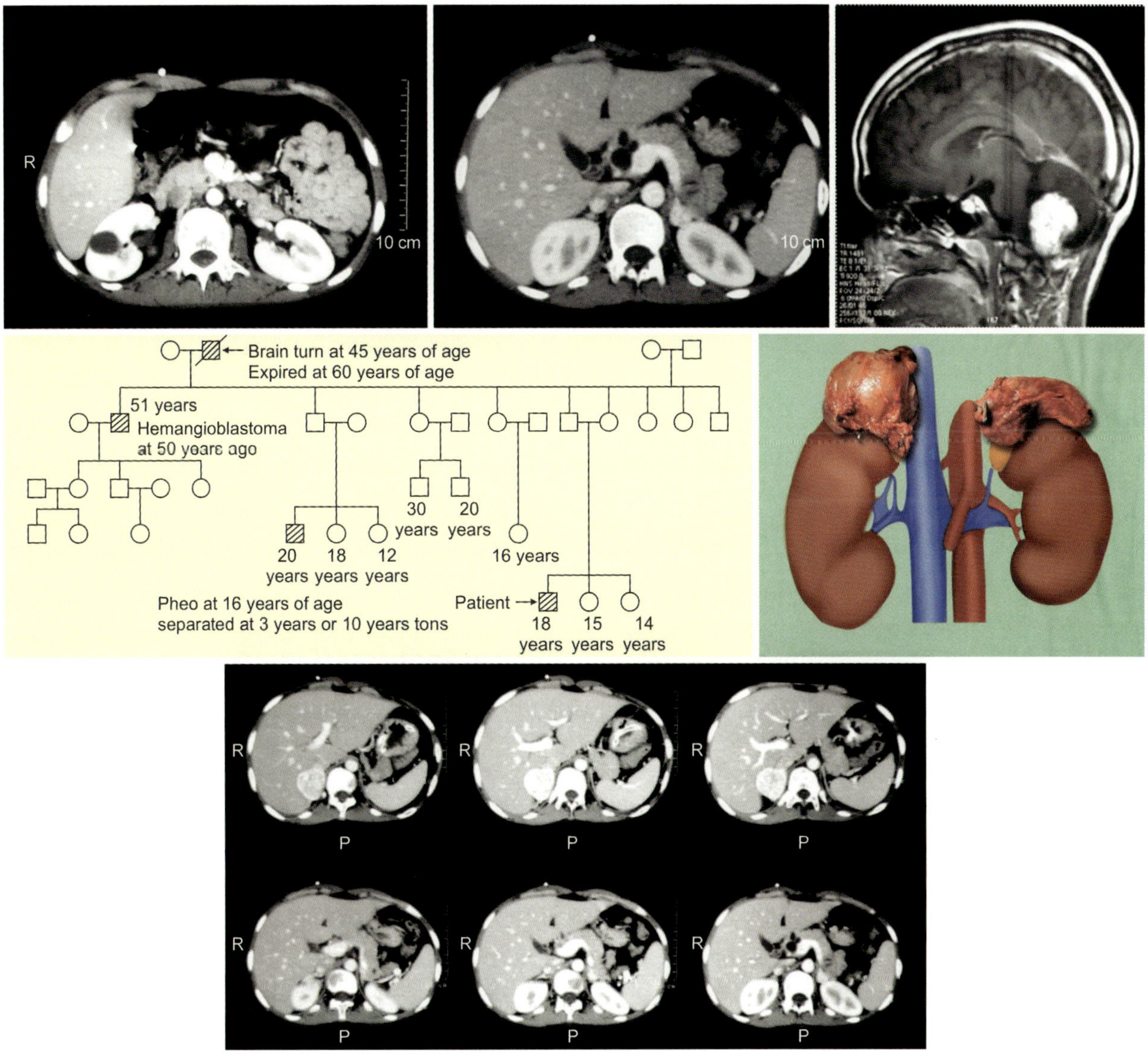

Fig. 4: *VHL:* Bilateral pheo, renal and pancreatic cysts. A 16-year-old boy developed quadriparesis. Subsequent CECT revealed a posterior fossa 4th ventricle tumor s/o hemangioblastoma; he was suspected of VHL and CECT abdomen was done which revealed bilateral adrenal lesions and pancreatic and renal cysts; he had a strong family history of HGB and PCC in family members subsequently, elevated urinary MN/NMN (5476 µg/mL) confirmed bilateral pheochromocytoma and he was taken up for bilateral adrenalectomy after adequate alpha-blockade. HPE of adrenal lesion revealed bilateral tumors without hyperplasia. Subsequently, he underwent complete excision of brainstem hemangioblastoma. Genetic mutation revealed heterozygous VHL: C277G known pathogenic variant.

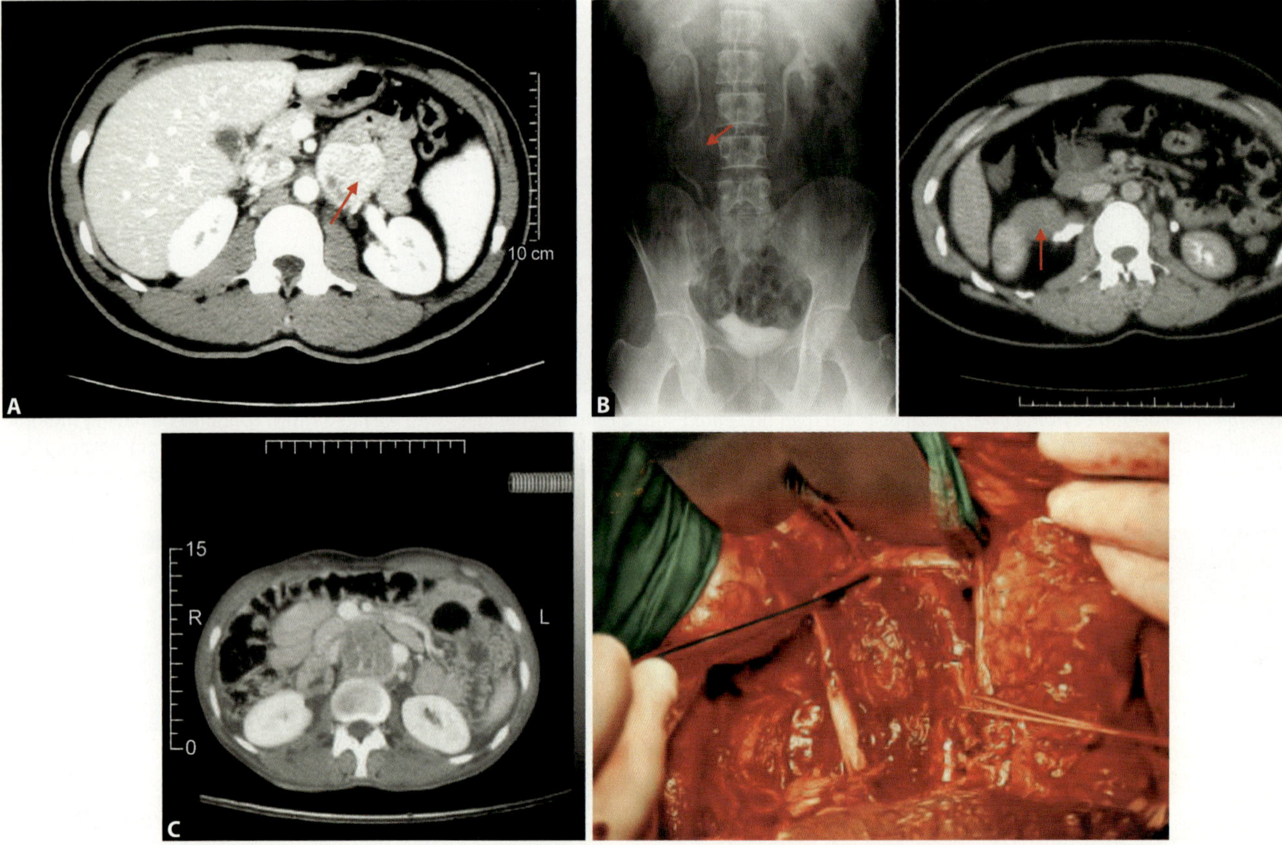

Figs. 5A to C: (A) Paraganglioma in the left para-aortic region at level L2-L3 superiorly limited by left renal vein; (B) Right infra-renal paraganglioma; (C) Inter-aortocaval paragnaglioma.

Box 1: Extra-adrenal locations of pheochromocytoma.

- Renal hilum
- Organ of Zuckerkandl
- Neck
- Urinary bladder
- Liver hilum
- Posterior mediastinum
- Intrapericardial

epinephrine by the phenylethanolamine N-methyltransferase enzyme, present only in the adrenal medulla and organ of Zuckerkandl. However, besides catecholamines, pheochromocytomas secrete other neurohormones such as dopamine, vasoactive intestinal peptide (VIP), adreno-corticotrophic hormones, and β-endorphins in different concentrations that may sometimes result in patients being normotensive instead of having the classical hypertension.

The hemodynamic (HD) pathophysiology of pheochromocytoma has the following features:

- There is no direct correlation between plasma levels of catecholamine and HD profile.
- The circulation in pheochromocytoma can be described as hyperdynamic, vasoconstrictive, and hypovolemic.
- Majority have left ventricular hypertrophy.
- Orthostatic hypotension

- *Types of hypertension in pheochromocytoma patients*:
  - *Type I hypertension*: Sustained hypertension (50%)
  - *Type IIA*: Paroxysmal hypertension (45%)
  - *Type IIB*: Normotensive (5%)
- Children have more sustained type of hypertension as compared to adults.
- 20% of patients with pheochromocytoma will have accompanying essential hypertension.

Clinical Features (Figs. 6 and 7)

About 90% of patients present with episodes of *"classical triad"* which include headache, palpitations, and sweating." Patients can have paroxysmal spells (five Ps: pressure—sudden increase in blood pressure; pain—headache, chest pain, abdominal pain; perspiration; palpitations; and pallor). Children usually present with complaints of profuse sweating and headache **(Tables 3 and 4)**.

- *Hypertension*: The most consistent presentation is hypertension which has three patterns:
  1. *Type A*: Episodic/paroxysmal hypertension
  2. *Type B*: Sustained hypertension
  3. *Type C*: Orthostatic hypotension with normotension/hypertension. Orthostatic hypotension is due to reduced intravascular volume as a result of chronic adrenergic stimulation.
- Cardiac disease in pheochromocytoma
- *Other symptoms (Table 4)*:

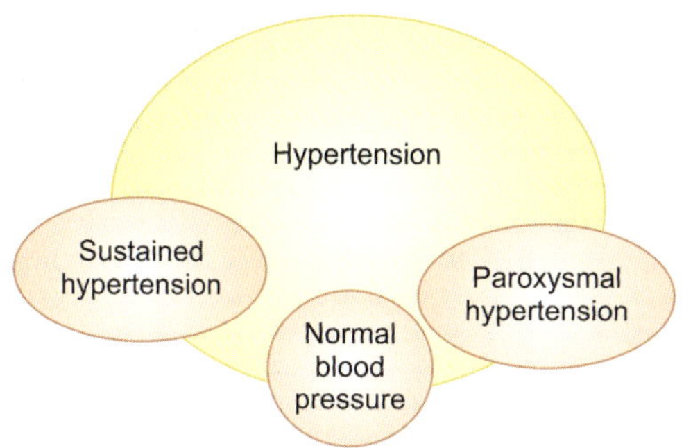

Fig. 6: Hypertension seen in pheochromocytoma.

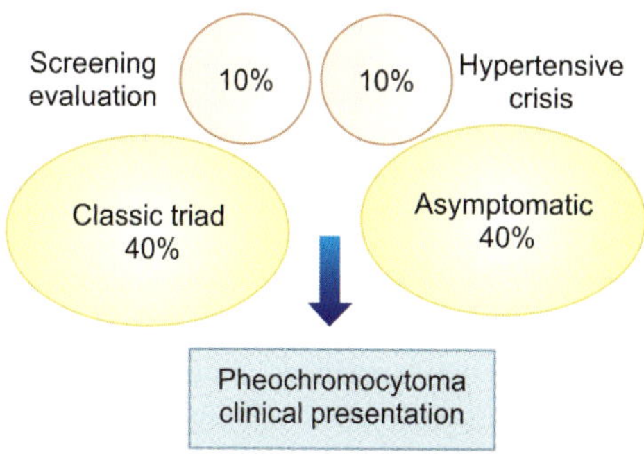

Fig. 7: Clinical features of pheochromocytoma.

Table 3: Signs and symptoms of pheochromocytoma.

Symptoms	Incidence	Signs	Incidence
Headache	76–100%	Hypertension	76–100%
Palpitations	51–75%	Tachycardia or reflex bradycardia	51–75%
Sweating	51–75%	Postural hypotension	51–75%
Anxiety/nervousness	26–50%	Hypertension, paroxysmal hypertension, weight loss	26–50%
Pain abdomen, chest	26–50%		
Fatigue or weakness	26–50%	Fasting hyperglycemia	26–50%
Dizziness	1–25%	Tremor	26–50%
Heat intolerance	1–25%		
Constipation	1–25%		
Breathlessness	1–25%	Psychosis	1–25%
Visual disturbances	1–25%	Flushing, paroxysmal	1–25%
Seizures, grand mal	1–25%		

Table 4: Atypical clinical manifestations of pheochromocytoma and paraganglioma.

Pathophysiology	Clinical manifestations and atypical presentations
Blood pressure	Normotension, shock
Vasospasm	Cyanosis, Raynaud's syndrome, gangrene
Cardiovascular	Chest pain, acute coronary syndrome, cardiomyopathy, heart failure, and cardiac paragangliomas
Gastrointestinal	Acute abdomen (intestinal ischemia); constipation, toxic megacolon
Metabolic	Hyperglycemia/diabetes, lactic acidosis, and fever
Neurologic	CVA, TIA, hemiplegia, hemianopsia, and seizure
Pulmonary	Pulmonary edema
Psychiatric	Anxiety attacks chronic fatigue; psychosis
Ectopic hormones	ACTH (Cushing's syndrome), VIP (Verner–Morrison syndrome); PTHrP (hypercalcemia), erythropoietin (erythrocytosis)
Children	More commonly have sustained hypertension, diaphoresis, visual changes, polyuria/polydipsia, seizures, edematous or cyanotic hands; more commonly harbor germline mutations, multiple tumors, and paragangliomas
Pregnancy	Hypertension mimicking eclampsia, hypertensive multisystem crisis during vaginal delivery, postpartum shock or fever

(ACTH: adrenocorticotropic hormone; CVA: cerebral vascular accident; PTHrP: parathyroid hormone-related protein; TIA: transient ischemic attack; VIP: vasoactive intestinal peptide)

- A patient can present with anxiety or panic attacks with a feeling of doomsday
- Unexplained stroke in a young patient or congestive heart failure or pulmonary edema
- It also may present with severe hypertensive crisis during or after a surgical procedure, following road-traffic accident, excessive exercise, some drug intake (corticosteroids, antibiotics—linezolid, glucagon, radiographic contrast dye, tricyclic antidepressants, metoclopramide, chemotherapeutic agents, or even micturition in the setting of bladder pheochromocytoma), and childbirth. Duration and frequency of intermittent symptoms are variable, ranging from a few seconds to several days and from several times daily to once every few weeks.

An unrecognized pheochromocytoma may lead to death as a result of a hypertensive crisis, arrhythmia, myocardial infarction, or multisystem crisis.

Pathology

Phaeochromocytomas are highly vascularized, with a cut surface appearing grayish-pink with areas of hemorrhage or necrosis. Microscopically, tumor cells are polygonal but the configuration varies considerably. Like all other endocrine malignancies, the differentiation between malignant and benign tumors is difficult. The following systems are used to predict malignancy on histopathology:

- High PASS (phaeochromocytoma of the adrenal gland scale score)
- *Grading system for adrenal pheochromocytoma and paraganglioma (GAPP)*

The following features are helpful in suggesting malignancy:

- High number of Ki-67-positive cells
- Vascular invasion
- Capsular invasion

Diagnosis

Pheochromocytoma can have diverse clinical manifestations and is therefore known as the great mimic. However, biochemical testing for a possible pheochromocytoma should be done in the following clinical settings:

- Paroxysmal hypertension
- Accelerated hypertension, especially in children and during the first two trimesters of pregnancy
- A paradoxical hypertensive response
- Hypertensive crisis during a surgical procedure or labor or angiography
- Unexplained heart failure
- Patients with a family history of VHL syndrome, MEN-2A or -2B, NF1, or inherited PG syndrome (due to mutation in one of the *SDH* genes)
- Labile hypertension or blood pressure refractory to standard drugs
- Orthostatic hypotension in the absence of antihypertensive drug therapy
- Adrenal incidentaloma
- Recent detection of hypertension in children and young individuals
- The diagnosis of pheochromocytoma is biochemical and relies on the demonstration of elevated levels of catecholamines or its metabolic products **(Table 4)**.
- A missed diagnosis of pheochromocytoma can be fatal, hence the need for a sensitive test. Usually, catecholamine or its metabolic products are measured either in blood or in urine.
- Measurements of plasma-free metanephrines or urinary fractionated metanephrines (normetanephrine and metanephrine separately) are the most sensitive tests for diagnosis **(Table 5)**. Plasma metanephrine measurement is more sensitive due to two reasons: (1) It measures the O-methylated metabolites whose production is continuous unlike the highly variable release of catecholamines; and (2) Not all tumors always release catecholamines. At least two measurements (preferably one urine based and one blood test) may be required because of episodic secretion.
- False-positive results can occur with drugs such as sympathomimetics, phenoxybenzamine, tricyclic antidepressants, and paracetamol.
- Urinary vanillylmandelic acid (VMA) also may be useful but has a low sensitivity. *Chromogranin A* has a sensitivity of 86% but poor diagnostic specificity.

Generally, biochemical levels of at least two-fold above the normal range are regarded as diagnostic.

Genetics

Triaging of genetic screening test is important to avoid excessive cost to the patient. In absence of a family history of a known mutation, triaging is decided by three things: tumor location, biochemical phenotype, and immunohistochemical evaluation for the presence of SDHB/A proteins. A simple way to do these tests in different settings has been described in **Table 6**.

If mutation is identified at any point in the testing algorithm, no further testing should be performed.

Utility of immunohistochemical (IHC) for SDHB: IHC testing with SDHB can also help to guide genetic testing. SDHx-related pheochromocytomas/PGs are associated with negative SDHB staining, thus signifying the presence of an SDHA mutation.

Differential Diagnosis

Many signs and symptoms of pheochromocytoma mimic other disorders and therefore pheochromocytoma is known as a great mimic. Common disorders which mimic pheochromocytoma include—thyrotoxicosis, anxiety disorders or panic attacks, carcinoid syndrome, pre-eclampsia, neuroblastoma, and insulinoma, acute clonidine withdrawal, hypoglycemia, renovascular hypertension, menopause, and migraine.

Table 5: Sensitivity/specificity for catecholamines and metabolites.

Test	Sensitivity (%)	Specificity (%)
Urinary catecholamines	86	88
Urinary-fractionated metanephrines	97	69
Plasma-free metanephrines	99	89
Urinary VMA	64	95
Dopamine	7	99
Serum chromogranin A	86	74

(VMA: vanillylmandelic acid)

Table 6: Simplified way of genetic testing in pheochromocytoma.

When to do genetic testing?	Rank of order
Unilateral pheochromocytomas in individuals <20 years	VHL > RET > SDHB = SDHD
Bilateral pheochromocytomas	VHL > RET > SDHB = SDHD
Sympathetic paragangliomas <20 years	VHL > SDHB > SDHD
Sympathetic paragangliomas ≥20 years	SDHB > VHL > SDHD
Elevated MN	RET > MAX, TMEM127
Elevated NMN (adrenal tumor)	VHL>SDHB, SDHD
Elevated NMN (extra-adrenal)	SDHB > SDHD > VHL
Elevated NMN (HNP)	SDHB > SDHD > SDHC, VHL, TMEM127
When not to do genetic testing?	**Age > 50 year**
Genetic testing is optional (not routinely recommended)	
Patients with unilateral pheochromocytomas, aged 20–50 years, and no suspicious clinical findings or family history for hereditary disease	SDHB > VHL > SDHD >>> RET

(RET: rearranged during transfection proto-oncogene; VHL: von Hippel–Lindau)

Localization

After clinical and biochemical diagnosis, the pheochromocytoma has to be localized. The frequency of anatomical location of pheochromocytoma is in the abdomen (97%), thorax (2–3%), and neck (1%). The most commonly used imaging procedure is the three-phase contrast CT.

CT Scan

It can detect up to lesions >1 cm in size. The typical appearance of pheochromocytomas is a homogeneous tumor with >20 Hounsfield units on an enhanced scan. Usually, there is a central unenhanced area due to cystic necrosis, thus giving a heterogeneous appearance **(Fig. 8)**. Even though the newer nonionic contrast media usually do not pose a risk of hypertensive crisis and can be used in a nonblocked patient, it is preferable to put the patient on α-blockade for a week before the CT examination.

Magnetic Resonance Imaging

Unlike CT, it provides a functional imaging typically appearing as hyperintense on T2-weighted imaging. It is the radiological investigation of choice for pregnant women and children and also for annual screening examinations (for patients with high-risk germline mutations) and any patient with a contrast allergy.

Metaiodobenzylguanidine

Metaiodobenzylguanidine (MIBG) is a norepinephrine analog, which accumulates in hyperfunctioning/tumorous chromaffin tissue. It is cumbersome to perform because prior to MIBG imaging, oral Lugol's iodine must be administered for at least 3 days to prevent uptake of radioactive iodine by the thyroid gland. MIBG scans have a low sensitivity but high specificity. It is now used only for detection of multifocal or metastatic disease.

Octreotide Scintigraphy

^{111}In-diethylenetriaminepenta-acetic acid (DTPA)-octreotide and ^{121}I-DTPA-octreotide are radiolabeled analogs of somatostatin and can be used to have a functional image of pheochromocytomas because of high density of somatostatin receptors in them.

Positron Emission Tomography Imaging

Positron emission tomography (PET) imaging with 18F-fluorodopamine, 18F-fluorodopa, 18F-dihydroxyphenylalanine, 11C-hydroxyephedrine, and 11C-epinephrine is highly specific for pheochromocytoma.

Management

Preoperative Preparation

Once the biochemical diagnosis is made, all patients are prepared with α-blockers to block the catecholamine excess to avoid or at least blunt the HD alterations during surgery. Majority of surgeons would like to use α-blockade; however, recently this concept has been challenged. The main goals of preoperative preparation are:

- Reasonable normalization of blood pressure and heart rate without significant orthostatic hypotension
- Restoration of volume depletion
- Prevention of any intraoperative hypertensive crisis and arrhythmia

Drugs used for preoperative preparation:
- α-blockers **(Table 7)**:
  - *Phenoxybenzamine (PBX):* It is a nonselective, long-acting, noncompetitive α-1 and α-2 receptor blocker with a long half-life of 24 hours. It is usually started as 10 mg twice-daily dose with increments of 10 mg every 2–3 days till 7–14 days and can go up to a maximum dose of 1 mg/kg/day. In children, 0.2 mg/kg orally once daily (maximum 10 mg) and increase by 0.2 mg/kg/day every 4 days. Maximum dosage of 240 mg/day may be required in an occasional patient. Significant side effects are postural hypotension with reflex tachycardia due to α2-receptor blockade, dizziness, syncope, and nasal congestion.

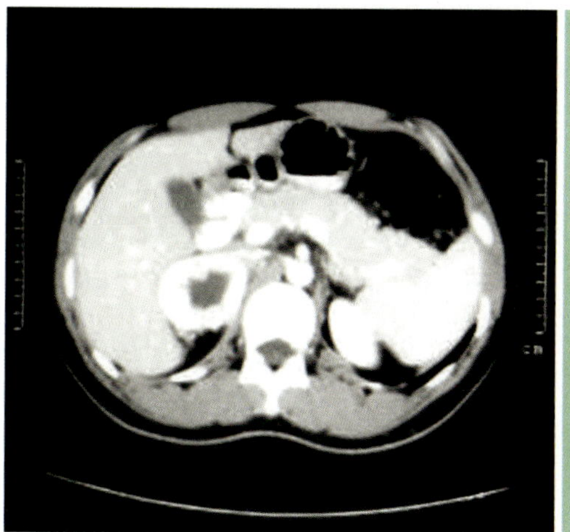
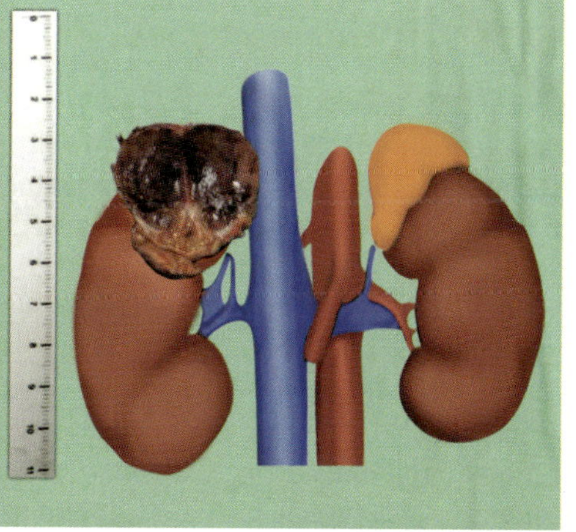

Fig. 8: CECT picture of unilateral pheochromocytoma showing central cystic area.

Table 7: Differences between the alpha-blockade produced by PBX and PZ.

Drug	Extent of blockade	Reversibility of blockade	Duration of blockade	Pre-operative side-effect	Post-operative side-effect
PBX	Complete	Irreversible	Prolonged	Tachycardia	Hypotension
PZ	Incomplete	Reversible	Short	No	No

- *Doxazosin, prazosin, and terazosin*: These are short-acting, selective, and competitive α-1 receptor blockers. *Dose*:
  - *Doxazosin*: 2–8 mg orally per day, maximum 16 mg/day
  - *Prazosin*: 2–5 mg orally two to three times a day, maximum: 20 mg/day
  - *Terazosin*: 2–5 mg orally per day, maximum 20 mg/day

They result in lesser postural hypotension, lesser reflex tachycardia, and lesser postoperative hypotension and are cheaper and easily available. However, they result in incomplete blockade as compared to phenoxybenzamine and patient may show HD alterations during surgery.

- *β-blockers*: These are added after adequate α-blockade has been achieved to avoid intraoperative tachyarrhythmia. If they are used prior to use of α-blockers, they can precipitate epinephrine-induced vasoconstriction and rebound hypertension by blocking the vasodilator component (β2-receptors). The nonselective β-receptor blocker propranolol (20–40 mg—three times a day) or cardioselective β1-blocker atenolol (25–50 mg per a day) is usually preferred. They can be added either when the patient develops tachycardia during α-blockade or may be added prophylactically 24 hours before operation in all patients.
- *Calcium-channel blockers*: They help to control hypertension and tachyarrhythmia by blocking norepinephrine-mediated calcium influx into vascular smooth muscle and they also prevent catecholamine-induced coronary vasospasm. The most commonly used agents are amlodipine 10–20 mg, nicardipine 60–90 mg/day, nifedipine SR 30–90 mg, and verapamil ER 180–540 mg/day. They may be used along with α-blockers, if hypertension is not being controlled but never as primary drugs for preparing patients for surgery.
- *Metyrosine*: It is a competitive inhibitor of tyrosine hydroxylase, the rate-limiting enzyme in catecholamine biosynthesis. Metyrosine is given in patients with extensive metastases. It is used in dose of 250 mg 8–12 hourly with increments by 250–500 mg every 2–3 day up to a maximum of 1.5–2 g/day.

In addition to all these drugs, the patients are also asked to take high-salt diet (15 g daily, usually 3 days after α-blockers are initiated) and expansion of blood volume by asking patients to take 4–5: of water per day to minimize postoperative hypotension.

Assessment of adequate alpha-blockade before surgery?
Roizen in 1982 defined certain criteria, which need to be applied 1 week prior to surgery:
- Blood pressure not >160/90 mm Hg
- Orthostatic hypotension not <80/45 mm Hg
- No more than one ventricular extrasystole every 5 minutes
- ECG without nonspecific ST-segment elevations or depression and T-wave inversions

However, these criteria are not universally followed.

Controversies over routine use of preoperative preparation: α-blockers have been routinely used for preoperative preparation in patients with pheochromocytoma. Based on a very long follow-up of 48-years, Goldstein et al. concluded that α-blockade led to a decrease in complications from 69 to 3%. However, with passing years, anesthesia techniques have vastly improved, more effective intraoperative drugs are now available, and minimally invasive surgery has been introduced. It is thought that because of these factors, it is not mandatory to put the patients on α-blockade and the patients may be taken up for surgery once a confirmed biochemical diagnosis is made. Groeben et al. conducted a consecutive case series study on 303 patients and concluded that there were no significant differences in maximum systolic blood pressure changes or any major complications in patients with and without use of α-blockers preoperatively. Hence, they challenged the routine use of α-blockers preoperatively.

Drugs used during intraoperative period: Intraoperative excess release of catecholamines can result in HD instability and sometimes death. Two major alterations—hypertension and tachycardia—require intervention. Intraoperative increase in blood pressures can occur at time of induction, intubation, and mechanical ventilation or while creating a pneumoperitoneum, direct tumor manipulation. Though there are no definitive predictive factors, certain features may predispose to intraoperative HD alteration, such as high NE levels, tumor size > 4 cm, a high BP at presentation, and after α-blockade [mean arterial pressure (MAP) >100 mm Hg] and postural drop (>10 mm Hg) in BP.

Drugs used during surgery to control blood pressure surges or tachycardia include **(Fig. 9)**:
- *Sodium nitroprusside (SNP)*: The main advantage of this drug is that it reduces both preload and afterload and has immediate onset as well as recovery in 1 minute, so titration is easier and fast.

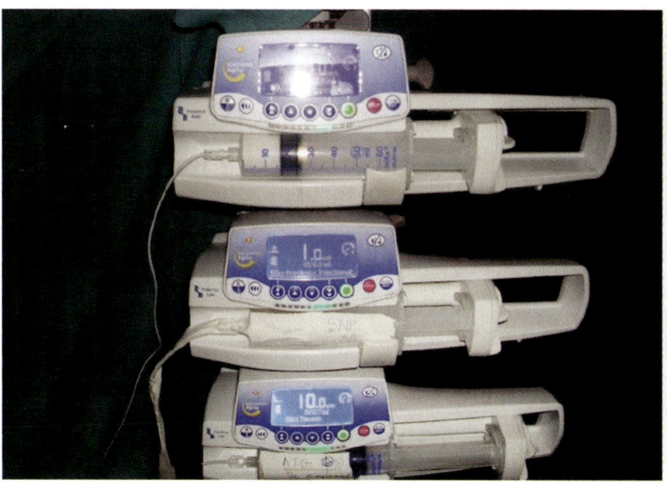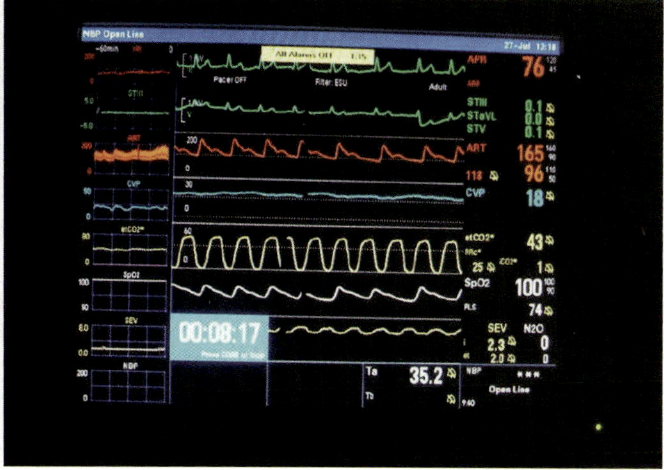

Fig. 9: Intraoperative hemodynamic alteration requiring SNP infusion.

- *Calcium-channel blockers*: They are powerful arterial vasodilators.
- *Magnesium sulfate*: Dual mode of action makes it particularly suitable for intraoperative use for surgery of pheochromocytoma. Besides inhibiting the release of catecholamine from the tumor, it has a direct vasodilatory effect on peripheral blood vessels.
- *Esmolol*: Esmolol hydrochloride, an intravenously administered cardioselective ultra-short-acting beta-1 receptor antagonist, is used when patients develop severe tachycardia or arrhythmias.
- *Nitroglycerin (NTG)—rapidly acting venodilator*:

It is a rapidly acting drug with a short duration and rapid titration and is thus the preferred drug. However, at higher doses, toxic metabolites, such as cyanide and thiocyanate, are a concern.

Surgery of Pheochromocytoma

Surgery is planned only after use of a selective α-adrenergic blocker (usually 7–14 days). The principles of surgery in pheochromocytoma are:
- Minimal tumor manipulation to avoid large surges in blood pressure
- Early control of adrenal vein if possible
- Adequate exposure to avoid other organ injuries

Numerous approaches can be made to the pheochromocytoma. The proper approach depends on:
- Size of the tumor
- Side of the tumor
- Habitus of the patient
- Experience and preference of the surgeon
  In today's era, the laparoscopic approach, if feasible, is the approach of choice.

Surgical technique: Certain concepts warrant attention:
- The adrenal glands lie high in the retroperitoneum and are located quite posterior; especially on the right side,

they tend to lie posterior to inferior vena cava (IVC), so adequate visualization is a must for a safe operation. Dissection may start in between the tumor and kidney progressing to lateral side and then freeing the gland superiorly from the liver and then dissecting the medial side of IVC to visualize the adrenal vein.
- The posterior surface is generally devoid of vasculature so it can be dissected by fingers.

Open surgical approaches:
- *Anterior transabdominal approach*: The anterior abdominal transperitoneal approach by subcostal incision for unilateral tumors and bucket handle incision or the Chevron incision for patients with bilateral pheochromocytoma is the most common approach.
- *Lateral flank approach*: This is a less favored approach.
- *Thoracoabdominal approach*: It is indicated for large tumors, usually >15 cm, or malignant pheochromocytoma involving adjacent organs, such as the kidney, pancreas, spleen, or inferior vena cava.

Laparoscopic adrenalectomy (LA): LA is the preferred option in sporadic pheochromocytomas (<10 cm) and majority of unilateral or bilateral syndromic pheochromocytomas (VHL, MEN, NF1).
- *Retroperitoneal approach*: The localized adrenal gland is accessed by retroperitoneoscopy after creation of a retroperitoneal space. Generally, three to four ports are required for introduction of the telescope, the dissector, the grasper, and a retractor. It is good for smaller tumors but has limited space to work and is done in a few centers only. The retroperitoneal approach has advantages in patients with previous abdominal surgery and those with enlarged liver. Repositioning is avoided in those requiring bilateral adrenalectomy. It has a shorter operative time and better cosmesis. However, it has a steep-learning curve.
- *Transperitoneal approach*: The transabdominal route has advantages of obvious and familiar anatomical landmarks

and wider operative space but has the potential for intraoperative injury to numerous surrounding organs and paralytic ileus.

Robotic adrenalectomy: Robotic adrenalectomy was first performed in 1999 by Piazza et al. and has overcome many of the drawbacks of the laparoscopic surgery such as compromised depth perception and camera syncing. It has been proposed as a safe, feasible, and effective approach more so in obese, larger lesions and when contemplating cortical sparing surgery. However, cost implications, loss of haptic feedback, and anesthetic perspective are some of the drawbacks. In spite of its many advantages, till date robotic adrenalectomy has not provided any distinct benefit over laparoscopy in terms of patient outcome and comfort.

*Bilateral adrenalectomy (**Fig. 10**):* This results in lifelong corticosteroid replacement with a high probability of mortality. Partial adrenalectomy performed first in 1996 via open method and 1998 via laparoscopy avoids postoperative steroid supplementation therapy in at least 50% of patients. For the remnant gland to retain corticotropic function, at least one-third of the adrenal grand has to be preserved. The risk of recurrence should be kept in mind, which ranges between 0 and 21%, especially in MEN2A patients, because of accompanying hyperplasia of the adrenal remnant. Endoscopic partial adrenalectomy results in a better outcome probably because of magnification. Cortical-sparing surgery has been advocated as the preferred method in MEN2/VHL-associated unilateral pheochromocytoma because 50% of such patients will develop contralateral metachronous pheochromocytoma.

Anesthetic and intraoperative considerations: Close, collegial communication between the surgeon and the anesthetist is crucial to the success of intraoperative management of patients undergoing pheochromocytoma resection. The following points need attention:

- *Anesthetic considerations*: An anxiolytic may be administered before the intra-arterial catheter is placed before induction. Place an intravenous catheter for antihypertensive administration (SNP, NTG) and place a central venous catheter for intravascular volume monitoring. Measurement of pulmonary capillary wedge pressure (PCWP) and cardiac output may be helpful especially in patients with heart disease because these patients may exhibit a discrepancy between right-sided and left-sided filling pressure. Depth of anesthesia is generally more important. Inhalation agents, such as halothane, result in severe arrhythmias and should be avoided but isoflurane, enflurane, and sevoflurane can be safely used. Induction with propofol or thiopental is safe. Ketamine and ephedrine should be avoided. Morphine causes histamine release, which is a known trigger of pheochromocytoma crisis. Droperidol should be avoided. Neuromuscular blockers, such as vecuronium, have little or no autonomic effects and do not release histamine and are the drug of choice.

The steps during surgery where the HD alterations are most likely to occur are:
- Induction of general anesthesia, when the myocardium is especially sensitized to the effects of catecholamine and endotracheal intubation
- Creating pneumoperitoneum in LA
- Excessive surgical manipulation of the tumor, due to increased release of catecholamines
- Ligation of the tumor blood supply, which may result in severe hypotension.

Intraoperative hypotension can result from:
- Massive vasodilation after excision of the tumor leading to sudden drop in catecholamine levels
- Residual effect of prolonged preoperative α-blockade, especially if PBX has been used.

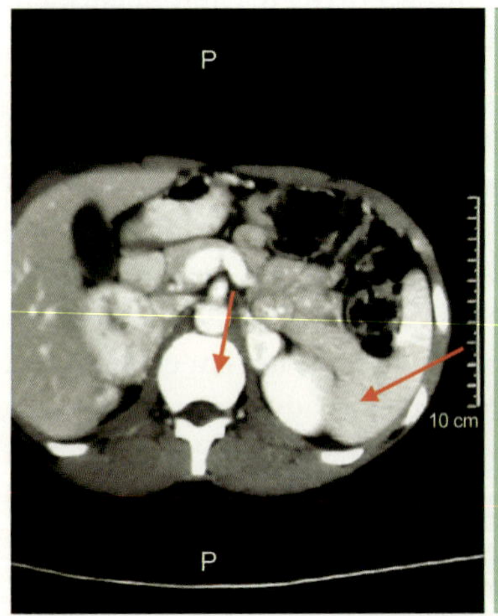

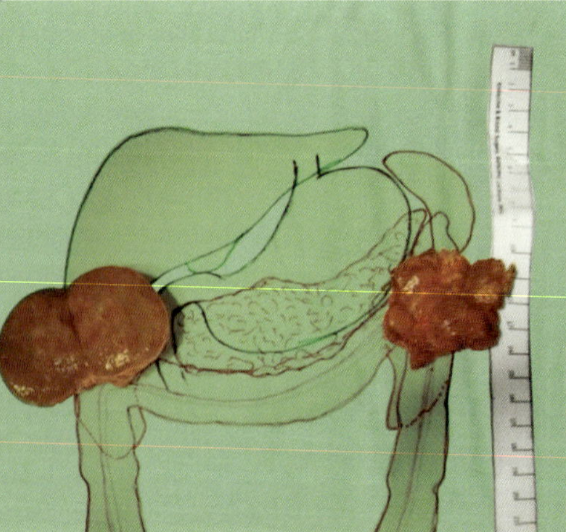

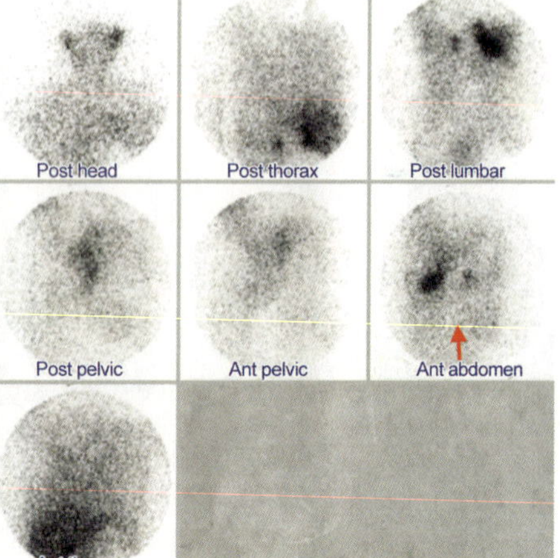

Fig 10: *Bilateral pheochromocytoma treated by unilateral and partial adrenalectomy:* A 27-year-old man diagnosed with bilateral pheochromocytoma. MIBG also suggested bilateral lesion; underwent right adrenalectomy with left partial adrenalectomy; later turned out to be sibling of VHL family.

- Excessive blood loss during surgery, myocardial infarction, and inadequate steroid replacement after bilateral adrenalectomy.

The complications that can happen during surgery of pheochromocytoma are summarized in **Table 8**.

Postoperative Care

Two important sequelae must be kept in mind:
- Patients may go into severe hypoglycemia due to relative increase in sensitivity to insulin after sudden withdrawal of the catecholamines, especially those patients who had abnormal glucose tolerance before surgery, so frequent monitoring (every 2 hours for the first 6 hours) of blood glucose is advisable.
- *Sustained hypotension*: The first step in managing this is to maintain intravascular volume by infusing colloids rather than crystalloids. If hypotension is persistent, then inotropes may be started which can usually be tapered and stopped over 12–24 hours. In refractory hypotension, vasopressin can be successfully used.

Follow-up

Patients are followed up with annual urinary metanephrine/normetanephrine estimations. If these are elevated, then further imaging is done to localize the recurrences/metastases. However, it must be kept in mind that 10–20% of patients will exhibit persistent hypertension without elevation of MN/NMN values. Metastatic disease may appear after several years. Metastatic disease is defined as the presence of catecholamine-secreting tissue (which is producing catecholamines or is imageable) in nonchromaffin-bearing organs.

Table 8: Complications following adrenal surgery.

Intraoperative complications	Postoperative complications following surgery
Hemorrhage/injury: • Inferior vena cava • Adrenal vein • Lumbar vein • Hepatic vein (in right adrenalectomy)	*Specific*: • Sustained hypotension • Persistent hypertension • Hypoglycemia
Vascular: • Ligation of renal artery branch • Ligation of mesenteric artery • IVC involvement	
Adjacent organ injury: • Pneumothorax • Pancreas, liver, and spleen • Stomach, colon, and kidney	
Complications related to HTN crisis: • Myocardial infarction • Pulmonary edema • Acute heart failure • Cerebral stroke	

(HTN: hypertension; IVC: inferior vena cava)

PHEOCHROMOCYTOMA CRISIS

Rarely, pheochromocytoma may present as an emergency in the form of hypertensive crisis (also known as pheochromocytoma crisis) which is an acute severe presentation of catecholamine-induced HD instability causing end-organ damage. It is often reversible with appropriate treatment. It can present in two forms:
1. *Type A crisis*: Hypertension but without sustained hypotension
2. *Type B crisis*: Severe crisis with sustained hypotension, shock, and multiorgan dysfunction

Pheochromocytoma crisis should be considered in any patient with unexplained shock, left ventricular failure, multiorgan failure, hypertensive crisis, or unexplained lactic acidosis.

Rather than rushing into an emergency surgery, such patients should be stabilized as early as possible and only then taken up for a semiemergent adrenalectomy.

MALIGNANT PHEOCHROMOCYTOMA

About 20% adrenal pheochromocytomas are malignant, especially extra-adrenal pheochromocytomas. It is very difficult to establish a preoperative diagnosis of malignant pheochromocytoma. However, elevated urinary dopamine is thought to be suggestive of a malignant pheochromocytoma. Complete surgical excision is the only potentially curative therapy for malignant pheochromocytoma, and aggressive surgical resection is indicated even if it entails removal of adjacent organs such as kidney or part of pancreas or spleen.

PHEOCHROMOCYTOMA IN PREGNANCY

An unsuspected pheochromocytoma in pregnancy can lead to hypertensive crisis with threat to both mother and unborn child. In a biochemically confirmed case, after adequate α-blockade, LA can be done in the second trimesters, while in the third trimester, a combined elective cesarean together with adrenalectomy should be planned.

CONCLUSION

Pheochromocytomas carry significant morbidity and mortality if untreated, but a successful outcome can be achieved by a correct biochemical diagnosis, precise tumor localization, optimal preoperative α-blockade, and unilateral or bilateral adrenalectomy. Even though few clinicians have questioned the need of preoperative blockade, it is still the standard of care in most centers. Though LA has become the standard of care for pheochromocytomas, the retroperitoneal approach is rapidly becoming an attractive option because it results in rapid recovery. Since familial pheochromocytoma is seen in as much as 30% cases and is now known to be associated with 18 susceptibility genes, it is important to keep a high index of suspicion for familial pheochromocytoma and the surgeon should triage the genetic testing based on factors such as clinical presentation, biochemical features, and family history.

◇ REFERENCES

1. Manger WM, Gifford RW. Pheochromocytoma. J Clin Hypertens. 2002:4:62-72.
2. Manger WM. An overview of pheochromocytoma: history, current concepts, vagaries, and diagnostic challenges. Ann NY Acad Sci. 2006;1073:1-20.
3. Pacak K. Preoperative management of the pheochromocytoma patient. J Clin Endocrinol Metab. 2007:92:4069-79.
4. Thomas RM, Ruel E, Shantavasinkul PC, Corsino L. Endocrine hypertension: an overview on the current etiopathogenesis and management options. World J Hypertens. 2015;5(2):14-27.
5. Lentschener C, Gaujoux S, Tesniere A, Dousset B. Point of controversy: perioperative care of patients undergoing pheochromocytoma removal-time for a reappraisal? Eur J Endocrinol. 2011;165(3):365-73.
6. Ramakrishna H. Pheochromocytoma resection: current concepts in anesthetic management. J Anaesthesiol Clin Pharmacol. 2015;31(3):317-23.
7. Goldstein RE, O'Neill JA Jr, Holcomb GW 3rd, Morgan WM 3rd, Neblett WW 3rd, Oates JA, et al. Clinical experience over 48 years with pheochromocytoma. Ann Surg. 1999;229(6):755-64; discussion 764-6.
8. Groeben H, Nottebaum BJ, Alesina PF, Traut A, Neumann HP, Walz MK. Perioperative α-receptor blockade in phaeochromocytoma surgery: an observational case series. Br J Anaesth. 2017;118(2):182-9.
9. Bruynzeel H, Feelders RA, Groenland TH, van den Meiracker AH, van Eijck CH, Lange JF, et al. Risk factors for hemodynamic instability during surgery for pheochromocytoma. J Clin Endocrinol Metab. 2010;95(2):678-85.
10. Bravo E. Evolving concepts in the pathophysiology, diagnosis, and treatment of pheochromocytoma. Endocr Rev. 1994;15(3):356-68.
11. Pacak K, Linehan WM, Eisenhofer G, Walther MM, Goldstein DS. Recent advances in genetics, diagnosis, localization, and treatment of pheochromocytoma. Ann Intern Med. 2001;134(4):315-29.
12. Manger WM, Gifford RW. Clinical and experimental pheochromocytoma, 2nd edition. Cambridge, MA: Blackwell Science; 1996.
13. Plouin PF, Degoulet P, Tugaye A, Ducrocq MB, Ménard J. Screening for phaeochromocytoma: in which hypertensive patients? A semilogical study of 2585 patients, including 11 with phaeochromcytoma. Nouv Presse Med. 1981;10(11):869-72.
14. Brouwers FM, Lenders JW, Eisenhofer G, Pacak K. Pheochromocytoma as an endocrine emergency. Rev Endocr Metab Disord. 2003;4:121-8.
15. Jafri M, Maher ER. The genetics of phaeochromocytoma: using clinical features to guide genetic testing. Eur J Endocrinol. 2012;166:151-8.
16. Havekes B, King K, Lai EW, Romijn JA, Corssmit EP, Pacak K. New imaging approaches to pheochromocytomas and paragangliomas. Clin Endocrinol. 2010;72:137-45.
17. Brandao LF, Autorino R, Laydner H, Haber GP, Ouzaid I, Sio MD, et al. Robotic versus laparoscopic adrenalectomy: a systematic review and meta-analysis. Eur Urol. 2014;65:1154-61.
18. Golden SH, Robinson KA, Saldanha I, Anton B, Ladenson PW. Clinical review: prevalence and incidence of endocrine and metabolic disorders in the United States—a comprehensive review. J Clin Endocrinol Metab. 2009;94(6):1853-78.
19. Lenders J, Eisenhofer G, Mannelli M, Pacak K. Phaeochromocytoma. Lancet 2005;366:665-75.
20. Gimenez-Roqueplo A, Dahia P, Robledo M. An update on the genetics of paraganglioma, pheochromocytoma, and associated hereditary syndromes. Horm Metab Res. 2012;44:328-33.
21. Scholz T, Eisenhofer G, Pacak K, Dralle H, Lehnert H. Clinical review: current treatment of malignant pheochromocytoma. J Clin Endocrinol Metab. 2007;92:1217-25.
22. Galan R, Kann H. Genetics and molecular pathogenesis of pheochromocytoma and paraganglioma. Clin Endocrinol (Oxf). 2013;78:165-75.
23. Pacak K, Eisenhofer G, Ahlman H, Bornstein SR, Gimenez-Roqueplo AP, Grossman AB, et al. International symposium on pheochromocytoma: recommendations for clinical practice from the first international symposium. Nat Clin Pract Endocrinol Metab. 2007;3:92-102.
24. Eisenhofer G, Goldstein DS, Walther MM, Friberg P, Lenders JWM, Keiser HR, et al. Biochemical diagnosis of pheochromocytoma: how to distinguish true from false positive test results. J Clin Endocrinol Metab. 2003;88:2656-66.
25. Goldstein DS, Eisenhofer G, Flynn JA, Wand G, Pacak K. Diagnosis and localization of pheochromocytoma. Hypertension. 2004;43:907-10.
26. Agrawal R, Mishra SK, Bhatia E, Mishra A, Chand G, Agarwal G, et al. Prospective study to compare peri-operative hemodynamic alterations following preparation for pheochromocytoma surgery by phenoxybenzamine or prazosin. World J Surg. 2013;38(3):716-23.
27. Agarwal A, Mehrotra PK, Jain M, Gupta SK, Mishra A, Chand G, et al. Size of the tumor and pheochromocytoma of the adrenal gland scaled score (PASS): can they predict malignancy? World J Surg. 2010;34(12):3022-8.
28. Bhargava PR, Mishra A, Agarwal G, Agarwal A, Verma AK, Mishra SK. Adrenal incidentalomas: experience from a developing country. World J Surg. 2008;32(8):1802-8.

Adrenocortical Carcinoma

Sendhil Rajan, Dhalapathy Sadacharan, Aromal Chekavar S

HISTORICAL PERSPECTIVE

Earlier in the 19th century, many cases were reported in autopsy studies and various terminologies have been used such as hypernephroma, fibromyxosarcoma, sarcoma, and carcinoma. The resolution of features of virilization following adrenal tumor excision was first documented in 1890. The first successful surgery was performed by Knowsley Thornton for a hirsute female patient with a left adrenal tumor.[1] In 1921, Collet described the resolution of virilization after resection of the adrenal tumor in a 2-year-old child.[2]

The association of Cushing's syndrome and adrenocortical carcinoma (ACC) was first described in 1934 at the Mayo Clinic. The mortality rate after adrenal surgeries was higher until the discovery of cortisone in 1949. Kendall, Hench, and Reichstein received the Nobel Prize in 1950 for the development of cortisone. In 1958, MacFarlane from London teaching hospitals described 55 patients which included 35 with hormonal and 25 with nonhormonal findings.[3] He was the first to propose an operative staging system based on tumor size, local invasion, and nodal and distant metastases. In 1961, Soffer described several cases of large malignant adrenal tumors with feminizing syndrome and widespread metastasis.[4]

In earlier days, surgery was considered as the only effective treatment for ACC and there were no additional systemic therapies for the metastatic and recurrent disease. The first adrenalytic agent tested was amphenone B [(1, 2-bis-(p-aminophenyl)-2-methyl propane-1], a derivative of dichlorodiphenyltrichloroethane (DDT) in 1950. Nelson and Woodward tested several other compounds such as DDD [2,2-bis(para chlorophenyl)-1,1-dichloroethane] and perthane which produced adrenocortical atrophy in dogs. The first major report of the National Cancer Institute evaluation of o,p'-DDD (mitotane) was by Hutter and Kayhoe in 1966.[5] In 1967, Eisenstein recommended DDD for patients with ACC, which was not amenable for complete surgical resection.[6] In 1982, Schteingart et al. described the effectiveness of mitotane as adjuvant therapy following surgery.[7] In 1983, Thompson described a combination of aggressive surgical treatment with adjuvant mitotane therapy in an earlier stage of disease which results in better treatment outcome.[8]

INTRODUCTION

Adrenocortical carcinoma is a rare disease with a reported incidence of 0.5–2 cases per million populations per year.[9] Majority of adrenal tumors are detected incidentally, among which ACC may account for up to 14%.[10] A more recent analysis of the SEER (surveillance, epidemiology, and end results) database indicated an annual age-adjusted incidence of 1.02 per million population.[11] ACCs may be sporadic or occur as part of a hereditary tumor syndrome. Recent Cancer Genome Atlas (TCGA) studies with the National Cancer Institute estimates 5–10% of patients with ACC have genetic predisposition syndromes. ACC can occur at any age but frequently been reported in the 4th and 5th decades with women being more commonly affected (female-to-male ratio of 1.6).[12] They can be both nonfunctional and functional tumors producing metabolic syndromes. ACC is an aggressive tumor with more than half of the cases having metastatic disease at the time of presentation. There is no general consensus on the diagnostic and therapeutic measures for ACC. Proper preoperative planning is required for complete resection of the tumor. The histopathological report should include Weiss score and Ki67 index. Mitotane is the only Food and Drug Administration (FDA) approved drug for treatment of ACC as adjuvant therapy and also as systemic therapy in metastatic disease. Recently, newer emerging therapies targeting genetic pathways, insulin-like growth factor (IGF), and Wnt/β-catenin pathways are under study. Even after extensive treatment, the prognosis is very poor with overall 5-year survival ranging between 16 and 44%.[13-15]

MOLECULAR PATHOGENESIS

The molecular mechanism in carcinogenesis in ACC is poorly understood. Most of the adrenocortical tumors are monoclonal, suggesting that an initial genetic or epigenetic alteration might occur in a single cell that acquires a selective advantage leading to tumor development. Alteration in various genetic pathways, especially Wnt/β-catenin and cyclic adenosine monophosphate (cAMP)/protein kinase A (PKA) ais being recognized in large cohorts of ACC **(Table 1)**.[16] Constitutive activation of β-catenin is the most frequent alteration in benign and malignant adrenocortical tumors.

The most frequently encountered molecular annotation is the activation of IGF2 signaling, occurring in up to 85% of cases.[17] Increase in IGF2 expression is being related to genetic alteration in 11p15 locus, and this is associated with a higher risk of tumor recurrence. Other growth factors involved in carcinogenesis include basic fibroblast growth factor 2 (FGF2), transforming growth factor (TGF)-α, TGF-β1, and vascular endothelial growth factor (VEGF). Multiple studies have shown that alterations in Wnt/β-catenin and p53 apoptosis/Rb1 cell cycle pathways are key molecular events in the pathogenesis of ACC.[17-19] TP53 mutations are found in 50–80% of children and in 20–35% of adults with sporadic ACC. Furthermore, the mutation in certain genes such as *PRKAR1A*, *RPL22*, *TERF2*, *CCNE1*, and *NF1* has also been encountered.[17] Upregulation of microRNAs, miR-483-5p, has recently been evaluated and their levels were predictive of more advanced disease stages.[20]

◇ GENETIC SYNDROMES ASSOCIATED WITH ADRENOCORTICAL CARCINOMA

Adrenocortical carcinoma is classically associated with familial cancer syndromes **(Table 2)**, and about 5–10% of ACC harbors germline mutations.[22]

Table 1: Genetic mutations associated with ACC.

Pathway affected	Genes affected	Frequency
Wnt/β-catenin signaling	ZNRF3	19–21%[17,19,21]
	CTNNB1	10–16%[17,19,21]
p53 apoptosis/Rb1 cell cycle	TP53	16–21%[17,19,21]
	CDKN2A	11–15%[17,19]
Chromatin remodeling/ maintenance	TERT	6–22%[17,19,21]
	MEN1	0–7%[17,19]
cAMP/PKA signaling	PRKAR1A	0–11%[17]

(ACC: adrenocortical carcinoma; cAMP: cyclic adenosine monophosphate; PKA: protein kinase A)

Li-Fraumeni Syndrome

Li-Fraumeni syndrome (LFS) is the most common syndromic association seen in children with ACC. The estimated prevalence varies from 1:20,000 to 1:1,000,000.[23] *TP53* is the most common mutation seen in children diagnosed with ACC and has an aggressive course of the disease.[24] Most often, ACC is the presenting malignancy in LFS, and hence all children diagnosed with ACC should be screened for LFS.

Lynch Syndrome

Lynch syndrome (LS) occurs due to germline mutations in DNA-mismatch repair (MMR) proteins PMS2, MSH2, MSH6, and MLH1.[23] In addition to ACC, ovarian, pancreatic, and sebaceous neoplasm, there is an increased risk for colorectal, endometrial, small bowel, and ureteric or renal pelvis tumors. If the diagnosis of LS is established in the index patient, the family members should undergo screening for germline mutation and, if positive, colorectal cancer screening should be performed.

Multiple Endocrine Neoplasia Type 1

Multiple endocrine neoplasia type 1 (MEN1) mutations are seen in 1–2% of all patients with ACC. On the contrary, the prevalence of ACC in MEN1-associated adrenal tumors is higher (13.8%).[25] Most of the MEN1-associated ACC arises from preexisting adrenal adenomas, and a majority of them are nonsecretory tumors.[25]

Familial Adenomatous Polyposis

The risk of ACC in familial adenomatous polyposis (FAP) is very low; hence, dedicated screening is not recommended.

Beckwith–Wiedemann Syndrome

Beckwith–Wiedemann syndrome (BWS) is often encountered in children with genetic alterations in IGF2 locus. ACC

Table 2: Genetic syndromes associated with ACC.[27]

Syndrome	Gene(s)	Prevalence of ACC	Other associated disease
Li-Fraumeni syndrome (LFS)	TP53 Chromosome 17p13	50–80% of children; 3–7% of adults	Brain cancer, breast cancer, lung cancer, sarcoma, leukemia, and choroid plexus tumor
Lynch syndrome (LS)	MSH2, MLH1, PMS2, MSH6, EPCAM	3% of adults	Colorectal, endometrial, small bowel, ureteral cancer, sebaceous carcinoma, pancreas cancer, and prostate cancer
MEN1	MENIN	1–2% of adults	Pituitary adenomas, primary hyperparathyroidism, pancreatic neuroendocrine tumors, other foregut neuroendocrine tumors, and adrenal adenomas
FAP	APC Chromosome 5q12-22	Rare, case reports	Colon cancer, duodenal adenomas, adrenal adenomas, and thyroid cancer
Beckwith–Wiedemann	IGF2 locus Chromosome 11p15	Rare, case reports; occur in childhood only	Cancers in childhood, Wilms' tumor, hepatoblastoma, rhabdomyosarcoma, neuroblastoma, benign adrenal cysts, and adenomas
Neurofibromatosis type 1	NF1	Rare, case reports, can occur in young children	Gliomas, malignant nerve sheath tumor, and benign neural tumors
Carney complex	PRKAR1A	Rare, case reports	PPNAD, pituitary and thyroid tumors, cardiac myxomas, schwannomas, and other tumors

(ACC: adrenocortical carcinoma; FAP: familial adenomatous polyposis; MEN1: multiple endocrine neoplasia type 1; PPNAD: primary pigmented nodular adrenocortical disease)

accounts for 1% of BWS whereas benign adrenal cysts and adenomas are more common. The risk of ACC and other cancers in BWS declines by adulthood.[26]

CLINICAL PRESENTATION

The initial presentation of ACC is due to symptoms and signs of hormonal excess, local compressive features by large mass, and complications of the metastatic disease. Some patients may have nonspecific manifestations such as fever, malaise, and weight loss. Recently, ACC is being discovered incidentally on imaging and frequency ranges from 13 to 17% in various series.[14,28]

Hormonal Excess

The majority of the tumors (50–60%) produces excess hormones, among which Cushing's syndrome is the most frequent presentation.[14] The key features of Cushing's syndrome in ACC are little or no weight gain, profound muscle atrophy, severe hypertension, glucose intolerance, profound depression, acute psychosis, and severe hypokalemia. The severity of the disease is because of the more rapid progression of the tumor and massive hypercortisolism.[29]

The second most frequent clinical presentation is based on coexisting hypersecretion of cortisol and adrenal androgens (~25%). Females with androgen excess develop acne, hirsutism, androgenetic effluvium, and oligomenorrhea. Less frequently, signs of virilization (clitoral enlargement, deepening of the voice, and baldness) were also seen. In males, estrogen-secreting tumors (5% of cases) leads to feminization, gynecomastia, loss of libido, and testicular atrophy. Recent-onset gynecomastia has been frequently reported as the initial manifestation.[30]

Aldosterone-secreting ACC is rare and accounts for <2% of patients with ACC. Majority of the patients present with hypertension and hypokalemia.[31] There were reports of tumor-induced hypoglycemia in patients with ACC, probably due to the paracrine release of IGF2, which acts on insulin receptors thereby increased glucose utilization.[32] In addition, ACC-secreting antidiuretic hormone (ADH), renin, erythropoietin, inhibin, and ectopic calcitonin have been reported.[33-37]

Locoregional Manifestation

Nonfunctioning tumors come to notice when a large tumor produces a mass effect such as abdominal fullness and pain, back pain, nausea, and vomiting.[38] Some patients may present with an acute abdomen or with retroperitoneal hemorrhage because of tumor rupture.[39] The tumor may invade inferior vena cava (IVC) and can extend up to the right atrium leading to impaired venous flow, leg edema, and respiratory distress.[40,41]

Symptoms related to Metastatic Disease

The most frequent sites of metastasis are lung, liver, and bone. Patients with advanced disease present with

Table 3: Hormonal work-up in patients with suspected ACC.[44]	
Glucocorticoid excess	• 1 mg dexamethasone suppression test or 24-h urinary free cortisol • Basal plasma ACTH
Sex steroids and precursors	• DHEAS • 17-OH-progesterone • Androstenedione • Testosterone (only in women) • 17-β-estradiol (in men and postmenopausal women) • 11-deoxycortisol
Mineralocorticoid excess	• Potassium • Aldosterone/rennin ratio (in patients with arterial hypertension and/or hypokalemia)
Exclusion of pheochromocytoma	Fractionated metanephrines in 24-h urine or plasma-free metanephrines

(ACC: adrenocortical carcinoma; ACTH: adrenocorticotropic hormone; DHEAS: dehydroepiandrosterone sulfate)

bone pain or fractures, paraplegia, hematuria, and urinary obstruction.[42,43]

HORMONAL EVALUATION

Detailed hormonal assessment is mandatory because the majority (50–60%) of the patients with ACC suffer from clinically evident hormonal excess **(Table 3)**.[44] An adrenal mass that cosecretes different types of steroids, especially glucocorticoids, in combination with sex hormones and its precursors is highly suspicious of ACC. In general, low dehydroepiandrosterone sulfate (DHEAS) suggests a benign adrenocortical tumor, whereas highly elevated DHEAS levels are indicative for ACC.[45] Moreover, preoperatively elevated hormones can serve as tumor markers during follow-up.

IMAGING

Nowadays, incidental adrenal lesions are frequently encountered due to the widespread use of high-resolution abdominal and thoracic imaging. Adrenal incidentaloma (AI) is present in approximately 4–6% of the imaged population in comparison with autopsy studies, where the overall frequency ranges from 1 to 32%.[46-48] The goal of an AI-screening protocol is to identify all patients with ACC as early as possible. Recommended guidelines suggest a radiographic re-evaluation of an AI at 3–6 months and then annually for 1–2 years with hormonal evaluation at the time of diagnosis and annually for a total of 5 years.[49]

Imaging of adrenal lesions has a role in the assessment of tumor characteristics and its extent to adjacent structures and also in the metastatic workup. The size of the lesion can predict malignancy and it can even contribute to prognostication. The risk of malignancy will increase from 2% for adrenocortical lesion ≤4 cm, 6% for a lesion 1–6 cm, and 25% for a lesion >6 cm.[50] Features that increase concern for a malignant adrenal neoplasm in imaging include heterogeneous enhancement, irregular margins, intratumoral necrosis, calcifications, hemorrhage, lipid content and intravenous washout characteristics, invasion into adjacent structures, venous extension, significant lymph nodes, and metastatic lesions.[49]

Contrast-enhanced Computed Tomography

The appearance of ACC on contrast-enhanced computed tomography (CECT) is a heterogeneous mass with necrosis, attenuation value >10 HU, displacement, or invasion of adjacent structures. Smaller ACC tumors may appear homogeneous but have a slower contrast washout than adenomas (APW <60%, RPW <40%).[51]

Magnetic Resonance Imaging

Magnetic resonance imaging (MRI) is superior to CT for the evaluation of invasion into adjacent structures and venous involvement.[52] The three major signs on the MRI, which are useful to confirm ACC, are the presence of isointense to hypointense signal on T1-weighted images, a hyperintense signal on T2-weighted images, and a heterogeneous signal drop on chemical shift. It can also detect tumor thrombus in the renal vein and IVC, regional lymphadenopathy, and distant metastasis.

¹⁸F-FDG PET-CT

The role of fluorodeoxyglucose (FDG) positron emission tomography (PET) in ACC is in preoperative treatment planning, postoperative surveillance, and evaluation and management in the metastatic setting. PET imaging will show high FDG uptake with a cutoff value of >1.45 for adrenal-to-liver maximum SUV. FDG PET combined with CECT has a sensitivity of 100% and a specificity of 87–97% for identifying malignant adrenal lesions. However, ¹⁸FFDG PET/CT cannot distinguish ACC from metastases, lymphoma, or pheochromocytoma, which also exhibits high metabolic activity. A newer PET tracer, 11C-metomidate, identifies lesions of adrenocortical origin with high tracer uptake, of which ACC has the highest uptake.[53]

◇ HISTOPATHOLOGICAL EVALUATION AND STAGING

Although biochemical and imaging evaluation points toward ACC, a definitive diagnosis requires confirmation by histopathological examination. When the definitive criteria for malignancy such as distant metastasis and local invasion are absent, the most commonly used tool to distinguish between benign and malignant adrenocortical tumors is Weiss criteria **(Box 1)**.[54] The presence of three or more out of nine criteria represents the high likelihood for malignancy.[55] The use of Ki67 immunohistochemistry marker is mandatory for every resected specimen of ACC.[45] In addition to this, there are several other markers such as steroidogenic factor-1 (SF-1), tumor protein P53, IGF-2, cyclin E, reticulin, and E3 ubiquitin-

Box 1: Weiss criteria.

- High nuclear grade (grade 3 or 4)
- Mitosis 6/50 high-powered field or higher
- Atypical mitosis
- Clear cells 25% or less
- Diffuse architecture 33% surface or more
- Confluent necrosis
- Venous invasion
- Sinusoidal invasion
- Capsular infiltration

The identification of the three or more of these above criteria strongly indicative of ACC.

(ACC: adrenocortical carcinoma)

Table 4: ENSAT staging.

T1 ≤ 5 cm	*Stage 1:* T1 N0 M0
T2 > 5cm	*Stage 2:* T2 N0 M0
T3—histologically proven tumor infiltration to surrounding periadrenal tissue	*Stage 3:* T1-2 N1 M0 T3-4 N0-1 M0
T4—tumor invasion of adjacent organs or venous tumor thrombus in vena cava or renal vein	*Stage 4:* T1-4 N0-1 M1
N0—no regional lymph node metastasis N1—metastasis in regional lymph nodes	
M0—no distant metastasis M1—presence of distant metastasis	

(ENSAT: European Network for the Study of Adrenal Tumors)

protein ligase (MIB-1), which are emerging nowadays but large-scale validation is still lacking.[56,57]

Staging is based on the European Network for the Study of Adrenal Tumors (ENSAT) classification, which is the widely accepted staging system **(Table 4)**.[44] In addition to this staging system, various other factors, such as hormone status, tumor resection status, Ki-67 index, and molecular markers, should be taken into account for better prognostication of the disease. The reported 5-year survival rates of stage I, II, III, and IV disease are 82%, 58%, 55%, and 18%, respectively.[58]

◇ TREATMENT

Surgery and Preoperative Planning

The mainstay of treatment in ACC is complete surgical resection of the tumor with curative intent and adjuvant therapies to decrease the chance of recurrence. Appropriate preoperative evaluation and operative planning are of the utmost importance. Surgery should be conducted only after appropriate preoperative diagnostic tests, including biochemical evaluation and imaging. Urinary or plasma metanephrines and normetanephrines should be measured to rule out pheochromocytoma before surgery to avoid potential intraoperative complications. Cortisol excess should be ruled out to prevent the life-threatening risk of postoperative adrenal insufficiency due to cortisol-secreting ACC.

Imaging studies help to guide the surgeon regarding the expected extent of resection required. Careful attention should be paid to the adjacent organs, the adrenal and renal veins, the inferior vena cava, and the aorta, including the takeoff of the celiac and superior mesenteric arteries. Imaging should be obtained as close as possible to the anticipated date of surgery due to rapid growth and fast infiltration of ACC, thereby altering the operative plan. In the case of thrombus, always evaluate the extent of the thrombus with imaging and other aides such as echocardiography, intravascular ultrasound, or venography. The European Society of Endocrine Surgeons and the European Network for the Study of Adrenal Tumors published summary guidelines in 2017 recommending preoperative imaging including CT chest-abdomen-pelvis and ^{18}F-FDG PET-CT within 6 weeks before planned adrenalectomy for suspected ACC. Additionally, gadolinium-enhanced MRI is recommended for patients in whom vascular invasion or hepatic metastasis is suspected.[59] Based on the extent of disease, ACC can be classified into localized, locally advanced, and metastatic disease.

Surgery for Localized Disease

For localized ACC, successful complete R0 resection is the only potentially curative treatment. The surgical plan is to achieve oncologically negative margins and en bloc resection, without disruption of the tumor capsule.[58] Open surgery was considered a standard of surgical treatment, but laparoscopic surgery can be considered in small (<6 cm) noninvasive tumors if negative margins and en bloc resection can be achieved.[44]

Surgery for Locally Advanced Disease

Surgical resection is the definitive treatment even for stage III disease with local invasion into the surrounding organs and vena cava involvement. En bloc resection of the adjacent solid organs, such as ipsilateral kidney, pancreas, spleen, stomach, or diaphragm, is often required to maintain capsule integrity and to achieve a good oncologic outcome.[58] For borderline resectable cases, there is a role for neoadjuvant therapy followed by surgery in select patient subgroups.[58,60]

In case of intracaval extension or tumor thrombosis which can be encountered in up to 25% of cases, tumor thrombectomy in the infrarenal IVC can be achieved by vascular control (via cross-clamping or hepatic vascular exclusion), followed by cavotomy and primary closure or vein resection and reconstruction with or without graft interposition. If the thrombus extends above the diaphragm or into the right atrium, cardiopulmonary bypass may be necessary.[60]

Surgery for Metastatic Disease

In metastatic disease, with limited intra-abdominal metastasis, adrenalectomy along with surgical resection of all lesions can be performed if feasible.[44,61] Even in case of limited extra-abdominal metastasis (≤2 organs involved), adrenalectomy

and therapy targeting other lesions can be considered.[44,61] However, adrenalectomy should not be performed in patients with widespread distant metastatic disease.[44]

In patients with severe hormone excess who cannot be controlled otherwise, surgical resection or debulking could be beneficial.[60,61] There are other therapeutic measures such as radiofrequency ablation, cryoablation, or chemoembolization, which can be adopted either in addition to surgery or alone depending on the type of lesion.[44]

Surgical Approach

The first operation is the best chance for long-term local control of malignancy due to lack of other effective treatment options such as radiotherapy or chemotherapy. So, following the oncological principles is the key to surgical cure in ACC. The principle of surgery is to follow a stepwise approach as follows: incision and exploration of the peritoneal cavity, evaluation of liver for metastasis, mobilization of organs adjacent to the tumor, en bloc resection, regional lymphadenectomy, provide intact en bloc specimen for pathological review, and mark field to facilitate postsurgical external beam radiation therapy (RT).

Even though few retrospective studies showed improved survival with formal lymph node dissections, there is no consensus regarding the extent of lymph node dissection in ACC.[62,63] The principle of lymphadenectomy follows the lymphatics along with the main arterial supply chain, which are the renal hilum and the origin of the celiac and mesenteric arteries. The recent European Society of Endocrinology clinical practice guidelines suggest that routine locoregional lymphadenectomy of periadrenal and renal hilum nodes should be performed along with adrenalectomy for highly suspected or proven ACC.[44]

Open versus Laparoscopic Approach

Even though laparoscopic surgery is the gold standard in adrenal surgeries for benign cases, open surgery is always preferred for ACC. This is because of increased rates of tumor capsule disruption leading to a higher chance for local recurrence and peritoneal carcinomatosis reported with laparoscopic resection.[58,64] Moreover, open surgery has the advantage of complete resection of the tumor along with adjacent organs if involved and regional lymph node dissection, which is important for accurate staging and further adjuvant treatment. However, in patients with a tumor <6 cm without any evidence of local invasion, laparoscopic adrenalectomy may be performed by an experienced surgeon, provided that all principles of oncologic surgery are followed.[58] There are few retrospective case series that suggest that both laparoscopic and open adrenalectomy are equally effective but insufficient to give a definitive conclusion because of the limited number of patients and lack of validation.[65,66] Due to these facts, the Society of Surgical Oncology (SSO), the European Society of Endocrine Surgeons (ESES), and the

European Network for the Study of Adrenal Tumors (ENSAT) all strongly recommend open surgery for known or suspected ACC as the gold standard approach.[44,59,67]

Adjuvant Treatment

In ACC, even after complete surgical resection, the estimated recurrence rate is 40–70%.[68] The main predictors of recurrence include advanced disease stage, incomplete surgical resection, certain genetic alterations, and high proliferation rate (Ki-67 proliferation index). Hence, an adjuvant treatment in a locally advanced disease aims at decreasing the high recurrence rates following surgical management. In the case of metastatic disease, the treatment is palliative rather than a cure. Treatment options are external beam radiation for palliation of local symptoms and better control of hormone excess, chemotherapy, and mitotane therapy.

Mitotane Therapy

Mitotane is a derivative of the insecticide DDT, which has both adrenolytic and adrenostatic properties.[69,70] Adjuvant mitotane therapy is recommended for patients who have a higher chance for a recurrent disease like those with stage III disease, incomplete tumor resection, and high-grade disease of any stage (Ki67 index >10%).[44] However for patients with low risk of recurrence and low-grade tumors (stages I–III and Ki67 <10% after R0 resection), the benefit of mitotane therapy is questionable, which will be addressed in an ongoing prospective randomized phase III trial (ADIUVO, NCT00777244).

Mitotane therapy generally is continued for approximately 2 years unless limited by severe or intolerable adverse events.[44] The most common adverse effects are nausea, vomiting, diarrhea, and generalized fatigue. Neurological complications such as ataxia, memory loss, lethargy, and depression can occur at higher doses. Other toxicity includes liver damage, hypercholesterolemia, pancytopenia, drug-induced skin rash, and hypothyroidism. Patients on mitotane should be supplemented with glucocorticoids to prevent adrenal insufficiency due to adrenolytic action of mitotane on contralateral normal adrenal gland.[44]

Radiation Therapy

There is limited data regarding the role of adjuvant RT for ACC. So, a decision regarding adjuvant RT should be on a case-by-case basis and must weigh the morbidity of treatment against the probability of tumor recurrence. If adjuvant RT is administered, the recommended dose is 50–60 Gy to the tumor bed given in fractionated doses of 2 Gy each.[44] Recent meta-analysis suggests that adjuvant RT significantly reduces the risk of local recurrence and also has a low rate of toxicity; therefore, it could be considered for high-risk ACC patients who had undergone surgical resection for stage II or III with positive margins and tumor > 10 cm.[71]

Chemotherapy

Adjuvant chemotherapy can be considered in selected patients who are at very high risk for recurrence and as palliation in the case of advanced metastatic disease.[44] A phase III randomized study FIRM-ACT (First International Randomized Trial in Locally Advanced and Metastatic Adrenocortical Carcinoma Treatment) trial showed the superiority of etoposide, doxorubicin, and cisplatin with mitotane over streptozocin with mitotane. Fassnacht and colleagues demonstrated a statistically significant improvement in progression-free survival for EDP-M compared with streptozocin–mitotane (5.3 months vs. 2.0 months).[72] Hence, the guidelines recommend the EDP-M scheme as the first line of therapy for advanced/metastatic ACC.[44] The second-line drugs—streptozocin plus mitotane or gemcitabine plus capecitabine with or without mitotane—can be used in patients with tumor progression after EDP-M treatment.

Future Directions

There are several ongoing clinical trials on immunotherapy with anti-CTLA4 and anti-PD-L1 agents. There are also several approaches to target the receptors for IGF1, VEGF, and epidermal growth factor as well as mammalian target of rapamycin (mTOR) inhibitors.[73-77] More recently, research aiming to investigate compounds that exert anticancer effect by suppressing Wnt/β-catenin pathways is under study.[78]

◇| SUMMARY

Adrenocortical carcinoma is a rare, aggressive malignancy that is usually diagnosed at an advanced stage. Preoperative assessment for hormonal hyperfunction and imaging to assess the extent of the disease are mandatory. The mainstay of therapy is complete surgical resection whenever possible. Surgical debulking has a role to reduce tumor burden and control of hormonal excess in certain cases. Mitotane therapy is recommended in high-grade, locoregional, and metastatic tumors. EDP with mitotane is the first-line regimen for systemic chemotherapy in advanced, metastatic disease. Studies on many targeted therapies and immunotherapies are ongoing. In advanced metastatic disease, the main focus of treatment is palliative care to improve the quality of life (QoL) by adequate control of hormonal symptoms, pain control, and prevention of fractures caused by bony metastasis as well as minimizing side effects from antineoplastic therapies.

◇| REFERENCES

1. Thornton JK. Abdominal nephrectomy for large sarcoma of the left suprarenal capsule: recovery. Trans Clin Soc London. 1890;23:150-3.
2. Welbourn RB. The history of endocrine surgery. New York: Praeger; 1990.

3. MacFarlane DA. Cancer of the adrenal cortex. Ann R Coll Surg Engl. 1958;23:155-62.

4. Soffer LJ. The human adrenal gland. Philadelphia, PA: Lea & Febiger; 1961.

5. Hutter MM Jr, Kayhoe DE. Adrenal cortical carcinoma. Results of treatment with o,p-DDD in 138 patients. Am J Med. 1966;41:581-9.

6. Eisenstein AB. The adrenal cortex. Boston, MA: Little, Brown and Company; 1967.

7. Schteingart DE, Motazedi A, Noonan RA, Thompson NW. The treatment of adrenal carcinoma. Arch Surg. 1982;117:1142-6.

8. Thompson NW. Adrenocortical carcinoma. In: Thompson NW, Vinik AI (Eds). Endocrine surgery update. New York: Grune and Stratton; 1983. pp 119-28.

9. Kebebew E, Reiff E, Duh QY, Clark OH, McMillan A. Extent of disease at presentation and outcome for adrenocortical carcinoma: have we made progress? World J Surg. 2006;30(5):872-8.

10. Mansmann G, Lau J, Balk E, Rothberg M, Miyachi Y, Bornstein SR. The clinically inapparent adrenal mass: update in diagnosis and management. SR Endocr Rev. 2004;25(2):309-40.

11. Sharma E, Dahal S, Sharma P, Bhandari A, Gupta V, Amgai B, et al. The characteristics and trends in adrenocortical carcinoma: A United States population based study. J Clin Med Res. 2018;10(8):636-40.

12. Mihai R. Diagnosis, treatment and outcome of adrenocortical cancer. Br J Surg. 2015;102(4):291-306.

13. Icard P, Goudet P, Charpenay C, Andreassian B, Carnaille B, Chapuis Y, et al. Adrenocortical carcinomas: surgical trends and results of a 253-patient series from the French Association of Endocrine Surgeons study group. World J Surg. 2001;25(7):891-7.

14. Abiven G, Coste J, Groussin L, Anract P, Tissier F, Legmann P, et al. Clinical and biological features in the prognosis of adrenocortical cancer: poor outcome of cortisol-secreting tumors in a series of 202 consecutive patients. J Clin Endocrinol Metab. 2006;91(7):2650-5.

15. Bellantone R, Ferrante A, Boscherini M, Lombardi CP, Crucitti P, Crucitti F, et al. Role of reoperation in recurrence of adrenal cortical carcinoma: results from 188 cases collected in the Italian National Registry for Adrenal Cortical Carcinoma. Surgery. 1997;122(6):1212-8.

16. Pittaway JFH, Guasti L. Pathobiology and genetics of adrenocortical carcinoma. J Mol Endocrinol. 2019;62(2):R105-R119.

17. Zheng S, Cherniack AD, Dewal N, Moffitt RA, Danilova L, Murray BA, et al. Comprehensive pan-genomic characterization of adrenocortical carcinoma. Cancer Cell. 2016;29(5):723-36.

18. Ragazzon B, Libé R, Gaujoux S, Assié G, Fratticci A, Launay P, et al. Transcriptome analysis reveals that p53 and {beta}-catenin alterations occur in a group of aggressive adrenocortical cancers. Cancer Res. 2010;70(21):8276-81.

19. Assié G, Letouzé E, Fassnacht M, Jouinot A, Luscap W, Barreau O, et al. Integrated genomic characterization of adrenocortical carcinoma. Nat Genet. 2014;46:607-12.

20. Salvianti F, Canu L, Poli G, Armignacco R, Scatena C, Cantini G, et al. New insights in the clinical and translational relevance of miR483-5p in adrenocortical cancer. Oncotarget. 2017;8(39):65525-33.

21. Juhlin CC, Goh G, Healy JM, Fonseca AL, Scholl UI, Stenman A, et al. Whole-exome sequencing characterizes the landscape of somatic mutations and copy number alterations in adrenocortical carcinoma. J Clin Endocrinol Metab. 2015;100(3):E493-502.

22. Else T. Association of adrenocortical carcinoma with familial cancer susceptibility syndromes. Mol Cell Endocrinol. 2012;351(1):66-70.

23. Else T, Kim AC, Sabolch A, Raymond VM, Kandathil A, Caoili EM, et al. Adrenocortical carcinoma. Endocr Rev. 2014;35(2):282-326.

24. Wasserman JD, Novokmet A, Eichler-Jonsson C, Ribeiro RC, Rodriguez-Galindo C, Zambetti GP, et al. Prevalence and functional consequence of TP53 mutations in pediatric adrenocortical carcinoma: a children's oncology group study. J Clin Oncol. 2015;33(6):602-9.

25. Gatta-Cherifi B, Chabre O, Murat A, Niccoli P, Cardot-Bauters C, Rohmer V, et al. Adrenal involvement in MEN1. Analysis of 715 cases from the Groupe d'etude des Tumeurs Endocrines database. Eur J Endocrinol. 2012;166(2):269-79.

26. Lapunzina P. Risk of tumorigenesis in overgrowth syndromes: a comprehensive review. Am J Med Genet. 2005;137(c1):53-71.

27. Petr EJ, Else T. Adrenocortical carcinoma (ACC): When and why should we consider germline testing? Presse Med. 2018;47(7-8 Pt 2):e119-25.

28. Fassnacht M, Libé R, Kroiss M, Allolio B. Adrenocortical carcinoma: a clinician's update. Nat Rev Endocrinol. 2011;7(6):323-35.

29. Koschker AC, Libé R, Kroiss M, Allolio B. Adrenocortical carcinoma: improving patient care by establishing new structures. Exp Clin Endocrinol Diabetes. 2006;114:45-51.

30. Gabrilove J, Sharma DC, Wotiz HH, Dorfman RI. Feminizing adrenocortical tumors in the male: a review of 52 cases including a case report. Medicine. 1965;44:37-9.

31. Seccia TM, Fassina A, Nussdorfer GG, Pessina AC, Rossi GP. Aldosterone-producing adrenocortical carcinoma: an unusual cause of Conn's syndrome with an ominous clinical course. Endocr Relat Cancer. 2005;12:149-59.

32. Hyodo T, Megyesi K, Kahn CR, McLean JP, Friesen HG. Adrenocortical carcinoma and hypoglycemia: evidence for production of nonsuppressible insulin-like activity by the tumor. J Clin Endocrinol Metab. 1977;44(6):1175-84.

33. Falchuk KR. Inappropriate antidiuretic hormone-like syndrome associated with an adrenocortical carcinoma. Am J Med Sci. 1973;266(5):393-5.

34. Yamanaka K, Iitaka M, Inaba M, Morita T, Sasano H, Katayama S. A case of renin-producing adrenocortical cancer. Endocr J. 2000;47(2):119-25.

35. Oka T, Onoe K, Nishimura K, Tsujimura A, Sugao H, Takaha M, et al. Erythropoietin-producing adrenocortical carcinoma. Urol Int. 1996;56(4):246-9.

36. Fragoso MC, Kohek MB, Martin RM, Latronico AC, Lucon AM, Zerbini MC, et al. An inhibin B and estrogen-secreting adrenocortical carcinoma leading to selective FSH suppression. Horm Res. 2007;67(1):7-11.

37. Pegoli W Jr, Kolbe A, Beaver BL, Chalew SA, Hill JL. Ectopic calcitonin in adrenocortical carcinoma: a new tumor marker. J Pediatr Surg. 1987;22(12):1183-4.

38. Allolio B, Hahner S, Weismann D, Fassnacht M. Management of adrenocortical carcinoma. Clin Endocrinol (Oxf). 2004;60:273-87.

39. Suyama K, Beppu T, Isiko T, Kanemitsu K, Hirota M, Baba H. Spontaneous rupture of adrenocortical carcinoma. Am J Surg. 2007;194(1):77-8.

40. Yeh MW, Lisewski D, Campbell P. Virilizing adrenocortical carcinoma with cavoatrial extension. Am J Surg. 2006;192(2):209-10.

41. Wright CB, Brennan L, Brophy P, Kirsh G, Shapiro M, Potter B, et al. Adrenocortical tumor with left renal vein, vena cava and intrahepatic venous extension. J Cardiovasc Surg (Torino). 2008;49(1):79-81.

42. Solans R, Vilardell M, Beatriz Vázquez A, Yagüe E. Bone metastases as presentation of adrenocortical carcinoma. Med Clin (Barc). 2001;116(2):767.

43. Macfarlane DA. Cancer of the adrenal cortex: the natural history, prognosis and treatment in a study of fifty-five cases. Ann RC Surg Engl. 1958;23(3):155-86.

44. Fassnacht M, Dekkers OM, Else T, Baudin E, Berruti A, de Krijger R, et al. European Society of Endocrinology Clinical Practice Guidelines on the management of adrenocortical carcinoma in adults, in collaboration with the European Network for the Study of Adrenal Tumors. Eur J Endocrinol. 2018;179(4):G1-G46.

45. Fassnacht M, Kenn W, Allolio B. Adrenal tumors: how to establish malignancy? J Endocrinol Invest. 2004;27(4):387-99.

46. Boland GW, Blake MA, Hahn PF, Mayo-Smith WW. Incidental adrenal lesions: principles, techniques, and algorithms for imaging characterization. Radiology. 2008;249(3):756-75.

47. Bovio S, Cataldi A, Reimondo G, Sperone P, Novello S, Berruti A, et al. Prevalence of adrenal incidentaloma in a contemporary computerized tomography series. J Endocrinol Invest. 2006;29(4):298-302.

48. Kloos RT, Gross MD, Francis IR, Korobkin M, Shapiro B. Incidentally discovered adrenal masses. Endocr Rev. 1995;16(4):460-84.

49. Young WF. Clinical practice. The incidentally discovered adrenal mass. N Engl J Med. 2007;356(6):601-10.

50. National Institutes of Health. NIH state-of-the-science statement on management of the clinically inapparent adrenal mass ("incidentaloma"). NIH Consens State Sci Statements. 2002;19(2):1-25.

51. Shin YR, Kim KA. Imaging features of various adrenal neoplastic lesions on radiologic and nuclear medicine imaging. Am J Roentgenol 2015;205(3):554-63.

52. Bharwani N, Rockall AG, Sahdev A, Gueorguiev M, Drake W, Grossman AB, et al. Adrenocortical carcinoma: the range of appearances on CT and MRI. Am J Roentgenol. 2011;196(6):W706-14.

53. Groussin L, Bonardel G, Silvéra S, Tissier F, Coste J, Abiven G, et al. 18F-Fluorodeoxyglucose positron emission tomography for the diagnosis of adrenocortical tumors: a prospective study in 77 operated patients. J Clin Endocrinol Metab. 2009;94(5):1713-22.

54. Weiss LM. Comparative histologic study of 43 metastasizing and nonmetastasizing adrenocortical tumors. Am J Surg Pathol. 1984;8(3):163-9.

55. Weiss LM, Medeiros LJ, Vickery AL Jr. Pathologic features of prognostic significance in adrenocortical carcinoma. Am J Surg Pathol. 1989;13(3):202-6.

56. Papotti M, Libè R, Duregon E, Volante M, Bertherat J, Tissier F. The Weiss score and beyond – histopathology for adrenocortical carcinoma. Horm Cancer. 2011;2(6):333-40.

57. Aubert S, Wacrenier A, Leroy X, Devos P, Carnaille B, Proye C, et al. Weiss system revisited: a clinicopathologic and immunohistochemical study of 49 adrenocortical tumors. Am J Surg Pathol. 2002;26(12):1612-9.

58. Sinclair TJ, Gillis A, Alobuia WM, Wild H, Kebebew E. Surgery for adrenocortical carcinoma: When and how? Best Pract Res Clin Endocrinol Metab. 2020;34(3):101408.

59. Gaujoux S, Mihai R. European Society of Endocrine Surgeons (ESES) and European Network for the Study of Adrenal Tumours (ENSAT) recommendations for the surgical management of adrenocortical carcinoma. Br J Surg. 2017;104:358-76.

60. Datta J, Roses RE. Surgical management of adrenocortical carcinoma: an evidence-based approach. Surg Oncol Clin N Am. 2016;25(1):153-70.

61. Livhits M, Li N, Yeh MW, Harari A. Surgery is associated with improved survival for adrenocortical cancer, even in metastatic disease. Surgery. 2014;156(6):1531-41.

62. Gaujoux S, Brennan MF. Recommendation for standardized surgical management of primary adrenocortical carcinoma. Surgery. 2012;152:123-32.

63. Reibetanz J, Jurowich C, Erdogan I, Nies C, Rayes N, Dralle H, et al. Impact of lymphadenectomy on the oncologic outcome of patients with adrenocortical carcinoma. Ann Surg. 2012;255:363-9.

64. Autorino R, Bove P, De Sio M, Miano R, Micali S, Cindolo L, et al. Open versus laparoscopic adrenalectomy for adrenocortical carcinoma: a meta-analysis of surgical and oncological outcomes. Ann Surg Oncol. 2016;23:1195-202.

65. Henry JF, Peix JL, Kraimps JL. Positional statement of the European Society of Endocrine Surgeons (ESES) on malignant adrenal tumors. Langenbecks Arch Surg. 2012;397:145-6.

66. Leboulleux S, Deandreis D, Al Ghuzlan A, Aupérin A, Goéré D, Dromain C, et al. Adrenocortical carcinoma: is the surgical approach a risk factor of peritoneal carcinomatosis? Eur J Endocrinol. 2010;162:1147-53.

67. Dickson PV, Kim L, Yen TWF, Yang A, Grubbs EG, Patel D, et al. Evaluation, staging, and surgical management for adrenocortical carcinoma: an update from the SSO Endocrine and Head and Neck Disease Site Working Group. Ann Surg Oncol. 2018;25:3460-8.

68. Glenn JA, Else T, Hughes DT, Cohen MS, Jolly S, Giordano TJ, et al. Longitudinal patterns of recurrence in patients with adrenocortical carcinoma. Surgery. 2019;165:186-95.

69. Schteingart DE. Adjuvant mitotane therapy of adrenal cancer: use and controversy. N Engl J Med. 2007;356:2415-8.

70. Sbiera S, Leich E, Liebisch G, Sbiera I, Schirbel A, Wiemer L, et al. Mitotane inhibits Sterol-O-Acyl transferase 1 triggering lipid-mediated endoplasmic reticulum stress and apoptosis in adrenocortical carcinoma cells. Endocrinology. 2015;156: 3895-908.

71. Viani GA, Viana BS. Adjuvant radiotherapy after surgical resection for adrenocortical carcinoma: a systematic review of observational studies and meta-analysis. J Cancer Res Ther. 2019;15(Supplement):S20-6.

72. Fassnacht M, Terzolo M, Allolio B, Baudin E, Haak H, Berruti A, et al. Combination chemotherapy in advanced adrenocortical carcinoma. N Engl J Med. 2012;366:2189-97.

73. Le Tourneau C, Hoimes C, Zarwan C, Wong DJ, Bauer S, Claus R, et al. Avelumab in patients with previously treated metastatic adrenocortical carcinoma: phase 1b results from the JAVELIN solid tumor trial. J Immunother Cancer. 2018;6:111.

74. Fassnacht M, Berruti A, Baudin E, Demeure MJ, Gilbert J, Haak H, et al. Linsitinib (OSI-906) versus placebo for patients with locally advanced or metastatic adrenocortical carcinoma: a double-blind, randomised, phase 3 study. Lancet Oncol. 2015;16: 426-35.

75. Lerario AM, Worden FP, Ramm CA, Hesseltine EA, Stadler WM, Else T, et al. The combination of insulin-like growth factor receptor 1 (IGF1R) antibody cixutumumab and mitotane as a first-line therapy for patients with recurrent/metastatic adrenocortical carcinoma: a multiinstitutional NCI-sponsored trial. Horm Cancer. 2014;5:232-9.

76. Naing A, Lorusso P, Fu S, Hong D, Chen HX, Doyle LA, et al. Insulin growth factor receptor (IGF-1R) antibody cixutumumab combined with the mTOR inhibitor temsirolimus in patients with metastatic adrenocortical carcinoma. Br J Cancer. 2013;108:826-30.

77. Rosen LS. Inhibitors of the vascular endothelial growth factor receptor. Hematol Oncol Clin North Am. 2002;16:1173-87.

78. Kahn M. Can we safely target the WNT pathway? Nat Rev Drug Discov. 2014;13:513-32.

CHAPTER 35

Techniques of Adrenalectomy and Approaches

Siddhartha Chakravarthy N, Anukriti Sood

SURGICAL ANATOMY AND ACCESS TO ADRENALS

Adrenals are two small yellowish bodies, flat anteroposteriorly, each situated immediately anterosuperior to each superior renal pole and surrounded by connective tissue containing perinephric fat and Gerota's fascia.

The right adrenal gland is an irregular tetrahedron, whereas the left is semilunar and usually larger and superior in level.[1,2]

Each measures around 50 mm vertically, 30 mm transversely, and 10 mm in anteroposterior dimension. The weight is about 5 g.

RELATIONS

Right Adrenal

Right adrenal is an irregular tetrahedron that lies posterior to the inferior vena cava (IVC) and right hepatic lobe and anterior to diaphragm and superior pole of the right kidney. Its inferior base adjoins the anteromedial aspect of the right superior renal pole. Below the apex, near the anterior border of the gland, is a short sulcal hilum where the right suprarenal vein emerges to join the IVC.

Posterior surface is divided into upper and lower areas by a curved transverse ridge, with upper convex area rests on the diaphragm; the lower concave contacts the superior pole and the adjacent anterior surface of the kidney.

Left Adrenal

Left adrenal is crescentic in shape with convexity present medially and concavity laterally. Its concavity is adapted to the medial side of the superior pole of the left kidney.

Anterior surface has a superior area covered by peritoneum of the omental bursa, which separates it from the cardiac end of the stomach.

Inferior surface is in contact with pancreas and splenic artery. Hilum faces ventrocaudallyd and is near the lowest part of anterior surface. The left suprarenal vein emerges to join the left renal vein.

Posterior surface is divided by a ridge into a lateral area adjoining the kidney and a smaller medial in contact with diaphragm's left crus.

Convex medial border is related to the left celiac ganglion which is inferomedial and to the left inferior phrenic and left gastric arteries which ascend on the left crus.

BLOOD SUPPLY

While the arterial blood supply is similar on both sides, the venous drainage is very different. The arterial blood supply consists of the superior adrenal artery (from the inferior phrenic artery), the middle adrenal artery (from the abdominal aorta), and the inferior adrenal artery (from the renal artery).

Medullary veins emerge from the hilum to form a suprarenal vein. The right adrenal vein is very short around 1 cm and drains into the posterolateral aspect of the IVC, while the left adrenal vein is longer about 2–3 cm and drains into the left renal vein.[3,4]

Lymph vessels end in lateral aortic nodes.

Identification and control of the adrenal veins are one of the most important parts of adrenalectomy.[5]

PREOPERATIVE MANAGEMENT

Preoperative preparation is particularly important in pheochromocytoma.

- *Preoperative α- and β-receptor blockade*: Its main aim is to prevent catecholamine-induced serious complications during surgery such as hypertensive crisis, cardiac arrhythmias, pulmonary edema, and cardiac ischemia.

α-adrenoceptor blockade can be achieved with either:

- Nonselective and noncompetitive α-adrenoceptor antagonist—phenoxybenzamine
- Competitive and selective α1-blockers, e.g., doxazosin, prazosin, and terazosin **(Table 1)**

After α-adrenoceptor blockade has been successfully established on day 2 or 3 of therapy with adequately controlled blood pressure, patients should be advised to add a plentiful amount of salt to their diet to restore the contracted intravascular volume and improve postural hypotension.

β-blockade should be initiated to control tachycardia and tachyarrhythmia induced by catecholamines or α-adrenoceptor blockers.

Table 1: Drugs used in pheochromocytoma.

Drug	Characteristics	Doses	Recommended use	Adverse effects
α-blockers (Begin 7–14 days prior to surgery):				
Phenoxybenzamine Prazosin Terazosin Doxazosin	Nonselective Selective	*Oral*: 1 mg/kg/day 2–5 mg/day	First-line therapy—normalizes BP and expands intravascular volume	Postural hypotension, reflex tachycardia, dizziness, and syncope
β-blockers (after α-blockers):				
Propranolol Metoprolol Atenolol	Nonselective Cardioselective	20–80 mg 25–50 mg 12.5–25 mg	Helps to control BP and tachycardia	Use in caution with airway, vascular disease
Calcium-channel blockers:				
Amlodipine Nicardipine Nifedipine	Extended-release action	10–20 mg/day 60–90 mg/day 30–90 mg/day	Useful in patients intolerant to α- and β-blockers	Headache, flushing, and edema
Catecholamine synthesis inhibitor:				
Metyrosine	Competitive inhibitor of tyrosine hydroxylase	250 mg every 8–12 hourly	Adjuvant treatment for metastatic and hyperactive tumors	Sedation, depression extrapyramidal signs, galactorrhea

It should never be administered prior to α-blockers due to the risk of exacerbating a hypertensive crisis resulting from the unopposed action of catecholamines on α-adrenoceptors (vasomotor reversal of Dale).

Roizen's criteria for adequate blockade:

- No in-hospital presurgical BP measuring >165/90 mm Hg, 24 hours before surgery
- No orthostatic hypotension with BP measuring <80/45 mm Hg
- No ECG showing ST-T changes 1 week prior to surgery
- No more than one premature ventricular contraction every 5 minutes
    - *Intraoperative preparation includes:*
        - Anesthetic considerations
        - Vasodilators
        - β-antagonists
        - Fluid management
- *Anesthetic considerations:*
    - Central venous catheter should be placed for intravascular volume monitoring.
    - *Inhalational agents:* Isoflurane, enflurane, and sevoflurane can be safely used. Halothane results in severe arrhythmia and should be avoided.
    - *Intravenous agents:* Induction with propofol or thiopental is safe. Ketamine and ephedrine should be avoided. Morphine causes histamine release which is a known trigger of pheochromocytoma crisis.
- *Vasodilators:* Sodium nitroprusside and nitroglycerin can be used in case of adrenergic crisis
- *β-antagonists:* Esmolol (short-acting) can be used to control tachyarrhythmia.

Choice of technique of adrenalectomy: The appropriate choice of procedure whether laparoscopic or open is determined by a number of factors, i.e.,

- Tumor size
- Presence of bilateral or unilateral disease
- Patient body habitus and anatomy
- Surgeon's experience with a given approach

Indications of open adrenalectomy:

- Adrenal malignancies
- Cortical tumors >6 cm as they carry high risk of malignancy. Very large benign lesions (>8–10 cm) are considered a relative indication for open adrenalectomy.
- Virilizing adrenal tumors as they have a 70–85% malignancy rate
- Recurrent adrenal tumor
- Evidence of local invasion found at time of laparoscopy necessitates conversion to an open approach
- Uncontrolled bleeding during a laparoendoscopic adrenalectomy

Approaches can be broadly classified as anterior and posterior approaches.

Anterior Approach

The anterior approach is one of the most commonly used approaches for an open adrenalectomy. Here, surgery can be performed through a single incision without the need to reposition the patient.

Steps

- *Position:* Patient positioning is similar for the transabdominal and thoracoabdominal approaches. For the transabdominal approach, the patient is placed supine on the operating table with the arms tucked or extended on arm boards at the sides.

For the thoracoabdominal approach, the patient should be placed on a beanbag with a shoulder roll placed vertically under the flank of the side of the adrenal tumor.

- *Incisions*: The anterior approach can be performed through a chevron, unilateral subcostal, or midline incision **(Fig. 1)**. A bilateral subcostal/chevron incision is preferred when excellent lateral, superior, and inferior exposure of both adrenals are required.

Right adrenalectomy:

a. The combined mobilization of the hepatic flexure of the colon and Kocher maneuver exposes the IVC, the right adrenal gland, and the upper pole of the right kidney.

b. The liver is mobilized by incising the lateral attachments of the right lobe of the liver, and the triangular ligament, facilitating superomedial retraction of the liver.

  i. It is important to remember to identify the middle hepatic vein and any inferior phrenic veins, which may be injured easily and cause rapid hemorrhage. If the liver is retracted too far medially, it may compress the IVC and decrease venous return, resulting in hypotension.

1. *To locate and ligate the right adrenal vein:* The right adrenal vein usually runs from the gland on its anterior surface near the superior medial margin and enters the IVC posteriorly. Suture ligation is more secure than simple free ties or clips. For pheochromocytomas, the vein should be ligated early to prevent release of catecholamines.

2. Dissection of the remainder of the gland, ligating any accessory venous branches and the arterial arcade.

3. Tumor thrombus, if present, is usually not adherent to the inner wall of the IVC and can be easily extracted through a small venotomy.

Left adrenalectomy:

1. Exposure of the left adrenal gland begins with mobilizing the splenic flexure of the colon at least one-third of the distance down the left paracolic gutter, along its lateral peritoneal attachments, and then across the gastrocolic ligament to the area of the inferior mesenteric vein.

  i. The peritoneum along with the inferior border of the pancreas is incised and the pancreas is reflected superomedially to expose the left adrenal gland.

2. To find the left adrenal vein, dissection should start at the inferolateral aspect of the gland. The vein, once identified, should be ligated early.

  i. Do not completely mobilize the inferior border of the adrenal at this point since it will allow the gland to retract cephalad, making the superior dissection more difficult.

3. Dissection of the superior pole and then proceed with downward retraction of the gland.

Advantages of Open Anterior Approach

It allows for complete exploration of the peritoneal cavity and en bloc resection of the adrenal and any adjacent structures that may be involved with malignant invasion.

Difficulties with Anterior Approach

- The medial posterior attachments of the liver contain the hepatic veins, which can be injured during liver mobilization and retraction.
- Excessive lateral retraction of the right adrenal gland, which may avulse the vein from the IVC.
- Excessive traction on the spleen during mobilization of the splenic flexure and superomedial retraction of the pancreas and spleen.
- Injury to the pancreatic parenchyma can lead to postoperative pseudocysts or pancreatic fistula. When identified, these injuries should be repaired with either ligation, transection, or wide drainage.
- The left adrenal gland extends inferomedially almost to the renal hilum, placing the renal vessels at risk of injury.

Thoracoabdominal/Lateral Transthoracic Approach

The thoracoabdominal approach is preferred for the following highly specific circumstances:

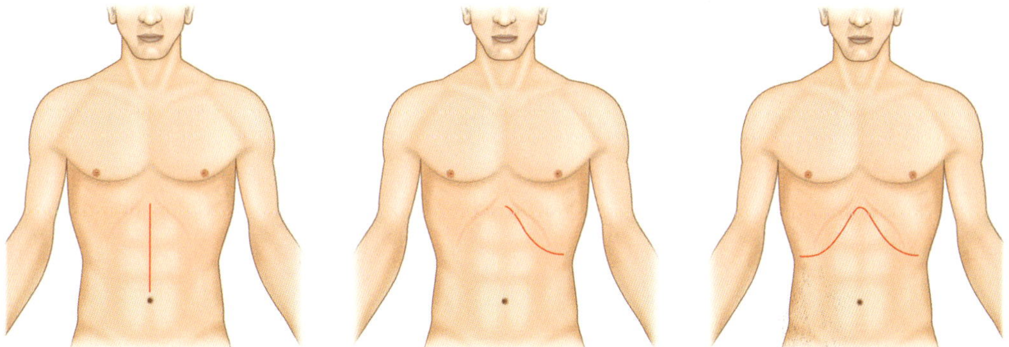

Fig. 1: Incisions for adrenalectomy through the anterior approach.

- Large tumors with substantial involvement of the surrounding structures (pancreas, spleen, and diaphragm on the left and liver, IVC, and diaphragm on the right).
- Access to the supradiaphragmatic vena cava for extensive tumor involvement of the vena cava is necessary.

Steps

Position: The patient is placed in either a full lateral or a semioblique (45° angle) position with the operative side up. The patient is placed on an operating table with the 10th rib superior to the center break in the table and the 12th rib inferior to it. The table is jackknifed to open the space between the ribs and stretch the chest wall.

Right adrenalectomy:

1. *Incision*: The incision for a right adrenalectomy begins over the right 10th rib and extended medially across the costal cartilage and then down toward the midline rectus muscle. The 10th rib is resected subperiosteally at its angle. The costal cartilage is divided and partially excised **(Fig. 2)**.
2. The diaphragm is divided along with the lateral wall to prevent injury to the phrenic nerve.
3. The lung is deflated and retracted superiorly.
4. The liver is fully mobilized and retracted superomedially, exposing the adrenal gland, and the supra- and infrahepatic vena cava.
5. Gerota's fascia is opened and the kidney retracted inferiorly and further dissection is same as in anterior approach.

Left adrenalectomy:

1. Here, the incision should begin over the 11th rib instead of the 10th rib.
2. To avoid entering the pleural cavity, parietal pleura should be dissected off the diaphragm.
3. The remainder of the dissection proceeds as described for the right thoracoabdominal and left anterior approaches.

A tube thoracostomy (under water chest drain) is placed in the pleural cavity (if the pleura is opened) and the muscle and fascia layers of the abdominal and chest walls are reapproximated.

Posterior/Retroperitoneal Approach

Earlier, it was popular for bilateral adrenalectomies or small, unilateral adrenalectomies and was a preferred approach for removing aldosteronomas. The posterior approach is effective for tumors of up to 5 cm in size.

The benefit of the posterior approach is that it is the most direct route to the adrenal glands, the peritoneal cavity is not entered, and hence there is a decreased rate of postoperative ileus.

Steps

Position: The patient is placed prone with the table break at the level of the 12th rib. Pillows are placed under the patient's abdomen and lower legs, and the table is jackknifed to increase the space between the rib cage and pelvis. Chest rolls or foam supports are placed under the chest. The knees are flexed and supported **(Fig. 3)**.

1. *Incision*: A hockey stick-shaped incision over the 10th rib, 5 cm lateral to the vertebral column, extending inferiorly and laterally to the iliac crest **(Fig. 4)**.

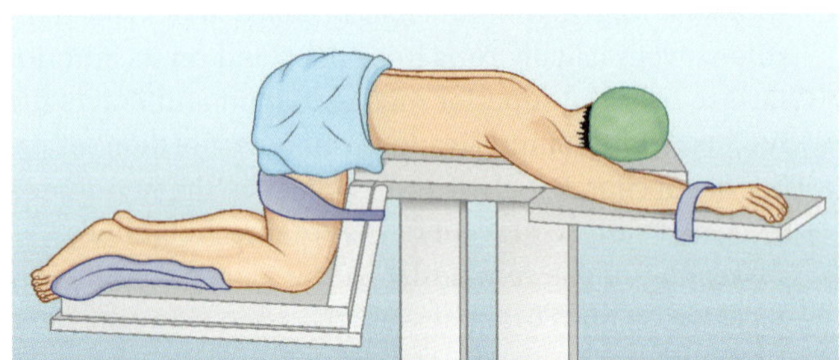

Fig. 3: Position for retroperitoneal/posterior adrenalectomy.

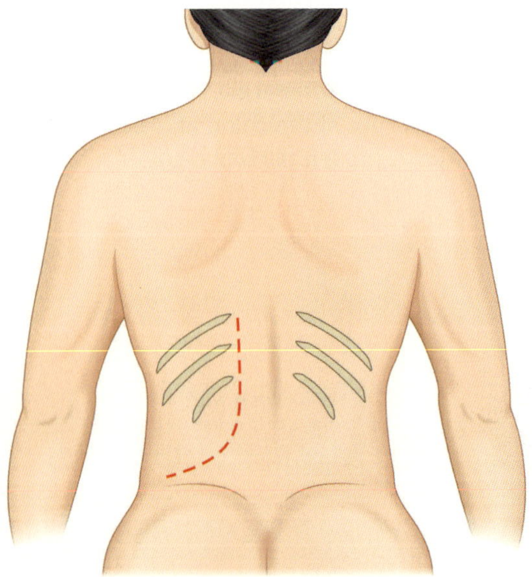

Fig. 4: Incision for open retroperitoneal adrenalectomy.

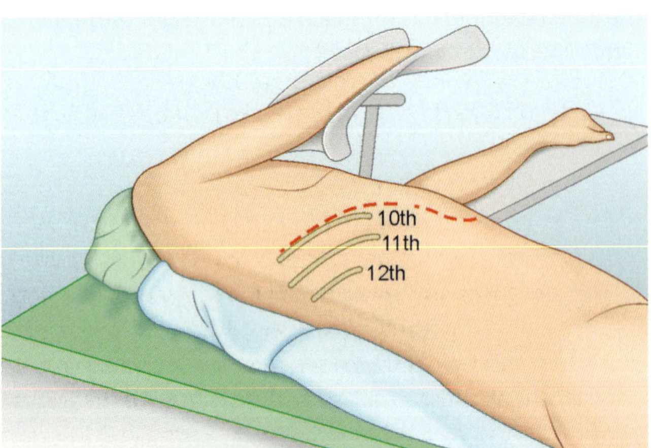

Fig. 2: Position and incision for right adrenalectomy through thoraco-abdominal approach.

2. The latissimus dorsi and sacrospinalis muscles are exposed and transected, exposing the 12th rib, and sacrospinalis is dissected off the 12th rib and retracted medially.
3. The lumbodorsal fascia under the sacrospinalis is incised, exposing the quadratus lumborum and transversalis fascia.
4. The periosteum of the 12th rib is then incised and stripped before the rib is resected subperiosteally. The 12th intercostal nerve is identified and preserved. The retroperitoneum is entered.
5. Dissection proceeds with the incision of Gerota's fascia to expose the kidney. Rotating the superior pole of the kidney inferiorly and posteriorly facilitates exposure of the adrenal gland.
6. The wound is closed in layers, taking care to avoid the neurovascular bundles around the ribs.

Flank Approach

Flank approach is a posterolateral extraperitoneal access to the adrenal.

It is useful in:
- Obese patients by allowing excess adipose tissue to fall away from the incision
- Large adrenal masses and in patients with extensive adhesions from prior abdominal surgery

Steps

Position: Patient is placed in the lateral decubitus position with the 10th rib superior to the center break in the operating table and the 12th rib inferior to the break.

1. *Incision*: The incision is made at the tip of the 11th rib on the right or 12th rib on the left at the midaxillary line and extends along the rib posteriorly **(Fig. 5)**. The latissimus dorsi, external and internal oblique, and intercostal muscles are transected.
2. The retroperitoneum is entered and dissection proceeds laterally to medially.
3. For the right adrenal gland, dissection starts superolaterally and proceeds in the direction of the adrenal vein. Release of the superior attachments facilitates inferior retraction of the adrenal gland and exposure of the adrenal vein.

For the left adrenal gland, the kidney is retracted medially, exposing the splenorenal ligament, which is divided to allow superomedial retraction of the pancreas and spleen.

The kidney is retracted inferiorly to expose the adrenal and dissection proceeds superomedially toward the adrenal vein.

Limitations

Only one adrenal gland can be evaluated at a time.

◇ POSTOPERATIVE MANAGEMENT

- *In case of pheochromocytoma*: Patients should be kept under close surveillance for the first 24 hours.
  Two important events one should be careful about are:
  1. *Hypotension*: Due to hemorrhage, sudden increase in venous capacitance, inadequate volume repletion, or residual effects of preparation of α-blockade (especially with phenoxybenzamine).
     Management is by giving fluids and if its not controlled to give pressor agents like noradrenaline.
  2. *Hypoglycemia*: Due to rebound hyperinsulinism that occurs when the inhibitory effect of norepinephrine on insulin secretion is suddenly gone and preoperative stimulation of glycogenolysis and lipolysis by catecholamine.
- *In case of bilateral adrenalectomy*: Steroids need to be replaced.
  Immediate postoperatively intravenous hydrocortisone is given for 5 days that is gradually replaced by life-long oral steroids.

Pearls

- Adrenal glands have very unique venous drainage with right adrenal vein of length around 1 cm only and left adrenal vein of around 3–4 cm.
- In case of pheochromocytoma, preoperative control of blood pressure and tachycardia is done by α-blockers followed by β-blockers.
- Laparoscopic adrenalectomy is the gold standard treatment for adrenal masses. Open adrenalectomy is preferred mostly in malignant adrenal diseases.
- Thoracoabdominal approach is preferred for tumors involving vena cava, especially supradiaphragmatic vena cava.
- Retroperitoneal approach has an advantage that it has a direct approach to adrenal gland without entering peritoneal cavity.

Laparoscopic Adrenalectomy

Indications

Laparoscopic adrenalectomy is the gold standard operation for most adrenal tumors. Gagner et al. popularized the transabdominal approach for this surgery.[6] This is an advanced laparoscopic technique and needs an expert

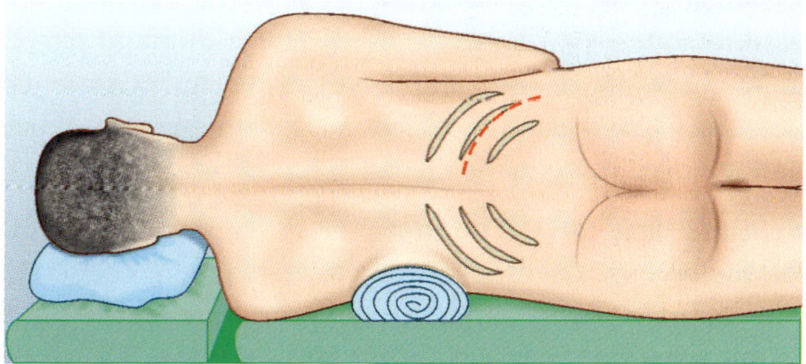

Fig. 5: Incision for open adrenalectomy through flank approach.

surgeon with a clear understanding of the anatomy and physiology of the adrenal gland.[7]

*Indications for surgery (**Box 1**):* Laparoscopic adrenalectomy can be safely performed on most tumors up to 8 cm in size and in experienced hands on tumors up to 12 cm in size.[8] However, laparoscopic adrenalectomy should be avoided when there is a suspicion of malignancy with vascular or local invasion or lymph nodal involvement.

Technique for Laparoscopic Adrenalectomy

We describe the commonly used transperitoneal lateral approach. The lateral approach has the advantage of using the gravity to retract the liver on the right and spleen and tail of pancreas on the left.

Surgical Equipment

The following equipment is needed for the surgery:
- Scope—30° 10-mm scope
- Three 10-mm ports/two 5-mm ports
- Laparoscopic vessel sealers (LigaSure/harmonic)
- L-hook cautery
- Suction
- Fan-shaped/liver retraction
- Bowel graspers

Preoperative Preparation and Positioning (Fig. 6)

Standard preoperative preparations for functional tumors have to be followed. The patient will need a nasogastric tube, urinary catheter, and an arterial line to monitor sudden fluctuations in blood pressure. Preoperative antibiotic prophylaxis is given as for clean cases.

The patient is placed in a lateral decubitus position on a bean bag with the operating side facing upward. The table is flexed at the lower chest near the 10th rib to open up the space between the hip and chest. The patient is positioned at a 10° posterior lean and taped at the hip, lower extremity, and chest.

Surgical Technique

Right adrenalectomy: Four ports are placed about two finger-breadths below the costal margin. The medial trocar is placed at the mid-clavicular line, either by an open port insertion technique or by Veress needle. The abdomen is thoroughly explored for any metastasis after insufflating to 15 mm Hg. Subsequent trocars are placed under direct vision preferably equidistant from each other (5–7 cm apart). The camera is inserted through the second port and the working instrument from the lateral two ports. The first step is to mobilize the liver by dividing the triangular ligament. After the liver is mobilized, the space between the liver and the retroperitoneum is opened. The IVC and adrenal gland are visible at this point and the dissection is continued in a superomedial direction lateral to the IVC. The right adrenal vein is typically short

<table>
<tr><td>Box 1: Indications for laparoscopic adrenalectomy.</td></tr>
</table>

Benign functioning lesions:
- Aldosteronoma
- Pheochromocytoma
- ACTH-independent Cushing's syndrome
- ACTH-dependent Cushing's syndrome

Benign nonfunctional masses:
- Adenoma
- Myelolipoma
- Cyst
- Ganglioneuroma
- Malignant adrenal tumors
- Metastasis

(ACTH: adrenocorticotropic hormone)

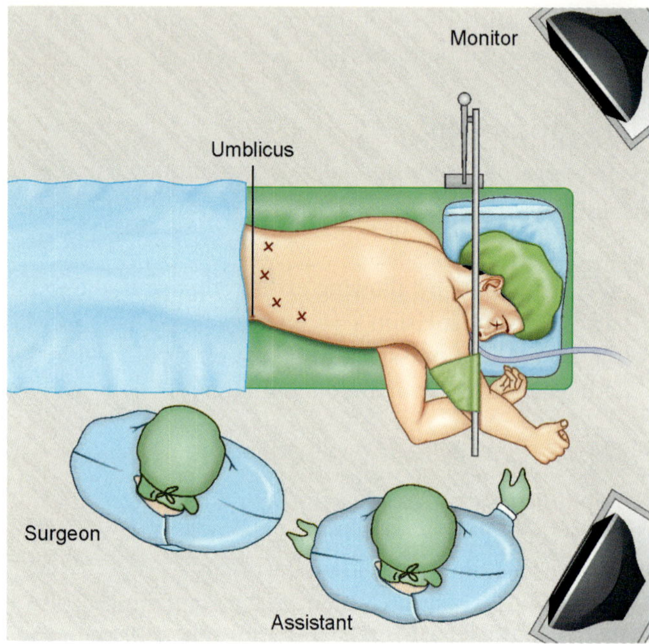

Fig. 6: Patient positioning in lateral transperitoneal adrenalectomy.

and enters the posterolateral aspect of the IVC. It has to be carefully dissected by sharp and blunt dissection and double clipped before cutting. After cutting the adrenal vein, the gland is retracted away from the IVC and the small branches are divided. Inferiorly, the gland is separated from the upper pole of the kidney. Care must be taken while dissecting near the renal vein, as in most patients, it is difficult to identify the junction of IVC to right renal vein, as the transition is a gradual curve. Finally, the avascular posterior and lateral attachments are divided and the adrenal gland is dissected out. The excised gland is placed in a specimen retrieval bag and removed through the medial 10-mm port.

Left adrenalectomy: The first port is placed in the mid-clavicular line 2 cm inferior to the costal margin. The rest of the ports are placed similar to the procedure on the right, 5 cm apart to prevent clashing. The initial step is to release the lateral attachments of the spleen and drop it anteromedially.

At this point, the tail of the pancreas can be seen, and has to be dissected anteriorly, and care must be taken as the splenic hilar vessels and tail of the pancreas are vulnerable to injury. In large adrenal tumors, the splenic flexure has to be mobilized inferiorly by dividing the splenocolic ligament. After identifying the adrenal gland and kidney, the dissection is continued medial to the adrenal gland. The avascular plane between the adrenal and the pancreas is opened until the fundus is visible. The adrenal gland is dissected from its superomedial aspect, proceeding caudally and ligating the middle adrenal arteries from aorta. The left adrenal vein is identified and dissected all around and clamped caudal to the inferior phrenic vein. The adrenal gland is dissected off from the kidney similar to the right side.

Complications

The described complications include bleeding from solid organs such as liver and spleen. If bleeding occurs from the slipped adrenal vein, then in most cases, it needs conversion to open technique. Other complications include hollow viscus perforation, pancreatic fistula, port-site infections, and metastasis.

Posterior Retroperitoneoscopic Adrenalectomy

This technique was initially popularized by Martin K Walz from Germany.[9] It combines the posterior approach with minimally invasive surgery and has the advantage of less blood loss, less pain, and a shorter hospital stay.

Indications and contraindications: This procedure is recommended for both functional and nonfunctional benign adrenal tumors up to 7 cm in size. Tumors as large as 10 cm can be removed using this technique, but during the initial learning phase, it is recommended to restrict the surgery to tumors up to 4 cm.[10] It is usually contraindicated in tumors >8 cm and in suspicious growths with ill-defined planes. It is not employed in patients with body mass index (BMI) >40 kg/m^2.

Technique: Posterior retroperitoneoscopic adrenalectomy is performed under general anesthesia in prone position. Arterial and central venous lines are usually kept to monitor blood pressure fluctuations particularly in pheochromocytomas.

A pillow is used for lifting the pelvis and another under the chest so that the abdomen is falling free. The hip joint and pelvis are bent to about 110° to increase the space between the 12th rib and iliac crest **(Fig. 7)**. The first 10-mm port is placed just inferior to the tip of the 12th rib, and the space is entered by sharp and blunt dissection. With a finger, we should then be able to feel the anterior surface of rib. Subsequently, blunt dissection is done in the retroperitoneal space and the second port (5 mm) is inserted under finger guidance 6–8 cm lateral and beneath the 11th rib. The retroperitoneal space is created with carbon dioxide and the pressure is maintained between 20 and 30 mm Hg. A 10-mm, 30° scope is inserted in the first port;

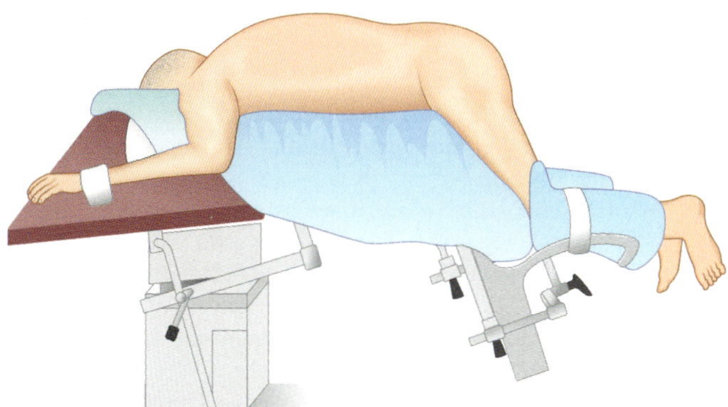

Fig. 7: Patient positioning in retroperitoneoscopic adrenalectomy.

the first view shows Gerota's fascia, which covers the kidney and the adrenal gland. The dissection should proceed in the superomedial direction as the adrenal gland is located toward the midline. All the fatty tissue from the posterior abdominal wall should be pushed down and the psoas muscle is visualized. The third 10-mm port is inserted 4–5 cm medial to the first port and 4 cm inferior to the 12th rib. The port is placed parallel to the spine and in a flat angle (30–45°). The camera is placed in the third port and the lateral two ports are the working ports.

The first step is to mobilize the perirenal tissue in the upper third of the kidney. This exposes the inferior aspect of the adrenal gland. The upper pole of the kidney is retracted and the inferior part of the adrenal gland is carefully separated from the kidney. On the right side, the adrenal is separated from the liver in a lateral to medial direction, carefully identifying and preserving the peritoneum. Near the medial edge, the IVC is identified and the adrenal gland is separated from the IVC. Laterally, the gland is lifted from Gerota's fascia and the adrenal vein is identified at the superomedial aspect of the gland where it drains into the IVC. The vein is carefully clipped or cauterized with LigaSure or harmonic and cut.

On the left side, the dissection proceeds from the lateral to medial direction until the lower pole is identified. The adrenal vein is identified near the adrenal gland dissected, clamped, and cut. After dissecting out the gland, the gland is delivered out through the first port.

Bilateral adrenalectomy can be done by this technique without need to change the position of the patient.

Postoperative Care

Intensive care unit care is required for patients with comorbidities, pheochromocytoma, and Cushing's syndrome. Patients are mobilized on the same day and diet is started by evening as the peritoneum is not opened. Paracetamol is used for analgesia and the patients can be discharged on the 2nd postoperative day.

◇| REFERENCES

1. Prinz RA, Madorin K. Open operative approaches to the adrenal gland. In: Clark OH (Ed). Textbook of Endocrine Surgery, 3rd edition. Philadelphia: Jaypee Brothers Medical Publishers; 2016. pp. 1081-8.

2. Dyson M. Endocrine System. In: Williams P, Bannister LH, Berry MM, Collins P, Dyson M, Dussek JE, Ferguson MW (Eds). Gray's Anatomy, 38th edition. Edinburgh: Churchill Livingstone; 2000. pp. 1900-5.

3. Elaraj DM, Duh QY. Technique of Open and Laparoscopic Adrenalectomy. In: Hubbard JGH, Inabnet WB, Lo CY (Eds). Endocrine Surgery Principles and Practice. London: Springer-Verlag; 2009. pp. 439-49.

4. Netter FH. Atlas of Human Anatomy, 6th edition. Philadelphia: Saunders; 2014. p. 320.

5. Image. http://higheredbcs.wiley.com/legacy/college/tortora/0470565101/hearthis_ill/pap13e_ch18_illustr_audio_mp3_am/simulations/figures/adrenal1.jpg. [Last accessed January, 2022].

6. Gagner M, Lacroix A, Bolté E. Laparoscopic adrenalectomy in Cushing's syndrome and pheochromocytoma. N Engl J Med. 1992;327(14):1033.

7. Godellas CV, Prinz RA. Surgical approach to adrenal neoplasms: laparoscopic versus open adrenalectomy. Surg Oncol Clin N Am. 1998;7(4):807-17.

8. Gagner M, Pomp A, Heniford BT, Pharand D, Lacroix A. Laparoscopic adrenalectomy: lessons learned from 100 consecutive procedures. Ann Surg. 1997;226(3):238-46; discussion 246-7.

9. Walz MK, Peitgen K, Krause U, Eigler FW. Dorsal retroperitoneoscopic adrenalectomy: a new surgical technique. Zentralbl Chir. 1995;120(1):53-8.

10. Walz MK, Alesina PF, Wenger FA, Deligiannis A, Szuczik E, Petersenn S, et al. Posterior retroperitoneoscopic adrenalectomy: results of 560 procedures in 520 patients. Surgery. 2006;140(6):943-8; discussion 948-50.

Pediatric Endocrine Tumors

Himagirish K Rao, Sapana Bothra Jain

◇ INTRODUCTION

The age-old dictum that "pediatric patients are not simply small adults with disease" definitely holds good for endocrine tumors as well. In comparison to other tumors, endocrine tumors are rare in normal population and far less incident in children. Tumors in children may differ in biological behavior from the same or similar tumors in adults. Growing children are more susceptible to oncogenic transformation than adults, due to the constant cell division and differentiation occurring in all tissues. Certain endocrine tumors can be more aggressive in children, e.g., adrenocortical cancer, whereas certain tumors, although may present with an advanced disease, may have an indolent course, e.g., papillary thyroid carcinoma (PTC). In this chapter, tumors of the major endocrine organs (thyroid, parathyroid, adrenals, and pancreas) in pediatric patients, their clinical presentation, and management are discussed.

◇ THYROID

Thyroid neoplasms—benign or malignant—present as nodules. These may be in the form of solitary thyroid nodule (STN), multinodular goiter (MNG), or diffuse enlargement of the thyroid.

Thyroid Nodules in Children

Epidemiology

Approximately 2% of the children have palpable thyroid nodules, but most of them are benign including inflammatory lesions or follicular adenomas. But in comparison to adults, thyroid nodules in children are associated with an increased risk of being malignant (5–10%, adult vs. 25%, children).[1] The Surveillance, Epidemiology, and End Results (SEER) registry data from 1973 to 2013 have reported an increasing incidence of thyroid cancer rising 3% per year over this 40-year period.[2]

Etiopathogenesis

Certain risk factors, including nutritional, genetic, and environmental, have been identified, which pose a greater risk of the development of thyroid nodules in children **(Box 1)**.

Radiation

There is enough evidence suggesting that thyroid gland in a child is more susceptible to the carcinogenic effects of radiation, be it external or internal. Children who have received external beam radiation for the treatment of Hodgkin's lymphoma and head and neck cancers have a higher incidence of development of thyroid nodules and thyroid cancer in adulthood. Children who survived nuclear accidents and nuclear attacks (Chernobyl disaster, Hiroshima and Nagasaki atomic blasts) are also at a higher risk of developing thyroid cancers. This risk is directly proportional to the dose of radiation and inversely proportional to the age of the child. Ironically radiation dose, which causes complete ablation of thyroid, do not increase the risk (e.g., treatment of Graves' disease).

Certain genetic mutations and syndromes are associated with an increased risk of developing thyroid cancers **(Table 1)**. Toxic adenomas due to mutations in thyroid-stimulating hormone (TSH) receptor mutations have also been reported in children.

Box 1: Risk factors for development of thyroid nodules and cancer.

- Iodine deficiency
- Prior radiation exposure
- Antecedent thyroid disease
- Genetic mutations

Table 1: Genetic syndromes associated with thyroid nodules and cancer.

Syndrome	Gene	Type of thyroid nodule
Gardner syndrome	APC	PTC
Carney complex	PRKAR1A	MNG, follicular adenoma, PTC, FTC
Cowden syndrome; Bannayan–Riley–Ruvalcaba syndrome	PTEN	MNG, follicular adenoma, FTC
Werner syndrome	WRN	PTC, FTC
MEN2A, MEN2B	RET	MTC
DICER 1 syndrome	DICER 1	MNG, thyroid cancer
–	TSH receptor	Toxic adenoma

(FTC: follicular thyroid carcinoma; MEN: multiple endocrine neoplasia; MNG: multinodular goiter; MTC: medullary thyroid carcinoma; PTC: papillary thyroid carcinoma; TSH: thyroid-stimulating hormone)

Clinical Manifestations

Most of the thyroid neoplasms in children present as asymptomatic thyroid nodules, detected incidentally on routine physical examination (palpable thyroid nodule) or an unrelated radiological examination (thyroid incidentaloma).

Toxic adenoma, although relatively rare, may present with signs and symptoms of hyperthyroidism—weight loss, sweating, anxiety, diarrhea, palpitations, and tremors.

Differentiated thyroid carcinoma (DTC) may have a varied presentation as an STN, recent rapid growth in a nodule, firm or hard fixed mass with features of compression such as dysphagia, dyspnea, hoarseness, or associated lymphadenopathy.

Medullary thyroid carcinoma (MTC) in children is usually associated with multiple endocrine neoplasia type 2A (MEN2A) and MEN2B and detected as an STN or a firm thyroidal mass or detected incidentally after a family member is diagnosed with MEN syndrome.

Diagnostic Algorithm

Thyroid nodules in children carry an increased risk of malignancy,[1] so all children with thyroid nodules should be evaluated, like in adults, using thyroid function tests (TFTs), ultrasonography (USG) of thyroid gland, and fine needle aspiration cytology (FNAC).

Thyroid function tests: Although majority will have normal TFTs, it is the initial evaluation to be done in all children with thyroid nodules. Patients with suppressed TSH (s/o hyperfunctioning nodule) should be evaluated further with nuclear scintigraphy and USG. Children with advanced disease are likely to have TSH above normal.

Thyroid scintigraphy: Radionuclide scan using technetium-99m or I^{123} is to be done in cases with suppressed TSH. Based on the uptake, the nodule is described as hot nodule (increased uptake), cold nodule (decreased uptake), and warm gland (diffuse increased uptake throughout). Most of the hyperfunctioning nodules are benign but based on a case series 8–29% may have associated PTC/follicular thyroid carcinoma (FTC).[3]

Neck ultrasound: The next step is a high-resolution ultrasonography (HRUS) of the neck with color Doppler. The ultrasound can detect the number of nodules, characterize them and improve the accuracy of FNAC while simultaneously evaluating the surrounding structures, mainly cervical lymph nodes, internal jugular vein (IJV), and carotid artery. Certain features which can differentiate between benign and malignant nodules are described in **Table 2**. Unlike in adults where the size of the nodule is used as a criterion to perform FNA of the nodule, the size alone cannot be used as a criterion for further evaluation in children as the thyroid gland in children is normally half the size of the adult. Both the clinical and radiological features should be considered in the decision-making for further evaluation.

Table 2: Sonographic features suggestive of a benign or malignant nodule.

Benign	Malignant
Homogeneous, spongiform	Heterogeneous
Hyperechoic, cystic	Hypoechoic
Increased peripheral vascularity	Increased central vascularity
Peripheral translucent halo	Incomplete halo
Egg-shell calcification, large coarse calcification	Microcalcifications
Smooth well-defined margin	Irregular margins
No cervical lymph nodes	Abnormal, enlarged, round lymph nodes
–	Documented enlargement of the nodule

Table 3: Bethesda classification 2017.

Bethesda class	Category	Risk of malignancy
I	Nondiagnostic/unsatisfactory	5–10%
II	Benign	0–3%
III	AUS/FLUS	10–30%
IV	Follicular neoplasm/suspicious of follicular neoplasm	25–40%
V	Suspicious for malignancy	50–75%
VI	Malignant	97–99%

(AUS: atypia of unknown significance; FLUS: follicular lesion of unknown significance)

Box 2: What is an adequate thyroid cytology specimen?

A cytology specimen containing at least six follicular cell groups, each containing 10–15 cells per group.

Fine needle aspiration cytology: It is the most accurate tool to diagnose a thyroid nodule. The size criterion to perform an FNAC in adults is >1 cm, but in children considering the volume of the gland is much lesser than that in adults. Any nodule even if <1 cm but with suspicious clinical or radiological features should be biopsied.

As per the American Thyroid Association (ATA) 2015 guidelines for the thyroid nodules and cancer in children, FNAC in children should be performed under ultrasound guidance to avoid sampling error. It is also preferable to do under guidance as co-operation could be an issue in children, especially in the prepubertal age group, some even requiring sedation or anesthesia. It is also advisable to do a bedside cytological examination to determine if the sample is adequate as obtaining repeat samples in children would be difficult and problematic. If there is a clinical or radiological evidence of enlarged cervical lymph nodes, they should also be subjected to FNAC. Thyroid FNAC like in adults is classified into six categories as per the Bethesda classification (updated in 2017) which estimates the risk of malignancy associated with the nodules, hence guiding further management **(Table 3 and Box 2)**.

Flowchart 1: Algorithm for the management of thyroid nodule in a child.

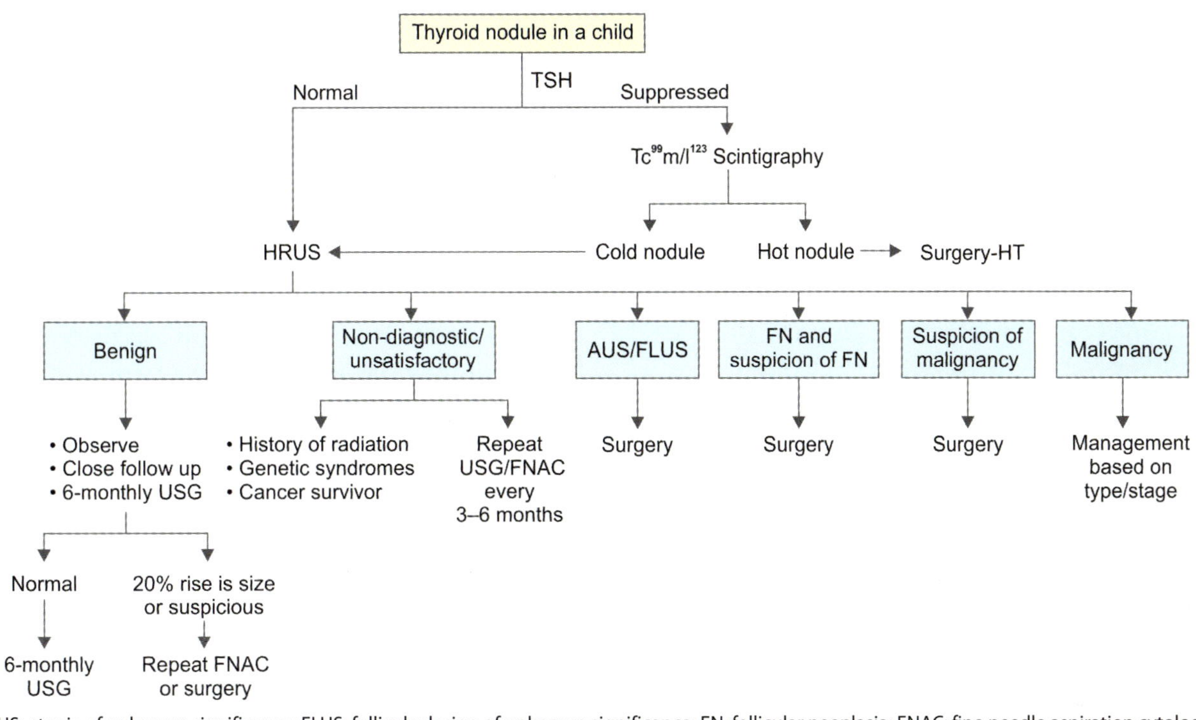

(AUS: atypia of unknown significance; FLUS: follicular lesion of unknown significance; FN: follicular neoplasia; FNAC: fine needle aspiration cytology; HRUS: high-resolution ultrasonography; HT: hemithyroidectomy; TSH: thyroid-stimulating hormone; USG: ultrasonography)

Molecular signatures: Molecular tests such as Gene Expression Classifier, Thyroseq, and Afirma have shown to aid in further diagnosis and management in adult thyroid nodules with indeterminate cytology. However, they are still not validated for use in pediatric population and hence not recommended by the ATA, suggesting a need for larger studies in this regard **(Flowchart 1)**.

Treatment

Benign thyroid neoplasms: The most common benign thyroid neoplasm in children is follicular adenoma (follicular neoplasm).[4] FNAC cannot differentiate between follicular neoplasm and FTC. There is 25–40% malignancy risk associated with follicular neoplasm, and hence surgery is the recommended treatment. Depending on the final histopathology, the patient may/may not require revision surgery.

Toxic adenomas are unlikely to resolve spontaneously. Surgical excision is the recommended treatment after achieving a euthyroid state with antithyroid medications.

When the FNA is suggestive of benign cytology, the nodule can be followed up with USG, and surgery is recommended if there is documented growth.

In children, 28% of atypia of unknown significance (AUS)/ follicular lesion of unknown significance (FLUS) lesions and 58% of suspicious follicular neoplasm are malignant and hence the ATA recommends surgery (hemithyroidectomy) over repeat FNAC for these lesions.[5]

Malignant thyroid tumors: Thyroid cancer, although rare in children, is the most common pediatric endocrine cancer, with PTC accounting for the majority of the cases (>90%). FTC is uncommon, while MTC, anaplastic thyroid carcinoma (ATC), and poorly differentiated thyroid carcinoma (PDTC) are extremely rare in young patients.[5] Most cases of pediatric thyroid carcinoma affect children in the second decade, with female-to-male preponderance [female to male ratio being (5:1)] which is not seen in children younger than 10 years of age. The risk factors and syndromes associated with the development of thyroid carcinoma have been discussed in **Box 1** and **Table 4**.

Molecular studies have shown that activation of RAS-RAF-MEK-ERK [MAPK] pathway is critical in the development of thyroid malignancies. BRAF point and RAS mutation are the most common cause of adult PTC and adult FTC, respectively.[6] In comparison to adult PTC, childhood PTC is associated with gene rearrangements, the most common being *RET*/PTC. It is well known that *RET* mutation is associated with the development of MTC in MEN2A and MEN2B syndromes both in children and in adults.

Papillary thyroid carcinoma: Papillary thyroid carcinoma most commonly presents as an asymptomatic thyroid nodule. It can also present as thyromegaly with cervical lymphadenopathy, or incidentally detected after imaging or surgery for an unrelated condition. It may infrequently develop in a remnant of thyroglossal duct or may be discovered in the thyroglossal cyst after surgery.

Papillary thyroid carcinoma is usually multifocal and bilateral. The histological variants are the same as those seen in adults, but uncommon variants that are solid and diffuse sclerosing variants are more common in children and tend to be more aggressive. Because of this, children usually have an advanced disease at presentation, with extrathyroidal extension in 20–60%, nodal disease in 40–80%, and disseminated lung metastasis in about 25% of the cases.[5] Children younger than 10 years have a high rate of recurrence as compared to adolescents.

Evaluation

These children should be evaluated with TFT, USG neck, and FNAC (nodule + lymph node) to confirm the diagnosis. Chest X-ray/contrast-enhanced computed tomography (CECT) of thorax should be considered for the evaluation of lung metastasis, especially in children who have extensive locoregional disease. CECT of neck with superior mediastinum should also be considered in children with extensive neck disease (large fixed neck masses, vocal cord paralysis, bulky metastasis) as the upper mediastinum and central compartment disease may be missed on USG neck.[5]

Treatment

Surgery is the mainstay of the treatment with total thyroid-ectomy being the procedure of choice as it facilitates radioactive iodine (RAI) therapy and follow-up with thyroglobulin easier. As per the ATA guidelines, if the central compartment lymph nodes are involved or there is extensive locoregional disease or extrathyroidal extension, the appropriate compartments need to be addressed. If there is no locoregional disease/extrathyroidal extension, the decision to perform central compartment lymph node dissection (CCLND) depends on the focality of the tumor and also the experience of the surgeon. All the lymph node dissections should be comprehensive and compartment focused. Berry picking is to be avoided strictly as it increases the chances of recurrence. Total thyroidectomy and central compartment dissections are associated with increased complications such as hypoparathyroidism and recurrent laryngeal nerve (RLN) injury, which can be minimized if the surgery is performed by an experienced high-volume endocrine surgeon.

Postoperative staging: Finally, the disease needs to be staged using the most recent American Joint Committee on Cancer (AJCC) tumor node metastasis (TNM) classification (as followed in adults) to describe the extent of the disease. Using the TNM classification, patients are categorized into three risk groups—low-, intermediate-, and high-risk groups. This risk categorization helps in identifying patients at risk of developing persistent disease who will need postoperative staging to screen for metastasis.

Postoperative staging/initial staging should be done within 12 weeks of surgery, to give adequate time for the recovery while simultaneously avoiding any delay in additional therapy. The main aim of postoperative staging is to identify patients who will need additional therapy—surgery or RAI therapy. The details of postoperative staging are given in **Table 4**.

Radioactive iodine: Traditionally adjunctive RAI therapy with I^{131} was given to all pediatric patients operated for PTC, to ablate any residual thyroid tissue and decrease the chances of recurrence. But with better risk stratification of patients and understanding of the potential side effects of RAI therapy, it is now advised to use RAI therapy selectively in patients (based on their risk to develop recurrent and persistent disease). This helps in minimizing the complications. RAI therapy is indicated in patients with iodine avid disease-local/locoregional (which cannot be resected) or iodine avid distant metastasis. I^{131} uptake by residual disease is facilitated by allowing TSH level to go >30 mIU/L. This can be achieved by withdrawing thyroxine for about 2 weeks along with low-iodine diet. Data regarding use of recombinant TSH (rTSH) in children is limited but can be used in situations in which endogenous hypothyroidism needs to be avoided (comorbidities) or when the child fails to mount an adequate TSH response.

Due to the differences in body size and iodine clearance in comparison to adults, it is preferred that all the I^{131} doses in children should be calculated by experts. This is based on the body surface area and body weight.

The main role of RAI therapy is to prevent recurrence and improve disease-free mortality. But it is challenging to identify children in whom the benefits of RAI therapy outweigh the risks. Parents and family should be involved in decision-making and be adequately informed about the benefits and complications including long-term follow-up.

Thyroid-stimulating hormone suppression: As per the ATA guidelines, the degree of TSH suppression using levothyroxine should be according to the risk stratification both during initial and dynamic assessment **(Table 4)**. But in children and growing adolescents, the thyroid suppression should be balanced with their development stages. Another issue is nonadherence to levothyroxine therapy which needs adequate monitoring and counseling.

Follow-up

Although children present with an advanced disease, the disease-specific mortality for children with DTC is very low. It is essential to follow these children lifelong as a larger proportion are at an increased risk of persistent and recurrent disease (risk of recurrence 30% and up to 30–40 years after the initial treatment).[5] Children are followed with periodic measurement of thyroglobulin (Tg) and antithyroglobulin (ATg). Routine neck USG, diagnostic RAI scans, and cross-sectional imaging should be done based on Tg and ATg values.

Table 4: Risk stratification, thyroid-stimulating hormone goal, and surveillance.

ATA risk level	Definition	Initial postoperative staging	TSH goal	Surveillance of patients with no e/o disease
Low	Disease grossly confined to thyroid or with micrometastasis in central lymph nodes	Suppressed Tg	0.5–1.0 mIU/l	USG at 6 months postoperatively and then annually suppressed Tg every 3–6 months for 2 years and then annually

Intermediate	Extensive N1a (central compartment lymph nodes) only or minimal N1b (ipsilateral lateral compartment) disease	Stimulated Tg, and DxWB RAI scan	0.1–0.5 mIU/L	• *USG neck:*
				  – 6 months
				  – 6–12 months for 5 years
				• Suppressed Tg every 3–6 months for 3 years and then annually
				• In patients treated with I^{131}, consider stimulated Tg and Dx WBRAI scan in 1–2 years

High	Extensive N1b disease or locally invasive disease with or without distant metastasis	Stimulated Tg, and DxWB scan in all patients	<0.1 mIU/L	• *USG neck:*
				  – 6 months
				  – 6–12 months for 5 years
				• Suppressed Tg every 3–6 months for 3 years and then annually
				• In patients treated with I^{131}, consider stimulated Tg and DxWB scan in 1–2 years

(ATA: American Thyroid Association; DxWB RAI: diagnostic whole-body radioactive iodine; Tg: thyroglobulin; TSH: thyroid-stimulating hormone)

Table 5: Difference between thyroid nodule and papillary thyroid carcinoma in adults and children.

	Thyroid nodule in adults	Thyroid nodules in children
Risk of malignancy	5–10%	25–50%
Indication for FNAC	Size of nodule >1 cm	Size along with ultrasonographic features and clinical context
	PTC in adults	**PTC in children**
Presentation	Less likely to present with an advanced disease	• Extrathyroidal extension in 20–60% • Locoregional disease in 40–80% disseminated lung metastasis in approximately 25% of the cases
Variant	Classical variant is most common	Solid and diffuse sclerosing variants are the most common
PFS	Less favorable	More favorable, low mortality rate
Genetic mutation	Point mutations of *BRAF* and *RAS* are the most common mutations, which cause genomic instability and dedifferentiation leading to decreased expression of Na/I symporter, and hence less RAI avid	RET/PTC rearrangement is the most common genetic abnormality; hence, better response to RAI therapy and explain their low mortality and rare progression to dedifferentiated tumors
Utility of rTSH	rTSH can be used for diagnostic and therapeutic RAI scans	Use of rTSH in children needs to be evaluated further with clinical trials
Treatment	Systemic therapy is recommended in patients with progressive disease	Needs further trials and studies

(FNAC: fine-needle aspiration cytology; PFS: progression-free survival; PTC: papillary thyroid carcinoma; rTSH: recombinant thyroid-stimulating hormone; RAI: radioactive iodine)

During each follow-up visit, patients should undergo a dynamic stratification based on their response to treatment and further managed according to their new class. Based on their clinical findings, Tg values, patients are restratified as having excellent response, biochemical incomplete response, structural incomplete response, or indeterminate response.

Surgical excision, if amenable, is the preferred management for persistent or recurrent disease. RAI therapy is advocated if surgery is not feasible as children tend to retain radioiodine avidity in contrast to adults **(Table 5)**. Children with progressive and life-threatening disease not amenable to surgery or further I^{131} should be considered for systemic therapy with oral tyrosine kinase inhibitors (TKIs). However, systemic therapy for advanced thyroid cancer is not yet studied and needs further clinical trials.

A discussion of the entire risk stratification is beyond the scope of this chapter. Children younger than 10 years treated with RAI are also at a risk of developing second malignancies such as leukemias, stomach, bladder, colon, salivary gland, and breast cancer, and hence associated symptoms should be managed with caution.

Like other cancers, parents consider children with DTC as vulnerable leading to overprotection and decreasing quality of life of the child. This can result in psychosocial consequences in the child, and hence supportive counseling is an important part in following up these patients.

Follicular Thyroid Carcinoma

There are no separate guidelines for FTC. Most of the guidelines include FTC under DTC along with PTC. FTC is rare and poorly studied malignancy in children representing <10% cases of thyroid cancer. Among the pediatric age group, FTC is more commonly diagnosed in adolescents. The female-to-male preponderance seen in PTC is not seen in FTC in adolescent age group. Iodine deficiency is a well-known risk factor.

RAS and PAX8/PPARγ mutations have been implicated in the development of FTC in adults, but somatic genetic mutations leading to pediatric FTC remain largely unstudied. A number of syndromes have been implicated with FTC with PTEN hamartoma being one of the most common **(Table 1)**. A high index of suspicion for PTEN hamartoma syndrome should always be kept in mind while managing children with FTC.

Follicular thyroid carcinoma in children can present as a thyroid nodule or a pulsatile bony lesion elsewhere. Pediatric FTC is less aggressive in comparison to PTC with fewer distant metastasis and lesser recurrence rates. It is typically a unifocal tumor, rarely metastasizing to regional lymph nodes, but can have early hematogenous metastasis at distant sites. Despite all these, FTC diagnosed in childhood has an excellent prognosis with a long-term survival.

The initial evaluation of these cases is more or less the same as that of a PTC. Cytopathological examination may miss FTC and hence a histopathology examination revealing capsular and vascular invasion is essential for diagnosis. Hurthle cell and clear cell variants are the two other variants of FTC. FNAC of these lesions could be in the form of follicular neoplasm, AUS/FLUS, or indeterminate lesion. These lesions should undergo hemithyroidectomy for confirmation of the diagnosis.

Depending upon the extent of invasion, FTC is classified as minimally invasive and widely invasive FTC. **Table 6** discusses the classification and the management of FTC.

Follow-up of patients with FTC is the same as that of PTC with the same risk stratification and follow-up protocol **(Table 4)**. However, routine neck ultrasound is not of much significance in patients post TT as the likelihood of regional disease is less likely **(Box 3)**.

Medullary Thyroid Carcinoma

Medullary thyroid carcinoma is a rare thyroid carcinoma arising from the calcitonin-producing parafollicular C-cells. Sporadic MTC is a disease of the fourth to fifth decade, comprising a minority of thyroid malignancies in children, and rarely diagnosed in adolescence with an incidence of 0.5 cases/million/year. Most cases of pediatric MTCs are hereditary due to gain-of-function mutation in the RET proto-oncogene. MTC in children is usually diagnosed in the course of a familial syndromic investigation—MEN2A, MEN2B, or FMTC.

Table 6: Classification and management of FTC.

Type	Definition	ATA risk	Treatment
Minimally invasive FTC	Only microscopic invasion of capsule but there is no penetration	Low risk	<4 cm-HT >4 cm-TT
Encapsulated angioinvasive FTC	• No capsular invasion • <4 foci of vascular invasion • >4 foci of vascular invasion	Low risk High risk	<4 cm-HT >4 cm-TT TT + WBRAI
Widely invasive	Gross invasion of capsule and extrathyroidal tissue with extensive vascular invasion	High risk	Total thyroidectomy + WBRAI

(ATA: American Thyroid Association; FTC: follicular thyroid carcinoma; HT: hemithyroidectomy; TT: total thyroidectomy; WBRAI: whole-body radioactive iodine)

Box 3: Genetic testing in children with FTC.

For children diagnosed with FTC, consideration should be given to genetic counseling and genetic testing for *PTEN* mutations, especially in children with macrocephaly or with a family history s/o PTEN hamartoma syndrome.

(FTC: follicular thyroid carcinoma)

Multiple Endocrine Neoplasia Type 2 Syndromes

Multiple endocrine neoplasia type 2A accounts for 90–95% of cases of MEN2 syndromes, with 90% of the carriers of the mutations developing MTC along with other features—pheochromocytoma (PCC) and hyperparathyroidism. MEN2A is associated with mutations in exon 10 (codons 609, 611, 618, and 620) and exon 11 (codon 634) of *RET* gene. There are four types of MEN2A—classical MEN2A, MEN2A and cutaneous lichen amyloidosis, MEN2A and Hirschsprung's disease, and FMTC. MEN2B is associated with mutations in exon 16 (codon 918T) of the RET oncogene. There is a well-established genotype–phenotype correlation with a specific mutation predicting disease aggressiveness.

MTC associated with MEN2A develops in the first two decades, while that associated with MEN2B develops in the first year of life and tends to be highly aggressive with lymph node metastasis.

The different types of MEN syndromes, associated features, and the risk categories of MTC based on codon mutations are the same as in adults, and a complete discussion is beyond the scope of this chapter. We will be discussing only the presentation and management of MTC in children.

Clinical Presentation and Diagnosis

Medullary thyroid carcinoma in children presents as a thyroid nodule like other thyroid cancers. MTC may also be diagnosed as a part of syndromic evaluation after a family member is diagnosed with MEN syndromes or the patient himself is diagnosed with other features of MEN2 syndromes.

All children with MTC should be considered to have associated genetic syndromes until unless proven otherwise. Hirschsprung's disease is almost always apparent at birth or shortly thereafter and 5–10% with Hirschsprung's disease have MEN2A syndrome.

Fifty percent of the patients with MEN2B have a unique physical appearance characterized by typical facies, ophthalmologic abnormalities including inability to make tears in infancy, thickened and everted eyelids, and prominent corneal nerves, marfanoid body habitus, and a generalized ganglioneuromatosis throughout the aerodigestive tract. However, an infant may not show a typical marfanoid habitus but may still have MTC. It is important to diagnose MTC in these patients at a stage when it is still curative. But practically most of the times, it is not possible to diagnose these patients until they present at an advanced stage of the disease.

A high degree of suspicion should be kept in mind in dealing with infants with the inability to produce tears and intestinal obstruction/constipation (ganglioneuromatosis) and should be considered for genetic analysis.

Hereditary MTC is typically multifocal, bilateral, and located at the junction of the upper one-third and the lower two thirds of thyroid lobes. C-cell hyperplasia is the initial stage of development, and there is an age-related progression of malignant disease. Lymph nodes are frequent, and distant metastasis occurs to mediastinal lymph nodes, lungs, liver, and bone marrow. Children with advanced disease and metastasis may present with flushing and diarrhea. Ectopic secretion of adrenocorticotropic hormone (ACTH) may present as Cushing's syndrome.

A child with thyroid nodule(s) should undergo a complete neck examination along with HRUS of neck and FNAC (thyroid nodule and lymph nodes). Once the FNAC is confirmatory of MTC, baseline serum calcitonin and serum carcinoembryonic antigen are assessed and are usually elevated. Additional cross-sectional imaging depends on the age of the child, disease presentation, and serum calcitonin.

Normally, children <3 years of age have higher calcitonin levels as compared to adults with a reference range of <40 ng/mL in children <6 months of age and <15 ng/mL in children aged 6 months to 3 years. There is no difference in values with adults' range after the age of 3 years. This should be kept in mind before labeling any child to have MTC.

Until the RET status is known, all children with MTC should be evaluated for PCC and should be offered genetic counseling and genetic analysis along with their parents.

Treatment

Surgery is the mainstay of the treatment even in patients with distant metastasis. This decreases the disease burden and makes follow-up easier. A total thyroidectomy along with level VI lymph node dissection is the recommended procedure. Lateral compartment should be addressed on a case-by-case basis. In patients with extensive locoregional disease, less aggressive treatment should be followed in order to preserve important functions such as speech, swallowing, and prevention of hypoparathyroidism. Hyperparathyroidism, if present, can be simultaneously addressed. A normal parathyroid which is devascularized during the procedure should be autotransplanted.

Prophylactic thyroidectomy is indicated in presymptomatic children who are RET positive. The timing of prophylactic thyroidectomy depends on the type of mutation. Children with MEN2B (918T) should have prophylactic thyroidectomy before the age of 1 year, and preferably in the first few months to increase the chances of cure. Children with other mutated codons should have a prophylactic thyroidectomy before the age of 5 years.[7]

Thyroid-stimulating hormone suppression: As parafollicular cells are not under the control of TSH, TSH suppression has no role in the management of MTC. Levothyroxine is only given as a replacement therapy after total thyroidectomy. Similarly, parafollicular cells do not trap RAI, and hence there is no role of RAI in MTC.

External beam radiotherapy: External beam radiotherapy (EBRT) is indicated only in patients with extensive neck or mediastinal disease who are at a high risk of local recurrence and airway obstruction.[7] Benefits should be weighed against the toxic side effects of radiation. EBRT is also useful in patients with painful bony metastasis.

Systemic therapy: In patients with significant tumor burden and progressive metastatic disease, systemic therapy with TKIs has shown some promising results. Vandetinib[8] and cabozantinib are Food and Drug Administration (FDA) approved for systemic therapy in these cases.[7]

Follow-up

Serum calcitonin, carcinoembryonic antigen (CEA), TFT, and neck USG are done at 6 months after surgery. Depending upon the calcitonin values, further follow-up in the form of frequent neck examination, cross-sectional imaging, and more frequent calcitonin monitoring is to be done. Calcitonin doubling time needs to be calculated in those wherein there is progressively increasing calcitonin values.

Local recurrence if amenable to surgery without causing excess morbidity should be excised.

Staging and Prognosis

Medullary thyroid carcinoma is staged as per the AJCC TNM classification followed in adults. Prognosis definitely depends on the type of codon mutated. MEN2B patients have the most aggressive course, while MEN2A have a comparatively milder course. Children who undergo a prophylactic thyroidectomy before the occurrence of MTC have the best prognosis and long-term survival.

Parathyroid Tumors

Primary Hyperparathyroidism due to Parathyroid Adenomas/Parathyroid Hyperplasia

Primary hyperparathyroidism (PHPT) affects all age groups but is extremely rare in children with an incidence of 2–5 cases/100,000/year, with more common involvement of older adolescents.[9] Familial cause accounts for 30–50% PHPT cases in children, chiefly MEN 1 syndrome.

Etiopathogenesis: Primary hyperparathyroidism in children has a bimodal age distribution—neonates and older adolescents. PHPT in neonates and infants occurs exclusively due to an inactivating mutation in calcium-sensing receptor (CaSR) which are inherited in an autosomal-dominant fashion. When the mutation is homozygous, it results in neonatal severe hyperparathyroidism (NSHPT) which presents with an extremely high parathyroid hormone (PTH) level causing osteoclastic activity resulting in hypercalcemia and severe bone disease and can be life-threatening. Children who have inherited heterozygous mutation present with a milder form of the disease referred to as familial hypocalciuric hypercalcemia (FHH). Patients with FHH have a mild hypercalcemia with low urinary calcium and do not usually require any treatment.

Primary hyperparathyroidism in older children and adolescents occurs due to adenoma or hyperplasia. It can be sporadic (65–70%) or familial (27–31%).[10] Parathyroid carcinoma in children is an extremely rare entity with only a few cases reported till now.[11]

The only identified risk factor for developing parathyroid disease in a sporadic setting is exposure to head and neck radiation with solitary parathyroid adenoma identified as the most common pathology.

Familial causes can present with multiple adenomas or multiglandular hyperplasia. Familial causes and their associated genes have been listed in **Table 7**. Among the familial causes, MEN1 accounts for 30–50% of pediatric patients with PHPT, with almost 100% penetrance by the age of 50 years. PHPT is the most common and often the earliest manifestation of MEN1. In comparison to sporadic cases PHPT occurs at an earlier age, usually 21–25 years and is typically a multiglandular disease. MEN1-related PHPT in

Table 7: Genetic causes of primary hyperparathyroidism.

Familial cause	Gene
MEN1	*MENIN*
MEN2A	*RET*
HPT-JT	*HRPT2/CDC73*
FIHPT	*MEN1/CaSR/HRPT2/CDC73*
FHH/NSHPT	*CaSR*

(FHH: familial hypocalciuric hypercalcemia; FIHPT: familial isolated hyperparathyroidism; HPT-JT: hyperparathyroidism jaw tumor syndrome; MEN: multiple endocrine neoplasia; NSHPT: neonatal severe hyperparathyroidism)

children is usually diagnosed after the age of 10 years but has been reported as early as 4 years of age.[12]

Multiple endocrine neoplasia type 2A accounts for 20% of cases of pediatric PHPT, often characterized by a single adenoma but multiglandular hyperplasia has also been described. PHPT in majority of the cases develops in the third or the fourth decade of life; however, it is reported in children below 5 years. Sometimes, it is diagnosed after total thyroidectomy when a parathyroid gland is removed accidentally along with the thyroid—either prophylactic or therapeutic.

Familial inherited hyperparathyroidism (FIHPT) and hyperparathyroidism jaw tumor syndrome are other rare inherited causes of PHPT in children. FIHPT is diagnosed when at least one family member is affected with PHPT in the absence of other endocrine disorders.

Clinical presentation: Children with NSHPT present within 6 months of life, mostly within the first few weeks. These children are almost always symptomatic with severe hypotonia, feeding difficulties, dehydration, constipation, lethargy, respiratory distress, failure to thrive, and delayed neuropsychological development. X-rays may show severe bone demineralization and subperiosteal resorption with fractures. NSHPT needs urgent parathyroidectomy to prevent fatality.

Older children with PHPT should be considered to be due to familial cause until proven otherwise. Unlike in adults where most are diagnosed during a routine investigation showing hypercalcemia, 80% of the children have symptoms and features of end-organ damage before diagnosis. This could be because symptoms in children are usually vague and nonspecific involving multiple systems. Symptoms can be in the form of loss of appetite, easy fatigability, weight loss, headache, nausea, vomiting, and irritability leading to a delayed diagnosis and often advanced presentation. It could also be because serum calcium is not a part of routine investigations in children.

Diagnosis: Biochemical diagnosis is made by demonstrating hypercalcemia with inappropriately high serum PTH. Routine evaluation in children with hypercalcemia includes renal function tests, vitamin D levels, and bone mineral density. Serum calcium should be done in all infants with hypotonia and failure to thrive at the earliest as NSHPT can be fatal without treatment. NSHPT presents with severe hypercalcemia (>15 mg/dL) with PTH elevated 10 times more than normal. Twenty-four-hour urinary calcium along with calcium–creatinine clearance ratio are to be done in all older children to rule out FHH, as this entity does not need any treatment.

As half of the cases of pediatric PHPT are due to genetic mutations, the role of genetic counseling and genetic testing is crucial in children. Present UK guidelines recommend genetic testing in all children with PHPT.[13] A positive genetic test aids in planning complete management and also helps in counseling the family for genetic screening. All neonates with hypercalcemia should undergo testing for CaSR mutations. Other mutations are tested for according to the associated symptoms. In case if there are no associated symptoms, testing should start with *MENIN* gene.

Imaging: Imaging modalities used to localize the parathyroid tumors include ultrasound neck, Tc-99m sestamibi scan with single-photon emission computed tomography (SPECT) imaging, four-dimensional computed tomography (CT), magnetic resonance imaging (MRI), and choline positron emission tomography (PET). The sensitivity of sestamibi decreases in the presence of multiglandular disease as is the feature in majority of familial syndromes.

Treatment: Once the diagnosis is made, hypercalcemia should be managed with hydration and diuretics. In cases with severe hypercalcemia, bisphosphonates and calcimimetic cinacalcet can be used as rescue therapy to buy time for surgery.

The most important factor in treating a parathyroid tumor is locating an experienced endocrine surgeon. Definitive treatment of PHPT includes surgical removal of the abnormal parathyroid glands. In neonates with NSHPT, surgery is the only lifesaving procedure. Imaging is usually negative in these cases and can be managed by total parathyroidectomy with autotransplantation in brachioradialis but with a caveat that autotransplantation is associated with a higher risk of persistent and recurrent hyperparathyroidism.

In cases in which a solitary parathyroid adenoma is localized on imaging with negative genetic testing, minimal invasive parathyroidectomy with intraoperative parathyroid hormone monitoring along with frozen section biopsy is the recommended procedure. The patient is said to be cured if PTH drops by >90% of the pre-excision or preincision value (Miami criteria).

In patients with negative localization studies, patients with genetic syndromes predisposed to multiglandular disease, exploration of all the four glands is the recommended procedure. In patients with MEN1, possible surgical approaches include subtotal parathyroidectomy, total parathyroidectomy, and total parathyroidectomy with autotransplantation in brachioradialis. These patients are at an increased risk of recurrence as compared to MEN2A patients. The surgical approach in MEN2A patients depends on the number of glands affected, but exploration of all four glands is a must.

There is no role of prophylactic parathyroid surgery even in patients with known genetic mutations. There is no appropriate timing and indications for surgery defined in pediatric age group with hereditary PHPT.[14]

Follow-up: Postoperatively, PTH and calcium drop significantly. These children should be monitored for hypocalcemia. Children with significant bone disease are at risk of developing hungry bone syndrome (hypocalcemia, hypophosphatemia, and hypomagnesemia) and should be managed with intravenous and oral calcium along with active vitamin D supplements.

Patients should be followed up with serum calcium and serum PTH at 6 weeks and then at 3 monthly intervals for the first year followed by 6 monthly monitoring for the second year and then annually. Children with positive genetic mutations should also be screened for other associated features. Bone mineral density should be done at 3 months to assess the improvement in bone function and then annually.

⬦ TUMORS OF THE ADRENAL GLANDS IN CHILDREN

Introduction

Diseases of the adrenal gland that require surgery are, invariably, masses of the adrenal medulla or cortex. Neuroblastoma is the most commonly observed neoplasm of the adrenal medulla. Adrenal cortical tumors, benign or malignant, are less frequent. Unlike adults, surgical resection is recommended in pediatric cases because of the higher prevalence of malignancy of adrenal masses. With regard to surgical approach, open surgery was widely preferred earlier, but laparoscopic adrenalectomy has gained favor over the past few years. At present, it is the standard of care. While the surgical approach has changed over time, the approach to management of adrenal tumors has not. The cornerstone of management is accurate functional assessment on the basis of biochemical tests, which must be followed by anatomical characterization with appropriate imaging. Only then can the surgical approach be contemplated. Regardless of whether it is an open or minimally invasive procedure, adrenal surgery warrants expertise and accrued knowledge.

Adrenal Anatomy

The adrenal cortex and medulla, which deal with steroid and catecholamine metabolism, respectively, have separate origins. In the 5th week of intrauterine life (IUL), mesothelial proliferation occurs between the root of the dorsal mesentery and the gonadal ridges. This tissue will develop into the fetal adrenal cortex. In due course, the cortex will come to envelop the medulla which develops from the neural crest. The adrenal gland is encapsulated by a layer of lateral plate mesoderm that separates it from the gonad and kidney that develop alongside.

By the 9th week of IUL, the adrenal cortex has differentiated into the definitive and the fetal zones.[15] The fetal cortex primarily produces androgens, which influence sexual differentiation of the fetus. By the 7th month of IUL, a third layer of adrenal cortex, the transitional zone, is formed. The definitive and transitional zones form the zona glomerulosa and fasciculata, which synthesize the mineralocorticoids and glucocorticoids, respectively. Over the first year of life, the fetal zone gradually involutes and the zona reticularis, the innermost layer, develops.[16]

At birth, the adrenal glands in the newborn are almost as big as the adult adrenal glands. In comparison to the adult body, they are 10–20 times larger in proportion.[17] This

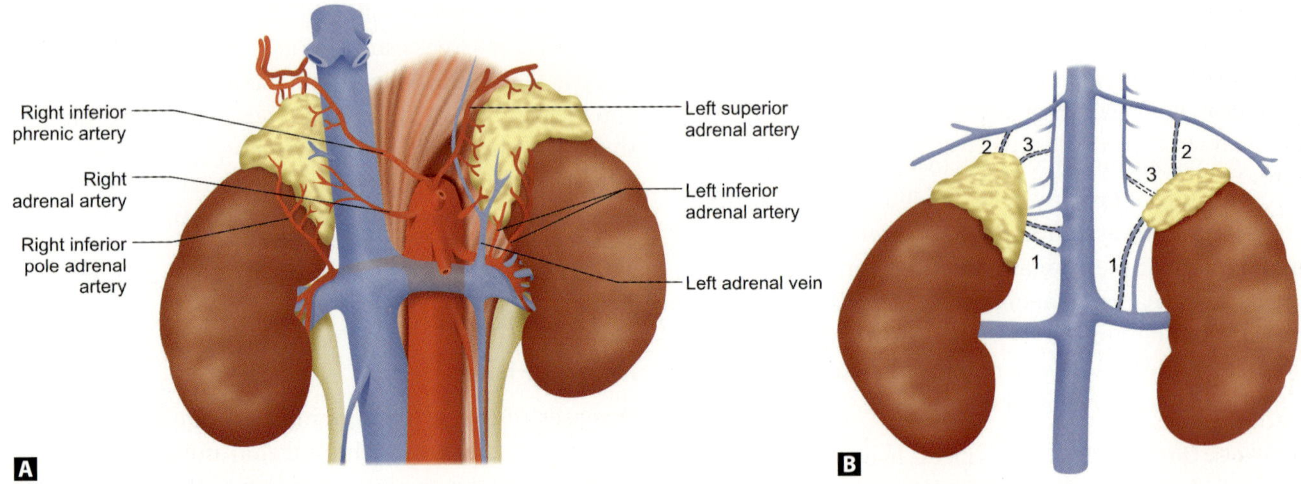

Figs. 1A and B: (A) Arterial supply to the adrenal glands; (B) Normally the adrenal vein drains into inferior vena cava on right side and reanal vein on left side. However, there can be anomalies like duplication of adrenal veins (1), drainage of the adrenal vein into the musculophrenic veins (2), or into the azygous system of veins (3)

factor is significant when identifying the glands on neonatal imaging studies: they appear to be about 30% of the size of the adjacent kidneys. In addition, retroperitoneal fat deposition is significantly scarce in children and so it is easier to identify the adrenal glands at surgery. Identification of adrenal glands, tumors, and even lymph node metastases at surgery is also aided by the distinct chrome yellow color of the glands, which is often retained in adrenocortical tumors (ACTs) and their metastases **(Figs. 1 and 2)**.

Physiology

The zona glomerulosa, the outermost layer of the adrenal cortex, produces and secretes aldosterone in response to activation of the renin–angiotensin system. Aldosterone affects sodium reabsorption and potassium secretion in the distal tubule of the kidney. Hyperaldosteronism (one of the causes of which is an aldosterone-secreting ACT) is characterized by hypertension (from the excess sodium absorbed), hypokalemia, and the associated clinical syndrome. The zona fasciculata, the middle and the most substantial layer of the cortex, synthesizes and secretes glucocorticoids (the foremost of them being cortisol). Regulation of cortisol secretion is multifactorial. The hypothalamo–pituitary–adrenal axis regulates it by means of a negative feedback loop. This phenomenon finds application in the biochemical diagnosis of Cushing's syndrome. In addition, stress response involves synchronous stimulation of the zona fasciculata and the adrenal medulla, resulting in enhanced secretion of corticosteroids as well as catecholamines. The zona reticularis, called so due to the reticulate appearance of chords of cells on histological examination, synthesizes and secretes the adrenal androgens, dehydroepiandrosterone (DHEA) and DHEA-sulfate (DHEA-S). The cells of zona reticularis appear darker than the rest of the adrenal cortex due to the pigment lipofuscin, which is synthesized in this layer.[20] Production of DHEA and DHEA-S is regulated by ACTH.[21]

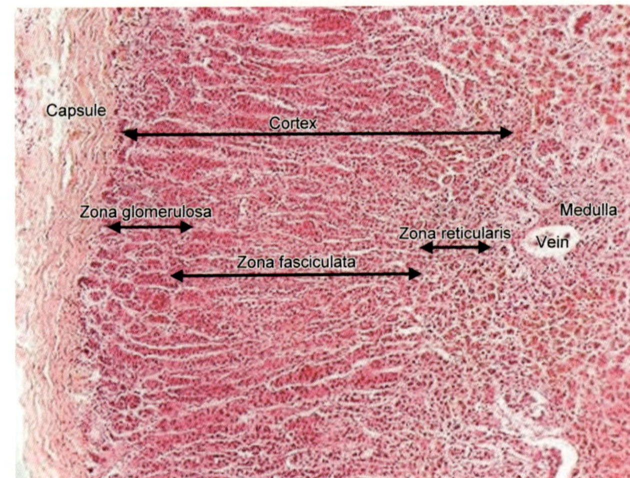

Fig. 2: Microscopic anatomy of normal adrenal gland.[18,19]

In states of ACTH-dependent stimulation of adrenal cortex, clinical features of virilization and feminization are seen. They are also seen in some patients with hypercortisolism due to the overlap of regulatory control. The neural crest, which gives rise to the chromaffin cells of the adrenal medulla, also gives rise to the chief cells of the paraganglia and the parafollicular cells of the thyroid. These cells are the cells of origin of PCCs, paragangliomas (PGLs), and neuroblastomas. They synthesize, secrete, and metabolize catecholamines. Estimation of catecholamines and their metabolites is the mainstay of biochemical diagnosis of these tumors.

PHEOCHROMOCYTOMA AND PARAGANGLIOMA

Pheochromocytoma or PGL is the cause of hypertension in 0.5–2% of pediatric hypertensive patients.[22] PCCs arise from the adrenal medulla and comprise 80–85% of catecholamine-secreting tumors while PGLs (15–20% of the tumors) arise from extra-adrenal locations. Sympathetic PGLs arise along the sympathetic chain in the chest, abdomen, and pelvis. Parasympathetic PGLs arise from parasympathetic tissue in the head and neck; these rarely secrete catecholamines. Tumors that originate within the adrenal medulla generally secrete epinephrine, while extra-adrenal tumors mostly secrete norepinephrine and dopamine.

Demographics, Epidemiology, and Clinical Features

The average age at presentation of PCCs and PGLs in pediatrics is 11–13 years, with a male preponderance of 2:1.[23] In contrast to adult patients, in whom paroxysmal hypertension is common, 60–90% of children with these tumors have sustained hypertension. Symptomatology may depend on the type of hormone being secreted. Individuals with epinephrine-secreting tumors can present with hypoglycemia and hypotensive shock, from excess catecholamine production and circulatory collapse. Dopamine-secreting tumors are usually asymptomatic, delaying diagnosis until the mass effect of the tumor is apparent. The mass effect from nonfunctional head and neck PGLs can lead to dysphagia, hoarseness, hearing disturbances, and pain **(Box 4)**.

Malignancy rates vary and are estimated to be between 12 and 47% based on small case series.[24-27] Those with succinate dehydrogenase B (SDHB) mutations have the highest prevalence for malignancy. With regard to risk for malignancy, a single-center retrospective review identified the following factors to be associated with an increased risk of malignancy: tumors >6 cm in the largest dimension, extra-adrenal location, and sporadic tumors.[24] In their study, the European-American Pheochromocytoma-Paraganglioma-Registry (EAPPR) reported malignant tumors in 30% of pediatric patients with PCC. Bilateral adrenal tumors have been reported in up to 40% of pediatric cases.[23]

Box 4: Clinical features of pheochromocytoma in children.

- Sustained hypertension
- Headaches
- Palpitations
- Sweating
- Pallor
- Nausea
- Flushing
- Anxiety
- Weight loss
- Visual disturbances
- Polyuria
- Polydypsia

Mass effects:
- Local pain
- Dysphagia
- Hoarseness
- Hearing disturbances

Genetics of Pheochromocytoma/ Paraganglioma in Children

Pheochromocytomas and PGLs occur sporadically as well as in the context of hereditary syndromes such as MEN2, von Hippel Lindau (VHL) type 2, neurofibromatosis type 1 (NF-1), and the PCC–PGL syndromes (PPGL, linked to the *SDHx* genes). Other susceptibility genes, not currently ascribed to syndromes, have been identified as well. As per data by the EAPPR, 80% of pediatric patients with PCC/PGL have a germline mutation in a gene associated with such tumors.[23] In addition to the known syndromic presentations of MEN2, NF-1, and VHL, germline succinate dehydrogenase (SDH) gene mutations form part of the familial PGL–PCC syndromes. SDH consists of the four subunits, A, B, C, and D. These syndromes are inherited in an autosomal-dominant fashion with varying penetrance. Carney's triad (gastrointestinal stromal tumors, PGLs, and pulmonary chondromas), Carney–Stratakis syndrome (diad of GIST and PGL/PCC), and Pacak–Zhuang syndrome (head and neck PGLs, polycythemia, and somatostatinoma) are rare syndromes with PGLs as one of the presenting features. The approach for genetic testing in PCC/PGL is outlined in **Flowchart 2**.

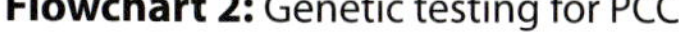

Flowchart 2: Genetic testing for PCC.

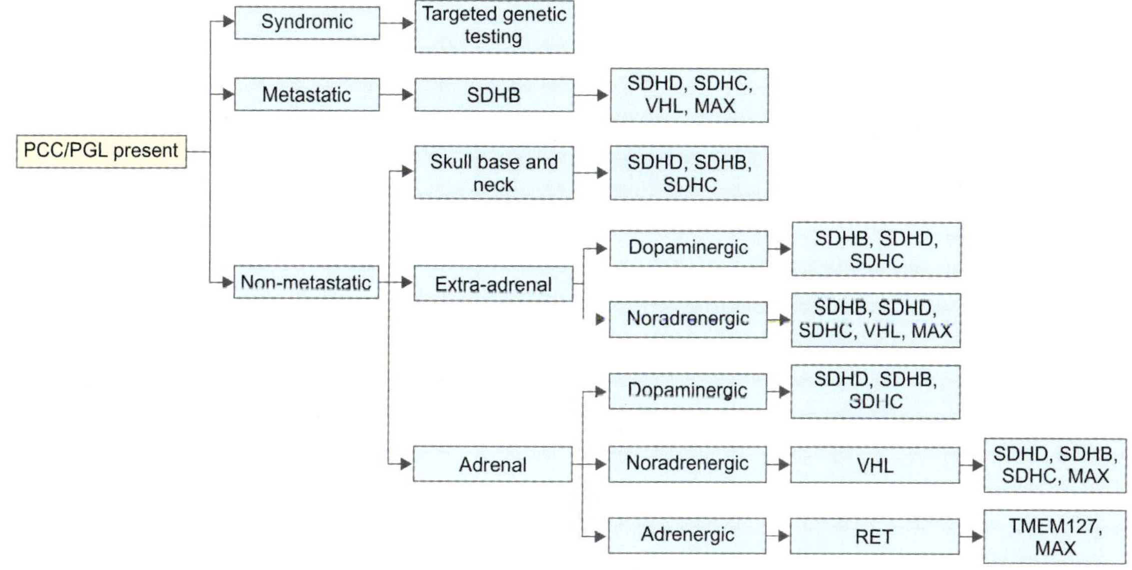

Work-up: Laboratory Testing

Once there is clinical suspicion for a PCC or PGL, the next step is biochemical confirmation of excess catecholamine secretion. Various metabolites are assessed in the urine as well as plasma **(Table 8)**. The gold standard for diagnosis, however, is the estimation of free metanephrines in the plasma.[28] The degree of elevation of catecholamine metabolites ought to be assessed when evaluating for catecholamine-secreting tumors, as shown in **Flowchart 3**. Values >4 times the upper limit of normal (ULN) are highly suggestive of a tumor[29] while values greater than ULN and lesser than 4 times the ULN need to be investigated further **Flowchart 3**. Chromogranin A (CgA), a protein present in chromaffin cells which controls secretion of hormones from secretory granules, may improve the sensitivity of diagnosing SDHB- and SDHD-related tumors with concomitant use of plasma metanephrines.[30] The algorithm for biochemical testing is outlined in **Flowchart 3**.

Imaging

Localization of catecholamine-secreting tumors must only be pursued after biochemical confirmation of diagnosis. In adults, the first modality of imaging is renal ultrasound. In children, however, USG is not very accurate, with sensitivity and specificity of 89%[31] and 61%[32], respectively. CT or MRI of the abdomen and pelvis has been the imaging modality of choice in pediatric cases given similar diagnostic sensitivities (90–100%) **(Fig. 3)**. Specificities of both are around 70–80%. MRI has been found to be more sensitive than CT for extra-adrenal tumors. In addition, the extent of invasion

Table 8: Metabolites assessed in the work-up of PCC/PGL.	
Metabolite	*Remarks*
Catecholamines (plasma, urine)	Secretion and release episodic
Vanillyl mandelic acid, AM (plasma, 24-hr urine)	Also produced by metabolic processes unrelated to PCC/PGL; less accurate
Metaneprhines (24-hr urine)	Constantly produced and released from the tumors; not influenced by episodic spikes of catecholamine secretion and release. Fractionated metanephrines in urine 95% sensitive and 99% specific for PCC/PGL
Metanephrines (plasma)	Estimation of free metanephrines is the gold standard

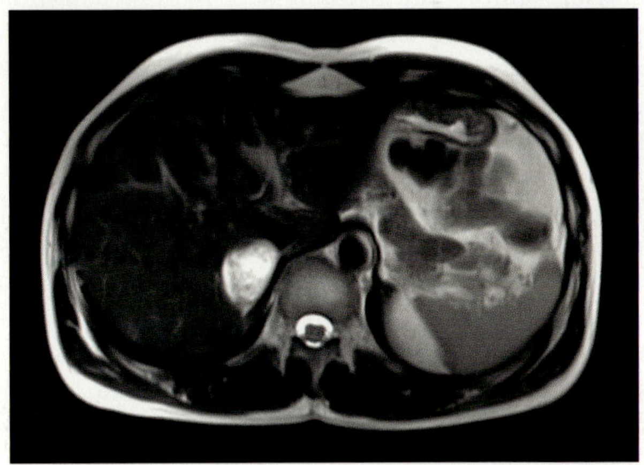

Fig. 3: MRI of Pheo.

Flowchart 3: Biochemical testing algorithm.

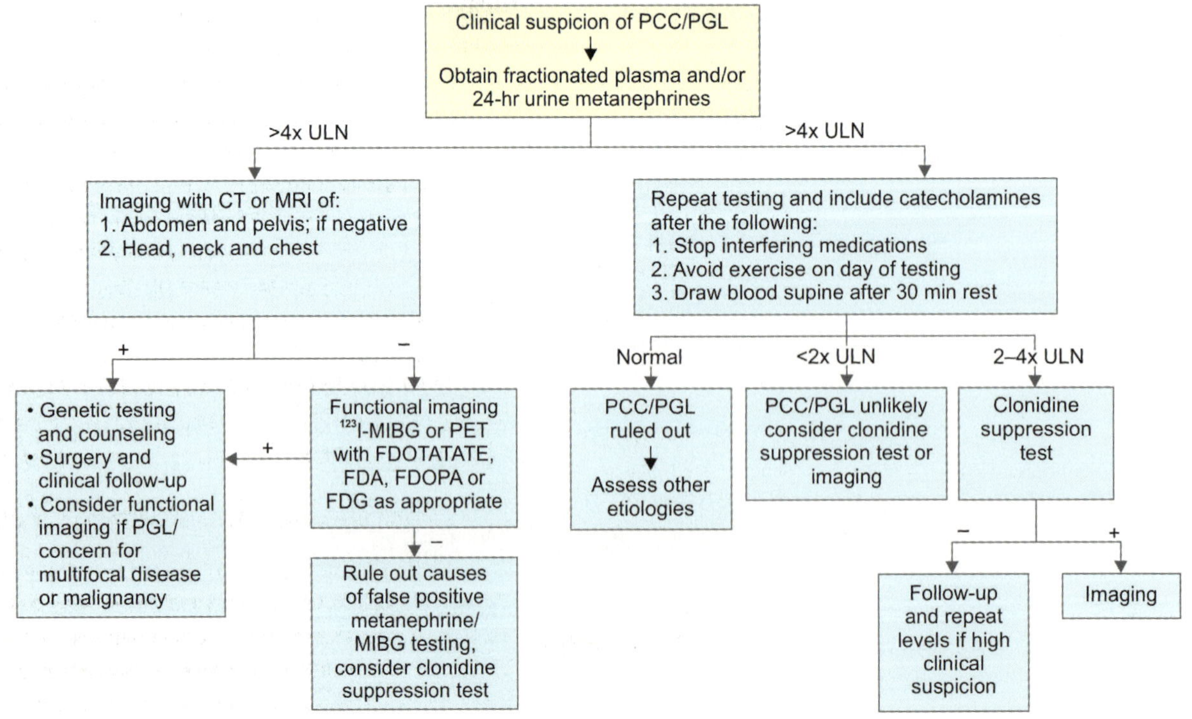

into the spinal canal and involvement of major vessels can be assessed accurately. Another obvious advantage of MRI over CT is that radiation exposure can be avoided. As neither study is as specific in discerning a PCC/PGL from other abdominal pathology, functional imaging studies need to be pursued if one has a high index of suspicion for PCCs or PGLs. These include the ^{123}I metaiodobenzylguanidine (^{123}I-MIBG) scan, PET with [18]fluorodopamine ([18]FDA), [18]fluorodeoxyglucose ([18]FDG), and [18]fluoro-dihydroxyphenylalanine (^{18}F-DOPA). The ^{123}I-MIBG scan has been used in conjunction with CT/MRI in some studies to locate and rule out multifocal disease, offering 95–100% specificity in localizing PCCs/PGLs.[33] Recent advances in functional imaging of PCCs/PGLs have led to the use of radiolabeled DOTA peptides, such as ^{68}Ga-DOTATATE PET, which has high affinity for somatostatin receptors type 2. Such receptors are known to be overexpressed in PCC/PGLs. Adult studies have demonstrated the superiority of ^{68}Ga-DOTATATE PET in localizing metastatic SDHB-associated PCCs/PGLs over the other functional imaging studies, excluding MIBG.[34] ^{68}Ga-DOTATATE PET was also the most sensitive test in detecting head and neck PGLs,[34,35] especially SDHD tumors but inferior to F-DOPA PET/CT in detecting PCCs[35] in sporadic cases.

Management

Sympathetic Blockade

Over the years, there has been a drastic decrease in perioperative complications with the use of sympathetic blockade **(Table 9)**. Beta-blockade is instituted following alpha-blockade to offset reflex tachycardia from alpha-2 receptor antagonism. Beta-blockade must never precede alpha-blockade. Once beta-1 and, more importantly, beta-2-mediated vasodilatation is blocked, unopposed alpha-receptor stimulation can cause the blood pressure to shoot up to alarming levels, potentially precipitating hypertensive crises. Dilated cardiomyopathy can develop from chronic catecholamine-induced hypertension and so preoperative echocardiography is valuable. Agarwal et al., in their study, found that postural hypotension related to use of alpha-blockers could be effectively prevented with a high sodium diet of 6–10 g and a fluid intake of at least 1.5 times the daily requirement.[36] Romero et al. have delineated a stepwise approach to the preoperative alpha-blockade in pediatric patients.[37]

Intraoperative Considerations

In this day and age, laparoscopic adrenalectomy has come to be the standard of care in adult patients **(Fig. 4)**. It has also been demonstrated to be safe in children and is an accepted approach for unilateral and bilateral adrenal pathology.[38] Laparoscopic resection and adrenal cortical-sparing procedures are now the preferred approach, the latter being important in patients with bilateral adrenal disease, to avoid cortisol deficiency. Intraoperative hypertension is controlled with a variety of agents including sodium nitroprusside or esmolol. Magnesium sulfate, dexmedetomidine, or nicardipine has also been used. Care should be exercised when giving fluids intraoperatively if patients are hypotensive, to avoid cardiopulmonary complications in the case of catecholamine-induced cardiomyopathy.[39] However, factors such as recurrence rates and the possibility of malignancy must be considered before opting for cortical-sparing surgery. Between 15% and 30% of the adrenal gland is needed to preserve function.[40] Given the potential complications of resecting such tumors, an experienced anesthesiologist and endocrine surgeon are essential to the care of these patients.

Postoperative Care

Use of phenoxybenzamine is associated with sustained postoperative hypotension. This effect is not seen with

Table 9: Drugs used in control of hemodynamics in PCC/PGL.

Class	Drug	Remarks
Alpha-blocker	Phenoxybenzamine	• Non-selective alpha-blocker; traditionally, the mainstay of alpha-blockade; • Crosses blood-brain barrier: headaches, nasal stuffiness • Reflex tachycardia due to blockade of alpha-2-mediated cardiac inhibition • First dose hypotension; may cause syncope • Sustained alpha-blockade may cause persistent hypotension postoperatively; volume replacement is more effective than pressors in postoperative BP recovery
	Prazosin/Doxazosin	• Alpha-1 selective blockade; newer agents; being increasingly used of late; shorter duration of action; postural hypotension and reflex tachycardia less likely (In theory) • First dose hypotension; first dose advised at bedtime
Tyrosine Hydroxylase inhibitor	Metyrosine	• Inhibits catecholamine synthesis • Advantages over blockade including better BP control, lesser intra-operative blood loss and lesser peroperative morbidity • Effects of overdose, including fatigue, anxiety, dry mouth, diarrhea, tremors and trismus, can be frightening.
Beta-blockers	Propranolol, esmolol	• Generally used after complete alpha-blockade • Stabilize the heart, suppress reflex tachycardia • Beta-blockade MUST NEVER be initiated before alpha-blockade • Standard usage 48–72 hours prior to surgery

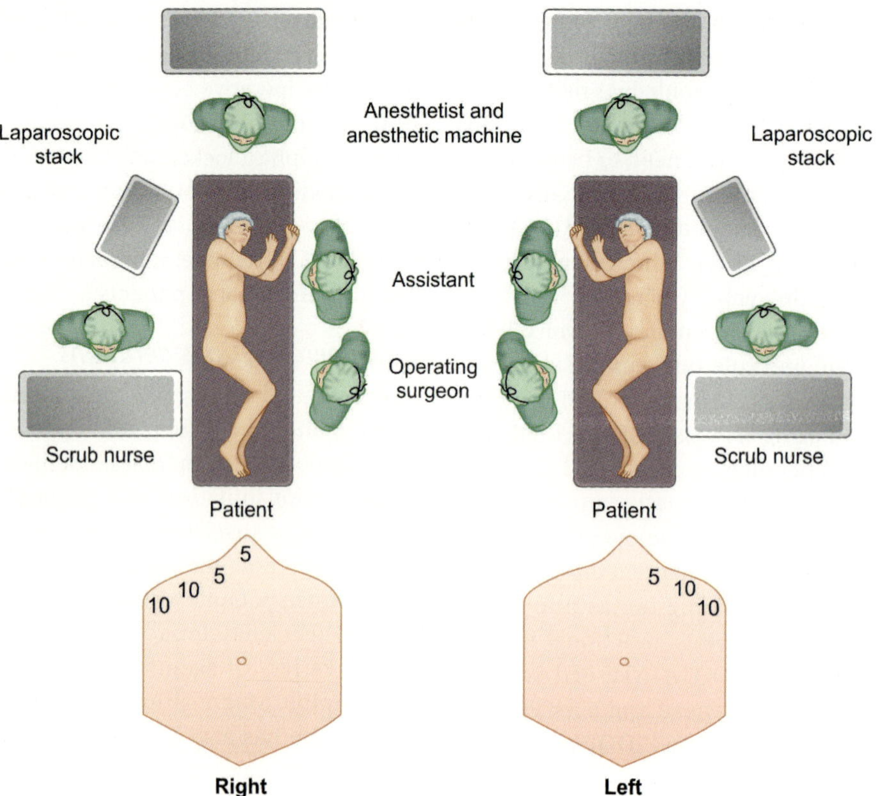

Fig. 4: OT scheme for laparoscopic adrenalectomy.

selective alpha-blockade.[41] Hypoglycemia can occur postoperatively due to rebound hyperinsulinism from a reduction of catecholamines.

Malignant Pheochromocytoma and Paraganglioma

Complete surgical resection is the curative therapy of PCCs and PGLs. In case of malignant tumors, adjuvant treatment for disease control is often required. ^{131}I-MIBG is currently used for malignant tumors and relies on the uptake of MIBG by the norepinephrine transporter. If the tumor uptake of this radioisotope is poor, peptide receptor radionuclide therapy with radiolabeled somatostatin analogs or ^{111}In-pentetreotide scintigraphy [somatostatin receptor scintigraphy (SRS)] may be performed.[42] Chemotherapy with cyclophosphamide, vincristine, and dacarbazine may be required too. The largest study to date has shown progressive disease in 52% (11 patients), while 4% (1 patient) had complete remission, 22% (5 patients) had partial response, and 22% (5 patients) had stable disease.[43] EBRT has been used to control metastatic PCCs and PGLs, with results of the largest retrospective study of 24 patients indicating symptomatic control in 81% of lesions and stable disease in 87% of lesions. A retrospective review shows that 17 patients with PGLs excluding head and neck PGLs were treated with EBRT with 76% of the patients achieving either local disease control or symptomatic relief.[44] Prospective studies would be useful to understand the long-term effects and outcomes of these therapies.

Prognosis

A retrospective chart review of 30 pediatric patients, from 1975 to 2005, showed that those who were classified as having benign disease had a 100% survival rate as compared to those with malignant disease, who had 5-, 10-, and 15-year survival rates of 78, 62, and 31%, respectively.[24] Malignant disease was classified as that with distant metastases, tumor unresectable due to local invasion of vital structures, or tumor recurrence regionally or distally after initial resection and initial negative microscopic margins. According to recent survival data of pediatric patients from the EAPPR, 8 out of 144 patients with hereditary disease (6%) died, with a follow-up mean range of 10–19 years (range 0–53 years).[10] Of these, three had VHL mutations, three had SDHB, two had NF-1, and one succinate dehydrogenase A (SDHA), with the cause of death being metastases in seven patients and cardiac failure in another patient. All 33 patients with sporadic disease, followed for a mean of 10 years (range 1–45 years), were alive at subsequent follow-ups. The overall mean life expectancy of hereditary disease was 62 years. Life expectancy was greatly reduced with SDHB-associated disease, at 47 years, while patients with VHL had the lowest life expectancy at 27 years.

Malignant PCCs and PGLs are defined by the World Health Organization (WHO) classification as the presence of metastases that does not include local invasion of a tumor. As such, a malignant tumor that has not yet metastasized may be classified as benign. Two classification systems exist to predict malignant potential of PCCs and PGLs, the PASS, or the Pheochromocytoma of the Adrenal Gland Scaled Score **(Box 5)**, and the GAPP, or the Grading system for Adrenal Pheochromocytoma and Paragangliomas **(Box 6)**. Given the lack of reliable markers to distinguish a benign lesion from a malignant one, lifelong follow-up of patients is required in the instance that metastases develop. Plasma methoxytyramine has been recognized as a biomarker for metastatic PCCs and PGLs. In the same study, extra-adrenal disease, tumor size >5 cm and SDHB mutation carriers have been reported to be associated with a high risk of malignancy.[45]

Long-term follow-up on patients with hereditary PCCs and PGLs cannot be stressed enough given the lifelong risk of recurrence and metastatic disease. Laboratory testing with serum/urine metanephrines should be performed yearly. The decision to advise follow-up imaging studies should be based on clinical features and/or positive laboratory testing. Generally, follow-up first at 6 weeks postoperatively is recommended, with repeat follow-up between 6 months and 1 year following initial surgery, followed by annual follow-up. If genetic analysis reveals involvement of genetic mutations, then the intensity and frequency of follow-up need to be increased. Recommendations of the EAPPR are to perform annual surveillance for the first 3 years after initial diagnosis of mutation carriers, followed by lifelong follow-up. However, since malignancy can occur much later in life too, constant and frequent follow-up is advisable in such patients.

Summary

- PCC/PGL is/are the cause in 2% of pediatric hypertensive patients.
- 80% of these tumors arise in the adrenal medulla.
- Majority of patients have sustained hypertension as opposed to paroxysms.
- Biochemical confirmation of diagnosis is essential before imaging tests. Gold standard is estimation of plasma metanephrines. However, fractionated metanephrines in a 24-hour urine sample are very sensitive and specific.
- CT or MRI of the abdomen affords localization and anatomical characterization. If they are not specific, then isotope scans are necessary.
- ^{68}Ga-DOTATATE PET is accurate for extra-adrenal tumors, especially head and neck tumors.
- Preoperative sympathetic blockade is essential. Beta-blockade MUST NOT precede alpha-blockade. Alpha-1 specific blockers are preferable. First-dose hypotension is common.
- Laparoscopic adrenalectomy is the standard of care for the surgical approach to PCC **(Fig. 5)**.
- Sustained postoperative hypotension might occur. Preoperative regimen of high salt diet can prevent this complication to an extent.
- 30% of these tumors have been reported to be malignant; often, the only evidence of malignancy is when the patient develops metastases or recurrence. Hence, lifelong follow-up is necessary.

◇ NEUROBLASTOMA

Although it was first recorded in the 19th century as "sarcoma of the adrenal gland" by Virchow, the term neuroblastoma was first used in 1910. One out of every ten solid tumors in the childhood is a neuroblastoma. While these tumors can

Box 5: Pheochromocytoma of the Adrenal Gland Scaled Score (PASS).

Parameter	Score
Diffuse cellular growth	2
Central or confluent tumour necrosis	2
High cellularity	2
Cell monotony	2
Narrowed tumor cells	2
Mitosis >3/10 HPF	2
Atypical mitosis	2
Invasion into fat	2
Invasion into vessels	2
Invasion into tumor capsule	1
Nuclear pleomorphism	1
Nuclear hyperchromasia	1

Score 4 or more corresponds to high metastatic potential

Box 6: Grading System of Adrenal Pheochromocytoma and Paragangliomas (GAPP).

Parameter	Score
Histological pattern	
Zellballen	0
Large/irregular cell nest	1
Pseudorosette	1
Cellularity	
Low (<150 cells/U)	0
Moderate (150–250 cells/U)	1
High (>250 cells/U)	2
Comedo necrosis	
Absent	0
Present	2
Vsacular/Capsular invasion	
Absent	0
Present	1
Ki-67 index	
<1%	0
1–3%	1
>3%	2
Catecholamine type	
Adrenaline type	0
Noradrenaline type	1
Nonfunctioning type	0

A score of 3 or more is associated with higher risk of metastasis

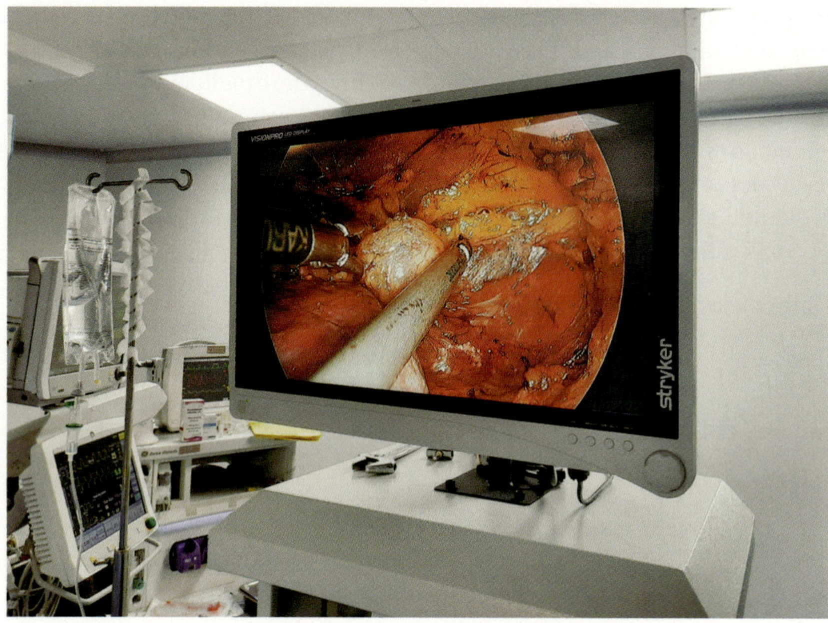

Fig. 5: Laparoscopic adrenalectomy.

occur in any structure that develops from the neural crest, they are most commonly seen in the adrenal medulla. The presentation includes a wide clinical spectrum. While in some children, the tumors disappear spontaneously, some children develop extensive metastases and succumb to the disease in spite of intensive, and often stage-appropriate, multimodal therapy. Bartlett performed the first recorded surgery for neuroblastoma in 1916.[46] It was the only known modality of treatment then. However, with the discovery of benefits of radiotherapy in the 1950s and chemotherapy later, the outlook for neuroblastoma has improved over time. A modest improvement in survival has been reported with the use of cyclophosphamide and vincristine for advanced disease.[47,48]

Clinical Features

It presents as a large mass in the abdomen. Effects of compression of adjacent structures can also be present, like paralysis resulting from spinal cord compression when the tumor invades the spinal canal. Clinical signs of distant metastasis include "raccoon eyes" (metastases in the orbit), "blue berry muffin sign (subcutaneous metastatic deposits), bone pain, hepatomegaly and respiratory embarrassment. Clinical features of excessive catecholamine metabolism include excessive sweating, tremors, hypertension, anxiety, and palpitations. Opsoclonus-myoclonus, or dancing eyes, is a disabling symptom which can rarely be a presenting feature. 60% of these tumors arise in the abdomen, with the thorax accounting for another 25%. 10% of the tumors arise in the pelvis and the remainder from other structures including the neck.

Investigations

Diagnosis is based on a high index of clinical suspicion. If no obvious cause is evident in a sick child who fails to thrive,

then the next step is ultrasound of the abdomen. If findings suggestive of a lesion show up on ultrasound, the next step is biochemical confirmation with a urine catecholamine assay, which is followed by further cross-sectional imaging (CECT or MRI) for more detailed anatomical characterization. Additional information about disease load can be obtained on CECT or MRI. Image-guided needle core biopsy of the lesion will enable tissue diagnosis as well as histopathological analysis. Sometimes, endoscopy may be necessary for this. Tissue ores thus obtained are better sent straight to the pathologist without adding any fixatives. Most tumors take up MIBG. MIBG gamma scanning is also performed to assess disease load and extent of spread.

Pathology and Molecular Pathology

In neuroblastoma too, like in other tumors, there is a wide spectrum of microscopic morphology. The well-differentiated tumors look very similar to mature neural elements, while some poorly differentiated tumors, which comprise small, blue cells, resemble embryonic blast cells and cannot be distinguished from other malignant tumors. According to the International Neuroblastoma Pathology Committee (INPC), there are three tumor types in ascending order of malignancy and from differentiated to undifferentiated: ganglioneuroma, ganglioneuroblastoma, and neuroblastoma.[49-51]

Tumors with diploid DNA have a worse prognosis than those with hyperdiploid. Other predictors of aggressive tumor behavior, and hence unfavorable prognosis, include amplification of the *MYCN* oncogene, deletion of the short arm of chromosome 1, loss of chromosome 11q, gain of chromosome arm 17q, and oncogenic mutations of anaplastic lymphoma kinase (ALK).

Staging and Risk-based Therapy

A risk-based approach to the management of the disease has resulted in a significant improvement of outcomes in terms of morbidity and mortality. In localized disease, surgery alone has been found to be curative.[52] In separate studies by workers from the Children's Cancer Study Group A (CCSG A) and Children's Hospital of Philadelphia, the outcome in patients of this disease was analyzed. The age of the patient and stage of the disease were found to be significant in prognosis.[53,54] A larger group of workers developed the staging principles further and published the International Neuroblastoma Staging System (INSS; **Box 7**).[55,56] As is evident, this system involved criteria which were predominantly postoperative. Later, the International Neuroblastoma Risk Group (INRG) complied data from more than 9,000 patients and devised a much more comprehensive staging system **(Box 8)**, which involves among other things, surgical risk factors (SRFs).[57] These SRFs are important to predict the risk and effectiveness of surgery in tumor excision.[58,59] SRFs have been assigned for each tumor site depending on the involvement and, therefore,

the risk of injury to the surrounding anatomical structures. In their study, the European Neuroblastoma Study Group (LNESG1) found that if SRFs were present, the rate of complete excision fell by 30% and the risk of surgical complications was found to be 12% higher than in cases with no SRFs. Hence, the presence of SRFs necessitates neoadjuvant therapy so that surgery can be more effective and safe. Patient age, tumor stage, histological grade, and molecular pointers including DNA ploidy, *MYCN* status and 11q status are the most important determinants of the outcome after therapy. On the basis of 5-year event-free survival (EFS) rates, four groups have been identified: group 1 (EFS of 85% or more), group 2 (EFS of 75–84%), group 3 (EFS of 50–74%), and group 4 (EFS <50%). Image-defined risk factors (IDRFs), similar to SRFs, have been identified on the basis of cross-sectional imaging **(Box 9)**. Staging of the tumor based on IDRF is as follows: L1—localized tumor with no IDRF; L2—localized tumor with IDRF; M—tumor with distant metastasis; MS—small primary tumor with metastasis confined to skin and liver in a patient less than 18 months of age.

Treatment Strategies

Surgical excision alone has been very effective for localized disease with no IDRFs (INSS stages 1 and 2, INRG stage L1),

---

Box 7: International Neuroblastoma Staging System (INSS).

This staging system is for postoperative patients and mainly for prognosis.

Stage 1
- Localized tumor with complete gross excision with or without microscopic residual disease
- Contralateral and representative ipsilateral regional lymph nodes negative for disease (nodes attached to and removed with primary tumor may be positive)

Stage 2a
- Localized tumor with incomplete gross excision
- Ipsilateral and contralateral nodes negative for tumor

Stage 2b
- Localized tumor with complete or incomplete resection
- Positive ipsilateral (non-adherent) nodes
- Contralateral nodes negative for tumor

Stage 3
- Unresectable lateral tumor that crosses the midline or
- Localized tumor with contralateral regional lymph node involvement
- Midline tumor with bilateral extension by infiltration or by lymph node involvement

Stage 4S ("special")
- <1 year of age
- Localized tumor (stage 1, 2A or 2B)
- Distant metastases confined to skin, liver and/or bone marrow

Stage 4
Distant metastases not fulfilling stage 4S

Box 8: International Neuroblastoma Risk Group Staging System (INRGSS).

The INRG was developed after INSS to formulate staging for preoperative neuroblastoma:[5,6]

Stage L1: Localized tumors confined to one body cavity and not involving image-defined risk factors (IDRFs)

Stage L2: Locoregional tumors involving one or more IDRFs

Stage M: Distant (remote) metastases (i.e. excludes metastases to local lymph node groups) excludes stage MS

Stage MS: Metastases in patients <18 months (some centers <12 months) confined to skin, liver and/or bone marrow

---

Box 9: Image-defined risk factors in neuroblastoma.

List of features that, if present, upstages a patient with local disease from L1 to L2.

Crossing/extending: From one compartment to another (e.g., chest to neck, abdomen to chest, abdomen to pelvis) through sciatic notch/foramen

Encasing vessels:
- Carotid artery
- Vertebral artery
- Internal jugular vein
- Subclavian artery/vein
- Aorta
- Superior or inferior vena cava
- Celiac artery
- Superior mesenteric artery (including branches at the mesenteric root)
- Iliac artery or vein

Compressing:
- Trachea
- Primary bronchi

Encasing nerves: Brachial plexus roots

Invading and infiltrating:
- To skull base into spinal canal—defined as:
  - >1/3 of canal involved on an axial section
  - Perimedullary leptomeningeal space not visible
  - Signal change in the adjacent spinal cord
- Costovertebral junction from T9 to T12
- Porta hepatis, hepatoduodenal ligament or liver
- Renal pedicle or kidney
- Pericardium
- Duodenopancreatic block
- Mesentery
- *Encasement:* In contact with >50% (artery or vein) or completely occluding a vein (n.b. <50% is "contact"; incomplete occlusion of a vein is "flattening")
  - *Compression:* Any cross-sectional narrowing of an airway
  - Synchronous and metachronous tumors should be staged separately

with reported 5-year relapse-free survival of 94% and overall survival (OS) of 99%.[60] For patients with INSS stage 3 or INRG stage L2 disease, primary surgery is contraindicated due to the unacceptably high risk of complications when compared to earlier stages (17 vs. 5%) and due to lesser chance of complete excision (46 vs. 75%).[58] These patients are benefitted by neoadjuvant chemotherapy with CADO regimen (carboplatin, etoposide, cyclophosphamide, vincristine, and doxorubicin). For metastatic disease in patients over 18 months of age (INSS stage 4, INRG stage M), the strategies involve: induction chemotherapy, surgical excision, and then consolidation therapy to deal with any residual disease. A combination of five drugs (COJEC—cisplatin, vincristine, carboplatin, etoposide, and cyclophosphamide) is administered for the induction. Stem cells from the peripheral blood are harvested at induction for bone marrow rescue, since these drugs cause significant bone marrow depression. Induction is followed by surgery, with a goal of complete tumor resection. Following surgery, high-dose adjuvant chemotherapy is given. After tumor excision, consolidation therapy involves retinoic acid and anti-GD2, a monoclonal antibody. Administration of consolidation therapy has afforded a significant improvement of outcomes with EFS of 66% and OS of 86% at 2 years.[61] In the case of metastatic "special" patients (age < 18 months; INSS stage 4S, INRG stage MS), the prognosis is very good, with an OS of 90%.[62] Treatment is started with chemotherapy using carboplatin and etoposide. While a single course of the regimen is often effective, persistence of symptoms necessitates more intensive chemotherapy. Surgical treatment by creation of an abdominal silo and/or ligation of the hepatic artery has been used in an emergency.

Radiation

Neuroblastoma is a radiosensitive tumor, but the use of this modality is avoided in infants due to the risk of long-term growth defects. While no benefit has been demonstrated in early stage disease (INSS stage 1 or 2), there has been some benefit seen in patients with stage 3 or 4 disease and bad biology. Targeted radiation with ^{131}I-MIBG may be useful, especially in recurrent disease.

Summary

- Neuroblastoma makes up 10% of all pediatric solid malignancies.
- The tumors are quite large, involving the trunk in 95% of cases.
- They synthesize and secrete catecholamines. Elevations of urinary catecholamine levels are the cornerstone of biochemical diagnosis.
- Tissue diagnosis is often necessary and can be obtained by image-guided FNAC.
- Most tumors take up ^{131}I-MIBG.
- Presence of hyperdiploidy is a molecular marker of favorable prognosis.

- Therapeutic approach is risk based. Surgical and image-guided risk factors have been defined and are regularly employed in prognostication and in treatment decisions.
- Prognostic staging includes preoperative estimation of disease load, SRFs, and IDRFs as well as the extent of surgery.
- This tumor is one of those amenable to all three modalities of treatment, including surgery, chemotherapy, and radiotherapy, with each modality having its place and indications depending on the risk stratification.

◇| ADRENOCORTICAL TUMORS

Adenomatous and carcinomatous tumors of the adrenal cortex are dealt with in this chapter together as ACTs, as it is difficult to distinguish between the two in terms of clinical features as well as histopathology in the absence of metastatic disease. Among the tumors of adrenal glands in children, the ACTs are less prevalent than neuroblastoma but more so than pheochromocytoma. Clinically and biologically, ACTs in childhood are distinct from those in adults.

Etiology

While most ACTs occur sporadically, there are some known risk factors such as mutations of the *p53* and insulin-like growth factor 2 (*IGF-2*) genes. The most well-known tumor syndrome that is associated with p53 mutation is the Li-Fraumeni, or SBLA (sarcoma, breast, leukemia, and adrenal gland), syndrome. Apart from ACTs, other possible elements of the syndrome include tumors of the brain, breast, larynx, and lung and sarcomas. ACTs are 100 times more common in this syndrome in comparison with the general population.

The Beckwith–Wiedemann syndrome results from overexpression of the *IGF-2* gene on chromosome 11q15. Also known as exophthalmos-macroglossia-gigantism (EMG) syndrome, the components include benign as well as malignant tumors such as ACTs, Wilms' tumor, and hepatoblastoma. ACTs can also be associated with certain other congenital abnormalities such as duplication of the renal collecting duct system and congenital adrenal hyperplasia and with neural tumors such as ganglioneuromas and ganglioneuroblastomas. It has been suggested that ACTs can also develop as an eventual outcome of environmental exposure to several agents.

Epidemiology

According to a recent SEER program study review, the incidence of adrenocortical carcinoma (ACC) in people under the age of 20 years is 0.21 per million.[63] Prevalence of ACTs in children may mimic prevalence of *p53* mutations, although other genetic and environmental factors may play a role. Typically, ACTs are seen in children under the age of 5 years. A biphasic distribution with respect to age has been reported, with peak incidence during infancy and adolescence.[64] The disease seems to affect girls more, with a female-to-male ratio of 3:2. This female preponderance is even more acute after adolescence (ratio of 6:1).[64]

Pathology

Adrenocortical tumors involve the right and the left adrenal gland with almost equal frequency. Bilateral involvement is seen in 1% of the patients. Ectopic sites have been described in spinal canal,[65] thoracic cavity,[66] and abdomen itself away from the adrenal glands. The ectopic occurrence can be explained by the close proximity of structures such as the celiac plexus, the kidneys, and the genitourinary tract during the development of the adrenal glands.

Adrenocortical adenomas are usually unilateral, solitary, round, well demarcated, have a smooth surface, and are smaller in size (typically, <50 g). They are yellow, or sometimes red-brown, in color. The tumor appears black if it contains large amounts of lipofuscin. ACCs are generally larger (>100 g in weight), although smaller tumors have been reported too. The shape is irregular, the surface is nodular and uneven, and they have coarse trabeculations. They appear yellow too, but the color is less uniform. There may be foci of hemorrhage that appear as darker patches. Areas of necrosis within the tumor are frequently seen. Cystic changes are seen more frequently in carcinomas than in adenomas.

On examination under the microscope, the appearance is similar to that of the normal zona fasciculata and glomerulosa. In adult patients in general, the adenomas are composed of mature, uniform cell types with a low nuclear:cytoplasmic ratio. Features like nuclear atypia, cellular polymorphism, hemorrhage, and necrosis are very sparse. In pediatric patients, however, these features are seen more commonly than in adults. In adult ACC specimens, a wide range of differentiation is evident, often within the same tumor. The cells can appear mature, like normal adrenocortical cells or like completely undifferentiated blast cells. The tumors are often separated into nodules by broad fibrous bands. Features such as hyperchromasia, bizarre giant cells, and vascular and capsular invasion are commonly seen on microscopy. In pediatric patients, however, these features are not exclusive to malignancy.

The tumor size, weight, and histological features may suggest malignant potential, but the only feature that is consistently associated with malignancy is the actual presence of distant metastases.[67] The most important determinant of aggressive tumor behavior is the mitotic rate.[68,69]

Clinical Features

In most cases, pediatric patients of ACTs present within the first year of life due to clinical features that are seen due to hormone secretion. Virilization, feminization, and Cushing's and Conn's syndromes are the most common presentations.

However, it is very rare for patients to present with classical and exclusive features of any particular syndrome, since ACTs usually secrete several hormones. Often, they present with clinical features of multiple syndromes.

Precocious puberty refers to the premature appearance of secondary sexual characters (SSCs) in girls before the age of 8 years and in boys before the age of 9 years. When gonadotropin-dependent, it is true precocious puberty. When independent of gonadotropins, it is pseudo-precocious puberty. When the SSCs are gender-appropriate, it is called isosexual precocious puberty. Otherwise, it is called heterosexual precocious puberty. ACTs usually synthesize and secrete androgens along with cortisol. Since the source of androgens and cortisol in functional ACTs are gonadotropin independent, ACTs present with Cushing's syndrome or pseudoprecocious puberty or both. Androgen secretion by the ACTs is reflected as deepening of acne, facial hair growth, deepening of voice, proliferation and excessive secretion from the sebaceous glands, and increased muscle mass in both genders. In males, features of isosexual precocious puberty are seen, such as early acne, development of pubic hair, and penile enlargement.[67] In females, heterosexual precocious puberty occurs, characterized by advanced bone age, hirsutism, pubic hair growth, clitorial enlargement, and amenorrhea.[67] Cushing's syndrome is seen in about 35% of the patients. Much like the adult cases, the clinical features include weight gain, centripetal obesity, moon facies, buffalo hump, plethora, striae, and hypertension. Aldosterone-producing tumors are rarely seen in pediatric patients. Clinical features include proximal muscle weakness, polyuria, headache, palpitations, a fast heartbeat, and hypertension. Overlapping manifestations of the various hormone excess states are more the rule than the exception.

Laboratory Testing

Biochemical testing must be done first to check for hormone function. It involves estimation of glucocorticoids, androgens, and their metabolites in body fluids. The most important marker for ACTs is the level of 17-ketosteroids (17-KS) in urine. Regardless of the clinical syndrome (Cushing's or virilization), urinary 17-KS levels are elevated. In about 90% of patients, DHEA-S levels are abnormal in plasma. 17-KS and DHEA-S are also excreted in urine and so estimation of these metabolites in urine is useful as well. While urinary 17-KS and DHEA-S are less sensitive compared to plasma levels, they are viable alternatives due to the ease of performing the test and wider availability. In case of Conn's syndrome, the negative feedback by the renin–angiotensin–aldosterone axis is disrupted. Therefore, biochemical evaluation in patients includes determination of urinary 17-KS and 17-OH, urinary or plasma cortisol (either baseline or suppressed), plasma DHEA-S, testosterone, androstenedione, 17-hydroxyprogesterone, aldosterone, renin activity, 11-deoxycorticosterone (DOC), and other 17-deoxysteroid precursors. In addition, estimation of serum electrolytes is useful. The hormone activity will not help differentiate benign from malignant lesions since both will have a significant elevation in these markers.

Imaging

Ultrasonography is often the first imaging procedure performed in children with abdominal masses, since it is simple, fairly painless, and hence does not necessitate sedation. The anatomical location and relationship to the surrounding vessels and organs, make-up (cystic or solid), vascularity, and associated liver metastases, if present, can be identified. However, a significant proportion of adrenocortical lesions tends to be small and, often, difficult to visualize. In case of malignant tumors with contiguous tumor thrombi in the adjacent vasculature [renal vein, inferior vena cava (IVC), right atrium], Doppler USG is helpful. On ultrasound, ACTs appear as round or ovoid lesions of variable size. Larger size, heteroechogenicity lobulated border, and central hypoechogenicity could suggest malignancy, although ACCs < 6 cm in size can appear homogeneous. Another characteristic, but uncommon, sign of ACCs is the scar sign, which refers to radiating linear echoes within the substance of the lesion.

The imaging modality of choice is the CECT. With CECT, it is possible to accurately assess tumor size, location, appearance, and relation to the surrounding structures. In addition, one can assess the surroundings or regional lymph node metastasis, tumor thrombi within adjacent vessels, and distant metastasis within the abdomen. Typically, ACTs are circumscribed, heterodense lesions, sometimes with a thin capsule.

Magnetic resonance imaging too affords accurate assessment of the anatomy of ACTs. In addition, it involves no radiation, displays different planes, and may better characterize tumor thrombus. The downside is that it may be more expensive than CT. ACTs have intermediate signal intensity on T1-weighted MR images and high signal intensity relative to the liver on T2-weighted images. MRI may help differentiate benign from malignant lesions based on the enhancement with gadolinium.

Positron emission tomography employs the differential metabolism of malignant lesions and thus helps in the assessment of disease load and in the setting of post-treatment follow-up.

Surgery for Adrenocortical Tumors

Estimation of the disease load and staging of the disease is the standard approach in oncology in general. In case of ACC, however, staging of the disease is based on preoperative assessment and imaging as well as on the extent of resection **(Table 10)**. Surgery is the cornerstone of treatment for ACT. The patient will be well served by careful operative planning, thorough preoperative assessment and appropriate perioperative support. It is safer to proceed

with the assumption that in all patients with functioning ACTs, the contralateral adrenal cortex is suppressed. Hence, supplementation with steroids in the perioperative period is almost a rule. Other aspects that need assiduous attention are maintenance of fluid and electrolyte balance, blood pressure, hemodynamics, wound care, and prevention of surgical site infection. In general, open laparotomy or a thoracoabdominal approach will afford the surgeon the best chance to completely excise the tumor. In a large majority of patients without distant metastasis at presentation, curative resection can be attempted. Complete and en bloc excision of the tumor has to be attempted even if it involves excision of a part or whole of contiguous structures (e.g., ipsilateral nephrectomy). The tumor tends to be vascular and friable and so the procedure is fraught with risks of tumor spillage, which has been reported in about 20% of initial operations, and in 43% of operations done for tumor recurrence.[70,71] In up to 20% of the patients, the IVC is infiltrated with tumor thrombus. This is a significant challenge to complete tumor excision. In cases of extensive vascular infiltration, when extensive thrombectomy and vascular reconstruction may be necessary, cardiopulmonary bypass may have to be performed to achieve the necessary vascular control.

In spite of apparently adequate surgery, tumor recurrence is possible and so these patients are kept on close follow-up with imaging and endocrine studies. Even in patients with distant metastasis, complete resection of the primary tumor is indicated and feasible due to the functional effects of the tumor. In cases in which resection is not possible, tumor ablation with ethanol injection may be the only option for local control. Lymph node metastases have been reported in up to 40% of the adult patients, but the pattern is not well documented in pediatric patients. Opinion is emerging that patients with large tumors (stage II) are better served by ipsilateral retroperitoneal resection along with complete excision of the primary tumor. Open laparotomy is still the approach of choice in ACC, but since laparoscopy is the standard of care for adrenalectomy in general, this approach has come to be used more and more in pediatric patients as well. The advantages of improved visualization and reduced postoperative pain are obvious, but it is suggested that laparoscopic adrenalectomy may be limited to patients with small, localized lesions.

Table 10: Staging of adrenocortical tumors.	
Stage	**Features**
I	• Tumor excised in toto with negative margins; weight <200 g; no evidence of metastasis; adrenal hormones return to normal levels postoperative • R0 resection
II	• Tumor excised in toto with negative margins; weight >200 g and/or persistently elevated adrenal hormone levels postoperative • R1 resection. Microscopic remnants
III	Gross residual tumor postoperative or Inoperable tumor
IV	Distant metastasis

Adjuvant Therapy

Mitotane, an insecticide derivative, inhibits the synthesis of corticosteroids and destroys the cells of the adrenal cortex. It has been used for chemotherapy in adults with advanced ACC. There have been occasional reports of complete response, but its use in pediatric patients has not been documented systematically. Although the impact on overall outcome is not significant, it should nevertheless be considered due to potential benefits in alleviation of symptoms. There have been reports of usage of a variety of anticancer drugs including platinum derivatives, etoposide, 5-fluorouracil, and ifosfamide. With regard to radiation, ACTs are generally radioresistant. In addition, radiation exposure in children with the Li–Fraumeni syndrome may increase the risk of developing other tumors. Recent advances in this field have thrown up many potential treatment options, including targeted radionuclide therapy with radiolabeled metomidate, epidermal growth factor inhibitors, inhibitors of vascular endothelial growth factor (VEGF)-mediated angiogenesis, IGF receptor inhibition, beta-catenin antagonists, steroidogenic factor inhibitors, and mammalian target of rapamycin (mTOR) antagonists. Gene therapy, including reactivation of tumor suppressor genes, or inhibition of tumorigenic genes and immunotherapy involving modulation of immune response against tumor cells are also being explored.

Outcomes

The overall outlook for ACC in children, especially in those under the age of 4 years, is better than that in adults.[72,73] Improvement of OS over the years may be a reflection of increase in diagnostic accuracy, refinements of surgical technique, and improved postoperative care.[9] According to a recent SEER review, the prognosis is more favorable in children under the age of 4 years compared to those aged between 5 and 19 years. In most patients with ACC, death occurs within 1–2 years of diagnosis. Metastases are found in the liver, lungs, and regional lymph nodes more often than in other organs.

Surgery of the primary tumor is the mainstay of successful treatment. There has been no significant improvement of OS with the use of mitotane and so it is not advisable to use it after complete surgical resection. In case of locoregional recurrence, it is advisable to attempt reoperation and removal of the recurrent tumor. In such patients, chemotherapy may be of benefit. Finally, an international registry has been established which may provide more insight into this rare tumor of childhood.

Summary

- It is often difficult to distinguish between benign and malignant ACTs, but the tumor mass affords a rough estimation of malignancy. Benign tumors often weigh <50 g, while malignant tumors weigh 100 g or more.

- Mutations and deletions of the p53 (Li-Fraumeni syndrome) and Beckwith-Wiedemann syndrome form important etiological factors.
- Most pediatric ACTs are functional tumors. The hormones secreted lead to clinical presentation within the first year of age. The most common syndrome is virilization syndrome.
- Estimation of 17-KS in urine is the cornerstone of laboratory testing.
- In unilateral tumors, the contralateral adrenal cortex is often suppressed. Perioperative supplementation of steroids is advised.
- While tumor spillage during surgery is harmful in any malignancy, it is particularly significant in ACTs.
- Often, the only treatment option is surgery. Hence, adequate exposure is of paramount significance. An open approach is advised for larger tumors even if extra-adrenal spread is not obvious on metastatic work-up.

◇ TUMORS OF THE ENDOCRINE PANCREAS

Pancreatic tumors are not common in the pediatric age group, but about 30% of those seen in the first two decades of life arise from the islets of Langerhans.[74] Generally, these tumors, referred to as pancreatic neuroendocrine tumors (PNETs) are indolent and asymptomatic. The second-most common manifestation of MEN1, PNETs are seen in up to 80% of patients with MEN1.[75]

Etiology

While the majority of these tumors occur sporadically, the association with inherited gene mutations is well established. MEN1, MEN2, VHL syndrome, neurofibromatosis 1 (NF1), and tuberous sclerosis are some of the associated syndromes.[76,77] In addition, PNETs have been identified with other novel mutations as well, including the mechanistic pathway of rapamycin (mTOR) genes (*TSC2*, *PTEN*, *PUK3CA*, etc.), the *ATRX* gene, and the *DAXX* gene, the latter two being part of a recently discovered pathway of molecular tumorigenesis.[78,79]

Pathology

It was previously thought that all neuroendocrine tumors (NETs), including PNETs, originated from the neural crest cells. Now, it is postulated that pluripotent stem cells develop into a neuroendocrine phenotype and give rise to NETs including PNETs.[80] In general, PNETs are indolent and slow-growing. The tumor cells demonstrate positive reactions to neuroendocrine markers like chromogranin (CG), neuron-specific enolase (NSE), and synaptophysin. These tumors can develop anywhere in the pancreas and are usually multiple. Benign as well as malignant tumors are seen. Benign tumors <5 mm are termed microadenomas, while larger benign tumors are called macroadenomas. Microadenomas are generally found in patients with hereditary cancer syndromes. The malignant tumors, the neuroendocrine carcinomas, can present with clinical features of distant metastasis.

Neuroendocrine tumors are classified on the basis of their degree of differentiation. Previously, they were classified into well-differentiated NETs, well-differentiated neuroendocrine carcinomas, and poorly differentiated neuroendocrine carcinoma. In 2010, a system of classification **(Table 11)** that included the tumor grade, mitotic count, and the Ki-67 index was formulated and endorsed by the WHO.[81,82] While the AJCC staging system was followed previously, the European Neuroendocrine Tumor Society (ENETS) has proposed a modified staging system,[83,84] which has been outlined in **Table 12**.

Clinical Presentation

Pancreatic neuroendocrine tumors can be functioning or nonfunctioning tumors. Functioning PNETs secrete pancreatic peptide hormones including gastrin, insulin, glucagon, or vasoactive intestinal polypeptide (VIP). Tumors may secrete more than one hormone, but generally, one of the hormones will be predominant, with the majority of clinical features corresponding to the main hormone that is secreted in excess. That said, the majority of PNETs in children are nonfunctional and are detected by chance or during the process of screening for MEN1.

Gastrinomas

Gastrinomas are the most common type of PNETs in pediatric patients. Refractory peptic ulceration along with diarrhea is the defining feature of the Zollinger–Ellison syndrome. Gastrinomas are seldom solitary. 90% of these tumors are found within a triangular area (Passaro's triangle) with vertices at the confluence of the cystic and common hepatic ducts superiorly, the junction of the second and third parts of the duodenum inferiorly and the neck of the pancreas medially. Overall, most of these tumors are located within the duodenal wall, while those associated with MEN1 occur mostly in the head of the pancreas.[85] At presentation, distant metastases are seen in up to two-thirds of the cases. Diagnosis is based on demonstration of elevated basal gastric acid output (BAO, acid output in the fasting state) with a gastric pH of 2.0 or less and a concomitant elevation of gastrin in serum. It is important to withhold proton-pump inhibitors and H_2-receptor blockers for at least a week before the test. Localization studies, including CECT, MRI, and functional imaging (PET/octreoscan/SPECT), may be performed afterward. While doing so, it is wise to evaluate the liver thoroughly to look for potential metastases.

Table 11: WHO 2010 Classification of PNETs.[82]

Grade	Features
I	2 or fewer mitoses/10 HPF and/or Ki-67 index of 2% or less
II	3–20 mitoses/10 HPF and/or Ki-67 index 3–20%
III	21 or more mitoses/10 HPF and/or Ki-67 index of 21% or more

Table 12: The AJCC and ENETS staging systems for PNETs.

TNM	ENETS		AJCC	
Tx	Primary cannot be assessed		Same as ENETS	
T1	Confined to pancreas, T <2 cm		Confined to pancreas, T <2 cm	
T2	Confined to pancreas, T 2–4 cm		Confined to pancreas, T >2 cm	
T3	Confined to pancreas, T >4 cm or invasion of duodenum and/or CBD		Peripancreatic spread, but without major vascular invasion (Celiac, SMA)	
T4	Invasion of adjacent organs or major vessels		Invasion of major vessels	
Nx	N status cannot be assessed		N status cannot be assessed	
N0	No regional node metastasis		No regional node metastasis	
N1	Positive regional node metastasis		Positive regional node metastasis	
Mx	M status cannot be assessed		M status cannot be assessed	
M0	No distant metastasis		No distant metastasis	
M1	Distant metastasis		Distant metastasis	
Stage	I	T1 N0 M0	IA	T1 N0 M0
			IB	T2 N0 M0
	IIA	T2 N0 M0	IIA	T3 N0 M0
	IIB	T3 N0 M0	IIB	T1-3 N1 M0
	IIIA	T4 N0 M0	III	T4 Any N M0
	IIIB	Any T N1 M0		
	IV	Any T Any N M1	IV	Any T Any N M1

Insulinomas

Insulinomas present with features of hyperinsulinism and hypoglycemia including weakness, confusion, sweating, and loss of consciousness. Characteristically, these symptoms are alleviated by feeding. Diagnosis is based on the demonstration of fasting hypoglycemia with a simultaneous finding of elevated plasma insulin and C-peptide levels. Whipple's triad, the cornerstone of diagnosis, refers to the triad of features including an episode of clinically overt hypoglycemia, demonstration of low blood glucose during the episode, and relief of symptoms on normalization of the blood glucose level.

Other Functioning Pancreatic Neuroendocrine Tumors

VIPomas, or tumors that secrete VIP, are characterized by the Verner–Morrison syndrome [watery diarrhea, hypokalemia and achlorhydria (WDHA)]. In children, these tumors are seldom found in the pancreas, unlike in the adults. Glucagonomas are characterized by hyperglycemia, anemia, weight loss, and necrolytic migratory erythema, a rash that typically affects the mouth and the lower limbs. Somatostatinoma are often asymptomatic, but some patients may present with diarrhea, steatorrhea, weight loss, and diabetes mellitus. Sporadically occurring glucagonoma and somatostatinomas have not been reported in children. Other rare forms of functioning PNETs have been reported to secrete corticotropin-releasing hormone (CRH), ACTH, growth hormone–releasing hormone (GHRH), parathyroid hormone-related peptide (PHRP), calcitonin [growth-hormone releasing factor (GRF)], or gonadotropin-releasing hormone (GnRH).

Nonfunctioning Pancreatic Neuroendocrine Tumors

Due to the absence of typical functional clinical features, PNETs often present late and are usually large. In about 50% of patients, distant metastases can be found by the time they present.[86] Most patients with symptoms have features of the mass effect of the tumor, with or without liver metastases. Kimura et al.[87] have reported that many of these tumors still produce subclinical amounts of hormones.[87]

Diagnosis

Diagnosis of these tumors is based on clinical features, demonstration of the products of these tumors (including the hormones and their metabolites) in circulation and localization of the tumors with the help of imaging techniques. Histopathological examination of the operated specimen is confirmatory. Those patients who have a significant family history or are known to have molecular risk factors should be screened for possible tumors. Tumor markers for PNETs include CgA, NSE, and pancreatic polypeptide (PP), which

is elaborated by more than one-third of PNETs.[88] Serum CgA may be elevated in other conditions too, such as atrophic gastritis, chronic renal insufficiency, and in patients on long-term proton-pump inhibitor (PPI) treatment.[89] With regard to imaging, a multimodality approach is indicated in most cases for accurate localization and staging. While the initial investigations ordered include CECT and MRI, SRS too is a useful tool in these patients, since most tumors possess these receptors. If SRS is negative for localization, MIBG scintigraphy is useful. Endoscopic ultrasound as a localizing tool is being used more and more in recent times. Intraoperative ultrasound is a useful adjunct on the operating table.

Surgical Management

The only curative option for PNETs is complete surgical excision, but when planning the surgery, it is advisable to consider that PNETs are often multifocal. Even when complete surgical extirpation is not possible, debulking surgery is a viable option, since it affords significant symptom relief and improvement in the quality of life and survival. Surgery for advanced disease has been aided in recent times by the increased application of novel techniques such as radiofrequency ablation (RFA) and cryotherapy. Recent advances in medical treatment, including hormone antagonism and monoclonal antibodies, have been encouraging in terms of post-treatment outcomes. Surgical enucleation of the tumor or a partial pancreatic resection is the aim of curative treatment for patients with functioning PNETs. Pancreatic resection is also beneficial for functioning glucagonomas and VIPomas. Surgery may be considered for nonfunctioning PNETs that are larger than 1 cm or those that demonstrate significant growth over a period of 6 months. In gastrinomas, however, the optimal surgical extent and approach remain controversial.[90] In most patients with gastrinomas, the tumors are small and multifocal and so cure is seldom achieved with surgery.

Nonoperative Management

The cornerstone of treatment in advanced disease (inoperable tumors, distant metastasis, etc.) is suppression of function with biotherapy (e.g., somatostatin analogs, interferons). Targeted therapy with radionuclides, chemotherapy, TKIs like sunitinib, and mTOR inhibitors like everolimus have also been reported to be effective.[91,92] In addition to symptom control, somatostatin analogs have also been reported to inhibit tumor biology and proliferation. Treatment with depot lanreotide (CLARINET, phase III trial) has been shown to halt progression of disease significantly in metastatic PNET.[93] PPIs and somatostatin analogs are employed for acid suppression in gastrinoma patients. These patients are also advised regular endoscopic surveillance for identification of peptic ulcers.

Outcomes and Prognosis

The TNM stage at the time of diagnosis, type of the PNET, degree of differentiation, and the proliferative activity are the main determinants of prognosis. Overall, PNETs are associated with a poorer prognosis among NETs of the gastrointestinal tract (GIT).[86] According to the SEER registry, the overall 5-year survival reported in PNETs in patients aged between 3 and 19 years was 78% (91% for localized tumors and 35% for tumors with distant metastasis).[94] Respective 5-year survival rates for grades 1, 2, and 3 are 96, 73, and 28%, respectively. With regards to TNM stage, the survival rates are 100, 90, 79, and 55% for stages I, II, III, and IV, respectively.[95]

Summary

- Thirty percent of the pancreatic tumors that present before the age of 20 years are PNETs. PNETs are the second-most common tumors in MEN1.
- They demonstrate positive reactions to neuroendocrine markers including NSE, CG, and synaptophysin.
- Gastrinomas and insulinomas comprise over half of PNETs.
- The classical presentation of gastrinoma is Zollinger–Ellison syndrome. They invariably are found within the gastrinoma triangle **(Fig. 6)**. Within this triangle, most tumors are duodenal. The MEN-associated gastrinomas, however, are predominantly intrapancreatic.
- 65% of the gastrinomas are metastatic by the time they present.
- The classical presentation of insulinoma is Whipple's triad.
- Most of the so-called nonfunctional PNETs secrete hormones in very small amounts.
- While cross-sectional imaging is important, most PNETs have somatostatin receptors and so SRS is a useful adjunct in the work-up.

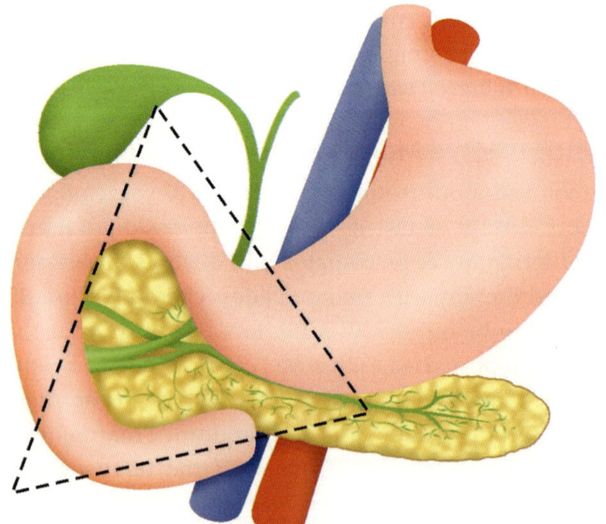

Fig. 6: Gastrinoma triangle. Unlike typical peptic ulcers, gastrinomas most commonly occur within this triangle (outlined by the hepatic portal vein, neck and body of the pancreas, and latter two-thirds of the duodenum) and hypersecrete gastrin—causing debilitating, recalcitrant acid reflux.

- Surgical resection is the primary modality of treatment.
- In metastatic disease, functional palliation is often effective in improving the quality of life.

◇ CONGENITAL HYPERINSULINISM

Congenital hyperinsulinism (CHI) refers to the congenital anomaly of excessive and unregulated insulin secretion from the beta cells of the pancreas. If untreated, the severe and profound hypoglycemia causes epilepsy, mental retardation, and cerebral palsy.[96] It is characterized by documentation of hyperinsulinemia during hypoglycemia.[97] Management includes avoidance of hypoglycemia and, if required, surgical excision by means of partial or subtotal pancreatectomy.

While the classic presentation is neonatal severe hypoglycemia, it can also present in a milder form in infancy and childhood. The incidence of CHI seems to be significantly high in communities with high rates of consanguinity (1 in 40,000 children in the general population and 1 in 2,500 in the latter).[97] Usually, normoglycemia can be maintained only with large volumes of concentrated dextrose infusions IV. Clinical features range from very severe (apnea, seizures, coma) to the mild (irritability, poor feeding, lethargy). The hyperinsulinemia is present in utero and so newborns are typically macrosomic. Other common features include hepatomegaly (increased hepatic glycogen storage) and hypertrophic cardiomyopathy. Typically, hypoglycemia occurs in the fasting state. In some cases, the hypoglycemia is provoked by protein loading or exercise.[97] Syndromic association of CHI is known too, e.g., Beckwith–Wiedemann syndrome.[98-]

Early diagnosis is vital to prevent irreversible brain injury. In the history, it is important to establish the duration of fasting and whether the hypoglycemia is precipitated by meals (protein sensitivity) or by exercise. Typically, the tolerance to fasting is very low (<1 hour). When the glucose requirement for maintenance of normoglycemia is very high (rate of IB infusion of 8 mg/kg/min or more, with the normal being 4–6 mg/kg/min), it is indicative of dysregulated insulin secretion. In addition, the serum levels of insulin and C-peptide are inappropriately high for the blood glucose level. Serum levels of ketone bodies and fatty acids are very low during the hypoglycemic episodes.[97] This metabolic profile (concomitant hypoglycemia, hypoketonemia, and low serum fatty acid levels) increases risk of brain damage.

The genes *ABCC8* and *KCNJ11* encode the proteins SUR1 and Kir6.2, which are instrumental in the glucose-mediated control of insulin secretion. Loss of function of these genes results in dysregulation of insulin secretion and is the most common cause of severe CHI.[99-101]

Depending on the pattern of involvement, there are two major subtypes, diffuse and focal CHI. In diffuse CHI, all the beta cells are affected. The disease can be sporadic or familial. The latter will involve recessively inherited or dominantly occurring mutations in the above said genes.

In focal CHI, there are islets of adenomatosis, 2–10 mm in size, with abnormal, dysfunctional, and dysregulated beta-cells that are surrounded by normal pancreatic tissue with normally functioning and regulated beta cells.[102] Focal CHI is not inherited genetically.[103]

Medical Management

In these patients, it is vital to maintain normoglycemia (blood glucose levels between 60 and 100 mg/dL) in order to prevent any damage to the CNS. In some patients, this is only possible with IV infusion of concentrated glucose which requires the insertion of a central venous catheter. The patient is maintained in the stable state with a combination of oral feeds with glucose polymers and infusions, while planning further procedures. In emergency situations when central venous access is difficult, glucagon can be administered as a temporizing measure. Glucagon acts as soon as it enters the bloodstream. It increases plasma glucose levels by releasing the stores of glycogen. It also stimulates the processes of gluconeogenesis, ketogenesis, and lipolysis. In older children, it can be given as an intramuscular injection bolus (0.5–1 mg). In infants and neonates, glucagon can be added to the IV glucose infusion, either alone or in combination with octreotide.

While the problem of enteral feeding can be reasonably addressed in adults with nasoenteral tubes, gastrostomy, or jejunostomy, the same is not feasible in infants due to certain specific problems. "Orality," or the inculcation of the natural feeding reflex, is vital. Long-term tube feeding might adversely affect orality. In addition, gastroesophageal reflux and motility disorders are common in infants with CHI.[97] In some cases, intervention with speech and language therapy may be required to establish a normal feeding pattern.[98]

Diazoxide, a drug that binds to the intact SUR1 component of the KAPT channels, acts by inhibition of insulin release from the beta cells. A single appropriate dose can act for as long as 8 hours. One important side effect is fluid retention (Na^+ as well as H_2O). To add to this, these patients necessarily receive large volumes of fluids, either IV or per orum. In neonates, it is administered along with chlorothiazide, a diuretic with additional hyperglycemic properties. In patients who do not respond to diazoxide, octreotide is given as the second-line therapy.-

Differentiating Focal from Diffuse Congenital Hyperinsulinism

If patients do not respond to diazoxide or other medical treatments, the next option is focal or near-total pancreatectomy, depending on whether the disease is focal or diffuse.[104] If the pattern of involvement is focal, then precise localization and surgical excision of these foci will result in cure. Focal lesions, which are usually 2–10 mm in size, are buried within the substance of the pancreas and are invisible to the naked eye.[105]

In patients with diffuse CHI, nothing less than near-total pancreatectomy will suffice. These patients will have to endure life-long implications, such as severe diabetes mellitus and exocrine insufficiency. Risk of diabetes mellitus is high even in patients on medical management.[106]

In infants, it is very difficult, if not impossible, to identify the pattern of involvement by clinical features or biochemical tests. In the past, the tools for identifying and localizing focal CHI included arterial calcium stimulation/venous sampling, testing of the acute insulin response intravenous glucose, calcium and tolbutamide, intrahepatic pancreatic portal venous sampling (PVS), and biopsy of the tail of the pancreas. These methods, while being technically challenging, are not very accurate. Conventional cross-sectional imaging (CECT, MRI) is not very useful either. However, recent advances in ^{18}F-DOPA-PET have helped revolutionize this aspect. The uptake of this isotope is markedly increased in cells with a high rate of insulin synthesis. It is possible to detect foci as small as 1 mm.[106] Integration of ^{18}F-DOPA-PET and CT has made it possible to appreciate the surrounding anatomy too, including the splenic vessels, portal vein, the mesenteric arteries, and the duodenum, apart from increasing the precision of localization.[107]

Furthermore, in case of inherited disease, since there is a consistent correlation between phenotype and genotype, genetic analysis helps to decide about ^{18}F-DOPA-PET/CT. The scan is indicated in those patients who have the genotype of a focal lesion (namely a paternally inherited mutation in *ABCC8* or *KCNJ11*) or have no mutations in the *ABCC8*/*KCNJ11* genes. If the patient has a homozygous or compound heterozygote mutation in *ABCC8* or *KCNJ11*, then this is likely to be associated with diffuse disease and an 18F-DOPA-PET/CT is not required these cases. The aim of the ^{18}F-DOPA-PET/CT is to allow preoperative localization of the focal domain. A recent review of ^{18}F-DOPA-PET/CT suggests that in focal lesions, 18F-DOPA-PET scan is useful in defining the site and dimension of the focal lesion in two third of the patients.[108]

Surgery for Congenital Hyperinsulinism

Surgery is indicated for cases of diffuse CHI which are medically unresponsive and in all cases of focal disease, provided that the focal lesion is accurately localized preoperatively. It should be done in centers of expertise which are equipped with all the relevant facilities and resources. While ^{18}F-DOPA-PET/CT is promising, limitations do remain with regard to the accuracy. Hence, it becomes necessary for frozen section examination of the excised specimen and histopathological confirmation of complete excision of the focus of CHI.

Surgery for Diffuse Congenital Hyperinsulinism

The goal of surgery would be to remove enough pancreatic tissue to enable independence from glucose infusions and maintenance of normoglycemia with the help of oral feeds, while avoiding the adverse effects of pancreatic insufficiency (both exocrine and endocrine). However, in the real world, it is a fine line between removing too much and leaving behind too much of pancreatic tissue. At present, the recommendation is near-total pancreatectomy or "95% pancreatectomy."[104] This involves excision of all visible pancreatic tissue except for a thin cuff of pancreas around the terminal part of the common bile duct (CBD) and a rim of tissue (about 2 mm thick) adjacent to the C loop of duodenum. This would avoid persistent hypoglycemia from too much of the hyperfunctioning beta cells, while ensuring enough functional pancreatic tissue to prevent diabetes mellitus and malabsorption sequelae.

Surgery for Focal Congenital Hyperinsulinism

In focal CHI, local resection of the involved focus is curative. Preoperative confirmation of focal CHI is essential and should involve a combination of genetic analysis and ^{18}F-DOPA-PET/CT imaging. Once imaging confirms the involved site, the appropriate procedure can be planned. However, the accuracy of ^{18}F-DOPA-PET/CT (approximately 70%) has to be borne in mind.[108] In addition, there are no reliable intraoperative adjuncts like postexcision blood glucose levels to confirm excision. Hence, it is essential to arrange for frozen section examination of the excised specimen and confirmation of excision of the hyperfunctioning focus. In case of proximal lesions, the head and neck of the pancreas are excised while preserving a cuff of tissue around the terminal CBD and a rim of tissue around the duodenal C loop, with a pancreaticojejunostomy to drain the distal pancreas. If the lesions are more distal, a distal pancreatectomy would suffice. While proximal surgery would necessarily be an open procedure, distal pancreatectomy could be performed either as an open procedure or with the help of the laparoscope.

Summary

- CHI is characterized by the inappropriate and unregulated secretion of insulin from the pancreatic β-cell. The severe and profound hypoglycemia is a major cause of mental retardation, epilepsy, and cerebral palsy.
- The patients suffer from severe hypoglycemia which is usually refractory to oral feeds. The disease presents in utero itself, with the majority of the affected babies being macrosomic.
- Affected newborns have markedly reduced fasting tolerance with hypoglycemia occurring in an hour following the last feed.
- During hypoglycemic attacks, levels of ketone bodies and fatty acids in the blood are markedly suppressed.
- There are two types of CHI on the basis of the extent of pancreatic involvement—diffuse and focal. In inherited CHI, there are distinct genetic alterations that code to these forms. Genetic assays are significant precursors of imaging studies for the assessment of type and extent of pancreatic involvement.
- In focal CHI, ^{18}F-DOPA-PET is a useful adjunct in localization of foci.
- Medical treatment of CHI includes administration of glucagon and diazoxide.
- Surgery for diffuse CHI often involves near-total pancreatectomy.

◇ CLINICAL PEARLS

Thyroid

- 1.2% of children have palpable thyroid nodules
- Papillary thyroid carcinoma is the most common pediatric thyroid cancer with solid and diffuse sclerosing variants predominating.
- In children, TSH suppressive dose should be balanced with their respective developing age/stage.
- Non-adherence to levothyroxine therapy is an important issue and needs adequate monitoring and counseling in children.

Parathyroid

- PHPT has a bimodal age presentation—neonates and older adolescents.
- PHPT in neonates and infants occurs exclusively due to CasR mutation.
- All neonates with hypercalcemia should undergo testing for CasR mutation.
- No role of prophylactic surgery even in patients with known genetic mutation.

Adrenal

- Adrenal tumors are relatively easier to locate in children when compared to adults due to the relatively sparse adipose tissue in general.
- Functioning paragangliomas and pheochromocytomas are the cause of hypertension in about 2% of pediatric hypertensive patients. Preoperative sympathetic blockade is essential. Laparoscopic adrenalectomy is the standard of care for the surgical approach to PCC. Often in the case of malignant tumors, the only evidence of malignancy is when the patient develops metastases or recurrence. Hence, life-long follow-up is necessary.
- Neuroblastoma makes up 10% of all pediatric solid malignancies. Elevations of urinary catecholamine levels are the cornerstone of biochemical diagnosis. Tissue diagnosis is often necessary and can be obtained by image-guided FNAC. Most tumors take up ^{131}I-MIBG. This tumor is one of those amenable to all three modalities of treatment including surgery—chemotherapy, and radiotherapy, with each modality having its place and indications depending on the risk stratification.

- It is often difficult to distinguish between benign and malignant ACTs, but larger tumors are more likely to be malignant. Most pediatric ACTs are functional tumors. The most common syndrome is virilization syndrome. Often, the only treatment option is surgery. In general, open adrenalectomy is advisable.

- 30% of the pancreatic tumors that present before the age of 20 years are pancreatic neuro-endocrine tumors (PNETs). Gastrinomas and insulinomas comprise over half of PNETs. The classical presentation of gastrinoma is Zollinger–Ellison syndrome. The classical presentation of insulinoma is Whipple's triad. Surgical resection is the primary modality of treatment. In metastatic disease, functional palliation is often effective in improving the quality of life.

◇| REFERENCES

1. Niedziela M. Pathogenesis, diagnosis and management of thyroid nodules in children. Endocr Relat Cancer. 2006;13: 427-53.

2. Qian ZJ, Jin MC, Meister KD, Megwalu UC. Paediatric thyroid cancer incidence and mortality trends in the United States, 1973–2013. JAMA Otolaryngol Head Neck Surg. 2019;145:617.

3. Niedziela M, Breborowicz D, Trejster E, Korman E. Hot nodules in children and adolescents in western Poland from 1996–2000: clinical analysis of 31 patients. J Paediatr Endocrinol Metab. 2002;15:823.

4. Schlumberger M, Pacini F. Thyroid tumours. Paris: Nucleon, 2003.

5. ATA guidelines for thyroid nodules and cancer in children.

6. Sobrinho-Simoes M, Máximo V, Rocha AS, Trovisco V, Castro P, Preto A, et al. Intragenic mutations in thyroid cancer. Endocrinol Metab Clin North Am. 2008;37(2): 333-62.

7. American Thyroid Association. (2015). ATA 2015 guidelines for MTC. [online] Available from https://www.thyca.org/download/document/814/MTC%20Guidelines%20ATA%202015%20031316.pdf [Last accessed December, 2021].

8. Fox E, Widemann BC, Whitcomb PO, Aikin A, Dombi E, Lodish M, Stratakis CA, Steinberg S, Wells Jr SA, Balis FM. Phase I/II trial of vandetanib in children and adolescents with hereditary medullary thyroid carcinoma. Journal of Clinical Oncology. 2009;27(15):10014.

9. Kollars J, Zarroug AE, van Heerden J, Lteif A, Stavlo P, Suarez L, et al. Primary hyperparathyroidism in paediatric patients. Paediatrics. 2005;115(4):974-80.

10. Alagratnam S, Kurzawinski TR. Aetiology, diagnosis and surgical treatment of primary hyperparathyroidism in children: new trends. Hormo Res Paediatr. 2015;83:365-75.

11. Hamil J, Maoate K, Beasley SW, Corbett R, Evans J. Familial parathyroid carcinoma in a child. J Paediatr Child Health. 2002;38:314-7.

12. Goudet P, Dalac A, Le Bras M, Cardot-Bauters C, Niccoli P, Lévy-Bohbot N, et al. MEN1 disease occurring before 21 years old: 160-patient cohort study from the Groupe d'etudedes Tumeurs Endocrines. J Clin Endocrinol Metab. 2015;100:1568-77.

13. Crowne E, Brain CB, et al. Hyperparathyroidism and pituitary tumours in association with multiple endocrine neoplasia 1(MEN1) syndrome. In: Spoudeas HA (Ed). Paediatric Endocrine Tumours. A Multi-disciplinary Consensus Statement of Best Practice from a Working Group Convened under the Auspices of the BSPED and UKCCG. Crawley: Novo Nordisk; 2005. pp. 107-20.

14. Brandi ML, Gagel RF, Angeli A, Bilezikian JP, Beck-Peccoz P, Bordi C, et al. Guidelines for diagnosis and therapy of MEN type 1 and type 2. J Clin Endocrinol Metab. 2001;86(12):5658-71.

15. Moore K, Persaud T. The Developing Human, 8th edition. New York: WB Saunders; 2008.

16. Basuyau JP, Mallet E, Leroy M, Brunelle P. Reference intervals for serum calcitonin in men, women, and children. Clin Chem. 2004;50:1828-30.

17. Misseri R. Adrenal surgery in the pediatric population. Curr Urol Rep. 2007;8:89-94.

18. Avisse C, Marcus C, Patey M, Ladam-Marcus V, Delattre JF, Flament JB. Surgical anatomy and embryology of the adrenal glands. Surg Clin North Am. 2000;80(1):403-15.

19. Brunt L, Cohen M. Adrenalectomy—open and minimally invasive. In: Fisher J, Bland K (Eds). Mastery of Surgery, 5th edition. Philadelphia: Lippincott Williams & Wilkins; 2007.

20. Silverman M, Lee A. Anatomy and pathology of the adrenal glands. Urol Clin North Am. 1989;16: 417-32.

21. Molina P. Endocrine Physiology, 3rd edition. New York: McGraw Hill; 2010.

22. Havekes B, Romijn JA, Eisenhofer G, Adams K, Pacak K. Update on pediatric pheochromocytoma. Pediatr Nephrol. 2009;24(5):943-50.

23. Bausch B, Wellner U, Bausch D, Schiavi F, Barontini M, Sanso G, et al. Long-term prognosis of patients with pediatric pheochromocytoma. Endocr Relat Cancer. 2014;21(1):17-25.

24. Pham TH, Moir C, Thompson GB, Zarroug AE, Hamner CE, Farley D, et al. Pheochromocytoma and paraganglioma in children: a review of medical and surgical management at a tertiary care center. Pediatrics. 2006;118(3):1109-17.

25. Ciftci AO, Tanyel FC, Senocak ME, Büyükpamukçu N. Pheochromocytoma in children. J Pediatr Surg. 2001;36(3):447-52.

26. Barontini M, Levin G, Sanso G. Characteristics of pheochromocytoma in a 4- to 20-year-old population. Ann N Y Acad Sci. 2006;1073(1):30-7.

27. Reddy VS, O'Neill JA Jr, Holcomb GW III, Neblett WW III, Pietsch JB, Morgan WM III, et al. Twenty-five-year surgical experience with pheochromocytoma in children. Am Surg. 2000;66(12):1085-91; discussion 1092.

28. Lenders JW, Pacak K, Walther MM, Linehan WM, Mannelli M, Friberg P, et al. Biochemical diagnosis of pheochromocytoma: which test is best? JAMA. 2002;287(11):1427-34.

29. Eisenhofer G, Goldstein DS, Walther MM, Friberg P, Lenders JW, Keiser HR, et al. Biochemical diagnosis of pheochromocytoma: how to distinguish true- from false-positive test results. J Clin Endocrinol Metab. 2003;88(6):2656-66.

30. Zuber S, Wesley R, Prodanov T, Eisenhofer G, Pacak K, Kantorovich V. Clinical utility of chromogranin A in SDHx-related paragangliomas. Eur J Clin Invest. 2014;44(4): 365-71.

31. Lucon AM, Pereira MA, Mendonça BB, Halpern A, Wajchenberg BL, Arap S. Pheochromocytoma: study of 50 cases. J Urol. 1997;157(4):1208-12.

32. Abrams HL, Siegelman SS, Adams DF, Sanders R, Finberg HJ, Hessel SJ, et al. Computed tomography versus ultrasound of the adrenal gland: a prospective study. Radiology. 1982;143(1):121-8.

33. Pacak K, Linehan WM, Eisenhofer G, Walther MM, Goldstein DS. Recent advances in genetics, diagnosis, localization, and treatment of pheochromocytoma. Ann Intern Med. 2001;134(4):315-29.

34. Janssen I, Blanchet EM, Adams K, Chen CC, Millo CM, Herscovitch P, et al. Superiority of [68Ga]-DOTATATE PET/CT to other functional imaging modalities in the localization of SDHB-associated metastatic pheochromocytoma and paraganglioma. Clin Cancer Res. 2015;21(17):3888-95.

35. Archier A, Varoquaux A, Garrigue P, Montava M, Guerin C, Gabriel S, et al. Prospective comparison of 68Ga-DOTATATE and 18F-FDOPA PET/CT in patients with various pheochromocytomas and paragangliomas with emphasis on sporadic cases. Eur J Nucl Med Mol Imaging. 2016;43(7): 1248-57.

36. Agarwal R, Mishra SK, Bhatia E, Mishra A, Chand G, Agarwal G, et al. Prospective study to compare peri-operative hemodynamic alterations following preparation for pheochromocytoma surgery by phenoxybenzamine or prazosin. World J Surg. 2014;38(3):716-23.

37. Romero M, Kapur G, Baracco R, Valentini RP, Mattoo TK, Jain A. Treatment of hypertension in children with catecholamine-secreting tumors: a systematic approach. J Clin Hypertens (Greenwich). 2015;17(9):720-5.

38. Castilho LN, Castillo OA, Dénes FT, Mitre AI, Arap S. Laparoscopic adrenal surgery in children. J Urol. 2002;168(1):221-4.

39. Bravo EL, Tagle R. Pheochromocytoma: state-of-the-art and future prospects. Endocr Rev. 2003;24(4):539-53.

40. Brauckhoff M, Stock K, Stock S, Lorenz K, Sekulla C, Brauckhoff K, et al. Limitations of intraoperative adrenal remnant volume measurement in patients undergoing subtotal adrenalectomy. World J Surg. 2008;32(5): 863-72.

41. Prys-Roberts C, Farndon JR. Efficacy and safety of doxazosin for perioperative management of patients with pheochromocytoma. World J Surg. 2002;26(8):1037-42.

42. van Hulsteijn LT, Niemeijer ND, Dekkers OM, Corssmit EP. ^{131}I-MIBG therapy for malignant paraganglioma and phaeochromocytoma: systematic review and meta-analysis. Clin Endocrinol. 2014;80(4):487-501.

43. Asai S, Katabami T, Tsuiki M, Tanaka Y, Naruse M. Controlling tumor progression with cyclophosphamide, vincristine, and dacarbazine treatment improves survival in patients with metastatic and unresectable malignant pheochromocytomas/paragangliomas. Horm Cancer. 2017;8(2):108-18.

44. Fishbein L, Bonner L, Torigian DA, Nathanson KL, Cohen DL, Pryma D, et al. External beam radiation therapy (EBRT) for patients with malignant pheochromocytoma and non-head and neck paraganglioma: combination with (131)I-MIBG. Horm Metab Res. 2012;44(5):405-10.

45. Eisenhofer G, Lenders JW, Siegert G, Bornstein SR, Friberg P, Milosevic D, et al. Plasma methoxytyramine: a novel biomarker of metastatic pheochromocytoma and paraganglioma in relation to established risk factors of tumour size, location and SDHB mutation status. Eur J Cancer. 2012;48(11):1739-49.

46. Lehman EP. Adrenal neuroblastoma in infancy—15 year survival. Ann Surg. 1932;95:473.

47. Leikin S, Evans A, Heyn R, Newton W. The impact of chemotherapy on advanced neuroblastoma: survival of patients diagnosed in 1956, 1962 and 1966–68 in Children's Cancer Study Group A. J Pediatr. 1974;84:131-4.

48. Sieber WK, Dibbins AW, Wiener ES. In: Ravitch MM, Welch KJ, Benson CD, Aberdeen E, Randolph JG (Eds). Paediatric Surgery, 3rd edition. Chicago: Yearbook Medical Publishers Inc; 1979. Chapter 99, p. 1095.

49. Shimada H, Ambros IM, Dehner LP, Hata J, Joshi VV, Roald B. Terminology and morphologic criteria of neuroblastic tumours: recommendations by the International Neuroblastoma Pathology Committee. Cancer. 1999;86:349-63.

50. Peuchmar M, d'Amore ES, Joshi VV, Hata J-I. Revision of the international neuroblastoma pathology classification: confirmation of the favourable and unfavourable diagnostic subsets in ganglioneuroblastoma, nodular. Cancer. 2003;98:2274-81.

51. Sano H, Bonadio J, Gerbing RB, London WB, Matthay KK, Lukens JN, et al. International neuroblastoma pathology classification adds independent prognostic information beyond the prognostic contribution of age. Eur J Cancer. 2006;42:1113-9.

52. O'Neill JA, Littman P, Blitzer P, Soper K, Chatten J, Shimada H. The role of surgery in localised neuroblastoma. J Pediatr Surg. 1985;20:708-12.

53. Evans AE, D'Angio GJ, Randolph J. A proposed staging system for children with neuroblastoma. Cancer. 1971;27:374-8.

54. Breslow N, McCann B. Statistical estimation of prognosis for children with neuroblastoma. Cancer Res. 1971;31: 2098-103.

55. Brodeur GM, Seeger RC, Barrett A, Berthold F, Castleberry RP, D'Angio G, et al. International criteria for diagnosis, staging and response to treatment in patients with neuroblastoma. J Clin Oncol. 1988;6:1874-81.

56. Brodeur GM, Pritchard J, Berthold F, Carlsen NL, Castel V, Castelberry RP, et al. Revisions of the international criteria for neuroblastoma diagnosis, staging, and response to treatment. J Clin Oncol. 1993;11(8):1466-77.

57. Monclair T, Brodeur GM, Ambros PF, Brisse HJ, Cecchetto G, Holmes K, et al. The International Neuroblastoma Risk Group (INRG) staging system: an INRG task force report. J Clin Oncol. 2009;27:298-303.

58. Cecchetto G, Mosseri V, Bernardi B, Helardot P, Monclair T, Costa E, et al. Surgical risk factors in primary surgery for localised neuroblastoma: the LNESG1 study of the European International Society of Pediatric Oncology Neuroblastoma Group. J Clin Oncol. 2005;23:8483-9.

59. Brisse HJ, McCarville MB, Granata C, Krug KB, Wootton-Gorges SL, Kanegawa K, et al. Guidelines for imaging and staging of neuroblastic tumors: consensus report from the International Neuroblastoma Risk Group Project. Radiology. 2011;261:243-57.

60. De Bernardi B, Mosseri V, Rubie H, Castel V, Foot A, Ladenstein R, et al. Treatment of localised resectable neuroblastoma. Results of the LNESG1 study by the SIOP Europe Neuroblastoma Group. Br J Cancer. 2008;99:1027-33.

61. Yu AL, Gilman AL, Ozkaynak MF, London WB, Kreissman SG, Chen HX, et al. Anti-GD2 antibody with GM-CSF, interleukin-2 and isotretinoin for neuroblastoma. N Eng J Med. 2010;363:1324-34.

62. Schleiermacher G, Rubie H, Hartmann O, Bergeron C, Chastagner P, Medinaud F, et al. Treatment of stage 4s neuroblastoma—report of 10 years' experience of French Society of Paediatric Oncology (SFOP). Br J Cancer. 2003;89:470-6.

63. McAteer JP, Huaco JA, Gow KW. Predictors of survival in pediatric adrenocortical carcinoma: a Surveillance, Epidemiology, and End Results (SEER) program study. J Pediatr Surg. 2013;48(5):1025-31.

64. Wieneke JA, Thompson LD, Heffess CS. Adrenal cortical neoplasms in the pediatric population: a clinicopathologic and immunophenotypic analysis of 83 patients. Am J Surg Pathol. 2003;27(7):867-81.

65. Kepes JJ, O'Boynick P, Jones S, Baum D, McMillan J, Adams ME. Adrenal cortical adenoma in the spinal canal of an 8-year-old girl. Am J Surg Pathol. 1990;14(5):481-4.

66. Medeiros LJ, Anasti J, Gardner KL, Pass HI, Nieman LK. Virilizing adrenal cortical neoplasm arising ectopically in the thorax. J Clin Endocrinol Metabol. 1992;75(6):1522-5.

67. Agrons GA, Lonergan GJ, Dickey GE, Perez-Monte JE. Adrenocortical neoplasms in children: radiologic-pathologic correlation. Radiographics. 1999;19(4):989-1008.

68. Weiss LM, Medeiros LJ, Vickery AL Jr. Pathologic features of prognostic significance in adrenocortical carcinoma. Am J Surg Pathol. 1989;13(3):202-6.

69. Ciftci AO, Senocak ME, Tanyel FC, Buyukpamukcu N. Adrenocortical tumors in children. J Pediatr Surg. 2001;36(4): 549-54.

70. Sandrini R, Ribeiro RC, DeLacerda L. Childhood adrenocortical tumors. J Clin Endocrinol Metabol. 1997;82(7):2027-31.

71. Michalkiewicz E, Sandrini R, Figueiredo B, Miranda ECM, Caran E, Oliveira-Filho AG, et al. Clinical and outcome characteristics of children with adrenocortical tumors: a report from the International Pediatric Adrenocortical Tumor Registry. J Clin Oncol. 2004;22(5):838-45.

72. Stojadinovic A, Ghossein RA, Hoos A, Nissan A, Marshall D, Dudas M, et al. Adrenocortical carcinoma: clinical, morphologic, and molecular characterization. J Clin Oncol. 2002;20(4):941-50.

73. Dehner LP. Pediatric adrenocortical neoplasms: on the road to some clarity. Am J Surg Pathol. 2003;27 (7):1005-7.

74. Jaksic T, Yaman M, Thorner P, Wesson DK, Filler RM, Shandling B. A 20-year review of pediatric pancreatic tumors. J Pediatr Surg. 1992;27 (10):1315-7.

75. Trump D, Farren B, Wooding C, Pang JT, Besser GM, Buchanan KD, et al. Clinical studies of multiple endocrine neoplasia type 1 (MEN1). QJM. 1996;89(9):653-69.

76. Jensen RT, Berna MJ, Bingham DB, Norton JA. Inherited pancreatic endocrine tumour syndromes: advances in molecular pathogenesis, diagnosis, management, and controversies. Cancer. 2008;113(7 suppl):1807-43.

77. Lodish MB, Stratakis CA. Endocrine tumours in neurofibromatosis type 1, tuberous sclerosis, and related syndromes. Best Pract Res Clin Endocrinol Metab. 2010;24(3):439-49.

78. Sobin LH, Gospodarowicz MK, Wittekind C (Eds). TNM Classification of Malignant Tumours. Oxford: Wiley-Blackwell; 2009.

79. Jiao Y, Shi C, Edil BH, de Wilde RF, Klimstra DS, Maitra A, et al. DAXX/ATRX, MEN1, and mTOR pathway genes are frequently altered in pancreatic neuroendocrine tumours. Science. 2011;331(6021):1199-203.

80. Kloppel G. Classification and pathology of gastroenteropancreatic neuroendocrine neoplasms. Endocr Relat Cancer. 2011;18:S1-16.

81. Sokmensuer C, Gedikoglu G, Uzunalimoglu B. Importance of proliferation markers in gastrointestinal carcinoid tumours: a clinicopathologic study. Hepatogastroenterology. 2001;48: 720-3.

82. Bosman FT, Carneiro F, Hruban RH, Theise ND. WHO classification of tumours of the digestive system. Lyon: IARC; 2010.

83. Rindi G, Falconi M, Klersy C, Albarello L, Boninsegna L, Buchler MW, et al. TNM staging of neoplasms of the endocrine pancreas: results from a large international cohort study. J Natl Cancer Inst. 2012;104(10):764-77.

84. Falconi M, Eriksson B, Kaltas G, Bartsch DK, Capdevilla J, Caplin M, et al. ENETS consensus guidelines update for the management of patients with functional pancreatic neuroendocrine tumors and non-functional pancreatic neuroendocrine tumors. Neuroendocrinology. 2016;103(2):153-71.

85. Pipeleers-Marichal M, Somers G, Willems G, Foulis A, Imrie C, Bishop AE, et al. Gastrinomas in the duodenums of patients with multiple endocrine neoplasia type 1 and the Zollinger-Ellison syndrome. N Engl J Med. 1990;322(11):723-7.

86. Ramage JK, Ahmed A, Ardill J, Bax N, Breen DJ, Caplin ME, et al. Guidelines for the management of gastroenteropancreatic neuroendocrine (including carcinoid) tumors (NETs). Gut. 2012;61:6-32.

87. Kimura W, Kurodan A, Morioka Y. Clinical pathology of endocrine tumors of the pancreas. Analysis of autopsy cases. Dig Dis Sci. 1991;36(7):933-42.

88. Eriksson B, Annibale B, Bajetta E, Mitry E, Pavel M, Platania M, et al. ENETS consensus guidelines for the standards of care in neuroendocrine tumors: chemotherapy in patients with neuroendocrine tumors. Neuroendocrinology. 2009;90(2): 214-9.

89. Maroun J, Koch W, Kvols L, Bjarnason G, Chen E, Germond C, et al. Guidelines for the diagnosis and management of carcinoid tumours. Part 1: the gastrointestinal tract. A statement from a Canadian national carcinoid expert group. Curr Oncol. 2006;13(2):67-76.

90. Thakker RV, Newey PJ, Walls GV, Bilezikian J, Dralle H, Ebeling PR, et al. Clinical practice guidelines for multiple endocrine neoplasia type 1 (MEN1). J Clin Endocrinol Metab. 2012;97(9): 2990-3011.

91. Raymond E, Dahan L, Raoul JL, Bang YJ, Borbath I, Lombard-Bohas C, et al. Sunitinib malate for the treatment of pancreatic neuroendocrine tumors. N Engl J Med. 2011;364(6):501-13.

92. Yao JC, Shah MH, Ito T, Bohas CL, Wolin EM, Van Cutsem E, et al. Everolimus for advanced pancreatic neuroendocrine tumors. N Engl J Med. 2011;364 (6):514-23.

93. Caplin ME, Pavel M, Ćwikła JB, Phan AT, Raderer M, Sedláčková E, et al. Lanreotide in metastatic enteropancreatic neuroendocrine tumors. N Engl J Med. 2014;371(3):224-33.

94. Allan B, David J, Perez E, Lew J, Sola J. Malignant neuroendocrine tumors: incidence and outcomes in paediatric patients. Eur J Paediatr Surg. 2013;23:394-9.

95. Pape UF, Jann H, Muller-Nordhorn J, Bockelbrink A, Berndt U, Willich SN, et al. Prognostic relevance of a novel TNM classification system for upper gastroenteropancreatic neuroendocrine tumors. Cancer. 2008;113:256-65.

96. Menni F, de Lonlay P, Sevin C, Touati G, Peigne C, Barbier V, et al. Neurologic outcomes of 90 neonates and infants with persistent hyperinsulinemic hypoglycemia. Pediatrics. 2001;107:476-9.

97. Aynsley-Green A, Hussain K, Hall J, Saudubray JM, Nihoul-Fékété C, De Lonlay-Debeney P, et al. The practical management of hyperinsulinism in infancy. Arch Dis Child Fetal Neonatal Ed. 2000;82:F98-107.

98. Hussain K, Nah SA, Pierro A. Congenital hyperinsulinism. In: Ledbetter DJ, Johnson PRV (Eds.). Endocrine Surgery in Children. Berlin: Springer; 2018. pp. 161-72.

99. Thomas P, Ye Y, Lightner E. Mutation of the pancreatic islet inward rectifier Kir6.2 also leads to familial persistent hyperinsulinemic hypoglycemia of infancy. Hum Mol Genet. 1996;5:1813-22.

100. Thomas PM, Cote GJ, Wohllk N, Haddad B, Mathew PM, Rabl W, et al. Mutations in the sulfonylurea receptor gene in familial persistent hyperinsulinemic hypoglycemia of infancy. Science. 1995;268(5209):426-9.

101. Dunne MJ, Kane C, Shepherd RM, Sanchez JA, James RF, Johnson PR, et al. Familial persistent hyperinsulinemic hypoglycemia of infancy and mutations in the sulfonylurea receptor. N Engl J Med. 1997;336:703-6.

102. Sempoux C, Guiot Y, Jaubert F, Rahier J. Focal and diffuse forms of congenital hyperinsulinism: the keys for differential diagnosis. Endocr Pathol. 2004;15(3):241-6.

103. Sempoux C, Guiot Y, Dahan K, Moulin P, Stevens M, Lambot V, et al. The focal form of persistent hyperinsulinemic hypoglycemia of infancy: morphological and molecular studies show structural and functional differences with insulinoma. Diabetes. 2003;52(3):784-94.

104. Fékété CN, de Lonlay P, Jaubert F, Rahier J, Brunelle F, Saudubray JM. The surgical management of congenital hyperinsulinemic hypoglycemia in infancy. J Pediatr Surg. 2004;39(3):267-9.

105. Rahier J, Sempoux C, Fournet JC, Poggi F, Brunelle F, Nihoul-Fekete C, et al. Partial or near-total pancreatectomy for persistent neonatal hyperinsulinaemic hypoglycaemia: the pathologist's role. Histopathology. 1998;32(1):15-9.

106. Gussinyer M, Clemente M, Cebrián R, Yeste D, Albisu M, Carrascosa A. Glucose intolerance and diabetes are observed in the long-term follow-up of nonpancreatectomized patients with persistent hyperinsulinemic hypoglycemia of infancy due to mutations in the *ABCC8* gene. Diabetes Care. 2008;31(6):1257-9.

107. Barthlen W, Blankenstein O, Mau H, Koch M, Höhne C, Mohnike W, et al. Evaluation of (18F)FDOPA PET-CT for surgery in focal congenital hyperinsulinism. J Clin Endocrinol Metab. 2008;93(3):869-75.

108. Zani A, Nah SA, Ron O, Totonelli G, Ismail D, Smith VV, et al. The predictive value of preoperative [18]Fluoro-L-DOPA-PET-CT scans in children with congenital hyperinsulinism of infancy. J Pediatr Surg. 2011. 2010;46(1):204-8.

Anish JC, MJ Paul

◇ ANATOMY AND PHYSIOLOGY OF THE ISLET OF LANGERHANS

The pancreas is a retroperitoneal organ that has a mixed exocrine and endocrine functions. The exocrine pancreas constitutes the bulk of the parenchyma. Interspersed among the acinar cells of the exocrine pancreas are the islets of Langerhans. The islets are arranged in clusters throughout the exocrine pancreas and are composed of four different cell types **(Table 1)**.

The islets of the pancreas comprise only about 2% of the pancreatic mass. Beta cells account for the majority (70%) of islet cells and are located in the center of the islets. These cells secrete insulin, a hormone that promotes storage of glucose thereby helping to conserve energy. The alpha, delta, and clear cells are located around the beta cells in the periphery of the islets. A few delta cells are also located centrally. Glucagon secreted by the alpha cells is responsible for the production of glucose resulting in increased levels in the bloodstream, thereby aiding in energy release. Therefore, the endocrine pancreas secretes hormones into the blood that aid in carbohydrate homeostasis to facilitate energy utilization and conservation.

Beta Cells and Insulin Secretion

Insulin is derived from chromosome 11 in the nucleus of the beta cells. It comprises two polypeptide chains and is composed of 56 amino acid sequences, the chains being connected by two disulfide bridges and a connecting peptide. Once formed, it is transported to the endoplasmic reticulum where the signal peptide is cleaved to form the precursor molecule—proinsulin. Proinsulin is transported to the Golgi apparatus where, in the secretory granules, the middle connecting portion, the C-peptide, is cleaved to release insulin. Insulin and C-peptide are secreted in equimolar amounts into the bloodstream through exocytosis.[1] The half-life of insulin is 4–6 minutes whereas the half-life of C-peptide is 11–14 minutes.[2] Insulin is rapidly destroyed in the liver while C-peptide is excreted by the kidneys.

◇ INCIDENCE AND DEMOGRAPHICS

Insulinomas are rare neuroendocrine tumors arising from the β-cells of the pancreas. They are the most common functioning neuroendocrine tumors of the pancreas. The reported annual incidence is approximately 1–4 people per million in the general population.[3] They commonly occur in the fifth decade of life with a slight female (60%) preponderance.[3,4] They may be either sporadic or hereditary. Hereditary forms (4–10%) are those that are associated with the multiple endocrine neoplasia type 1 (MEN1) syndrome.[5] Unlike the sporadic insulinomas, which are typically solitary lesions, hereditary forms present much earlier and are associated with multiple tumors. Malignancy is rare accounting for <10% of all insulinomas.

◇ ETIOLOGY

Insulinoma may occur sporadically or in association with MEN1 syndrome. Mutations in the *MEN1* gene located on chromosome 11q13 result in MEN1 syndrome, which is an autosomal dominant disorder. The presence of MEN1 germline mutations along with loss of heterozygosity at 11q13 is observed in patients with MEN1 syndrome.[6,7] This phenomenon has suggested a role of MEN1 as a tumor suppressor gene, requiring inactivation of alleles for both clonal expansion and tumor development. In addition, sporadic pancreatic insulinomas have also expressed somatic mutations and loss of heterozygosity of the MEN1 alleles, demonstrating that the *MEN1* gene may play the same role in nonhereditary endocrine tumors.[6-9] Very rarely, insulinomas may develop in patients with tuberous sclerosis and neurofibromatosis type 1.[10]

Table 1: Islet cell types.		
Cell type	Substance produced	Percentage of all islet cells (%)
Alpha cells	Glucagon	20
Beta cells	Insulin	70
Delta cells	Somatostatin, gastrin, and pancreatic polypeptide	5–10
Clear cells	Unknown	<5

A 63-year-old gentleman presented with recurrent episodes of tiredness, giddiness, and weakness over the past 1 year. These episodes occurred mostly following a morning walk. He had recorded his blood sugars during these episodes and it was found to be between 60 and 70 mg%. To avoid these symptoms, he started taking snacks early morning before his walk and every 3–4 hours during the day. He has noticed a gain of 6 kg of weight over the past 1 year. 1 month ago, he forgot to take a snack and ventured on his morning walk and thus suffered a transient loss of consciousness. He was subsequently admitted for evaluation of his symptoms. The evaluation and management of this patient will be detailed in the appropriate sections of this chapter.

CLINICAL FEATURES

Glucose Homeostasis

The control of insulin secretion from the beta cells of the pancreas in normal individuals is controlled by the blood glucose levels. Insulin is secreted from the pancreas as the blood glucose levels rise while its secretion is decreased as blood glucose levels fall.

Physiological Response to Hypoglycemia

As the brain cannot synthesize or store glucose, maintenance of brain function requires a continuous supply of glucose from the circulation. Therefore, the plasma glucose levels have to be maintained within the physiological range because blood to brain glucose transport is a direct function of the arterial plasma glucose concentration. The major source of glucose to the body is from the diet. Between meals and during a fast, the plasma glucose levels are maintained by:
- Breakdown of glycogen from the hepatic stores
- Gluconeogenesis

The normal physiological responses to counter a fall in blood glucose levels include:
1. Decrease in insulin secretion when the blood glucose levels fall to <80 mg/dL

   As the glucose levels reach the hypoglycemic range (<70 mg/dL), counterregulatory hormones are released.
2. *Glucagon*: This is the first and most important hormone to be released, which helps to increase glycogenolysis and gluconeogenesis.
3. *Epinephrine*: When glucagon is insufficient, epinephrine is released to promote gluconeogenesis and in addition, it limits glucose utilization in the peripheral tissue by sensitizing insulin.
4. *Growth hormone and cortisol*: With prolonged hypoglycemia, these hormones are released to further decrease glucose utilization and support its production.

   If plasma glucose levels continue to fall despite the above mechanisms which are typically seen in patients with insulinomas, they will start to develop clinical symptoms.

Symptoms and Signs

Symptoms of insulinoma can be broadly classified into two categories:

Table 2: Symptoms and signs of insulinoma.

Neuroglycopenic	Adrenergic/autonomic
Apathy	Palpitation
Dizziness	Chest pain
Clouded sensorium	Dry mouth
Behavioral disturbance	Tremor
Blurred vision/diplopia	Warmth
Seizure	Sweating
Focal neurological deficit	Tachycardia
Coma	Hunger
	Nausea and vomiting

1. Neuroglycopenic
2. Adrenergic/autonomous (the result of sympathoadrenal discharge in response to hypoglycemia)

As glucose is an obligate fuel for the brain, deprivation of plasma glucose (levels <50 mg/dL) will affect the brain leading to neuroglycopenic symptoms. In addition, the sympathoadrenal discharge in response to the fall in plasma glucose (<60 mg/dL) manifests as the autonomic symptoms **(Table 2)**. Among the symptoms, the neuroglycopenic symptoms are the most frequent.

The symptoms classically present after an episode of fasting or exercise and hence are commonly seen in the morning before breakfast and late afternoon. With time, patients find that they can prevent these symptoms by eating more frequent meals which result in weight gain. Therefore, these patients are generally obese.

In the majority of patients, there is a delay in diagnosis which may be several months to even years. This diagnostic delay has been attributed to the nonspecific nature, variability, and severity of the clinical presentation and also to the lack of awareness of the physician—insulinoma being a very rare entity.

DIFFERENTIAL DIAGNOSIS

The causes of hypoglycemia are listed in **Box 1**. The most common cause of hypoglycemia is related to drug intake. Critically ill patients are also prone to hypoglycemia. Therefore, a detailed history, especially the medications taken by the patient, would help to exclude these causes for hypoglycemia. In addition, a careful, detailed history would also exclude accidental or surreptitious causes for hypoglycemia.

Large mesenchymal tumors [synovial sarcomas, myxoid liposarcomas, malignant peripheral nerve sheath tumors, chondrosarcomas, Ewing's sarcoma, and gastrointestinal stromal tumors (GISTs)] account for the nonislet cell tumors that cause hypoglycemia due to the overproduction of incompletely processed insulin-like growth factor 2 (IGF-2) or IGF-1.[11,12]

Box 1: Causes of hypoglycemia.

Drugs:
- Insulin or insulin secretagogue
- Alcohol

Critical illness:
- Hepatic, renal, or cardiac failure
- Sepsis

Hormone deficiency:
- Cortisol
- Glucagon
- Epinephrine

Non-islet cell tumors
- Synovial sarcoma
- Myxoid liposarcoma
- Malignant peripheral nerve sheath tumors
- Chondrosarcomas
- Ewing's sarcoma
- GIST

Endogenous hyperinsulinism:
- Insulinoma
- *Functioning β-cell disorders:*
  - Noninsulinoma pancreatogenous hypoglycemia syndrome (NIPHS)
  - Postgastric bypass hypoglycemia
- Insulin autoimmune hypoglycemia
- Antibody to insulin
- Antibody to insulin receptor

Congenital deficiencies of enzymes of carbohydrate metabolism:
- Glycogen storage disorders
- Hereditary fructose intolerance

Accidental or surreptitious

Nesidioblastosis, in which there is diffuse hypertrophy and sometimes hyperplasia of the pancreatic islets cells resulting in the noninsulinoma pancreatogenous hypoglycemia syndrome (NIPHS), presents with hypoglycemia typically 2–4 hours after a meal.[13-15] A similar postprandial hypoglycemia due to nesidioblastosis may be witnessed in patients following a Roux-en-Y gastric bypass for obesity.[16-18]

People with a history of autoimmune disorders may develop antibodies to native insulin. In these patients, the insulin bound to the circulating antibodies dissociates from the antibody in an unregulated manner following a meal. Thus, symptomatic hypoglycemia is witnessed in the late postprandial period. Though a rare entity, very high insulin levels during hypoglycemia should alert the physician to this cause.[19]

◇| INVESTIGATIONS

As depicted above, hypoglycemia can result from a multitude of causes. Unless the evaluation is directed to patients with the highest probability of having an insulinoma, patients may be exposed to unnecessary evaluation, cost, and potential harm. Therefore, the American Endocrinology Society recommends evaluation of adult hypoglycemic disorders only in patients with documented Whipple's triad.[19]

The evaluation for most endocrine disorders follows two basic principles:
1. Confirmation of the diagnosis by biochemical testing
2. Localization of the lesion with imaging

Patients suspected to have an insulinoma on clinical evaluation are subjected to a similar evaluation process.

◇| CONFIRMATION OF THE DIAGNOSIS

The diagnosis of an insulinoma requires the demonstration of clinical/laboratory evidence of hypoglycemia combined with an inappropriate elevation of insulin. In addition, other causes for hypoglycemia need to be excluded.

Whipple's Triad

Historically, in the 1930s, it was discovered that hypoglycemic symptoms were due to increased production of insulin. Some of these patients were cured of their symptoms following surgery to the pancreas whereas others were not. Biochemical tests were rudimentary and imaging was nonexistent; hence, a diagnosis of insulinoma had to be made on clinical judgment. Allen O Whipple in 1938 proposed a clinical criterion for the diagnosis of insulinoma to avoid unnecessary operations on the pancreas.[20] These criteria include:
- Symptoms and signs of hypoglycemia occur during a period of fasting.
- Blood sugar level ≤45 mg/dL at the time of symptoms
- Symptoms recover following the administration of oral/intravenous glucose.

Prolonged Fasting (72-Hour Fast) Test

In practice, a spontaneous hypoglycemic episode is unlikely to be observed. Therefore, to confirm the diagnosis, one must recreate the circumstances in which symptomatic hypoglycemia is likely to occur. Therein, the prolonged fasting test was formulated. It is performed to document an episode of fasting hypoglycemia associated with an inappropriately elevated insulin and thus confirms a diagnosis of insulinoma. Currently, this is considered the gold standard test for establishing the diagnosis of an insulinoma.

The patient is admitted and an intravenous access is started. Initially, blood samples are collected for the estimation of glucose, insulin, and C-peptide levels. The patient then begins to fast (all food and fluids containing calories are withheld) and blood glucose levels are monitored every 6 hours until the glucose drops to 60 mg/dL or the patient develops hypoglycemic symptoms following which the frequency of testing is increased to every 1–2 hours. Simultaneous insulin and C-peptide levels are estimated along with blood glucose at this time. The fast is concluded when the blood glucose levels fall to 40 mg/dL or less. At this time, blood is drawn for insulin, proinsulin, C-peptide, β-hydroxybutyrate, and sulfonylurea.

It has been observed that hypoglycemic symptoms occur in 33% of patients within 12 hours, in 80% within 24 hours, in 90–95% within 48 hours, and in 98–100% by 72 hours.[21] Hence, majority of patients would be able to discontinue the test by 48 hours.

◇| INTERPRETATION

Plasma Blood Glucose

In healthy individuals, symptoms of hypoglycemia develop when plasma glucose levels fall to <55 mg/dL. However, this glycemic threshold shifts to a lower plasma glucose concentration in patients with recurrent hypoglycemia. Therefore, documented blood glucose levels ≤45 mg/dL during fasting would indicate the presence of hypoglycemia.

Plasma Insulin Levels

Plasma insulin levels ≥6 µU/mL by radioimmunoassay or ≥3 µU/mL by immunometric assay when plasma glucose is <45 mg/dL are suggestive of an excess of insulin.

C-Peptide Levels

Insulin and C-peptide are released together in equal amounts from the secretory granules. Exogenously administered insulin does not contain C-peptide. Therefore, measuring the C-peptide levels helps to distinguish endogenous from exogenous hyperinsulinemia. A plasma C-peptide value of ≥0.6 ng/mL in the presence of hyperinsulinemia is indicative of an endogenous cause.

Proinsulin Levels

In a normal individual, circulating proinsulin levels are <20% of the total immunoreactive insulin. In patients with an insulinoma, proinsulin levels are elevated. A proinsulin value ≥5 pmol/L is indicative of an insulinoma.

β-Hydroxybutyrate Levels

β-hydroxybutyrate is a ketone body. Insulin is an antiketogenic agent, hence β-hydroxybutyrate levels are very low (≤2.7 mmol/L) in patients with insulinoma.

Sulfonylurea

A number of recent oral hypoglycemic agents (sulfonylureas) release insulin and C-peptides from the pancreas resulting in hypoglycemia. These may be taken in excess surreptitiously. Therefore, one must rule this out by screening for sulfonylureas prior to diagnosing a patient with an insulinoma.

Plasma Insulin–Glucose Ratio

In patients with an insulinoma, despite the fall in blood glucose levels, the insulin levels remain high. Therefore, it is speculated that the ratio of insulin:glucose (I:G) may aid in the diagnosis of an insulinoma. A ratio of <0.4 is observed in normal individuals, whereas in patients with an insulinoma, this ratio is ≥1. Though this test has not found favor in many institutions, some centers still endorse this criterion for the diagnosis of an insulinoma. A recent study by Ahn et al. has depicted >90% sensitivity and specificity for this test in diagnosing insulinoma.[22]

◇| LOCALIZATION

Virtually, all insulinomas are found within the pancreas. They are small tumors, approximately 82% being <2 cm, while 47% are <1 cm.[23] Therefore, localization of these lesions within the pancreas can be challenging. It has been estimated that approximately 10–27% of lesions may not be detected following extensive preoperative imaging.[24,25] In addition, some centers have documented intraoperative identification of lesions previously not visualized on imaging. In view of the above, some researchers have questioned the role of preoperative localization studies.[26,27] However, preoperative imaging for localization is considered essential for several reasons:

- It distinguishes between a solitary lesion and multiple pancreatic lesions.
- It enables planning the appropriate surgery—enucleation versus resection.
- It aids in determining the surgical approach—laparoscopic versus open approach.
- Awareness of the location of the lesion helps the surgeon in preventing injury to major vascular structures.
- It shortens the operating time as the surgical approach can be focused and thereby reduces the associated morbidity.
- Metastatic disease may also be detected.

Further, approximately 10% of insulinomas are not detected on intraoperative evaluation. Therefore, following documentation of hyperinsulinemic hypoglycemia, preoperative localization is recommended.[23,28] Localization techniques may be either noninvasive or invasive.

Noninvasive Localization

Transabdominal Ultrasonography

Insulinomas appear as a small hypoechoic solid mass on ultrasonogram (USG). Though this modality is readily available, safe, noninvasive, inexpensive, and rapid, it has a poor detection rate with reports ranging from 9 to 66%.[5,10,24,29] Factors limiting the detection rate include the small tumor size, interference from bowel gas and other intra-abdominal organs, patient obesity, operator dependence, and location of the lesion in the pancreas.

Computed Tomography

The reported sensitivity of a conventional CT scan is 30–70%.[5,24,25,30] The advent of helical CT and, more recently, the multidetector CT (MDCT) has revolutionized preoperative imaging, as they have overcome the limitations of conventional CT. The faster imaging capability of the advanced CT enables biphasic imaging of the pancreas in the arterial phase and portal venous phase, using thin sections, thus greatly increasing the detection rates of these lesions.

The enhanced scan acquisition speed and high spatial resolution due to thin collimation in the MDCT enable precise imaging as well as the ability to reconstruct images in multiple planes, enhancing lesion detection and its relationship to vital structures, thereby facilitating preoperative planning. This is due to the fact that MDCT enables multiple slices to be imaged at the same time depending on the number of detectors present. Hence, the scan acquisition time of one region can be greatly shortened by enabling multiphase imaging, or the same area scanned using thinner sections which allows higher spatial resolution. These recent modalities have increased the detection rate of insulinomas to >90%.[31,32]

Majority of insulinomas are isodense with the pancreas on precontrast images and become hypervascular on arterial phase images **(Figs. 1A and B)**. Occasionally, these lesions may be better detected on portal venous phase images and rarely may have calcifications. Lesions that are pedunculated, hypovascular, or are adjacent to major vessels may lead to false-negative results.[33]

Thus, in view of the above reasons and in addition, as helical CT and MDCT are safe, simple, widely available, have the ability to delineate relationship of the lesion to surrounding structures, and can identify metastasis, this modality has become the first-line imaging in the preoperative localization of insulinomas.

Magnetic Resonance Imaging

Magnetic resonance imaging (MRI) may be used to confirm lesions identified on the CT or to localize lesions missed on CT. Improved accuracy of detecting insulinoma has been reported when both modalities are used.[30] In addition, MRI is useful in delineating the relationship of the insulinoma with the main pancreatic duct as well as the detection of hepatic metastasis. Hence, its role is complementary to CT.

Insulinomas appear hypointense on T1-weighted images and hyperintense on T2-weighted images **(Figs. 2A and B)**. Lesions containing abundant fibrous tissue may show low-signal intensity in both T1- and T2-weighted sequences.[10,34] The availability, cost, and operator dependence are limitations to its use. In addition, the size of the lesion affects detection rates by both CT and MRI. >70% of lesions ≥3 cm are detected whereas <50% of lesions <1 cm may be detected.[28]

Invasive Methods for Localization

Invasive modalities, such as endoscopic ultrasound (EUS) and arteriography, have been shown to be highly accurate in the preoperative localization of insulinomas. They have frequently been shown to be superior to noninvasive localization techniques.

Endoscopic Ultrasound

The transabdominal USG for detection and evaluation of disorders of the gastrointestinal lumen and pancreas was impeded by a low-resolution secondary to the intervening gas and bone. This led to the development of the endoscopic ultrasound, the underlying hypothesis being that EUS could simultaneously visualize the gastrointestinal lumen and accomplish high-resolution scans of adjacent structures such as the pancreas.

Endoscopic ultrasound is currently the investigation of choice in many developed countries with sensitivity of 80–100% being reported in expert hands.[10,19,22,28,31] The appearance of an insulinoma on EUS is quite characteristic, with most

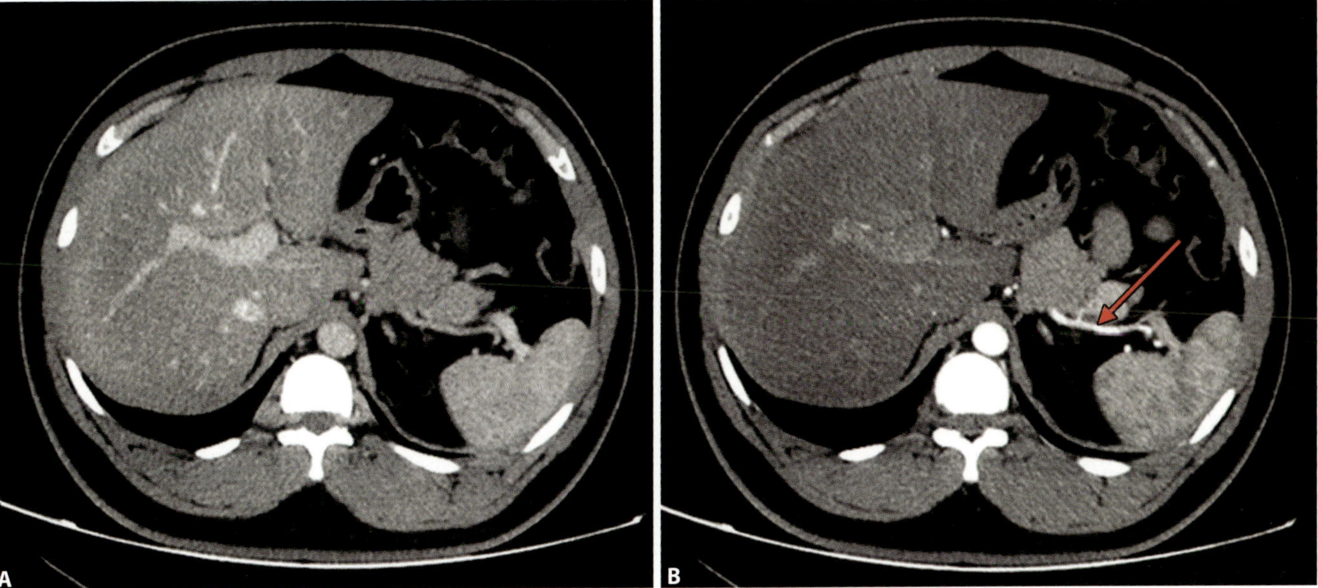

Figs. 1A and B: (A) Depicting an isodense lesion on the superior margin of the tail of the pancreas in the venous phase which becomes hyperdense on arterial phase—arrow pointing to the lesion (B).

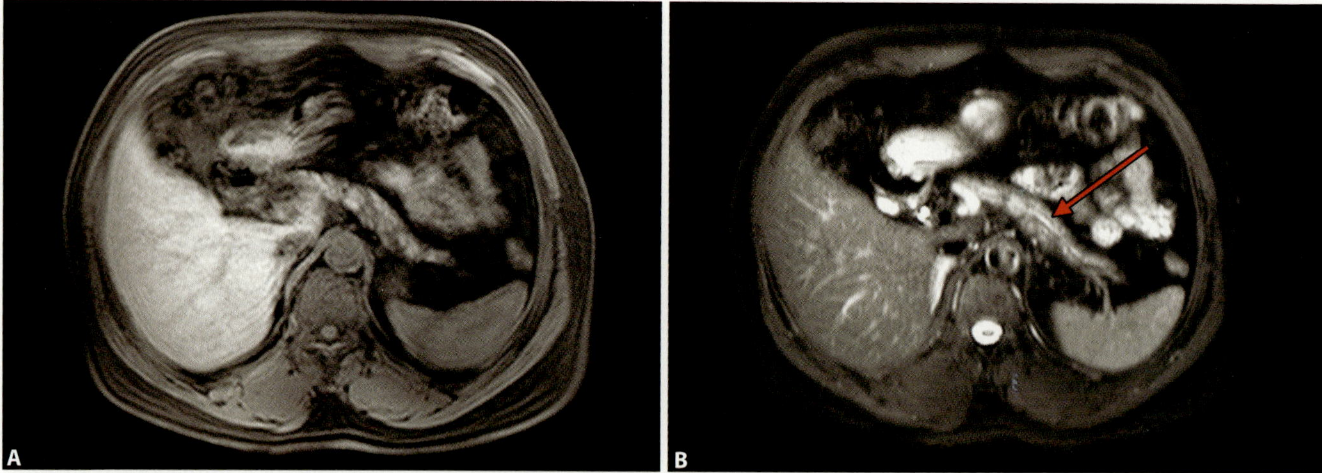

Figs. 2A and B: (A) An isointense lesion in the body of the pancreas in the T2-weighted image which becomes hyperintense on SPAIR (Spectral Adiabatic Inversion Recovery)—arrow pointing to the lesion (B).

tumors homogeneously hypoechoic and rounded in shape with distinct margins **(Fig. 3)**. This modality can detect other lesions within the pancreas if present as well as delineate the relationship of the lesion with the main pancreatic duct and surrounding vessels. In addition, EUS offers the advantage of performing a guided fine-needle aspiration cytology (FNAC) from the lesion, if required.

Although EUS is a highly reliable procedure for the preoperative localization of insulinomas, there are several problems associated with the detection of these tumors using EUS: (1) EUS is an invasive procedure which requires sedation. (2) It is highly dependent on the experience of the user; (3) Some insulinomas are missed by preoperative EUS because they are completely isoechoic. A low body mass index, female gender, and young age may be risk factors for negative imaging; (4) Pancreatic nodularities may be mistaken for insulinomas resulting in a false-positive image; (5) The sensitivity of EUS for insulinomas depends on the location and size of the tumor; sensitivity is greatest for tumors in the head of the pancreas and lowest for those in the tail of the pancreas.[10,24]

Arteriography/Angiography

Insulinomas are highly vascular tumors and produce a characteristic blush on angiography. This feature has prompted clinicians to use angiography for localization of insulinoma. Sensitivity of up to 80% has been reported with this modality.[35] As with other invasive procedures, the results depend upon the experience of the radiologist.

Arterial Stimulation Venous Sampling and Percutaneous Transhepatic Portal Venous Sampling

These two invasive techniques regionalize the insulinoma to a specific part of the pancreas but cannot localize the lesion to a specific site. Percutaneous cannulation of the portal vein through the liver carries its own morbidity and hence percutaneous transhepatic portal venous sampling (PTPVS)

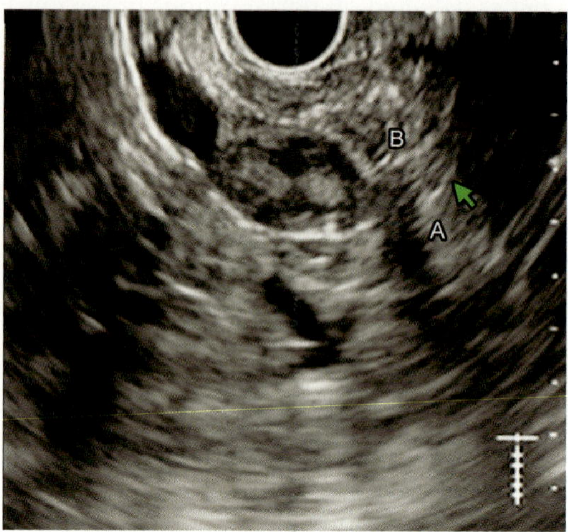

Fig. 3: Depicting a hypoechoic lesion in the tail of the pancreas (A) and its relationship with the splenic vein (B).

is rarely used at present. Arterial stimulation venous sampling (ASVS) relies on the fact that calcium is a potent stimulant for the release of insulin, thereby regionalizing the tumor by verifying hormonal function. ASVS is a potent method for localization of atypical insulinomas as well as those not localized by other noninvasive techniques. The accuracy of ASVS in localizing insulinomas has been reported to range from 94 to 100%.[24]

Somatostatin Receptor Scintigraphy

Nuclear imaging with somatostatin receptor scintigraphy (SRS) is based on the fact that all endocrine tumors contain somatostatin receptors. However, insulinomas contain a low density of somatostatin receptors, expressing the somatostatin subtypes-2 and -5 in only 50% of the tumors. This has resulted in the reported low sensitivity of SRS for localization of insulinomas (20–50%), limiting its role in the localization of lesions.[10,19,23,30] However, in patients with a malignant insulinoma with systemic metastasis, a positive SRS would aid in therapy.

Recently, several studies have demonstrated that when ^{68}Ga-labeled somatostatin analog positron emission tomography (PET) is combined with CT, sensitivity for detecting a neuroendocrine tumor is higher than with SRS alone.[23,36,37] Thus, ^{68}Ga-DOTA-TATE PET/CT may be used in patients with negative radiologic localization studies or as an alternative to invasive methods.

[11]C-Methionine PET

As essential amino acids are crucial for protein synthesis and tumor growth, methionine accumulates in tumors via the L-type amino acid transporter 1 (LAT1). This property was the basis for ^{11}C-methionine PET scan. However, high ^{11}C-methionine uptake is seen in normal pancreas as well resulting in the limited utility of this scan in locating the pancreatic tumor.[38]

Glucagon-like Peptide-1 Receptor Imaging

As discussed earlier, somatostatin receptor expression is low in benign insulinomas resulting in low detection rates. This led to investigation into other receptor-targeted imaging techniques for this type of neuroendocrine tumor. Glucagon-like peptide-1 (GLP-1) and its analogs, liraglutide and exenatide, have been shown to enhance insulin secretion by β-cells. Further, data from in vitro studies suggest that GLP-1 receptors are expressed in about 97% of insulinomas resulting in this being used as specific target for in vivo receptor imaging. Preliminary reports on GLP-1R imaging have shown 95% sensitivity for the detection of insulinomas indicating that this modality may play an important role for the localization in the future.[38,39]

◇| INTRAOPERATIVE ADJUNCTS

Intraoperative USG

This modality was first used for the detection of an insulinoma in 1982. The ability to directly image the pancreas without the interference of the overlying organs or gas has increased the detection rates. Prior knowledge of tumor location with other localization techniques enables a focused ultrasound scanning and limits the pancreatic mobilization required.[40] Lobulated lesions can be well appreciated with an intraoperative USG (IOUS) allowing adequate enucleation and in addition, important anatomical structures, such as the main pancreatic duct and major vessels, can be clearly visualized intraoperatively.

Intraoperative USG may be performed either during a laparotomy or a laparoscopic approach. Laparoscopic USG can detect about 90% of insulinomas, and its sensitivity is comparable to that of manual palpation along with IOUS during open surgery.[41]

Frozen Section

Frozen section may be used intraoperatively to confirm the nature of the lesion identified, whether normal pancreatic parenchyma or neuroendocrine tumor when there is a doubt.

Manual Palpation

Though most insulinomas can be detected on intraoperative palpation, reported sensitivities range from 75 to 95%; this depends upon extensive mobilization of the pancreas and the experience of the surgeon.[35] Therefore, once the lesion has been identified preoperatively, intraoperative manual palpation can aid as an adjunctive tool to identify the lesion.

Intraoperative Glucose Monitoring

Combination of Methods

As is evident, every localization method has its own advantage and disadvantage accompanied with its own detection rates. However, multiple studies have shown higher detection rates when a combination of preoperative localization methods was used rather than a single modality alone, some even showing rates close to 100%.[23,30,31] Therefore, it may be prudent to use at least two modalities for preoperative localization of an insulinoma.

The patient discussed earlier underwent a 72-hour fast to confirm a diagnosis of hyperinsulinemic hypoglycemia. Within 4 hours, he developed hypoglycemic symptoms with the following biochemistry:
RBS: 35 mg%; *C-peptide*: 4.43 ng/mL; *Insulin:* 38.6 mU/mL

Confirming the diagnosis of hyperinsulinemic hypoglycemia. Further evaluation was done to localize the endogenous source of insulin. A contrast-enhanced computed tomography (CECT) (with pancreatic protocol), EUS, and MRI did not localize the lesion. Therefore, he underwent ^{68}Ga DOTA-TATE PET-CT which was also negative.

He was started on medical management with diazoxide with which his symptoms improved and planned for a repeat assessment in 6 months' time. A repeat MRI on follow-up detected a 9-mm lesion in the body of the pancreas on SPAIR and diffusion-weighted images **(Fig. 4)**.

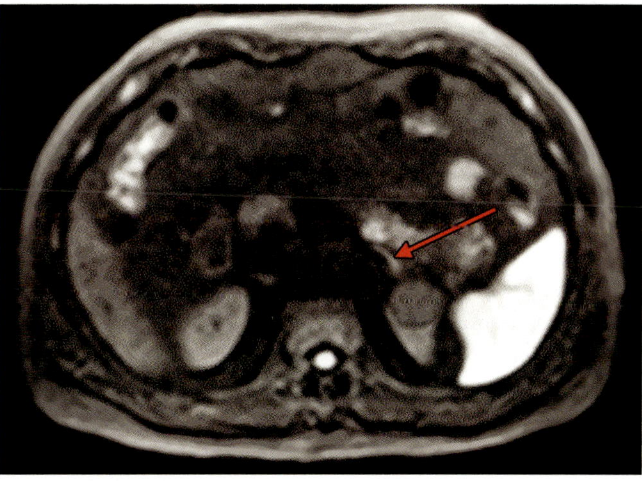

Fig. 4: SPAIR MRI with arrow pointing to a lesion in the body of pancreas.

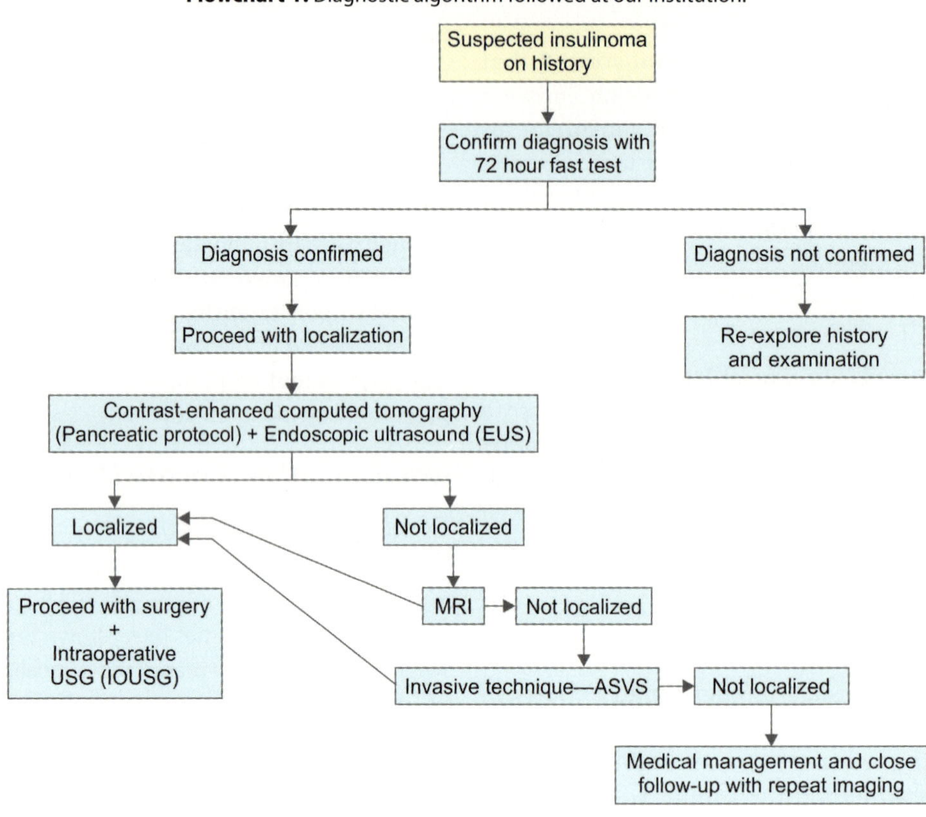

Flowchart 1: Diagnostic algorithm followed at our institution.

From the above discussion, it is clear that there are multiple localization modalities available for insulinomas. Imaging techniques are constantly being evaluated, upgraded, and improved resulting in increased detection rates. However, most modalities are user dependent. Therefore, ultimately the localization technique used by the treating physician/surgeon depends upon the available expertise and resources.

The diagnostic management protocol followed at our institution is depicted in **Flowchart 1**.

WHEN TO SUSPECT/EVALUATE FOR MEN-1?

Approximately 5–10% of insulinoma may be genetically acquired as part of the MEN-1 syndrome. Patients with an insulinoma in whom one should suspect and evaluate for the MEN-1 syndrome include:[23]

- Young age of presentation (<40 years)
- Those with a personal or family history of any endocrinopathy, especially hyperparathyroidism
- A concomitant gastrinoma or other rare functional tumors [glucagonomas, VIPomas, somatostatinomas, GRHomas, ACTHomas, pancreatic neuroendocrine tumors (pNETs) causing carcinoid syndrome or hypercalcemia (PTHrPomas)]
- Those with a nonfunctional pNET
- Presence of multiple insulinomas or recurrent disease

PATHOLOGY

Insulinomas are tumors that arise from the β-cells of the pancreas. They are the most common functioning tumor of the pancreas. The lesions are equally distributed in the head, body, and tail of the pancreas. The majority (90%) are sporadic, single, small (<2 cm), and benign. The familial forms associated with MEN-1 syndrome account for 5–10%.[5,42-45] MEN1-related insulinomas tend to occur in younger patients and are multiple. Insulinomas with local invasion to the surrounding structures lymph node/distant metastasis are deemed malignant as there are no definitive histological criteria to diagnose malignancy. The WHO in 2017 has revised the classification of tumors of endocrine organs. Based on their classification, pancreatic neuroendocrine neoplasms (PNENs) are now divided into well-differentiated and low-grade PNEN (grades 1 and 2), well-differentiated and high-grade PNEN (grade 3), and poorly differentiated and high-grade pancreatic neuroendocrine carcinoma (grade 3) according to their histomorphologic characteristics **(Table 3)**.[46]

IMMUNOHISTOCHEMISTRY

Well-differentiated PNEN is characterized by the cytoplasmic neuroendocrine granules, and currently, synaptophysin and chromogranin A are reliable markers for the same. Well-differentiated PNEN tends to show stronger and more diffuse

Table 3: WHO classification (2017) and grading of pancreatic neuroendocrine neoplasms (PNEN).

Classification	Grade	Mitosis	Ki-67
Well-differentiated and low-grade PNEN	1	<2 mitosis/10 HPF	<3%
Well-differentiated and low-grade PNEN	2	2–20 mitosis/10 HPF	3–20%
Well-differentiated and high-grade PNEN	3	>20 mitosis/10 HPF	>20%
Poorly differentiated and high-grade pancreatic neuroendocrine carcinoma	3	>20 mitosis/10 HPF	>20%

staining with these neuroendocrine markers than poorly differentiated PNEN. The mitotic count and the Ki-67/MIB-1 labeling index are the most reliable prognostic markers for PNEN.

◇| MANAGEMENT

Once the diagnosis is confirmed and the lesion is localized, surgery should be planned. Surgery remains the only proven curative treatment of insulinoma.

Preoperative Management

Prior to surgery, prevention of hypoglycemia is the management objective. Frequent meals and minimizing prolonged exercise are methods used for the same. The night before the surgery, once oral intake is stopped, intravenous glucose should be administered.

Intraoperative Management

During the operation, blood sugar levels need to be monitored every 30 minutes till excision and several hours postexcision of the insulinoma. Once the lesion is excised, the intravenous glucose is stopped and normal saline initiated. A rebound hyperglycemia indicates successful excision. Some centers estimate the peripheral insulin levels 10 minutes after excision—a 50% drop indicating a curative surgery.

Postoperative Management

After removal of the tumor, blood sugar has to be closely monitored as an initial period of hyperglycemia may ensue. This may be immediate or up to 1 hour following excision. Insulin may have to be administered for the management of postexclsion hyperglycemia in some patients. This period of hyperglycemia usually resolves in 1 week to 10 days. In patients with underlying diabetes, the hyperglycemia persists for >10 days.

Surgical Management

Excision of an insulinoma may be performed either by a minimal resection—enucleation or a more extended resection of the pancreas. The type of surgery depends upon:

- Size of the tumor
- Location of the tumor
- Number of lesions
- Proximity to the pancreatic duct and splenic vessels
- Benign or malignant

Localized Solitary Lesion

Enucleation of a solitary lesion should be performed, wherever possible to minimize the risks of exocrine insufficiency. Factors that are considered favorable to perform an enucleation are:[10,44]

- Single lesion <2 cm in size
- Tumor located on the surface of the pancreas
- Distance between the lesion and the pancreatic duct >2–3 mm
- Benign insulinomas

Lesions that do not fulfill the above criteria or have an ill-defined plane between the lesion and the pancreatic parenchyma would require a pancreatic resection. Depending on the location of the lesion, this would entail either a distal pancreatectomy, spleen preserving or with splenectomy (for lesions in the pancreatic body or tail), or a pancreaticoduodenectomy (for lesions within the pancreatic head). Similar outcomes for both enucleation and resection of the pancreas in patients with neuroendocrine tumors have been reported.[40,47,48] The surgical approach, open via a subcostal/midline incision, or laparoscopic depends upon the experience of the surgeon.

Intraoperatively, these lesions can be seen as a cherry red lesion on the surface of the pancreas. Deep-seated lesions may be palpable. An intraoperative ultrasound is of paramount value as it can help to localize the lesion, rule out other lesions, and confirm the relationship of the lesion with the pancreatic duct and splenic vessels and thus help in the surgical decision making.

Associated with MEN-1

MEN-1-associated insulinomas tend to be multiple; therefore, a thorough exploration of the entire pancreas—visual, palpatory, and IOUS—is of paramount importance. The extent of surgery for MEN-1 patients with an insulinoma would depend upon the number and location of the lesions. Though total pancreatectomy would be curative, it is considered to be an extreme modality of treatment for this condition with the associated morbidity. The operation recommended is a subtotal pancreatectomy with enucleation of lesions within the pancreatic head as this procedure potentially decreases the likelihood of a recurrence and in addition may prevent exocrine insufficiency.

Non-localized Lesion

Earlier, a blind distal pancreatectomy was recommended when no lesion was localized preoperatively or intraoperatively. This recommendation is no longer justified due to the morbidity associated with such a procedure and the associated high rates of failure to cure the disease. In addition, with the advancements in localization studies, almost all insulinomas can be detected. Currently, in this situation, it is recommended to refer the patient to a specialized center. The first step would then be to reconfirm the diagnosis. Once the diagnosis is confirmed, the patient may be either medically managed or an attempt should be made to localize the lesion after 3–6 months. An alternative strategy would be to attempt invasive localization methods such as ASVS.

Surgical Morbidity and Mortality

The morbidity and mortality rates depend upon the type of surgery performed. The most common morbidity following pancreatic surgery is a pancreatic fistula, occurring in 3–60% of patients. Other complications include intra-abdominal abscess (4.8–6.6%), pulmonary complication (3.5–10%), wound infection (2.5–8%), delayed gastric emptying (1–5%), intra-abdominal bleed (1–3.5%), and acute pancreatitis (0.5–5.5%).[10,32,49,50] Pancreatic exocrine deficiency and diabetes mellitus occur in 60% of patients following a pancreaticoduodenectomy, 5–10% following a left-sided pancreatectomy, and almost never after an enucleation. Mortality following an enucleation is rare, while it may reach 1–2% for left-sided pancreatectomy and up to 4–5% following a pancreaticoduodenectomy.[10]

Medical Management

Though surgical excision is the only curative treatment modality, some patients may require medical management to prevent the hypoglycemic episodes. These patients include:

- Those in whom the lesion is not localized
- Are at a high risk for surgical intervention
- Malignant insulinoma

The options for medical management are limited. Currently, the drug of choice is diazoxide, a potassium-channel activator. It acts by inhibiting insulin release from the β-cells via stimulation of α-adrenergic receptors. In addition, it inhibits cyclic adenosine monophosphate phosphodiesterase resulting in enhanced glycogenolysis. Common adverse effects of diazoxide include hirsutism, edema, gastrointestinal discomfort, and weight gain.[51]

The somatostatin analogs, octreotide and lanreotide, have been used in the past with limited benefits as the somatostatin receptors 2 and 5 are found in <50% of insulinomas. Octreotide binds these receptors inhibiting insulin secretion. In addition, octreotide induces the arrest of cell cycle in G1 phase resulting in the arrest of growth of the tumor. This antiproliferative and moderate antitumoral property has encouraged some researchers to use these agents in the management of malignant insulinomas.[24,51]

Other drugs reportedly used with varying results for the medical management of insulinoma are phenytoin, verapamil, diltiazem, propranolol, glucocorticoids, and glucagon.[5,52-55]

Ablative Methods

The morbidity and mortality associated with pancreatic surgery may preclude an operation in high-risk patients; in addition, some patients may refuse surgery. In this subset of patients, alternative treatment modalities have been explored which have been shown to be feasible and safe. However, long-term outcomes are yet to be reported.[56-61] The methods tried include:

- EUG-guided alcohol ablation
- CT- radiofrequency ablation (RFA)
- Embolization

Management of Malignant Insulinoma

Malignant insulinoma is a rare condition accounting for only 5–10% of insulinomas. Malignant insulinomas are usually single, large tumors and the most common sites of metastasis include lymph nodes and liver. The management of these patients poses a challenge as it involves control of tumor progression as well as the control of hypoglycemia.

Patients with a reasonable performance status, minimal extrahepatic disease, and a resectable primary tumor are candidates for cytoreductive surgery. Metastasectomy, if possible, may be added as this would alleviate the hypoglycemic symptoms. Unfortunately, cytoreductive surgery is effective in <10% of all patients with metastatic insulinoma.[51]

Palliative interventional measures include RFA and hepatic embolization of visceral metastatic lesions. Radionuclide therapy with targeting peptide receptors can be used. Lastly, palliative therapy includes diazoxide and chemotherapy (streptozocin, doxorubicin, and 5-flurouracil).

The chemotherapeutic agents, everolimus and sunitinib, have been recently approved for the management of advanced insulinoma, with promising progression-free survival and overall survival. Everolimus inhibits mammalian target of rapamycin (mTOR), a serine-threonine kinase, that stimulates cell growth, proliferation, and angiogenesis, thereby inhibiting a pathway implicated with tumor proliferation of pancreatic neuroendocrine tumors. Adverse effects of everolimus include stomatitis, rash, diarrhea, fatigue, anemia, and hyperglycemia. Sunitinib, a multitargeted receptor tyrosine kinase inhibitor, has shown delayed tumor growth in pancreatic neuroendocrine tumors by inhibiting vascular endothelial growth factor (VEGF) and platelet-derived growth factor (PDGF) receptors. The most frequent side effects of sunitinib are diarrhea, nausea, vomiting, asthenia, and fatigue.[62,63]

Our patient underwent an open enucleation of the lesion. Intraoperatively, the lesion was visualized after pancreatic mobilization and confirmed with an IOUS (**Figs. 5A and B**). Following enucleation, blood sugars rose necessitating insulin injections. The blood sugars normalized in 10 days. He developed a low output pancreatic fistula in the postoperative period which was conservatively managed with a drain placed at surgery.

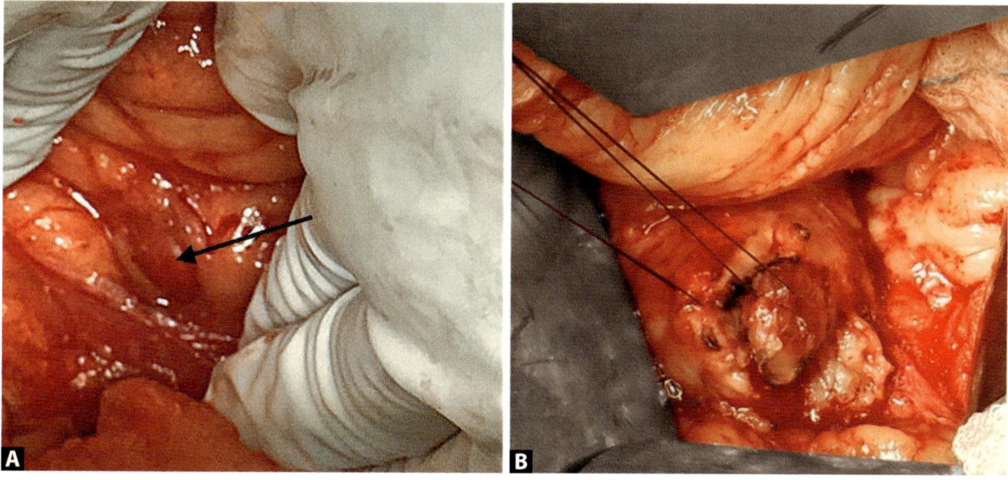

Figs. 5A and B: (A) An intraoperative picture depicting the insulinoma (arrow pointing the lesion) and being enucleated (B).

PROGNOSIS AND OUTCOMES

Factors that influence the prognosis and outcomes of insulinoma include:

- Size of the tumor
- Grade
- Number of mitosis
- Proliferative index
- Local invasion
- Presence of metastasis

Benign insulinomas have a very favorable prognosis with an estimated 10-year survival rate close to 100%. On the other hand, the reported 10-year survival rate for malignant lesions drops to 30%.[10,23]

CLINICAL PEARLS

- Insulinomas are the most common functional neuroendocrine tumors of the pancreas.
- Majority (90%) are sporadic, small (<2 cm), single, and benign.
- The familial form is associated with MEN-1 syndrome and these are usually multicentric.
- The clinical diagnosis is based on eliciting Whipple's triad.
- Evaluation of patients suspected to have an insulinoma involves biochemically confirming the diagnosis (72-hour fast test) followed by localizing the lesion.
- The operative approach depends upon the size, location, and relationship of the lesion to the pancreatic duct and splenic vessels.
- Enucleation is the procedure of choice for most sporadic insulinomas, while subtotal pancreatectomy is the procedure of choice for MEN-associated insulinomas.
- Malignant lesions are rare accounting for ~10% of insulinomas.
- Benign insulinomas carry an excellent prognosis while that of malignant insulinomas are poor.

REFERENCES

1. Molinete M, Irminger JC, Tooze SA, Halban PA. Trafficking/sorting and granule biogenesis in the beta-cell. Semin Cell Dev Biol. 2000;11(4):243-51.
2. Starr JI, Rubenstein AH. Metabolism of endogenous proinsulin and insulin in man. J Clin Endocrinol Metab. 1974;38(2):305-8.
3. Service FJ, McMahon MM, O'Brien PC, Ballard DJ. Functioning insulinoma—incidence, recurrence, and long-term survival of patients: a 60-year study. Mayo Clin Proc. 1991;66(7):711-9.
4. Nikfarjam M, Warshaw AL, Axelrod L, Deshpande V, Thayer SP, Ferrone CR, et al. Improved contemporary surgical management of insulinomas: a 25-year experience at the Massachusetts General Hospital. Ann Surg. 2008;247(1):165-72.
5. Shin JJ, Gorden P, Libutti SK. Insulinoma: pathophysiology, localization and management. Future Oncol. 2010;6(2):229-37.
6. Ludwig L, Schleithoff L, Kessler H, Wagner PK, Boehm BO, Karges W. Loss of wild-type MEN1 gene expression in multiple endocrine neoplasia type 1-associated parathyroid adenoma. Endocr J. 1999;46(4):539-44.
7. Shen HCJ, He M, Powell A, Adem A, Lorang D, Heller C, et al. Recapitulation of pancreatic neuroendocrine tumors in human multiple endocrine neoplasia type I syndrome via Pdx1-directed inactivation of MEN1. Cancer Res. 2009;69(5):1858-66.
8. Libutti SK, Crabtree JS, Lorang D, Burns AL, Mazzanti C, Hewitt SM, et al. Parathyroid gland-specific deletion of the mouse *MEN1* gene results in parathyroid neoplasia and hypercalcemic hyperparathyroidism. Cancer Res. 2003;63(22):8022-8.
9. Chandrasekharappa SC, Guru SC, Manickam P, Olufemi SE, Collins FS, Emmert-Buck MR, et al. Positional cloning of the gene for multiple endocrine neoplasia-type 1. Science. 1997;276(5311):404-7.
10. Vezzosi D, Bennet A, Maiza JC, Buffet A, Grunenwald S, Fauvel J, et al. (2011). Diagnosis and treatment of insulinomas in the adults. [online]. Available from https://www.intechopen.com/books/basic-and-clinical-endocrinology-up-to-date/diagnosis-and-treatment-of-insulinomas-in-the-adults. [Last accessed December, 2021].
11. Fukuda I, Hizuka N, Ishikawa Y, Yasumoto K, Murakami Y, Sata A, et al. Clinical features of insulin-like growth factor-II producing non-islet-cell tumor hypoglycemia. Growth Horm IGF Res. 2006;16(4):211-6.

12. Nauck MA, Reinecke M, Perren A, Frystyk J, Berishvili G, Zwimpfer C, et al. Hypoglycemia due to paraneoplastic secretion of insulin-like growth factor-I in a patient with metastasizing large-cell carcinoma of the lung. J Clin Endocrinol Metab. 2007;92(5):1600-5.

13. Service FJ, Natt N, Thompson GB, Grant CS, van Heerden JA, Andrews JC, et al. Noninsulinoma pancreatogenous hypoglycemia: a novel syndrome of hyperinsulinemic hypoglycemia in adults independent of mutations in *Kir6.2* and *SUR1* genes. J Clin Endocrinol Metab. 1999;84(5):1582-9.

14. Thompson GB, Service FJ, Andrews JC, Lloyd RV, Natt N, van Heerden JA, et al. Noninsulinoma pancreatogenous hypoglycemia syndrome: an update in 10 surgically treated patients. Surgery. 2000;128(6):937-4; discussion 944-5.

15. Won JGS, Tseng HS, Yang AH, Tang KT, Jap TS, Lee CH, et al. Clinical features and morphological characterization of 10 patients with noninsulinoma pancreatogenous hypoglycaemia syndrome (NIPHS). Clin Endocrinol (Oxf). 2006;65(5):566-78.

16. Service GJ, Thompson GB, Service FJ, Andrews JC, Collazo-Clavell ML, Lloyd RV. Hyperinsulinemic hypoglycemia with nesidioblastosis after gastric-bypass surgery. N Engl J Med. 2005;353(3):249-54.

17. Patti ME, McMahon G, Mun EC, Bitton A, Holst JJ, Goldsmith J, et al. Severe hypoglycaemia post-gastric bypass requiring partial pancreatectomy: evidence for inappropriate insulin secretion and pancreatic islet hyperplasia. Diabetologia. 2005;48(11):2236-40.

18. Goldfine AB, Mun E, Patti ME. Hyperinsulinemic hypoglycemia following gastric bypass surgery for obesity. Curr Opin Endocrinol Diabetes. 2006;13(5):419-24.

19. Cryer PE, Axelrod L, Grossman AB, Heller SR, Montori VM, Seaquist ER, et al. Evaluation and management of adult hypoglycemic disorders: an Endocrine Society Clinical Practice Guideline. J Clin Endocrinol Metab. 2009;94(3):709-28.

20. Allan FN, Boeck WC, Judd ES. The surgical treatment of hyperinsulinism. J Am Med Assoc. 1930;94(15):1116-9.

21. van Heerden JA, Edis AJ, Service FJ. The surgical aspects of insulinomas. Ann Surg. 1979;189(6):677-82.

22. Ahn CH, Kim LK, Lee JE, Jung CH, Min SH, Park KS, et al. Clinical implications of various criteria for the biochemical diagnosis of insulinoma. Endocrinol Metab. 2014;29(4):498.

23. Jensen RT, Cadiot G, Brandi ML, de Herder WW, Kaltsas G, Komminoth P, et al. ENETS Consensus Guidelines for the management of patients with digestive neuroendocrine neoplasms: functional pancreatic endocrine tumor syndromes. Neuroendocrinology. 2012;95(2):98-119.

24. Okabayashi T. Diagnosis and management of insulinoma. World J Gastroenterol. 2013;19(6):829.

25. Abboud B, Boujaoude J. Occult sporadic insulinoma: localization and surgical strategy. World J Gastroenterol. 2008;14(5):657-65.

26. Hashimoto LA, Walsh RM. Preoperative localization of insulinomas is not necessary. J Am Coll Surg. 1999;189(4):368-73.

27. Van Heerden JA, Grant CS, Czako PF, Service FJ, Charboneau JW. Occult functioning insulinomas: which localizing studies are indicated? Surgery. 1992;112(6):1010-5.

28. Kulke MH, Anthony LB, Bushnell DL, de Herder WW, Goldsmith SJ, Klimstra DS, et al. NANETS treatment guidelines: well-differentiated neuroendocrine tumors of the stomach and pancreas. Pancreas. 2010;39(6):735-52.

29. McAuley G, Delaney H, Colville J, Lyburn I, Worsley D, Govender P, et al. Multimodality preoperative imaging of pancreatic insulinomas. Clin Radiol. 2005;60(10):1039-50.

30. Druce MR, Muthuppalaniappan VM, O'Leary B, Chew SL, Drake WM, Monson JP, et al. Diagnosis and localisation of insulinoma: the value of modern magnetic resonance imaging in conjunction with calcium stimulation catheterisation. Eur J Endocrinol. 2010;162(5):971-8.

31. Gouya H, Vignaux O, Augui J, Dousset B, Palazzo L, Louvel A, et al. CT, endoscopic sonography, and a combined protocol for preoperative evaluation of pancreatic insulinomas. Am J Roentgenol. 2003;181(4):987-92.

32. Mehrabi A, Fischer L, Hafezi M, Dirlewanger A, Grenacher L, Diener MK, et al. A systematic review of localization, surgical treatment options, and outcome of insulinoma. Pancreas. 2014;43(5):675-86.

33. Tucker ON, Crotty PL, Conlon KC. The management of insulinoma. Br J Surg. 2006;93(3):264-75.

34. Matos C, Mathieu A, Closset J, Bali MA, Metens T. Successful preoperative localization of a small pancreatic insulinoma by diffusion-weighted MRI. JOP. 2009;10(5):528-31.

35. Böttger TC, Junginger T. Is preoperative radiographic localization of islet cell tumors in patients with insulinoma necessary? World J Surg. 1993;17(4):427-32.

36. Nockel P, Babic B, Millo C, Herscovitch P, Patel D, Nilubol N, et al. Localization of insulinoma using 68Ga-DOTATATE PET/CT scan. J Clin Endocrinol Metab. 2016;102(1):195-9.

37. Tuzcu SA, Pekkolay Z, Kılınç F, Tuzcu AK. 68Ga-DOTATATE PET/CT can be an alternative imaging method in insulinoma patients. J Nucl Med Technol. 2017;45(3):198-200.

38. Kyrilli A, Igoillo-Esteve M, Féry F, Grieco FA, Eisendrath P, Blocklet D, et al. Insulinoma localization by glucagon-like peptide-1 receptor imaging after 18 years of hypoglycemia. AACE Clin Case Rep. 2015;1(3):e187-93.

39. Christ E, Wild D, Ederer S, Béhé M, Nicolas G, Caplin ME, et al. Glucagon-like peptide-1 receptor imaging for the localisation of insulinomas: a prospective multicentre imaging study. Lancet Diabetes Endocrinol. 2013;1(2):115-22.

40. Jaroszewski DE, Schlinkert RT, Thompson GB, Schlinkert DK. Laparoscopic localization and resection of insulinomas. Arch Surg. 2004;139(3):270-4.

41. Wu M, Wang H, Zhang X, Gao F, Liu P, Yu B, et al. Efficacy of laparoscopic ultrasonography in laparoscopic resection of insulinoma. Endosc Ultrasound. 2017;6(3):149-55.

42. Demeure MJ, Klonoff DC, Karam JH, Duh QY, Clark OH. Insulinomas associated with multiple endocrine neoplasia type I: the need for a different surgical approach. Surgery. 1991;110(6):998-1004; discussion 1004-5.

43. Doherty GM, Doppman JL, Shawker TH, Miller DL, Eastman RC, Gorden P, et al. Results of a prospective strategy to diagnose, localize, and resect insulinomas. Surgery. 1991;110(6):989-96; discussion 996-997.

44. Finlayson E, Clark OH. Surgical treatment of insulinomas. Surg Clin North Am. 2004;84(3):775-85.

45. Paul TV, Jacob JJ, Vasan SK, Thomas N, Rajarathnam S, Selvan B, et al. Management of insulinomas: analysis from a tertiary care referral center in India. World J Surg. 2008;32(4):576-82.

46. Fukushima N. Neuroendocrine neoplasms of the pancreas: the pathological viewpoint. JOP. 2018;S(3):328-34.

47. Hu M, Zhao G, Luo Y, Liu R. Laparoscopic versus open treatment for benign pancreatic insulinomas: an analysis of 89 cases. Surg Endosc. 2011;25(12):3831-7.

48. Drymousis P, Raptis DA, Spalding D, Fernandez-Cruz L, Menon D, Breitenstein S, et al. Laparoscopic versus open pancreas resection for pancreatic neuroendocrine tumours: a systematic review and meta-analysis. HPB. 2014;16(5):397-406.

49. Strobel O, Cherrez A, Hinz U, Mayer P, Kaiser J, Fritz S, et al. Risk of pancreatic fistula after enucleation of pancreatic tumours. BJS. 2015;102(10):1258-66.

50. Crippa S, Zerbi A, Boninsegna L, Capitanio V, Partelli S, Balzano G, et al. Surgical management of insulinomas: short- and long-term outcomes after enucleations and pancreatic resections. Arch Surg. 2012;147(3):261-6.

51. Taye A, Libutti SK. (2015). Diagnosis and management of insulinoma: current best practice and ongoing developments. [online] Available from https://www.dovepress.com/diagnosis-and-management-of-insulinoma-current-best-practice-and-ongoi-peer-reviewed-fulltext-article-RRED. [Last accessed December, 2021].

52. Blum I, Rusecki Y, Doron M, Lahav M, Laron Z, Atsmon A. Evidence for a therapeutic effect of dl-propranolol in benign and malignant insulinoma: report of three cases. J Endocrinol Invest. 1983;6(1):41-5.

53. Ulbrecht JS, Schmeltz R, Aarons JH, Greene DA. Insulinoma in a 94-year-old woman: long-term therapy with verapamil. Diabetes Care. 1986;9(2):186-8.

54. Stehouwer CD, Lems WF, Fischer HR, Hackeng WH. Malignant insulinoma: is combined treatment with verapamil and the long-acting somatostatin analogue octreotide (SMS 201-995) more effective than single therapy with either drug? Neth J Med. 1989;35(1-2):86-94.

55. Shaklai M, Aderka D, Blum I, Laron Z, Asherov J, Doron M, et al. Suppression of hypoglycemic attacks and insulin release by propranolol in a patient with metastatic malignant insulinoma. Diabete Metab. 1977;3(3):155-8.

56. Dąbkowski K, Gajewska P, Walter K, Londzin-Olesik M, Białek A, Andrysiak-Mammos E, et al. Successful EUS-guided ethanol ablation of insulinoma, four-year follow-up: case report and literature review. Endokrynol Pol. 2017;68(4):472-9.

57. Jürgensen C, Schuppan D, Neser F, Ernstberger J, Junghans U, Stölzel U. EUS-guided alcohol ablation of an insulinoma. Gastrointest Endosc. 2006;63(7):1059-62.

58. Qin S, Lu X, Jiang H. EUS-guided ethanol ablation of insulinomas: case series and literature review. Medicine (Baltimore). 2014;93(14):e85.

59. Procházka V, Hlavsa J, Andrašina T, Starý K, Můčková K, Kala Z, et al. Laparoscopic radiofrequency ablation of functioning pancreatic insulinoma: video case report. Surg Laparosc Endosc Percutan Tech. 2012;22(5):e312-5.

60. Limmer S, Huppert PE, Juette V, Lenhart A, Welte M, Wietholtz H. Radiofrequency ablation of solitary pancreatic insulinoma in a patient with episodes of severe hypoglycemia. Eur J Gastroenterol Hepatol. 2009;21(9):1097-101.

61. Moore TJ, Peterson LM, Harrington DP, Smith RJ. Successful arterial embolization of an insulinoma. JAMA. 1982;248(11):1353-5.

62. Yao JC, Shah MH, Ito T, Bohas CL, Wolin EM, Van Cutsem E, et al. Everolimus for advanced pancreatic neuroendocrine tumors. N Engl J Med. 2011;364(6):514-23.

63. Raymond E, Dahan L, Raoul J-L, Bang Y-J, Borbath I, Lombard-Bohas C, et al. Sunitinib malate for the treatment of pancreatic neuroendocrine tumors. N Engl J Med. 2011;364(6):501-13.

Familial Endocrine Syndromes

Mallika Dhanda, Suneel Mattoo, Amit Agarwal

◇ INTRODUCTION

The familial endocrine predisposition syndromes include the following:

- Multiple endocrine neoplasia syndrome type 1 (MEN-1)
- Multiple endocrine neoplasia syndrome type 2 (MEN-2)
- Hereditary pheochromocytoma/paraganglioma syndrome (PPGL)
- Hereditary thyroid cancer syndromes
- Hyperparathyroid-jaw tumor (HPT-JT) syndrome

These fascinating syndromes have been well characterized in the past 30 years following identification of their molecular mechanisms, and genetic testing plays an indispensable role in surveillance and clinical management of index patients as well as their asymptomatic kindreds. MEN-1 probably has the widest pleiotropy of any hereditary cancer syndrome and MEN-2 is notable for remarkably precise genotype–phenotype correlations at the level of the codon and even amino acid level that determines timing of surgical intervention and age for starting surveillance.

Clinicians need to recognize the main clinical features of MEN syndrome because the MEN patients are at risk for multiple conditions, require complex management and life-long follow-up, have to apply new paradigm in surgery, have to adequately address the risk of disease in relatives, and have to develop a tailored surveillance protocol.

The endocrine surgeon who recognizes these syndromes and uses a multidisciplinary approach can take advantage of valuable opportunities for early and presymptomatic diagnosis, reduction of morbidity and mortality, avoidance of surgical misadventures, and even cure.

- Familial hyperparathyroidism syndromes
- Hereditary medullary thyroid carcinoma (MTC)
- Pheochromocytoma/paraganglioma syndromes
- Pancreatic neuroendocrine tumors (pNET)

When to suspect hereditary parathyroid disease?

Recognition of MEN1:

Before surgery:

- HPT <30 years of age
- Multiglandular disease
- Recurrent HPT in patients <30 years (either because of inadequate surgery done thinking it is a sporadic adenoma or after a subtotal parathyroidectomy)

At the time of surgery: If multiple enlarged glands are found. Therefore, a detailed family history should be obtained before any surgery for HPT, especially in younger patients.

Recognition of MEN2A: Only 20% of MEN2A patients present with HPT. Since there is a genotype–phenotype correlation in MEN2A, the presence of codon 634 mutation should alert the surgeon to an increased risk of HPT in the index case and family.

Recognition of familial isolated hyperparathyroidism (FIHPT): Hypercalcemia in family members without manifestations typical of MEN1 syndrome or other endocrinopathies should arise suspicion of FIHP.

Recognition of HPT-JT syndrome: The following should raise suspicion for HPT-JT syndrome:

- A cystic parathyroid adenoma
- HPT associated with fibro-osseus lesions of maxilla or mandible
- Parafibromin-negative parathyroid tumors

Thus, clinical findings s/o hereditary HPT in a patient of hypercalcemia include:

- Early onset of HPT <30 years
- Recurrent HPT especially <30 years
- Family history of hypercalcemia
- Presence of skin lesions (lipomas, facial angiofibromas, and collagenomas)
- Associated pituitary adenoma
- Associated pheochromocytoma or adrenal adenoma
- 634 codon mutation
- Jaw tumors, especially associated with renal cysts or cystic parathyroid tumors
- Parathyroid carcinoma <30 years
- Hypercalcemia with hypercalciuria, especially the if calcium:creatinine ratio is <0.01

When to suspect hereditary pheochromocytoma/paraganglioma syndrome?

- *Clinical presentation*:
  - *If metastatic on presentation*: Suspect presence of *SDHB* mutation
  - *If multiple abdominal paragangliomas (PGLs)*: *SDHD*
  - *If multiple/bilateral pheochromocytoma (PCC)*: *TMEM127*

- *If multiple PGLs + pNET (somatostatinoma)*: Hypoxia-inducible factor 2α (HIF2α)
- *Tumor location*:
  - *Head and neck (H and N) PGLs*: SDHD, SDHC, and SDHB
  - *H and N PGLs with strong FH of H and N PGLs*: SDHAF2
- *Biochemical phenotype*:
  - *Dopamine*: SDHB
  - *Methoxytyramine*: SDHx tumors
- *Syndromic/familial stigmata: If features of MEN or von Hippel–Lindau (VHL)*
- *Histological features: Negative SDHB immunohistochemistry (IHC) indicates presence of SDHx-related PCC/PGLs*
- *Metastases: SDHB and SDHD*

When to suspect pNET being part of MEN1?
- Renal colic with pNET
- Any patient of Zollinger–Ellison syndrome (ZES)
- Young age onset of a functional pNET
- Multiple pNETs
- pNET with hypercalcemia, especially with parathyroid hyperplasia or MGD

◇ MULTIPLE ENDOCRINE NEOPLASIA SYNDROME-TYPE 1

It is an inherited autosomal-dominant disorder and is characterized by predisposition to develop endocrine tumors/hyperplasia in pituitary, parathyroid, and pancreas. In the absence of treatment, endocrine tumors are associated with an earlier mortality in patients with MEN1. Untreated patients with MEN1 have a decreased life expectancy with a 50% probability of death by the age of 50 years, and the cause of death in 50–70% of patients with MEN1 is usually a malignant tumor process or sequelae of the disease. Recently, there has been a shift in MEN1-associated mortality; now, malignant pNET and thymic carcinoid tumors are associated with a marked increase in risk of death. Hence, it is imperative to treat MEN1 as early as possible. However, the treatment outcomes are not as successful as those in non-MEN1 patients because **(Table 1)**.

Genetics of MEN1

The *MEN*-gene is a tumor suppressor gene and has been localized to the long arm of chromosome 11 (11q13) and is composed of 10 exons. It encodes a 610 amino acid nuclear protein called *MENIN* mutation in *MEN-1* gene and results in truncation of the menin protein which in turn results in DNA instability. *MENIN* has the unique property of promoting oncogenesis in hemopoietic lineage but suppressing tumorigenesis in endocrine lineage.[1]

Definition of Familial MEN-1

A diagnosis of MEN-1 can be established by one of the following criteria:[2,3]
- If an individual has two or more primary MEN-1 endocrine tumors [parathyroid adenoma/hyperplasia; gastroenteropancreatic (GEP) tumors, pituitary adenoma]
- Discovery of one of the MEN-1 tumors in first-degree relative
- Identification of MEN-1 mutation

Clinical Manifestations of MEN-1

Penetrance is usually 100% by the age of 50 years **(Figs. 1A to F)**:
- *Primary HPT (adenoma/hyperplasia)*: 90–100%
- *Pancreatic endocrine tumors*: 20–70%
- *Pituitary adenoma*: 20–65%

Besides the primary lesions, other associated lesions commonly seen in MEN-1 are:
- *Adrenal tumors*: 10–75%
- Thyroid benign adenomas
- Carcinoid tumors (thymic, gastric, and bronchial)
- Skin and subcutaneous lesions (facial angiofibromas, collagenomas, lipomas, and café-au-lait macules)
- Central nervous system (CNS) tumors (meningiomas and schwannomas)
- Smooth muscle tumors (leiomyomas and leiomyosarcomas)

Parathyroid Disease

It is the most common and first to appear and reaches 100% penetration by 50 years. The clinical presentation is no different from sporadic HPT, except that there is no female preponderance and hypercalcemia is usually mild.[3-5] Imaging studies are not useful because all four glands are involved, and therefore a bilateral exploration is the approach of choice. The timing of surgery has been a matter of debate—early surgery may obviate the deleterious biochemical effects of HPT on target organs; on the other hand, waiting for surgery may make the parathyroid glands enlarge further and make the identification at operation easier. Even though all four glands are enlarged, the enlargement is asymmetrical as they are independent clonal adenomas. The extent of gland removal has also been debated: operations range from three gland, three and half gland, or four gland removal with or without autotransplantation. Nonetheless, the preferred operation is subtotal parathyroidectomy (three and half gland resection) along with thymectomy. Recurrence rates are higher if less than three and half gland parathyroidectomy and can be in the range of 40–60%.[6,7]

Table 1: Reasons why treatment outcomes in MEN-1 are poor.

- MEN1-associated tumors (except pituitary tumors) are usually multiple, thereby making it difficult to achieve a successful surgical cure.
- Occult metastatic disease is more prevalent in MEN1 patients.
  - Metastases in 50% versus 10% in sporadic tumors
- MEN1-associated tumors may be larger, more aggressive, and more resistant to treatment
  - *Pituitary macroadenomas*: 85% versus 64%
  - *Parasellar extension*: 30% versus 10%
  - *Persistent disease*: 45% versus 20%

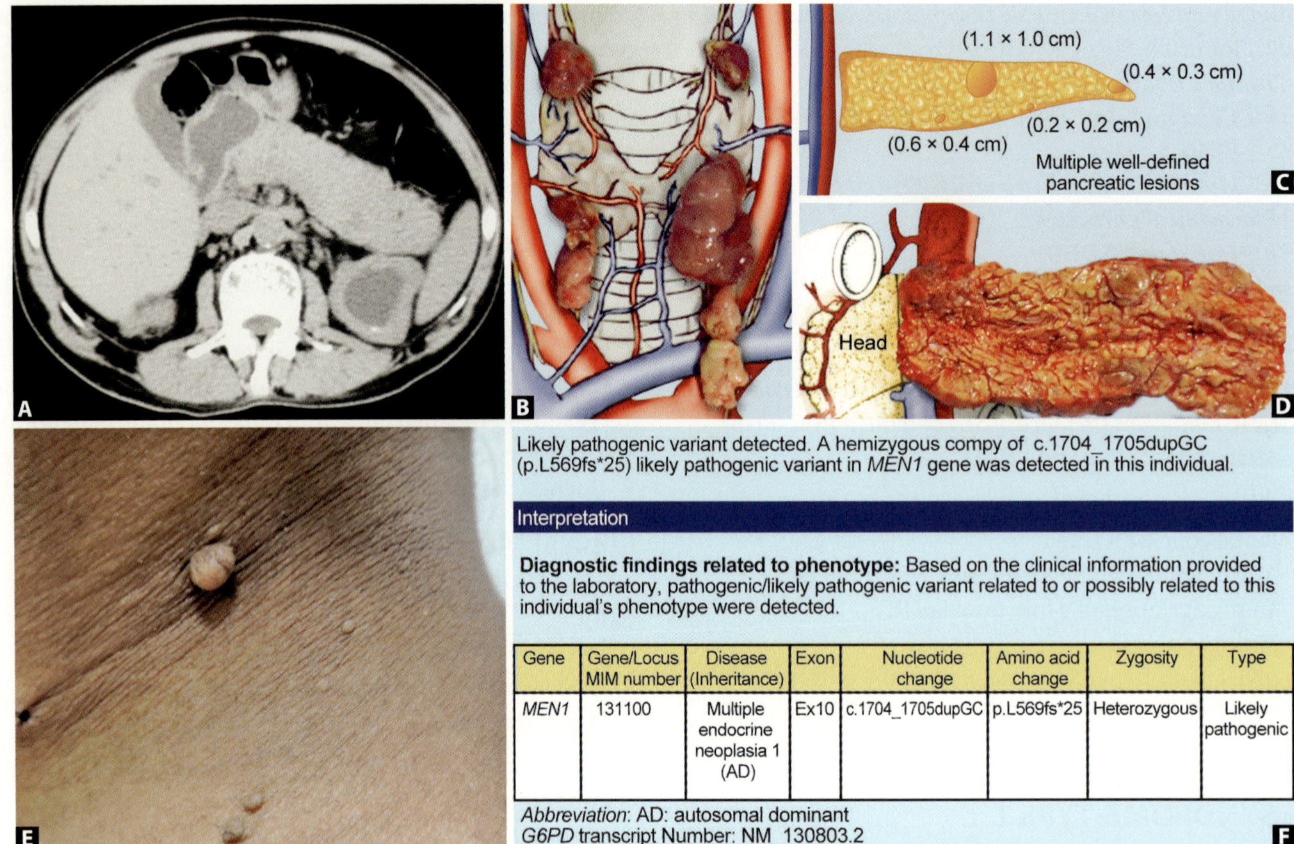

Likely pathogenic variant detected. A hemizygous compy of c.1704_1705dupGC (p.L569fs*25) likely pathogenic variant in *MEN1* gene was detected in this individual.

Interpretation

Diagnostic findings related to phenotype: Based on the clinical information provided to the laboratory, pathogenic/likely pathogenic variant related to or possibly related to this individual's phenotype were detected.

Gene	Gene/Locus MIM number	Disease (Inheritance)	Exon	Nucleotide change	Amino acid change	Zygosity	Type
MEN1	131100	Multiple endocrine neoplasia 1 (AD)	Ex10	c.1704_1705dupGC	p.L569fs*25	Heterozygous	Likely pathogenic

Abbreviation: AD: autosomal dominant
G6PD transcript Number: NM_130803.2

Figs. 1A to F: Case of multiple endocrine neoplasia type 1 (MEN-1). A 42-year-old male presented with hypercalcemic crisis along with altered sensorium. Investigations revealed serum calcium >14 mg%, FBS of 55 mg% with insulin levels of 64.77 pmol/L. USG showed enlargement of all four glands and CECT of abdomen revealed multiple lesions in body and tail of pancreas (A). He underwent three-and-half-gland parathyroidectomy (B); with thymectomy and subtotal pancreatectomy (C and D); He also had collagenomas of the skin (E); Exome analysis revealed pathogenic mutation in *MEN1* gene (F). (CECT: contrast-enhanced computed tomography; FBS: fasting blood sugar; USG: ultrasonography)

Pancreatic Neuroendocrine Tumor

MEN-1-associated pNET may be functional or nonfunctional. pNETs associated with MEN-1 present with *special challenges* because:

- They are multiple, multicentric, and multifocal.
- They have earlier age of onset.
- They are frequently malignant.
- They secrete multiple hormones.
- They may not result in a distinct clinical syndrome despite secreting a number of peptides, thus causing diagnostic dilemma.
- Tumors may vary from microadenomas to macroadenomas to carcinomas. In fact, the most characteristic MEN-1 lesion is the presence of diffuse microadenomatosis (0–5 mm).
- Surgery is seldom curative as they have high lymph node (LN) metastases (45–95%) by the time they are detected.

Frequency of lesions:
- *Gastrinomas*: 55%
- *Insulinomas*: 20%
- *Glucagonomas*: 5%
- *Somatostatinomas*: 1%

Imaging Studies

Cross-sectional imaging such as computed tomography (CT), magnetic resonance imaging (MRI), and ultrasonography (USG) tends to miss tumors <2 cm. Gallium DOTATATE is the most sensitive imaging method to pick up the small pNETs. Endoscopic ultrasound (EUS) can also pick up lesions as small as 0.1–0.2 cm.

Surgical Treatment

Because the natural history of ZES or NF-pNET is unclear, it is difficult to analyze the risk–benefit ratio for taking a decision for surgery in these patients. Over the decades, the primary reason for mortality in patients with MEN1 has shifted from gastric acid hypersecretion to malignant carcinoids and again to the present thinking of metastatic pNET as the main cause of death in MEN1 patients. Thus, the following factors make the role of surgery difficult to elucidate—unknown natural history, low cure rates with less aggressive surgery, excellent prognosis for small pNETs in ZES and NF-PNET, good medical control of functional pNETs, and increased morbidity and mortality of aggressive surgery.

Zollinger–Ellison syndrome: MEN1 patients typically have multiple, small duodenal gastrinomas with associated LN metastases in almost 50% cases. The choice of operation is either a local removal of duodenal gastrinomas by duodenotomy (which of course is associated with increased recurrence rates) or Whipple's operation (which, though curative, is associated with major morbidity and also obviates the future possibility of gastric carcinoid).[8-10]

Insulinoma: Patients with MEN-1 have multiple tumors dispersed throughout the pancreas with a dominant (>2 cm) pNET in the body or tail of pancreas. Again, the choice is between a resection and enucleation.

Nonfunctional pNETS: NF is usually asymptomatic and not associated with a clinical syndrome, or there may be only minor elevations of pancreatic hormones. Because of the increased sensitivity of recent radiological methods (CT, MRI, PET, and EUS), there is an increased identification rate of NF-pNET to the extent of 55%.[11] Management of NF-pNET, even though they being asymptomatic, is of concern because metastases from malignant pNET are the most common cause of death in MEN-1 patients and the detection of NF-PNET is delayed as they are asymptomatic. Surgical management of NF-pNET is controversial. Most studies take size as the criteria for surgical decision-making. Tumors <1 cm or <2 cm can be followed-up with EUS and intervention is done whenever growth occurs. Other factors that have been taken into decision-making include Ki-67 rates of the EUS biopsy from NF-NET. Thus, it is recommended that surgical exploration should be done only for tumors >2 cm.[8,9] Options range from distal/subtotal pancreatectomy with intraoperative ultrasound (IOUS)-directed enucleation of tumors from head of pancreas to Whipple's procedure.

Carcinoid tumors: Occur in 3% of MEN-1 patients:
- *Gastric carcinoids*: 35%
- *Bronchial carcinoids*: 8%
- *Thymic carcinoids*: 8%

Gastric carcinoids: These are usually type 2 ECL carcinoids and are usually asymptomatic. They are usually very aggressive, either locally or metastatic, by the time they are detected during an endoscopic or imaging procedure. Treatment includes endoscopic excision to subtotal to total gastrectomy with D-2 LN dissection and additional treatments with long-standing sandostatin analogs. In order to detect gastric carcinoids early, it is recommended that all patients with MEN-1 undergo annual endoscopic evaluations.

Thymic carcinoids: Unlike the MEN-1-associated bronchial carcinoids, thymic carcinoids are usually nonfunctional and locally aggressive and metastasize early, thus requiring radical thymectomy. It is more common in males and smokers. Though recommendation of routine thymectomy during parathyroid surgery for MEN-1-associated HPT does reduce the risk of subsequent development of thymic carcinoid, continued surveillance is still required. After pNET, thymic carcinoids are the major cause of death in MEN-1 patients.[12]

Pituitary Tumors

They can be the presenting manifestation in as much as 25% of MEN-1 cases.[13-15] Unlike sporadic cases, these are plurihormonal and are bigger (macroadenomas). The most common pituitary tumor in MEN-1 is prolactinoma, others being growth hormone (GH)-secreting tumors and ACTH-producing tumors. Patients may present with loss of peripheral vision or features of acromegaly or Cushing's disease. However, the results of medical treatment or even trans-sphenoidal surgery are not encouraging as compared to those seen in sporadic pituitary tumors.

Mutation Analysis in MEN-1

65% of germline mutations in MEN1 are frameshift or truncated mutations and 23% are missense mutations.[16] Mutational analysis of *MEN1* gene for diagnostic purposes unlike *MEN2A* mutational analysis is difficult because of several reasons: (1) There is a wide diversity of mutations in the coding region of *MEN1* gene (there are >1,300 mutations which are not clustered but spread across the 1830-bp coding region); (2) There is no genotype–phenotype correlation in MEN1; (3) Because of large gene deletions, mutations may not be detected; (4) Due to the presence of phenocopies. Mutational analysis is helpful in clinical practice by confirming the clinical diagnosis and offering/starting early treatment of index case as well as screened family members and can also help avoid the unpleasant life-long annual testing for the 50% family members who are not harboring the mutation. The analysis should be offered as early as possible (even in children as young as 5 years).

Familial Isolated Hyperparathyroidism

It is a variant of MEN1 (**Fig. 2**). Some kindreds of a family may just show isolated hypercalcemia only without evidence of involvement of other endocrine organs. Such a condition is known as *FIHPT*. The concepts and explanation for FIHPT have undergone changes and reversals over the last eight decades.[17] Between 1960 and 1980, it was thought that FIHPT was due to incomplete expression of MEN1 syndrome and absence of *MEN* mutation was necessary to make a diagnosis of FIHPT. Then, there was a reversal of concept and it was suggested that with longer follow-up, most of these FIHPT kindreds would express one or more syndromal extraparathyroid features of MEN1 and FIHPT with mutation in one of the *MEN1*, *CDC73*, or *CASR* genes could still be termed FIHPT. The most recent concept incorporates presence of *GCM2* mutation in FIHPT.

◇ MULTIPLE ENDOCRINE NEOPLASIA TYPE 2A

- Genetics of MEN2A
- MTC in MEN2A
- HPT in MEN2A
- PCC in MEN2A

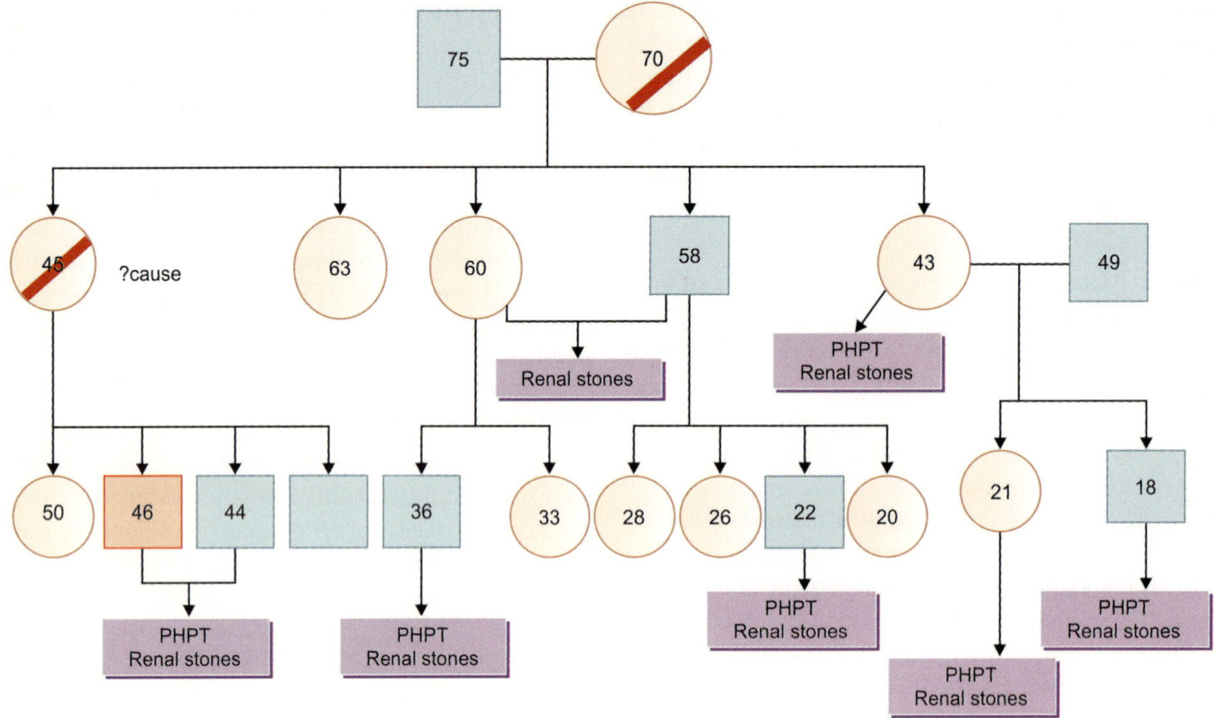

Fig. 2: Pedigree of family of familial isolated hyperparathyroidism (FIHPT). Seven members of a family across two generations and spread over 15 years presented only with renal stones and found to be having hyperparathyroidism with no evidence of involvement of pancreas or pituitary gland. (PHPT: primary hyperparathyroidism).

- Genotype–phenotype relationship
- Rare codon mutations
- Genetic testing and screening in MEN2A
- Effect of genetic testing in clinical outcome

Differences from MEN1/Sporadic Tumors

- Age is younger than sporadic.
- Female preponderance in MEN2A
- Strong genotype–phenotype relationship
- Specific genetic test with 95% accuracy
- *Pathology:*
  - *Single adenoma*: 25–35%
  - *Double adenoma*: 15%
  - *Multiglandular disease*: 50%
  - *Ectopic/supernumerary*: 15%/8%

Genetics of MEN2A

It is also known as Sipple's syndrome. It consists of MEN2A, MEN2B, and FMTC. They are all due to germline mutations in *RET* proto-oncogene and are inherited as autosomal dominant disorder.

RET oncogene has 21 exons and encodes for the trans-membrane tyrosine kinase which as a role in cell growth and normal embryogenesis, especially of neural crest cells. 90% of mutations are located in exons 10-11 and 13-15 of the *RET* oncogene. Among the codons, 85% of mutations were thought to be in codon 634 of exon 10, though now mutations are also detected in the so-called rare exons such as 10, 13, 14, and 15.

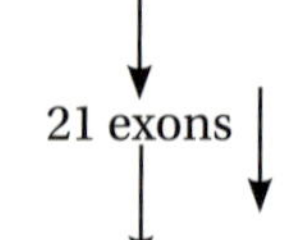

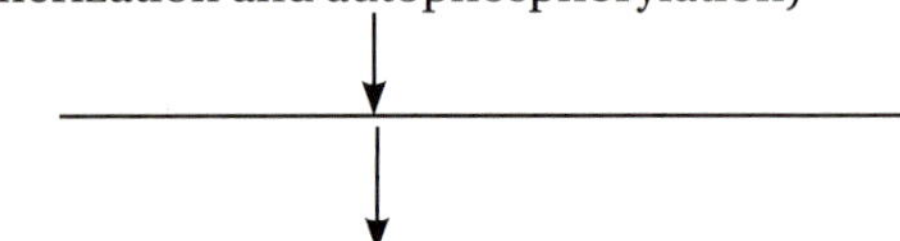

- *Extracellular domain:*
  - 4 cadherin-rich regions
  - 1 cysteine-rich region
- Trans-membrane domain (codon 636-657)
- *Intra-cellular domain:*
  - Juxtramembrane region
  - 2 Tyrosine kinase regions

RET is activated by ligand binding, and the most common ligands belong to glial cell-derived neurotrophic factor (GDNF) family. However, majority of the mutations involve ligand-independent dimerization and activation of mutated RET, especially in exons 10 and 11, which fall within the extracellular cysteine-rich domain of RET protein. The cysteine-rich domain is considered to stabilize the normal tertiary structure of the RET protein through the formation of disulfide bonds between cysteine residues in the region. Changing one of the cysteine residues to another amino acid (as happens in mutations) results in unpaired cysteine which may form aberrant bonds with other cysteines within the same molecule or between abnormal RET molecules.[18,19] This results in ligand-independent dimerization and persistent intracellular signaling by RET, which in turn stimulates multiple downstream pathways such as ATK and PI3K.

Clinical Features of MEN2A (Table 2 and Figs. 3A to H)

MEN2A-Hyperparathyroidism

Unlike MEN1-HPT, MEN2A-associated HPT is milder and often asymptomatic. They usually present as a synchronous lesion with MTC and PCC (75%), or present after a previous total thyroidectomy for MTC (20%), and rarely as the first presenting manifestation (5%). Surgery is the treatment of choice and is undertaken in two situations: symptomatic MEN2A-HPT and in asymptomatic patients when at the time of surgery for MTC, one or more parathyroid glands are found to be enlarged. Prophylactic parathyroidectomy at the time

Table 2: Features of familial syndromes.

Syndrome	Prevalence	Endocrine tumors (%)	Associated features/variants
MEN2A	75%	MTC: 90–100 PCC: 50 HPT: 20–30	CLA and HD
MEN2B	10%	MTC: 100 PCC: 50	Marfanoid habitus, mucosal neuromas, intestinal ganglioneuromatosis
FMTC	15%	MTC: 95	–

(FMTC: familial medullary thyroid cancer; HPT: hyperparathyroid; MEN: multiple endocrine neoplasia; MTC: medullary thyroid carcinoma; PCC: pheochromocytoma)

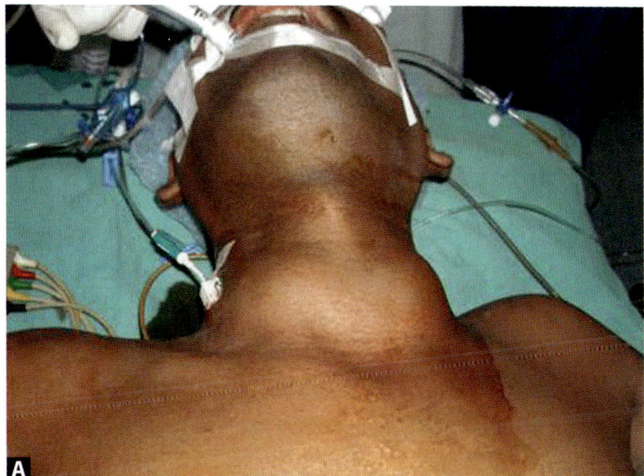

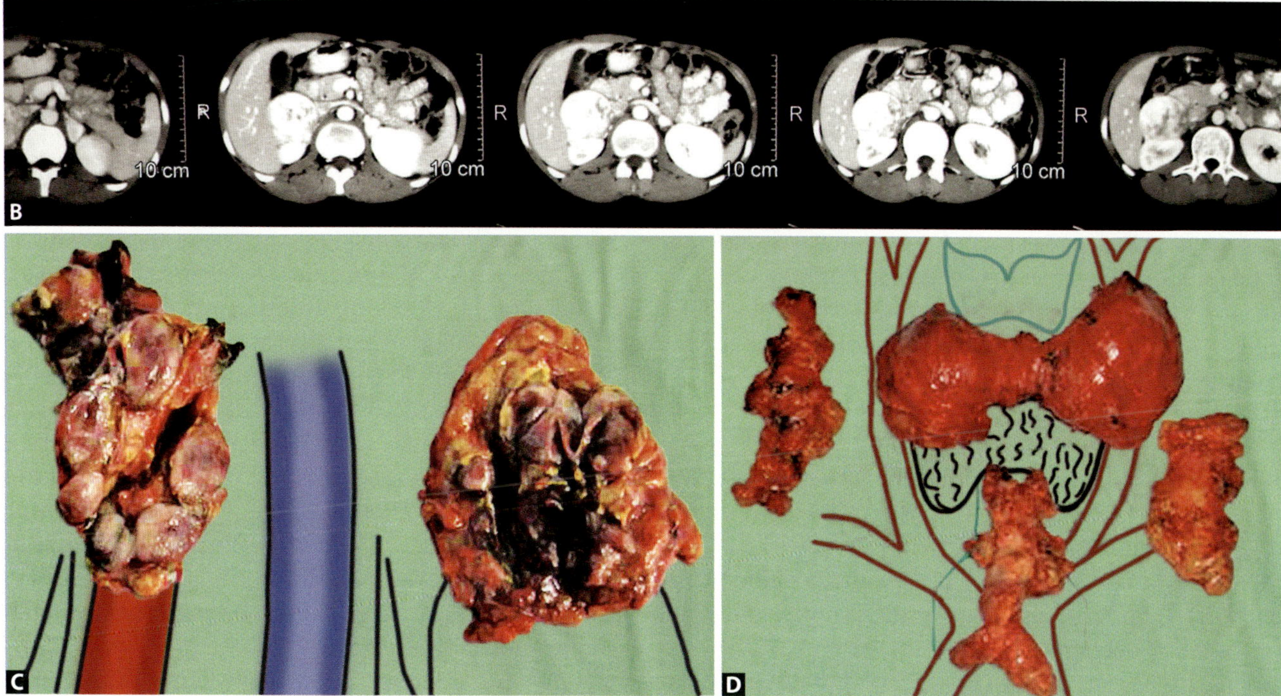

Figs. 3A to D: Multiple endocrine neoplasia type 2A (MEN-2A). A 35-year-old normotensive male patient was referred for surgery for MTC (A). On evaluation, his 24-hour urinary NMN was found to be elevated (>1,000 μg) and subsequent adrenal imaging revealed bilateral pheochromocytomas (B). He underwent bilateral adrenalectomy (C) followed by total thyroidectomy with bilateral CCLND and bilateral MRND (D).

Name of test	: **Medullary Thyroid Carcinoma**
Specimen	: **Blood**
Method	: DNA was isolated using standard protocol. Direct sequencing of the PCR products was used to detect mutations in the various exons of the *RET* gene.

Test Results

Exon Number	Codon	Presence of mutation
Exon 10	600 / 603 / 606 / 609 / 611 / 618 / 620	Not detected
Exon 11	634	Detected
Exon 13	767 / 768 / 777 / 778 / 781 / 790 / 791	Not detected
Exon 14	804 / 813 / 836 / 844	Not detected
Exon 15	873 / 891 / 893 / 897 / 904 / 907	Not detected
Exon 16	918 / 921 / 922	Not detected

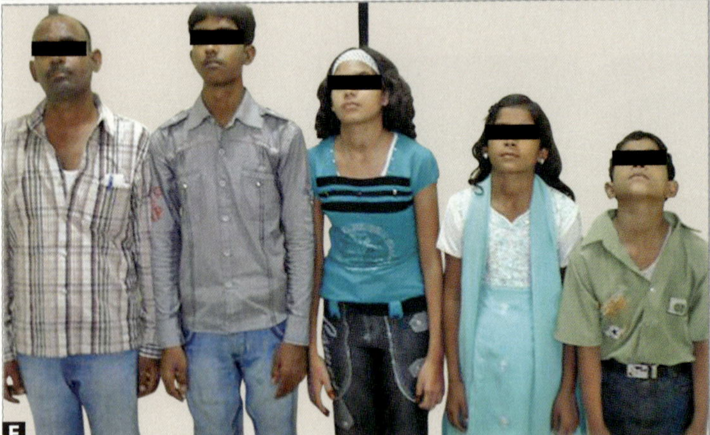
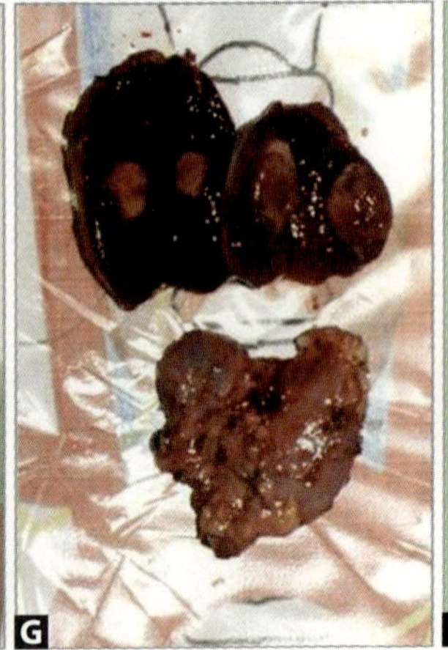
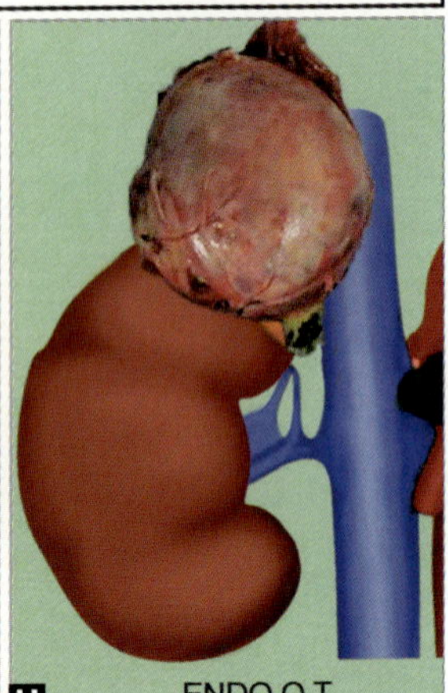

Figs. 3E to H: Genetic analysis revealed 634 mutations (E). On evaluation, three of his four siblings were found to be having elevated serum calcitonin levels and mutation in RET oncogene with normal urinary MN/NMN (F). All of them underwent total thyroidectomy with bilateral CCLND (G). All siblings were on annual follow-up with urinary MN/NMN and calcium/PTH. One of the female siblings developed elevated NMN and underwent adrenalectomy for a right pheochromocytoma (H). (CCLND: central compartment lymph node dissection; SLND: modified neck dissection; NMN: normetanephrine; PTH: parathyroid hormone)

of surgery for MTC is not justified. Operation of choice is an MIP and excision of only macroscopically enlarged glands. This approach results in minimal complications such as permanent hypocalcemia as well as low rates of recurrent/persistent hypercalcemia. The other option is a subtotal or total parathyroidectomy. The dictum is that it is easier to manage a mild recurrent/persistent hypercalcemia than a permanent hypocalcemia. 5-year recurrence rates range from 0 to 12%.[20-23]

Management of MEN2A-MTC

The term prophylactic thyroidectomy is used when a thyroidectomy is performed in an RET carrier who has a normal calcitonin level and clinical or imaging evidence of MTC. However, despite no preoperative evidence of malignancy, the histopathology of the prophylactic total thyroidectomy may range from no evidence of MTC, C cell hyperplasia (CCH), micro-MTC, or frankly invasive MTC. It should be kept in mind that the parents of the child may become concerned if the specimen does not show any evidence of MTC; hence, proper counseling before operation

is necessary. Prophylactic thyroidectomy in children with RET mutation has been shown to be of great benefit in reducing the mortality. In the study by Skinner et al.[24] published in 2005, there was no persistent or recurrent disease in 88% of children at a follow-up of 5 or more years after prophylactic total thyroidectomy. Thus, the usefulness of prophylactic thyroidectomy is no longer debatable; nevertheless, the point of continuing debate is at what age the prophylactic thyroidectomy should be performed. In the study by Jeniffer et al.[25] after a mean follow-up of 7 years, the authors concluded that recurrent disease was observed only in patients with mutations in codon 634 and 918; these children had not undergone prophylactic thyroidectomy at an appropriate age. The recent American Thyroid Association (ATA) guidelines have suggested the following:

- *ATA-HST category*: Prophylactic thyroidectomy within 1st year, preferably within first 6 months
- *ATA-high category*: Prophylactic thyroidectomy at 5 years or earlier based on detection of calcitonin levels. If calcitonin > 40 pg/mL, then add central compartment lymph node dissection (CCLND).

- *ATA-moderate category*: Screening with USG, a calcitonin level should begin at 5 years. Whenever calcitonin levels start rising, total thyroidectomy should be done to avoid the continuous long-term annual evaluation.

Pheochromocytoma in MEN2A

There is enough evidence that there is a very strong genotype–phenotype relationship between different RET mutations and clinical presentation (penetrance, biochemistry, etc.) and outcome.[26] Not only different codons, even different amino acid substitutions within each codon may be associated with variable rates of PCC **(Box 1)**.

Most studies suggest that annual screening for PCC should begin at 11 years for ATC-HST and ATA-H and by age of 16 years in ATA-MOD categories of mutation.[27,28]

Treatment

In a patient with a unilateral lesion, partial or total unilateral adrenalectomy is the operation of choice. Since only 50% of

patients with unilateral MEN2A-associated PCC will develop a contralateral PCC and this may take as long as 10 years, upfront or prophylactic bilateral adrenalectomy in the absence of image-localized bilateral lesion is not advisable because of the high risk of steroid dependence and possible mortality due to steroid deficiency.

Cortical-sparing adrenalectomy: It is a recommended option for MEN2A-associated PCC done either at the time of initial surgery when the patient presents with bilateral tumors or at the time when the patient develops a contralateral tumor after a previous unilateral adrenalectomy. At least, a third of one adrenal gland should be preserved to avoid the development of Addison's disease[29] **(Figs. 4A to C)**. In a multinational observational retrospective population-based study which compiled data on 563 patients of PCC associated with MEN2A, recurrence was seen in only 4 (3%) of 153 cortical sparing surgery after 6–13 years.[1] 47 (57%) of 82 patients with bilateral PCC who underwent cortical sparing did not become steroid dependent. **Table 3** shows the results of recent and older studies of cortical sparing adrenalectomy for hereditary PCC. One point that emerges out of Castennati study[30] is that the recurrence is lower in recent studies which have used an endoscopic approach which provides better magnification to achieve a technically better cortical sparing adrenalectomy.

◇ PHEOCHROMOCYTOMA/ PARAGANGLIOMA SYNDROMES

Pheochromocytomas and PGLs are chromaffin cell tumors derived from adrenal or extra-adrenal sympathetic/parasympathetic paraganglia and referred together as PPGLs. Up to 40% of these have a germline mutation in a known susceptibility gene, more than any other solid tumor. More than 20 susceptibility genes and 12 different genetic syndromes have been identified till date. Despite extensive heterogeneity found among the various syndromes of hereditary PPGLs, these genes and syndromes can still be

BOX 1: Variable penetration of pheochromocytoma with different codons and aminoacid substitutions.	
Mutation:	*Penetrance of PCC (50%)*
634	50
618	33
620	14
609	7
Amino acid substitution expressing PCC	*Penetrance(%)*
C634S	100
C634G	40
C634R	50
C634Y	50
C609G	50
C609Y	0
C618G	24
C618F	0
C618Y	0

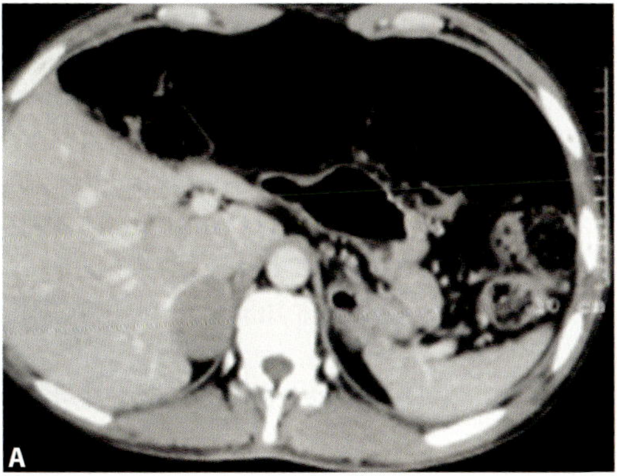
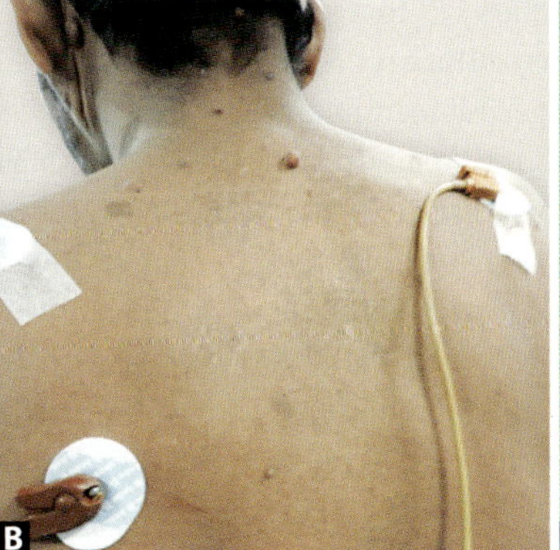
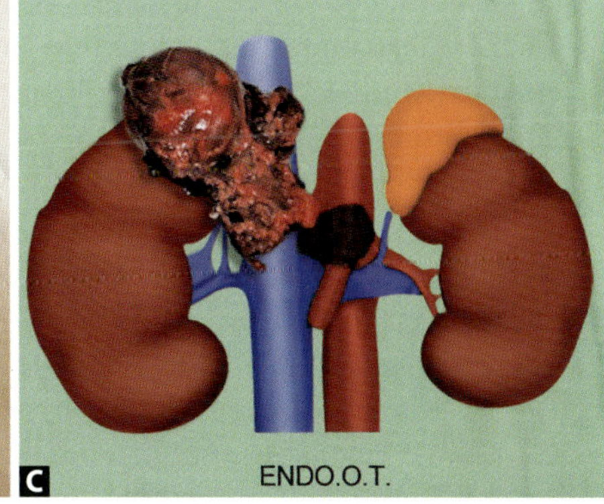

Figs. 4A to C: Neurofibromatosis (NF). *Familial pheochromocytoma (NF-1):* A 26-year-old man presented with hypertension and was found to be having a right adrenal mass with elevated NMN (A); He was also found to be having multiple cafe-au-lait patches over neck and trunk (3 of them >15 mm in diameter) along with multiple neurofibromatosis (1–3 mm) (B); Slit-lamp examination revealed >2 Lisch nodules (≥2 mm), thus fulfilling three criteria to make a clinical diagnosis of NF-1. He underwent right adrenalectomy (C).

Table 3: Results of recent and older studies of cortical sparing adrenalectomy for hereditary PCC.

Author	Patients	Hereditary disorder	Approach	Recurrence	Steroid independent	Follow-up
Kittah et al.[31]	18	MEN, VHL	Endoscopic and open	3	56%	8.5 years
Neuman et al.[32]	324	MEN, VHL	Endoscopic and open	33 (13%)		8 years
Castinetti et al.[33]	114	MEN2	Endoscopic and open	3%	57%	10 years
Grubbs et al.[34]	33	MEN2, VHL	Endoscopic and open	7%	58%	8 years
Alesina et al.[35]	57	MEN2A, VHL	Retroperitoneoscopic and endoscopic	0%	91%	4 years
Lee et al.[36]	14	MEN2A, VHL	Open	21%	93%	11.6 years

(MEN: multiple endocrine neoplasia; PCC: pheochromocytoma; VHL: von Hippel–Lindau)

divided into four clusters based on their similar pathogenesis and biology. Clustering of different genetic mutations helps in personalized care and treatment of such a complex entity as PPGL. These are heterogeneous group of tumors and exhibit different attributes in the following aspects **(Table 4)**:

- Origin
- *Pathogenesis:* Functional, pathogenesis-based classification allows a better understanding of actual tumorigenesis, biochemical profiles, tumor location, and malignant potential. This functional classification of currently established susceptibility genes consists of *four* major groups: the pseudohypoxia group (further subdivided into two groups: the *VHL/EGLN1/EPAS1* related and the tricarboxylic acid cycle related), the kinase signaling group, the Wnt signaling group, and the disease-modifying gene group.
- *Clinical presentation:* PPGLs from PH cluster have less symptoms related to catecholamine excess and instead have signs and symptoms related to local growth such as pain and cranial nerve palsies
- Biochemical profile
- *Location:* Sympathetic PGLs are distributed from base of skull to pelvis; however, parasympathetic PGLs are commonly limited to head and neck area
- Imaging features
- Gene susceptibility
- *Malignancy rates:* Prediction of malignancy is difficult and metastases may develop as late as 20 years.[37,38] Increased risk of malignancy is seen in tumors >5 cm, those secreting methoxytyramine, and those with *SDHB* germline mutation. Pheochromocytoma of the Adrenal Gland Scaled Score (PASS) score is not found to be sensitive enough to predict malignancy; however, GAPP grading is more useful.[39]
- *Metastatic potential:* The management of metastases includes the following:
  - *Metaiodobenzylguanidine (MIBG) therapy:* In two studies,[40,41] mean progression-free survival (PFS) time increased only to 23.1 and 28.5 months. Ultratrace [131]MIBG is thought to be more effective than standard MIBG.
  - *Chemotherapy:* The most common is the CVD regime (cyclophosphamide, vincristine, and dacarbazine).[42]

A study tried to link genomic information with treatment regimes.[43] They replaced dacarbazine with temozolomide (CTD regime) in SDHB-associated PPGL (these tumors lack the enzyme needed to repair DNA alkylating damage caused by temozolomide)

- *Glutaminase inhibitors* in SDH-associated tumors
- *Drugging of hypoxia signaling pathways*—by hypoxia-inducible factor 1α (HIF1α)-inhibitors such as sunitinib and other tyrosine kinase inhibitors (TKIs).
- *90Y or 177 Lu peptide receptor radionuclide therapy (PPRT):* Pseudohypoxic TCH cycle-related PPGLs are unique in having a relatively high expression of type 2 SSTR receptors.
- Long-acting somatostatin analogs such as lanreotide[44]
- *Immune checkpoint inhibitors* such as CTLA4 and PD-L antibodies[45]

Summary

- PPGLs have 40% germline mutations in >20 susceptibility genes.
- All patients with PPGLs should be sent for genetic testing.
- PPGLs are a heterogeneous group of tumors.
- Personalized newer therapies based on genetic mutation are the future.

◇ HPT-JT SYNDROME

It is an autosomal-dominant disorder and is characterized by:

- *HPT (70%):* Unlike other familial HPT disorders, there are some striking features in HPT-JT syndrome. Usually, it is caused by a single adenoma (80%), is frequently cystic, has high incidence of parathyroid carcinoma (20–30%), has underlying CDC73 mutation in as much as 80% cases, and results in complete loss of nuclear parafibromin expression on IHC.[46,47]
- Benign fibro-osseous lesions in mandible and maxilla (25–50%)
- *Benign and malignant uterine lesions (75%):* Polyps, hamartomas, endometrial hyperplasia, endometrial carcinoma, and leiomyomas

- *Renal tumors, renal cysts, renal cell carcinoma, Wilms tumors*: Infrequent

Genetics

The HPT-JT syndrome results from a truncating or mis-sense mutation of *CDC73* gene (cell division cycle 73, formerly known as *HRPT2* gene), which encodes for parafibromin, a 531 amino acid protein with antiproliferative activities. Thus, loss of nuclear parafibromin staining by IHC in any parathyroid adenoma or carcinoma should prompt suspicion for presence of underlying *CDC73* mutation especially in a young child or adolescent patient.[48,49]

Surveillance

Surveillance for carriers of *CDC73* mutation should begin as early as age 5–10 years and should include: (1) Annual biochemical screening for hyperparathyroidism; (2) Dental panoramic films every 5 years; (3) Renal ultrasound every 5 years. Women of reproductive age should be advised to undergo routine gynecologic assessment with uterine ultrasound as clinically indicated (i.e., with menorrhagia or abnormal uterine bleeding).[50]

Management

Management is multidisciplinary including an endocrinologist, a high-volume endocrine surgeon, and a relevant subspecialist for associated lesions. For HPT, surgery is the treatment of choice but the extent and approach of surgery are controversial. From the earlier concept of bilateral exploration and subtotal/total parathyroidectomy, the concept has changed to a more focused and limited parathyroidectomy. Fibrous lesions of maxilla and mandible even though benign have a tendency to grow and cause functional limitations; hence, they need to be surgically treated.[51,52]

◇| HEREDITARY THYROID CANCER

Familial nonmedullary thyroid cancer (FNMTC) is more aggressive than sporadic nonmedullary thyroid cancer (NMTC), being associated with early age of onset, an increased incidence of multiple benign thyroid nodules, multifocality, nodal involvement, LN metastasis, shorter disease-free survival period, and recurrence, among others. Though total thyroidectomy is the treatment of choice, there is no role of prophylactic thyroidectomy. It can be divided into:

- *Familial PTC (FNMTC) (95%)*: The underlying genetic susceptibility is less well defined.
- *Genetic syndromes involving NMTC (5%):* It has well-defined driver mutations.

Familial PTC

The familial non-medullary papillary thyroid cancer (FNMTC) accounts for about 6% of patients with papillary thyroid carcinomas and 10.5% of patients with follicular cell origin thyroid carcinomas. Hereditary features that indicate FNMTC include three or more affected relatives in a kindred, early onset disease, or cancer in men (female predilection is generally observed). Various putative susceptibility genes have been mapped to several chromosomal loci.[53,54]

Genetic Syndromes Involving NMTC

Hereditary NMTC may occur as a minor component of familial cancer syndromes; even though rare, it is important to recognize them to initiate surveillance of family members.

- *Cowden syndrome (multiple hamartoma syndrome, pTEN)*: Follicular thyroid carcinoma is the predominant histopathologic subtype in Cowden syndrome, along with multicentric follicular adenomas, adenomatous nodules, and microadenomas.[55]
- *Familial adenomatous polyposis (FAP; APC)*: Papillary thyroid carcinoma is an extracolonic manifestation of FAP syndrome. The lifetime risk in APC mutation carriers is about 2–12%; young female carriers face about a 160-fold increased risk. Most cases present as bilateral and multifocal cancer and the rare cribriform-morular variant is suggestive of FAP.
- *Carney complex type 1 (Carney complex type 1 PRKAR1), and Carney complex type II with an unknown gene at chromosomal locus 2p16)*: Multiple thyroid nodules, primarily follicular, are seen in up to 75% of individuals with the Carney complex, and papillary or follicular thyroid cancer may occur.
- McCune–Albright syndrome (GNAS1 mosaic)
- Werner syndrome (WRN)[56]

◇| CONCLUSION

It is recommended that patients with MEN syndrome and their families be cared for by centers with expertise such as a multidisciplinary team of endocrinologists, endocrine surgeons, pituitary surgeons, oncologists, gastroenterologists, and geneticists. These patients need special care and have to be given sufficient time in outpatients. They require life-long follow-up. One major issue, particularly in developing countries is to convince the parents of the asymptomatic child to give consent for prophylactic surgery and thus require special handling and counseling. Development of national MEN registries and collaborations to collect important information such as natural history of adrenal lesion in MEN1, geographically prevalent amino acid and codon-based genotype and phenotype correlation, and role of surgery in nonfunctioning pNETs will also help in developing protocols.

Table 4: Features of various PPGL syndromes (Fig. 5).

S. No.	Groups and genes	%	Pathogenesis	Clinical presentation	Biochemistry	PCC >50% Adrenal extra adrenal PCC	High head and neck PGL	Prevalence of malignancy	Treatment	Newer therapy	High SPG	Specific imaging technique
A	*Pseudohypoxia group:* 1. VHL/EGLN-1/ EPAS-1 related	35% 20%		VHL disease Polycythemia PG genes	NMN	High High		1%		HIF-2£ PT2399 R 59949	EPAS High	(hematoma) (genetics) FDG (VHL) DOPA E-pass
	2. Tricarboxylic acid cycle related	15%		PGL syndrome	NMN, Methoxy-tyramine CGA							DOTA-TATE
	SDH complex genes		The mitochondrial enzyme SDH has dual function. It converts succinate to fumarate in tricarboxylic acid (TCA), and participates as a complex II in the respiratory electron transfer within the mitochondrial membrane. Subsequently, FH converts fumarate to malate within the same TCA cycle. Accumulated TCA metabolites—succinate, fumarate, and malate—have oncogenic properties and inhibit enzymes involved in cell signaling and chromatin maintenance	PGL syndrome								
	SDHA		Catalytic subunit	PGL syndrome								
	SDHB	10%	Catalytic subunit	PGL syndrome				High > 50%				
	SDHC		Anchoring subunit	PGL syndrome								
	SDHD	5%	Anchoring subunit	PGL syndrome			High					
	SDHAF2 (SDH5)		Cofactor for complex II leading to flavination of SDHA	PGL syndrome		High						
	FH	<1%	TCA cycle enzyme, which converts fumarate to malate	Handling								
	MDH2			RCC PCC/PGL								

Contd...

Contd...

S. No.	Groups and genes	%	Pathogenesis	Clinical presentation	Biochemistry	PCC>50% Adrenal extra adrenal PCC	High head and neck PGL	Prevalence of malignancy	Treatment	Newer therapy	High SPG	Specific imaging technique
B	**Kinase-signaling**	**60%**										*DOPA PET*
	RET	5%		MEN 2A/2B		....	High	5%				
	NF1	1%		NF1 syndrome		....	Low	10%				
	MAX		MAX is a transcription factor heterodimerizes with MYC to control cellular proliferation, differentiation, and apoptosis	PCC-bil			High					
	TMEM127		The protein is a negative regulator of mTOR, which is a PI3K kinase, and associated with increased cell proliferation and angiogenesis.				High					
	HRAS	—		PCC/ EAPGL			High					
	EPAS1		An increase in the transcriptional activity of HIF-2 alpha genes (VEGF), but the actual transcriptional signature different from the one associated with VHL									
	MDH2		TCA cycle enzyme which converts malate to oxaloacetate further down in the TCA cycle									
	NF-1		Its main function as a tumor suppressor is RAS GTPase which deactivates RAS, thus preventing activation of the oncogenic RAS-RAF-MEK signaling cascade			....						
	RET		Prevents tumorigenesis through activation of the tyrosine kinase, which signals through the PI3K pathway			....						
	VHL		The product of VHL is a von Hippel–Lindau tumor suppressor protein (pVHL), which serves as a component of an E3 ubiquitin ligase complex 3E which inactivates hypoxia-inducible factors to control transcription of genes involved in angiogenesis such as GLUT-1, VEGF									

(MEN: multiple endocrine neoplasia; PCC: pheochromocytoma; PGL: paraganglioma; SDH: succinate dehydrogenase; VEGF: vascular endothelial growth factor)

◇ REFERENCES

1. Yokoyama A, Cleary ML. Menin critically links MLL proteins with LEDGF on cancer-associated target genes. Cancer Cell. 2008;14:36-46.

2. Thakker RV, Newey PJ, Walls GV, Bilezikian J, Dralle H, Ebeling PR, et al. Clinical Practice Guidelines for Multiple Endocrine Neoplasia Type 1 (MEN1). J Clin Endocrinol Metab. 2012;97(9):2990-3011.

3. Brandi ML, Gagel RF, Angeli A, Bilezikian JP, Beck-Peccoz P, Bordi C, et al. Guidelines for diagnosis and therapy of MEN type 1 and type 2. J Clin Endocrinol Metab. 2001;86:5658-71.

4. Thakker RV. Multiple endocrine neoplasia type 1. In: De Groot L, Jameson JL (Eds). Endocrinology, 6th edition. Philadelphia: Elsevier; 2010. pp. 2719-41.

5. Machens A, Schaaf L, Karges W, Frank-Raue K, Bartsch DK, Rothmund M, et al. Age-related penetrance of endocrine tumours in multiple endocrine neoplasia type 1 (MEN1): a multicentre study of 258 gene carriers. Clin Endocrinol (Oxf). 2007;67:613-22.

6. Schreinemakers JM, Pieterman CR, Scholten A, Vriens MR, Valk GD, Rinkes IH. The optimal surgical treatment for primary hyperparathyroidism in MEN1 patients: a systematic review. World J Surg. 2011;35:1993-2005.

7. Waldmann J, Lóʹpez CL, Langer P, Rothmund M, Bartsch DK. Surgery for multiple endocrine neoplasia type 1-associated primary hyperparathyroidism. Br J Surg. 2010;97: 1528-34.

8. Jensen RTCG, Brandi ML, de Herder WW, Kaltsas G, Komminoth P, Scoazec JY, et al. ENETS consensus guidelines for the management of patients with digestive neuroendocrine neoplasms: functional pancreatic endocrine tumor syndromes. Neuroendocrinology. 2012;95(2):98-119.

9. Kulke MHAL, Bushnell DL, de Herder WW, Goldsmith SJ, Klimstra DS, Marx SJ, et al. NANETS treatment guidelines: well-differentiated neuroendocrine tumors of the stomach and pancreas. Pancreas. 2010;9(6):735-52.

10. Kunz PLR-LD, Anthony LB, Bertino EM, Brendtro K, Chan JA, Chen H, et al. Consensus guidelines for the management and treatment of neuroendocrine tumors. Pancreas. 2013;42(4): 557-77.

11. Thomas-Marques L, Murat A, Delemer B, Penfornis A, Cardot Bauters C, Baudin E, et al. Prospective endoscopic ultrasonographic evaluation of the frequency of nonfunctioning pancreaticoduodenal endocrine tumors in patients with multiple endocrine neoplasia type 1. Am J Gastroenterol. 2006;101:266-73.

12. Teh BTMJ, Chan SP, Menon J, Hartley L, Pullan P, Ho J, et al. Clinicopathologic studies of thymic carcinoids in multiple endocrine neoplasia type 1. Medicine. 1997;76:21-9.

13. Melmed S. Pathogenesis of pituitary tumors. Nat Rev Endocrinol. 2011;7:257-66.

14. Beckers A, Betea D, Valdes Socin H, Stevenaert A. The treatment of sporadic versus MEN1-related pituitary adenomas. J Intern Med. 2003;253:599-605.

15. Burgess JR, Shepherd JJ, Parameswaran V, Hoffman L, Greenaway TM. Spectrum of pituitary disease in multiple endocrine neoplasia type 1 (MEN 1): clinical, biochemical, and radiological features of pituitary disease in a large MEN 1 kindred. J Clin Endocrinol Metab. 1996;81:2642-6.

16. Lemos MC, Thakker RV. Multiple endocrine neoplasia type 1 (MEN1): analysis of 1336 mutations reported in the first decade following identification of the gene. Hum Mutat. 2008;29:22-32.

17. Marx SJ. New concepts about familial isolated hyperparathyroidism. J Clin Endocrinol Metab. 2019;104: 4058-66.

18. Asai N, Iwashita T, Matsuyama M, Takahashi M. Mechanism of activation of the ret proto-oncogene by multiple endocrine neoplasia 2A mutations. Mol Cell Biol. 1995;15:1613-9.

19. Kjaer S, Kurokawa K, Perrinjaquet M, Abrescia C, Ibanez CF. Self-association of the transmembrane domain of RET underlies oncogenic activation by MEN2A mutations. Oncogene. 2006;25:7086-95.

20. O'Riordain DS, O Brian T, Grant CS, Weaver A, Gharib H, van Heerden JA. Surgical management of primary hyperparathyroidism in multiple endocrine neoplasia type 1 and 2. Surgery. 1993;114:1031-9.

21. Kraimps JL, Denizot A, Carnaille B, Henry JF, Proye C, Bacourt F, et al. Primary hyperparathyroidism in multiple endocrine neoplasia type IIa: retrospective French multicentric study. Groupe d'Etude des Tumeurs á Calcitonine (GETC, French Calcitonin Tumors Study Group), French Association of Endocrine Surgeons. World J Surg. 1996;20(7):808-12.

22. Raue F, Kraimps JL, Dralle H, Cougard P, Proye C, Frilling A, et al. Primary hyperparathyroidism in multiple endocrine neoplasia type 2A. J Intern Med. 1995;238(4):369-73.

23. Herfarth KK, Bartsch D, Doherty GM, Wells SA Jr, Lairmore TC. Surgical management of hyperparathyroidism in patients with multiple endocrine neoplasia type 2A. Surgery. 1996;120(6):966-73.

24. Skinner MA, Moley JA, Dilley WG, Owzar K, DeBenedetti MK, Wells SA. Prophylactic thyroidectomy in multiple endocrine neoplasia type 2. N Engl J Med. 2005;353:1105-13.

25. Schreinemakers JM, Vriens MR, Valk GD, de Groot JW, Plukker JT, Bax K, et al. Factors predicting outcome of total thyroidectomy in young patients with multiple endocrine neoplasia type 2: a nationwide long-term follow-up study. World J Surg. 2010;34:852-60.

26. Quayle FJ, Fialkowski EA, Benveniste R, Moley JF. Pheochromocytoma penetrance varies by RET mutation in MEN 2A. Surgery. 2007;142:800-5.

27. Wells SA Jr, Asa SL, Dralle H, Elisei R, Evans DB, Gagel RF, et al. Revised American Thyroid Association guidelines for the management of medullary thyroid carcinoma. Thyroid. 2015;25(6):567-610.

28. Machens A, Brauckhoff M, Holzhausen HJ, Thanh PN, Lehnert H, Dralle H. Codon-specific development of pheochromocytoma in multiple endocrine neoplasia type 2. J Clin Endocrinol Metab. 2005;90:3999-4003.

29. Brauckhoff M, Gimm O, Thanh PN, Bar A, Ukkat J, Brauckhoff K, et al. Critical size of residual adrenal tissue and recovery from impaired early postoperative adrenocortical function after subtotal bilateral adrenalectomy. Surgery. 2003;134:1020-7; discussion 1027-8.

30. Castinetti F, Taieb D, Henry JF, Walz M, Guerin C, Brue T, et al. Outcome of adrenal sparing surgery in heritable pheochromocytoma. Eur J Endocrinol. 2016;174:R9-R18.

31. Kittah NE, Gruber LM, Bancos I, Hamidi O, Tamhane S, Iñiguez-Ariza N, et al. Bilateral pheochromocytoma: clinical characteristics, treatment and longitudinal follow-up. Clin Endocrinol (Oxf). 2020;93(3):288-95.

32. Neumann HPH, Tsoy U, Bancos I, Amodru V, Walz MK, Tirosh A, et al. Comparison of pheochromocytoma-specific morbidity and mortality among adults with bilateral pheochromocytomas undergoing total adrenalectomy vs cortical-sparing adrenalectomy. JAMA Netw Open. 2019;2(8):e198898.

33. Castinetti F, Qi XP, Walz MK, Maia AL, Sansó G, Peczkowska M, et al. Outcomes of adrenal-sparing surgery or total adrenalectomy in phaeochromocytoma associated with multiple endocrine neoplasia type 2: an international retrospective population-based study. Lancet Oncol. 2014;15(6):648-55.

34. Grubbs EG, Rich TA, Ng C, Bhosale PR, Jimenez C, Evans DB, et al. Long-term outcomes of surgical treatment for hereditary pheochromocytoma. J Am Coll Surg. 2013;216:280-9.

35. Alesina PF, Hinrichs J, Meier B, Schmid KW, Neumann HP, Walz MK. Minimally invasive cortical-sparing surgery for bilateral pheochromocytomas. Langenbeck's Arch Surg. 2012;397:233-8.

36. Lee JE, Curley SA, Gagel RF, Evans DB, Hickey RC. Cortical-sparing adrenalectomy for patients with bilateral pheochromocytoma. Surgery. 1996;120:1064-70; discussion 1070-61.

37. Chen H, Sippel RS, O'Dorisio MS, Vinik AI, Lloyd RV, Pacak K, et al. The North American Neuroendocrine Tumor Society consensus guideline for the diagnosis and management of neuroendocrine tumors: pheochromocytoma, paraganglioma, and medullary thyroid cancer. Pancreas. 2010;39(6):775-83.

38. Pacak K. Preoperative management of the pheochromocytoma patient. J Clin Endocrinol Metab. 2007;92(11):4069-79.

39. Kimura N, Takayanagi R, Takizawa N, Itagaki E, Katabami T, Kakoi N, et al. Pathological grading for predicting metastasis in phaeochromocytoma and paraganglioma. Endocr Relat Cancer. 2014;21:405-14.

40. van Hulsteijn LT, Niemeijer ND, Dekkers OM, Corssmit EPM. ^{131}I-MIBG therapy for malignant paraganglioma and phaeochromocytoma: systematic review and meta-analysis. Clin Endocrinol (Oxf). 2014;80:487-501.

41. Yoshinaga K, Oriuchi N, Wakabayashi H, Tomiyama Y, Jinguji M, Higuchi T, et al. Effects and safety of ^{131}I-metaiodobenzylguanidine (MIBG) radiotherapy in malignant neuroendocrine tumors: results from a multicenter observational registry. Endocr J. 2014;61:1171-80.

42. Niemeijer ND, Alblas G, van Hulsteijn LT, Dekkers OM, Corssmit EPM. Chemotherapy with cyclophosphamide, vincristine and dacarbazine for malignant paraganglioma and pheochromocytoma: systematic review and meta-analysis. Clin Endocrinol (Oxf). 2014;81:642-51.

43. Hadoux J, Favier J, Scoazec JY, Leboulleux S, Al Ghuzlan A, Caramella C, et al. SDHB mutations are associated with response to temozolomide in patients with metastatic pheochromocytoma or paraganglioma. Int J Cancer. 2014;135:2711-20.

44. Caplin ME, Pavel M, Cwikla JB, Phan AT, Raderer M, Sedlackova E, et al. Lanreotide in metastatic enteropancreatic neuroendocrine tumors. N Engl L Med. 2014;371:224-33.

45. Mandal R, Chan TA. Personalized oncology meets immunology: the path toward precision immunotherapy. Cancer Discov. 2016; 6:703-13

46. Kutcher MR, Rigby MH, Bullock M, Trites J, Taylor SM, Hart RD. Hyperparathyroidism-jaw tumor syndrome. Head Neck. 2013;35(6):E175-7.

47. Juhlin CC, Haglund F, Obara T, Arnold A, Larsson C, Höög A, et al. Absence of nucleolar parafibromin immunoreactivity in subsets of parathyroid malignant tumours. Virchows Arch Int J Pathol. 2011;459:47-53.

48. Gill AJ, Clarkson A, Gimm O, Keil J, Dralle H, Howell VM, et al. Loss of nuclear expression of parafibromin distinguishes parathyroid carcinomas and hyperparathyroidism-jaw tumor (HPT-JT) syndrome-related adenomas from sporadic parathyroid adenomas and hyperplasias. Am J Surg Pathol. 2006;30(9):1140-9.

49. Cetani F, Ambrogini E, Viacava P, Pardi E, Fanelli G, Naccarato AG, et al. Should parafibromin staining replace HRTP2 gene analysis as an additional tool for histologic diagnosis of parathyroid carcinoma? Eur J Endocrinol. 2007;156(5): 547-54.

50. Wasserman JD, Tomlinson GE, Druker H, Kamihara J, Kohlmann WK, Kratz CP, et al. Multiple endocrine neoplasia and hyperparathyroid-jaw tumor syndromes: clinical features, genetics, and surveillance recommendations in childhood. Clin Cancer Res. 2017;23(13):e123-32.

51. Iacobone M, Barzon L, Porzionato A, Masi G, Macchi V, Viel G, et al. The extent of parathyroidectomy for HRPT2-related hyperparathyroidism. Surgery. 2009;145(2):250-1.

52. Iacobone M, Camozzi V, Mian C, Pennelli G, Pagetta C, Ide EC, et al. Long-term outcomes of parathyroidectomy in hyperparathyroidism-jaw tumor syndrome: analysis of five families with CDC73 mutations. World J Surg. 2020;44(2): 508-16.

53. Pal T, Vogl FD, Chappuis PO, Tsang R, Brierley J, Renard H, et al. Increased risk for nonmedullary thyroid cancer in the first-degree relatives of prevalent cases of nonmedullary thyroid cancer: a hospital-based study. J Clin Endocrinol Metab. 2001;86:5307-12.

54. Hemminki K, Eng C, Chen B. Familial risks for nonmedullary thyroid cancer. J Clin Endocrinol Metab. 2005;90:5747-53.

55. Harach HR, Soubeyran I, Brown A, Bonneau D, Longy M. Thyroid pathologic findings in patients with Cowden disease. Ann Diagn Pathol. 1999;3:331-40.

56. Yang SP, Ngeow J. Familial non-medullary thyroid cancer: unraveling the genetic maze. Endocr Relat Cancer. 2016;23(12):R577-95.

CHAPTER 39

Laboratory Evaluation of Endocrine Tumors

Pooja Ramakant, Manish Gutch, Chanchal Rana, Shreyamsa M, Sasi Mouli

INTRODUCTION

Laboratory evaluation of all the endocrine tumors begins with biochemical evaluation. To localize the tumor, anatomical and functional imaging methods are used. We will describe the full comprehensive workup of various endocrine tumors including thyroid, parathyroid, adrenal, pancreas, and pituitary.

LABORATORY EVALUATION OF A PATIENT PRESENTING WITH A THYROID NODULE

The laboratory evaluation of a patient presenting to our outpatient clinic with a thyroid nodule begins with testing of thyroid function, which is an indispensable part of the investigative battery. Along with function, the laboratory investigations also aim at assessing the structural changes, extent of disease, and response to treatment.

PHYSIOLOGICAL BASIS OF THE THYROID FUNCTION TESTS

Thyroid homeostasis is maintained by hypothalamic-pituitary-thyroid axis.[1] The biochemical investigations use this pathway to assess the thyroid functioning. The thyroid hormones [triiodothyronine (T3) and thyroxine (T4)] are produced by the follicular cells of the gland under stimulation of thyrotropin [thyroid-stimulating hormone (TSH)] from the pituitary. TSH secretion is regulated by a hypothalamic hormone thyrotropin-releasing hormone (TRH). T3 and T4 inhibit production of TSH and TRH by means of a negative feedback loop. The thyroid hormones are present in the blood in two forms, bound and free. The bound form makes up nearly 99.6% of all thyroid hormones and the binding occurs with thyroxine-binding globulin (TBG), transthyretin (TTR), and albumin.[2] Protein-bound hormones are incapable of crossing plasma membranes and are hence inactive while the free form can act on target receptors bringing about physiological changes. In addition to these hormones, parafollicular cells produce calcitonin (Ctn), a hormone involved in calcium metabolism.[3]

THYROID FUNCTION TESTS

Thyroid function tests are the most commonly used diagnostic tests in evaluation of endocrine disorders.[4] These tests serve the following functions:

- Screening
- Diagnosis of euthyroid state, hypothyroidism, or hyperthyroidism
- Assess adequacy of treatment
- Follow-up in patients diagnosed with having thyroid cancer.

These tests also assess the associated pathophysiological processes **(Table 1)**.

Measurement of TSH and T4 [in the form of free thyroxine (fT4)] forms the core thyroid function tests. T3 is also frequently measured. These tests are mostly based on automated immunoassays, but recently liquid chromatography-tandem mass spectrometry (LC-MS/MS) techniques have also been used for measuring the free thyroid hormones and urinary iodine.[5] It is generally difficult to measure free hormones as they require assays that are free from interference by much higher concentration of total hormones.[6,7] The measurement of serum concentrations of total hormones and thyroglobulin (Tg) have standardized reference values while those for TSH, free hormones and urinary iodine still remain challenging.[8]

Table 1: Various tests used to assess the function of pathophysiological processes.

Function assessed	Tests
Hypothalamic-pituitary-thyroid axis	• Thyroid-stimulating hormone (TSH) • Serum total triiodothyronine • Serum total thyroxine • Serum free thyroxine • Serum free tri-iodothyronine • Thyrotropin-releasing hormone
Autoimmunity of thyroid	• TSH receptor antibody • Thyroglobulin antibody • Thyroid peroxidase antibody
Surveillance/follow-up	• Serum thyroglobulin • Serum calcitonin
Iodine uptake/metabolism	• Radioactive iodine uptake study • Urinary iodine

Thyroid-stimulating Hormone

Thyroid-stimulating hormone is a 28-kDa glycoprotein hormone secreted by thyrotrophs of anterior pituitary. Structurally, it consists of α and β subunits that are covalently bound.[9] The testing of thyroid function usually starts with TSH, as minimal changes in peripheral hormones result in exponential TSH response, which can be measured. This renders TSH a valid indicator of thyroid functional status, but a suboptimal measure of disease severity.

The accuracy and sensitivity of tests measuring TSH have improved considerably over time. The "first-generation" assays employed radioimmunoassay (RIA) techniques and carried a sensitivity of 1 mIU/L, but this was not enough to determine the lower limits to identify hyperthyroidism, especially in mild thyrotoxicosis.[10] These TSH-RIAs cross-reacted with gonadotropins and human chorionic gonadotropin (hCG) due to the shared α subunits and hence their clinical utility was restricted to the diagnosis of primary hypothyroidism. The immunometric assays (IMAs) which used monoclonal antibodies for detection of TSH replaced the RIA methods, forming the "second generation" of tests. These tests detected TSH at level 0.1 mIU/L and reliably detected low TSH values.[11] With further improvements in monoclonal antibody technology and changes in IMA techniques, the "third-generation" (ultrasensitive) assays are able to detect serum TSH as low as 0.01 mIU/L. Automated third-generation IMA-TSH assays are the standard of care at present. Fourth and fifth assays, which carry a sensitivity of 0.001 mIU/L, have been developed, but not widely available yet.

The sensitivity of current TSH assays very uncommonly suffer artifact interference due to heterophilic antibodies in the presence of contamination the sample or animal immunoglobulins used on the assay.[12] Many drugs used for related or unrelated conditions also affect the TSH levels in an individual **(Table 2)**.[13] Pregnancy also affects TSH measurements in the first trimester due to hCG stimulation of TSH. Normal levels of TSH still remain a debatable topic. Large population studies have found that ethnicity, gender,

body mass index, and iodine intake status can affect TSH levels.[14] The American Thyroid Association (ATA) and the American Association of Clinical Endocrinologists (AACE) recommend a value of 0.4–4 mIU/L as normal reference range for measurement of TSH.[15,16] However, an age-based reference would be ideal.

Current guidelines recommend that serum TSH should be used as first-line test for all nodular diseases and overt or subclinical thyroid dysfunction (hypothyroidism or hyperthyroidism) in a patient assumed to have an intact hypothalamic and pituitary function.[17,18] In a patient with nodular disease, patients with normal TSH levels do not require any further laboratory investigations, but will need imaging and cytological investigations. When TSH is beyond normal levels, further workup in the form of hormonal assessment is imperative. In patients with hypothalamic or pituitary abnormalities, serum TSH will be found within normal limits and concomitant evaluation of thyroid hormones is necessary for evaluation of the underlying disease.

Thyroid Hormones

- *Total thyroid hormones*: Approximately 0.04% of all T4 and 0.4% of all T3 in serum are found in an unbound form while the remaining majority is protein bound.[4] TBG binds 75% of all available T4 while TTR binds 20% and albumin about 5–10%.[19] Protein binding helps in distribution of the hormones throughout the body and releasing the hormones by unbinding at tissue sites based on the need.[20] T4 under physiological conditions is present at concentrations about tenfold higher than T3. Like the TSH assays, techniques of thyroid hormone measurements have also undergone tremendous improvements over time starting from RIA to the currently available LC-MS/MS. These tests for estimation of total hormone levels are adequately accurate and specific, but not always reliable, as factors affecting binding protein concentrations interfere with the tests yielding false levels **(Table 3)**.[21,22] These binding protein abnormalities affect the use of total hormones as stand-alone tests. Whenever possible, total hormones should be accompanied by a test for assessment of binding protein status.
- *Free thyroid hormones*: The free (unbound) fraction is responsible for biological activity of thyroid hormones; hence, it should reflect the biological effects of thyroid hormones better than the total hormone levels, but the extremely low concentrations of free hormones in the serum make measurement of these a challenging task, even with modern techniques and methods. The methods for measurement of free hormones are broadly classified into two types.[5,23] *Direct methods* (equilibrium dialysis, ultrafiltration) employ physical separation technique of free and bound hormones. These methods are expensive and technically challenging. They can be influenced by endogenous inhibitors of binding proteins, dilution, and

Table 2: Drugs used to decrease or increase thyroid-stimulating hormone (TSH).	
Drugs that decrease TSH	*Drugs that increase TSH*
• Thyroid hormones • Somatostatin analogs • Glucocorticoids • Dopamine analogs • Cytokines • Serotonin antagonists • Selective serotonin reuptake inhibitors • Rexinoids • Histamine receptor blockers • Alpha-adrenergic blockers • Benzodiazepines	• Thyrotropin-releasing hormone • Opioids • Dopamine receptor antagonists • Amphetamines • Ephedrine • Theophylline • Glucocorticoid synthesis inhibitors (ketoconazole, mitotane, and aminoglutethimide) • Haloperidol • Chlorpromazine

Table 3: Factors affecting the binding protein concentration.

	Increased TBG	*Decreased TBG*	*TTR or albumin abnormalities*
Drugs	• Estrogens • Selective estrogen receptor modulators • 5-fluorouracil • Clofibrate • Nicotinic acid	• Antiandrogens • Anabolic steroids • L-asparaginase	–
Physiological conditions	Pregnancy	–	Pregnancy
Pathological conditions	• Hypothyroidism • Hepatitis • Adrenal insufficiency • Acute intermittent porphyria • Acquired immunodeficiency syndrome	• Hyperthyroidism • Sepsis • Diabetic ketoacidosis • Nephrotic syndrome • Chronic alcoholism • Acromegaly • Cushing's syndrome • Malnutrition	• Nonthyroidal illnesses • Malnutrition
Familial/congenital conditions	TBG excess (X-linked)	• *TBG* gene defects • Carbohydrate-deficient glycoprotein syndrome (type I)	• Familial dysalbuminemic hyperthyroxinemia • TTR-associated hyperthyroxinemia

(TBG: thyroxine-binding globulin; TTR: transthyretin)

heat leading to false results.[24] *Estimate testing* methods (two test index, free hormone immunoassay) physically separate free from bound hormones before measuring free hormones by immunoassays. These tests are protein dependent, hence prone to errors if binding protein abnormalities exist. No single method is universally validated for all clinical utilization.

From a clinical perspective, in a patient with low serum TSH suggestive of hyperthyroidism, an fT4 measurement should be performed. When elevated, it confirms thyrotoxicosis. A total T4 assay is generally avoided due to risk of binding protein abnormalities. Similarly, in a case of nodular disease, increased fT4 suggests an autonomously functioning nodule, a hyperfunctioning gland, or a toxic multinodular goiter. A radioiodine uptake scan will help diagnosing the above.[25] fT3 measurement in a regular scenario is usually unnecessary, since fT4 along with TSH adequately assesses thyroid hormone deficiency or excess. fT3 measurement is useful where fT4/TSH assays are discordant and in states characterized by peripheral T3 secretion, viz., Graves' disease or toxic adenoma.[26]

◇ TESTS IN AUTOIMMUNE CONDITIONS OF THYROID

The response of immune cells to thyroid antigens can result in autoimmune thyroid diseases (AITDs). Tests for these antibodies are vital to the diagnosis of AITDs. Patients with Graves' disease have elevated TSH receptor antibodies (TSHRAbs), which are a type of thyroid-stimulating immunoglobulins (TSIs). Thyroid peroxidase antibodies (TPOAbs) as well as the thyroglobulin antibodies (TgAbs) are responsible for autoimmune hypothyroidism.

Thyroid-stimulating Hormone Receptor Antibodies

Binding of TSH to its receptors activates cyclic adenosine monophosphate production and in turn stimulation of thyrocyte. Two major types of TSHRAb are found, namely (1) the thyroid-stimulating antibodies (TSAbs) and (2) the thyroid blocking antibodies (TBAbs). Presence of a neutral type of antibodies has also been described.[27] Graves' disease is typically confirmed with a TSHRAb titer. Two methods are used to assess the TSHRAbs, namely (1) the bioassays and (2) the receptor assays. Bioassays assess the functionality of antibodies and, hence, distinguish between TSIs and TBAbs. The receptor (binding) assays detect antibodies at receptor, but do not measure their functionality, hence do not distinguish between the two types. However, assays for TBAbs are not available for routine clinical use. A TSHRAb titer of <1.5 IU/L is considered as normal.[28] Patients with a titer of >12 IU/L at diagnosis are known to be at risk for relapses after therapy.

Thyroid Peroxidase Antibodies

Thyroid peroxidase, a glycoprotein, catalyzes iodination of tyrosine residues and their subsequent coupling that finally leads to the formation of the thyroid hormones. TPOAbs are a characteristic finding of autoimmune thyroiditis (AT) and very uncommonly in few normal individuals.[29] They can be detected in the serum of 90–95% of AT patients (Hashimoto's disease), approximately 80% of patients with Graves' disease, and 10–15% of patients with non-AITD.[30] TPOAbs are usually not associated with malignancy. TPOAb assessment is performed when AT is clinically suspected. However, the absence of TPOAb does not exclude thyroiditis as they are undetectable in a small subgroup of patients.

Thyroglobulin Antibodies

Thyroglobulin antibodies are present in 70–80% of patients with AT, 30–40% of patients with Graves' disease, and 10–15% of patients with nonthyroid autoimmune diseases.[30] Mere presence of TgAb does not correlate with abnormal TSH levels, hence it is not recommended to test for TgAb in AITD screening.[31] In patients with indications of AITD, however, testing both TPOAb and TgAb is found to be beneficial.[32] TgAb interferes with Tg tests, even the ultrasensitive ones. This effect is relevant for interpretation of the test in patients with differentiated thyroid cancer, wherein Tg is a critical marker and monitoring tool postsurgery.[31]

◇ TESTS IN SURVEILLANCE/FOLLOW-UP OF THYROID MALIGNANCIES

Thyroglobulin

Thyroglobulin is a glycoprotein which forms the backbone of thyroid hormone synthesis. It is stored in colloid and some amount of Tg is always released into the circulation during hormone synthesis, hence detectable in most individuals. In a normal individual, the levels of serum Tg is generally 20–25 ng/mL (1 ng/mL per 1 g of thyroid mass).[33] Concentrations of Tg in the serum reflect three factors: (1) thyroid mass, (2) possible injury to thyroid, and (3) extent of TSH stimulation. After ablation or extirpation of thyroid for differentiated thyroid carcinoma (DTC), Tg should be undetectable. Its subsequent appearance signifies either persistent or recurrence.

Serum Tg is useful in the follow-up management of DTC as it is a sensitive marker of recurrence. In patients with DTC, the levels of serum Tg is directly proportional to the mass of malignant tissue. The Tg secretion also depends on TSH.[34] When the levels of serum TSH are stable during follow-up, any changes in serum Tg levels reflect a change in the tumor mass. Typically, a serum Tg level <0.2 ng/mL in absence of TSH stimulation and <1 ng/mL with withdrawal of TSH suppression are acceptable in patients with DTC on follow-up (ATA guidelines).

Calcitonin

Calcitonin, a 32 amino acid linear polypeptide hormone, is produced by parafollicular C cells. It is a tumor marker of medullary thyroid carcinoma (MTC) and correlates with tumor burden. Serum Ctn levels may be elevated in patients with chronic renal failure, hyperparathyroidism (HPT), AT, small cell and large cell lung cancers, prostate cancer, mastocytosis, and various enteric and pulmonary neuroendocrine tumors,[35] but the serum Ctn levels in these conditions do not increase in response to calcium or pentagastrin stimulation. When compared to MTC, the non-MTC lesions usually produce less Ctn per gram of tissue.[36] Depending on the type of assay used, 56–88% of normal persons have serum Ctn levels below the functional sensitivity while 3–10% have Ctn levels >10 pg/mL.[37] Increasing levels of Ctn are directly proportional to aggressiveness of the disease.

Fine-needle Aspiration

Fine-needle aspiration cytology (FNAC) of thyroid lesions has now been established as an essential investigation worldwide in determining the nature of thyroid lesions.[38] This is a rapid method of diagnosis and not only avoids unnecessary surgeries thereby relieving the psychological as well as financial burden to the patients, especially in benign nodules, but also helps the surgeons to appropriately triage the patients with malignant condition for appropriate interventions. FNA is safe and accurate as a diagnostic tool in thyroid lesions with sensitivity of 93.4%, positive predictive value of malignancy 98.6%, and specificity of 74.9%.[39,40] FNA using ultrasound guidance is favored for nodules that are nonpalpable, located deeply/posteriorly in the thyroid bed, or have a predominantly cystic component.[41]

Indications

Fine-needle aspiration in thyroid lesion is primarily indicated in following scenario:[42,43]

- Nodules ≥1 cm in greatest dimension with high-to-intermediate suspicion sonography pattern.
- Nodules with ≥1.5 cm and ≥2 cm in greatest dimension for low and very low suspicion ultrasonography pattern, respectively.
- For confirmation and, characterization of clinically obvious thyroid malignancy
- To provide material for ancillary genetic tests.

There is generally no contraindication for thyroid FNAC. Local hemorrhage may happen occasionally due to needling; however, complications like carotid hematoma, transient vocal cord paralysis, acute suppurative thyroiditis, chemical neuritis, and puncture of trachea are uncommon and rare.[44-47] Use of fine caliber needle and gentle needling technique may further avoid these complications and make the procedure safer and comfortable for patients.

Limitation of Thyroid Fine-needle Aspiration

Cytodiagnosis is generally accurate in most of the situations, except for the inability to differentiate between follicular adenoma and carcinoma. FNA thyroid has certain limitations and can have false-positive or false-negative results. The common causes of false-negative results are: follicular adenoma mistaken for adenomatous goiter, cystic lesions harboring malignancy, low- and intermediate-grade lymphomas in background of lymphocytic thyroiditis, malignancies with marked necrosis, and focal involvement of glands or inadequate. Performing FNA under ultrasound guidance can minimize the false-negative rate.[48,49]

A false-positive diagnosis can be also be given in situations like cellular colloid goiter mistaken for follicular neoplasm or chronic lymphocytic thyroiditis misdiagnosed for malignant lymphoma.[50]

Cytological Reporting of Thyroid Diseases

Thyroid nodule FNAC should be reported as per the Bethesda System for Reporting Thyroid Cytopathology (TBSRTC). In 2007, the National Cancer Institute (NCI) hosted a conference in Bethesda and *TBSRTC* was developed, thereby developing a uniform terminologies for reporting thyroid cytology.[51]

In 2017, this system has been revised with addition of molecular testing as an adjunct to FNAC. With TBSRTC, the thyroid lesions are categorized in six diagnostic categories each of which has its own implied risk of malignancy **(Table 4)**.[52] TBSTRC is now the most robust and widely used reporting system for thyroid lesions.

Core Needle Biopsy

Core needle biopsy (CNB) was introduced in 1990s.[53] With the advent of thinner needle, automatic devices, improved techniques, and high-resolution ultrasound machines, CNB may be useful in patients with previous FNA results of nondiagnostic and atypia of undetermined significance.[54,55] Studies have documented significantly lower inadequacy rates in CNB as compared to FNAC.[56,57]

Advantages of Core Needle Biopsy

- The tissue obtained by CNB provides more robust material than FNA cytology.
- We can also do along with a histologic examination, immunohistochemistry, and molecular testing when required.
- Lymphoma, MTC, anaplastic thyroid carcinoma, and parathyroid lesions can be diagnosed with CNB based on histologic morphology in conjunction with immunohistochemistry.

- Useful in situations with paucicellular FNA due to presence of calcified/degenerating nodules, marked fibrosis, sclerosis, etc.

Limitations of Core Needle Biopsy[58]

- Inability to differentiate between follicular adenoma and carcinoma.
- Inability to differentiate between noninvasive follicular thyroid neoplasm with papillary-like nuclear features and invasive follicular variant of PTC.
- Costly, more technical, and lengthy reporting procedure as compared to FNA.

Role of Specialized Techniques in Thyroid Pathology

In recent years, objective measures that differentiate benign from malignant lesions mainly include immunohistochemical markers and molecular markers, using gene expression, somatic mutation, and microRNA analyses.[58]

- *Immunohistochemistry*: Immunohistochemical markers can be divided into organ-specific marker as well as markers used for differential diagnosis. In poorly differentiated or undifferentiated tumor, immunohistochemical biomarkers play an active diagnostic role.

  Table 5 enumerated the various markers commonly used in context with diagnostic dilemma in thyroid nodules.[58,59]

  The most commonly proposed panel is galectin-3 (GAL-3), Hector Battifora mesothelial-1 (HBME-1), and cytokeratin 19 (CK19) to differentiate between benign and malignant lesions of thyroid. Tg and thyroid transcription factor-1 (TTF-1) may be used to identify thyroidal origin at metastatic site.[60]

- *Molecular diagnostics in thyroid neoplasm:* The role of molecular testing in thyroid is to minimize overtreatment in indeterminate thyroid nodules and to provide prognostic information thereby leading to proper surgical and therapeutic decisions. **Table 6** gives brief review of various genetic abnormalities along with their average incidence on different types of thyroid cancers.[60,61]

	Risk of malignancy if NIFTP ≠ CA (%)	Risk of malignancy if NIFTP = CA (%)	Usual management
Diagnostic category			
Nondiagnostic or unsatisfactory	5–10	5–10	Repeat FNA with ultrasound guidance
Benign	0–3	0–3	Clinical and sonographic follow-up
Atypia of undetermined significance or follicular lesion of undetermined significance	6–18	~10–30	Repeat FNA, molecular testing, or lobectomy
Follicular neoplasm or suspicious for a follicular neoplasm	10–40	25–40	Molecular testing, lobectomy
Suspicious for malignancy	45–60	–75	Near-total thyroidectomy or lobectomy
Malignant	94–96	97–99	Near-total thyroidectomy or lobectomy

Table 4: The 2017 Bethesda System for Reporting Thyroid Cytopathology: Implied risk of malignancy and recommended clinical management.

(FNA: fine-needle aspiration; NIFTP: noninvasive follicular thyroid neoplasm with papillary-like nuclear features ; CA: carcinoma)

Table 5: Various markers commonly used in context with diagnostic dilemma in thyroid nodules.

Markers	Property	Use	Limitations and sensitivity/specificity
Thyroglobulin	Thyroid hormone precursor	Thyroid organ-specific differentiation	• Benign and malignant thyroid lesions cannot be differentiated • May be negative in poorly or undifferentiated thyroid carcinomas
TTF-1	Plays vital role in organogenesis and differentiation of thyroid and lung lesions	Thyroid organ-specific differentiation	• Also expressed in lung, colorectal, ovarian, breast, endometrial, and endocervical adenocarcinomas • Cannot differentiate between benign and malignant thyroid lesions • May be negative in poorly or undifferentiated thyroid carcinomas
Hector Battifora mesothelial-1 (HBME-1)	Membrane antigen found in microvilli of mesothelial cells, normal tracheal epithelium, and adenocarcinoma of the lung, pancreas, and breast	• Overexpression/diffuse expression in malignant thyroid neoplasm, especially PTC • Virtually no expression in normal thyroid tissue • Negative in hyalinizing trabecular tumors of thyroid	• Negative or weakly positive in Hurthle cell neoplasm • 78.8% for thyroid cancer, 87.3% for PTC, and 65.2% for FTC • Specificity ~82.1%
Cytokeratin 19 (CK19)	Low-molecular-weight cytokeratin found in simple or glandular epithelia, both normal and their neoplastic counterpart	• Absent or weak focal positivity in normal follicular epithelium • CK19 overexpression is indicator for PTC	• Low sensitivity for FTC • Sensitivity of CK19 is 79.3% for malignancy, 82.2% for PTC, and 44.3% for FTC • Specificity is ~63.1%
Galectin-3 (GAL-3)	Member of a family of beta-galactoside-binding animal lectins involved in tumor progression/metastasis	• Diffuse overexpression in well-differentiated follicular-derived thyroid carcinomas • Focal positivity in benign lesions	• GAL-3 sensitivity is 84.6% for malignancy, 87.5% for PTC, and 72.6% for FTC • Specificity is ~83.6%
Thyroperoxidase (TPO)	Thyroid-specific enzyme reflecting normal thyroid function	• Diffusely expressed in normal follicular epithelial cells • Lack of expression signifies malignancy	• Sensitivity 90% for PTC, 76% for FTC • Specificity of ~88%

(FTC: follicular thyroid carcinoma; PTC: papillary thyroid carcinoma; TTF-1: thyroid transcription factor-1)

Table 6: Genetic alteration in thyroid neoplasms.[60,61]

Genetic alteration	Pathway activated	Prevalence	Interesting facts
• *RET/PTC rearrangement* • 11 RET/PTC rearrangements are reported • Three forms RET/PTC1, RET/PTC2, and RET/PTC3 are more common	Mitogen-activated protein kinase (MAPK) pathway	• *Adult sporadic PTC:* 10–20% • *History of radiation exposure:* 50–80% • *Children and young adults:* 40–70%	• Clonal RET/PTC is of significance • RET/PTC1 most common (60–70%) of positive cases • RET/PTC3 in 20–30% of positive cases • RET/PTC2 in <5% of positive cases • RET/PTC1 is associated with favorable prognosis • RET/PTC3 is associated with more aggressive behavior and dedifferentiation
• *BRAF mutation* • Point mutation is most common genetic alteration • Involve nucleotide 1,799 and result in a valine-to-glutamate substitution at residue 600 (V600E)	MAPK pathway	40–45%	• Typically present in classical/tall cell variant PTC • Rare in follicular variant • Absent in benign thyroid nodule, hence a very specific molecular marker • Associated with worse prognosis and less responsiveness to radioiodine therapy
• *RAS mutation* • Human *RAS* gene includes: *KRAS, HRAS,* and *NRAS* genes • *NRAS codon 61* and *HRAS codon 61* are most commonly associated with thyroid tumors	• MAPK pathway • Phosphoinositide 3-kinase (PI3K) pathway • AKT pathway	• 40–50% in conventional follicular carcinoma • 20–40% in follicular adenomas • Also expressed in 10–20% of FV-PTC	• Provide strong evidence of neoplasia, but does not establish the diagnosis of malignancy • May be associated with less favorable prognosis, increased chances of metastasis and dedifferentiation

Contd...

Contd…

Genetic alteration	Pathway activated	Prevalence	Interesting facts
PAX8/PPARγ rearrangement	t(2;3)(q13;p25)	30–40% of conventional follicular carcinoma	• Associated with younger age, smaller size, and more frequent vascular invasion • Detection of PAX8/PPARγ should prompt pathologist to perform an exhaustive search for vascular or capsular invasion
CTNNB1 mutation	CTNNB1 proto-oncogene encodes a member of Wnt signaling pathway	• ~25% of PDTC • ~60% of ATC	• Thyroid neoplasm is associated with somatic CTNNB1 mutation • Very rare in well-differentiated thyroid cancer, mainly associated with cribriform-morular variant PTC
TP53	TP53/p53 is a tumor suppressor gene that plays role in cell cycle regulation and DNA repair	• 10–40% of PDTC • 50–80% of ATC	Inactivating mutation in TP53 is a late event in thyroid cancer progression, which determines tumor dedifferentiation

(ATC: anaplastic thyroid carcinoma; DNA: deoxyribonucleic acid; FV-PTC: follicular variant of papillary thyroid carcinoma; PDTC: poorly differentiated thyroid carcinoma; PPARγ: peroxisome proliferator-activated receptor γ ; CTNNB1: Mutations of the beta-catenin gene; TP53: tumor protein p53)

LABORATORY EVALUATION OF HYPERPARATHYROIDISM

Hyperparathyroidism may be asymptomatic or can manifest with a variety of symptoms ranging from mild fatigue, muscle cramps to classical "painful bones, renal stones, abdominal groans, psychic moans, and fatigue overtones" to more severe acute hypercalcemic crisis. High clinical suspicion is necessary for further workup, diagnosis, and prompt treatment.

◇ BIOCHEMICAL EVALUATION

The diagnosis of primary hyperparathyroidism (PHPT) is essentially biochemical, components include increased or inappropriate levels of parathyroid hormone (PTH), hypercalcemia, hypophosphatemia, with some patients having high urinary calcium levels.[62] Another entity, normocalemic primary hyperparathyroidism (NCPHP), includes persistently normal levels of albumin corrected serum total calcium (Ca) and ionized calcium (iCa) after ruling out all possible causes of secondary HPT that has a prevalence of 1–17% among the surgically treated PHPT patients.[63-65]

Serum Parathyroid Hormone

Parathyroid glands secrete PTH, an 84 amino acid polypeptide, as a positive feedback for low serum calcium levels in normal individuals. It results in overall increase in serum calcium by bone resorption, gut absorption of calcium, and reducing renal calcium excretion. PTH with vitamin D plays major role in calcium homeostasis. First-generation PTH assay measures inactive C-terminal of PTH, which may be high in any etiology of chronic hypercalcemia. Parathyroid hormone-related peptide (PTHrP), cross-reacts with this type of assay, gives false-positive results in humoral hypercalcemia of malignancy (HHM). In 1987, Nussbaum et al. described-second generation PTH assay that measures intact (1–84)

PTH (iPTH) by using two-site immunoradiometric assay.[66] Subsequently, third-generation PTH assay, i.e., "whole" PTH that measures the bioactive PTH levels also were developed. With regard to diagnosis of PHPT, the sensitivity is similar for second- and third-generation PTH assays and is higher than first-generation PTH assay.[67,68] PTHrP is 146 amino acid single chain polypeptide having first 13 amino-terminal amino acids homologous to PTH, which avidly binds to PTH receptors and is responsible for subsequent effects similar to PTH.[69] Biotin interferes with PTH assay, so it is mandatory to repeat PTH levels after discontinuing biotin.[70]

Intraoperative Parathyroid Hormone

Second-generation PTH assay, described by Nussbaum et al. in 1987, was modified using chemiluminescent assay in 1994 by Irvin et al. to provide quick results to the operating surgeon within 10–15 minutes to assess the biochemical cure of HPT and limit the parathyroid dissection. Various criteria for determining biochemical cure are given in **Table 7** and their accuracy rates when used for curative intent are described in **Table 8**.[71]

Serum Calcium

Total calcium comprises protein bound (50%), ionized (40%), and calcium complexed with inorganic and organic anions (10%). Hence, serum albumin corrected total calcium levels give the degree of hypercalcemia. The textbook formula for correction of calcium is calculated by:

Corrected serum calcium = Serum calcium (mg/dL) + 0.8 × [4 – serum albumin (g/dL)]

Usually primary HPT presents with mild hypercalcemia (i.e., 1-2 mg/dL higher than the upper normal range).

Table 7: Various criteria used for IOPTH and their definitions for biochemical cure.

Name	Definition of the criteria
Miami (1996)	≥50% PTH fall from either highest preincision or preexcision level at 10 minutes after all hypersecreting glands are excised that denotes a successful operation in most patients
Halle (2006)	PTH level falls into the low normal range (<35 ng/L) within 15 minutes of removing all hyperfunctioning parathyroid glands
Vienna (2007)	PTH level fall = 50% from the baseline PTH level at 10 minutes from gland resection that indicates a successful operation
Rome (2008)	PTH level fall = 50% from the highest preexcision PTH level and/or a PTH level within the reference range at 20 minutes postexcision and/or a PTH level 7.5 ng/L lower than the 10 minutes postexcision level

(IOPTH: intraoperative parathyroid hormone; PTH: parathyroid hormone)

Table 8: Intraoperative parathyroid hormone (IOPTH) accuracy rates in predicting postoperative serum calcium values when using different criteria.

Criteria	Sensitivity	Specificity	Positive predictive value	Negative predictive value	Accuracy
Miami	97.6	93.3	99.6	70	97.3
Vienna	92.2	93.3	99.6	60.9	92.3
Rome	82.9	100	100	26.3	83.8
Halle	62.9	100	100	14.2	65

Clinical features of hypercalcemia manifest more often when the corrected calcium levels >12 mg/dL or with a rapid increase in the calcium levels.[72] In contrast, parathyroid carcinoma present with higher levels of calcium >14 mg/dL as well as a palpable neck mass in 30–76% of these patients.[73-75] A well-accepted criteria for hypercalcemic crisis is albumin corrected calcium levels >14.5 mg/dL associated with acute clinical features which are usually reversible with correction of hypercalcemia.[76] Thiazide reduces calcium loss from renal tubules (secondary HPT) thereby normalizing serum calcium and PTH levels, hence differentiates it from PHPT, where thiazides unmask PHPT.[77]

25-hydroxy Vitamin D

25-hydroxy vitamin D (i.e., calcidiol), produced by liver, circulates in nanomolar range, with a longer half-life than the active form, i.e., 1,25-dihydroxyvitamin D (calcitriol) which is formed by proximal convoluted tubule of kidney, i.e., in picomolar range. In PHPT, under the influence of raised PTH, there is increased conversion of 25-hydroxy vitamin D to 1,25-dihydroxyvitamin D, resulting in normal or low-normal range of 25-OH vitamin D with increased $1,25(OH)_2$ vitamin D.[78] Also, the calcium and PTH levels should be always vitamin D corrected (>30 ng/mL) in order to rule out vitamin D deficiency-induced secondary HPT.

Urinary Calcium Excretion and Calcium-creatinine Clearance Ratio

About 30–40% of patients with PHPT have high normal levels of urinary calcium (>100 mg/day) and few present with overt hypercalciuria (>400 mg/day). For those patients with urine calcium levels >400 mg/day, mandate further renal stone profile workup.[11] To diagnose FHH, with hypocalciuria, it

Box 1: Essential investigations for evaluation of patients with primary hyperparathyroidism.

- *Serum*: Intact parathyroid hormone, total calcium, phosphorus, albumin, 25-hydroxy vitamin D, renal function tests, and alkaline phosphatase
- 24-hour urinary calcium and creatinine
- Three-site bone mineral density (lumbar spine, hip, and distal third forearm)
- Stone risk profile (if urinary calcium >400 mg/day)
- Abdominal imaging
- Vertebral spine assessment

has 87% sensitivity and 72% specificity. Calcium-creatinine clearance ratio (CCCR) differentiates PHPT (CCCR >0.02) from familial hypocalciuric hypercalcemia (FHH) (CCCR <0.001) with 80% sensitivity and 88% specificity.[79,80] Those patients with CCCR between 0.01 and 0.02 would benefit by genetic testing.

CCCR = (24-hour urine calcium × plasma creatinine)/(24-hour urine creatinine × plasma total calcium)

Box 1 enlists investigations essential for evaluation of PHPT.[81] Differential diagnosis includes secondary/tertiary HPT, drugs, FHH, and HHM. **Table 9** enumerates biochemical differences between these conditions. The optional tests include high-resolution peripheral quantitative computed tomography (HR-pQCT) (which is available only at few research centers), trabecular bone score (TBS) by dual-energy X-ray absorptiometry (DXA) that needs a specific software in addition to DXA, which identifies few aspects of bone quality from lumbar spine DXA.[82,83]

Humoral Hypercalcemia of Malignancy

This entity can be biochemically differentiated from PHPT by very high levels of serum calcium, high levels of

Table 9: Biochemical parameters in various conditions.

| Parameters | PHPT | NCPHP | Secondary HPT | | | Tertiary HPT | FHH |
			Vitamin D deficiency	*Urinary calcium leak*	*Malabsorption syndromes*		
Albumin corrected total calcium	High	Normal	Normal	Normal or low	Low or normal	High	Normal or high
Phosphorus	Normal or low-normal	Normal or low-normal	Variable	High	Variable	Usually high	Normal
Intact parathyroid hormone	High	High	High	High	High	High (moderately elevated)	Normal or high
25-hydroxy vitamin D	Low or normal	Normal	Low	Normal	Low	Normal	Normal
1,25-dihydroxy vitamin D	High-normal or high	Variable but not low	Low	Low	High	Low	Normal
24-hour urine calcium	Normal or high	Usually normal, can be high	Normal	High	Normal	Low	Low with CCCR* < 0.010
Bone mineral density	Usually low at cortical sites	Can be low at cortical sites	Low in long standing	Low in long standing	Low in long standing	Often low	Normal

*CCCR is calculated as mentioned above in the text.
(CCCR: calcium-creatinine clearance ratio; FHH: familial hypocalciuric hypercalcemia; HPT: hyperparathyroidism; NCPHP: normocalcemic primary hyperparathyroidism; PHPT: primary hyperparathyroidism)

bicarbonate, and hypophosphatemia, with mild hypokalemic hypochloremic alkalosis. Contrasting features of PHPT include low or normal phosphorus, high chloride, and low bicarbonate with mild acidosis. Other laboratory investigations for HHM would usually reveal reduced PTH, increased PTHrP. Hematological malignancies have extrarenal conversion of 25-hydroxy vitamin D to active form 1,25-hydroxy vitamin D thereby resultant hypercalcemia, hence making measurements of 1,25-dihydroxyvitamin D indispensable.[83,84]

PARATHYROID PATHOLOGY

The role of FNAC in parathyroid lesions is limited as a diagnostic modality because of better imaging modalities and localizing scans such as methoxy isobutyl isonitrile (MIBI) technetium 99. However, FNAC is useful for locating incidentally detected lesions in asymptomatic patient presenting as cystic masses or when the lesions are present in abnormal locations.[85] The differentiation of parathyroid hyperplasia, adenoma, and carcinoma is almost impossible on FNAC and it is in fact not required. However, some studies have attempted to do so.[86,87]

On histopathology, parathyroid adenoma is encapsulated, cellular, homogeneous lesions, rarely papillary, and composed of chief cells with some oxyphil cells in delicate capillary network. Rim of normal parathyroid may be seen at the periphery. Parathyroid carcinoma can be differentiated by presence of high proliferative index, capsular and/or vascular invasion, and/or invasion in surrounding parenchyma. There has been a steady and substantial increase in the knowledge of the genetics of parathyroid tumors. Several genetic abnormalities have been detected in parathyroid adenomas, most of which are sporadic but can also occur as part of several hereditary syndromes. The primary genetics drivers known to date include somatic alteration of *MEN1* and *CCND1/PRAD*.[88]

LABORATORY EVALUATION OF ADRENAL AND PARAGANGLIOMA TUMORS

Adrenal tumors and paragangliomas can be functional or nonfunctional. Pathologically, they can be benign or malignant. According to cells of origin, paragangliomas are seen in sympathetic/parasympathetic ganglions and adrenal tumors can be arising either from adrenal cortex or medulla leading to various disorders as enumerated here:
- Cushing's syndrome
- Conn's adenoma or bilateral adrenal hyperplasia (micro-/macronodular)
- Pheochromocytoma (PCC)—mostly benign, rarely malignant
- Adrenocortical carcinoma
- Adrenal cysts
- Teratoma
- Myelolipoma.

◇ WORKUP FOR HYPERALDOSTERONISM (IDIOPATHIC HYPERALDOSTERONISM AND ALDOSTERONE-PRODUCING ADENOMAS)

Biochemical Evaluation

- Serum potassium
- Plasma aldosterone concentration (PAC)
- Plasma renin activity (PRA)
- Plasma aldosterone concentration/PRA ratio—20:1 to 50:1 ng/dL per ng/mL/h, >555 pmol/L per ng/mL/h, and PAC >15 ng/dL (≥416 pmol/L)—suggestive of hyperaldosteronism.

Drugs needed to be withhold during these tests are:
- Spironolactone
- Eplerenone
- Amiloride.

Hypokalemia needs to be corrected prior to start of these tests.

Timing of tests: Morning in ambulatory seated patients.

Four confirmatory tests are:
1. Captopril stimulation test
2. Fludrocortisone suppression test
3. Saline infusion test
4. Oral sodium loading test.

Saline suppression test: 2 L of isotonic saline is infused over 4 hours duration [take caution in patients with severe hypertension (HTN)/heart failure] and if PAC >10 ng/dL (not suppressed), then it is suggestive of hyperaldosteronism.

Oral sodium loading test: Patients are told to consume high salt in food for 3–4 days and at 3rd day morning, following tests are done:
- 24 hours urinary aldosterone, sodium, and creatinine.
- If 24 hours urinary sodium excretion is >200 mEq, then it means that patient consumed adequate salt intake.

- If urinary aldosterone fails to be suppressed <12 µg, then it is confirmatory of primary hyperaldosteronism.

How to differentiate between idiopathic hyperaldosteronism (IHA) and aldosterone-producing adenoma (APA)?
The differentiating features between IHA and APA are described in **Table 10**.

Imaging Protocols[89]

The imaging protocols for hyperaldosteronism are given in **Flowchart 1**.

Adrenal Venous Sampling

Primary hyperaldosteronism can be caused either by unilateral lesion or bilateral pathology. Distinction between

Table 10: Major differences between IHA and APA.

	APA	IHA
Age	Younger	Older patients
HTN	Severe not responding to medications and mostly present with hypokalemia	–
Treatment	Surgery	Medical
PAC and urinary aldosterone	Higher	–
Response to spironolactone	Better	
	• Unresponsive to renin-angiotensin-aldosterone system • PAC may decrease with normal circadian rhythm	• Highly sensitive to slight increase in angiotensin II in upright posture • PAC may rise after standing for 4 hours

(APA: aldosterone-producing adenoma; HTN: hypertension; IHA: idiopathic hyperaldosteronism; PAC: plasma aldosterone concentration)

Flowchart 1: Imaging protocols for hyperaldosteronism

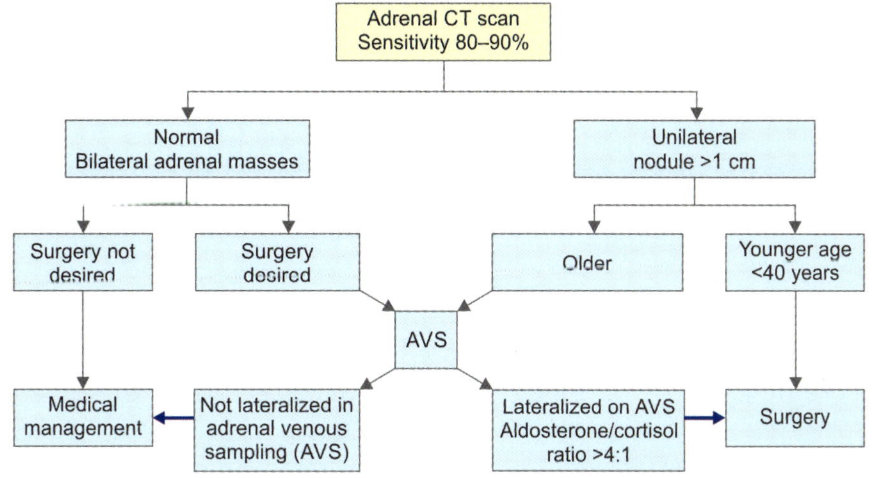

the two is very critical as unilateral lesions are managed by surgery and bilateral lesions are managed medically. Adrenal venous sampling (AVS) is the gold standard test to differentiate the two conditions.

This procedure is technically challenging and costly, hence done in few dedicated endocrine centers only.

Procedure Details

Sampling is done from bilateral adrenal veins and inferior vena cava. Cosyntropin, a synthetic analog of adrenocorticotropic hormone (ACTH), is infused 30 minutes prior to sampling as it stimulates adrenal gland to secrete cortisol and aldosterone and also increases the sensitivity and specificity of AVS. Catheter is inserted in common femoral vein and directed to each adrenal vein.

Interpretation of the Results

Cortisol levels in adrenal veins: peripheral veins = 3:1 with cosyntropin stimulation and 2:1 without stimulation.

Complications related to this procedure are rare:
- Adrenal hemorrhage
- Adrenal vein thrombosis.

◇| WORKUP FOR CUSHING'S SYNDROME

Screening Tests

At least two out of three tests if positive then it is considered as confirmatory.[90]
- 24-hour urinary-free cortisol (95% sensitivity and 98% specificity)
- *1 mg overnight dexamethasone suppression*: 1 mg dexamethasone tablet given to the patients at 11 PM and blood sample is collected next morning 8 AM.

- Late night salivary cortisol level (11 PM to midnight sample in saliva, sensitivity and specificity in diagnosis are 86% and 100%).

Serum ACTH levels—to differentiate between ACTH-dependent (ACTH >15 pg/mL) and non-ACTH (ACTH <5 pg/mL)-dependent CS.

Imaging Tests

The imaging tests for Cushing's syndrome are described in **Table 11**.

Inferior Petrosal Sinus Sampling Procedure

The intervention radiologist inserts a catheter in inferior petrosal sinuses and samples for ACTH are taken from both sides simultaneously at basal, after intravenous (IV) injection of 100 µg of corticotropin-releasing hormone (CRH) 3, 5, and 10 minutes and same time a peripheral blood sample is also taken.

Interpretation

At basal level, inferior petrosal sinus sample: Peripheral sample >2 or after stimulation >3 is diagnostic of Cushing disease.

Complications of the Procedure

- Vascular damage to brainstem
- Deep venous thrombosis
- Pulmonary emboli
- Cranial nerve palsies.

CT Scan Characteristics of Adrenal Tumors (Table 12)

Absolute washout = 100% × (attenuation in early phase–attenuation in delayed phase)/(attenuation in early phase – unenhanced attenuation)

Table 11: Imaging tests for Cushing's syndrome.		
For pituitary lesions	• MRI scan of brain • Picks lesion in up to 60% of patients as most lesions are microadenomas <10 mm	• If MRI is negative/inconclusive, then can do IPSS bilateral • High sensitivity (95–99%) and specificity for Cushing disease and diagnostic accuracy >90%
For ectopic ACTH-secreting tumors	CECT or MRI of thorax and abdomen	• Somatostatin receptor scintigraphy • ^{18}F-FDG or ^{68}Ga-somatostatin receptor PET/CT
For adrenal lesions	CECT or MRI of abdomen	–

(ACTH: adrenocorticotropic hormone; CECT: contrast-enhanced computed tomography; FDG: fluorodeoxyglucose; IPSS: inferior petrosal sinus sampling; PET: positron emission tomography)

Table 12: CT scan characteristics of adrenal tumors.		
Characteristics	**Benign adenomas**	**Malignancy**
Intracellular lipid content	• Rich mostly (70%) • 30% may be lipid poor	Poor
HU on noncontrast CT scan	• <10 • High specificity 98% and sensitivity 71%	>10
Enhancement in early phase and washout in delayed phase of contrast injection	Enhance in early phase mostly and rapid washout in delayed phase	Rapid enhancement but slow washout

(HU: Hounsfield unit)

Relative washout = 100% × (attenuation in early phase – attenuation in delayed phase)/attenuation in early phase

An absolute enhancement washout >60% or relative washout >40% is diagnostic for adrenal adenoma with high sensitivity (>86% for absolute washout and >96% for relative washout) and high specificity (>92% for absolute washout and 100% for relative washout).

Functional Imaging

The functional imaging methods are especially useful for detecting occult ectopic ACTH-secreting neuroendocrine tumors when anatomical imaging methods fail to detect the lesions.

- Octreotide scan
- Fluorodeoxyglucose-positron emission tomography (FDG-PET)
- ^{68}Ga-somatostatin receptor PET/CT.

◇ WORKUP FOR PHEOCHROMOCYTOMA/ PARAGANGLIOMA[91]

Biochemical Tests to Confirm Diagnosis

- 24 hours urinary fractionated metanephrines (uMNs)/ normetanephrine levels.
  Method: High-performance liquid chromatography (HPLC), tandem mass spectromctry.
- Plasma-free metanephrines (pMNs)—blood samples collected in resting supine position.
  Drug interference: Acetaminophen, tricyclic antidepressants, and phenoxybenzamine.
  Sensitivity/specificity: 94%/93% and 91%/93% for measurement of pMNs and uMNs using HPLC or IA methods, respectively.[92]
  The diagnostic efficacy was as follows: Normetanephrine fraction sensitivity 87.3% [95% confidence interval (CI) 79.4–92.4] and specificity 95.0% (92.5–96.8); metanephrine fraction sensitivity 56.9% (47.2–66.1) and specificity 95.0% (92.5–96.8); and elevation of either normetanephrine or metanephrine fraction sensitivity 97.1% (91.7–99.0) and specificity 91.1% (87.9–93.5).

Imaging Methods for Localization (Table 13)

Functional imaging methods have both diagnostic as well as therapeutic roles especially in cases of:

Table 13: Imaging methods for localization.

Anatomical imaging	CT scan or MRI of abdomen/pelvis
Functional imaging	^{123}I-MIBG scan 60% of PCC/PGL are MIBG avid

(MIBG: metaiodobenzylguanidine; PCC: pheochromocytoma; PGL: paraganglioma)

- Malignant lesions with metastases
- Young patients with hereditary syndromes.[93]

◇ PATHOLOGICAL EVALUATION OF ADRENAL NEOPLASMS

- *Role of fine-needle aspiration*: FNAC of adrenal gland is a less frequently performed technique.[94] However, there are studies, which have demonstrated that FNA biopsy of adrenal glands is a specific and sensitive procedure in the evaluation of adrenal lesions.[94,95] FNA not only allows the confirmation of surgical conditions like primary and metastatic malignancies, benign neoplasms, and cystic lesions, but also helps to diagnose the medical disorders which can be managed medically like infections, e.g., tuberculosis (TB) and histoplasmosis.[96]

The cytological evaluation of adrenal may pose diagnostic challenges in certain scenario:

- Pleomorphism and hypercellularity are not the reliable features to distinguish between adrenal adenoma and adrenocortical carcinoma.
- Typing of malignant small round cell tumors.
  The overall sensitivity of adrenal FNA in diagnosing malignancy has been up to 85%. However in study performed by us, the FNA was 100% specific for malignant lesions and correctly diagnosed 83.3% of the adrenal masses.[96]
- *Histopathological evaluation of adrenal neoplasm*: Histopathological specimens can be received in the form of CT-guided CNB or as final resection specimens. The utility of CNB has been scantly studied.[97] However, its primary role remains in differentiating primary from metastatic disease and also in the workup of incidentalomas.[98]

With the development of more sophisticated imaging techniques, an increasing number of small adrenocortical neoplasms are being discovered and therefore adrenocortical neoplasms not associated with ominous macroscopic features are increasing in number. Hence, distinction between benign and malignant in such scenario has become one of the most diagnostic difficulties encountered. Also, there are no single diagnostic histological criteria that can efficiently and reliably differentiate between benign and malignant neoplasms. Many systems had been developed so far, incorporating histological and/or nonhistological criteria. The most favored by pathologists so far, which included only the histopathological features, had been proposed by Weiss in 1984 which was later modified in 2002.[99,100] In the original criteria, there were nine parameters, which were reduced to five when modified **(Table 14)**.

Presence of metastasis is the only absolute criterion for malignancy in patients with PCC. Several scoring systems considering invasion, histologic growth patterns,

Table 14: Original Weiss criteria versus modified Weiss criteria for malignancy.

Original Weiss criteria for malignancy	Modified Weiss criteria
• Nuclear grade III or IV based on *Fuhrman criteria* • >Five mitotic figures/50 HPF (40X objective) *(counting 10 random fields in area of greatest number of mitotic figures on five slides with greatest number of mitoses)* • Presence of atypical mitotic figures *(abnormal distribution of chromosomes or excessive number of mitotic spindles)* • Clear or vacuolated cells comprising 25% or less of tumor • Diffuse architecture *(more than one-third of tumor forms patternless sheets of cells; trabecular, cord, columnar, alveolar, or nesting pattern is not considered to be diffuse)* • Microscopic necrosis • Venous invasion *(veins must have smooth muscle in wall; tumor cell clusters or sheets forming polypoid projections into vessel lumen or polypoid tumor thrombi are covered by endothelial layer)* • Sinusoidal invasion *(sinusoid is endothelial-lined vessel in adrenal gland with little supportive tissue; consider only sinusoids within tumor)* • Capsular invasion *(nests or cords of tumor extending into or through capsule with a stromal reaction, either incomplete or complete)*	• Mitotic rate >5 per 50 high-power fields (HPFs) • Cytoplasm (clear cells comprising 25% or less of the tumor) • Abnormal mitoses • Necrosis • Capsular invasion
• Each criterion is scored 0 when absent and 1 when present in the tumor • Score >3 suggests malignancy • Above criteria may not apply to childhood tumors	• Each criterion is scored 0 when absent and 1 when present in the tumor • *Calculate*: 2 × mitotic rate criterion + 2 × clear cytoplasm criterion + abnormal mitoses + necrosis + capsular invasion • Score of 3 or more suggests malignancy

Table 15: Pheochromocytoma of the Adrenal Gland Scaled Score.

Histomorphological parameters	Score
Nuclear hyperchromasia	1
Profound nuclear pleomorphism	1
Capsular invasion	1
Vascular invasion	1
Extension into periadrenal adipose tissue	2
Atypical mitotic figures	2
Greater than three mitotic figures/10 high-power field	2
Tumor cell spindling	2
Cellular monotony	2
High cellularity	2
Central or confluent tumor necrosis	2
Large nests or diffuse growth (>10% of tumor volume)	2
Total	20

and mitotic activity have been used to stratify the risk. One of the most utilized score is Pheochromocytoma of the Adrenal gland Scaled Score (PASS) proposed by Thompson in 2002 **(Table 15)**.[101]

A PASS score <4 or ≥4 suggests benign versus malignant lesion, respectively.

■ *Role of immunohistochemistry in adrenal neoplasm*: The neoplasms arising from adrenal can be divided into: those arising from cortex (adrenocortical neoplasm) and arising from medulla (neuroblastoma and PCC). The major diagnostic problems which surgical pathologists face in

adrenocortical pathology at this juncture are whether resected lesions are benign or not and if malignant whether primary or metastatic. The discussion below focuses on how the various immunohistochemical markers can be helpful in different scenarios:

• *Adrenocortical adenoma versus adrenocortical carcinoma*: Both adrenocortical adenomas and carcinomas show similar immunohistochemical profiles and express the same cortical lineage markers including synaptophysin, inhibin, melan-A, and SF-1.[102,103] However, these markers are expressed with lower sensitivity in adrenocortical carcinomas. Only the analysis of cell proliferation using Ki67 or MIB1 and topoisomerase II alpha antibodies can provide any additional meaningful information to carefully performed histopathological analysis. The adrenocortical neoplasms with >5–6% of MIB1 labeling index can be considered as adrenocortical malignancy.

• *Neuroblastoma versus other small round blue cell tumors*: Neuroblastoma, depending on the level of differentiation, expresses variable proportion of neuroblasts, Schwannian stroma as well as ganglion cells. Hence, markers pertaining to these component are helpful in diagnosis **(Table 16)**.[104]

PHOX2B is now considered as the most specific and sensitive markers for neuroblastoma.[105]

• *Adrenocortical carcinoma versus metastaic carcinoma*: Positivity for SF-1, inhibin, Melan-A (Mart-1, A103), and synaptophysin favors adrenocortical lineage. d4BP/SF-1 immunoreactivity has demonstrated

Table 16: Cellular components along with their markers.

Cellular components	Immunohistochemical (IHC) markers
Neuroblasts	• Neuron-specific enolase (NSE) • CD57/Leu7 • CD56 • Protein gene product 9.5 (PGP 9.5), synaptophysin • Chromogranin • Neurofilament protein • ALK1 • PHOX2B
Schwannian stroma	S100
Ganglion cells	• S100 • Synaptophysin, neurofilament protein • Glial fibrillary acidic protein (GFAP) • PGP 9.5 • Type IV collagen

Table 17: Major genetic differences between adrenocortical carcinoma and adrenocortical adenoma.

	Adrenocortical carcinoma	Adrenocortical adenoma
Chromosomal abnormalities	• Loss of heterozygosity (LOH) at 2p16, 11q13, and 17p13 • Loss of 1p21-31, 2q, 3q, 6q, 9p, and 11q14-qter • Gain of 5q12, 9q32-qter, 12q, and 20q	Loss of 17q, 17p, and 9q32-qter
Genetic abnormalities	• Upregulation of IGF (2, 2R, 3, and BP6) • Upregulation of UFD1L • Downregulation of CXCL10, RARRES2, ALD1f1A1, CYBRD1, and GSTA4	–

in almost all the tumor cells of adrenocortical carcinoma, both histological sections and cytology specimens regardless of the degrees of differentiation, but not in renal cell carcinoma, hepatocellular carcinoma, malignant melanoma, ovarian and uterine clear cell carcinoma, large cell carcinoma of the lung, and pheochromocytoma.[105]

- *Role of molecular diagnostics in adrenal neoplasm*: Most adrenocortical adenomas can be distinguished from carcinomas by permanent section microscopy based on well-defined, uniformly agreed-upon pathologic criteria. Various comparative genomic hybridization and gene profiling studies have documented different chromosomal and genetic abnormalities which may differentiate benign from malignant adrenal neoplasm. **Table 17** shows the common genetic differences between an adenoma and carcinomas.[106-109]

Studies have documented similar pattern in pediatric adrenal neoplasm. Few microRNA profiling studies have demonstrated difference in microRNA expression in benign and malignant neoplasms. The miR-335 and miR675 have been found to be upregulated in malignant lesions.[110] The number of cases are still small and significance of findings require further validation.

◇ WORK-UP FOR PITUITARY TUMOR[111-116]

Growth Hormone Stimulation Tests

Confirmation of growth hormone (GH) deficiency is done by two different stimulation tests, unless there is a setting for GH deficiency like trauma, surgery, etc., in which case one test may suffice.

Prerequisites

- Systemic causes of short stature are ruled out.
- Euthyroid state is documented by T4 or fT4 and not TSH.
- *Priming*: It is required if the child has reached the age of normal puberty and is still prepubertal (<stage 3 of puberty).
- *Male*: Injection testosterone enanthate 100 mg intramuscular (IM) 2–5 days before testing.
- *Female*: Oral conjugated equine estrogen (Premarin®) 1.25 mg OD for 3 days *or* estradiol (Lynoral®) 50–100 µg OD for 3 days.
- Give an appointment for admission and prime if required.

Clonidine Stimulation Test

Contraindications:
- Sick sinus syndrome
- Low IV volume.

Requirements: Tablet clonidine (Arkamine®) 100 µg, injection normal saline, IV drip set, scalp vein set, injection heparin/Hep-Lock, and disposable syringes.

Procedure:
- Record height, weight, and calculate body surface area (BSA). Test is conducted in a fasting state (water is allowed).
- Collect baseline sample for GH.
- Administer tablet clonidine 150 µg/m² orally (maximum 300 µg). Collect samples at 30 minutes interval (30, 60, 90, and 120 minutes).

Monitoring:
- Watch for drowsiness.
- Monitor blood pressure (BP) every 15 minutes.
- If BP <80 mm Hg, start normal saline drip but continue sampling.
- Once the test is over, ask the child to eat in your presence. He/she is allowed to leave only when he/she is fully conscious, ambulatory, and BP is normal without any postural fall.
- Warn parents about excessive sleepiness and tiredness.

Insulin Tolerance Test

This test has been recommended as the diagnostic test in adults by the Growth Hormone Research Society.

This test can also be used to assess hypothalamic-pituitary-adrenal (HPA) axis simultaneously.

Note: The concerned resident should be present throughout the test.

Contraindications:
- Presence or history of seizure disorder
- Electrocardiogram (ECG) evidence or history of ischemic heart disease.

Requirements: Injection plain insulin 40 U/mL, insulin syringes (U40), fluoride vials for blood glucose, 25% dextrose, scalp vein set, injection heparin/Hep-Lock, glucometer, strips, and disposable syringes.

Procedure:
- Test is conducted in fasting state. One dedicated IV line is kept ready for glucose infusion if it is needed.
- Take baseline samples for GH and blood sugar and measure capillary blood glucose. Administer plain insulin in the dose of 0.1 U/kg body weight (BW) as an IV bolus.
- If panhypopituitarism or hypocortisolism is suspected, then the insulin dose is halved to 0.05 U/kg BW.
- Check capillary blood glucose every 15 minutes.
- Further samples are collected at 15, 30, 45, 60, and 90 minutes for GH and capillary blood glucose (laboratory confirmation of hypoglycemia is must).
- Collect serum for cortisol at 60 minutes with the GH sample (if simultaneous assessment of HPA axis is to be done).
- Hypoglycemia is defined as blood glucose <40 mg/dL or <2.2 mmol/L.
- If blood sugar is not low even at 30 minutes, repeat insulin injection (0.1 U/kg) and restart sample collection after the second injection.
- If child is symptomatic (drowsiness, convulsions), terminate hypoglycemia with IV dextrose 0.5 g/kg BW but continue to collect samples for GH.
- Ask the child to eat breakfast in your presence after completion of the test.
- Allow the patient to go only when he/she has been ambulatory for half an hour without any symptoms.

Interpretation:
- Provided adequate hypoglycemia is achieved, this test differentiates GH deficiency from the reduced GH secretion that accompanies normal aging and obesity.
- The normal response for plasma cortisol (60 minutes) is >20 µg/dL (550 nmol/L).

Glucagon Test

Contraindication: Chronic liver disease.

Requirements: Injection glucagon, scalp vein set, injection heparin/Hep-Lock, and disposable syringes.

Procedure:
- Collect baseline sample for GH.
- Administer glucagon in the dose of 0.1 mg/kg BW (maximum 1 mg) IM or subcutaneous (SC). Collect samples for GH at 30, 60, 90, 120, 150, and 180 minutes.

Monitoring: Watch for nausea, vomiting, and pain in abdomen. Hypoglycemia can occur toward the end of the test.

L-dopa Propranolol Test

Contraindication: Cardiac arrhythmia.

Requirements: Tablet propranolol, tablet L-dopa, injection normal saline, IV drip set, scalp vein set, injection heparin/Hep-Lock, and disposable syringes.

Procedure:
- Test is conducted in a fasting state. Collect baseline sample for GH.
- Administer propranolol in the dose of 0.75 mg/kg of BW (maximum 40 mg) PO and L-dopa.
- PO in the dose as given below:
  - *Body weight < 15 kg*: 125 mg
  - *15–35 kg*: 250 mg
  - *>35 kg*: 500 mg.
- Collect samples for GH at 30, 60, and 90 minutes.

Monitoring:
- Monitor pulse and BP every 15 minutes.
- If BP < 80 mm Hg, start normal saline drip and continue to collect samples. Watch for nausea, vomiting, vertigo, fatigue, and headache.
- Once test is over, ask the child to eat in your presence and allow him/her to leave only when BP is normal and child is ambulatory.

Arginine Infusion Test

Requirements: L-arginine hydrochloride, injection normal saline, injection 25% dextrose, scalp vein set, injection heparin/Hep-Lock, and disposable syringes.

Procedure:
- Collect baseline sample for GH.
- L-arginine hydrochloride is administered in the dose of 0.5 g/kg BW (maximum 30 g) as an infusion in normal saline over 30 minutes.
- Collect samples for GH at 15, 30, 45, 60, and 90 minutes.

Monitoring: May cause insulin release, so monitor for hypoglycemia.

Growth Hormone-releasing Hormone Test

This test is most useful to distinguish between hypothalamic and pituitary disease because growth hormone-releasing hormone (GHRH) acts at the pituitary level.

Requirements: Injection GHRH, scalp vein set, injection heparin/Hep-Lock, and disposable syringes.

Procedure:

- Collect baseline sample for GH.
- Inject GHRH in the dose of 1 µg/kg BW as an IV bolus.
- Collect samples for GH at 0, 15, 30, 60, 90, and 120 minutes.

Side effect: Flushing.

Interpretation of Growth Hormone Stimulation Tests

Growth hormone deficiency is *likely* in children if the peak serum GH concentration is <5 ng/mL and *possible* if the peak response is 5–10 ng/mL in monoclonal antibody immunoradiometric assay (IRMA) and more advanced assays.

In adults, GH deficiency is likely if the peak serum GH concentration is <3 ng/mL and possible if the peak response is 3–5 ng/mL.

◇ GROWTH HORMONE SUPPRESSION TEST[117-120]

Indications

- Suspected case of acromegaly or gigantism
- Workup of a case of nonfunctioning pituitary adenoma.

Requirement

Glucose powder anhydrous 75 g (hydrous 82.5 g).

Prerequisite

Normal plasma glucose or controlled diabetes.

Procedure

- Test is done after an overnight fast.
- Do not give insulin on the morning of the test. Collect baseline sample for GH.
- Administer 1.75 g/kg BW (maximum 75 g) anhydrous glucose in water.
- Collect serum samples for GH at 30, 60, 90, and 120 minutes.

Monitoring

Not required.

Interpretation

- *Normal response*: GH is suppressed to <1 ng/mL.
- However, with the use of ultrasensitive GH assays (i.e., detection threshold of 0.05 ng/mL), postglucose suppression level of 0.3 ng/mL is considered normal.
- *Acromegaly*: GH level >1 ng/mL.

◇ INSULIN-LIKE GROWTH FACTOR-1 SAMPLE[121,122]

- It is a precise screening test for acromegaly.
- The sensitivity of insulin-like growth factor-1 (IGF-1) for the diagnosis of GH deficiency ranges from 47 to 100% in

various studies (and the specificity from 48 to 98%), limiting its use as a screening test. However, IGF-1 is a valuable tool as an ancillary test in the diagnosis of GHD, apart from clinical and auxologic criteria and GH provocative testing.

- Single random sample is collected.
- Results have to be compared with age and gender-matched normal values.

◇ WATER DEPRIVATION TEST[121-125]

Indication

To evaluate a case of polyuria suspected to have diabetes insipidus (DI).

Prerequisites

- Document polyuria a couple of time.
- Polyuria is defined as urine output >40 mL/kg/24 h in adults, >2,500 mL/m^2 BSA in infants, and >1,500 mL/m^2 BSA in children. Normal urine output in children is 30 mL/kg/day.
- Patient should be euthyroid and eucortisolemic prior to performing the test.
- Rule out osmotic diuresis. Baseline tests like fasting blood sugar, renal function, potassium, and calcium should be done as renal disease; hypercalcemia or hypokalemia can impair urinary concentrating ability.

Requirements

Weighing machine, desmopressin (DDAVP) injection (Desmopressin® 4 µg/mL) or desmopressin spray (Minirin® 100 µg/mL) or aqueous vasopressin (Cpressin-P® 20 units/mL).

Procedure

- The patient must be admitted for conducting the test and the laboratory must be informed in advance about the test.
- The patient should be closely supervised to avoid surreptitious access to water during the test.

Preparation Phase

- If the patient is on DDAVP, stop the drug at least 24 hours before the test. Patient should have free access to fluids night before the test.
- A light breakfast can be given on the morning of the test. Avoid caffeine and smoking.
- Measure fluid intake and urine output from midnight until the start of test.
- Weigh the patient at the start of the test, calculate 95% of his weight, and record on the chart.

Dehydration Phase

- *When to start dehydration depends on the urine output. If patient has mild polyuria <4 L/day, then dehydration can be started the previous night, but test should start in the morning (8.00 AM) if patient has massive polyuria 6–10 L/day.*

- Measure plasma, urine osmolality, and urine volume at 8.00 AM or at the start of dehydration phase.
- Restrict all fluids till adequate dehydration is achieved. Weigh patient, monitor pulse and BP, and urine volume hourly.
- Urine osmolality is measured every 2 hours.
- If measured osmolality is not available, then we can calculate the osmolality on the basis of serum sodium, blood glucose, and blood urea nitrogen (BUN).
- *End the test when*: Weight loss exceeds 5% of the basal weight, or thirst is intolerable, or clinical signs of dehydration appear, or serum sodium > 148 mEq/L, or serum osmolality > 295 mOsmol/L in the phase of dilute urine (<300 mOsmol/L), or three stable urine osmolalities are achieved. Take urine and serum samples and inject vasopressin/DDAVP.
- A chart is maintained as follows:

Time	Pulse	Blood pressure	Weight	Serum osmolality	Urine osmolality	Serum sodium	Urine output

Desmopressin Phase

- Inject DDAVP SC or IV in a dose of 0.5 µg/m² BSA (maximum 5 µg).
- Intranasal dose of DDAVP is 10 times the IV dose, i.e., 5 µg/m² BSA (maximum 20 µg). Aqueous vasopressin is given IV in a dose of 0.1 unit/kg BW (maximum 5 units).
- Allow the patient to eat and drink up to 1.5–2.0 times the volume of urine output during the dehydration phase.
- Beware of water intoxication.
- Measure plasma, urine osmolality, and urine output hourly for the next 4 hours.

Interpretation

- *Normal response*: Urine osmolality rises and urine volume and free water clearance fall progressively with water deprivation. Plasma osmolality rises but remains below 295 mOsmol/kg but simultaneous urine osmolality of >750 rules out DI.
- *Central DI*: Urine osmolality fails to rise appropriately and urine volume remains inappropriately high in spite of rising plasma osmolality. More than 50% increase in urine osmolality after DDAVP injection confirms central DI.
- *Nephrogenic DI*: Plasma osmolality rises and urine osmolality fails to rise appropriately as in central DI, but urine fails to concentrate after DDAVP, <9% rise in urine osmolality after DDAVP injection.
- *Primary polydipsia*: Maximum plasma osmolality <295 mOsmol/kg, urine osmolality > 290 mOsmol/kg before DDAVP, and no further rise in urine osmolality after DDAVP.
- *Partial, central, or nephrogenic DI*: Plasma osmolality rises to >295 mOsmol/kg and urine osmolality fails to rise appropriately as in complete DI, but urine osmolality rises between 9 and 50% after DDAVP.

- Rise in urine osmolality between 9 and 50% can be seen in partial central DI, nephrogenic DI, or primary polydipsia and all three conditions difficult to differentiate conclusively.

Limitations

Many patients with partial defects and mild forms of hypothalamic DI, nephrogenic DI, and primary polydipsia cannot always be differentiated by this test. Furthermore, prolonged polyuria from any cause leads to partial resistance to the antidiuretic action of vasopressin because of dilution of the renal medullary interstitium.

◇ GONADOTROPIN-RELEASING HORMONE TEST[126-130]

Indications

To distinguish central precocious puberty (CPP) from peripheral precocious puberty (PPP), delayed puberty from hypogonadotropic hypogonadism.

Principle

"Primed" pituitary gland responds to gonadotropin-releasing hormone (GnRH) with a brisk elevation of gonadotropins.

Procedure

It can be carried out at any time of the day. Insert a cannula prior to test. Basal sample is taken at 0 minute. An IV bolus of 100 µg/m² BSA (100 µg) GnRH (Factrel/Gonadorelin) is injected and samples are drawn at 30, 60, and 90 minutes after injection. The serum has to be stored at –20ºC, if not assayed within 24 hours.

Alternatively, GnRH can be given SC in a dose of 100 µg and single sample is taken 40 minutes after injection.

Interpretation

Gonadotropin-releasing Hormone Stimulation Test Response in Normal Children

Gonadotropin-releasing hormone stimulation test response in normal children is given in **Table 18**.

Tanner stage	LH		FSH	
	Male	*Female*	*Male*	*Female*
Prepubertal	1.8 ± 1.3 IU/L	1.8 ± 1.3 IU/L	–	–
1	3.2 ± 3.0 IU/L	2.0 ± 1.5 IU/L	4.7 ± 2.2 IU/L	21 ± 5.5 IU/L
2, 3	15 ± 6.3 IU/L	21 ± 17 IU/L	3.4 ± 2.2 IU/L	10 ± 5.0 IU/L
4, 5	42 ± 23 IU/L	33 ± 20 IU/L	11 ± 5.6 IU/L	11 ± 3.3 IU/L

Table 18: GnRH stimulation test response in normal children.

(GnRH: gonadotropin-releasing hormone; FSH: follicle-stimulating hormone; LH: luteinizing hormone)

Gonadotropin-releasing Hormone Stimulation Test Response in Children with Central Precocious Puberty (CPP)

Gonadotropin-releasing hormone stimulation test response in children with CPP is described in **Table 19**.

A pubertal response to GnRH stimulation is classically characterized by a pattern of luteinizing hormone (LH) predominance indicating an elevation of LH above that of follicle-stimulating hormone (FSH) whereas a prepubertal response is marked by a minimal increase in LH, if any, but may elicit an FSH response above baseline. An intermediate response typified by an FSH predominant response is seen in early central puberty and in premature thelarche.

◇ GONADOTROPIN-RELEASING HORMONE ANALOG TEST[131]

Indications and prerequisite are same as for GnRH testing.

Procedure

Basal sample is taken at 0 minute. Triptorelin in a dose of 0.1 mg is given SC and sample is collected at 1 and 2 hours after LH and FSH. Some authors have also collected sample at 4 hours after the bolus.

Interpretation

It is the same as for GnRH testing.

◇ ORAL GLUCOSE TOLERANCE TEST[132-134]

Indications

Diagnosis of diabetes.

Prerequisite

3 days of unrestricted physical activity and diet (>150 g carbohydrate per day) and after an overnight fast of 8–14 hours.

Method

Fasting blood glucose is measured followed by oral ingestion of 75 g of anhydrous glucose (equivalent to 82.5 g of hydrous glucose) in 250–300 mL of water over 5 minutes.

For children, the dose is 1.75 g/kg maximum up to 75 g of glucose. Blood sample is collected 2 h after the load for glucose estimation. Subject should remain seated and refrain from smoking throughout the test.

World Health Organization Criteria

The World Health Organization (WHO) criteria for estimating oral glucose tolerance test (OGTT) are given in **Table 20**.

◇ GESTATIONAL DIABETES MELLITUS

Screening Strategy for Detecting Gestational Diabetes Mellitus

Gestational diabetes mellitus (GDM) risk—should be ascertained at the first prenatal visit.

Low-risk patients require no testing. Low-risk status is limited to women meeting all of the following criteria:

- Age < 25 years
- Weight normal before pregnancy
- Member of an ethnic group with a low prevalence of GDM
- No family history of diabetes in first-degree relatives
- No history of abnormal glucose metabolism
- No history of poor obstetric outcome.

Average-risk patients (all patients who fall between low and high risk) should be tested at 24–28 weeks of gestation by either:

- *One-step procedure*: Diagnostic oral GTT is performed in all individuals.
  - The 100-g OGTT is the most commonly used standard test. Two or more of the glucose concentrations indicated in **Table 21** must be met or exceeded for a positive diagnosis.
  - Alternatively, a 75-g OGTT can be performed, but it is not as well-validated as the 100 g test.
- *Two-step procedure*: The first step is a 50-g oral glucose load (the patient needs not be fasting) followed by a plasma glucose determination at 1 hour. A plasma glucose value >7.8 mmol/L (140 mg/dL) indicates the need for definitive testing.

Table 20: World Health Organization criteria for estimating oral glucose tolerance test.

	*Fasting**	*2 hours*
Impaired glucose tolerance	100–125 (5.6–6.9)	140–199 (7.8–11.0)
Diabetes	≥126 (≥7.0)	≥200 (≥11.1)
Normal	<100 (5.6)	<140 (<7.8)

*Any single abnormal value should be repeated on a separate day for confirmation.

Table 21: Diagnosis of gestational diabetes mellitus (GDM) 100 g oral glucose load.

	*Carpenter-Coustan plasma glucose oxidase (mg/dL)**
Fasting	95
1 hour	180
2 hours	155
3 hours	140

*Two or more values must be met or exceeded for a positive diagnosis of GDM.

Table 19: GnRH stimulation test response in children with CPP.*

	CPP	*Non-CPP*
Peak LH after IV GnRH	26 ± 13 IU/L	2.9 ± 2.6 IU/L
LH after SC GnRH	30 ± 18 IU/L	2.8 ± 2.4 IU/L

*Ultrasensitive chemiluminometric assay.
(CPP: central precocious puberty; GnRH: gonadotropin-releasing hormone; IV: intravenous; LH: luteinizing hormone; SC: subcutaneous)

- *High-risk patients* should undergo immediate testing. They are defined as having:
  - Marked obesity
  - Personal history of GDM
  - Glycosuria
  - Strong family history of diabetes.

If test is normal, it should be repeated at 24–28 weeks or at any time the patient has symptoms or signs suggestive of hyperglycemia.

The WHO recommends using the 75-g OGTT and the same criteria as used to diagnose impaired glucose tolerance or diabetes as in the nonpregnant state (fasting ≥ 126 mg/dL and 2-hour value ≥140 mg/dL) and one or more glucose value must meet threshold.

◇| C-PEPTIDE[135]

Indications

Measurement of C-peptide response to IV glucagon or glucose can aid in the rare cases in which it is difficult to differentiate between type 1 and type 2 diabetes mellitus.

To diagnose the etiology of hypoglycemia due to hyper-insulinism, especially to differentiate between endogenous cause versus factitious hyperinsulinism. For diagnosis of fasting hypoglycemia (especially in beta-cell tumor with intermittent hyperinsulinism as C-peptide having longer half-life may be high, even if insulin levels are low). It can be used to monitor results of pancreatic surgery. C-peptide should be undetectable after radical pancreatectomy and should increase after a successful pancreas or islet cell transplantation.

Prerequisite

12-hour fasting

Method

Place a syringe in refrigerator to cool. Collect blood in cold syringe and transport it to the laboratory in a beaker of ice at 2–8°C. Sample should be centrifuged as soon as possible (at the most within 2 hours of collection). Serum/plasma can be stored at 2–8°C for 24 hours but at –20°C for longer periods.

Interpretation

Serum levels of C-peptide are age dependent **(Table 22)**.

Table 22: Serum levels of C-peptide as per different age groups.		
Age groups	*Mean (nmol/L)*	*Range (nmol/L)*
Cord blood	0.24	0.10–0.49
Neonates (36–60 hours)	0.12	0.03–0.24
Infants	0.22	0.13–0.40
1–6 years	0.18	0.08–0.36
6–12 years	0.41	0.17–0.85
Adults	0.39	0.18–0.79

◇| AUTONOMIC FUNCTION TESTING[136]

Cardiovascular Tests

Indications

To diagnose autonomic damage caused by diabetes mellitus and other disorders.

There is no consensus regarding when and how frequently to perform these tests. Tests for cardiovascular autonomic functions are performed in presence of symptoms suggestive of autonomic neuropathy or if there is significant postural fall in blood pressure.

Requirements

Sphygmomanometer, electrocardiogram machine, aneroid manometer, and handgrip dynamometer.

Prerequisites

- Should be performed in morning after 8 hours fast after the patient has been supine for 30 minutes in a quite relaxed atmosphere
- Should refrain from smoking
- Should not have performed vigorous exercise in the past 24 hours and has not had recent episode of hypoglycemia.
- Should not receive short-acting insulin in the last 8 hours. If on long-acting insulin/pump, maintain the dose.

Procedure

- *Heart rate response to Valsalva maneuver*: The patient blows into a mouthpiece connected to an aneroid manometer or a modified sphygmomanometer and holds it at a pressure of 40 mm Hg for 15 seconds while an ECG is recorded throughout the procedure. The maneuver is performed three times with 1-minute interval in between. Valsalva ratio = Longest R-R interval after maneuver: Shortest R-R interval during maneuver.
  Calculate the mean of three cycles for a final value.

  Test is contraindicated if patient has proliferative retinopathy. Heart rate response is altered in the presence of congestive heart failure.
- *Heart rate response (R-R interval) to deep breathing*: Patient while sitting breathes deeply at rate of 6 breaths/min (5 seconds in and 5 seconds out) and ECG is recorded continuously.

  The maximum and minimum R-R interval during each breathing cycle is measured with a ruler and converted to beats a minute. The result is then expressed as the mean of the difference between maximum and minimum heart rates for the six cycles in beats a minute.
- *Blood pressure response to sustained handgrip*: Patient squeezes a handgrip dynamometer to maximum in sitting position and then maintains at 30% of maximum for as long as possible or up to 5 minutes. BP is measured three times before and at 1-minute interval during handgrip. Calculate

Table 23: Interpretation of autonomic function testing.

	Normal	Borderline	Abnormal
Heart rate tests			
Valsalva ratio*	≥1.21	1.11–1.20	≤1.10
R-R interval variation during deep breathing*	≥15 beats/min	11–14 beats/min	≤10 beats/min
30:15 ratio*	≥1.04	1.01–1.03	≤1.00
Blood pressure (BP) tests			
Postural fall in systolic BP**	<10 mm Hg	11–29 mm Hg	≥30 mm Hg
Diastolic response to sustained handgrip**	≥16 mm Hg	11–15 mm Hg	≤10 mm Hg

*Tests reflecting parasympathetic function.
**Tests reflecting sympathetic function.

the difference between the highest diastolic pressure during handgrip and mean of three diastolic readings before squeezing.

- *Heart rate response to standing*: Patient lies on a couch, stands unaided while ECG is being recorded continuously. The point of starting to stand is marked on ECG.

  30:15 ratios = Longest R-R interval at 30th beat: Shortest R-R interval at 15th beat after standing.

- *Blood pressure response to standing*: Patient lies on a couch and blood pressure is measured and again 3 minutes after standing.

  If the patient is unable to stand, then orthostatic may be done after the patient has risen to a sitting position with feet dangling over the edge of the bed.

  Postural fall = Difference between lying and standing/sitting systolic blood pressure is noted.

Interpretation

The interpretation is given in **Table 23**.

◇ DIAGNOSTIC FAST[137-139]

Test is to be done under close supervision as this test is potentially dangerous.

Indication

In many conditions, hypoglycemia occurs episodically, usually during periods of low calorie intake or starvation. It may therefore be necessary to perform a diagnostic test if suitable specimen has not been obtained during the episode of hypoglycemia.

Prerequisite

Patient should be hospitalized 1 day prior to testing. Reports of liver and renal function tests should be available. All nonessential drugs should be stopped.

Requirements

25% dextrose, cold drink, glucose powder, heparin, fluoride vials, cold syringe, cold tube, glass tubes, injection glucagon 1 mg, and ice box/pack for transportation.

Procedure

- Secure IV cannula containing heparinized saline to correct hypoglycemia by administering dextrose.
- The maximum duration of fast should be decided before starting based on the age of the child and the maximum interval that he/she normally has between the feeds at home. For infants, who are fed every 4–6 hours, the fast involves omitting only one or at the most two feeds. For older children, who are normally not fed during the night at home, the fast begins after the evening meal. Using this protocol, most children will be at risk of hypoglycemia when they are awake between 10.00 AM and 6.00 PM (i.e., after 16–24 hours fasting).
- Allow the patient to drink calorie-free, caffeine-free beverages (like soda water and lemon water). Ensure that the patient is active during waking hours.
- Blood glucose, free fatty acids, ketone bodies, lactate, and alanine should be monitored serially throughout the test, from the time of what would have been the last feed in babies and from 6 to 12 hours starvation onward in children older than 1 year.
- Depending on the history and the age of the patient, monitoring may be at 2-hour intervals initially, but thereafter should be at 1-hour intervals. More frequent sampling is indicated if symptoms develop.
- Sampling without venous stasis should be possible through the IV cannula.
- Doctor and nurse should be available in the ward to monitor vital parameters and symptoms and signs of hypoglycemia (palpitations, sweating, headache, giddiness, tremor, and increasing sleepiness/obtundation).
- If blood glucose <45 mg/dL or sign/symptoms of hypoglycemia occur, the concentration of all metabolites and hormones listed in **Table 24** are measured and hypoglycemia is terminated by IV dextrose.
- If no sign/symptom or hypoglycemia occur, these specimens should be taken at the end of the fast anyway (maximum 72 hours).
- Inject glucagon 0.03–0.1 mg/kg body weight (maximum 1 mg) IV or IM with sampling for plasma glucose at 5, 15, 30, 45, 60, and 90 minutes.
- Patient must be fed before being discharged.

Table 24: Intermediary metabolites and hormones of importance in the diagnosis of hypoglycemia.

Metabolite and hormone	Aspects of sampling	Laboratory method
Blood		
Glucose	1–2 mL blood in fluoride	
Lactate		
Pyruvate	• 0.5 mL blood (without venestasis) into perchloric acid • Store deep frozen	
3-hydroxybutyrate		Fluoroenzymatic assays
Acetoacetate		
Glycerol		
Free fatty acids	Plasma	Spectrophotometric enzyme-linked assay
Amino acids	• 1–2 mL blood into lithium heparin • Store plasma deep frozen	Automated column chromatography
Free and acylcarnitine		Radioenzymatic methods
Acylcarnitine profile*	Blood on Guthrie card	Tandem mass spectrometry
Insulin		
C-peptide		
Glucagon	Plasma or serum	Radioimmunoassay
Growth hormone		
Cortisol		
Urine		
Ketones	• Next urine sample produced after hypoglycemic episode or urine collected during diagnostic fast • Store deep frozen	Acetest tablets
Dicarboxylic acids		Gas chromatography
Glycine conjugates		Mass spectrometry
Reducing substances (galactose, fructose)		Sugar chromatography
Carnitine derivatives		• Gas chromatography • Mass spectrometry

*This is best taken when child is not hypoglycemic.

Interpretation

Table 25 lists the levels of various metabolites and hormones in fasting healthy children.

In normal persons, on fasting, insulin levels fall to a very low <5 µU/mL (RIA) or undetectable levels. In patients with insulinoma, on fasting, plasma glucose falls below 45 mg/dL with elevated plasma insulin >6 µU/mL (RIA) or >3 µU/mL [immunochemiluminometric assay (ICMA)], C-peptide levels >0.2 nmol/mL (ICMA), and proinsulin levels >5 pmol/mL (ICMA).

In most normal children (after glucagon injection), the blood glucose rises by about 2 mmol/L. In hyperinsulinism, there is an exaggerated hyperglycemic response. Measurement of this parameter is valid only when plasma glucose is 60 mg/dL or lower at the end of the fast.

The pattern of plasma glucose and beta-cell polypeptides in sulfonylurea-induced hypoglycemia is identical to that observed in patients with insulinoma except that these patients have elevated levels of serum sulfonylurea levels.

◇ DIAGNOSTIC FAST IN CHILDREN[137,139]

Test should be done under close supervision as this test is potentially dangerous.

Indications

It is used in the diagnosis of conditions causing persistent or recurrent hypoglycemia in children when symptoms of hypoglycemia are absent and blood sugar is normal. Examples of such conditions include:

- Hyperinsulinism
- Glycogen storage disorders
- Fatty acid oxidation disorders
- Amino acid and organic acid disorders
- Carnitine deficiency.

Prerequisite

Patient should be hospitalized 1 day prior to testing.

The hazards are greatest in defects of long-chain fatty acid oxidation, which carries a risk of arrhythmia as well as hypoglycemia. If such defect is possible, fasting should be avoided until cardiomyopathy is excluded by echocardiography.

Requirements

25% dextrose, cold drink, glucose powder, heparin, fluoride vials, cold syringe, cold tube, glass tubes, injection glucagon 1 mg, and ice box/pack for transportation.

Table 25: Reference ranges for intermediary metabolites and hormones in normal children after overnight starvation*.

Metabolite/hormone	mmol/L
Lactate	0.4–2.0
Pyruvate	0.03–0.16
Ratio of lactate to pyruvate	5.9–25
3-hydroxybutyrate	0.01–0.34
Acetoacetate	0.01–0.15
Glycerol	0.03–0.10
Alanine	0.18–0.48
Glucose	4.1–5.5
Free fatty acids	0.2–1.2
Triglycerides	0.45–1.8
Cholesterol	3.6–7.3
	μmol/L
Free carnitine	23–60
Short-chain carnitine	5–18
Long-chain carnitine	7–13
Total carnitine	38–81
Acylated carnitine (%)	24–56%
Insulin	2.8–13.5 mU/L**
C-peptide	0.18–0.52 nmol/L**
Plasma cortisol (midnight)	220 nmol/L
Plasma cortisol (8.00 AM)	120–720 nmol/L

*Ranges are likely to vary substantially according to age and duration of fasting.
**Depending on blood glucose level.

Procedure

- For younger children, maintain a separate IV line in addition to heparin lock.
- The maximum duration of fast should be decided before starting based on the age of the child and the maximum interval that he/she normally has between feeds at home. For infants, who are fed every 4–6 hours, the fast involves omitting only one or at the most two feeds. For older children, who are normally not fed during the night at home, the fast begins after the evening meal. Using this protocol, most children will be at risk of hypoglycemia when they are awake between 10.00 AM and 6.00 PM (i.e., after 16–24 hours fasting).
- In case of infants on IV glucose infusion, the test may involve stopping the infusion and testing blood glucose every 15 minutes.
- Depending on the history and the age of the patient, glucose monitoring may be at 2-hourly intervals initially, but thereafter should be at 1-hour intervals. More frequent sampling is indicated if symptoms develop. More frequent monitoring (15–30 minutes) is needed in case of neonates and young infants.

Terminate the fast if:
- Glucose < 50 mg/dL
- Worrisome signs of hypoglycemia
- Bicarbonate (HCO_3) <15 mEq (even in absence of hypoglycemia)
- Completion of the duration of the fast.

If severe symptoms develop, administer 5 mL/kg of 10% dextrose.

If hyperinsulinism is suspected, give glucagon 30 μg/kg (maximum 1 mg) by slow IV push at the termination of the test and test for rise in glucose.

The serum sample during hypoglycemia should be assessed for glucose, insulin, C-peptide, cortisol, GH, lactate, ammonia, free fatty acid (FFA), β-hydroxybutyrate, and electrolytes.

All urine or the urine sample produced after the hypoglycemic episode is collected and assessed for ketones and other tests as in **Table 24**.

General Considerations

- Frequent assessment of patient for symptoms and signs of hypoglycemia. Maintain a flowsheet of vitals, glucose, and urine ketones.
- Patient can drink water freely.
- Glucagon may cause vomiting hence child to be kept in lateral position.
- Keep fluoride vials handy for taking glucose samples to prevent red blood cell (RBC) metabolism and cause falsely low blood sugar.

Interpretation

- Episodes of hypoglycemia are considered abnormal at any time throughout the test.
- *Any detectable insulin* in the presence of hypoglycemia (>2–5 μU/mL) favors hyperinsulinism. GH secretion >5–10 ng/mL usually follows the hypoglycemic episode.
- Serum cortisol secretion is increased to >20 μg/dL during fast.

ARTERIAL STIMULATION AND VENOUS SAMPLING

Indication

Cases with biochemical diagnosis of endogenous hyperinsulinemia with negative pancreatic imaging.

Prerequisite

It is done more than 2 hours following oral intake. Prerequisites are: nomral prothrombin time (PT), activated partial thromboplastin time (APTT), and creatinine.

Procedure

- Glucose 5% is infused through a peripheral vein.
- Sampling catheter is placed transfemorally in the right hepatic vein close to its junction with the inferior vena cava.

- Celiac trunk and the superior mesenteric artery (SMA), hepatic artery, the gastroduodenal artery (GDA), and the splenic artery (SA) are catheterized.
- Digital subtraction arteriogram of these arteries is obtained prior to stimulation.
- Each artery is stimulated with calcium gluconate 0.025 mEq Ca/kg body weight (1 mg/kg) diluted to a 5-mL bolus.
- Blood sample is drawn from right hepatic vein at 0, 30, 60, and 120 seconds after the intra-arterial injection of calcium.
- At least 5 minutes interval should be between successive calcium injections.

Interpretation

- Gastroduodenal artery—pancreatic head and secondarily the uncinate process.
- Superior mesenteric artery—uncinate process and secondarily the pancreatic head.
- Splenic artery—primarily the body and tail of the pancreas.

More than two- to threefold rise in insulin levels within 30–120 seconds after the injection of calcium localizes insulin-secreting tumor in the vascular territory of the artery stimulated. No response from normal cells.

◇| REFERENCES

1. Ortiga-Carvalho TM, Chiamolera MI, Pazos-Moura CC, Wondisford FE. Hypothalamus-pituitary-thyroid axis. In: Terjung R (Ed). Comprehensive Physiology. Hoboken: John Wiley & Sons, Inc.; 2016. pp. 1387-428.
2. Grebe SKG. Laboratory testing in thyroid disorders. In: Luster M, Duntas LH, Wartofsky L (Eds). The Thyroid and Its Diseases. Cham: Springer International Publishing; 2019. pp. 129-59.
3. Hirsch PF, Baruch H. Is calcitonin an important physiological substance? Endocrine. 2003;21(3):201-8.
4. Ceccarini G, Santini F, Vitti P. Tests of thyroid function. In: Vitti P, Hegedüs L (Eds). Thyroid Diseases: Pathogenesis, Diagnosis, and Treatment. Cham: Springer International Publishing; 2018. pp. 33-55.
5. Soldin OP, Soldin SJ. Thyroid hormone testing by tandem mass spectrometry. Clin Biochem. 2011;44(1):89-94.
6. Welsh KJ, Soldin SJ. Diagnosis of endocrine disease: How reliable are free thyroid and total T3 hormone assays? Eur J Endocrinol. 2016;175(6):R255-63.
7. Baloch Z, Carayon P, Conte-Devolx B, Demers LM, Feldt-Rasmussen U, Henry JF, et al. Laboratory medicine practice guidelines. Laboratory support for the diagnosis and monitoring of thyroid disease. Thyroid. 2003;13(1):3-126.
8. Faix JD, Miller WG. Progress in standardizing and harmonizing thyroid function tests. Am J Clin Nutr. 2016;104 Suppl 3: 913S-7.
9. Gordon DF, Ridgway EC. (2019). Thyroid-Stimulating Hormone: Physiology and Secretion. [online] Available from https://www.clinicalkey.com/#!/content/book/3-s2.0-B9780323189071000743?scrollTo=%23hl0000431. [Last accessed April, 2020].
10. Spencer CA, Nicoloff JT. Improved radioimmunoassay for human TSH. Clin Chim Acta. 1980;108(3):415-24.
11. van Heyningen V, Abbott SR, Daniel SG, Ardisson LJ, Ridgway EC. Development and utility of a monoclonal-antibody-based, highly sensitive immunoradiometric assay of thyrotropin. Clin Chem. 1987;33(8):1387-90.
12. Ross HA, Menheere PP: Endocrinology Section of SKML (Dutch Foundation for Quality Assessment in Clinical Laboratories), Thomas CM, Mudde AH, Kouwenberg M, et al. Interference from heterophilic antibodies in seven current TSH assays. Ann Clin Biochem. 2008;45(Pt 6):616.
13. Barbesino G. Drugs affecting thyroid function. Thyroid. 2010;20(7):763-70.
14. Hollowell JG, Staehling NW, Flanders WD, Hannon WH, Gunter EW, Spencer CA, et al. Serum TSH, T4, and thyroid antibodies in the United States Population (1988 to 1994): National Health and Nutrition Examination Survey (NHANES III). J Clin Endocrinol Metab. 2002;87(2):489-99.
15. Jonklaas J, Bianco AC, Bauer AJ, Burman KD, Cappola AR, Celi FS, et al. Guidelines for the Treatment of Hypothyroidism: Prepared by the American Thyroid Association Task Force on Thyroid Hormone Replacement. Thyroid. 2014;24(12):1670-751.
16. Garber JR, Cobin RH, Gharib H, Hennessey JV, Klein I, Mechanick JI, et al. Clinical practice guidelines for hypothyroidism in adults: cosponsored by the American Association of Clinical Endocrinologists and the American Thyroid Association. Endocr Pract. 2012;18(6):988-1028.
17. Haugen BR, Alexander EK, Bible KC, Doherty GM, Mandel SJ, Nikiforov YE, et al. 2015 American Thyroid Association Management Guidelines for Adult Patients with Thyroid Nodules and Differentiated Thyroid Cancer: The American Thyroid Association Guidelines Task Force on Thyroid Nodules and Differentiated Thyroid Cancer. Thyroid. 2016;26(1):1.
18. Ross DS, Burch HB, Cooper DS, Greenlee MC, Laurberg P, Maia AL, et al. 2016 American Thyroid Association Guidelines for Diagnosis and Management of Hyperthyroidism and Other Causes of Thyrotoxicosis. Thyroid. 2016;26(10):1343-421.
19. Pappa T, Ferrara AM, Refetoff S. Inherited defects of thyroxin-binding proteins. Best Pract Res Clin Endocrinol Metab. 2015;29(5):735-47.
20. Janssen OE, Golcher HMB, Grasberger H, Saller B, Mann K, Refetoff S. Characterization of T4-Binding Globulin Cleaved by Human Leukocyte Elastase. J Clin Endocrinol Metab. 2002;87(3):1217-22.
21. Sarne D. Effects of the environment, chemicals and drugs on thyroid function. In: Feingold KR, Anawalt B, Boyce A, Chrousos G, Dungan K, Grossman A (Eds). South Dartmouth: MDText.com, Inc.; 2000.
22. Stockigt JR, Lim CF. Medications that distort in vitro tests of thyroid function, with particular reference to estimates of serum free thyroxine. Best Pract Res Clin Endocrinol Metab. 2009;23(6):753-67.
23. van Deventer HE, Mendu DR, Remaley AT, Soldin SJ. Inverse log-linear relationship between thyroid-stimulating hormone and free thyroxine measured by direct analog immunoassay and tandem mass spectrometry. Clin Chem. 2011;57(1): 122-7.
24. Toldy E, Lőcsei Z, Szabolcs I, Bezzegh A, Kovács GL. Protein interference in thyroid assays: an in vitro study with in vivo consequences. Clin Chim Acta. 2005;352(1-2):93-104.
25. Al-Muqbel KM, Tashtoush RM. Patterns of thyroid radio-iodine tptake: Jordanian experience. J Nucl Med Technol. 2010;38(1):32-6.

26. Smith TJ, Hegedüs L. Graves' disease. N Engl J Med. 2016;375(16):1552-65.

27. Michalek K, Morshed SA, Latif R, Davies TF. TSH receptor autoantibodies. Autoimmun Rev. 2009;9(2):113-6.

28. Tun NNZ, Beckett G, Zammitt NN, Strachan MWJ, Seckl JR, Gibb FW. Thyrotropin receptor antibody levels at diagnosis and after thionamide course predict Graves' disease relapse. Thyroid. 2016;26(8):1004-9.

29. Jung SJ, Kim DW. Ultrasonographic and cytopathological features of an inflammatory pseudonodule in the thyroid gland. Diagn Cytopathol. 2016;44(9):725-30.

30. Carvalho GA, Perez CL, Ward LS. The clinical use of thyroid function tests. Arq Bras Endocrinol Metabol. 2013;57(3):193-204.

31. Spencer C, Petrovic I, Fatemi S. Current thyroglobulin Autoantibody (TgAb) assays often fail to detect interfering TgAb that can result in the reporting of falsely low/undetectable serum Tg IMA values for patients with differentiated thyroid cancer. J Clin Endocrinol Metab. 2011;96(5):1283-91.

32. Aras G, Gültekin SS, Küçük NO. The additive clinical value of combined thyroglobulin and antithyroglobulin antibody measurements to define persistent and recurrent disease in patients with differentiated thyroid cancer. Nucl Med Commun. 2008;29(10):880-4.

33. Indrasena BSH. Use of thyroglobulin as a tumour marker. World J Biol Chem. 2017;8(1):81-5.

34. Francis Z, Schlumberger M. Serum thyroglobulin determination in thyroid cancer patients. Best Pract Res Clin Endocrinol Metab. 2008;22(6):1039-46.

35. Bevilacqua M, Dominguez LJ, Righini V, Valdes V, Vago T, Leopaldi E, et al. Dissimilar PTH, gastrin, and calcitonin responses to oral calcium and peptones in hypocalcuric hypercalcemia, primary hyperparathyroidism, and normal subjects: A useful tool for differential diagnosis. J Bone Miner Res. 2006;21(3):406-12.

36. Wells SA, Asa SL, Dralle H, Elisei R, Evans DB, Gagel RF, et al. Revised American Thyroid Association Guidelines for the Management of Medullary Thyroid Carcinoma: The American Thyroid Association Guidelines Task Force on Medullary Thyroid Carcinoma. Thyroid. 2015;25(6):567-610.

37. d'Herbomez M, Caron P, Bauters C, Cao CD, Schlienger JL, Sapin R, et al. Reference range of serum calcitonin levels in humans: influence of calcitonin assays, sex, age, and cigarette smoking. Eur J Endocrinol. 2007;157(6):749-55.

38. Castro MR, Gharib H. Thyroid fine-needle aspiration biopsy: progress, practice, and pitfalls. Endocr Pract. 2003;9(2):128-36.

39. Sangalli G, Serio G, Zampatti C, Bellotti M, Lomuscio G. Fine needle aspiration cytology of the thyroid: a comparison of 5469 cytological and final histological diagnoses. Cytopathology. 2006;17(5):245-50.

40. Ravetto C, Colombo L, Dottorini ME. Usefulness of fine-needle aspiration in the diagnosis of thyroid carcinoma: a retrospective study in 37,895 patients. Cancer. 2000;90(6):357-63.

41. Popoveniuc G, Jonklaas J. Thyroid nodules. Med Clin North Am. 2012;96(2):329-49.

42. Haugen BR, Sawka AM, Alexander EK, Bible KC, Caturegli P, Doherty GM, et al. American Thyroid Association Guidelines on the Management of Thyroid Nodules and Differentiated Thyroid Cancer Task Force Review and Recommendation on the Proposed Renaming of Encapsulated Follicular Variant Papillary Thyroid Carcinoma Without Invasion to Noninvasive Follicular Thyroid Neoplasm with Papillary-Like Nuclear Features. Thyroid. 2017;27(4):481-3.

43. Orell SR, Sterrett G. Orell and Sterrett's Fine Needle Aspiration Cytology, 5th edition. Philadelphia: Churchill Livingstone; 2011.

44. Park MH, Yoon JH. Anterior neck hematoma causing airway compression following fine needle aspiration cytology of the thyroid nodule: a case report. Acta Cytol. 2009;53(1):86-8.

45. Alkan S, Koŝar AT, Erdurak SC, Dadaŝ B. Transient vocal cord paralysis following ultrasound-guided fine-needle aspiration biopsy for a thyroid nodule. J Otolaryngol. 2009;38(1):E14-5.

46. Nishihara E, Miyauchi A, Matsuzuka F, Sasaki I, Ohye H, Kubota S, et al. Acute suppurative thyroiditis after fine-needle aspiration causing thyrotoxicosis. Thyroid. 2005;15(10):1183-7.

47. La Rosa GL, Belfiore A, Giuffrida D, Sicurella C, Ippolito O, Russo G, et al. Evaluation of the fine needle aspiration biopsy in the preoperative selection of cold thyroid nodules. Cancer. 1991;67(8):2137-41.

48. Hsu C, Boey J. Diagnostic pitfalls in the fine needle aspiration of thyroid nodules. A study of 555 cases in Chinese patients. Acta Cytol. 1987;31(6):699-704.

49. Malheiros DC, Canberk S, Poller DN, Schmitt F. Thyroid FNAC: Causes of false-positive results. Cytopathology. 2018;29(5):407-17.

50. Cibas ES, Ali SZ. The Bethesda system for reporting thyroid cytopathology. Thyroid. 2009;19(11):1159-65.

51. Cibas ES, Ali SZ. The 2017 Bethesda system for reporting thyroid cytopathology. Thyroid. 2017;27(11):1341-6.

52. Baek JH. Current status of core needle biopsy of the thyroid. Ultrasonography. 2017;36(2):83-5.

53. Burman DR. Core needle biopsy of adrenal neoplasm-A study of diagnostic efficacy of combination of A103 and AE1/AE3. J Dent Med Sci. 2017;16(10):5-11.

54. Na DG, Kim J, Sung JY, Baek JH, Jung KC, Lee H, et al. Core-needle biopsy is more useful than repeat fine-needle aspiration in thyroid nodules read as nondiagnostic or atypia of undetermined significance by the Bethesda system for reporting thyroid cytopathology. Thyroid. 2012;22(5):468-75.

55. Suh CH, Baek JH, Lee JH, Choi YJ, Kim KW, Lee J, et al. The role of core-needle biopsy in the diagnosis of thyroid malignancy in 4580 patients with 4746 thyroid nodules: a systematic review and meta-analysis. Endocrine. 2016;54(2):315-28.

56. Jung CK, Baek JH. Recent advances in core needle biopsy for thyroid nodules. Endocrinol Metab. 2017;32(4):407-12.

57. Yoon JH, Kim EK, Kwak JY, Moon HJ. Effectiveness and limitations of core needle biopsy in the diagnosis of thyroid nodules: review of current literature. J Pathol Transl Med. 2015;49(3):230-5.

58. Liu H, Lin F. Application of immunohistochemistry in thyroid pathology. Arch Pathol Lab Med. 2014;139(1):67-82.

59. Baloch Z, Mete O, Asa SL. Immunohistochemical Biomarkers in Thyroid Pathology. Endocr Pathol. 2018;29(2):91-112.

60. Goldblum JR, Lamps LW, McKenney JK, Myers JL, Ackerman LV, Rosai J. Rosai and Ackerman's Surgical Pathology, 11th edition. Philadelphia: Elsevier; 2018.

61. Ferrari SM, Fallahi P, Ruffilli I, Elia G, Ragusa F, Paparo SR, et al. Molecular testing in the diagnosis of differentiated thyroid carcinomas. Gland Surg. 2018;7(Suppl 1):S19-29.

62. AACE/AAES Task Force on Primary Hyperparathyroidism. The American Association of Clinical Endocrinologists and the American Association of Endocrine Surgeons position statement on the diagnosis and management of primary hyperparathyroidism. Endocr Pract. 2005;11(1):49-54.

63. Cusano NE, Silverberg SJ, Bilezikian JP. Normocalcemic primary hyperparathyroidism. J Clin Densitom. 2013;16(1):33-9.

64. Harvey A, Hu M, Gupta M, Butler R, Mitchell J, Berber E, et al. A new, vitamin D-based, multidimensional nomogram for the diagnosis of primary hyperparathyroidism. Endocr Pract. 2012;18(2):124-31.

65. Jin J, Mitchell J, Shin J, Berber E, Siperstein AE, Milas M. Calculating an individual maxPTH to aid diagnosis of normocalcemic primary hyperparathyroidism. Surgery. 2012;152(6):1184-92.

66. Nussbaum SR, Zahradnik RJ, Lavigne JR, Brennan GL, Nozawa-Ung K, Kim LY, et al. Highly sensitive two-site immunoradiometric assay of parathyrin, and its clinical utility in evaluating patients with hypercalcemia. Clin Chem. 1987;33(8):1364-7.

67. Eastell R, Arnold A, Brandi ML, Brown EM, D'Amour P, Hanley DA, et al. Diagnosis of asymptomatic primary hyperparathyroidism: Proceedings of the Third International Workshop. J Clin Endocrinol Metab. 2009;94(2):340-50.

68. Glendenning P. Diagnosis of primary hyperparathyroidism: controversies, practical issues and the need for Australian guidelines. Intern Med J. 2003;33(12):598-603.

69. Edelson GW, Kleerekoper M. Hypercalcemic crisis. Med Clin North Am. 1995;79(1):79-92.

70. Piketty ML, Prie D, Sedel F, Bernard D, Hercend C, Chanson P, et al. High-dose biotin therapy leading to false biochemical endocrine profiles: validation of a simple method to overcome biotin interference. Clin Chem Lab Med. 2017;55(6): 817-25.

71. Barczynski M, Konturek A, Hubalewska-Dydejczyk A, Cichon S, Nowak W. Evaluation of Halle, Miami, Rome, and Vienna intraoperative iPTH assay criteria in guiding minimally invasive parathyroidectomy. Langenbecks Arch Surg. 2009;394(5):843-9.

72. Bilezikian JP. Primary hyperparathyroidism. J Clin Endocrinol Metab. 2018;103(11):3993-4004.

73. Shane E. Parathyroid carcinoma. J Clin Endocrinol Metab. 2001;86(2):485-93.

74. Fahey T. Parathyroid carcinoma: A 43-year outcome and survival analysis. Yearbook Surg. 2012;2012:180-1.

75. Stack JBC, Bodenner DL. Medical and Surgical Treatment of Parathyroid Diseases: An Evidence-based Approach. Cham: Springer International Publishing; 2018.

76. Eisner BH, Ahn J, Stoller ML. Differentiating primary from secondary hyperparathyroidism in stone patients: the "thiazide challenge". J Endourol. 2009;23(2):191-2.

77. Insogna KL. Primary hyperparathyroidism. N Engl J Med. 2018;379(11):1050-9.

78. Christensen SE, Nissen PH, Vestergaard P, Heickendorff L, Brixen K, Mosekilde L. Discriminative power of three indices of renal calcium excretion for the distinction between familial hypocalciuric hypercalcemia and primary hyperparathyroidism: a follow-up study on methods. Clin Endocrinol. 2008;69(5):713-20.

79. Shinall M, Dahir K, Broome J. Differentiating familial hypocalciuric hypercalcemia from primary hyperparathyroidism. Endocr Pract. 2013;19(4):697-702.

80. Silva BC, Bilezikian JP. Trabecular bone score: perspectives of an imaging technology coming of age. Endocrinol Metab. 2014;58(5):493-503.

81. Silva BC, Broy SB, Boutroy S, Schousboe JT, Shepherd JA, Leslie WD. Fracture rick prediction by non-BMD DXA measures: the 2015 ISCD official positions. Part 2: trabecular bone score. J Clin Densitom. 2015;18(3):309-30.

82. Kebebew E, Clark OH. Parathyroid adenoma, hyperplasia, and carcinoma: localization, technical details of primary neck exploration, and treatment of hypercalcemic crisis. Surg Oncol Clin North Am. 1998;7(4):721-48.

83. Mudde AH, van den Berg H, Boshuis PG, Breedveld FC, Markusse HM, Kluin PM, et al. Ectopic production of 1,25-dihydroxyvitamin D by B-cell Lymphoma as a cause of hypercalcemia. Cancer. 1987;59(9):1543-6.

84. Hewison M, Kantorovich V, Liker HR, Herle AJV, Cohan P, Zehnder D, et al. Vitamin D-mediated hypercalcemia in lymphoma: evidence for hormone production by tumor-adjacent macrophages. J Bone Min Res. 2003;18(3): 579-82.

85. Layfield LJ. Fine needle aspiration cytology of cystic parathyroid lesions: a cytomorphologic overlap with cystic lesions of the thyroid. Acta Cytol. 1991;35(4):447-50.

86. Tseng FY, Hsiao YL, Chang TC. Ultrasound-guided fine needle aspiration cytology of parathyroid lesions: a review of 72 cases. Acta Cytol. 2002;46(6):1029-36.

87. Kumari N, Mishra D, Pradhan R, Agarwal A, Krishnani N. Utility of fine-needle aspiration cytology in the identification of parathyroid lesions. J Cytol. 2016;33(1):17-21.

88. Giordano TJ. Parathyroid glands. In: Goldblum J, Lamps L, McKenney J, Myers J (Eds). Rosai and Ackerman's Surgical Pathology, 11th edition. Philadelphia: Elsevier; 2017. pp. 357-8.

89. McKenzie TJ, Lillegard JB, Young WF, Thompson GB. Aldosteronomas—state of the art. Surg Clin North Am. 2009;89(5): 1241-53.

90. Wagner-Bartak NA, Baiomy A, Habra MA, Mukhi SV, Morani AC, Korivi BR, et al. Cushing syndrome: Diagnostic workup and imaging features, with clinical and pathologic correlation. AJR Am J Roentgenol. 2017;209(1):19-32.

91. Kimura N, Takekoshi K, Naruse M. Risk stratification on pheochromocytoma and paraganglioma from laboratory and clinical medicine. J Clin Med. 2018;7(9):E242.

92. Därr R, Kuhn M, Bode C, Bornstein SR, Pacak K, Lenders JWM, et al. Accuracy of recommended sampling and assay methods for the determination of plasma-free and urinary fractionated metanephrines in the diagnosis of pheochromocytoma and paraganglioma: a systematic review. Endocrine. 2017;56(3): 495-503.

93. Fishbein L. Pheochromocytoma and paraganglioma: Genetics, diagnosis, and treatment. Hematol Oncol Clin North Am. 2016;30(1):135-50.

94. Jhala NC, Jhala D, Eloubeidi MA, Chhieng DC, Crowe DR, Roberson J, et al. Endoscopic ultrasound-guided fine-needle aspiration biopsy of the adrenal glands: analysis of 24 patients. Cancer. 2004;102(5):308-14.

95. Fassina AS, Borsato S, Fedeli U. Fine needle aspiration cytology (FNAC) of adrenal masses. Cytopathology. 2000;11(5):302-11.

96. Rana C, Krishnani N, Kumari N. Spectrum of adrenal lesions on fine needle aspiration cytology. Indian J Pathol Microbiol. 2012;55(4):461-6.

97. Villelli NW, Jayanti MK, Zynger DL. Use and usefulness of adrenal core biopsies without FNA or on-site evaluation of adequacy: A study of 204 cases for a 12-year period. Am J Clin Pathol. 2012;137(1):124-31.

98. Harisinghani MG, Maher MM, Hahn PF, Gervais DA, Jhaveri K, Varghese J, et al. Predictive value of benign percutaneous adrenal biopsies in oncology patients. Clin Radiol. 2002;57(10): 898-901.

99. Weiss LM. Comparative histologic study of 43 metastasizing and nonmetastasizing adrenocortical tumors. Am J Surg Pathol. 1984;8(3):163-9.

100. Aubert S, Wacrenier A, Leroy X, Devos P, Carnaille B, Proye C, et al. Weiss system revisited: a clinicopathologic and immunohistochemical study of 49 adrenocortical tumors. Am J Surg Pathol. 2002;26(12):1612-9.

101. Thompson LDR. Pheochromocytoma of the adrenal gland scaled score (PASS) to separate benign from malignant neoplasms: a clinicopathologic and immunophenotypic study of 100 cases. Am J Surg Pathol. 2002;26(5):551-66.

102. Busam KJ, Iversen K, Coplan KA, Old LJ, Stockert E, Chen YT, et al. Immunoreactivity for A103, an antibody to melan-A (Mart-1), in adrenocortical and other steroid tumors. Am J Surg Pathol. 1998;22(1):57-63.

103. Renshaw AA, Granter SR. A comparison of A103 and inhibin reactivity in adrenal cortical tumors: distinction from hepatocellular carcinoma and renal tumors. Mod Pathol. 1998;11(12):1160-4.

104. Papotti M, Duregon E, Volante M, McNicol AM. Pathology of the adrenal cortex: a reappraisal of the past 25 years focusing on adrenal cortical tumors. Endocr Pathol. 2014;25(1):35-48.

105. Wirnsberger GH, Becker H, Ziervogel K, Höfler H. Diagnostic immunohistochemistry of neuroblastic tumors. Am J Surg Pathol. 1992;16(1):49-57.

106. Hung YP, Lee JP, Bellizzi AM, Hornick JL. PHOX2B reliably distinguishes neuroblastoma among small round blue cell tumours. Histopathology. 2017;71(5):786-94.

107. Bielinska M, Parviainen H, Kiiveri S, Heikinheimo M, Wilson DB. Origin and Molecular Pathology of Adrenocortical Neoplasms. Vet Pathol. 2009;46(2):194-210.

108. US National Library of Medicine. (2019). Evaluation of Molecular Markers in Adrenal Tumors. [online] Available from https://clinicaltrials.gov/ct2/show/NCT01348698. [Last accessed April, 2020].

109. Zhao J, Speel EJ, Muletta-Feurer S, Rütimann K, Saremaslani P, Roth J, et al. Analysis of genomic alterations in sporadic adrenocortical lesions. Gain of chromosome 17 is an early event in adrenocortical tumorigenesis. Am J Pathol. 1999;155(4):1039-45.

110. Schmitz KJ, Helwig J, Bertram S, Sheu SY, Suttorp AC, Seggewiß J, et al. Differential expression of microRNA-675, microRNA-139-3p and microRNA-335 in benign and malignant adrenocortical tumours. J Clin Pathol. 2011;64(6):529-35.

111. Dattani MT, Hindmarsh PC. Growth hormone deficiency in children. In: DeGroot LJ, Jemeson JL, de Kretser D, Grossman AB, Marshall JC, Melmed S, Potts JT, Weir GC (Eds). Endocrinology, 5th edition. Philadelphia: Elsevier Saunders; 2006. pp. 733-54.

112. Ho KKY. Growth hormone deficiency in adults. In: DeGroot LJ, Jemeson JL, de Kretser D, Grossman AB, Marshall JC, Melmed S, Potts JT, Weir GC (Eds). Endocrinology, 5th edition. Philadelphia: Elsevier Saunders; 2006. pp. 754-65.

113. Sizonenko PC, Clayton PE, Cohen P, Hintz RL, Tanaka T, Laron Z. Diagnosis and management of growth hormone deficiency in childhood and adolescence. Part 1: diagnosis of growth hormone deficiency. Growth Horm IGF Res. 2001;11(3):137-65.

114. Growth Hormone Research Society. Consensus guidelines for the diagnosis and treatment of growth hormone (GH) deficiency in childhood and adolescence: summary statement of the GH Research Society. GH Research Society. J Clin Endocrinol Metab. 2000;85(11):3990-3.

115. Molitch ME, Clemmons DR, Malozowski S, Merriam GR, Shalet SM, Vance ML, et al. Evaluation and treatment of adult growth hormone deficiency: an Endocrine Society Clinical Practice Guideline. J Clin Endocrinol Metab. 2006;91(5):1621-34.

116. Ho KK, 2007 GH Deficiency Consensus Workshop Participants. Consensus guidelines for the diagnosis and treatment of adults with GH deficiency II: a statement of the GH Research Society in association with the European Society for Pediatric Endocrinology, Lawson Wilkins Society, European Society of Endocrinology, Japan Endocrine Society, and Endocrine Society of Australia. Eur J Endocrinol. 2007;157(6):695-700.

117. Melmed S. Acromegaly. In: DeGroot LJ, Jemeson JL, de Kretser D, Grossman AB, Marshall JC, Melmed S, Potts JT, Weir GC (Eds). Endocrinology, 5th edition. Philadelphia: Elsevier Saunders; 2006. pp. 411-28.

118. Fisher DA, Carlton E. Endocrine testing. In: DeGroot LJ, Jemeson JL, de Kretser D, Grossman AB, Marshall JC, Melmed S, Potts JT, Weir GC (Eds). Endocrinology, 5th edition. Philadelphia: Elsevier Saunders; 2006. pp. 3605-33.

119. Giustina A, Barkan A, Casanueva FF, Cavagnini F, Frohman L, Ho K, et al. Criteria for cure of acromegaly: a consensus statement. J Clin Endocrinol Metab. 2000;85(2):526-9.

120. Chang-DeMoranville BM, Jackson IMD. Diagnosis and endocrine testing in acromegaly. Endocrinol Metab Clin North Am. 1992;21(3):649-68.

121. Ball SG, Baylis PH. Vasopressin, diabetes insipidus, and syndrome of inappropriate antidiuresis. In: DeGroot LJ, Jemeson JL, de Kretser D, Grossman AB, Marshall JC, Melmed S, Potts JT, Weir GC (Eds). Endocrinology, 5th edition. Philadelphia: Elsevier Saunders; 2006. pp. 537-56.

122. Czernichow P. Testing water regulation. In: Ranke MB (Ed). Diagnostics of Endocrine Function in Children and Adolescents, 2nd edition. Germany: Johann Ambrosius Barth Verlag; 1996. pp. 230-40.

123. Edelmann CM, Barnett HL, Stark H, Boichis H, Soriano JR. A standarized test of renal concentrating capacity in children. Am J Dis Child. 1967;114(6):639-44.

124. Frasier SD, Kutnik LA, Schmidt RT, Smith FG. A water deprivation test for the diagnosis of diabetes insipidus in children. Am J Dis Child. 1967;114(2):157-60.

125. Miller M, Dalakos T, Moses AM, Fellerman H, Streeten DH. Recognition of partial defects in antidiuretic hormone secretion. Ann Intern Med. 1970;73(5):721-9.

126. Eckert KL, Wilson DM, Bachrach LK, Anhalt H, Habiby RL, Olney RC, et al. A single-sample, subcutaneous gonadotropin-releasing hormone test for central precocious puberty. Pediatrics. 1996;97(4):517-9.

127. Roger M, Lahlou N, Chaussain JL. Gonadotropin-releasing hormone testing in pediatrics. In: Ranke MB (Ed). Diagnostics of Endocrine Function in Children and Adolescents, 2nd edition. Germany: Johann Ambrosius Barth Verlag; 1996. pp. 346-69.

128. Neely EK, Hintz RL, Wilson DM, Lee PA, Gautier T, Argente J, et al. Normal ranges for immunochemiluminometric gonadotropin assays. J Pediatr. 1995;127(1):40-6.

129. Eugster EA, Pescovitz OH. Precocious puberty. In: DeGroot LJ, Jemeson JL, de Kretser D, Grossman AB, Marshall JC, Melmed S, Potts JT, Weir GC (Eds). Endocrinology, 5th edition. Philadelphia: Elsevier Saunders; 2006. pp. 2831-46.

130. Alberti KG, Zimmet PZ. Definition, diagnosis and classification of diabetes mellitus and its complications. Part 1: diagnosis and classification of diabetes mellitus provisional report of a WHO consultation. Diabet Med. 1998;15(7):539-53.

131. Poomthavorn P, Khlairit P, Mahachoklertwattana P. Subcutaneous gonadotropin-releasing hormone agonist (triptorelin) test for diagnosing precocious puberty. Horm Res. 2009;72(2):114-9.

132. Metzger BE, Coustan DR. Summary and recommendations of the Fourth International Workshop-Conference on Gestational Diabetes Mellitus. The Organizing Committee. Diabetes Care. 1998;21 Suppl 2:B161-7.

133. Metzer BE, Purdy LP, Phelps RL. Diabetes mellitus and pregnancy. In: DeGroot LJ, Jemeson JL, de Kretser D, Grossman AB, Marshall JC, Melmed S, Potts JT, Weir GC (Eds). Endocrinology, 5th edition. Philadelphia: Elsevier Saunders; 2006. pp. 3419-35.

134. Metzger BE, Buchanan TA. Summary and recommendations of the Fifth International Workshop-Conference on Gestational Diabetes Mellitus. Diabetes Care. 2007;Suppl 2: S251-60.

135. Knip M, Akerblom HK. Plasma C-peptide and insulin in neonates, infants, and children. J Pediatr. 1981;99(1):103-5.

136. Ewing DJ, Clarke BF. Diagnosis and management of diabetic autonomic neuropathy. Br Med J. 1982;285(6346):916-8.

137. Soltesz G, Aynsley-Green, Morris A. Approach to the diagnosis of hypoglycemia in infants and children. In: Ranke MB (Ed). Diagnostics of Endocrine Function in Children and Adolescents, 2nd edition. Germany: Johann Ambrosius Barth Verlag; 1996. pp. 275-98.

138. Soltesz G, Aynsley-Green A. Hyperinsulinism in infancy and childhood. In: Brandis M, Frick P, Kochsiek K, Martini GA, Prader A (Eds). Ergebnisse der innerenMedizin und KinderneilKunde. Berlin: Springer; 1984. pp. 152-202.

139. Gerich JE. Hypoglycemia. In: DeGroot LJ, Jemeson JL, de Kretser D, Grossman AB, Marshall JC, Melmed S, Potts JT, Weir GC (Eds). Endocrinology, 5th edition. Philadelphia: Elsevier Saunders; 2006. pp. 1203-29.

Endocrine Radiology

Archana Gupta, Pankaj Sharma

◇ INTRODUCTION

Endocrine radiology is a subspecialty of radiology, in which diagnostic and interventional radiology principles are applied, for management of patients with endocrinopathies. By endocrinopathies, we mean disorders, which result from a pathological source of hormone production.[1-3] Whenever we encounter a patient with endocrinopathy, we first try to evaluate the patient using noninvasive imaging, along with laboratory investigation and clinical presentation. Invasive intervention, in the form of endocrine venous sampling, is done only when the source of endocrinopathy is not detected using noninvasive methods.[4] Moreover, endocrine venous sampling helps us in localizing disease, by detecting relative elevation of hormone, in organ of interest. Management of endocrinopathy requires team approach between laboratory medicine, endocrine radiologist, interventional radiologist, medical endocrinologist, and endocrine surgeon.

The human endocrine system includes the following organs:
- Pineal gland
- Pituitary–hypothalamic axis
- Thyroid and parathyroid glands
- Thymus
- Pancreas
- Adrenals
- Testes (in males)
- Ovaries (in females)

Endocrine disorders occur in two conditions:
1. *If there is too much hormone*: In this condition, we first try to detect the source of excess hormone production. Thereafter, we try to suppress this excess hormone production.
2. *If there is too less hormone*: In this condition, we try to find the cause of hormone deficiency and then we try to stimulate gland to increase hormone production.

Endocrine disorder may primarily be due to dysfunction at three important levels:
1. *Central level*: Hypothalamic/pituitary axis
2. *Peripheral level*: Dysfunction of peripheral glands
3. *Receptor/postreceptor level*: Target cell insufficiency or low sensitivity to hormone action

◇ CLINICAL PRESENTATION

Majority of insulinomas are small (<1 cm) and solitary.[5] Insulinomas are multiple in MEN1 and Von Hippel–Lindau disease. Postexercise or postfasting hypoglycemia, neuroglycopenic symptoms, and relief after eating or intravenous glucose supplementation constitute the Whipple triad of insulinoma.

◇ LABORATORY INVESTIGATIONS

Whenever there is an endocrine disorder, we first do the following laboratory investigations:
- *Standard biochemistry*: Sodium, potassium, and glucose
- Plasma hormone level
- Hormone diurnal rhythm
- Urinary hormones/metabolites
- Stimulatory/inhibitory tests

Adrenal hemorrhage: Serum cortisol level of >18 µg/dL is often used to exclude adrenal insufficiency in situations of severe stress.

If hypertension is present, we measure plasma aldosterone concentration and plasma renin activity. An appropriate screening test in this condition is a random aldosterone to renin activity ratio that is >30.

Plasma metanephrines have similar sensitivity and specificity for pheochromocytoma as urine-fractionated metanephrines and may be considered as the first screening test.

Routine hormonal evaluation of all adrenal incidentalomas (AIs) will be costly and is not routinely performed. Biochemical evaluation should be considered only if there are clinical signs or symptoms of adrenal hyperfunction.

For all adrenal tumors, hormonal evaluation should be performed at the time of diagnosis and then annually for 5 years.

◇ FUNCTIONAL TESTS

First of all, we try to detect hormone levels in blood or urine. We also try to check hormone diurnal rhythm. But very often, the basal hormone level does not allow us to establish a diagnosis of hypofunction or hyperfunction. So, we have to resort to stimulatory test, if we suspect hypofunction, as this helps us to quantify functional reserve of the endocrine gland.

Few stimulatory tests used for patient management are as follows:

- Gonadotropin-releasing hormone (GnRH) test
- Corticotropin-releasing hormone (CRH) test
- Insulin hypoglycemia test
- Thyrotropin-releasing hormone (TRH) test
- Metyrapone test
- Levodopa test
- Arginine infusion test

If we suspect hyperfunction, then we do inhibitory tests to quantify the response of endocrine glands to these inhibitory factors.

Few inhibitory tests used for patient management are as follows:

- Dexamethasone test
- *Dopaminergic drugs test:*
  - Physiological stress → hypothalamus releases CRH → triggers release of adrenocorticotropic hormone (ACTH) from anterior pituitary → stimulates release of cortisol from adrenal cortex → promotes gluconeogenesis, fat mobilization, and protein mobilization → downregulates further release of CRH and ACTH

◇ IMAGING TECHNIQUES

Imaging techniques are used in endocrinopathy, for two indications:

1. To localize endocrine active tumors, adenomas, hyperplasia, or ectopic hormonal producing lesions
2. To evaluate systemic complications of these endocrinopathies

Modalities used for noninvasive imaging are as follows:

- X-rays
- Ultrasonography (USG)
- Computed tomography (CT)
- Magnetic resonance imaging (MRI)
- Scintigraphy

X-rays

X-ray examination is the first investigation done in many endocrinopathies, such as:

1. Increased parathyroid activity leading to characteristic subperiosteal resorption in hands and salt, and pepper skull.
   - Osteolysis of sella turcica as a late manifestation of large pituitary tumors. These tumors are appreciated in the early stage by MRI
   - Arachnodactyly
   - Thyroid masses may incidentally be detected on chest radiography
   - Thoracic inlet view may demonstrate tracheal compression, caused by thyroid mass.

- Adrenal gland calcification may be seen on abdominal X-ray, in some conditions such as in Addison disease.

Ultrasonography

High-resolution USG of thyroid is done for characterizing focal and diffuse thyroid nodules, using a 7–12 MHz linear probe. For obese patients, patients with short neck and large thyroid gland (goiter, low-frequency probe is required. On ultrasound, we can differentiate between solid and cystic components, by using gray-scale with Doppler. Moreover, USG can be used for image-guided fine-needle aspiration cytology (FNAC)/biopsy of thyroid nodules.

We use American College of Radiology (ACR) Thyroid Imaging Reporting and Data System (TIRADS) for characterizing focal thyroid nodules and for recommending management decisions.[6] In ACR TIRADS, we characterize focal thyroid nodules, based on the following imaging five characteristics:

1. *Composition*: 0–2 points
2. *Echogenicity*: 0–3 points
3. *Shape*: 0–3 points
4. *Margin*: 0–3 points
5. *Echogenic foci*: 0–3 points

The final score is addition of scores for each imaging characteristic, and based on the final score, each nodule is assigned a category TR1 or TR2, or TR3 or TR4, or TR5. In each category (TR1 to TR5), the management decision is recommended based on the maximum diameter of the thyroid nodule. A maximum of four thyroid nodules are assigned category TR1 to TR5 and a maximum of two thyroid nodules are selected for FNAC/biopsy, based on most suspicious features, or higher assigned category: TR1 to TR5. Significant enlargement of thyroid nodule in ACR TIRADS is said to occur, if there is:

- 20% increase in at least two nodule dimensions or minimal increase of 2 mm
- 50% or greater increase in volume.

Minimal follow-up period in ACR TIRADS for a suspicious thyroid nodule is 1 year. Imaging can stop at 5 years if there is no change in size. The follow-up interval for different thyroid nodules is as follows:

- *TR5*: Scanning every year for up to 5 years
- *TR4*: 1, 2, 3, and 5 years
- *TR3*: 1, 3, and 5 years

If all thyroid nodules show a similar echogenic pattern, then no follow-up is required according to ACR TIRADS.

The ACR TIRADS has a few limitations:

- Neck nodes are not evaluated.
- Elastography is not included.
- T5 is a broad category, with scores ranging from 7 to 15, and needs further subcategorization.

Neck nodes are considered suspicious for malignancy, if the following features are seen:
- Loss of the normal echogenic hilum
- Globular shape
- Presence of peripheral rather than central flow
- Heterogeneity with cystic components
- Punctate echogenic foci that may represent micro-calcification

For histological examination of thyroid nodules (especially for deeply located nodules, cystic nodules, and nonpalpable nodules), we do USG-guided FNAC. The complication rate for USG-guided FNAC varies from 0 to 8.6%, and these include hematoma around thyroid gland, edema of the thyroid gland, and temporary changes in voice. USG-guided core needle biopsy (CNB) is an alternative to FNAC, if previous USG-guided FNAC result comes as nondiagnostic.[7-9] An important technical tip for avoiding injury in the recurrent laryngeal nerve is to start from isthmus and then going into the thyroid gland for a deeply seated suspicious thyroid nodule. If there is a large cystic-solid nodule, then sometimes we may have to aspirate cystic components, before targeting a solid portion of the nodule for FNAC.

High-resolution USG is sometimes used for localizing and characterizing parathyroid adenomas.[10,11] These parathyroid adenomas are generally seen as well-defined, round to oval, hypoechoic lesions, posterior to the thyroid gland and medial to the carotid vessels. But, sometimes, parathyroid adenoma may be seen anterior or anterolateral to carotid vessels.

USG is also useful for localizing adrenal gland and endocrine pancreatic lesions.[12,13] But these lesions are better characterized on cross-sectional imaging—CT/MRI. USG is used for detecting large adrenal masses.

Intraoperative USG is done as work-up for pancreatic insulinomas, both for diagnosis and as guidance for biopsy. However, the limitation is a long learning curve, along with limited evaluation of pancreatic tail and nodal sites. Insulinoma is generally seen in the pancreas as a well-defined, round hypoechoic lesion, with smooth margins. Combined sensitivity of multidetector computed tomography (MDCT) + endoscopic ultrasound (EUS) is 95–100%.

90% gastrinomas are seen in the gastrinoma triangle.[14,15] The boundaries of gastrinoma triangle are as follows:
- Junction of common and cystic duct
- Junction of neck and body of pancreas
- Junction of second and third segments of duodenum
  70–80% gastrinomas are sporadic and 20–25% gastrinomas are associated with multiple endocrine neoplasia type 1 (MEN1) syndrome. In MEN1 syndrome, gastrinomas are more often multicentric, extrapancreatic, and benign. Gastrinomas can be associated with liver and nodal metastasis.

Nonfunctioning pancreatic neuroendocrine tumor (pNET) accounts for 50–70% pNET, and most are solitary, sporadic, and large, with symptoms from mass effect.[16,17]

Most nonfunctioning pNETs have no syndrome, can secrete hormones such as pancreatic polypeptide, and can be metastatic to liver and nodes at presentation. Nonfunctioning pNET can invade pancreatic ducts and 33% have venous thrombosis.

Predictors of nodal metastasis in pNET are primary tumor size >4 cm and radiologically detectable lymph nodes.

Computed Tomography

Computed tomography is an imaging modality of choice for detecting adrenal lesions, as small as 3–4 mm, and for characterizing calcification. CT has an important role to play in characterizing adrenal lesions, especially AIs.[18-20] AIs are adrenal lesions of size 1 cm or more in diameter, which are discovered on imaging for indications, exclusive to adrenal conditions. The first question we ask on seeing AI is whether AI is functioning or not. Then, we measure attenuation of AI in Hounsfield unit (HU) on a precontrast scan. If HU is <10 HU, then adrenal lesion is lipid-rich adenoma. If HU is >10 HU on precontrast scans, then this lesion needs further characterization. We do postcontrast scans and measure HU of adrenal lesion at 1 and 15 minutes. Then, we measure absolute coefficient (AC) and relative coefficient (RC) as follows:

Adrenal lesion AC	$\dfrac{HU\ at\ 1\ min - HU\ at\ 15\ min \times 100\%}{HU\ at\ 1\ min - HU\ on\ precontrast\ scan}$
Adrenal lesion RC	$\dfrac{HU\ at\ 1\ min - HU\ at\ 15\ min \times 100\%}{HU\ at\ 1\ min}$

Lipid-poor adenomas show AC 60% or more and RC 40% or more. These adenomas are generally followed by and surgery is only done if there is confirmed hormonal activity [ACTH-independent hypercortisolemia or primary hyperaldosteronism (PH)].

Pheochromocytomas follow the 10% rule:[21,22] 10% malignant, 10% bilateral, 10% extra-adrenal, and 10% pediatric. Pheochromocytoma diagnosis is based on biochemistry and CT is used for localizing pheochromocytomas, if size is >1 cm. Most pheochromocytomas show intense contrast enhancement, with AC <60% and RC <40%. Approximately 35% of pheochromocytomas may have signal hypointensity on CT, and these pheochromocytomas show AC >60% and RC >40%.

Intravenous administration of nonionic contrast material for CT is a safe practice for patients with pheochromocytoma and related tumors, even without α-1-blocking medication.

Any adrenal lesion that increases in size on a 6-month scan is considered malignant. Benign adrenal lesions can show an increase in size in the following two conditions:
1. Traumatic or spontaneous hemorrhage in adrenal gland
2. Adenomas and myelolipomas

If AIs are stable in size on two imaging, 6 months apart, and if these AIs do not exhibit hormonal hypersecretion over 4 years, then further follow-up is not warranted.

Adrenal cortical carcinomas (ACCs) are generally >4 cm in size and show evidence of large necrotic areas.[23,24] Calcification is seen in 30% of ACC.

Adrenal metastasis generally shows homogeneous appearance, similar to adenomas. But metastasis has AC <60% and RC <40%.

Adrenal metastasis is most commonly from lung, breast, stomach, kidney, melanomas, and lymphomas.[25-27] Adrenal metastasis is seen in 33% of patients with bronchogenic carcinoma. The possibility of an adrenal nodule being malignant in patients with known malignancy is 25–36%. However, this probability reduces to <0.5% in patients without known malignancy. Metastasis is usually homogeneous and similar in appearance to adenomas, especially when small in size.

Imaging workup for an androgen-secreting tumor should include CT or MR imaging of both the adrenal gland and the pelvis to evaluate for an ovarian tumor.[28-30] Androgen-secreting tumors arising from the adrenal gland are usually >1.5 cm and are well visualized at CT, whereas the majority of androgen-secreting ovarian tumors are relatively small (<2 cm) and can be missed at pelvic examination, diagnostic laparoscopy, and/or US.

In Addison disease, adrenal atrophy with calcification can be seen as an evidence of tuberculosis.[31]

In Cushing disease, 80% cases have bilateral hyperplasia due to pituitary (75%) or paraneoplastic (5%) ACTH overproduction.[32,33]

Adrenal myelolipomas contain macroscopic fat.[34,35]

For thyroid lesions, CT is not as good as USG, at resolving lesions within the thyroid. However, CT is good for detecting calcification and for assessing mediastinal disease.

For neuroendocrine tumors (NET), including insulinomas and gastrinomas, we do multiphasic pancreatic CT (noncontrast, early arterial, pancreatic parenchymal, and portal venous phase), with NET detected best in early arterial phase. Multiphasic CT is also useful to access venous involvement and to detect liver metastasis. Most insulinomas are detected in pancreas and are octreotide negative whereas most gastrinomas are detected in the gastrinoma triangle. Dual-energy CT has been found useful for NET, with sensitivity 87–96% for dual-energy, dual-phase CT.

Liver metastasis is detected in pNET on multiphase imaging.[36] While classically metastases are hyperintense on arterial phase imaging and hypointense on portovenous phase imaging, metastasis can be very varied in the same patient and between studies.

Magnetic Resonance Imaging

Magnetic resonance imaging has an advantage of better soft-tissue resolution and is radiation free. MRI is useful for differentiation of pituitary tumors and hemangioma. MRI is also good for localization of parathyroid glands in cases of recurrent/persistent hyperparathyroidism.

Cushing syndrome (CS) results from prolonged exposure to an elevated cortisol level. CS resulting from pituitary oversecretion is called Cushing disease, and the majority of these cases are due to ACTH-secreting pituitary adenomas. Pituitary adenomas are usually seen in young patients, with a 3.5:1 female-to-male ratio. Imaging consists of dedicated pituitary protocol MRI. However, up to 40% of scans are falsely negative.

The adrenal gland shows low-to-intermediate signal intensity on T1- and T2-weighted images. MRI techniques which are sensitive to the presence of lipid are as follows:[37,38]

- Dixon method (in-phase and out-of-phase imaging)
- Short tau inversion recovery (STIR) sequence
- Phase-contrast sequence
- Radiofrequency-selective fat suppression

Lipid-rich adrenal adenomas show loss of signal on out-of-phase imaging, as compared with the corresponding in-plane imaging.

An MRI may help in differentiating between subacute hemorrhage and fat-containing adrenal masses, as both these lesions can show high-signal intensity on T1-weighted spin-echo images.

Diffusion-weighted imaging (DWI) along with apparent diffusion coefficient (ADC) plays an important complementary role in differentiating benign from malignant adrenal lesions.

For thyroid lesions, MRI is better for differentiating fibrosis from residual tumor.

For detecting insulinomas, we use the following methods:
- Fat-suppressed T1-weighted sequence
- Dynamic postcontrast fat-saturated T1-weighted images
- Fat-suppressed T2-weighted images
- Diffusion-weighted imaging

MRI has an evolving role in detection and grading of insulinoma, along with detection of unexpected metastasis, and for nodal status. It is best for detecting liver metastasis, especially when we use liver-specific agents.

Diffusion-weighted imaging may aid in detection of gastrinoma, in evaluating tumor grade, and in differential diagnosis.

MRI sequences for detecting nodal disease in pNET are T2-weighted sequence, diffusion and black blood sequence for vessels. Poorly differentiated pNETs have lower ADC values than well-differentiated pNET.

MRI has more sensitivity than CT and octreotide for detecting liver metastasis in pNET. MRI sensitivity for detecting liver metastasis in pNET on different sequences is as follows—diffusion 72%, T2-weighted sequence 57%, and dynamic scan 48%.

Scintigraphy[39-41]

Scintigraphy refers to application of isotope and its uptake in functional parenchyma of endocrine glands. Ideal radiopharmaceutical is cheap, readily available, localizes only in organ of interest, is easy to prepare, is easily incorporated without altering behavior, and has half-life of elimination from body similar to duration of test.

Different radiopharmaceuticals are used in endocrine radiology and they emit radiation as follows:

- ^{131}I: β + γ-emitter
- ^{125}I: γ-emitter
- $^{99m}Tc\text{-}MIBI$: γ-emitter
- $131I\text{-}MIBEG$: β + γ-emitter
- $^{99m}Tc\text{-}octreotide$: γ-emitter

Thyroid Scintigraphy[42-44]

For thyroid, the following three radiopharmaceuticals are used: ^{99m}Tc-pertechnetate, ^{123}I, and ^{131}I.

^{99m}Tc-pertechnetate is a cheap and readily available radiopharmaceutical, competes with iodide for uptake, is trapped in the thyroid gland, but not organified. Moreover, it shows poor image quality and can be misleading, if there is activity in esophagus or vascular structures.

^{123}I and ^{131}I are expensive, cyclotron-generated and better for retrosternal goiter. Moreover, both ^{123}I and ^{131}I are trapped and organified in the thyroid gland. ^{131}I has a large radiation dose. Hence, ^{131}I is used only when treatment with ^{131}I is planned. Both ^{123}I and ^{131}I require a long scanning time, as long as 24 hours for delayed scans.

An important point we will like to highlight here is that iodinated contrast should not be given 10 days prior to thyroid scintigraphy, as it blocks the uptake of radiopharmaceutical. After thyroid scintigraphy, the thyroid nodule can be hot or cold. If the thyroid nodule is hot, then the risk of malignancy is 4%. However, if the thyroid nodule is cold, then the risk of malignancy is 16%.

In toxic nodular goiter and in diffuse toxic goiter (Graves), we see an increase in thyroid radionuclide uptake. In thyroiditis, we see a decrease in thyroid radionuclide uptake.

Here, we will like to reemphasize that the first investigation for thyroid nodule is cytology and ultrasound. Radionuclide imaging is used for investigation of hyperthyroidism, especially for detecting location of ectopic thyroid disease.

Parathyroid Scintigraphy[45]

Primary hyperparathyroidism is in 80% cases due to parathyroid adenoma, in 15% cases due to parathyroid hyperplasia, and in 1% cases due to carcinoma.

Uncomplicated primary hyperparathyroidism has 90–95% surgical success without imaging. However, for recurrent/persistent hyperparathyroidism, surgical success without imaging is only 50%. We use combined radionuclide imaging along with MRI for recurrent/persistent hyperparathyroidism, with a surgical success rate, as high as 90%.

For parathyroid imaging, we use the following radio-pharmaceuticals:

- ^{99m}Tc/^{201}Tl subtraction scans
- ^{99m}Tc-MIBI early/late scans

Both the above-mentioned scintigraphy techniques are good for detection of ectopic parathyroids, with false-positive results in thyroid pathology and false-negative results in parathyroid hyperplasia.

Adrenal Scintigraphy[46,47]

Both radiological and scintigraphy imaging methods of the adrenal glands are necessary and, therefore, should be considered complementary.

Adrenal cortical radionuclide imaging: We use radiolabeled cholesterol esters (^{75}seleno-methyl-norcholesteorol, ^{131}I-6B iodomethyl-19-norcholesterol) and do imaging at 4 and 7 days. >50% difference in activity between sides is abnormal.

- In ACTH-dependent (pituitary/ectopic) CS, we see an increase in activity in bilateral adrenal glands.
- In ACTH-independent CS, with bilateral adrenal nodular hyperplasia, we see an increase in activity in bilateral adrenal glands.
- However, in ACTH-independent CS, with adrenocortical adenoma, we see an increase in activity in the unilateral adrenal gland.
- In adrenocortical carcinoma, we see a decrease in activity in bilateral adrenal glands.
- In CS, radionuclide imaging is used for detecting residual functioning of adrenal remnants, if there is residual disease after prior bilateral adrenalectomy.

Adrenal medullary radionuclide imaging: We use metaiodo-benzylguanidine (MIBG), as it localizes in catecholamine storage vesicles of adrenergic nerve endings **(Table 1)**.

- In primary aldosteronism, radionuclide imaging is used along with dexamethasone suppression test to detect tumors as small as 1 cm.
- Adrenal visualization before 5 days is abnormal (bilateral/unilateral).
- For functioning AI, diagnosis is based on clinical features and biochemistry. However, confirmation is done using radionuclide imaging.
- Somatostatin receptor (SSTR) scanning is used for detecting the source of ectopic ACTH, especially from small bronchial carcinoid tumors.

Neuroendocrine Tumor Scintigraphy[48,49]

In-111 octreotide imaging:

- It is an analog of somatostatin and binds strongly to receptors 2 and 5 and weakly to receptor 3.
- It binds well to well-differentiated noninsulinoma pNET, but not to poorly differentiated PNET.

Table 1: MIBG scanning.	
Diseases	*Senstivity*
Pheochromocytoma	95%
Neuroblastoma	80–90%
Carcinoid	70%
MTC	40%

(MIBG: metaiodobenzylguanidine)

- *Overall sensitivity*: 60–90%
- Sensitivity for glucagonomas is 100%, for VIPomas is 88%, and for gastrinomas is 73%.
- Sensitivity for insulinomas is only 50–70%, because they express predominantly SSTR3.
- Imaging is done at 4 and 24 hours, with single-photon emission computed tomography (SPECT) and fusion with CT.
- Well-differentiated nonfunctioning pNETs are octreotide positive.
- *Fused octreotide*: SPECT/CT improves specificity for detection of nodal disease in pNET.

Future directions: Positron emission tomography (PET) agents and Ga-DOTA-NoC

Positron Emission Tomography[50-55]

- PET has a sensitivity of 96% for insulinomas.
- Sensitivity of ^{18}F-FDG PET-CT for nonfunctioning pNET is approximately 58%, and this is complementary to octreotide.
- ^{18}F-FDG PET-CT is more likely to show uptake when it is a poorly differentiated nonfunctioning PNET.
- Poorly differentiated nonfunctioning PNET may show atypical enhancement.
- Poorly differentiated nonfunctioning pNET is hypovascular or shows enhancement more in portal venous phase than arterial phase enhancement.
- Standard unit value (SUV) predicts overall survival and progression-free survival in nonfunctioning pNET, exceeding that of Ki67, liver metastasis, and chromogranin A levels.
- Poorly differentiated pNET has a poorer prognosis and a higher incidence of liver metastasis, lymph node metastasis, and necrosis.
- Radiopharmaceuticals such as norcholesterol, MIBG, and fluorodeoxyglucose (FDG) may provide significant functional information for tissue characterization in adrenal lesions.
- In order to localize tumors causing catecholamine excess, ^{18}F-DOPA PET is superior to ^{123}I-MIBG scintigraphy and CT/MRI.

Invasive Imaging[56-61]

Melbey et al. first proposed the idea of adrenal venous sampling in 1970. Invasive venous sampling is required when surgery is planned and we are not sure that from which site or side, excess hormone production is there. We can check local hormone concentration by doing selective venous catheterization, with selective blood sample collection.

- *Catheterization of inferior sinus petrosus:* In this method, we collect blood samples selectively from venous drainage of pituitary gland.

Principle: Local concentration of ACTH (before and after stimulation with CRH) may distinguish pituitary and paraneoplastic CS.

10% of the normal subjects will have a nonfunctioning pituitary tumor or incidentaloma at MRI. The interventional radiologist may be consulted in cases with equivocal imaging findings and/or biochemical test results.

- *Catheterization of inferior vena cava:* In this method, we collect blood samples selectively from abdominal veins.
- *Principle*: Localization of small (CT/MRI undetectable) abdominal tumor (carcinoid, insulinoma, etc.) due to high local concentration of hormone.
- *Primary hyperaldosteronism*: It is seen in 5–10% of screened hypertensive patients. 62.5% of PH patients have potentially curable adenoma as the underlying etiology. Adrenal venous sampling is the criterion standard to distinguish between unilateral and bilateral adrenal disease in patients with PH. The technical success rate of catheterizing all four vessels (both adrenal and both gonadal veins) for the workup of hyperandrogenism is quite low, with success rates ranging from 27 to 45%.

Surgical intervention for hyperaldosteronism on the basis of imaging alone leads to unacceptably high rates of wrong-sided adrenalectomy or exclusion from later curative surgery.[34,35] To date, adrenal venous sampling is the only widely available and reliable method to identify a lateralizing adrenal source of inappropriate aldosterone production.

If imaging evaluation fails to localize an adrenal or ovarian tumor, adrenal and ovarian venous sampling can be performed.

Image-guided FNAC/Biopsy

Image-guided FNAC/biopsy is done in cases of focal thyroid nodules, as per the ACR TIRADS scoring system and recommendation. We target two most suspicious nodules only. We have to avoid the calcific/cystic/necrotic part of nodule. An important technical point which we have to keep in mind while targeting focal thyroid nodules is that we enter the needle through thyroid isthmus and then enter the thyroid gland to target nodule. This has to be done to avoid injury to recurrent laryngeal nerve. In almost 30–50% cases, thyroid nodule FNAC will come as inconclusive. Then, we can either repeat FNAC with cytotechnician on site or better would be to do CNB using 18- or 20-G biopsy gun.

In some cases, we may have to do adrenal mass biopsy. We can do adrenal lesion biopsy using USG guidance, if the lesion size is >1 cm and if we can see needle along the entire tract during USG-guided biopsy. If the lesion is not seen properly on USG, then it is better to approach the adrenal lesion under CT guidance, in prone position, using the retroperitoneal approach.

Endocrine Radiology

Archana Gupta, Pankaj Sharma

INTRODUCTION

Endocrine radiology is a subspecialty of radiology, in which diagnostic and interventional radiology principles are applied, for management of patients with endocrinopathies. By endocrinopathies, we mean disorders, which result from a pathological source of hormone production.[1-3] Whenever we encounter a patient with endocrinopathy, we first try to evaluate the patient using noninvasive imaging, along with laboratory investigation and clinical presentation. Invasive intervention, in the form of endocrine venous sampling, is done only when the source of endocrinopathy is not detected using noninvasive methods.[4] Moreover, endocrine venous sampling helps us in localizing disease, by detecting relative elevation of hormone, in organ of interest. Management of endocrinopathy requires team approach between laboratory medicine, endocrine radiologist, interventional radiologist, medical endocrinologist, and endocrine surgeon.

The human endocrine system includes the following organs:
- Pineal gland
- Pituitary–hypothalamic axis
- Thyroid and parathyroid glands
- Thymus
- Pancreas
- Adrenals
- Testes (in males)
- Ovaries (in females)

Endocrine disorders occur in two conditions:
1. *If there is too much hormone*: In this condition, we first try to detect the source of excess hormone production. Thereafter, we try to suppress this excess hormone production.
2. *If there is too less hormone*: In this condition, we try to find the cause of hormone deficiency and then we try to stimulate gland to increase hormone production.

Endocrine disorder may primarily be due to dysfunction at three important levels:
1. *Central level*: Hypothalamic/pituitary axis
2. *Peripheral level*: Dysfunction of peripheral glands
3. *Receptor/postreceptor level*: Target cell insufficiency or low sensitivity to hormone action

CLINICAL PRESENTATION

Majority of insulinomas are small (<1 cm) and solitary.[5] Insulinomas are multiple in MEN1 and Von Hippel–Lindau disease. Postexercise or postfasting hypoglycemia, neuroglycopenic symptoms, and relief after eating or intravenous glucose supplementation constitute the Whipple triad of insulinoma.

LABORATORY INVESTIGATIONS

Whenever there is an endocrine disorder, we first do the following laboratory investigations:
- *Standard biochemistry*: Sodium, potassium, and glucose
- Plasma hormone level
- Hormone diurnal rhythm
- Urinary hormones/metabolites
- Stimulatory/inhibitory tests

Adrenal hemorrhage: Serum cortisol level of >18 µg/dL is often used to exclude adrenal insufficiency in situations of severe stress.

If hypertension is present, we measure plasma aldosterone concentration and plasma renin activity. An appropriate screening test in this condition is a random aldosterone to renin activity ratio that is >30.

Plasma metanephrines have similar sensitivity and specificity for pheochromocytoma as urine-fractionated metanephrines and may be considered as the first screening test.

Routine hormonal evaluation of all adrenal incidentalomas (AIs) will be costly and is not routinely performed. Biochemical evaluation should be considered only if there are clinical signs or symptoms of adrenal hyperfunction.

For all adrenal tumors, hormonal evaluation should be performed at the time of diagnosis and then annually for 5 years.

FUNCTIONAL TESTS

First of all, we try to detect hormone levels in blood or urine. We also try to check hormone diurnal rhythm. But very often, the basal hormone level does not allow us to establish a diagnosis of hypofunction or hyperfunction. So, we have to resort to stimulatory test, if we suspect hypofunction, as this helps us to quantify functional reserve of the endocrine gland.

Few stimulatory tests used for patient management are as follows:

- Gonadotropin-releasing hormone (GnRH) test
- Corticotropin-releasing hormone (CRH) test
- Insulin hypoglycemia test
- Thyrotropin-releasing hormone (TRH) test
- Metyrapone test
- Levodopa test
- Arginine infusion test

If we suspect hyperfunction, then we do inhibitory tests to quantify the response of endocrine glands to these inhibitory factors.

Few inhibitory tests used for patient management are as follows:

- Dexamethasone test
- *Dopaminergic drugs test:*
  - Physiological stress → hypothalamus releases CRH → triggers release of adrenocorticotropic hormone (ACTH) from anterior pituitary → stimulates release of cortisol from adrenal cortex → promotes gluconeogenesis, fat mobilization, and protein mobilization → downregulates further release of CRH and ACTH

◇ IMAGING TECHNIQUES

Imaging techniques are used in endocrinopathy, for two indications:

1. To localize endocrine active tumors, adenomas, hyperplasia, or ectopic hormonal producing lesions
2. To evaluate systemic complications of these endocrinopathies

Modalities used for noninvasive imaging are as follows:

- X-rays
- Ultrasonography (USG)
- Computed tomography (CT)
- Magnetic resonance imaging (MRI)
- Scintigraphy

X-rays

X-ray examination is the first investigation done in many endocrinopathies, such as:

1. Increased parathyroid activity leading to characteristic subperiosteal resorption in hands and salt, and pepper skull.
   - Osteolysis of sella turcica as a late manifestation of large pituitary tumors. These tumors are appreciated in the early stage by MRI
   - Arachnodactyly
   - Thyroid masses may incidentally be detected on chest radiography
   - Thoracic inlet view may demonstrate tracheal compression, caused by thyroid mass.

- Adrenal gland calcification may be seen on abdominal X-ray, in some conditions such as in Addison disease.

Ultrasonography

High-resolution USG of thyroid is done for characterizing focal and diffuse thyroid nodules, using a 7–12 MHz linear probe. For obese patients, patients with short neck and large thyroid gland (goiter, low-frequency probe is required. On ultrasound, we can differentiate between solid and cystic components, by using gray-scale with Doppler. Moreover, USG can be used for image-guided fine-needle aspiration cytology (FNAC)/biopsy of thyroid nodules.

We use American College of Radiology (ACR) Thyroid Imaging Reporting and Data System (TIRADS) for characterizing focal thyroid nodules and for recommending management decisions.[6] In ACR TIRADS, we characterize focal thyroid nodules, based on the following imaging five characteristics:

1. *Composition*: 0–2 points
2. *Echogenicity*: 0–3 points
3. *Shape*: 0–3 points
4. *Margin*: 0–3 points
5. *Echogenic foci*: 0–3 points

The final score is addition of scores for each imaging characteristic, and based on the final score, each nodule is assigned a category TR1 or TR2, or TR3 or TR4, or TR5. In each category (TR1 to TR5), the management decision is recommended based on the maximum diameter of the thyroid nodule. A maximum of four thyroid nodules are assigned category TR1 to TR5 and a maximum of two thyroid nodules are selected for FNAC/biopsy, based on most suspicious features, or higher assigned category: TR1 to TR5. Significant enlargement of thyroid nodule in ACR TIRADS is said to occur, if there is:

- 20% increase in at least two nodule dimensions or minimal increase of 2 mm
- 50% or greater increase in volume.

Minimal follow-up period in ACR TIRADS for a suspicious thyroid nodule is 1 year. Imaging can stop at 5 years if there is no change in size. The follow-up interval for different thyroid nodules is as follows:

- *TR5*: Scanning every year for up to 5 years
- *TR4*: 1, 2, 3, and 5 years
- *TR3*: 1, 3, and 5 years

If all thyroid nodules show a similar echogenic pattern, then no follow-up is required according to ACR TIRADS.

The ACR TIRADS has a few limitations:

- Neck nodes are not evaluated.
- Elastography is not included.
- T5 is a broad category, with scores ranging from 7 to 15, and needs further subcategorization.

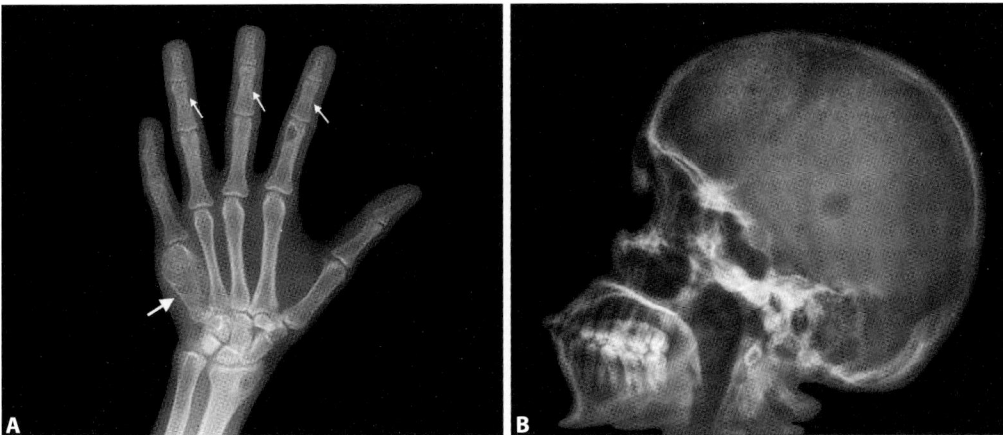

Figs. 1A and B: Hyperparathyroidism. (A) Radiograph of the anteroposterior (AP) view of the hand of a 35-year-old patient with hyperparathyroidism secondary to parathyroid adenoma shows an expansile lytic lesion involving fifth metatarsal (thick arrow) suggestive of brown tumor. Another tiny lytic lesion is seen in proximal phalanx of second digit. Note is made of subperiosteal resorption on the radial aspect of second, third, and fourth digits (thin arrows); (B) Radiograph of the lateral view of the skull of a 45-year-old male patient with hyperparathyroidism shows the classic salt and pepper skull.

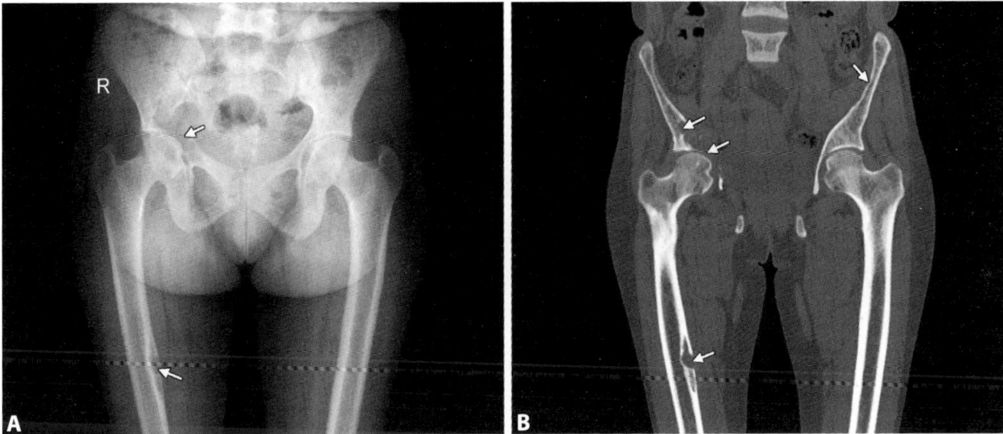

Figs. 2A and B: A 35-year-old patient with hyperparathyroidism and parathyroid adenoma. (A) Anteroposterior (AP) radiograph of pelvis with proximal thigh shows lytic lesion involving right acetabulum. Another cortical-based lytic lesion involving proximal right femur is seen; (B) Coronal CT section of pelvis with proximal thigh (bone window) shows two lytic lesions in right acetabulum and proximal femur as seen on radiograph. In addition, another lytic lesion causing scalloping of the left ilium is seen. All the lytic lesions described represented brown tumors associated with hyperparathyroidism.

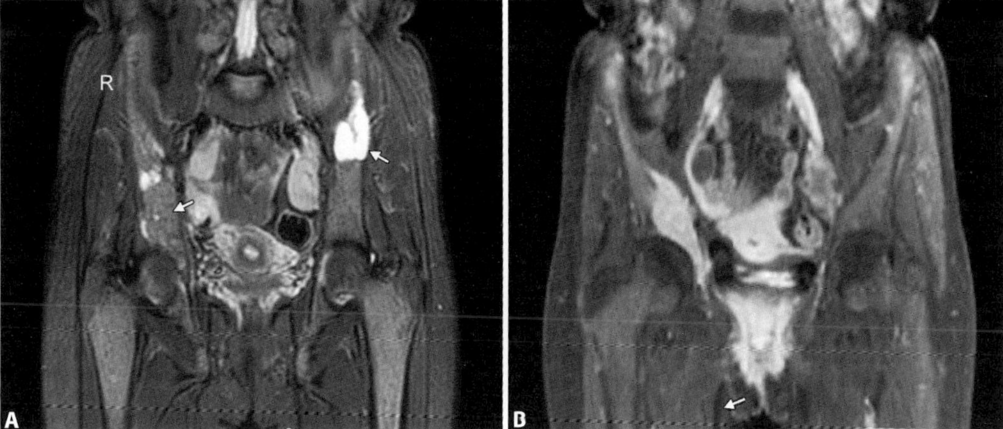

Figs. 3A and B: A 35-year-old patient with hyperparathyroidism and parathyroid adenoma. (A) Coronal STIR section of pelvis shows hypointense soft-tissue component in the lesion in the right acetabulum. The lesion in the left iliac bone shows hyperintense cystic components; (B) Coronal postcontrast section of pelvis shows intense postcontrast enhancement in soft tissue associated with acetabular lesion. All the lytic lesions described represented brown tumors associated with hyperparathyroidism.

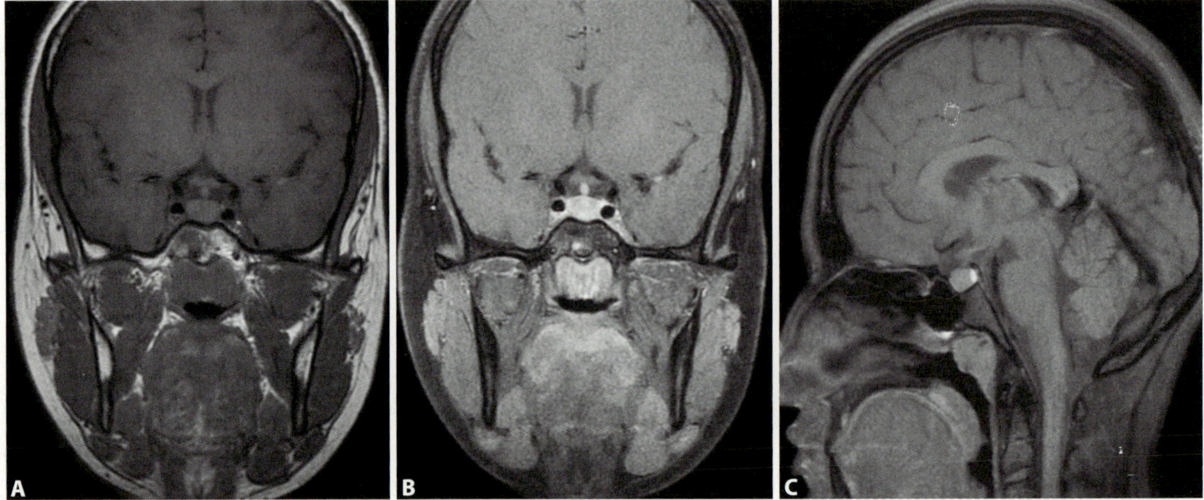

Figs. 4A to C: Coronal T1WI (A); Corresponding postcontrast T1WI (B); and sagittal T1WI (C) of a 16-year-old female with history of oligomenorrhea and hyperprolactinemia show a homogeneously enhancing enlarged pituitary gland (10.5 × 11.4 × 10 mm—TR × AP × CC) with upward convexity of the superior borders. A thickened central pituitary stalk is seen which shows homogeneous postcontrast enhancement. A posterior pituitary bright spot is maintained. Features are suggestive of autoimmune hypophysitis.

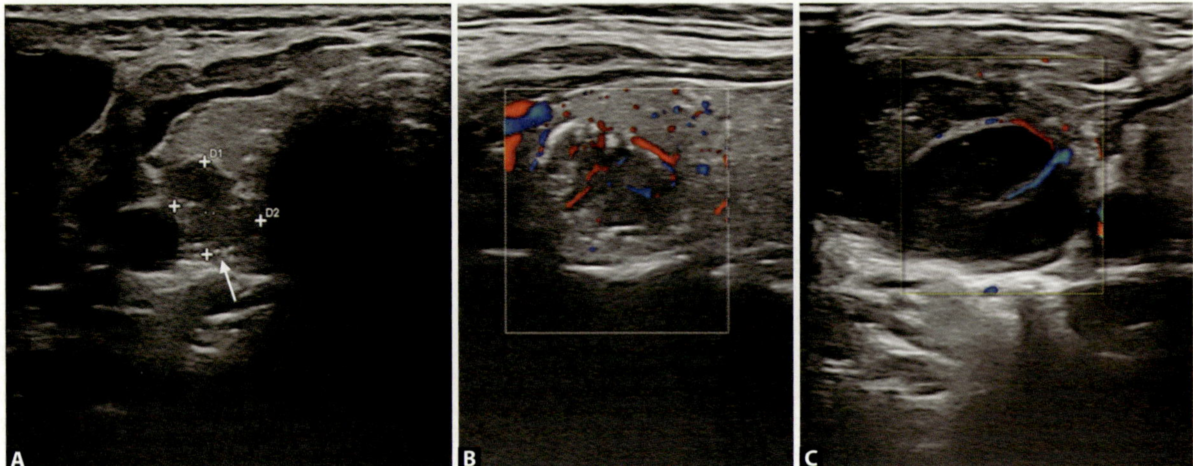

Figs. 5A to C: (A) Transverse ultrasound section of the right lobe of thyroid of a 24-year-old female shows a solid, taller than wider hypoechoic nodule (arrow) with peripheral microcalcifications suggestive of TIRADS V nodule; (B) Longitudinal ultrasound section of the right lobe of thyroid shows increased vascularity in the nodule on color Doppler. (C) Transverse ultrasound section of neck of the patient shows enlarged level III lymph node.

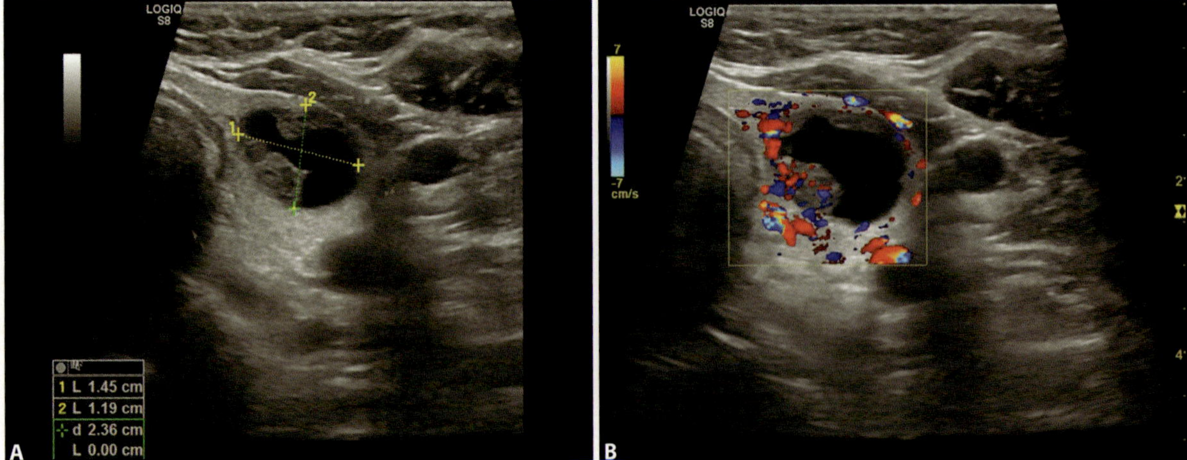

Figs. 6A and B: (A) Transverse ultrasound section of the left lobe of thyroid of a 45-year-old female shows a cystic nodule with an internal solid component in the left lobe of thyroid; (B) Color Doppler image shows increased vascularity in the solid component and in the periphery of the nodule.

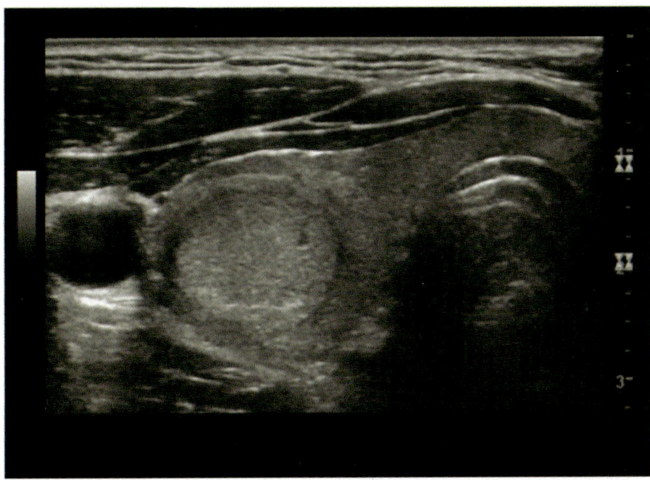

Fig. 7: Ultrasound (US) image showing a ACR TIRADS T3 nodule. Note the presence of solid nodule (2 point), hyperechoic (1 point), wider than tall (0 point), smooth margin (0 point), and no echogenic foci (0 point). Total score 3 points, corresponding to TR3. With size more than 2.5 cm, fine-needle aspiration cytology (FNAC) was recommended as per ACR TIRADS guidelines.

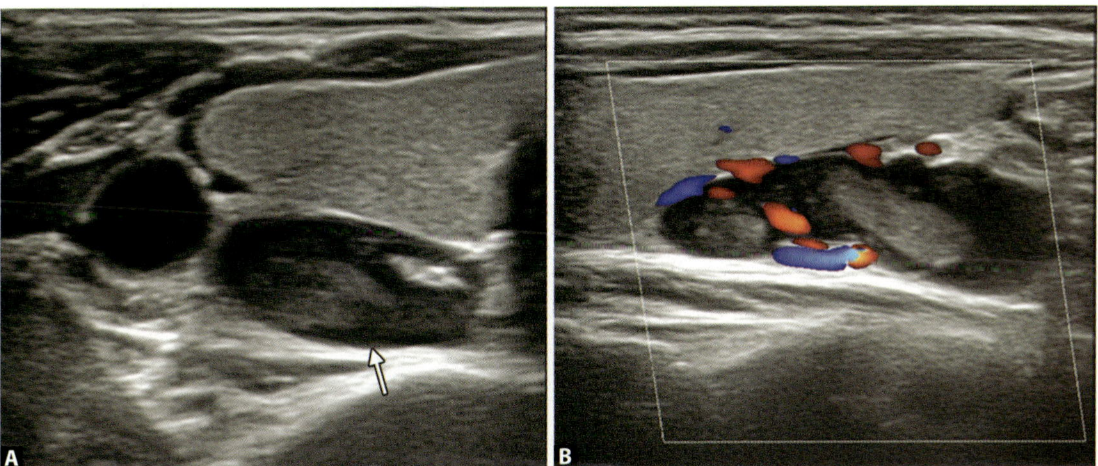

Figs. 8A and B: (A) Transverse ultrasound section through the right lobe of thyroid of a 35-year-old female with high serum parathormone levels shows a well-defined hypoechoic solid lesion (arrow) behind the thyroid; (B) Longitudinal ultrasound section through the right lobe of thyroid shows that the hypoechoic lesion is behind the inferior pole of the right lobe of thyroid and the lesion shows moderate internal vascularity. The final diagnosis of parathyroid adenoma was made.

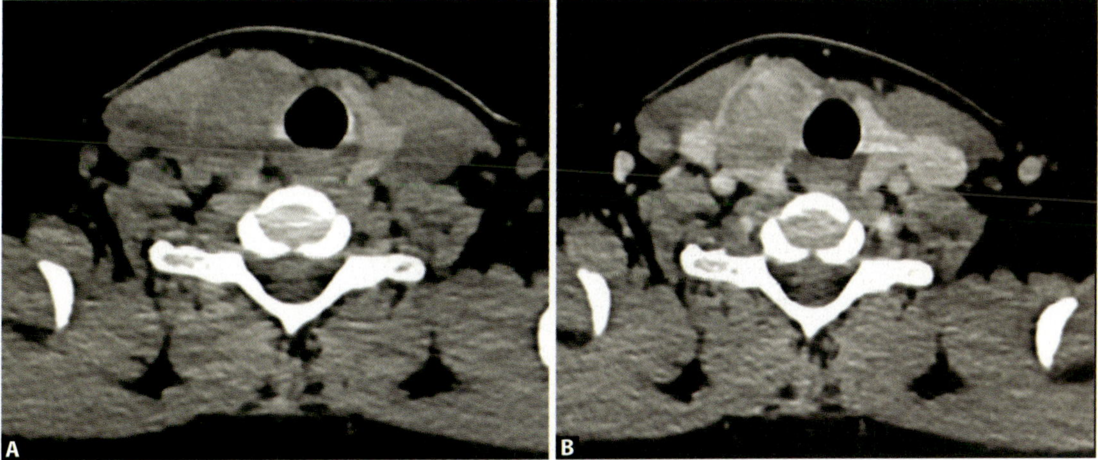

Figs. 9A and B: Axial noncontrast and corresponding postcontrast axial CT sections of neck of a 36-year-old female with a known case of papillary carcinoma thyroid show well-defined hypodense, heterogeneously enhancing nodule replacing the right lobe of thyroid. No calcifications or cystic components are seen within the nodule.

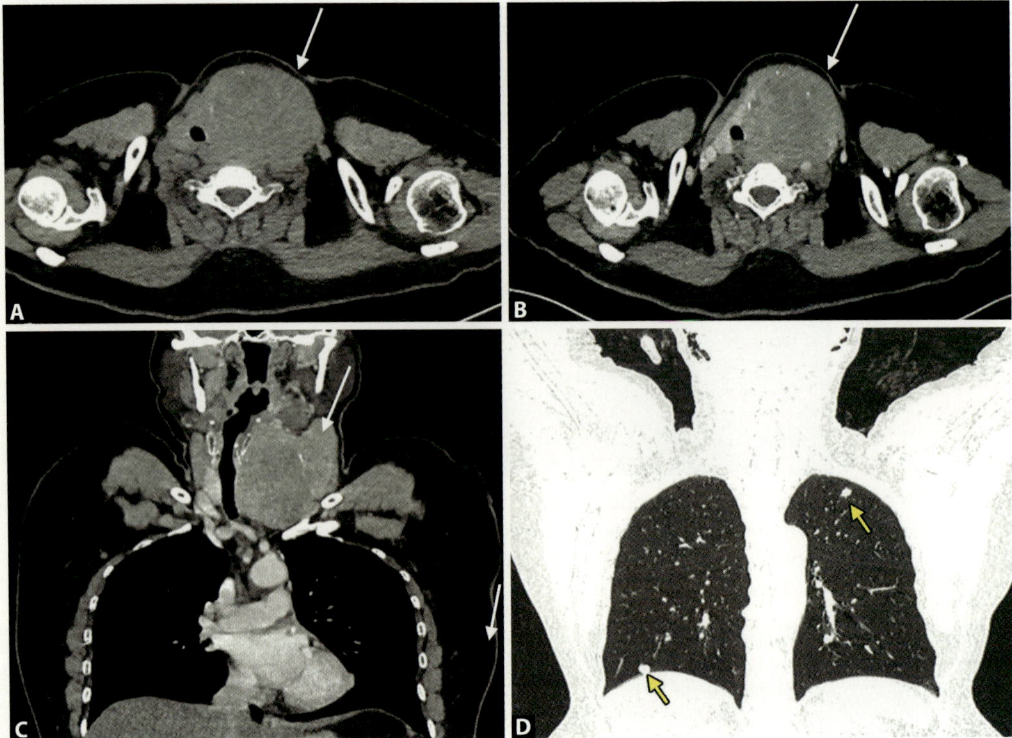

Figs. 10A to D: (A and B) Axial noncontrast and corresponding postcontrast axial sections of neck of a 49-year-old female show heterogeneously enhancing mass lesion replacing left lobe and isthmus of thyroid and causing mass effect on trachea, extrathyroidal and prevertebral extension; (C) Coronal postcontrast CT section of neck and thorax show the thyroid mass exerting mass effect on trachea; (D) Coronal CT section (lung window) shows two well-defined nodules in both lungs. Diagnosis of neoplastic mass in thyroid was confirmed on thyroidectomy with follicular carcinoma as the histopathological variant.

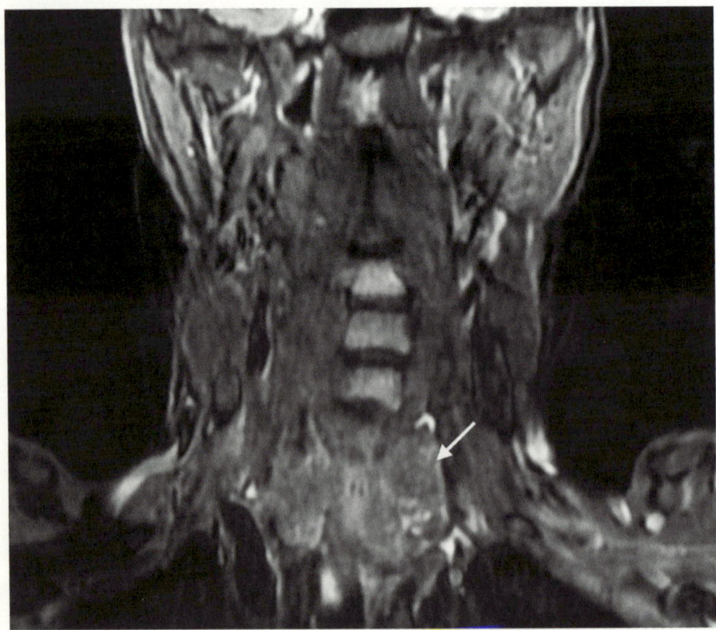

Fig. 11: Coronal STIR image of a 55-year-old female with known multinodular goiter shows enlarged thyroid lobes and isthmus which are replaced by multiple hypointense nodules.

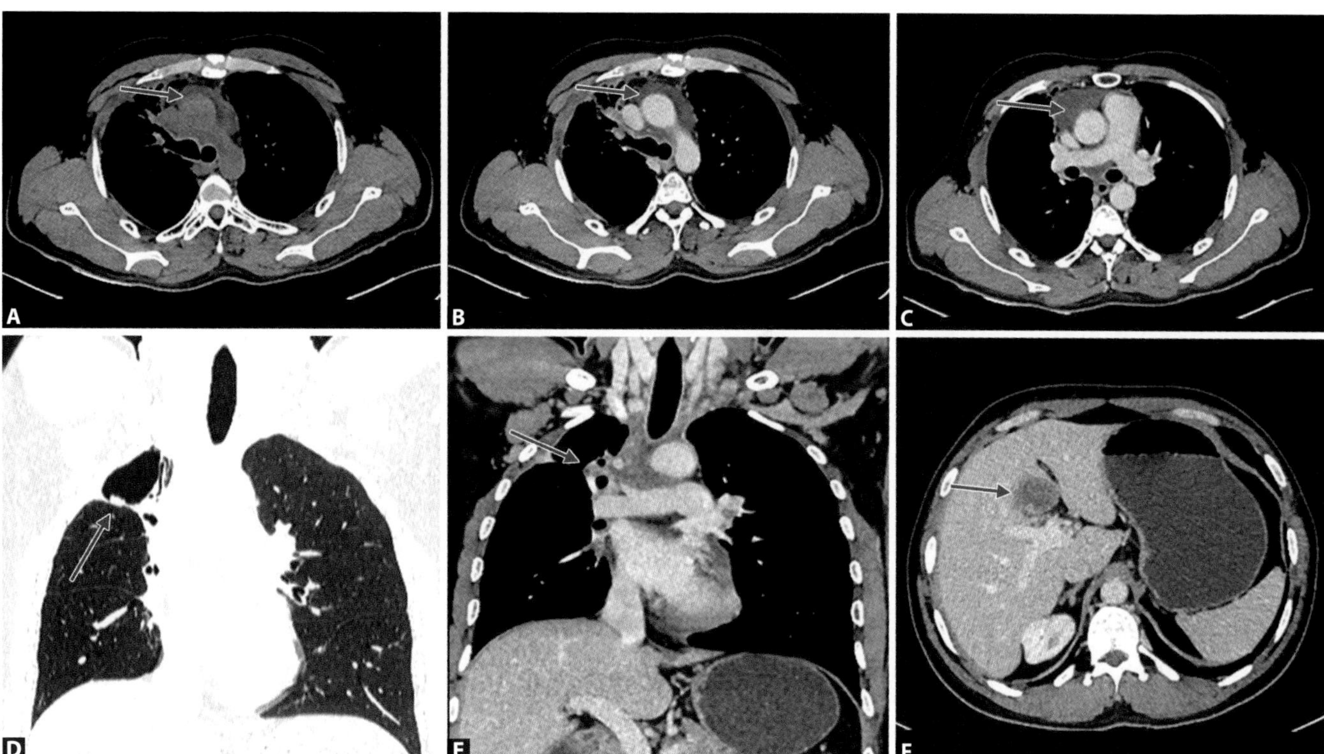

Figs. 12A to F: (A and B) Axial noncontrast and corresponding postcontrast CT sections of thorax of a 30-year-old male show a hypodense, heterogeneously enhancing lesion in the anterior and middle mediastinum; (B and C) The lesion is abutting the arch of aorta, ascending aorta, main pulmonary trunk, and trachea; (D) Coronal lung window sections of thorax show an irregularly walled cavity in the right upper lung lobe adjacent to the lesion; (E) Coronal postcontrast CT sections of thorax show that the lesion is encasing azygos vein (arrow) and abutting major vessels and trachea; (F) Axial postcontrast section of the upper abdomen shows a heterogeneously enhancing lesion in liver suggestive of metastasis. A diagnosis of large-cell neuroendocrine tumor of mediastinum was confirmed on histopathology.

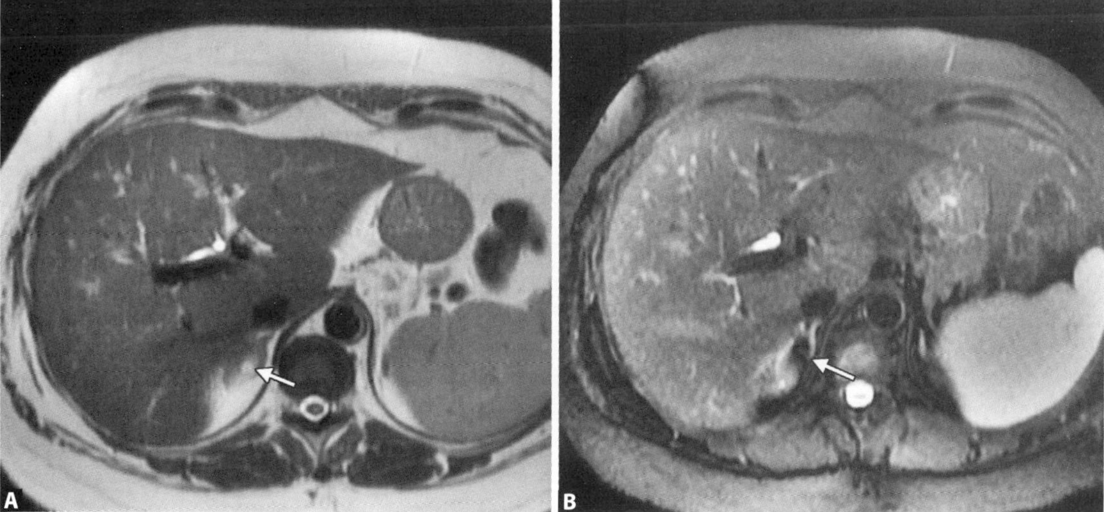

Figs. 13A and B: Axial T2W image (A) and corresponding T2W fat-saturated image (B) of the abdomen of a 44-year-old female show an incidentally detected tiny (<10 mm) T2W hyperintense lesion along the medial limb of the right adrenal gland (arrow) which shows suppression on fat-saturated image suggestive of lipid-rich adenoma.

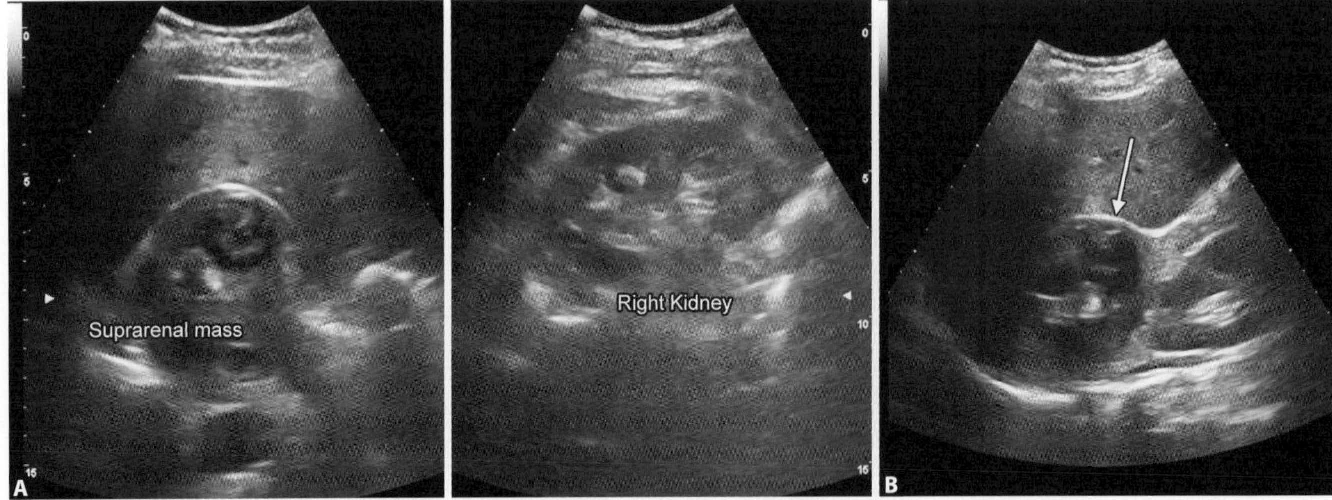

Figs. 14A and B: Longitudinal ultrasound images of a 47-year-old hypertensive male show a right suprarenal mass compressing but separate from right kidney (arrow). Final diagnosis came out to be pheochromocytoma.

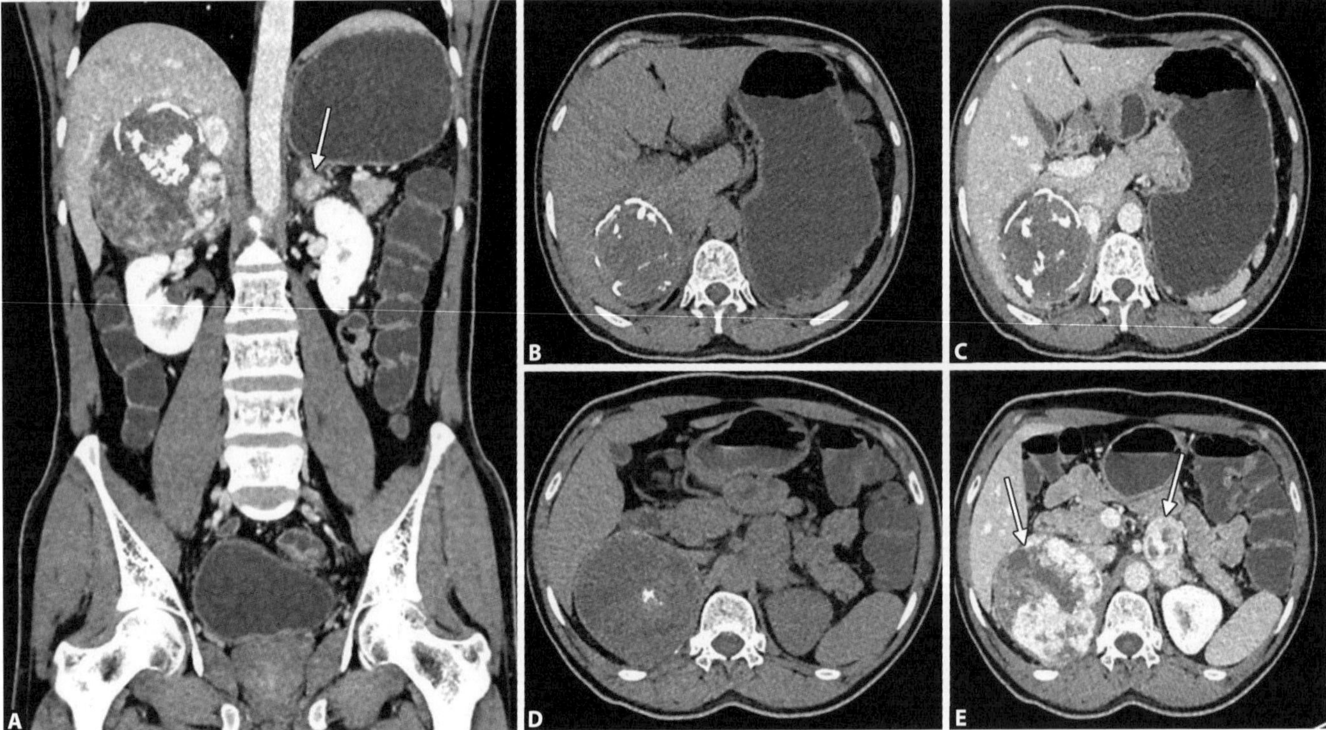

Figs. 15A to E: (A) Coronal postcontrast CT sections of abdomen of a 40-year-old male with known *3p* gene mutation and positive history of von Hippel–Lindau disease show heterogeneously enhancing large right suprarenal mass and a smaller left adrenal mass (arrow); (B to E) Contiguous axial sections (noncontrast and corresponding postcontrast) show calcifications in the right suprarenal mass. Heterogeneous postcontrast enhancement is seen (E: arrow). A diagnosis of bilateral adrenal pheochromocytomas was made.

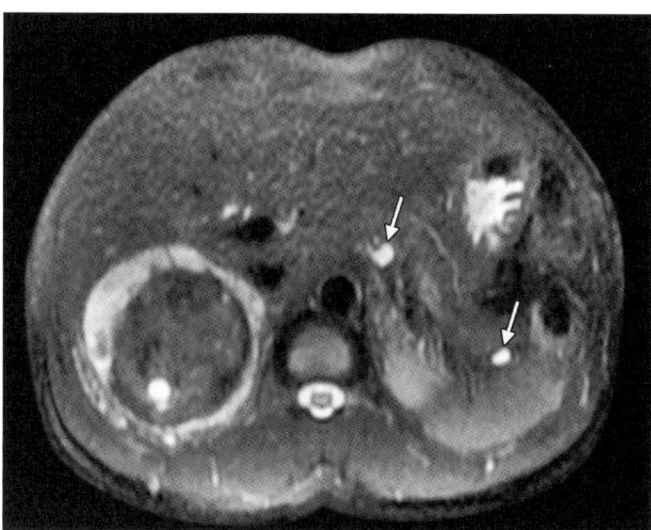

Fig. 16: Axial T2WI fat-saturated image of the abdomen of a 40-year-old male, with known *3p* gene mutation and a positive history of von Hippel–Lindau disease, shows heterogeneous signal intensity in right suprarenal mass and two tiny pancreatic cysts (arrows).

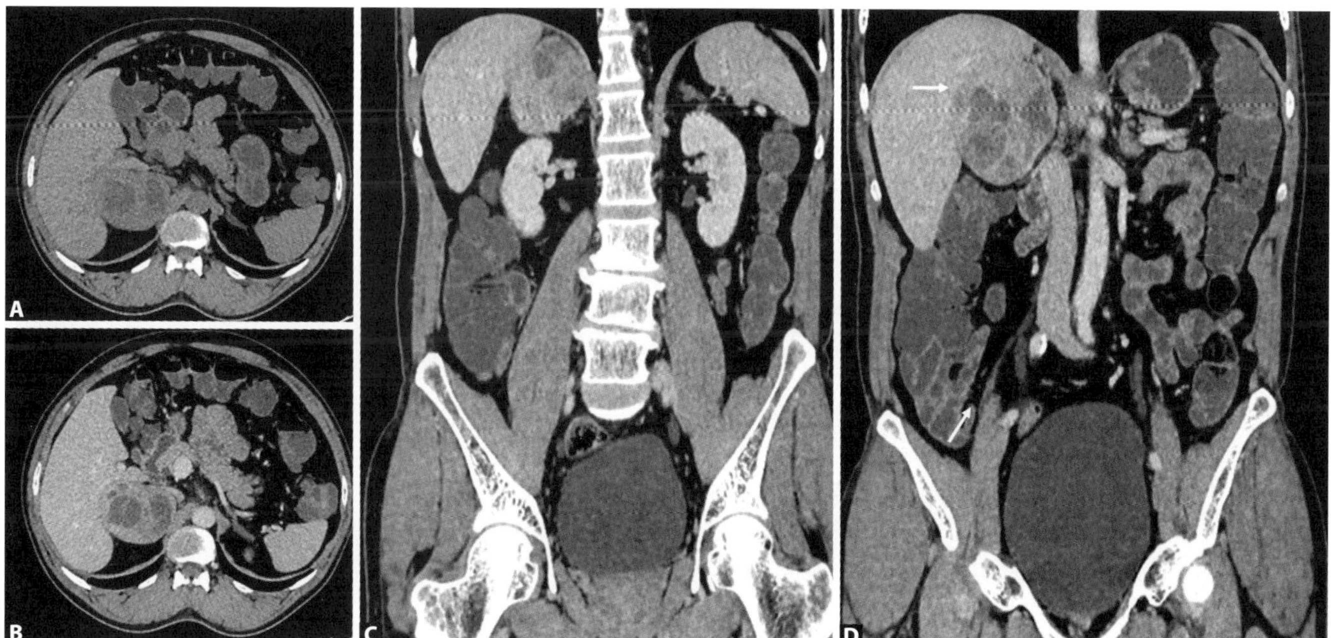

Figs. 17A to D: Axial noncontrast (A) and corresponding postcontrast CT; (B) sections of abdomen of a 43-year-old hypertensive male show a heterogeneously enhancing mass in right suprarenal region. Right adrenal is not visualized separately; (C) Coronal postcontrast image shows that the mass has maintained fat planes with right kidney; (D) Coronal postcontrast image shows that the mass shows loss of fat planes with segment VI of liver superiorly. Diagnosis of pheochromocytoma was made which correlated with raised urine metanephrine levels.

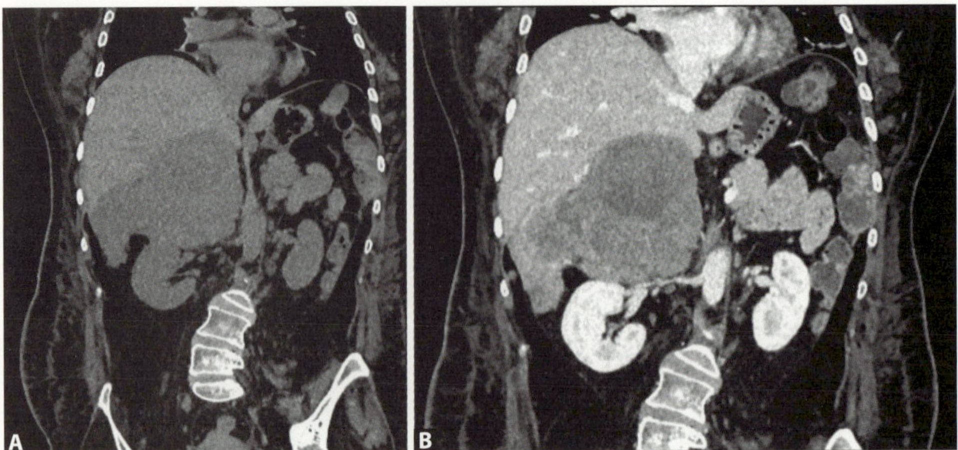

Figs. 18A and B: Coronal noncontrast (A) and corresponding postcontrast (B) CT images of upper abdomen of a 34-year-old female show a large heterogeneously enhancing right suprarenal mass with infiltration into surrounding liver parenchyma. Right adrenal is not separately visualized. The mass is compressing the right kidney inferiorly. Diagnosis of adrenocortical carcinoma was confirmed with a pathological diagnosis.

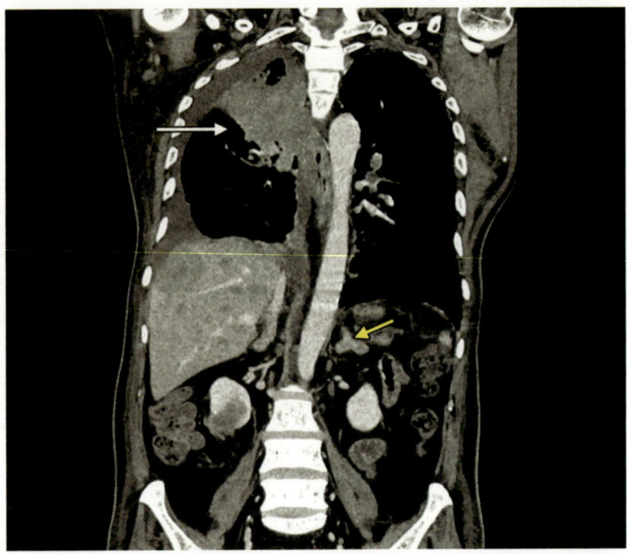

Fig. 19: Coronal postcontrast CT sections of thorax and abdomen of a 49-year-old male, who is a known case of carcinoma right lung shows right upper lobe lung mass (arrow) with bulky left adrenal gland (yellow arrow) suggestive of metastasis.

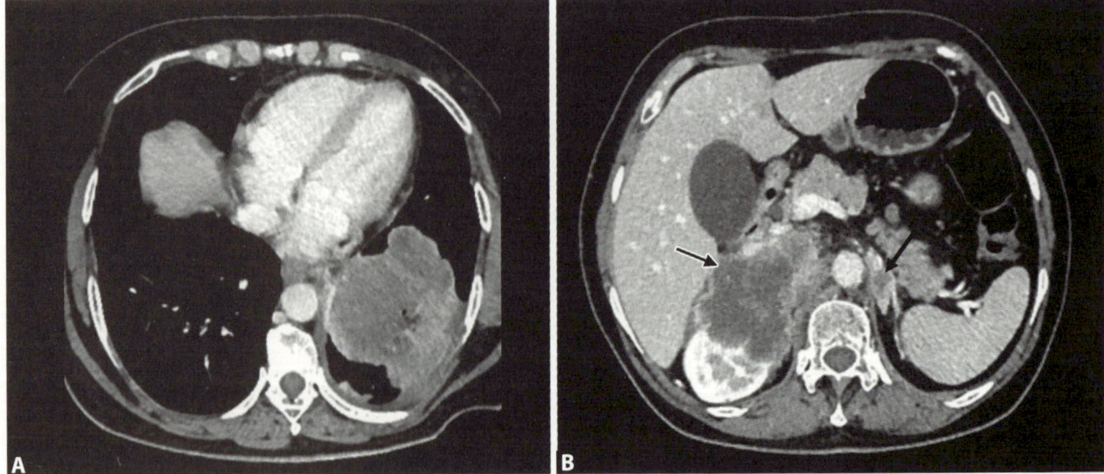

Figs. 20A and B: (A) Axial postcontrast image of thorax of a 45-year-old female with known carcinoma of left lung shows a heterogeneously enhancing necrotic lesion in left lower lobe; (B) Axial postcontrast sections of upper abdomen show heterogeneously enhancing lesion in right suprarenal region with no separate visualization of adrenal gland (thick arrow). Another smaller lesion is seen involving body and medial limb of left adrenal gland (thin arrow). Features are suggestive of bilateral adrenal metastasis.

◇ REFERENCES

1. Chaudhary V, Bano S. Imaging of pediatric pituitary endocrinopathies. Indian J Endocrinol Metab. 2012;16(5):682-91.

2. Gupta AK, Kandasamy D. Imaging in endocrine disorders. Indian J Med Res. 2018;147(3):323-4.

3. Dingman JF, Thorn GW. Role of radiology in endocrine diagnosis. Radiol Clin North Am. 1967;5(2):187-91.

4. Monroe EJ, Carney BW, Ingraham CR, Johnson GE, Valji K. An interventionist's guide to endocrine consultations. Radiographics. 2017;37:1246–67.

5. Okabayashi T, Shima Y, Sumiyoshi T, Kozuki A, Ito S, Ogawa Y, et al. Diagnosis and management of insulinomas. World J Gastroenterol. 2013;19(6):829–37.

6. Tessler FN, Middleton WD, Grant EG. Thyroid imaging reporting and data system (TI-RADS): a user's guide. Radiology. 2018;287(1):29-36.

7. Baek JH. Current status of core needle biopsy of the thyroid. Ultrasonography. 2017;36:83-5.

8. Suh CH, Baek JH, Kim KW, Sung TY, Kim TY, Song DE, et al. The role of core-needle biopsy for thyroid nodules with initially nondiagnostic fine-needle aspiration results: a systemic review and meta-analysis. Endocr Pract. 2016;22(6):679-88.

9. Jung CK, Baek JH. Recent advances in core needle biopsy for thyroid nodules. Endocrinol Metab (Seoul). 2017;32(4):407-12.

10. Piciucchi S, Barone D, Gavelli G, Dubini A, Oboldi D, Matteuci F. Primary hyperparathyroidism: imaging to pathology. J Clin Imaging Sci. 2012;2:59.

11. Tsai K, Liang TZ, Grant EG, Swanson MS, Barnett B. Optimal imaging modality for diagnosis of parathyroid adenoma: case report and review of the literature. J Clin Transl Endocrin. 2020;17:00065.

12. Lewis RB, Lattin GE, Paal E. Pancreatic endocrine tumors: radiologic-clinicopathologic correlation. Radiographics. 2010;30:1445-64.

13. Tamm EP, Bhosale P, Lee JH, Rohren E. State-of-the-art imaging of pancreatic neuroendocrine tumors. Surg Oncol Clin N Am. 2016;25(2):375-400.

14. Yang RH, Chu YK. Zollinger-Ellison syndrome: revelation of the gastrinoma triangle. Radiol Case Rep. 2015;10(1):827.

15. Hubbard H. Evaluation of possible gastrinoma. Med Gen Med. 2007;9(1):31.

16. Bar-Moshe Y, Mazeh H, Grozinsky-Glasberg S. Non-functioning pancreatic neuroendocrine tumors: surgery or observation? World J Gastrointest Endosc. 2017;9(4):153-61.

17. Bartolini I, Bencini L, Risaliti M, Ringressi MN, Moraldi L, Taddei A. Current management of pancreatic neuroendocrine tumors: from demolitive surgery to observation. Gastroenterol Res Prac. 2018;22(2018):9647247.

18. Garrett RW, Nepute JC, Hayek ME, Albert SG. Adrenal incidentalomas: clinical controversies and modified recommendations. Am J Roent. 2016;206:1170-8.

19. Sahdev A. Recommendations for the management of adrenal incidentalomas: what is pertinent for radiologists? Br J Radiol. 2017;90(1072):20160627.

20. Kilcoyne A, McDermott S, Blake MA. (2017). MR imaging of adrenal lesions. [online] Available from https://appliedradiology.com/communities/MR-Community/mr-imaging-of-adrenal-lesions. [Last accessed December, 2021].

21. Čtvrtlík F, Koranda P, Schovánek J, Škarda J, Hartmann I, Tüdös Z, et al. Current diagnostic imaging of pheochromocytomas and implications for therapeutic strategy. Exp Ther Med. 2018;15(4):3151-60.

22. Leung K, Stamm M, Raja A, Low G. Phaeochromocytoma: the range of appearances on ultrasound, CT, MRI, and functional imaging. Am J Roent. 2013;200:370-8.

23. Bharwani N, Rockall AG, Sahdev A, Gueorguiev M, Drake W, Grossman AB, et al. Adrenocortical carcinoma: the range of appearances on CT and MRI. Am J Roent. 2011;196:706-14.

24. Panda A, Das CJ, Dhamija E, Kumar R, Gupta AK. Adrenal imaging (Part 1): imaging techniques and primary cortical lesions. Ind J Endocrin Metabol. 2015;19(1):8-15.

25. Choi YA, Kim CK, Park BK, Kim B. Evaluation of adrenal metastases from renal cell carcinoma and hepatocellular carcinoma: use of delayed contrast-enhanced CT. Radiology. 2013;266(2):514-20.

26. Tu W, Verma R, Krishna S, McInnes MDF, Flood TA, Schieda N. Can adrenal adenomas be differentiated from adrenal metastases at single-phase contrast-enhanced CT? Am J Roentgenol. 2018;211:1044-50.

27. Dhamija E, Panda A, Das CJ, Gupta AK. Adrenal imaging (Part 2): Medullary and secondary adrenal lesions. Ind J Endocrin Metabol. 2015;19(1):16-24.

28. Cordera F, Grant C, Heerden JV, Thompson G, Young W. Androgen-secreting adrenal tumors. Surgery. 2003;134(6):874-80.

29. Padilla SL. Androgen producing tumors in children and adolescents. J Ped Adol Gyne. 1989;2(3)135-42.

30. Zhou W, Chen N, Liolescents C. A rare case of pure testosterone-secreting adrenal adenoma in a postmenopausal elderly woman. BMC Endocr Disord. 2019;19:14.

31. Guo YK, Yang ZG, Li Y, Ma ES, Deng YP, Min PQ, et al. Addison's disease due to adrenal tuberculosis: contrast enhanced CT features and clinical duration correction. Eur J Rad. 2007;62(1):126-31.

32. Rockall AG, Babar SA, Sohaib SAA, Isidori AM, Diaz-Cano S, Monson JP, et al. CT and MR imaging of the adrenal glands in ACTH-independent Cushing Syndrome. Radiographics. 2004;24:435-52.

33. Wagner-Bartak NA, Baiomy A, Habra MA, Mukhi SV, Morani AC, Korivi BR, et al. Cushing syndrome: diagnostic workup and imaging features, with clinical and pathological correlation. Am J Roent. 2017;209:19-32.

34. Khater N, Khauli R. A myelolipomas and other fatty tumours of the adrenals. Arab J Urol. 2011;9(4):259-65.

35. Venyo AKG. Myelolipoma of the adrenal gland: a review and update of the literature. Pulsus J Surg Res. 2018;2(2):50-63.

36. Dromain C, Déandréis D, Scoazec JY, Goere D, Ducreux M, Baudin E, et al. Imaging of neuroendocrine tumors of the pancreas. Diagn Interv Imaging. 2016;97(12):1241-57.

37. Seo JM, Park BK, Park SY, Kim CK. Characterization of lipid-poor adrenal adenoma : chemical-shift MRI and washout CT. Am J Roentgenol. 2014;202:1043-50.

38. Schieda N, Siegelman ES. Update on CT and MRI of adrenal nodules. AJR. 2017;208:1206-17.

39. Sharma P, Kumar R. Nuclear medicine imaging in the evaluation of endocrine hypertension. Indian J Endocrinol Metab. 2012;16(5):706-12.

40. Becker D, Charkes ND, Dworkin H, Hurley J. Procedure guideline for thyroid scintigraphy:1.0. J Nucl Med. 1996;37(7):1264-6.

41. Iglesias P, Cardona J, Diez JJ. The pituitary in nuclear medicine imaging. Eur J Inter Med. 2019;68:6-12.

42. Intenzo CM, dePapp AE, Jabbour S, Miller JL, Kim SM, Capuzzi DM, et al. Scintigraphic manifestations of thyrotoxicosis. Radiographics. 2003;23:857-69.

43. Ramos CD, Wittmann DEZ, Etchebehere ECSC, Tambascia MA, Silva CAM, Camargo EE, et al. Thyroid uptake and scintigraphy using 99mTc pertechnetate: standardization in normal individuals. Sao Paulo Med J/Rev Paul Med. 2002;120(2):45-8.

44. Giovanella L, Avram AM, Iakovou I, Kwak J, Lawsone SA, Lulaj E, et al. EANM practice guideline/SNMMI procedure standard for RAIU and thyroid scintigraphy. Eur J Nuc Med Mol Imag. 2019;46:2514-25.

45. Eslamy HK, Ziessman HA. Parathyroid scintigraphy in patients with primary hyperparathyroidism: 99mTc Sestamibi SPECT and SPECT/CT. Radiographics. 2008;28:1461-76.

46. Maurea S, Mainenti PP, Romeo V, Mollica C, Salvatore M. Nuclear imaging to characterize adrenal tumors: comparison with MRI. World J Radiol. 2014;6(7):493-501.

47. Freitas JE. Adrenal cortical and medullary imaging. Semin Nucl Med. 1995;25(3):235-50.

48. Al-Nahhas A. Nuclear medicine imaging of neuroendocrine tumours. Clin Med (Lond). 2012;12(4):377-80.

49. Maxwell JE, Howe JR. Imaging in neuroendocrine tumors: an update for the clinician. Int J Endocr Oncol. 2015;2(2):159-68.

50. Becherer A, Vierhapper H, Pötzi C, Karanikas G, Kurtaran A, Schmaljohann J, et al. FDG-PET in adrenocortical carcinoma. Cancer Biother Radiopharm. 2001;16(4):289-95.

51. Launay LN, Silvera S, Tenenbaum F, Groussin L, Tissier F, Audureau E, et al. Value of 18-F-FDG PET/CT and CT in the diagnosis of indeterminate adrenal masses. Int J Endocrinol. 2015;2015:213875.

52. Mittal B, Kumar R, Jois A, Singh H, Ashwani Sood, Anish Bhattacharya, et al. F-18 FDG PET/CT in patients with adrenocortical carcinoma: a tertiary care centre experience. J Nucl Med. 2017;58(1):122.

53. Guerin C, Pattou F, Brunaud L, Lifante JC, Mirallié E, Haissaguerre M, et al. Performance of 18F-FDG PET/CT in the characterization of adrenal masses in noncancer patients: a prospective study. J Clin Endo Metabol. 2017;102(7):2465-72.

54. Dong A, Cui Y, Wang Y, Zuo C, Bai Y. 18F-FDG PET/CT of adrenal lesions. Am J Roentgenol. 2014;203:245-52.

55. Assen S, Chan D, Pasieka JL. The addition of 18F-FDG PET/CT in the assessment of indeterminate adrenal incidentalomas. Clin Oncol. 2017;2:1180.

56. Daunt N. Adrenal vein sampling: how to make it quick, easy, and successful. Radiographics. 2005;25:143-58.

57. England RW, Geer EB, Deipolyi AR. Role of venous sampling in the diagnosis of endocrine disorders. J Clin Med. 2018;7(5):114.

58. Valji K. Adrenal vein sampling: How I do it? Arab J Intervent Radiol. 2019;3:44-9.

59. Harsha A, Trerotola SO. Technical aspects of adrenal vein sampling. J Vas Interv Radiology. 2015;26(2):239.

60. Zampetti B, Grossrubatscher E, Ciaramella PD, Boccardi E. Bilateral inferior petrosal sinus sampling. Endocr Connect. 2016;5(4):12-25.

61. Gandhi CD, Meyer SA, Patel AB, Johnson DM, Post KD, et al. Neurologic complications of inferior petrosal sinus sampling. Am J Neuroradiol. 2008;29:760-5.

CHAPTER 41

Suvradeep Mitra, Niraj Kumari, Munita Menon Bal, Santosh Menon, Narendra Krishnani

Pathology of Diseases of Endocrine Organs

◇ INTRODUCTION

The endocrine organs of the human body regulate the metabolism in various ways. Therefore, the homeostasis is disrupted in the endocrine diseases. The pathology of the endocrine organs is both intriguing and challenging from diagnostic and prognostic angles. The pathologist plays an important role in the management of endocrine diseases. While histopathology is the gold standard of the disease diagnosis, biopsy/resection and histopathology are not always a feasible option. Therefore, fine-needle aspiration cytology (FNAC) is often used for the preoperative tissue diagnosis. Besides, intraoperative frozen sections often provide a fair idea about the diagnosis to the surgeons and help in the decision-making.

Both neoplastic and non-neoplastic lesions can affect the endocrine organs. While the neoplastic lesions often need surgical resection, the non-neoplastic lesions often are medically managed. Therefore, the preoperative distinction into neoplastic and non-neoplastic pathology often aids in the decision-making and prevents unnecessary intervention. This has an immense psychological, social, psychosocial, and economic significance apart from its medical values.

The addition of ancillary techniques to the repertoire of cytology and histopathology both strengthens the diagnostic prowess and adds to the prognostic value. Techniques such as immuno(cyto)histochemistry, in situ hybridization, and molecular techniques also provide an insight into the disease pathogenesis and help in the future dream of personalized medicine.

In brief, the role of pathologists in the management of endocrine disorders is immense. A good liaison and understanding between the surgeon and the pathologist is required for the adequate management of the endocrine disorders. Therefore, we aim to discuss the pathology of the endocrine disorders in this chapter with highlights on the neoplastic pathology. We tend to discuss the thyroid, parathyroid, adrenal, pancreas, and pituitary pathology in the index chapter. This chapter aims to provide a brief overview into the pathology of the above-mentioned organ systems to the practicing surgeons.

◇ THYROID NEOPLASMS

Introduction

Thyroid neoplasms can be broadly categorized as: (1) tumors of thyroid follicular epithelium, (2) tumors of parafollicular C-cell, and (3) miscellaneous tumors. Any combination of the former two groups is possible. Thyroid follicular epithelium, also known as thyrocyte, is responsive to thyroid-stimulating hormone (TSH) and secretes thyroxine that helps to regulate various metabolic activities of the body. The secreted product of the follicular epithelium accumulates within the thyroid follicle as eosinophilic proteinaceous material known as colloid. Thus, the thyroid follicles are rounded structures lined by the thyrocytes (cuboidal cells) containing colloid material. The large majority of the primary thyroid neoplasms including follicular neoplasms, noninvasive follicular thyroid neoplasm with papillary-like nuclear features (NIFTP), papillary carcinoma, poorly differentiated thyroid carcinoma (PDTC), and undifferentiated/anaplastic carcinoma arises from the follicular epithelium. The C-cells are polygonal or spindle-shaped cells that remain adjacent to the follicles and release calcitonin, a key molecule in the calcium homeostasis. Medullary carcinoma of thyroid shows C-cell differentiation. The miscellaneous group of thyroid tumors includes hematolymphoid neoplasms, mesenchymal neoplasms, neoplasms with thymic differentiation, neoplasms arising from the intrathyroid parathyroid gland, and metastatic malignancies **(Flowchart 1)**.[1]

Role of the Pathologist

The pathologists play a pivotal role in the diagnosis and management of the thyroid lesions by (1) ascertaining its neoplastic character and distinguishing it from reactive conditions and (2) classifying and categorizing the neoplastic lesions. The interpretation of a cytopathologist is crucial in distinguishing a neoplastic lesion from a reactive one as FNAC is often employed as the stepping stone in the diagnosis of the thyroid lesions. FNAC can also categorize and diagnose the exact nature of the lesion with a fair degree of accuracy, though a few limitations exist. The distinction of follicular adenoma from follicular carcinoma is not possible by FNAC,

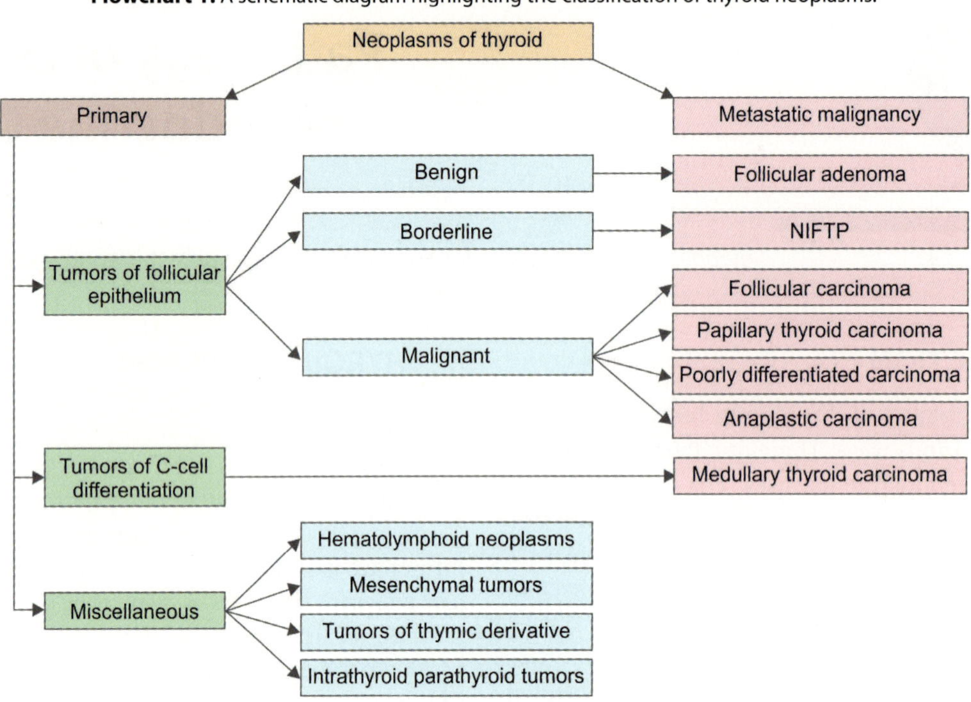

Flowchart 1: A schematic diagram highlighting the classification of thyroid neoplasms.

(NIFTP: noninvasive follicular thyroid neoplasm with papillary-like nuclear features)

Table 1: The Bethesda System of Reporting Thyroid Cytopathology: categories, risk of malignancy, and management.[2]

Category	Name of the category	Lesions included in the category (meaning in common parlance)	Risk of malignancy	Management
I	Unsatisfactory/nondiagnostic	Only cyst fluid/acellular specimen (no-minimal cellular component to ascertain the benignity/malignancy of the lesion. This could be due to a cystic lesion/sampling error)	5–10	Repeat FNAC under ultrasound guidance
II	Benign	Consistent with lymphocytic (Hashimoto thyroiditis), granulomatous thyroiditis, benign follicular nodule (adequately cellular smears to ascertain the benignity of the lesion)	0–3	Clinicoradiological follow-up
III	Atypia/follicular lesion of undetermined significance	The cytopathologist is unsure about the character of the lesion; the lesion mostly looks benign although few cells look atypical; these cells could be reactive or neoplastic	~10–30	Repeat FNAC/ molecular testing/ lobectomy
IV	Follicular neoplasm/ suspicious for a follicular neoplasm	Follicular/Hürthle cell adenoma and carcinoma (the distinction between an adenoma and carcinoma can only be done by histopathology)	25–40	Molecular testing/ lobectomy
V	Suspicious for malignancy	The lesion looks malignant although the cellularity may be a bit low to make the cytopathologist certain	50–75	Lobectomy/near-total thyroidectomy
VI	Malignant	Papillary thyroid carcinoma, poorly differentiated carcinoma, anaplastic carcinoma, medullary carcinoma, non-Hodgkin lymphoma, etc. (The cytopathologist is sanguine about the diagnosis of malignancy)	97–99	Lobectomy/near-total thyroidectomy

(FNAC: fine-needle aspiration cytology)

and a surgical specimen with adequate sampling is required. Therefore, a histopathologist requires the surgically resected specimen of thyroid for the final diagnosis. This, though crucial for the postsurgical management and prognosis of the thyroid neoplasms, cannot decide the cases that require a surgical/medical treatment. Thus, the report issued by an experienced cytopathologist aids in the surgical decision making.

Cytopathology of Thyroid

The cytopathologists follow The Bethesda System (TBS) of Reporting Thyroid Cytopathology (TBSRTC), a comprehensive and universal format of reporting thyroid cytology. The details of TBSRTC are given in **Table 1**. The clinicians and surgeons need to be well acquainted with TBS for interpretation of the cytopathology report and decision-making.[2]

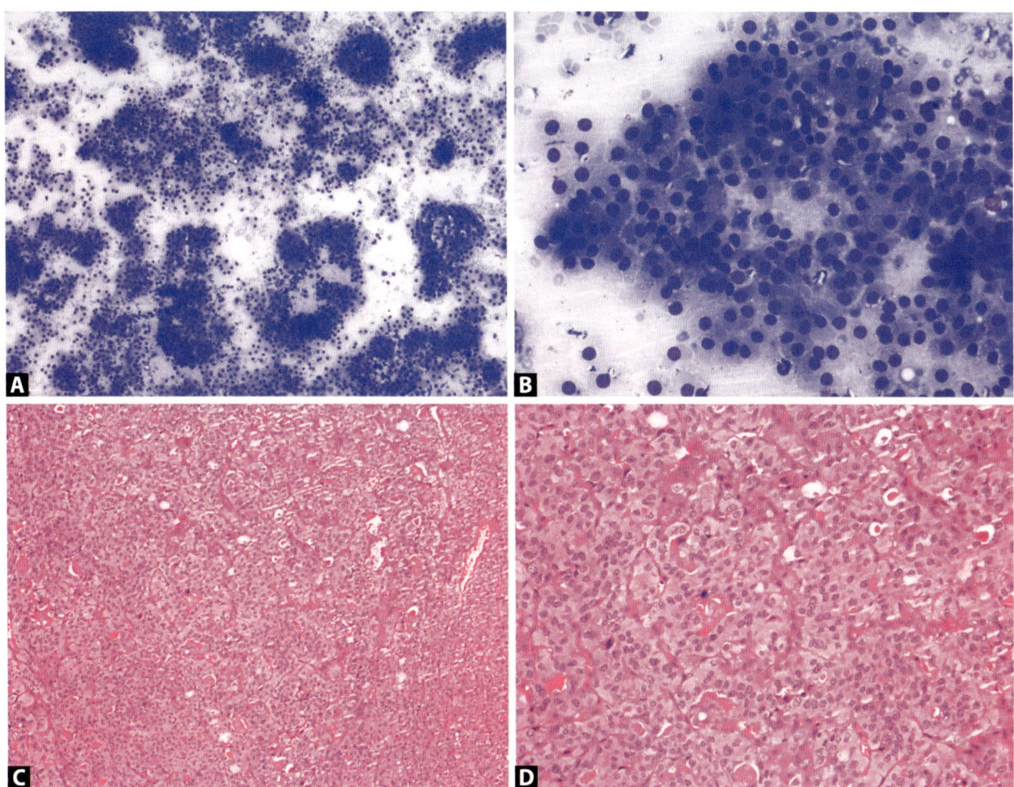

Figs. 1A to D: *Cytology and histomorphology of a follicular neoplasm (adenoma)*: The cytology smears were cellular (A, May-Grünwald-Giemsa, 100×) and contained diffuse sheets and repetitive microfollicles (B, May-Grünwald-Giemsa, 400×). Note the absence of the nuclear features of papillary carcinoma. The histology showed numerous microfollicles (C, H and E, 100×) corresponding to the cytology smears. Note the absence of the nuclear features of papillary carcinoma (D, H and E, 200×).

The six categories depicted in TBSRTC primarily ascertain the adequacy of the sampling. Therefore, a nondiagnostic/unsatisfactory sampling (Category I) does not obviate the risk of malignancy. These categories also accept a chance of false-negative cytopathology reports. This is reflected in the 0–3% risk of malignancy with category II (benign lesions). The risk of malignancy gradually increases with categories III, IV, V, and VI. Besides, TBSRTC also provides the protocol for usual management following the diagnosis of a category. Irrespective of its high sensitivity and specificity, thyroid cytology fails to diagnose a few cases conclusively. This is especially true for the category III lesions where a cytopathologist is unsure of the true nature of the lesion. Besides, the follicular neoplasms (category IV) cannot be further classified into follicular adenoma and carcinoma. Nevertheless, thyroid cytopathology aids in the definite primary decision-making.

Cytological Features and Histomorphology of Various Neoplasms of Thyroid

Follicular Adenoma and Follicular Carcinoma

Follicular adenoma mostly occurs as a cold painless nodule in an adult or young adult women. Only occasional adenomas are hyperfunctioning and appear "hot" on radionuclide scans.

In contrast, the patients of follicular carcinoma are older and can present either as an anterior neck mass or the features of distant metastasis. Thus, FNAC/biopsy of a bony mass and detection of metastatic follicular carcinoma are not unusual.[3]

The characteristic feature of follicular neoplasm is the presence of the follicular architectural pattern in the absence of the characteristic nuclear features of papillary thyroid carcinoma (PTC). FNAC smears show moderate to marked cellularity contributed by numerous microfollicles, repetitive microfollicles, diffuse sheets, and singly scattered follicular epithelial cells. These follicular epithelial cells are typically monomorphic with only occasional/mild atypia **(Figs. 1A and B)**.

Grossly, follicular adenoma is seen as a well-circumscribed and well-encapsulated mass with a fleshy tan to brown cut surface. Follicular carcinoma may not appear well encapsulated depending on its degree of invasion.

Histopathology of follicular adenoma shows an encapsulated mass with dominantly microfollicular pattern, though an admixture with macrofollicles, normal-sized follicles, and trabeculae is usual. These follicles are composed of monomorphic population of tumor cells. These cells lack in the nuclear features of PTC (described below) **(Figs. 1C and D)**. Invasion of the capsule or the vessels is the only reliable criterion to distinguish follicular carcinoma from adenoma.

This can only be assessed during histopathological examination. Multiple sections are taken from the tumor-native parenchyma interface to ascertain the capsular invasion. It is usually seen as a tongue-like or mushroom-like protrusion of the tumor that completely penetrates and breaches the capsule. The vascular invasion is assessed in the vessels located within or outside the capsule in the form of a tumor mass within the vessels that are either endothelialized or show accumulation of fibrin over it.[4,5]

The presence of oncocytes (Hürthle cells) is common in follicular neoplasms. These are seen as large cells with centrally placed nuclei, conspicuous to prominent nucleoli, and abundant amount of eosinophilic cytoplasm, the latter being attributed to the abundance of mitochondria. Hürthle cell neoplasm refers to a follicular neoplasm containing a predominant population (>75%) of Hürthle cells.

Follicular neoplasms show immunopositivity for PAX8 (nuclear), thyroglobulin (cytoplasmic), and thyroid transcription factor-1 (TTF-1) (nuclear), the latter two being markers of follicular differentiation. Carcinoembryonic antigen (CEA) and calcitonin (marker of C-cell) are consistently negative. PAX8–peroxisome proliferator-activated receptor γ (PPARγ), RAS, and PTEN pathways are commonly implicated in the molecular pathogenesis of follicular neoplasms.[6,7]

Papillary Thyroid Carcinoma

Papillary thyroid carcinoma is the most common malignancy affecting thyroid. It affects individuals of all ages and has a striking female preponderance. The most common presentation is the occurrence of a painless mass in the thyroid. Cervical lymphadenopathy due to metastatic deposits occurs in approximately one-third individuals at presentation. Occasionally, the nodal enlargement can occur in the absence of a palpable anterior neck mass.

The FNAC and the cell block show highly cellular smears arranged in monolayered sheets and papillae **(Fig. 2A)**. The nuclear features of PTC are characteristic with enlargement, overlapping, crowding, nuclear grooving, nuclear clearing (Orphan–Annie eye), and nuclear pseudoinclusions. The presence of psammomatous calcification is often considered pathognomonic of this tumor **(Fig. 2B)**. FNAC can be performed from the primary (thyroid) as well as metastatic site (cervical lymph node). This is of particular importance in the unsuspected cases of PTC. The aspiration of colloid material from a cervical lymph node often provides the necessary allusion to an astute cytopathologist.

The gross specimen of PTC usually shows an infiltrative and poorly circumscribed mass. The cut surface is gray–white in color with firm to hard consistency. Granularity/papillary excrescences can be visualized on close observation. Grittiness while cutting is a common feature and occurs due to the abundance of psammomatous calcification.[8] The tumor is multifocal in approximately two-third cases.

The histopathology shows a tumor with an infiltrative margin. The predominant architectural pattern is papillary and micropapillary although other patterns, especially follicular, are also noted **(Fig. 2C)**. The tumor shows a fibrous stroma owing to the desmoplastic reaction. The tumor cells are cuboidal, columnar, or hobnail in morphology and show the characteristic nuclear features described above **(Fig. 2D)**. Foamy macrophages are often seen in abundance.

Papillary thyroid carcinoma can show multiple variant morphologies. These morphological variants are important from diagnostic and prognostic points. Tall cell, columnar cell, micropapillary, and dedifferentiated variants show an aggressive clinical course. Cribriform-morular variant is associated with familial adenomatous polyposis. Besides, the majority of these variants does not show the classical morphology, described above, or show them only focally and thus is difficult to diagnose.

The immunoprofile of PTC is similar to follicular neoplasm, both showing follicular differentiation. Rearranged in transformation (RET)–PTC fusion, *BRAF V600E* mutation, and *RAS* mutation are all implicated in the molecular pathogenesis of PTC.[9,10]

Poorly Differentiated Thyroid Carcinoma

Poorly differentiated thyroid carcinoma shows an intermediate differentiation between well-differentiated papillary and follicular carcinoma and undifferentiated anaplastic thyroid carcinoma. It commonly affects elderly ladies who present with anterior neck mass, and the features of extrathyroidal extension are not uncommon.

Fine-needle aspiration cytology smears are moderately to markedly cellular. Three-dimensional groups surrounded by spindle-shaped endothelial cells or capillary fragments represent the insular pattern. Only occasional foci show a follicular pattern. Individual tumor cells have a high nucleocytoplasmic ratio and are relatively monomorphic **(Figs. 3A and B)**. The presence of mitosis, apoptosis, and necrosis can be observed.

The tumor usually has an infiltrative margin and a firm, grayish–white cut surface. Occasionally, partial encapsulation of the tumor is also noted.

Histologically, Turin criteria have been proposed for the diagnosis of PDTC. The tumors usually have an insular (large solid nests) and/or noninsular (solid and trabecular) pattern **(Fig. 3C)**. The characteristic nuclear features of PTC are absent. The individual cells are relatively monomorphic with hyperchromatic nuclei and scant amount of cytoplasm. The presence of convoluted nuclei, mitosis ≥3/10 high-power fields, and tumor necrosis is usual and has been emphasized in Turin criteria.[11,12] Stromal desmoplasia and extensive lymphovascular emboli can be observed.

PAX8, TTF-1 **(Fig. 3D)**, and thyroglobulin immunopositivity are seen in this tumor, although the positivity of thyroglobulin

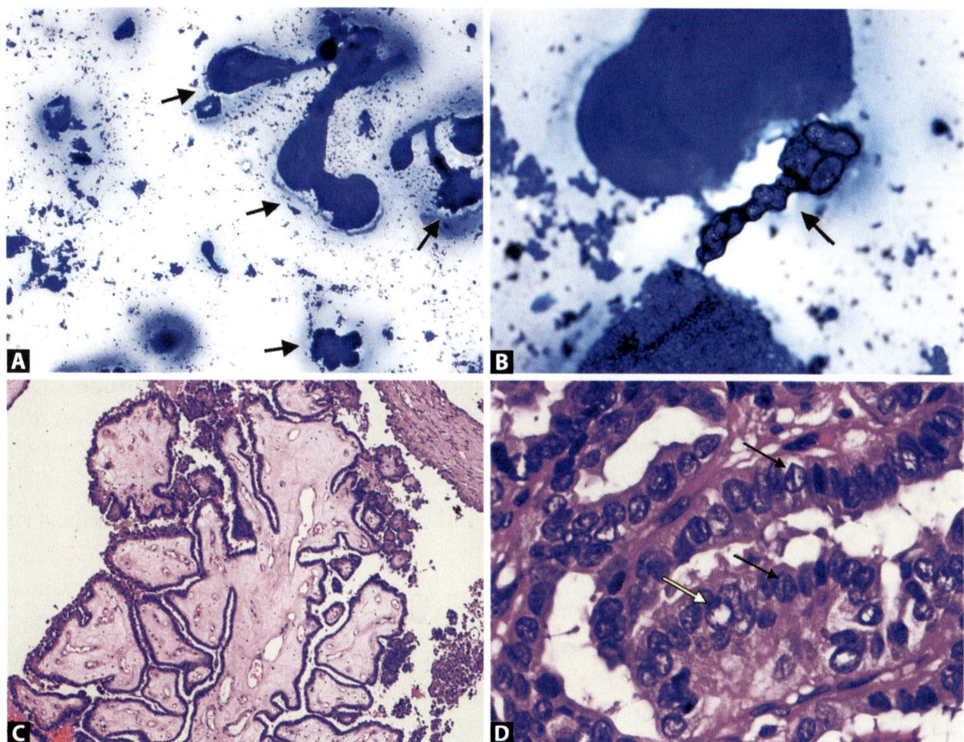

Figs. 2A to D: *Cytology and histomorphology of a papillary thyroid carcinoma (PTC)*: The characteristic papillae (A, May-Grünwald-Giemsa, 100×) (black arrows) and psammomatous calcification (B, May-Grünwald-Giemsa, 400×) (black arrow) was noted in cytosmears. The papillary architecture with central fibrovascular core was also noted in histology section (C, H and E, 100×). The characteristic nuclear features included crowding and overlapping, grooving (black arrows), and nuclear pseudoinclusion (white arrow) (D, H and E, 1000×).

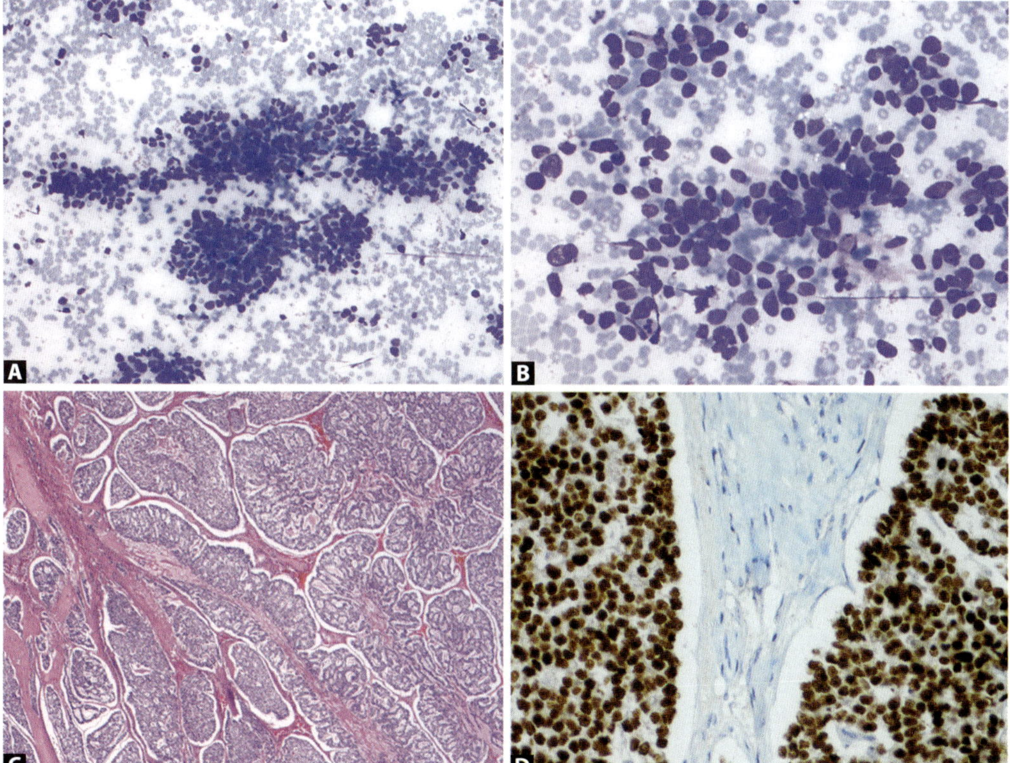

Figs. 3A to D: *Cytology and histomorphology of a poorly differentiated thyroid carcinoma*: The cytosmears were highly cellular (A, May–Grünwald–Giemsa, 200×). Individual tumor cells were relatively monomorphic with a high nucleocytoplasmic ratio (B, May–Grünwald–Giemsa, 400×). The characteristic insular pattern was noted in histology (C, H and E, 40×). Thyroid transcription factor-1 (TTF-1) immunostain showed diffuse strong nuclear positivity in the tumor cells (D, 400×).

can be very focal to absent. Typically, calcitonin immunostain is negative which distinguishes it from the medullary carcinoma of thyroid. Ki-67-labeling index is high. *TP53* and β-catenin molecular pathways are implicated in a subset of PDTC cases.

Undifferentiated/Anaplastic Thyroid Carcinoma

Undifferentiated thyroid carcinoma (UTC) is one of the most aggressive thyroid malignancies. It usually affects elderly ladies who present with a rapidly growing anterior neck mass with or without the history of long-standing goiter. It often infiltrates the adjacent structures and causes dysphagia, dyspnea, pain, and hoarseness of voice.[13]

Fine-needle aspiration cytology shows a variable degree of cellularity depending on the degree of stromal desmoplasia. The tumor cells are often pleomorphic and are either polygonal or spindle-shaped or both. Small-cell morphology, giant cell, bizarre cell, rhabdoid cell, plasmacytoid cell, and squamoid cells are common. Enlarged nuclei with vesicular chromatin and prominent nucleoli are seen. A brisk mitosis and extensive areas of necrosis are common. The background can show a neutrophil-predominant inflammation **(Fig. 4A)**. Engulfment of the neutrophils by the tumor cells is also noted. Notably, FNAC could be the only modality of tissue diagnosis feasible, owing to the rapid growth and extrathyroidal extension of the UTC.

Surgical resection is often not possible in UTC. The gross specimen of thyroid often shows a large mass infiltrating the thyroid and extrathyroidal tissue. The cut surface is firm to hard in consistency and gray–white in color.

The histopathology shows variable morphology of an infiltrative mass. The tumor cells are highly pleomorphic and show spindle-cell (sarcomatoid) and/or epithelioid (polygonal cell) morphology **(Fig. 4B)**. The sarcomatoid areas can mimic poorly differentiated sarcoma. Squamoid areas, giant cells, mitotic figures, and areas of coagulative necrosis are seen. The tumor cells may show aggregates of intracytoplasmic neutrophils.[13]

PAX8 is usually positive though it can be focal. In contrast, the tumor tends to lose TTF-1 and thyroglobulin, the markers of follicular differentiation, rendering these markers to be immunonegative. Pancytokeratin and vimentin are positive in a variable number of cases albeit focally. *TP53*, β-catenin, and RAS pathways are involved in the molecular pathogenesis of this tumor.[14]

Noninvasive Follicular Thyroid Neoplasm with Papillary-like Nuclear Features

Noninvasive follicular thyroid NIFTP is a newly recognized entity that shows a combination of follicular growth pattern and follicular differentiation along with the nuclear features of PTC. This tumor is either well-circumscribed or well-encapsulated and does not show any evidence of invasion, follicular growth pattern, papillary architecture, and nuclear features of PTC. Besides, this tumor has <30% solid, trabecular, or insular growth pattern, no capsular or vascular invasion, no necrosis, and low mitosis (<3/10 high-power field).[15]

The diagnosis of NIFTP by FNAC is difficult. Therefore, NIFTP is variably categorized into category IV, V, and III lesions.[15]

Medullary Thyroid Carcinoma

Medullary thyroid carcinoma (MTC) is a malignancy arising from the parafollicular C-cells. The tumor shows neuroendocrine differentiation. Three-fourth of the MTCs are sporadic whereas the rest are familial. A slight female preponderance is noted although it is not as evident as the tumors showing follicular differentiation. The age of presentation of sporadic MTC is in the fourth to fifth decade although presentation as early as second decade is well known, especially among the patients of multiple endocrine neoplasia (MEN).[16]

Fine-needle aspiration cytology smears are moderate-to-hypercellular with singly scattered population of tumor cells having plasmacytoid, polygonal, and/or spindle-cell appearance. Occasional clustering of the tumor cells is also seen. The nuclei of the tumor cells are round to oval that are eccentrically placed and the nuclear chromatin shows fine to coarse granularity (salt and pepper chromatin). Moderate-to-abundant cytoplasm occasionally contains fine granules.

The gross morphology of MTC is that of an infiltrative mass although well circumscription is not uncommon. The cut surface of the tumor is gray–white to tan and firm in consistency.

Histomorphologically, the tumor shows architectural pattern of a neuroendocrine tumor (NET) in the form of nests, cords, packets, and trabeculae surrounded by delicate fibrovascular septa. The individual tumor cells are relatively monomorphic with round to oval nuclei, stippled chromatin, and inconspicuous nucleoli. Intranuclear inclusions are often prominent. This tumor often shows a peculiarity of producing intratumoral amyloid **(Fig. 4C)** that can be demonstrated by Congo red staining and apple–green birefringence under polarizing microscopy.[17]

Thyroid transcription factor-1 is positive in this tumor and PAX-8 is variable. Thyroglobulin is negative. The tumor shows diffuse strong granular cytoplasmic positivity for the neuroendocrine markers (synaptophysin, chromogranin, and neurospecific enolase). Cytoplasmic positivity for CEA and calcitonin **(Fig. 4D)** often clinches the diagnosis of MTC. Both sporadic and heredofamilial MTCs show mutation in the *RET* proto-oncogene. The sporadic MTC can also show mutation in the *RAS* proto-oncogene in the absence of *RET* mutations.[18,19]

Other Epithelial Malignancies

Mucoepidermoid carcinoma, sclerosing mucoepidermoid carcinoma with eosinophilia, mucinous carcinoma, and squamous cell carcinoma can occur in thyroid. Rarely, a

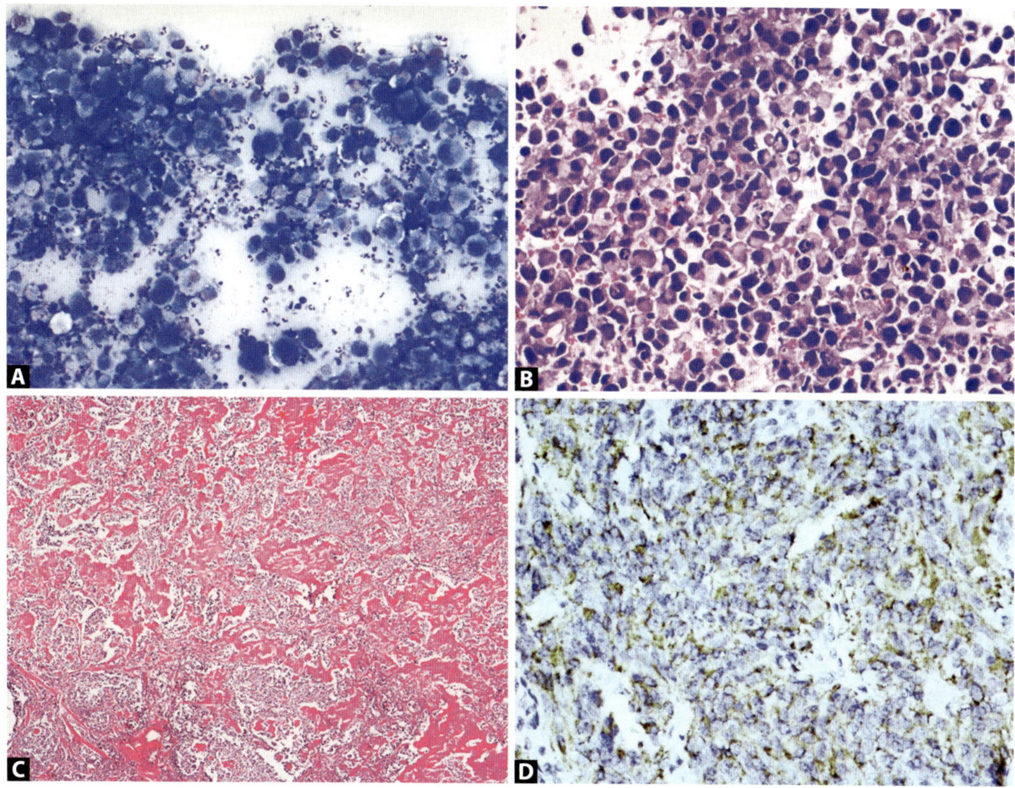

Figs. 4A to D: Cytology and histomorphology of an undifferentiated thyroid carcinoma (A and B) with diffuse sheets of rhabdoid/epithelioid cells along with scattered neutrophils (A, May–Grünwald–Giemsa, 200×) (B, H and E, 200×); Histomorphology of medullary thyroid carcinoma showing an organoid pattern of tumor cells having interspersed intratumoral amyloid (C, H and E, 100×). Immunostain for calcitonin in the same case of medullary carcinoma showing diffuse strong cytoplasmic positivity (400×).

combination of MTC and follicular carcinoma is seen (mixed medullary and follicular thyroid carcinoma).

Miscellaneous Lesions

The histomorphology of intrathyroidal parathyroid adenoma or ectopic thymoma is similar to their native counterparts. Various indolent and malignant hematolymphoid neoplasms involve the thyroid gland of which extranodal marginal zone lymphoma (Maltoma), diffuse large B-cell lymphoma, Rosai–Dorfman disease, Langerhans cell histiocytosis, and extramedullary plasmacytoma are common. Various other tumors such as paraganglioma, solitary fibrous tumor, smooth muscle neoplasms, peripheral nerve sheath tumors, and vascular tumors occur in thyroid. Occasionally, germ cell neoplasms and metastatic malignancies can also be seen.[1]

Grossing of Resected Thyroid Specimen

There are various protocols for grossing a resected specimen of thyroid. The basic principles are as follows:
- Orientation of the specimen and weighing
- Inking the external aspect of the whole specimen for the assessment of the resection limits
- Serial slicing of the individual lobes to expose the maximum cut surface (preferably, these are transverse slices)

- Identification of the mass followed by its measurement, assessment of laterality (if both lobes are resected), focality, color, consistency, and cut surface
- Photographic documentation of the mass lesion
- Multiple sections (at least 10) obtained (for blocks) from the lesion including the interface between the lesion and the native thyroid parenchyma
- The inked surface of the thyroid needs to be adequately sampled. This should include the areas where the lesion is closest to the resection limits
- Sectioning of the grossly uninvolved lobe to identify any microscopic area of tumor and the background pathology, if any.

◇ PARATHYROID

Normal Anatomy and Histology

The parathyroid glands range between 1 and 12 in number; however, in majority of the cases, they are present as four oval structures located on the posterior surface of thyroid designated as a pair of superior and inferior parathyroid glands. They may occur at abnormal locations such as carotid bifurcation, lateral to inferior pole of thyroid gland, pharyngeal wall, retropharyngeal, and retroesophageal spaces. The superior pairs develop from fourth and inferior pairs from the third branchial pouches. Normally, each gland measures between 2 and 7 mm, and larger than this is considered abnormal. The maximum normal weight of the individual gland is 30 or 120 mg in aggregate of all four glands. Single gland weighing >60 mg is considered abnormal. The amount of intraglandular stromal fat in a normal parathyroid is on an average 17% but may reach up to 50% and is little more in females than males. Exceptions include lipoadenoma and in children with a large amount of stromal fat.

The individual gland is covered by a thin fibrous capsule and is composed of admixture of epithelial cells arranged in cords, nests, and small sheets embedded in richly vascularized and fatty stroma **(Figs. 5 and 6)**. Intraglandular fat increases from puberty till the age of 25–30 years and is also related to nutritional status. Epithelial component consists of chief, oxyphil, water clear and transitional forms **(Figs. 7A to C)**.

Chief cells are round to polygonal, 6–10 μ in diameter, with central nuclei and pale granular cytoplasm. Oxyphil cells are few in young and increase with age in the form of irregular nodules. These cells are large measuring about 20 μ in diameter having eosinophilic granular cytoplasm. Another type of epithelial cell is water clear cell that shows abundant clear cytoplasm with sharply defined cell borders. Transitional cells have appearances intermediate between chief cells, oxyphil cells, and water clear cells. These cells are more commonly seen in hyperfunctioning parathyroid.

Lesions of Parathyroid

Parathyroid Hyperplasia

Hyperplasia of parathyroid glands involves enlargement of more than one gland; usually, all four glands having variable sizes and weight. Microscopically, glands of hyperplasia

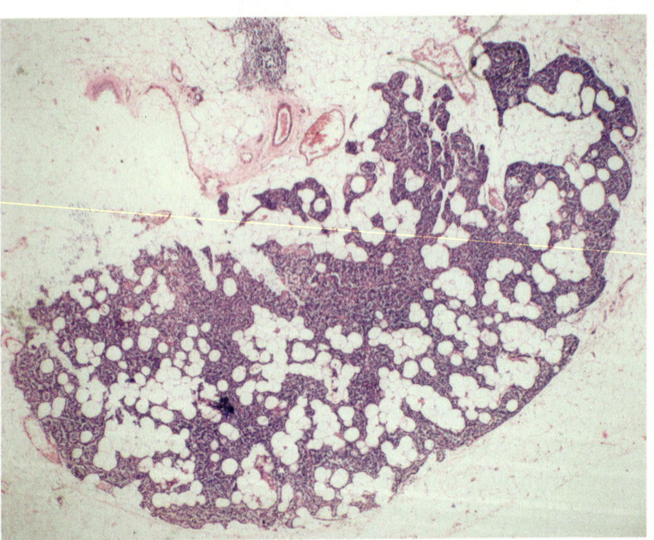

Fig. 5: Low-power photomicrograph of a normal parathyroid gland composed of epithelial cells along with intraglandular fat (H and E stain; 40× magnification).

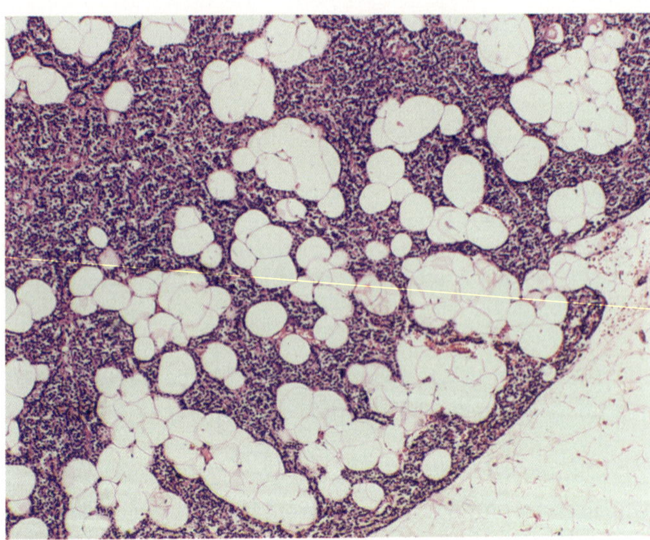

Fig. 6: Normal parathyroid gland composed largely of chief cells arranged in nests and cords intermixed with significant amount of intraglandular fat (H and E stain; 200× magnification).

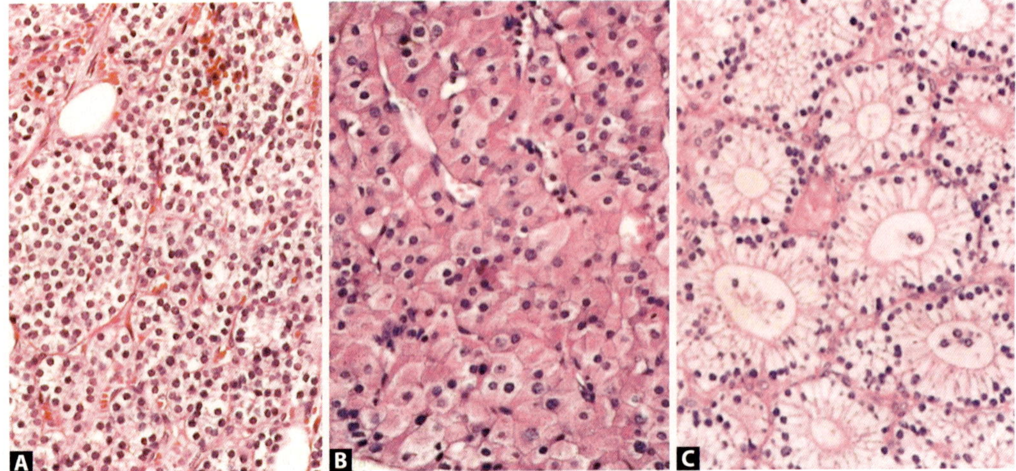

Figs. 7A to C: A panel of high-power photomicrograph composed of: (A) Chief cells; (B) Oxyphil cells having abundant granular cytoplasm; (C) Water clear cells having pale cytoplasm.

consist of similar composition of cells as in adenoma; however, fat content may be more and variable than adenoma. The enlarged glands also appear multinodular rather than uninodular on histology. Patients of parathyroid hyperplasia should always be worked for MEN and secondary causes of hyperplasia should be ruled out.

Parathyroid Adenoma

Incidence: Parathyroid adenoma accounts for 80–85% cases of primary hyperparathyroidism (PHPT). Parathyroid hyperplasia is responsible for 6.5–15% and carcinoma in <1– 6% cases for PHPT.[20,21]

Gross pathology: Parathyroid adenoma weighs <1 g to several grams. In general, the more severe the hypercalcemia, the larger the adenoma. The gland is enlarged, soft, and appears brown to reddish yellow with hemorrhage and cystic degeneration on cut surface.

Microscopic pathology: Microscopically, the gland is hypercellular with usually presence of a compressed rim of normal parathyroid at the periphery **(Fig. 8)**. The cell types comprise chief, clear, and oxyphil cells with variable amounts of transitional cells arranged in sheets, cords, acini, follicles, or microglandular pattern **(Figs. 9A to D)**. Stromal fat is either absent or generally present as a small cluster in the periphery. Exception includes lipoadenoma. The nuclei are larger than normal, with mild anisonucleosis, as they appear largely monomorphic and hyperchromatic. Mitosis is generally scarce

and occasional. Rarely, some nodular foci may occur and contain cells with high proliferative index. Secondary changes such as edema, fibrous bands, and cystic degeneration may be seen. Parathyroid adenoma also exists as few morphological variants such as lipoadenoma, water clear adenoma, follicular adenoma, and oxyphil adenoma.

Morphological variants: Lipoadenoma shows fat content of about 20–90%. Its adenomatous nature is recognized

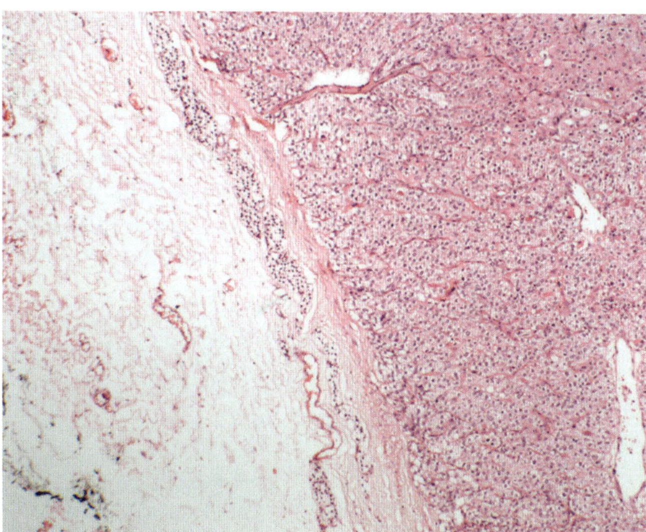

Fig. 8: Low-power photomicrograph of parathyroid adenoma displaying compressed normal parathyroid gland outside the capsule of adenoma at the periphery.

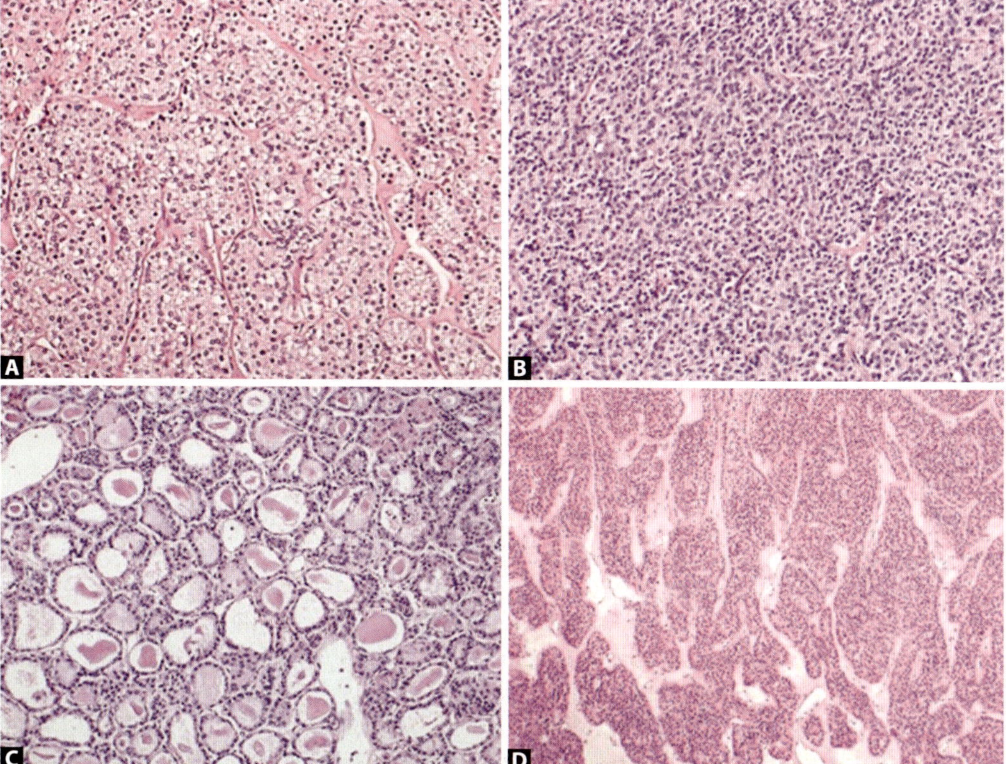

Figs. 9A to D: A panel of microphotographs composed of chief cells, clear and oxyphil cells with variable numbers of transitional cells arranged in: (A) Nests; (B) Sheets; (C) Microglandular; (D) Follicular pattern in trabeculae.

by circumscription and large size (1–15 cm). The cellular composition is similar to classical adenoma with the exception of having abundant adipocytes **(Fig. 10)**. About 50% of lipoadenoma cases are associated with hypercalcemia.[22] Certain histological features irrespective of malignancy are seen in cases of hyperparathyroidism causing hypercalcemic crisis. These include microcystic patterns, intracytoplasmic vacuoles, intratumoral broad fibrous bands, and thickened capsules **(Figs. 11 to 14)**.[23] Water clear adenomas are rare and show prominent water clear cells **(Fig. 15)**.[24] Oxyphil adenomas contain prominent oxyphil cells **(Fig. 16)** and are usually nonfunctioning. They are associated with lesser degrees of hypercalcemia. There are occasional case reports of functioning oxyphil adenoma causing hyperparathyroidism leading to osteitis fibrosa cystica.[25] Parathyroid adenomas with a prominent follicular pattern may be confused with follicular neoplasm;

however, attention to the cytoplasmic character of cells having admixture of clear, oncocytic, clear, and transitional cells may help to arrive at a diagnosis.

In Indian patients, the clinical, biochemical, and pathological characteristics do not differ between parathyroid hyperplasia, adenoma, and carcinoma except for significantly higher tumor weight in carcinomas.[26,27]

Double Adenoma

It is a controversial and rare entity yet acknowledged with a prevalence of 1.7–12% of all PHPT. The criteria for diagnosis include: (1) two enlarged glands that are histologically hypercellular, (2) a confirmation that the remaining two glands are normal (preferably on histology), (3) no clinical or family history of MEN or familial hyperparathyroidism, and (4) permanent cure of hypercalcemia after excision of two enlarged glands.[28-30] However, with more and more approach

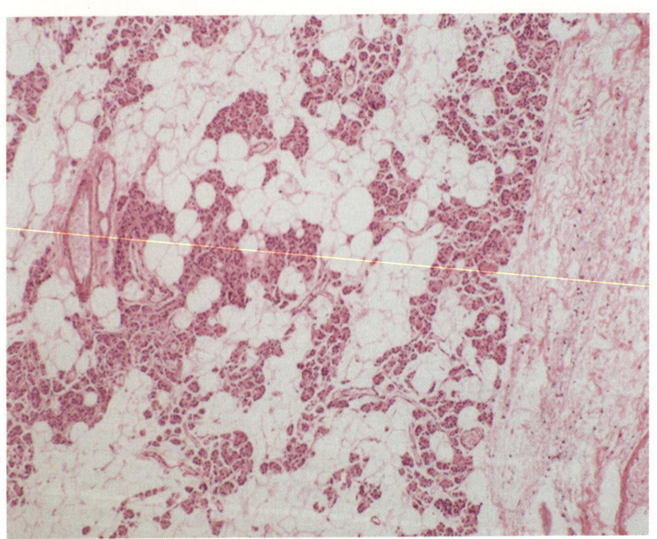

Fig. 10: Lipoadenoma composed of abundant mature adipocytes and cellular composition similar to classical adenoma.

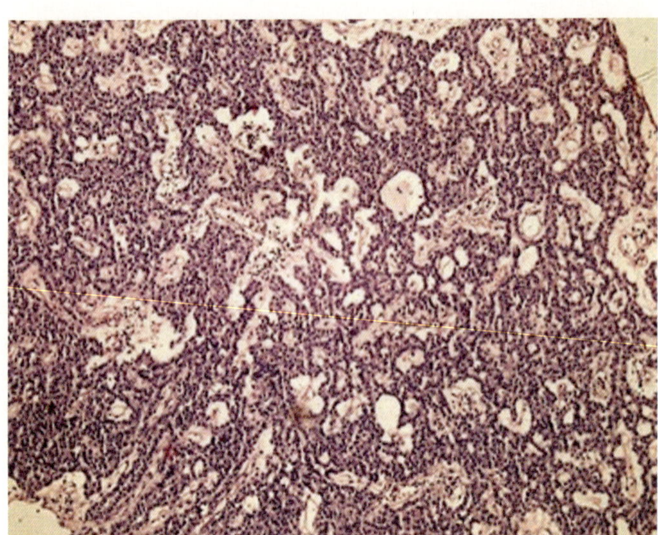

Fig. 11: Microcystic pattern in parathyroid adenoma presenting with hypercalcemic crisis.

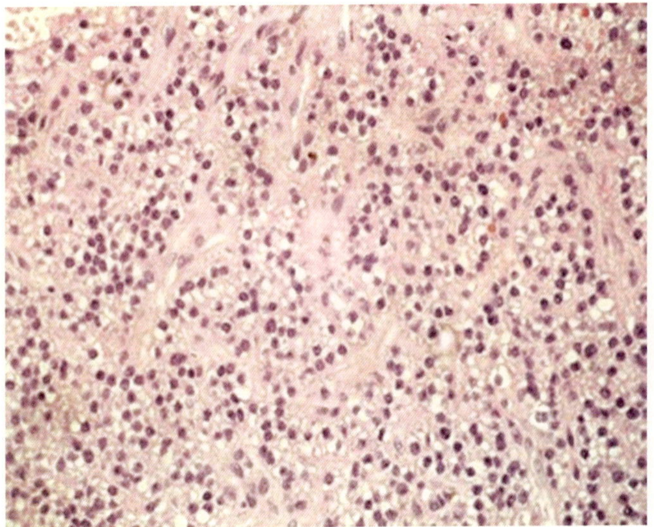

Fig. 12: Parathyroid adenoma displaying predominant intracytoplasmic vacuoles.

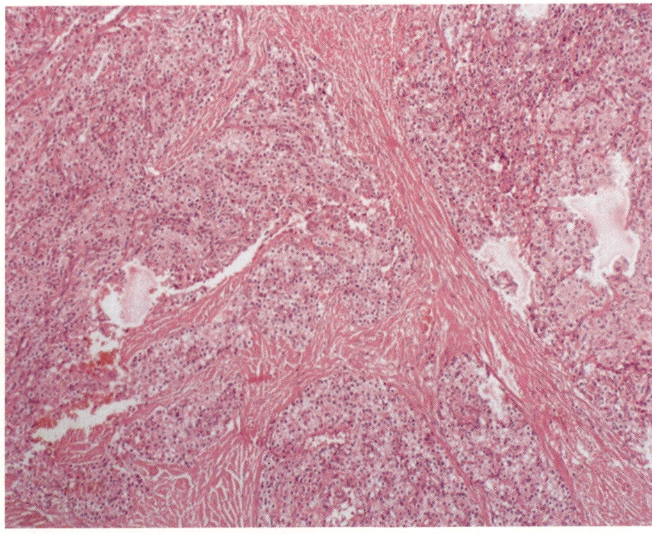

Fig. 13: Parathyroid adenoma presenting with hypercalcemic crisis shows broad intratumoral fibrous.

of focused parathyroidectomy, double adenoma is hardly being reported now.

Parathyroid Carcinoma

Parathyroid carcinoma generally affects patients a decade younger than adenoma. Grossly, it shows a gray–white, firm mass which is rarely accompanied with necrosis and calcification.

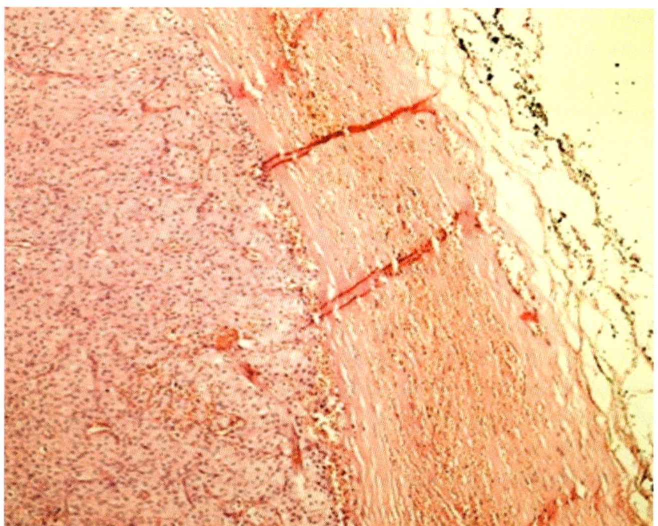

Fig. 14: Parathyroid adenoma displaying thickened broad capsule seen in patients presenting with hypercalcemic crisis.

Microscopically, carcinomas show thick capsules with cytological features similar to adenoma; however, they may show pronounced nuclear pleomorphism, high nuclear-cytoplasmic ratio, and increased cellularity. In the absence of distant metastasis, histopathology alone or with immunohistochemistry (IHC) is the only modality to diagnose a case of parathyroid mass lesion as carcinoma. The latest histological criteria for assessing the risk of malignancy in a parathyroid mass lesion are given in **Table 2** and shown in **Figures 17A to D**.

Parathyroid Neoplasm of Uncertain Potential (Atypical Adenoma)

The parathyroid masses that histologically resemble an adenoma but harbor three or more worrisome features on histology are labeled as atypical adenoma. These tumors generally follow a benign course. Follow-up with serum calcium monitoring is helpful in these cases.

Ancillary studies in parathyroid neoplasms:
Immunohistochemistry:

- Cells of parathyroid neoplasm usually stain for classical neuroendocrine markers such as chromogranin and synaptophysin in addition to cytokeratin, parathormone (PTH), and GATA3.

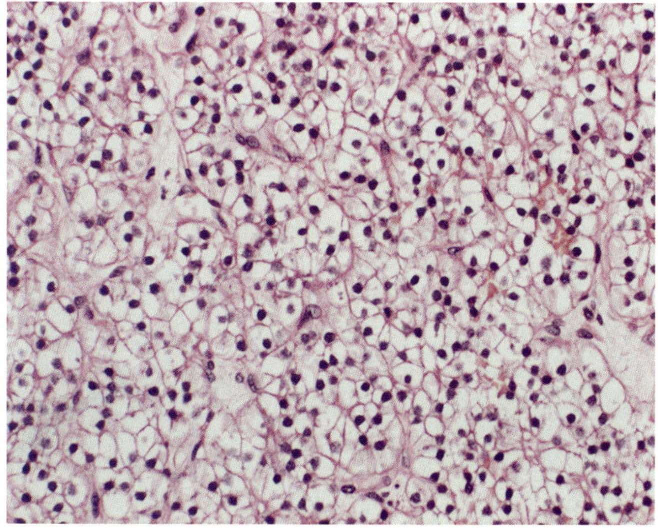

Fig. 15: A parathyroid adenoma composed predominantly of water clear cells having small central nuclei and abundant clear cytoplasm.

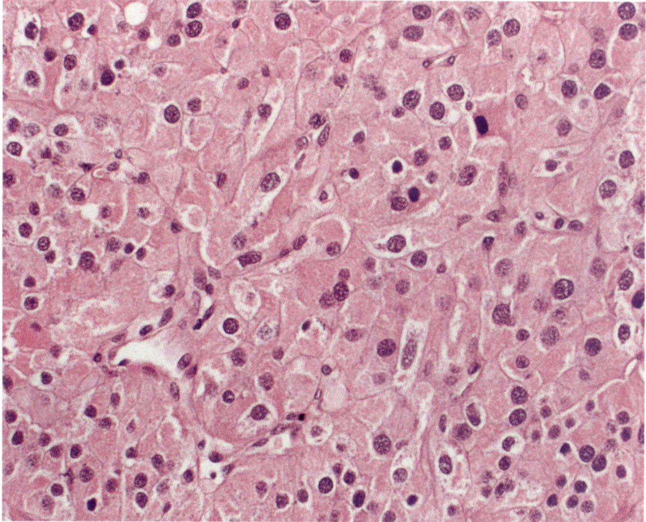

Fig. 16: Photograph from oxyphil adenoma composed of large polygonal cells having abundant granular brightly eosinophilic cytoplasm.

Table 2: Histological criteria for diagnosis for malignancy in parathyroid neoplasms.[30-34]	
*Absolute criteria of malignancy**	*Features associated with malignancy†*
• Invasion into the surrounding soft tissues • Invasion of surrounding vital structures—thyroid, esophagus, pharynx, larynx, trachea, recurrent laryngeal nerve, and carotid artery • Vascular invasion • Perineural invasion • Histologically documented regional or distant metastasis	• Capsular invasion without extension into the surrounding soft tissues • Mitosis >5/10 hpf • Broad intratumoral fibrous bands forming expansile nodules • Coagulative tumor necrosis • Diffuse sheet-like monotonous small cells with high N:C ratio • Diffuse cellular atypia • Macronucleoli present in many tumor cells

*Presence of *any one* of the following features qualifies for diagnosis of parathyroid carcinoma
†Presence of *four or more* of these features qualifies for parathyroid carcinoma while *one to three* of these features qualifies for diagnosis of atypical adenoma.

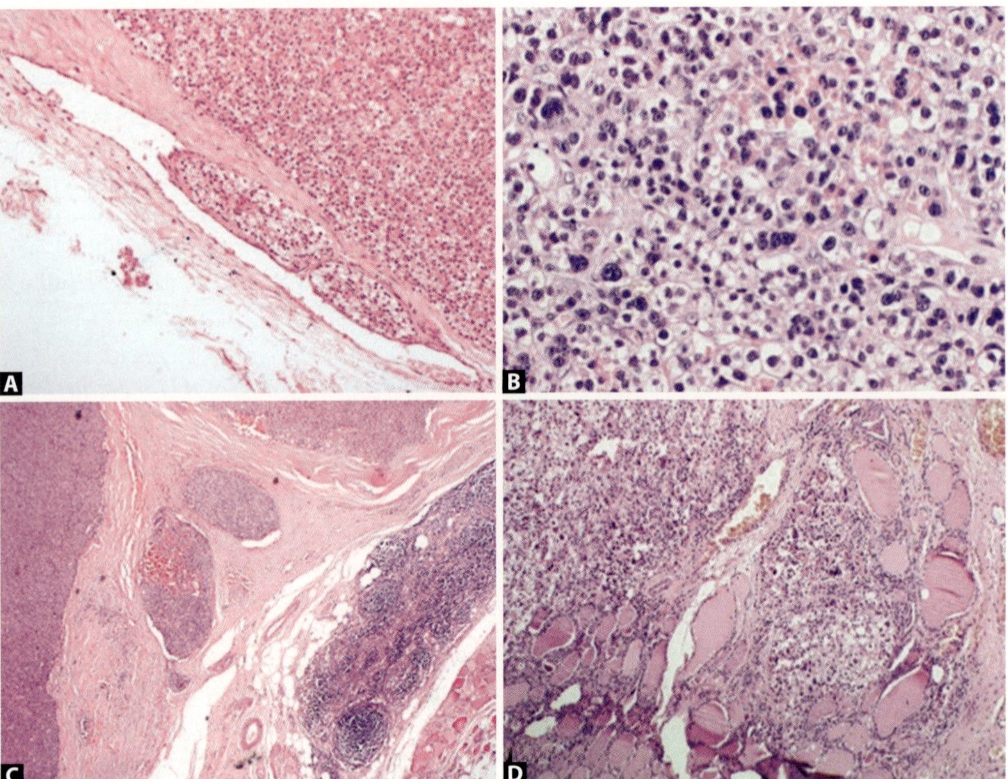

Figs. 17A to D: A panel of microphotographs from the case of parathyroid carcinoma displaying (A) vascular invasion outside the tumor capsule; (B) Macronucleoli displaying prominent nucleolus within cells; (C) Foci of capsular invasion; (D) Intrathyroidal infiltration by parathyroid carcinoma cells.

- *CyclinD1 (PRAD1/CCND1)*: Translocation of *cyclin D1* gene with *PTH* gene resulting from inversion of chromosome 11 occurs in a small subset of cases of adenoma. This results in overexpression of *cyclin D1* by IHC, which is generally seen in >91% of adenomas.[30,35,36]

- *Ki-67 proliferation index*: A high Ki-67 index suggests carcinoma; however, a low index does not exclude malignancy. Ki-67 index in parathyroid neoplasms varies between 0.4 and 26%, with an average range of 6.05–8.4%. Adenomas show Ki-67 index in the range of 0.5–5.1% (mean 2.03–3.28%). Patients with Ki-67 index of >5% should be subjected to close follow-up **(Fig. 18)**.

- *Parafibromin (PF)*: It is the protein product of *HRPT2 (hyperparathyroidism-2)* tumor suppressor gene and has role in the regulation of various cell cycle processes. PF is expressed in certain normal tissues including parathyroid, adrenal, kidneys, pancreas, heart, and skeletal muscle.[37] Its loss is invariably associated with mutational inactivation of *HRPT2* gene. Complete and partial loss of PF expression **(Figs. 19A and B)** has been observed in hyperparathyroidism-jaw tumor (HPT-JT) and cancers of parathyroid, breast, lung, gastric, and colorectum. Its expression is shown to be associated with tumor size, pathologic stage, and lymphovascular invasion as well as prognosis in different cancer. The sensitivity and specificity of PF loss in carcinoma have been reported in the range of 4.5–100% and 89.5–100%, respectively, in

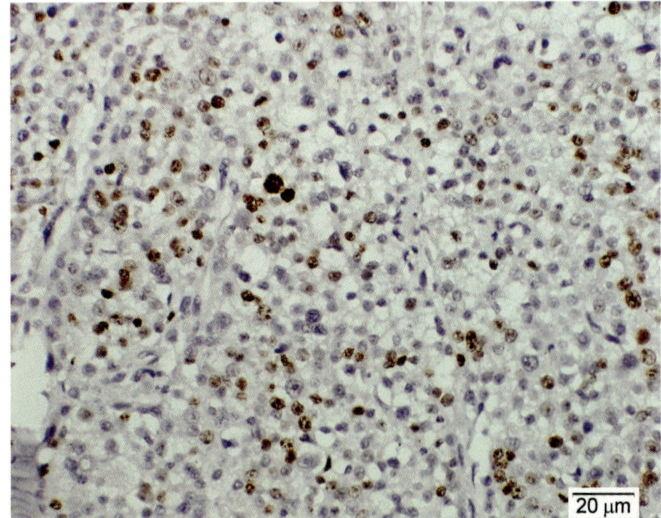

Fig. 18: High nuclear expression of Ki-67 (proliferation marker) in case of parathyroid carcinoma.

different studies.[31,38-46] Absence of PF immunoreactivity suggests either parathyroid adenoma or carcinoma with underlying genetic alteration of *HRPT2* gene. However, positive PF immunoreactivity strongly suggests benign tumor.[42,47] According to Brown et al., presence of PF staining in histologically atypical adenoma confirms a diagnosis of benign adenoma whereas if it is absent, it suggests adenoma having some malignant potential.

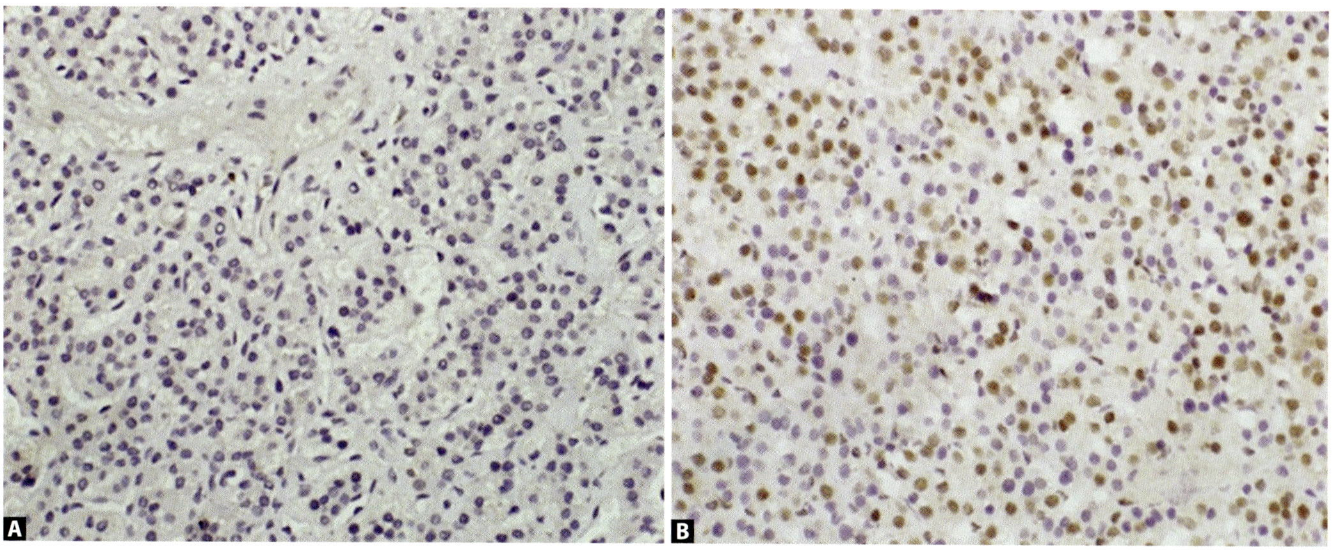

Figs. 19A and B: *Parafibromin immunostaining*: (A) Complete absence of parafibromin; (B) Partial expression of nuclear parafibromin.

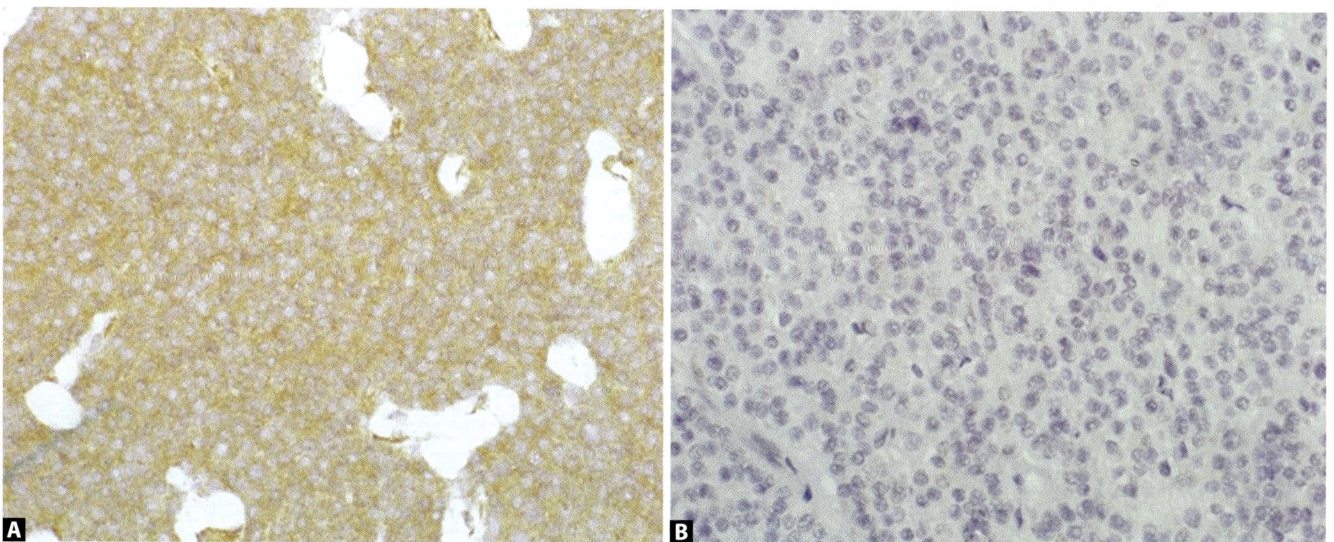

Figs. 20A and B: *Immunostaining of APC (adenosis Polyposis coli protein)*: (A) Cytoplasmic expression of APC; (B) Loss of APC expression.

On the contrary, in a histologically malignant tumor, presence of PF indicates low-grade malignant tumor and absence indicates malignant tumor with a more aggressive course.[48]

- *Adenomatous polyposis coli (APC)*: APC is a tumor suppressor gene which is a member of Wnt signaling pathway and has been shown to have role in distinguishing parathyroid adenoma from carcinoma with high specificity and sensitivity. It is expressed in adenomas but usually absent in atypical adenomas and carcinoma **(Figs. 20A and B)**. Juhlin et al. showed 75% sensitivity and 100% specificity of loss of APC immunoreactivity in parathyroid carcinoma.[49]

- *Galectin-3*: Gal-3 is another IHC marker that is involved in cell–cell and cell–matrix interactions, cell growth, damage, and repair mechanisms. These proteins regulate cell cycle and apoptosis.[50] Gal-3 is associated with anti-apoptosis, leading to cancer cell survival, tumor progression, and

invasive behavior.[31] Gal-3 is expressed in various cancers such as thyroid (follicular and papillary), colorectal, breast, gastric and hepatocellular, brain tumors, large cell lymphoma, and melanoma.[46,50,51] It is seen to be overexpressed in majority of parathyroid carcinoma and in some adenoma, and parathyromatosis **(Figs. 21A and B)**. The sensitivity and specificity of Gal-3 expression in parathyroid carcinoma are reported in the range of 54.2–93.3% and 73.7–100% respectively in different studies.[31,44,46,50,51]

- *Combined protein gene product 9.5 (PGP9.5)*: PGP9.5 is a neuron-specific protein that serves both as ubiquitin carboxyl-terminal hydrolase and as ligase.[52] It is one of the protein products of UCHL-1 (ubiquitin carboxyl-terminal esterase L1), the overexpression of which is known to be strongly associated with parathyroid carcinoma and HPT-JT-related tumors. It is normally

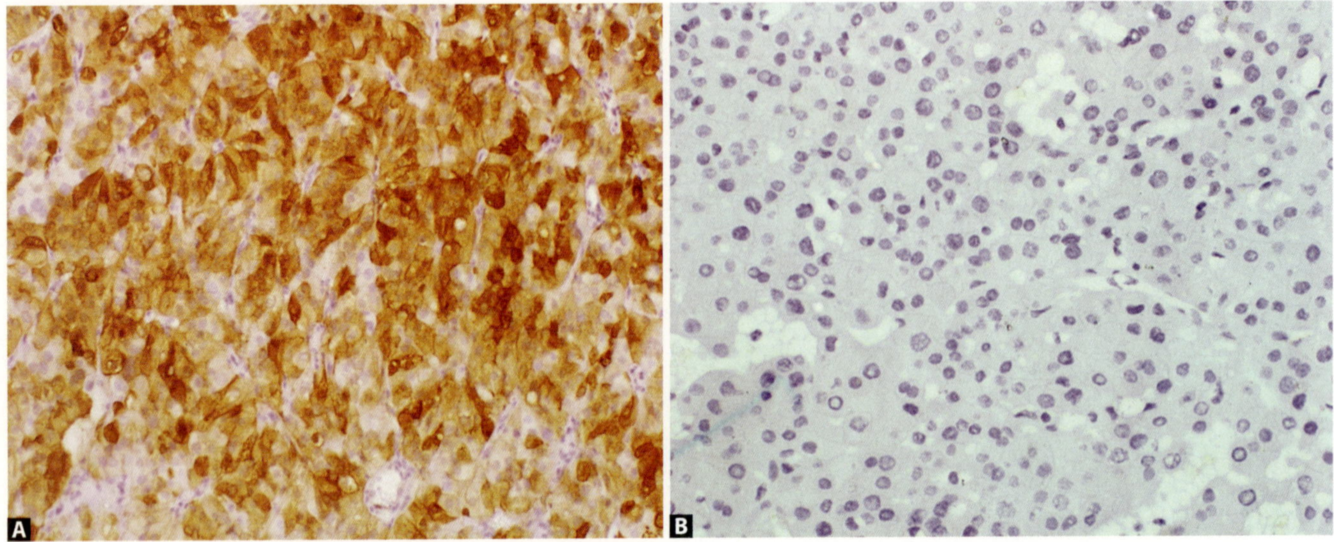

Figs. 21A and B: (A) Cytoplasmic and membranous expression, of galectin; (B) Negative galectin expression.

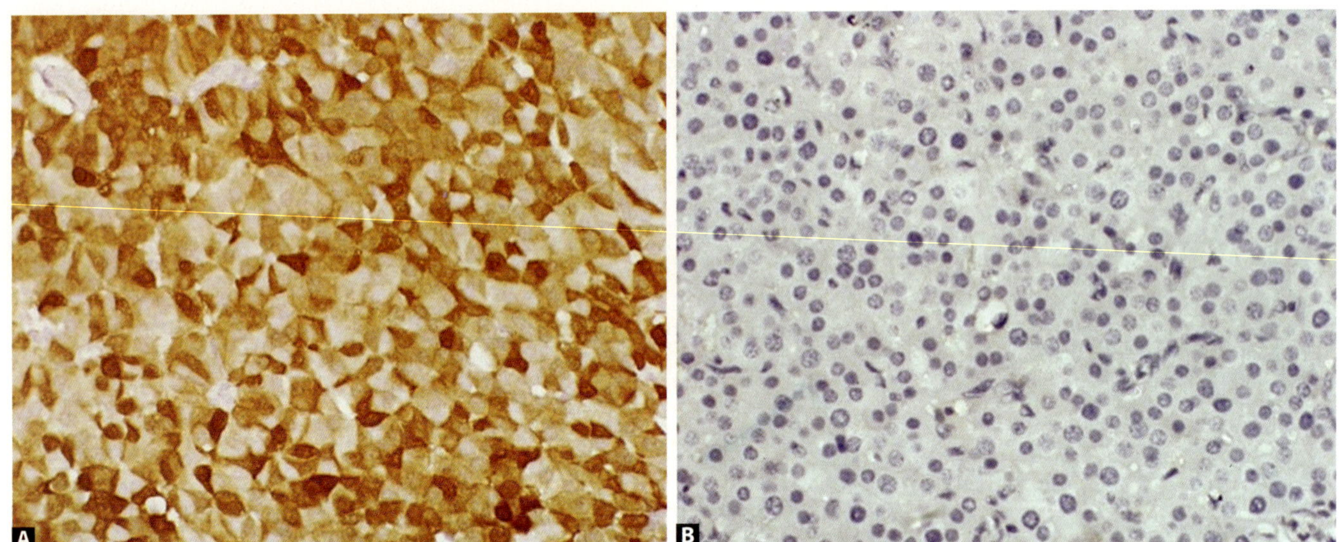

Figs. 22A and B: (A) Cytoplasmic and membranous expressions of PGP9.5; (B) Negative PGP9.5 expression.

expressed in neuronal as well as neuroendocrine tissues. Its overexpression causes increased cellular proliferation and is seen in vast majority of human cancers including pancreatic, colorectal, non-small-cell lung, medullary thyroid, renal cell carcinoma metastasis, myeloma, and mesenchymal neoplasms, where it is associated with invasive features.[45,53-56] PGP9.5 is an equally sensitive and specific marker as complete loss of nuclear expression of PF in identifying cases of parathyroid carcinoma **(Figs. 22A and B)**. In addition, PGP9.5 is also positive in parathyroid tumors associated with missense mutation in HPT-JT.[57] The sensitivity and specificity of PGP9.5 expressions in parathyroid carcinoma are reported in the range of 33.3–78% and 100%, respectively, in different studies.[44,45] PGP9.5 reactivity with loss of PF reactivity increases the sensitivity and specificity of these markers for diagnosis of parathyroid carcinoma.

In the author's own study, complete loss of PF, overexpression of Gal-3, and PGP9.5 were found to have significantly higher expression in parathyroid carcinoma (50.0%, 42.8%, and 64.3%, respectively) than adenomas (9.8%, 9.8% and 14.9%, respectively) (p-value <0.001). Complete loss of PF showed moderate sensitivity (50.0%) and high specificity (90.2%) for PC with a predictive accuracy of 87.5%. APC loss was seen in only 9% carcinomas, and this antibody served no diagnostic utility. Combination of PF, Gal-3, and PGP9.5 showed 50% sensitivity, 97.9% specificity, and 95.4% predictive accuracy for carcinoma.[58,59]

Molecular genetics:

HRPT2 (hyperparathyroidism-2) mutation: PF is the protein product of *HRPT2* gene and mutation in HRPT2 results in loss of PF expression on IHC. Partial loss of PF immunostaining is not always associated with *HRPT2* mutations. There have been cases with intact PF staining present with *HRPT2* mutation and vice versa. Immunostaining of PF being economical can act as a screening tool for atypical adenomas and parathyroid carcinomas and unequivocal cases may be subjected to *HRPT2* mutation analysis.[41] Somatic *HRPT2* mutation occurs in 66–100% of parathyroid carcinomas resulting in absent expression of PF in atypical adenomas and carcinomas.[47,60] Tan et al. showed absence of PF in adenomas related to HPT-JT syndrome suggesting absence of PF immunoreactivity as indicative of *HRPT2* mutation.[39] Few studies have shown reduced PF reactivity and *HRPT2* mutation in sporadic parathyroid adenomas.[41,61]

Unusual Parathyroid Lesions

- *Cysts*: These are usually unilocular, smooth-lined cysts. Some of them may be functional, however, majority are nonfunctional.
- *Parathyromatosis*: It refers to multiple hyperplastic parathyroid tissue found in soft tissues of neck usually lying close to parathyroid gland, in mediastinum and various other sites. It is more common in females and is believed that developmental rests of parathyroid gland occur at these sites, which become hyperplastic in patients of parathyroid hyperplasia. Diagnosis of parathyromatosis becomes challenging as it closely mimics metastasis or recurrence of parathyroid carcinoma.
- *Histiocytosis*: Rarely, primary hypoparathyroidism has been observed in cases of Langerhans histiocytosis.[62]

Role of Intraoperative Diagnosis (Frozen Section) in Parathyroid

The conventional approach of distinguishing adenoma and hyperplasia of parathyroid glands is a frozen-section approach during surgery, which has an accuracy of around 99%. It is generally used for confirmation of parathyroid tissue and to distinguish between adenoma or hyperplasia. With the advent of newer technologies, minimally invasive parathyroidectomy along with intraoperative PTH estimation has become a standard practice. Since PTH has a very short half-life of about 5 minutes, a rapid decrease in levels of serum PTH after removal of abnormal parathyroid gland/glands provides an evidence in favor of adenoma or hyperplasia.

◇| PANCREAS

Introduction

Pancreatic neuroendocrine neoplasms (PanNENs) are defined as pancreatic neoplasms with neuroendocrine differentiation. The first description of PanNEN, "simple islet cell adenoma," appeared in 1902 as an incidental autopsy finding.[63] Subsequently, the similarities and differences were recognized between PanNEN and the gastrointestinal (GI) NETs. Not long ago, a nomenclature of "gastroenteropancreatic neuroendocrine tumors" was coined to replace the earlier nomenclature of carcinoid tumors for all NET of GIT, including those of the pancreas.

Pancreatic endocrine neoplasms are relatively uncommon with an annual incidence of <1 case per 100,000 per year.[64,65] They constitute 2–5% of all pancreatic tumors.[64-66] They are indolent neoplasms and often remain undetected till late stages. This is reflected by their higher incidence of 0.8–10% in different autopsy studies.[65,67] Fraenkel et al. reviewed the surveillance epidemiology and end result registry and the European database of pancreatic NET and found a higher incidence in males and African–American ethnicities as compared to the Whites.[64] Halfdanarson et al. in their meta-analysis also found a higher incidence in males.[65]

Association with Genetic Syndromes

Pancreatic neuroendocrine neoplasms are associated with four genetic syndromes—MEN1 syndrome, von Hippel–Lindau (VHL), neurofibromatosis-1 (NF1), and tuberous sclerosis (TSC1/2).[68-71] All these syndromes have an autosomal dominant pattern of inheritance and the causative genes *MEN1, VHL, NF1, TSC1/2* act as tumor suppressor genes **(Table 3)**.[68-71]

Table 3: Genetic syndromes associated with PanNEN.[68-71]

	MEN1	*VHL*	*NF1*	*TSC*
Gene	Menin	VHL	NF1	TSC1; TSC2
Chromosome	11q13	3p25-26	17q11.2	
Inheritance	Autosomal dominant	Autosomal dominant	Autosomal recessive	Autosomal dominant
Role	Tumor suppressor gene	Tumor suppressor gene	Tumor suppressor gene	Tumor suppressor gene
Tumors/lesions	Parathyroid tumor and hyperplasia, pancreatic NET, and pituitary adenoma	• Hemangioblastomas of the retina and central nervous system • Renal cell carcinoma and renal cysts, pancreatic NET (11–17%) • Pheochromocytomas, endolymphatic sac tumors	Café-au-lait macules (>99%), neurofibromas (cutaneous >99%, deep-seated—44%), skin-fold freckling (85%), iris Lisch nodules (iris hamartomas seen on slit-lamp 17 examination) (>95%), optic pathway gliomas (15%), and bony dysplasia (sphenoid wing and bowing of long bones of the bones)	Hamartomas, benign tumors, and rarely, malignant tumors in multiple organs including the brain, heart, eyes, kidney, skin, and lungs

(MEN1: multiple endocrine neoplasia 1; NF1: neurofibromatosis 1; TSC: tuberous sclerosis; VHL: von Hippel–Lindau)

Pathologic Features

Majority of the PanNENs are well-differentiated neoplasms. Only a small subset of PanNEN is poorly differentiated; these are labeled as poorly differentiated NECs.

Gross Features

Grossly, majority of well-differentiated PanNENs present as solitary, well-circumscribed, with absent to variable encapsulation, mass lesions that may occur in part of the pancreas. PanNENs that are <0.5 cm are defined as microadenomas. All microadenomas have a malignant potential. Larger NF-PanNENs tend to be more heterogeneous and can have infiltrative borders. Majority are solid while in a few, cystic changes can also occur.[72] The latter is more frequently associated with MEN1 syndrome and is less aggressive than the solid variant. Cystic PanNENs are more frequent in the pancreatic tail as compared to the solid tumors, which are more common in the head region. Two-thirds of the surgically resected nonfunctioning PanNENs occur in the head of pancreas. Tumors in the tail are clinically asymptomatic and are incidentally detected.[73] Multicentric tumors may be observed in MEN1 syndrome.

Histologic Features

Histologically, PanNENs are divided into three broad types:
1. Well-differentiated neuroendocrine tumor (WDNET)
2. Poorly differentiated neuroendocrine carcinoma (PDNEC)
3. Mixed neuroendocrine non-neuroendocrine neoplasms (MiNENs)

Well-differentiated Neuroendocrine Tumor

These are neuroendocrine neoplasms composed of cells of uniform size, moderate amount of pale eosinophilic cytoplasm, round nuclei with stippled chromatin showing minimal atypia, arranged in a nested or organoid pattern, lacking geographic necrosis, with diffuse expression of synaptophysin and usually chromogranin.[74]

The tumors show a variety of growth patterns and architecture such as nested, trabecular, gyriform, pseudoglandular, cords, and solid patterns.[74] The tumor stroma may range from minimal to extensively hyalinized. Some tumors exhibit amyloid-like stroma and stromal calcifications may be seen. There can be morphologic variants of WDNET.

Clear cell type: These cells show clear cytoplasm owing to intracytoplasmic lipid or glycogen deposits. This type is seen especially in VHL syndrome patients, but cases also have been reported in general population and patients with MEN1 syndrome.[75] These tumors can mimic conventional clear cell type of renal cell carcinoma.

Oncocytic: The tumor cells contain abundant, finely granular, eosinophilic granular cytoplasm due to the presence of numerous mitochondria in the cytoplasm. However, the neoplastic cells have round to oval nuclei and finely stippled nuclear chromatin typical of NET. Oncocytic PanNENs can be mistaken for metastatic, adrenocortical carcinoma (ACC), hepatocellular carcinoma, and other neoplasms.

PanNENs with dense stromal fibrosis: A few PanNENs, about 10%, are characterized by dense stromal fibrosis, small nests or tubules, and an infiltrative growth pattern. Serotonin production by these tumors has been implicated in producing stromal fibrosis leading to pancreatic duct stenosis resulting in the dilatation of the main pancreatic duct/pancreatic atrophy. These tumors have an infiltrative growth pattern. Even small pancreatic endocrine neoplasm can produce upstream ductal dilatation and/or pancreatitis out of proportion to the size of the tumor.

Cystic PanNENs: On imaging, these may mimic other cystic lesions of the pancreas. Enhancement of cyst wall rim with contrast is a helpful feature of cystic PanNENs.[72] Microscopically, the tumor is cystic and delineated by a thin fibrinous band. According to the WHO 2019, the WDNET is divided into three grades: grades 1–3 based on proliferation marker, Ki67, and mitotic rate.

According to the WHO 2019, the WDNET is divided into three grades: Grades 1–3 based on proliferation marker, Ki-67, and mitotic rate.

Poorly Differentiated Neuroendocrine Carcinoma

These are histologically poorly differentiated NETs, composed of closely packed, small-to-intermediate sized cells with brisk mitosis, geographic necrosis, and marked atypia.[76] They are histologically of two types:
1. Small cell type
2. Large cell type

Small cell type: These are microscopically similar to the pulmonary small cell carcinoma counterpart. They are characterized by small-sized cells with a scant cytoplasm, inconspicuous nucleoli, and frequent crushing. The term "small cells" is actually a misnomer as the cells are—two to four times the lymphocyte size, with a high nucleus-to-cytoplasmic ratio, stippled nuclear chromatin, inconspicuous nucleoli, and nuclear molding.[76] There are usually areas of necrosis, brisk apoptosis cells, and frequent mitoses.

Large cell type: In contrast to the small cell type, these are composed of polygonal or rounded cells with moderate amounts of cytoplasm and rounded nuclei, vesicular chromatin, and prominent nucleoli. These cells are in sheets, nests, or organoid patterns. Apoptosis and mitoses are numerous. Expression of neuroendocrine markers is essential for a diagnosis of large cell NEC.[76] According to the WHO 2019, PDNEC is classified as NEC, G3 (grade 3).

Mixed Neuroendocrine Non-neuroendocrine Neoplasms

Mixed neuroendocrine non-neuroendocrine neoplasms are rare tumors composed of a combination of a neuroendocrine and a non-neuroendocrine component. The criteria to make a diagnosis of MiNEN are stringent, i.e., each component must be discretely identifiable, morphologically as well as immunohistochemically, and constitutes >30% of the neoplasm.[77]

A neoplasm should not be regarded as MiNEN, if:
- The cells of a non-neuroendocrine neoplasm merely show immunohistochemical expression of neuroendocrine markers, without the morphology.
- The non-neuroendocrine counterpart is a precursor or preinvasive lesion.
- Both the counterparts arise in the same organ independently (not clonally related), even if they juxtapose each other.
- The carcinoma was treated with neoadjuvant chemotherapy, unless the diagnosis is based on a pretreatment specimen as the neuroendocrine counterpart in treated cases may not show prognostic significance like in a de novo scenario.

Gross Features

Macroscopically, MiNENs present as solitary, polypoidal or infiltrative, solid mass lesions, ranging in size from 0.4 to 14 cm in greatest dimension.

Histologic Features

MiNENs can display significant pathologic heterogeneity in the individual component, sometimes in site-specific distribution. The non-neuroendocrine counterpart may comprise a non-gland forming entity, such as squamous cell carcinoma, acinic cell carcinoma, and carcinosarcoma while the neuroendocrine component may be a high-grade neuroendocrine (small cell/large cell) carcinoma or a low-grade NET.

Immunohistochemistry

The commonly used immunohistochemical markers include:
- Synaptophysin (as a small vesicle antigen)
- Chromogranin A (a component of neurosecretory granules)
- Insulinoma-associated protein (INSM1)
- CD56 [neural cell adhesion molecule (N-CAM)]
- Protein gene product (PGP) 9.5
- Neuron-specific enolase (NSE)

Immunohistochemistry for Diagnosis

Small vesicle-associated markers: Synaptophysin is an integral membrane glycoprotein of 38,000 MW that occurs in presynaptic vesicles of neurons and small clear vesicles of normal and neoplastic neuroendocrine cells. It is expressed independently of the other neuroendocrine markers; notably secretory granule products synapsin, synaptotagmin, SV2, or synaptobrevin have been identified as further components of the small clear vesicles.[78]

Secretory granule-associated markers: Chromogranins A, B, and C (secretogranin II) are a group of acidic monomeric proteins of various sizes. They constitute a family of soluble proteins localized to the matrix of secretory granules of neuroendocrine cells. The chromogranins serve as powerful universal markers for neuroendocrine tissue and tumors.[79]

Transcription factor: INSM1 is a zinc finger transcription factor originally isolated from pancreatic insulinomas. It plays a key role in the development of normal neuroendocrine cells and controls the development of neuroendocrine differentiation in different neoplasms. It is a very sensitive and specific IHC marker of NE differentiation.[80]

Cytosolic markers: NSE-gamma dimer of the glycolytic enzyme enolase is the best-known marker of cells with neuroendocrine differentiation.[79] The advantage of NSE as a marker is that its reactivity is unrelated to the content of secretory granules in the cells. Its disadvantage is that it may also stain some non-NET tissues such as solid-cystic (papillary-cystic) tumor of the pancreas, Schwannoma, carcinoma and fibroadenoma of the breast, renal cell carcinoma, chordoma, giant cell tumor of the tendon sheet, and certain malignant lymphomas. These findings, therefore, advise caution in using NSE positivity as a neuroendocrine marker reaction in tumor diagnosis.

Protein gene product 9.5 (PGP9.5)—also known as ubiquitin carboxyl-terminal hydrolase-1 (UCH-L1)—is a 27-kDa protein and a cytoplasmic protease originally extracted from brain tissue and found to be a marker of neuronal cells as well as neuroendocrine cells.[56]

IHC of Specific Hormones

Using IHC, hormones (somatostatin, gastrin, insulin, serotonin, pancreatic polypeptide, vasoactive intestinal peptide, etc.) can be detected in the tumor cells. Their expression can be quite variable and differs with the cell type, site, and differentiation of the tumor. These can be performed to confirm the source of a clinical symptomatology. However, IHC expression and tumor's hormonal secretion may not always correlate; IHC expression may occur without hormone secretion or there may be no IHC expression even with hormonal secretion. Higher grade tumors may be nonsecretory. While specific hormonal IHC may add prognostic information, its advantage independent of the WHO grading and staging are not evident.

IHC Markers Associated with Prognosis

Pancreatic neuroendocrine neoplasms expressing CK19 and KIT have higher metastatic potential and an aggressive course.[81] KIT expression is seen in embryonic and fetal pancreas and is not expressed in the adult pancreas. Thus, KIT expression is considered to be a stem cell feature.[81]

The CK19 is one of a 20-member cytokeratin family that encompasses the intermediate filaments of epithelial cells.

It is strongly expressed only in the early embryonic life.[81] Overexpression of CK19 has been associated with poor prognosis.

These markers (CK19, CD99, etc.) are still under investigation and currently employed mainly for research and are at present not recommended for routine use.

IHC for Grading

Immunohistochemistry for Ki-67 (MIB-1) is mandatory for tumor grading. IHC for Ki-67 (MIB1), a cell cycle proliferation antigen, is routinely used for evaluating the tumor grade.

Grading

The grade of a tumor refers to its inherent aggressiveness. It is a reliable measure of tumors aggressiveness. As per the WHO 2019,[82] grading is based on two factors:

1. Histologic differentiation
2. Rate of proliferation, which is assessed by calculating the mitotic count and Ki-67 index in histologic material.

Well-differentiated NETs are subclassified into three grades: grade 1 (G1), grade 2 (G2), and grade 3 (G3) NETs. These are well differentiated on histology, i.e., are recognizable as NETs on histology, and generally show diffuse and strong immunoreactivity for neuroendocrine IHC markers, especially in the G1 and G2 tumors.

In contrast, the term "carcinoma" is used for tumors with poor differentiation, showing either a morphology of small cell carcinoma or large cell neuroendocrine carcinoma. These are accompanied by increased mitosis, presence of necrosis, and high Ki-67 labeling >20%.

Two important measurements that are required for grading of PanNENs are: (1) mitotic index and (2) Ki-67 labeling index.

Mitotic Index Assessment

Mitotic index is based on evaluation of mitoses in 50 high-power field (0.2 mm^2) in areas of highest density and expressed per 10 HPF.

Ki-67 Index Assessment

Ki-67 (MIB1), a cell cycle proliferation antigen, is seen as nuclear stain and is mandatory for tumor grading by the WHO 2019 classification.

The Ki-67 index is assessed in the hot spots on 2,000 cells (minimum of 500 cells for biopsies). Manual counting of camera-captured images was found to be the most reliable method by Reid et al.[83] and Tang et al.[84] when compared to other methods such as eyeballing, eye counting, and digital analyzers. It has drawbacks of being expensive and personnel dependent. The different methods of Ki-67 assessment have been enumerated in **Table 4**.

There may be interlaboratory variability in Ki-67 due to the variability in tissue fixation, processing, and reagents used and in the pre-treatment procedures. External standardization

Table 4: Methods of Ki-67 evaluation.[83,84]

Method	Time taken	Comments
Eyeballing or eyeball estimation	<1 minute	Fastest method but poorest reliability and reproducibility
Eye counting of cells	6 minutes	Poor reproducibility
Manual counting through camera-captured images	8.1 minutes	Most reliable method
Digital analyzer	5 minutes	Least practical—expensive, personnel dependent, miscalculation because of the inclusion of lymphocytes fibroblasts as tumor cells

Table 5: WHO 2019 Classification of Pancreatic Neuroendocrine Tumors.[82]

Terminology	Differentiation	Grade	Mitotic rate (mitoses/2 mm2)	Ki-67 index
NET, G1	Well differentiated	Low	<2	<3%
NET, G2		Intermediate	2–20	3–20%
NET, G3		High	>20	>20%
SCNEC	Poorly differentiated	High	>20	>20%
LCNEC			>20	>20%
MiNEN	Well to poorly differentiated	Variable	Variable	Variable

(LCNEC: large cell neuroendocrine carcinoma; MiNEN: mixed neuroendocrine non-neuroendocrine neoplasm; NET: neuroendocrine tumor; SCNEC: small cell neuroendocrine carcinoma)

may help in increasing reliability and reproducibility. Another problem in the evaluation of Ki-67 is intratumoral heterogeneity which can occur synchronously within the same tumor or metachronously as higher-grade metastasis developing in the course of the disease.[85]

The WHO classification is depicted in **Table 5**.

Molecular Landscape

The WDNET and PDNEC harbor contrasting molecular profiles further establishing their distinction at the molecular genetic level. **Table 6** highlights the differences in the molecular alterations in the WDNET and PDNEC.

The most commonly mutated genes in WDNET are those involved in chromatin remodeling such as *MEN1*, *DAXX* (death domain-associated protein gene), and ATRX (alpha-thalassemia mental retardation X-linked).[86,87] Additionally, 5% PanNENs harbor mutation in phosphatidylinositol 3-kinase (PI3K) Akt/mammalian target of rapamycin (mTOR) signaling pathway, especially those with VHL syndrome and tuberous sclerosis.[88,89]

The WDNET lacks mutation in p53 and Rb1 found in PDNEC.[90] Yachida et al. in 2012 found that alterations in p53 and Rb were frequent in both small-cell and large-cell NECs, whereas *SMAD4/DPC4*, *DAXX*, and *ATRX* labeling was retained in virtually all the PDNEC.[91] In contrast, *DAXX* and *ATRX* labeling was lost in 45% of WDNETs, whereas p53

Table 6: Molecular profile of PanNEN.[91]

Gene	PDNEC small cell	PDNEC large cell	WDNET	Pan ductal adenocarcinoma
KRAS	25%	33%	0%	>90%
CDKN2A	11%	50%	0%	80–95%
TP53	100%	90%	4%	75%
SMAD4	0%	10%	0%	55%
RB1	89%	50%	0%	13%
DAXX/ATRX	0%	0%	43%	0%
MEN1	0%	0%	44%	0%

(MEN1: multiple endocrine neoplasia type 1; PanNEN: pancreatic neuroendocrine neoplasms; PDNEC: poorly differentiated neuroendocrine carcinoma; WDNET: well-differentiated neuroendocrine tumor)

Box 1: Weiss system for separating benign from malignant adrenocortical neoplasm.[106]

- High nuclear grade (grade 3 or 4 according to criteria of Fuhrman et al.[108])
- Mitotic rate >5/50 high-power fields (hpf)
- Atypical mitosis
- Clear cell comprising 25% or less of the tumor
- Diffuse architecture (greater than one-third of tumor)
- Necrosis
- Invasion of venous structures
- Invasion of sinusoidal structures
- Invasion of capsule of tumor

Note: Each factor is given a score of 1 if present and 0 when absent. Presence of three or more criteria (score 3 or more) correlated with subsequent malignant behavior.

and Rb were intact in these same cases. Overexpression of Bcl-2 protein was observed in all small-cell NECs and in 50% of large-cell NECs in their study. Bcl-2 overexpression was significantly correlated with a higher mitotic rate and Ki-67 labeling index in neoplasms in which it was present. Small-cell NECs are genetically similar to large-cell NECs and are distinct from WDNET.[91]

The molecular alterations in pancreatic neuroendocrine neoplasms are enlisted in **Table 6**.

◇| ADRENAL

Adrenocortical Carcinoma

Introduction

Adrenocortical carcinoma is a rare endocrine malignancy of adrenal cortex. The reported incidence is approximately 0.02%.[92] Females are more likely to be affected than males.[93] This disease tends to be highly aggressive with a 5-year mortality rate of approximately 75–90%. The main treatment of ACC is the complete surgical removal of the tumor. The poor prognosis of ACC is explained in part by its relative unresponsiveness to chemotherapy and external beam radiation.[94,95]

The differential diagnosis between malignant and benign tumors of the adrenal cortex can be a difficult task for both clinicians and pathologists. The definitive criteria for malignancy are distant metastasis and/or local invasion. The increasing discovery of incidental adrenal masses by radiologic studies performed for unrelated reasons has made the prediction of malignancy an increasingly important challenge in clinical practice.

Gross Features

Adrenocortical carcinomas have a nodular appearance with individual nodules varying from pink to yellow-tan, depending on lipid content. Functioning ACC associated with feminization or virilization tends to be red-brown, whereas those associated with Cushing syndrome are more often yellow-tan. Foci of hemorrhage, necrosis, and calcification are common, particularly in large tumors.

Histomorphology of Adrenocortical Carcinoma

Adrenocortical carcinoma has different growth patterns that include trabecular, solid, alveolar, and mixtures of these patterns are common.[96-98] Large tumors often show extensive necrosis. Foci of myxoid change, pseudoglandular pattern, and spindle cell growth may be prominent in some tumors. Histological variants of ACC include myxoid adrenocortical carcinoma, oncocytic adrenocortical carcinoma, carcinosarcoma, and adenosquamous carcinoma.[99-105]

Criteria for Malignancy in Adrenocortical Tumor

It may be extremely difficult to distinguish between benign and malignant adrenocortical tumors, and different authors have used a variety of parameters to differentiate these neoplasms. In 1979, Hough et al. proposed a system based on combination of a nonhistopathologic and histopathologic index of a malignancy to separate malignant from benign cortical tumors.[93]

In 1984, Lawrence Weiss proposed a system for evaluating adrenocortical malignancy based on nine histopathologic criteria found to be associated with adrenal cortical tumors that had metastasized or locally recurred.[106]

The Weiss System and the Modified Weiss System for Diagnosis of Adrenocortical Carcinoma (Boxes 1 and 2)

- The Weiss system appears to be the most utilized system, because of its simplicity and reliability.[106] However, only a few studies have tried to evaluate its diagnostic and discriminatory utility to differentiate benign and malignant adrenal neoplasms. Moreover, the interpretation and the application of Weiss histopathologic criteria are sometimes difficult or subjective. In 2002, Aubert et al.[107] proposed simplifying the Weiss system by eliminating criteria that were considered to be more subjective or difficult to interpret. Using a stepwise regression analysis, a modified scoring system was generated using five histopathologic criteria which elucidated in **Box 2**.

Box 2: Modified Weiss system for separating benign from malignant adrenocortical neoplasms.[107]

- Mitotic rate (5 per 50 hpf)
- Cytoplasm (clear cells comprising 25% or less of the tumor)
- Abnormal mitoses
- Necrosis
- Capsular invasion

Note: Modified Weiss scoring system = (2 × mitotic rate) + (2 × cytoplasm) + abnormal mitoses + necrosis + capsular invasion.
A score of 3 or greater correlates with subsequent malignant behavior.
hpf: high-power fields.

Box 3: Armed Forces Institute of Pathology criteria for separating benign from malignant adrenocortical neoplasms in pediatric patients.[113]

- Tumor weight >400 g
- Tumor size >10.5 cm
- Extension into periadrenal soft tissues and/or adjacent organs
- Invasion into vena cava
- Venous invasion
- Capsular invasion
- Presence of tumor necrosis
- >15 mitoses per 20 hpf
- Presence of atypical mitotic figures

Note: The presence of up to two criteria is associated with benign outcome; three criteria are considered indeterminate for malignancy; and four or more criteria are associated with malignancy.
hpf: high-power fields.

A given adrenocortical tumor is assigned a numeric score according to the number of the aforementioned histologic features present. The individual histologic parameters in the Weiss system are not weighted and carry equal value; individual criterion is simply given a score of 1 if present and 0 if absent, yielding an overall score which ranges from 0 to 9.

Several authors have felt recognition and interpretation of some of the histologic criteria of the Weiss system to be difficult and subject to interobserver variability.[109,110] In 2002, Aubert et al.[107] proposed simplifying the Weiss system by eliminating criteria that were considered to be more subjective or difficult to interpret. Using a stepwise regression analysis, a modified scoring system was generated using five criteria which included mitotic rate, cytoplasmic character, abnormal mitosis, necrosis, and capsular invasion. These were then assigned a weighted multiplication factor.

These five histologic criteria that finally were incorporated in this system were based on high interobserver agreement as measured by κ values and discarding the variable, which had poor interobserver agreement from the original Weiss criteria. For an individual tumor, each criterion is given a score of 0 when absent and 1 when present, yielding an overall score that can range from 0 to 7. Similar to the original Weiss system, a score of 3 or greater is considered indicative of malignancy. This modified system correlated well with the original Weiss system and was easier to use in practice because only five histologic features are assessed rather than nine.[111]

Some Special Variants of Adrenocortical Tumors and their Criteria for Malignancy

Oncocytic adrenocortical carcinoma: Bisceglia et al.[99] have reviewed the criteria for the distinction of benign and malignant adrenocortical oncocytic tumors. According to these authors, the major criteria for malignancy include high mitotic rate, atypical mitosis, and venous invasion whereas minor criteria include large tumor size, necrosis, capsular invasion, and sinusoidal invasion. The presence of one major criterion is sufficient for diagnosis of malignancy, whereas one minor criterion was sufficient for diagnosis of tumor of uncertain malignant potential. The absence of any of the criteria correlated with benign behavior.

Myxoid adrenocortical neoplasm: In the study of myxoid adrenocortical tumor by Papotti et al.,[112] 8 out of 10 cases fulfilled Weiss criteria for malignancy (score >3). The authors concluded that a myxoid adrenocortical tumor represents a rare but histologically and phenotypically distinct entity exhibiting malignant behavior. However, these are so rare that many larger series may be required before these are characterized categorically.

Pediatric adrenocortical neoplasm: In the pediatric age group, features associated with an increase in probability of malignancy include tumor weight >400 g, size >10.5 cm, vena cava invasion, necrosis, severe nuclear atypia, capsular and/or vascular invasion, extension into periadrenal soft tissue, >15 mitosis per 20 HPF, and the presence of atypical mitotic figures[113] **(Box 3)**.

Immunohistochemistry

Immunohistochemically, the cells of ACC are positive for vimentin, synaptophysin, inhibin, and Melan-A. They also stain for *BCL2*, calretinin, and keratin. They are negative for epithelial markers such as epithelial membrane antigen (EMA) and CEA. Many studies also proved the importance of Ki-67 IHC in distinguishing adrenocortical adenoma from carcinoma and also categorizing low-grade and high-grade ACC.[114-116]

Pheochromocytoma

Introduction

Pheochromocytoma (PCC) is an intra-adrenal sympathetic paraganglioma arising from the medulla. Both PCC and sympathetic paraganglioma (called PPGL together) are catecholamine-producing tumors, which often have a common genetic basis and functional similarities. They may clinically present as refractory hypertension or hypertensive crisis. In some patients, there may be other subtle symptoms of catecholamine excess such as tachycardia, sweating, and anxiety.[117,118]

Pathology

Pheochromocytomas are circumscribed, usually unencapsulated, with pink, gray-tan cut surface. Microscopically, the classical nested pattern of tumor cells with capillary network, "the Zellballen" pattern, is a prominent feature of most PCCs. The tumor cells are usually monomorphic punctuated by sudden anisonucleosis or sudden pleomorphism of tumor nuclei.[118] PCCs in MEN2 can be either multiple or single and often show abundant hyaline globules. VHL-related tumors may have a thick vascular capsule, edematous stroma, small-to-medium-sized cells that lack nuclear atypia and mitoses, have amphophilic cytoplasm, and lack hyaline globules.[118,119] NF1-related tumors usually lack the marked vascularity of VHL tumors. In succinate dehydrogenase (SDH)-deficient PCC, the cells may have a pseudorosette arrangement of tumor cells, sometimes with vacuolated cytoplasm, and may lack sheet-like architecture. The tumor cells are positive for neuroendocrine markers (chromogranin-A, synaptophysin, INSM1), tyrosine hydroxylase, and negative for keratin. The supporting, sustentacular cells are S100 and SOX10 positive. Loss of SDHB immunoreactivity occurs with mutation in any SDH subunit.[118-120]

There are no universally acceptable histologic criteria predicting metastasis. Based on the clinical follow-up data, the WHO Endocrine Tumor Classification, 4th edition, deduced that all PPGLs have some metastatic potential and eliminated the previous categories of benign and malignant tumors in favor of an approach based on risk stratification.[121] Pheochromocytoma of the Adrenal Gland Scaled Score (PASS), comprising 12 histological parameters and scores up to 20 points, was initially used to risk stratify the tumors. A PASS score ≥4 is deemed to stratify tumors with increased metastatic potential, whereas those with a score <4 were considered benign.[122] Owing to the poor reproducibility and utility of PASS scoring, Kimura et al. then developed another scoring system, Grading of Adrenal Pheochromocytoma and Paraganglioma (GAPP), based on the presence or absence of six parameters including cellularity, comedonecrosis, capsular/vascular invasion, Ki67-labeling index, and catecholamine phenotype.[123] GAPP could be utilized for clinical decision-making and has been validated for the prediction of metastatic potentiality.[124]

◁| PITUITARY GLAND

Pituitary Gland Lesions

Pituitary gland and seller tumors constitute around 15% of central nervous system tumors. Pituitary adenomas are the most common tumors. Rarely, pituitary carcinoma and pituitary blastoma are primary pituitary tumors. Other tumors are neuronal and paraneuronal tumors such as gangliocytoma, neurocytoma, paraganglioma, and neuroblastoma. The posterior pituitary tumors are nonendocrine low-grade and consist of pituicytoma, granular cell tumor of neurohypophysis, spindle cell oncocytoma, and seller ependymoma. All posterior pituitary tumors express nuclear TTF-1 suggesting a morphological spectrum

of single entity and originating from variants of pituicytes. Craniopharyngioma are also not uncommon tumors in sellar region. Other rare tumors of seller region are germ cell tumors, mesenchymal tumors, and hematological tumors.[125] The non-neoplastic lesions are Rathke cleft cyst and lymphocytic hypophysitis.

Pituitary adenomas are a group of heterogeneous tumors having varied presentations and invasive tendency, hormone secretion, and sometime histomorphological features. The WHO 2017 classification is based on tumor hormonal content assessed by IHC and presence of transcription factors in tumor differentiation according to cell lineages and regulation of specific pituitary hormones production **(Table 7)**.[126]

Pituitary tumors type depends on largest dimension: microadenoma (<1 cm), macroadenoma (1–4 cm), or giant adenoma (>4 cm).

Association of Hereditary and Familial Conditions in Pituitary Adenoma

Most of the pituitary adenomas are sporadic. Rarely, adenomas are associated with hereditary or familial syndromes including MEN syndrome, MEN1 and MEN4, Carney's complex, the McCune–Albright syndrome, the *SDH* gene-associated hereditary PCC and paraganglioma syndrome, the familial isolated pituitary adenoma syndrome, and X-linked acrogigantism. Most of the hereditary and familial syndrome-associated pituitary adenomas predominantly secrete GH and/or PRL; however, some are nonfunctioning adenomas.[127]

Ancillary Techniques for Pituitary Lesions

Reticulin stain is used to find microadenoma where reticulin disruption is evident on a background of preserved reticulin framework of normal pituitary gland. It is also useful to differentiate hyperplasia from adenoma where an intact and expanded reticulin pattern is seen. Application of periodic acid–Schiff (PAS) stain is useful to identify adrenocorticotropic hormone (ACTH)-positive secretory granules.

The new classification is based mainly on IHC and electron microscopy is not required as an ancillary tool. Ultrastructure study is rarely required in pituitary adenomas. To classify pituitary adenoma, hormone IHC along with application of transcription factors IHC is applied. Transcription factors play an important role in classifying pituitary tumors such as null cell adenoma, plurihormonal Pit-1-positive adenoma. GH, PRL, and TSH hormone cells express Pit-1, T-pit transcription factor in ACTH hormone-producing cells, and steroidogenic factor 1 (SF-1) in gonadotroph hormone expressing cells. GATA2 is also expressed in gonadotroph and thyrotrophs cell lineage. Expression of ERα is seen in PRL and gonadotroph-secreting cells. Low-molecular-weight cytokeratin IHC is helpful to identify sparsely granulated somatotroph adenoma (SGSA) from densely granulated somatotroph adenoma and

Table 7: WHO Classification of Pituitary Adenomas (2017).

Adenoma types	Morphological variants	Pituitary hormone IHC	Transcription factors/co-factors
Somatotroph adenomas			
	Densely granulated somatotroph adenoma	GH, α-subunit	Pit-1
	Sparsely granulated somatotroph adenoma	GH	Pit-1
	Mammosomatotroph adenoma	GH + PRL (in same cells) + α-subunit	Pit-1, ERα
	Mixed somatotroph-lactotroph adenoma	GH + PRL (in different cells) + α-subunit	Pit-1, ERα
Lactotroph adenomas			
	Sparsely granulated lactotroph adenoma	PRL	Pit-1, ERα
	Densely granulated lactotroph adenoma	PRL	Pit-1, ERα
	Acidophil stem cell adenoma	PRL, GH (focal and variable)	Pit-1, ERα
Thyrotroph adenoma		β-TSH, α-subunit	Pit -1, GATA2
Corticotroph adenomas			
	Densely granulated corticotroph adenoma	ACTH	T-pit
	Sparsely granulated corticotroph adenoma	ACTH	T-pit
	Crooke's cell adenoma	ACTH	T-pit
Gonadotroph adenoma		β-FSH, β-LH, and α-subunit	SF-1, GATA2, and ERα
Null cell adenoma		None	None
Plurihormonal adenomas			
	Pit-1-positive plurihormonal adenoma	GH, PRL, β-TSH ± α-subunit	Pit-1
	Adenomas with unusual immunohistochemical combinations	Various combinations	

(ACTH: adrenocorticotropic hormone; FSH: follicle-stimulating hormone; IHC: immunohistochemistry; SF-1: steroidogenic factor 1; TSH: thyroid-stimulating hormone)

also evaluation of Crooke's hyaline change in tumor and nontumor areas. Other immunohistochemical markers, though not required for classifying adenoma, are used for assessment of aggressive behavior or as predictive markers such as somatostatin receptor (SSTR-2 AND SSTR-5), methylguanine-DBA methyltransferase (MGMT), MSH6, Ki-67, and p53. Most of the pituitary adenomas display gland histological features with rare mitotic figures, <3% Ki-67 index in most of pituitary tumors.[128-130]

Clinically Aggressive Pituitary Tumors

Clinically aggressive tumors are assessed by a frequent mitotic count, high proliferative Ki-67 index, and evidence of invasion on MRI and/or intraoperative impression. High-risk pituitary adenomas which require regular follow-up are mainly SGSA, lactotroph adenoma in men, Crooke's cell adenoma, silent corticotroph adenoma, and plurihormonal adenoma.[131]

Pituitary blastoma has recently been introduced in WHO 2017 classification. Most of the pituitary blastoma is encountered in <2 years of age with signs and symptoms of Cushing's syndrome. The tumor consists of primitive cells, epithelial glands with rosette-like formations, and larger secretory epithelial cells. Pituitary blastoma is associated with DICER1 syndrome or pleuropulmonary blastoma familial tumor where heterozygous germline mutation in the *DICER1* gene is found.[132]

Pituitary carcinoma is a rare pituitary tumor with frequency of <1%. There are no morphological features which can differentiate locally aggressive from pituitary carcinoma if the tumor is limited within the confine of sella. Invasion in dura or bone is commonly present; however, it is also not diagnostic of carcinoma. The definitive diagnosis of pituitary carcinoma is rendered if there is systemic metastasis or craniospinal dissemination. Most of the pituitary carcinomas, approximately 80–85%, are prolactin secreting or ACTH secreting.

Somatotroph Adenoma

Somatotroph adenoma accounts for 10–15% of neuroendocrine pituitary tumors. Pure somatotroph adenoma has only somatotroph cells consisting of densely granulated somatotroph adenomas (DGSAs) and SGSAs. Other somatotroph adenomas include mixed somatotroph and lactotroph adenomas, mammosomatotroph adenomas, and plurihormonal adenomas with expression of GH and Pit-1 on IHC.[133,134]

Densely granulated somatotroph adenomas present as acromegaly whereas mammosomatotroph adenomas predominantly present as gigantism. Most somatotroph tumors are macroadenomas. DGSAs most often respond to somatostatin analogs. SGSAs are usually larger and invasive and usually do not respond to somatostatin analogs. Minority of somatotroph adenomas are associated with hereditary or familial syndromes. Morphologically, deeply eosinophilic tumor cells are characteristics of DGSAs and show diffuse positivity for GH, α-subunit, and perinuclear staining pattern with low molecular weight keratin (LWMK). SGSAs display small lightly eosinophilic or chromophobic cells and negative to variably positive for GH, negative for α-subunit and LWMK express juxtanuclear fibrous bodies. Most DGSAs respond to somatostatin analogs whereas

SGSAs usually do not respond to somatostatin analogs and are associated with a more aggressive behavior.

Mammosomatotroph adenomas express both GH and PRL with variable intensity along with α-subunit and ERα. Mixed somatotroph and lactotroph adenomas are composed of a dual cell population. Positivity for PRL and ERα and negativity for α-subunit distinguish lactotroph adenoma component. Rare examples of GH-producing plurihormonal adenomas can present with a DGSA phenotype with variable thyrotroph and mammosomatotroph differentiation.[133,134]

Lactotroph Adenoma

Lactotroph adenoma is immunohistochemically positive for PRL and arises from Pit-1 lineage cells and expresses Pit-1 and ERα. Morphologically, lactotroph adenoma includes sparsely granulated lactotroph adenomas (SGLA), densely granulated lactotroph adenomas (DGSA), and acidophil stem cell adenomas (ASCA). Lactotroph adenoma accounts for approximately 30–50% of pituitary adenoma and is the most common functioning tumor. It usually presents as mass effect in males and females and as galactorrhea–amenorrhea syndrome. Some individuals with lactotroph adenoma have a genetic susceptibility. SGLA is the most common subtype of lactotroph adenoma and responds well to dopamine agonists. SGLAs are composed of chromophobic cells whereas DGLAs and ASCAs usually show a diffuse cytoplasmic reactivity for PRL. ASCAs show oncocytic cell morphology of tumor cells containing dilated or giant mitochondria. Few fibrous bodies can be identified in ASCAs. Dopamine agonist-treated tumors can mimic as lymphocytic hypophysitis and small round-cell tumors including hematolymphoid neoplasms; therefore, the application of PRL along with Pit-1 and ERα IHC is useful to differentiate from lymphocytic hypophysitis.[133,134]

Thyrotroph Adenomas

Thyrotroph adenoma is the least common tumor and usually detected as invasive macroadenomas. It is usually chromophobic composed of elongated angular or irregular cells with cytoplasmic processes and desmoplastic stroma. Variable β-TSH and α-subunit of the glycoprotein positivity are seen on IHC. Thyrotroph adenomas also express nuclear Pit-1 lineage.[133,134]

Corticotroph Adenomas

Corticotroph adenoma accounts approximately 15% of pituitary adenomas. It arises from adenohypophyseal T-pit cell lineage and expresses ACTH and other proopiomelanocortin-derived peptides on IHC. Histologically identified subtypes are densely granulated corticotroph adenomas (DGCA), sparsely granulated corticotroph adenomas (SGCA), and Crooke cell adenomas. DGCA is the most common and usually seen as microadenomas. Approximately 20% of corticotroph tumors are nonfunctional. Type 1 silent corticotroph adenomas refer to silent DGCAs, and type 2 silent corticotroph adenomas refer to silent SGCAs. Crooke cell adenomas and both silent corticotroph adenomas usually present aggressive clinical behavior.

Corticotroph tumors express T-pit and low molecular weight keratin (LMWK). DGCAs cells appear basophilic and are densely PAS-positive and ACTH-expressing secretory granules. SGCAs cells are usually chromophobic and weakly positive for PAS and ACTH. Crooke cell adenomas display a ring-like characteristic LMWK and relocation of PAS-positive and ACTH-containing secretory granules to the periphery of the cell membrane as well as to the paranuclear zone. The identification of Crooke hyaline change of the nontumorous corticotroph is a consequence of negative feedback suppression due to an autonomous glucocorticoid excess. Silent corticotroph adenomas do not display Crooke hyaline change of the nontumorous corticotrophs.

Up to 60% of corticotroph tumors harbor somatic mutations in *USP8 (ubiquitin-specific protease 8)* gene. Aggressive forms of corticotroph tumors with absent or low MGMT expression respond to temozolomide.[133,134]

Gonadotroph Adenomas

Gonadotroph adenomas are uncommon tumors and secrete the gonadotropins follicle-stimulating hormone (β-FSH) and luteinizing hormone (β-LH). The hormone production is efficient to cause a clinically active tumor, and most of the symptoms are due to local mass effect of tumor due to the compression on optic chiasm and suprasellar extension leading to visual field loss, headache, hypopituitarism, loss of libido, and cranial nerve palsies.

Most gonadotroph adenomas are arranged in a diffuse pattern and sometimes papillary arrangement of tumors and predominantly composed of chromophobic cells. The papillary pattern looks like perivascular pseudorosette formation. There is variable expression of β-FSH, β-LH, and α-subunit or combinations on IHC. Complementary immunostain for the steroidogenic factor (SF-1), when pituitary hormones immunostaining is equivocal or negative in gonadotroph adenomas. ERα is also expressed in these tumors as expressed in PRL-secreting tumor cells.[133,134]

Null Cell Adenoma

Diagnosis of null cell adenomas can be made when there is absent immunohistochemical evidence, pituitary transcription factors differentiation, and all anterior pituitary hormones.

Plurihormonal Adenomas

Plurihormonal adenoma expresses more than one adenohypophyseal hormone with exception of synchronous expression of GH and PRL or β-FSH and β-LH hormones. Plurihormonal pituitary adenoma can express one or more than one cell lineage transcription factors. The prototype of monomorphous plurihormonal adenoma is the silent subtype III adenoma. Initially considered as the third variant of silent corticotroph adenoma, silent subtype III pituitary adenomas have been recognized as biologically aggressive tumors. Double adenoma is considered when two distinct tumors with two different cell types occur simultaneously and multiple adenomas are labeled when there is coexistence of more than two separate tumors in the pituitary gland, and this should not be confused with plurihormonal pituitary adenoma. The characteristic finding is the expression of Pit-1 and presence of nuclear inclusions on light microscopy. Plurihormonal tumors are usually associated with MEN1 syndrome and seen in younger age. Plurihormonal tumors often show a distinct immunohistochemical staining characterized by very focal or scattered positivity for one or more Pit-1 family hormones including GH, PRL, and β-TSH along with variable expression for ERα and α-subunit. It is useful to differentiate these aggressive tumors from other pituitary NETs, since these tumors are radiosensitive and also respond to temozolomide.

Pituitary Blastoma

Pituitary blastoma was first described by Scheithauer et al. (2008).[132] Pituitary blastoma is a rare neonatal or early childhood tumor consisting of cells, which appear similar to primordial Rathke epithelium, small folliculostellate cells, and a limited range of partially differentiated secretory adenohypophyseal cells. Most of the pituitary blastomas are associated with Cushing disease. Pituitary blastomas show germline mutation in *DICER1*.

Pituitary blastomas are composed of varying proportions of small undifferentiated blastemal-like chromophobic cells, larger pattern-less epithelial cells, and cuboidal to columnar cells with attempt at gland formation.

Immunoreactivity with ACTH or growth hormone may be seen. The variability of Ki-67 proliferation index from case to case indicates the occurrence of both low-grade and high-grade pituitary blastoma.

◇ NEURONAL AND PARANEURONAL TUMORS

Gangliocytoma and Mixed Gangliocytoma Adenoma

Gangliocytoma and mixed gangliocytoma adenoma are rare tumors and account for 0.25–1.26% with female predominance. The most common component is somatotroph adenoma followed by corticotroph adenoma in mixed gangliocytic and mixed adenomatous tumors. These tumors on histology display mature ganglionic cells, intermediate cells, and with or without admixed prolactin, or ACTH hormone-positive pituitary adenoma cells. Intrasellar growth hormone-releasing hormone (GHRH)-secreting pure gangliocytomas are extremely rare.[126]

Neurocytoma

Extraventricular sellar neurocytoma of the hypothalamic-pituitary area is rarely reported. The tumor is composed of monotonous population of round cells with neuronal differentiation in a background of fibrillary stroma and expresses neuronal/neuroendocrine markers on IHC.[126]

Paraganglioma and Neuroblastoma

Both tumors are extremely rare tumors and morphological features are similar to paraganglioma and neuroblastoma arising from other locations.[126]

Tumors of Posterior Pituitary

Posterior pituitary tumors are morphological spectrum originating from pituicytes, the specialized glia of posterior pituitary which includes pituicytoma, granular cell tumor of the sellar region, spindle cell oncocytoma, and sellar ependymoma. IHC expresses TTF-1 in pituicytomas, spindle-cell oncocytoma, and granular cell tumors, suggesting morphological spectrum of single nosological entity. All tumors of the posterior pituitary are negative for chromogranin A, synaptophysin, adenohypophyseal hormones, and variably positive for GFAP, S100, vimentin, CD68, and EMA. Genomic copy number imbalances, including losses on chromosome arms 1p, 14q, and 22q and gains on 5p, have been identified in pituicytomas. Most of posterior pituitary tumors have favorable outcome with low Ki-67 index. However, recurrent tumors show an increased Ki-67 proliferation index.[126]

Tumor-like Proliferative/Inflammatory Conditions

This includes lymphocytic hypophysitis, granulomatous hypophysitis, xanthomatous hypophysitis, and inflammatory pseudotumors. Lymphocytic hypophysitis is inflammatory condition of pituitary gland. Pituitary gland or stalk may be secondarily involved by Langerhans cell histiocytosis, Erdheim–Chester disease, sarcoidosis, Wegener granulomatosis, Sjögren, or Rathke cleft cyst syndrome. Lymphocytic or granulomatous hypophysitis may coexist with germ cell tumors, pituitary adenoma, or craniopharyngioma. Primary hypophysitis is an autoimmune disorder, usually present as pure lymphocytic, granulomatous, or xanthomatous inflammation without any associated underlying conditions.[135] Xanthomatous hypophysitis can occur due to rupture of Rathke's cyst, and xanthogranulomatous inflammation can be seen in response to craniopharyngioma. Inflammatory pseudotumor of pituitary gland is due to systemic syndrome known as IgG4-related disease.[136]

Major Update in Pituitary Lesion[136]

- Now, all pituitary adenomas are labeled as pituitary neuroendocrine tumors because aggressiveness is not predictable by morphology.

- Use of lineage-specific markers and reclassifying hormone-negative tumors based on transcription factor expression.
- Inclusion of new lesions including pituitary blastoma.
- Hypophysitis due to immunotherapy, IgG4-disease, and xanthomatous hypophysitis as the cause of inflammatory pseudotumor.
- Posterior pituitary tumors have common thyroid transcription factor-1 in pituicytoma variants including granular cell tumor and spindle cell oncocytoma.

◇ REFERENCES

1. Lloyd RV, Osamura RY, Klöppel G, Rosai J. Chapter 2: Tumours of the thyroid gland. WHO Classification of Tumours of Endocrine Organs, 4th edition. Lyon: International Agency for Research on Cancer; 2017. p. 66.
2. Baloch ZW, Cooper DS, Gharib H, Alexander EK. Overview of diagnostic terminology and reporting. In: Ali SZ, Cibas ES (Eds). The Bethesda system of reporting thyroid cytopathology. Definitions, criteria, and explanatory notes, 2nd edition. New York: Springer International Publishing; 2018. pp. 1-6.
3. Gupta P, Bardia A, Rajwanshi A, Nijhawan R, Srinivasan R, Gupta N, et al. Cytodiagnosis of distant metastases from follicular thyroid carcinoma. Diagn Cytopathol. 2016;44(2): 108-12.
4. Franssila KO, Ackerman LV, Brown CL, Hedinger CE. Follicular carcinoma. Semin Diagn Pathol. 1985;2(2):101-22.
5. Mete O, Asa SL. Pathological definition and clinical significance of vascular invasion in thyroid carcinomas of follicular epithelial derivation. Mod Pathol. 2011;24(12):1545-52.
6. Oyama T, Vickery AL Jr, Preffer FI, Colvin RB. A comparative study of flow cytometry and histopathologic findings in thyroid follicular carcinomas and adenomas. Hum Pathol. 1994;25(3):271-5.
7. Nikiforova MN, Lynch RA, Biddinger PW, Alexander EK, Dorn GW 2nd, Tallini G, et al. RAS point mutations and PAX8-PPAR gamma rearrangement in thyroid tumors: evidence for distinct molecular pathways in thyroid follicular carcinoma. J Clin Endocrinol Metab. 2003;88(5):2318-26.
8. Vickery AL Jr, Carcangiu ML, Johannessen JV, Sobrinho-Simoes M. Papillary carcinoma. Semin Diagn Pathol. 1985;2(2):90-100.
9. Nikiforov YE. RET/PTC rearrangement in thyroid tumors. Endocr Pathol. 2002;13(1):3-16.
10. Ciampi R, Nikiforov YE. Alterations of the *BRAF* gene in thyroid tumors. Endocr Pathol. 2005;16(3):163-72.
11. Volante M, Collini P, Nikiforov YE, Sakamoto A, Kakudo K, Katoh R, et al. Poorly differentiated thyroid carcinoma: the Turin proposal for the use of uniform diagnostic criteria and an algorithmic diagnostic approach. Am J Surg Pathol. 2007;31(8):1256-64.
12. Asioli S, Erickson LA, Righi A, Jin L, Volante M, Jenkins S, et al. Poorly differentiated carcinoma of the thyroid: validation of the Turin proposal and analysis of IMP3 expression. Mod Pathol. 2010;23(9):1269-78.
13. Carcangiu ML, Steeper T, Zampi G, Rosai J. Anaplastic thyroid carcinoma: a study of 70 cases. Am J Clin Pathol. 1985;83(2):135-58.
14. Garcia-Rostan G, Tallini G, Herrero A, D'Aquila TG, Carcangiu ML, Rimm DL. Frequent mutation and nuclear localization of beta-catenin in anaplastic thyroid carcinoma. Cancer Res. 1999;59(8):1811-5.
15. Nikiforov YE, Ghossein RA, Kakudo K, LiVolsi V, Papotti M, Randolph GW, et al. Non-invasive follicular thyroid neoplasm with papillary-like nuclear features. In: Lloyd RV, Osamura RY, Klöppel G, Rosai J (Eds). WHO classification of tumours of endocrine organs, 4th edition. Lyon, France: International Agency for Research on Cancer; 2017. pp. 78-80.
16. Mulligan LM, Kwok JB, Healey CS, Elsdon MJ, Eng C, Gardner E, et al. Germ-line mutations of the RET proto-oncogene in multiple endocrine neoplasia type 2A. Nature. 1993;363(6428):458-60.
17. Uribe M, Fenoglio-Preiser CM, Grimes M, Feind C. Medullary carcinoma of the thyroid gland. Clinical, pathological, and immunohistochemical features with review of the literature. Am J Surg Pathol. 1985;9(8):577-94.
18. Elisei R, Cosci B, Romei C, Bottici V, Renzini G, Molinaro E, et al. Prognostic significance of somatic RET oncogene mutations in sporadic medullary thyroid cancer: a 10-year follow-up study. J Clin Endocrinol Metab. 2008;93(3):682-7.
19. Moura MM, Cavaco BM, Pinto AE, Leite V. High prevalence of RAS mutations in RET-negative sporadic medullary thyroid carcinomas. J Clin Endocrinol Metab. 2011;96(5):E863-8.
20. Pradeep PV, Jayashree B, Mishra A, Mishra SK. Systematic review of primary hyperparathyroidism in India: The past, present and the future trends. Int J Endocrinol. 2011;2011:921814.
21. Baloch ZW, LiVolsi VA. Thyroid and parathyroid. In: Mills SE (Ed). Sternberg's Diagnostic Surgical Pathology, 6th edition. Philadelphia: Wolters Kluwer; 2015. pp. 1114-251.
22. Weiland LH, Garrison RC, ReMine WH, Scholz DA. Lipoadenoma of the parathyroid gland. Am J Surg Pathol. 1978;2:3-7.
23. Singh DN, Gupta SK, Kumari N, Krishnani N, Chand G, Mishra A, et al. Primary hyperparathyroidism presenting as hypercalcemic crisis: Twenty-year experience. Indian J Endocr Metab. 2015;19:100-5.
24. Prasad KK, Agarwal G, Krishnani N. Water clear cell adenoma of the parathyroid gland: a rare entity. Indian J Pathol Microbiol. 2004;47:39-40.
25. Prasad KK, Agarwal G, Mishra SK, Krishnani N. Oxyphil cell adenoma of parathyroid resulting in primary hyperparathyroidism and osteitis fibrosa cystic: a case report. Indian J Pathol Microbiol. 2006;49:448-50.
26. Agarwal G, Prasad KK, Kar DK, Krishnani N, Pandey R, Mishra SK. Indian primary hyperparathyroidism patients with parathyroid carcinoma do not differ in co-investigative characteristics from those with benign parathyroid pathology. World J Surgery. 2006;30:732-42.
27. Agrawal R, Agarwal A, Kar DK, Agarwal G, Jain M, Krishnani N, et al. Parathyroid carcinoma. J Assoc Physician India. 2001;49:990-3.
28. Verdonk CC, Edias AJ. Parathyroid "double adenomas": fact or fiction? Surgery. 1981;90:523-6.
29. Bartsch D, Nies C, Hasse C, Willuhn J, Rothmund M. Clinical and surgical aspects of double adenoma in patients with primary hyperparathyroidism. Br J Surg. 1995;82:926-9.
30. Chan JKC. Tumors of the thyroid and parathyroid glands. In: Fletcher CDM (Ed). Diagnostic Histopathology of Tumors, 5th edition. Philadelphia: Elsevier; 2020. pp. 1340-61.
31. Fernandez-Ranvier GG, Khanafshar E, Jensen K, Zarnegar R, Lee J, Kebebew E, et al. Parathyroid carcinoma, atypical parathyroid adenoma, or parathyromatosis? Cancer. 2007;110:255-64.
32. Christakis I, Bussaidy N, Clarke C, Kwatampora LJ, Warneke CL, Silva AM, et al. Differentiating atypical parathyroid neoplasm from parathyroid cancer. Ann Surg Oncol. 2016;23:2889-97.

33. Chan JKC, Tsang WY. Endocrine malignancies that may mimic benign lesions. Semin Diagn Pathol. 1995;12:45-63.

34. DeLellis RA. Parathyroid tumors and related disorders. Mod Pathol. 2011;24:S78-93.

35. Shi Y, Hogue J, Dixit D, Koh J, Olson JA Jr. Functional and genetic studies of isolated cells from parathyroid tumors reveal the complex pathogenesis of parathyroid neoplasia. Proc Natl Acad Sci USA. 2014;111:3092-7.

36. Hsi ED, Zukerberg LR, Yang WI, Arnold A. Cyclin D1/PRAD1 expression in parathyroid adenomas: an immunohistochemical study. J Clin Endocrinol Metab. 1996;81:1736-9.

37. Juhlin C, Larsson C, Yakoleva T, Leibiger I, Leibiger B, Alimov A, et al. Loss of parafibromin expression in a subset of parathyroid adenomas. Endocr Relat Cancer. 2006;13:509-23.

38. Cui C, Lal P, Master S, Ma Y, Baradet T, Binq Z. Expression of parafibromin in major renal cell tumors. Eur J Histochem. 2012;56:e39.

39. Tan MH, Morrison C, Wang P, Yang X, Haven CJ, Zhang C, et al. Loss of parafibromin immunoreactivity is a distinguishing feature of parathyroid carcinoma. Clin Cancer Res. 2004;10:6629-37.

40. Gill AJ, Clarkson A, Gimm O, Keil J, Dralle H, Howell VM, et al. Loss of nuclear expression of parafibromin distinguishes parathyroid carcinomas and hyperparathyroidism-jaw tumor (HPT-JT) syndrome-related adenomas from sporadic parathyroid adenomas and hyperplasias. Am J Surg Pathol. 2006;30:1140-9.

41. Cetani F, Ambrogini E, Viacava P, Pardi E, Fanelli G, Naccarato AG, et al. Should parafibromin staining replace *HRTP2* gene analysis as an additional tool for histologic diagnosis of parathyroid carcinoma? Eur J Endocrinol. 2007;156:547-54.

42. Juhlin CC, Villablanca A, Sandelin K, Haglund F, Nordenström J, Forsberg L, et al. Parafibromin immunoreactivity: its use as an additional diagnostic marker for parathyroid tumor classification. Endocr Relat Cancer. 2007;14:501-12.

43. Kim HK, Oh YL, Kim SH, Lee DY, Kang HC, Lee JI, et al. Parafibromin immunohistochemical staining to differentiate parathyroid carcinoma from parathyroid adenoma. Head Neck. 2012;34:201-6.

44. Truran PP, Johnson SJ, Bliss RD, Lennard TWJ, Aspinall SR. Parafibromin, Galectin-3, PGP9.5, Ki67, and Cyclin D1: using an immunohistochemical panel to aid in the diagnosis of parathyroid cancer. World J Surg. 2014;38:2845-54.

45. Howell VM, Gill A, Clarkson A, Nelson AE, Dunne R, Delbridge LW, et al. Accuracy of combined gene product 9.5 and parafibromin markers for immunohistochemical diagnosis of parathyroid carcinoma. J Clin Endocrinol Metab. 2009;94:434-41.

46. Wang O, Wang CY, Shi J, Nie M, Xia WB, Li M, et al. Expression of Ki-67, galectin-3, fragile histidine triad, and parafibromin in malignant and benign parathyroid tumors. Chinese Med J. 2012;125:2895-901.

47. Shattuck TM, Valimaki S, Obara T, Gaz RD, Clark OH, Shoback D, et al. Somatic and germ-line mutations of the HRPT2 gene in sporadic parathyroid carcinoma. N Engl J Med. 2003;349:1722-9.

48. Brown S, O'Neill C, Suliburk J, Sidhu S, Sywak M, Gill A, et al. Parathyroid carcinoma: increasing incidence and changing presentation. ANZ J Surg. 2011;81:528-32.

49. Juhlin CC, Haglund F, Villablanca A, Forsberg L, Sandelin K, Bränström R, et al. Loss of expression for the Wnt pathway components adenomatous polyposis coli and glycogen synthase kinase 3-beta in parathyroid carcinomas. Int J Oncol. 2009;34:481-92.

50. Bergero N, De Pompa R, Sacerdote C, Gasparri G, Volante M, Bussolati G, et al. Galectin-3 expression in parathyroid carcinoma: immunohistochemical study of 26 cases. Hum Pathol. 2005;36:908-14.

51. Saggiorato E, Bergero N, Volante M, Bacillo E, Rosas R, Gasparri G, et al. Galectin-3 and Ki-67 expression in multiglandular parathyroid lesions. Am J Clin Pathol. 2006;126:59-66.

52. Tezel E, Hibi K, Nagasaka T, Nakao A. PGP9.5 as a prognostic factor in pancreatic cancer. Clin Cancer Res. 2000;6:4764-7.

53. Yamazaki T, Hibi K, Takase T, Tezel E, Nakayama H, Kasai Y, et al. PGP 9.5 as a marker for invasive colorectal cancer. Clin Cancer Res. 2002;8:192-5.

54. Hibi K, Westra WH, Borges M, Goodman S, Sidransky D, Jen J. PGP9.5 as a candidate tumor marker for non-small-cell lung cancer. Am J Pathol. 1999;155:711-5.

55. Sasaki H, Yukiue H, Moriyama S, Kobayashi Y, Nakashima Y, Kaji M, et al. Expression of the protein gene product 9.5, PGP9.5, is correlated with T-status in non-small cell lung cancer. Jpn J Clin Oncol. 2001;31:532-5.

56. Campbell LK, Thomas JR, Lamps LW, Smoller BR, Folpe AL. Protein gene product 9.5 (PGP 9.5) is not a specific marker of neural and nerve sheath tumors: an immunohistochemical study of 95 mesenchymal neoplasms. Modern Pathol. 2003;16:963-9.

57. Sharretts JM, Kebebew E, Simonds WF. Parathyroid cancer. Semin Oncol. 2010;37:580-90.

58. Kumari N, Chaudhary N, Pradhan R, Agarwal A, Krishnani N. Role of histological criteria and immunohistochemical markers in predicting risk of malignancy in parathyroid neoplasms. Endocr Pathol. 2016;27:87-96.

59. Kumari N, Chaudhary N, Mishra P, Agarwal A, Krishnani N. Association of biochemical and histological features with parafibromin, Galectin-3 or PGP9.5 in parathyroid neoplasms. World J Endocr Surg. 2019;11:6-14.

60. Schantz A, Castleman B. Parathyroid carcinoma. A study of 70 cases. Cancer. 1973;31:600-5.

61. Cetani F, Pardi E, Borsari S, Viacava P, Dipollina G, Cianferotti L, et al. Genetic analyses of the *HRPT2* gene in primary hyperparathyroidism: germline and somatic mutations in familial and sporadic parathyroid tumors. J Clin Endocrinol Metab. 2004;89:5583-91.

62. Priyambada L, Bhatia V, Krishnani N, Agarwal V, Bhattacharyya A, Jain S, et al. Primary hypothyroidism, precocious puberty and hypothalamic obesity in Langerhans cell histiocytosis. Indian J Pediatr. 2011;78:351-3.

63. Nicholls AG. Simple adenoma of the pancreas arising from an Island of Langerhans. J Med Res. 1902;8(2):385-95.

64. Fraenkel M, Kim MK, Faggiano A, Valk GD. Epidemiology of gastroenteropancreatic neuroendocrine tumours. Best Pract Res Clin Gastroenterol. 2012;26(6):691-703.

65. Halfdanarson TR, Rubin J, Farnell MB, Grant CS, Petersen GM. Pancreatic endocrine neoplasms: epidemiology and prognosis of pancreatic endocrine tumors. Endocr Relat Cancer. 2008;15(2):409-27.

66. Yadav S, Sharma P, Zakalik D. Comparison of demographics, tumor characteristics, and survival between pancreatic adenocarcinomas and pancreatic neuroendocrine tumors: a population-based study. Am J Clin Oncol. 2018;41(5):485-91.

67. Kimura W, Kuroda A, Morioka Y. Clinical pathology of endocrine tumors of the pancreas. Analysis of Autopsy Cases. Dig Dis Sci. 1991;36(7):933-42.

68. Jensen RT, Berna MJ, Bingham DB, Norton JA. Inherited pancreatic endocrine tumor syndromes: advances in molecular pathogenesis, diagnosis, management, and controversies. Cancer. 2008;113(7 Suppl):1807-43.

69. Larsson C, Skogseid B, Oberg K, Nakamura Y, Nordenskjold M. Multiple endocrine neoplasia type 1 gene maps to chromosome 11 and is lost in insulinoma. Nature. 1988;332(6159):85-7.

70. Corcos O, Couvelard A, Giraud S, Vullierme MP, Dermot OT, Rebours V, et al. Endocrine pancreatic tumors in von Hippel-Lindau disease: clinical, histological, and genetic features. Pancreas. 2008;37(1):85-93.

71. Larson AM, Hedgire SS, Deshpande V, Stemmer-Rachamimov AO, Harisinghani MG, Ferrone CR, et al. Pancreatic neuroendocrine tumors in patients with tuberous sclerosis complex. Clin Gen. 2012;82(6):558-63.

72. Ligneau B, Lombard-Bohas C, Partensky C, Valette PJ, Calender A, Dumortier J, et al. Cystic endocrine tumors of the pancreas: clinical, radiologic, and histopathologic features in 13 cases. Am J Surg Pathol. 2001;25(6):752-60.

73. Kent RB, van Heerden JA, Weiland LH. Nonfunctioning islet cell tumors. Ann Surg. 1981;193(2):185-90.

74. Klöppel G, Heitz PU. Pancreatic endocrine tumors. Pathol Res Pract. 1988;183(2):155-68.

75. Nunobe S, Fukushima N, Yachida S, Shimada K, Kosuge T, Sakamoto M. Clear cell endocrine tumor of the pancreas which is not associated with von Hippel-Lindau disease: report of a case. Surg Today. 2003;33(6):470-4.

76. Basturk O, Tang L, Hruban RH, Adsay V, Yang Z, Krasinskas AM, et al. Poorly differentiated neuroendocrine carcinomas of the pancreas: a clinicopathologic analysis of 44 cases. Am J Surg Pathol. 2014;38(4):437-47.

77. La Rosa S, Sessa F, Uccella S. Mixed Neuroendocrine-Nonneuroendocrine Neoplasms (MiNENs): unifying the concept of a heterogeneous group of neoplasms. Endocr Pathol. 2016;27(4):284-311.

78. Buffa R, Rindi G, Sessa F, Gini A, Capella C, Jahn R, et al. Synaptophysin immunoreactivity and small clear vesicles in neuroendocrine cells and related tumours. Mol Cell Probes. 1987;1(4):367-81.

79. Lloyd RV, Mervak T, Schmidt K, Warner TF, Wilson BS. Immunohistochemical detection of chromogranin and neuron-specific enolase in pancreatic endocrine neoplasms. Am J Surg Pathol. 1984;8(8):607-14.

80. Goto Y, De Silva MG, Toscani A, Prabhakar BS, Notkins AL, Lan MS. A novel human insulinoma-associated cDNA, IA-1, encodes a protein with "zinc-finger" DNA-binding motifs. J Biol Chem. 1992;267(21):15252-7.

81. Son E-M, Kim JY, An S, Song K-B, Kim SC, Yu E, et al. Clinical and prognostic significances of cytokeratin 19 and KIT expression in surgically resectable pancreatic neuroendocrine tumors. J Pathol Transl Med. 2015;49(1):30-6.

82. Nagtegaal ID, Odze RD, Klimstra D, Paradis V, Rugge M, Schirmacher P, et al. WHO classification of tumours editorial board. Histopathology. 2020;76(2):182-8.

83. Reid MD, Bagci P, Ohike N, Saka B, Erbarut Seven I, Dursun N, et al. Calculation of the Ki-67 index in pancreatic neuroendocrine tumors: a comparative analysis of four counting methodologies. Mod Pathol. 2015;28(5):686-94.

84. Tang LH, Gonen M, Hedvat C, Modlin IM, Klimstra DS. Objective quantification of the Ki-67 proliferative index in neuroendocrine tumors of the gastroenteropancreatic system: a comparison of digital image analysis with manual methods. Am J Surg Pathol. 2012;36(12):1761-70.

85. Yang Z, Tang LH, Klimstra DS. Effect of tumor heterogeneity on the assessment of Ki-67 labeling index in well-differentiated neuroendocrine tumors metastatic to the liver: implications for prognostic stratification. Am J Surg Pathol. 2011;35(6):853-60.

86. Jiao Y, Shi C, Edil BH, de Wilde RF, Klimstra DS, Maitra A, et al. DAXX/ATRX, MEN1, and mTOR pathway genes are frequently altered in pancreatic neuroendocrine tumors. Science. 2011;331(6021):1199-203.

87. Heaphy CM, de Wilde RF, Jiao Y, Klein AP, Edil BH, Shi C, et al. Altered telomeres in tumors with ATRX and DAXX mutations. Science. 2011;333(6041):425.

88. Missiaglia E, Dalai I, Barbi S, Beghelli S, Falconi M, della Peruta M, et al. Pancreatic endocrine tumors: expression profiling evidences a role for AKT mTOR pathway. J Clin Oncol. 2010;28(2):245-55.

89. Speisky D, Duces A, Bieche I, Rebours V, Hammel P, Sauvanet A, et al. Molecular profiling of pancreatic neuroendocrine tumors in sporadic and Von Hippel-Lindau patients. Clin Cancer Res. 2012;18(10):2838-49.

90. Hu W, Feng Z, Modica I, Klimstra DS, Song L, Allen PJ, et al. Gene amplifications in well-differentiated pancreatic neuroendocrine tumors inactivate the p53 pathway. Genes Cancer. 2010;1(4):360-8.

91. Yachida S, Vakiani E, White CM, Zhong Y, Saunders T, Morgan R, et al. Small cell and large cell neuroendocrine carcinomas of the pancreas are genetically similar and distinct from well-differentiated pancreatic neuroendocrine tumors. Am J Surg Pathol. 2012;36(2):173-84.

92. Dackiw AP, Lee JE, Gagel RF, Evans DB. Adrenal cortical carcinoma. World J Surg. 2001;25(7):914-26.

93. Hough AJ, Hollifield JW, Page DL, Hartmann WH. Prognostic factors in adrenal cortical tumors: a mathematical analysis of clinical and morphologic data. Am J Clin Pathol. 1979;72(3):390-9.

94. Gröndal S, Cedermark B, Eriksson B, Grimelius L, Harach R, Kristoffersson A, et al. Adrenocortical carcinoma: a retrospective study of a rare tumor with a poor prognosis. Eur J Surg Oncol. 1990;16(6):500-6.

95. Markoe AM, Serber W, Micaily B, Brady LW. Radiation therapy for adjunctive treatment of adrenal cortical carcinoma. Am J Clin Oncol. 1991;14(2):170-4.

96. Page DL, DeLellis RA, Hough AJ. Tumors of the adrenal. Washington, DC: Armed Forces Institute of Pathology; 1986.

97. Lack EE. Pathology of the adrenal glands. London, UK: Churchill Livingstone; 1990.

98. Tischler AS. Pheochromocytoma and extra-adrenal paraganglioma: updates. Arch Pathol Lab Med. 2008;132(8):1272-84.

99. Bisceglia M, Ludovico O, Di Mattia A, Ben-Dor D, Sandbank J, Pasquinelli G, et al. Adrenocortical oncocytic tumors: report of 10 cases and review of the literature. Int J Surg Pathol. 2004;12(3):231-43.

100. Hoang MP, Ayala AG, Albores-Saavedra J. Oncocytic adreno-cortical carcinoma: a morphologic, immunohistochemical and ultrastructural study of four cases. Mod Pathol. 2002;15(9):973-8.

101. Lin BT-Y, Bonsib SM, Mierau GW, Weiss LM, Medeiros LJ. Oncocytic adrenocortical neoplasms: a report of seven cases and review of the literature. Am J Surg Pathol. 1998;22(5):603-14.

102. Barksdale SK, Marincola FM, Jaffe G. Carcinosarcoma of the adrenal cortex presenting with mineralocorticoid excess. Am J Surg Pathol. 1993;17(9):941-5.

103. Decorato JW, Gruber H, Petti M, Levowitz BS. Adrenal carcinosarcoma. Surg Oncol. 1990;45(2):134-6.

104. Fischler DF, Nunez C, Levin HS, McMahon JT, Sheeler LR, Adelstein DJ. Adrenal carcinosarcoma presenting in a woman with clinical signs of virilization a case report with immunohistochemical and ultrastructural findings. Am J Surg Pathol. 1992;16(6):626-31.

105. Drachenberg C, Lee HK, Gann D, Wong-You-Cheong J, Papadimitriou J. Adrenal cortical carcinoma with adenosquamous differentiation. Report of a case with immunohistochemical and ultrastructural studies. Arch Pathol Lab Med. 1995;119(3):260-5.

106. Weiss LM, Medeiros LJ, Vickery Jr AL. Pathologic features of prognostic significance in adrenocortical carcinoma. Am J Surg Pathol. 1989;13(3):202-6.

107. Aubert S, Wacrenier A, Leroy X, Devos P, Carnaille B, Proye C, et al. Weiss system revisited: a1 clinicopathologic and immunohistochemical study of 49 adrenocortical tumors. Am J Surg Pathol. 2002;26(12):1612-9.

108. Fuhrman SA, Lasky LC, Limas C. Prognostic significance of morphologic parameters in renal cell carcinoma. Am J Surg Pathol. 1982;6(7):655-64.

109. Gandour MJ, Grizzle WE. A small adrenocortical carcinoma with aggressive behavior. An evaluation of criteria for malignancy. Arch Pathol Lab Med. 1986;110(11):1076-9.

110. Volante M, Buttigliero C, Greco E, Berruti A, Papotti M. Pathological and molecular features of adrenocortical carcinoma: an update. J Clin Pathol. 2008;61(7):787-93.

111. Van't Sant H, Bouvy N, Kazemier G, Bonjer H, Hop W, Feelders R, et al. The prognostic value of two different histopathological scoring systems for adrenocortical carcinomas. Histopathology. 2007;51(2):239-45.

112. Papotti M, Volante M, Duregon E, Delsedime L, Terzolo M, Berruti A, et al. Adrenocortical tumors with myxoid features: a distinct morphologic and phenotypical variant exhibiting malignant behavior. Am J Surg Pathol. 2010;34(7):973-83.

113. Wieneke JA, Thompson LD, Heffess CS. Adrenal cortical neoplasms in the pediatric population: a clinicopathologic and immunophenotypic analysis of 83 patients. Am J Surg Pathol. 2003;27(7):867-81.

114. Zhang H, Bu H, Chen H, Wei B, Liu W, Guo J, et al. Comparison of immunohistochemical markers in the differential diagnosis of adrenocortical tumors: immunohistochemical analysis of adrenocortical tumors. Appl Immunohistochem Mol Morphol. 2008;16(1):32-9.

115. Cho EY, Ahn GH. Immunoexpression of inhibin α-subunit in adrenal neoplasms. Appl Immunohistochem Mol Morphol. 2001;9(3):222-8.

116. Schmitt A, Saremaslani P, Schmid S, Rousson V, Montani M, Schmid D, et al. IGFII and MIB1 immunohistochemistry is helpful for the differentiation of benign from malignant adrenocortical tumours. Histopathology. 2006;49(3): 298-307.

117. Kimura N, Takekoshi K, Naruse M. Risk stratification on pheochromocytoma and paraganglioma from laboratory and clinical medicine. J Clin Med. 2018. 27;7(9):242.

118. Turchini J, Cheung VKY, Tischler AS, De Krijger RR, Gill AJ. Pathology and genetics of phaeochromocytoma and paraganglioma. Histopathology. 2018;72(1):97-105.

119. Koch CA, Mauro D, Walther MM, Linehan WM, Vortmeyer AO, Jaffe R, et al. Pheochromocytoma in Von Hippel-Lindau disease: distinct histopathologic phenotype compared to pheochromocytoma in multiple endocrine neoplasia type 2. Endocr Pathol. 2002;13(1):17-27.

120. Cheung VKY, Gill AJ, Chou A. Old, new, and emerging immunohistochemical markers in pheochromocytoma and paraganglioma. Endocr Pathol. 2018;29(2):169-75.

121. Kimura N, Capella C. Extraadrenal paraganglioma. In: Lloyd RV, Osamura RY, Kloppel G, (Eds). WHO Classification of Tumors of Endocrine Organs, 4th edition. Lyons, France: IARC Press; 2017. pp. 190-5.

122. Thompson LD. Pheochromocytoma of the Adrenal gland Scaled Score (PASS) to separate benign from malignant neoplasms: a clinicopathologic and immunophenotypic study of 100 cases. Am J Surg Pathol. 2002;26(5):551-66.

123. Kimura N, Takayanagi R, Takizawa N, Itagaki E, Katabami T, Kakoi N, et al. Pathological grading for predicting metastasis in phaeochromocytoma and paraganglioma. Phaeochromocytoma Study Group in Japan. Endocr Relat Cancer. 2014; 21(3):405-14.

124. Koh JM, Ahn SH, Kim H, Kim BJ, Sung TY, Kim YH, et al. Validation of pathological grading systems for predicting metastatic potential in pheochromocytoma and paraganglioma. PLoS One. 2017;12(11):e0187398.

125. Louis DN, Ohgaki H, Wiestler OD, Cavenne C. WHO Classification of Tumours of the Central Nervous System, revised 4th edition. Lyons, France: IARC Press; 2016.

126. Ricardo VL, Osamura RY, Gunter Kloppel G, Rosai J. Chapter 1, Tumours of Pituitary Gland. WHO Classification of Tumours of Endocrine Organs, 4th edition. Lyon France: International Agency for Research on Cancer; 2017. pp. 11-63.

127. Duan K, Mete O. Hereditary endocrine tumor syndromes: the clinical and predictive role of molecular histopathology. AJSP. 2017;22:246-68.

128. Asa SL. Tumors of the Pituitary Gland. AFIP Atlas of Tumor Pathology, Series 4, Fascicle 15. Silver Spring: ARP Press; 2011.

129. Gomez-Hernandez K, Ezzat S, Asa SL, Mete Ö. Clinical implications of accurate subtyping of pituitary adenomas: perspectives from the treating physician. Turk Patoloji Derg. 2015;31(Suppl 1):4-17.

130. Mete O, Asa SL. Therapeutic implications of accurate classification of pituitary adenomas. Semin Diagn Pathol. 2013;30:158-64.

131. Mete O, Gomez-Hernandez K, Kucharczyk W, Ridout R, Zadeh G, Gentili F, et al. Silent sub-type 3 pituitary adenomas are not always silent and represent poorly differentiated monomorphous plurihormonal Pit-1 lineage adenomas. Mod Pathol. 2016;29:131-42.

132. Scheithauer BW, Kovacs K, Horvath E, Kim DS, Osamura RY, Ketterling RP, et al. Pituitary blastoma. Acta Neuropathol. 2008;116:657-66.

133. Mete O, Lopes MB. Overview of the 2017 WHO Classification of Pituitary Tumours. Endocr Pathol. 2017;28:228-43.

134. Manojlovic-Gacic E, Engström, BE, Casar-Borota O. Histopathological classification of non-functioning pituitary neuroendocrine tumours. Pituitary. 2018;21:119-29.

135. Rosai J. Chapter 29: Pituitary gland. In: Kleinschmidt-DeMasters BK (Ed). Rosai and Ackerman's Surgical Pathology, 10th edition. Amsterdam: Elsevier; 2011. pp. 2459-60.

136. Asa SL, Mete O. What's new in pituitary pathology? Histopathology. 2018:72:133-41.

CHAPTER 42

Role of Nuclear Medicine in Endocrine Surgery

CS Bal, Saurabh Arora

◇| NUCLEAR ENDOCRINOLOGY

The first applications of radiotracers were in endocrinology to study the functioning of the thyroid gland using radioactive isotopes of iodine in the 1930s. Subsequently, radioiodine was used in the treatment of hyperthyroidism and well-differentiated thyroid cancer in 1942. Thus, nuclear thyroidology has made nuclear medicine and endocrinology as conjoint twins. The next best applications of nuclear endocrinology are in the detection or localization of parathyroid adenoma. For adrenal medullary tumors namely pheochromocytoma and paraganglioma (PGL) and neuroendocrine tumors like insulinoma, glucagonoma, gastrinoma, and VIPoma, they are recent applications of radiopharmaceuticals in diagnosis and in the therapy of these tumors. The foray of nuclear medicine for the diagnosis of ectopic adrenocorticotropic hormone (ACTH) producing Cushing's syndrome and the detection of tumor-induced osteomalacia (TIO) are a few new applications and the list is ever increasing. Some of the above pathologies are amenable to therapeutic applications too when surgery is not possible or no suitable medical treatments are available.

◇| INTRODUCTION

Nuclear endocrinology is a subspecialty of nuclear medicine that involves the application of radiopharmaceuticals for diagnosis and therapy of endocrine disorders.

In general, radiopharmaceutical consists of two parts: (1) radionuclide and (2) pharmaceutical. When used for diagnosis, it is called a tracer and when used for therapeutic applications, it is called a drug. Few radionuclides namely sodium pertechnetate ($^{99m}TcO_4$) or thallium (^{201}Tl) chloride can directly be used for diagnostic purposes and interestingly, ^{131}I is for both diagnostic and therapeutic purposes; otherwise, it is radiopharmaceuticals commonly used in nuclear medicine departments.

Radionuclide or radioisotope is the radioactive component of the radiopharmaceutical. It is the unstable atom (having excess nuclear energy) which converts to stable atom by releasing excess energy called radioactive decay in the form of gamma-ray photon/alpha particle/beta particle/positron particles depending on the type of element and its decay characteristics.

- Gamma photon can be detected externally either by different nonimaging devices like counting probe [e.g., thyroid uptake probe for radioactive iodine uptake (RAIU)], or well counter, etc., or by imaging devices like gamma camera imaging.
- Beta and alpha particles deposit almost all of its energy in the tissue in a short distance; hence, they are used for therapeutic applications. Often particulate emissions are associated with gamma-ray emission that can be suitably used for dosimetry (quantity of radiation energy deposited in the organ/tissue is called radiation absorbed dose).
- The radiation imaging instruments are based on the type of emission that is being imaged.
- The planar imaging device is called a gamma camera. When gamma camera acquires the images in 360° and image reconstruction is done in the three-dimensional (3D) mode, it is called single-photon emission computed tomography (SPECT) camera. The radiotracers used are technetium (Tc-99m), iodine (I-123/131), Lu-177, etc., gamma photons.
- Positron emission tomography (PET) scans twin photons released by an annihilation (positron interacts with electron) process—fluorine (F-18), carbon (C-11), gallium (Ga-68), etc.

◇| THYROID GLAND

Elemental iodine is the raw material for thyroid hormone synthesis; the thyroid cells have the ability to trap iodine using sodium iodide symporter (NIS). The beauty is that NIS can trap iodine from the blood pool against a concentration gradient. The whole processes of iodide trapping and synthesis of hormones are primarily under thyroid-stimulating hormone (TSH) regulation. TSH is a pituitary hormone that stimulates both of these thyroid functions. RAI enters thyroid cells by a similar mechanism and hence can be used for diagnosis and therapy of hyperthyroidism and thyroid cancer.

Thyroid Scan

Radiopharmaceuticals

- Tc-99m pertechnetate (TcO_4^-, 2–10 mCi IV)
- I-123 (200–400 μCi orally) (Note: I-123 is not available in India till date).

Figures 1A to D show the patterns of uptake on thyroid scan in a patient with thyrotoxicosis.

The simple pertechnetate thyroid scan at 20 minutes can easily distinguish these four causes of thyrotoxicosis in 90–95% of the time without any additional imaging or laboratory investigations.

Toxic adenoma (TA) [autonomously functioning thyroid nodule (AFTN)] is characterized by focal increased uptake in the hyperfunctioning nodule/adenoma with suppressed radioiodine distribution in the surrounding and contralateral thyroid lobe.

Toxic multinodular goiter (TMNG) shows areas of focal increased in functional nodules and intervening thyroid tissue having suppressed uptake. If nodules are small in size and large in numbers in TMNG patients, in the thyroid scan, it may be difficult to differentiate from that of Graves' disease (GD).

Graves' disease shows the classic diffuse tracer distribution pattern with suppression of surrounding salivary gland uptakes. Rarely, there could be coexistent nodules in a small number of patients and such nodule in Graves' gland needs evaluation to rule out malignancy.

Subacute thyroiditis or viral thyroiditis is usually accompanied by a history of sore throat. On scanning, it shows a complete absence or minimal uptake of tracer in the thyroid bed with the toxic thyroid hormone profile. The thyroid scan is particularly helpful in the absence of pain and tenderness over the thyroid region to distinguish from GD.

Radioactive Iodine Uptake

Radioactive iodine uptake measures the amount of tracer uptake that is taken by the thyroid gland at prefixed intervals after the administration. Two types of radioiodine used—the ideal one is I-123; unfortunately, I-123 is not available in India; thus, we use I-131 for RAIU measurement. The I-123 is given 200–400 µCi or 5–10 µCi of iodine-131. A special uptake probe measures the RAIU. The timing of measurement varies from institution to institution; however, the same has to be compared against the institutional standard uptake values obtained from healthy volunteers free of any thyroid diseases. The standard uptake times are 2 hours and 24 hours or 4 hours and 24 hours.

Indications

Radioactive iodine uptake, a simple test, is elegantly used to distinguish various causes of thyrotoxicosis. Thyrotoxic patients are classified into two groups—(1) having elevated or normal uptake and (2) those with near-absent uptake.

The former ones are GD, TA or TMNG, trophoblastic disease, isolated TSH-producing pituitary adenomas, and resistance to thyroid hormone (T3 receptor beta mutation, THRß).

The later ones are painless (silent) thyroiditis, type II amiodarone-induced thyroiditis, de Quervain's thyroiditis, overtreatment with thyroxine supplementation (iatrogenic thyrotoxicosis), factitious thyrotoxicosis, struma ovarii, and rarely well-differentiated thyroid cancer with extensive functioning metastases.

Radioactive iodine uptake over the pelvis and whole-body RAI scanning are useful in the diagnosis of struma ovarii and functioning metastases, respectively.

How it is calculated: RAIU% = (Neck – Thigh counts/Neck phantom counts – Background counts) × 100.[1] Indian normal uptake values determined in the early 1970s used to be 2 hours 5–15% and 24 hours 15–35%; however, a recent study after

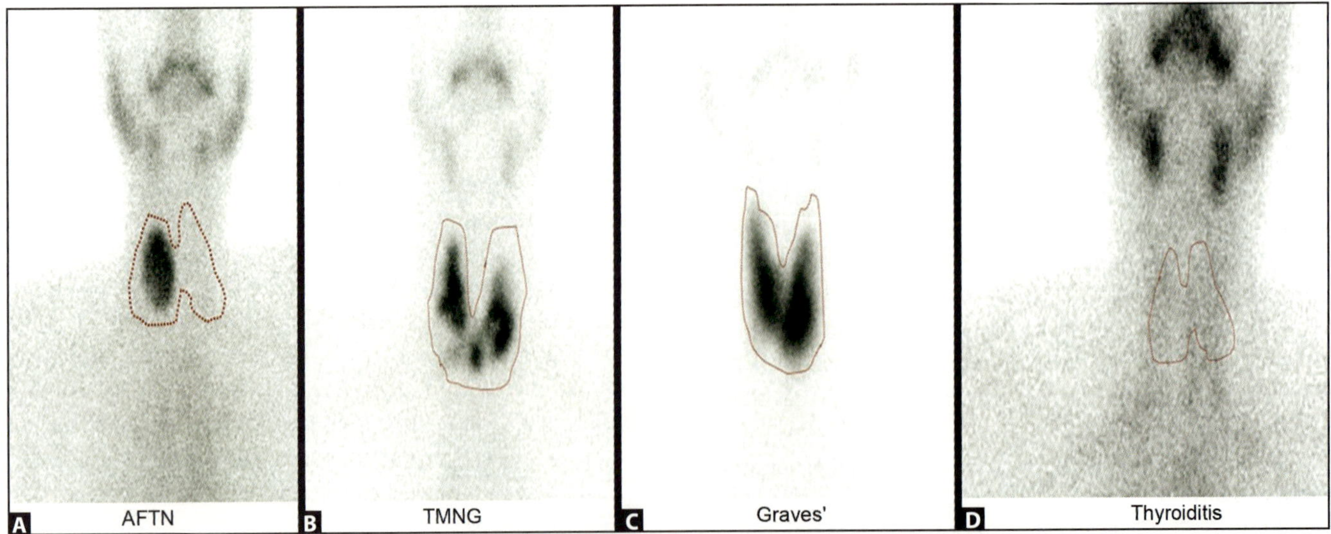

Figs. 1A to D: Different patterns of thyrotoxicosis on ⁹⁹ᵐTc thyroid scan. (A) The scan shows solitary hyperfunctioning thyroid nodule in the right lobe with suppressed uptake in the left lobe (AFTN); (B) Enlarged gland with heterogeneous areas of increased and decreased tracer uptake corresponding to TMNG; (C) Enlarged gland with diffusely increased tracer uptake (GD); (D) Suppressed uptake in the region of the thyroid gland suggesting thyroiditis.
(AFTN: autonomously functioning thyroid nodule; GD: Graves' disease; TMNG: toxic multinodular goiter)

30 years of successful universal salt iodization program in India has reestablished the normal reference range: 2 hours: 1–7%, 24 hours: 7–18%.[2]

When interpreting RAIU, one should always rule out cold iodine contamination from various sources namely exposure to iodinated contrast exposure in the preceding 1–2 months or ingestion of diet rich in iodine (seaweed soup, kelp, and drugs like amiodarone) that interferes with the uptake.

Technetium uptake: Along with thyroid scan, technetium ($^{99m}TcO_4^-$) uptake measurements at 20 minutes can be evaluated using a camera-based method. It is a poor cousin of classic RAIU; however, pertechnetate uptake shows the trapping function of the thyroid gland, but not organification (hormone synthesis).

In good old days, pertechnetate thyroid scan was used as the mainstay of investigation in the workup of euthyroid solitary thyroid nodule (STN) for detection of "cold nodule"; however, now entirely was replaced by ultrasonography (USG) with color Doppler studies.

Treatment of Hyperthyroidism by Radioactive Iodine: I-131

Saul Hertz started radioactive iodine treatment of hyperthyroidism from Massachusetts General Hospital (MGH) in 1942 and interestingly, it is still a popular form of definitive treatment of GD, AFTN, and TMNG.

Contraindications: Definite contraindication is pregnancy and relative contraindications are lactation, incontinence, and individuals unable to comply with safety guidelines (mentally challenged).

- *Graves' disease*: Recommendations of the American Thyroid Association (ATA) 2016 for appropriate use of RAI in GD include patients with contraindications to antithyroid drug (ATD) use or failure to achieve euthyroidism during 18 months of adequate treatment with ATDs. Other indications of I-131 are patients who had earlier subtotal thyroidectomy with relapse, patients with comorbidities that enhances surgical risk, or had a history of neck irradiation. Other suitable candidates for RAI therapy are patients with thyrocardiac disease namely periodic thyrotoxic hypokalemic paralysis, atrial fibrillation, and congestive heart failure.

  Dose of RAI: Two options are available—(1) empiric activity of I-131 should be administered 5–15 mCi (185–555 MBq) as a single dose or (2) by adjusting for the gland size and the trapping ability of RAI to render the patient hypothyroid.[3,4] In good old days, the gland size was determined by palpation; however, currently based on the neck ultrasound that is more accurate.

  Management in children: RAI therapy should be avoided in children below 5 years of age. When given, sufficient I-131 should be administered in a single dose (fear of developing

malignancy later life in sublethally damaged thyrocytes) to render the patient hypothyroid. Interestingly, to date, long-term studies enumerating the incidence of nonthyroidal malignancies of children treated with RAI have not been published.[5,6]

Precautions in patients with Graves' orbitopathy (GO): As per the European Group on Graves' Orbitopathy (EUGOGO), GO is considered active in patients with a clinical activity score (CAS) > 3. In patients with GD "without" GO or who have "mild active" orbitopathy and if no other known risk factors that predict deterioration of their eye disease, I-131 treatment is a good, acceptable option. However, long-term ATDs or total thyroidectomy should be considered as equally acceptable therapeutic options. In patients with mild eye disease CAS 1–3, RAI should be given under steroid cover for 3–6 weeks in tapering doses. In the case of "moderate-to-severe" or sight-threatening GO, it is being recommended that no RAI therapy should be attempted. In such a situation, surgery or long-term ATD is preferred treatment options for GD in this subset of patients.

- *Toxic adenoma or TMNG*: Patients with overtly TMNG or toxic AFTN can be treated with I-131 or total thyroidectomy in former and lobectomy in later. Specific factors that favor I-131 include advanced age, life-threatening comorbidities, prior surgery, small gland size, and most importantly, RAIU sufficient to allow therapy.

  Dose of RAI: Conventionally, the activity of I-131 used to treat "TMNG" is roughly usually higher than that needed to treat GD. Besides, the RAIU values for TMNG may be lower and goiter size is larger as compared to GD, necessitating an increase in the applied activity of RAI. Around 15–25 mCi activity is used for the treatment of TMNG. For TA, a fixed activity of I-131, approximately 10–20 mCi (370–740 MBq), is administered after adjusting for nodule size and corrected for 24 hours uptake values.

THYROID CANCERS

Radiotracers Useful in Imaging and Treatment

- *Both for well and poorly differentiated thyroid cancer (DTC)*: I-131 (imaging and therapy), ^{18}F-fluorodeoxyglucose (^{18}F-FDG) (for radioiodine negative cases).
- *Medullary thyroid cancer (MTC)*: Host of radiotracers are available for imaging namely ^{18}F-FDG, ^{18}F-6-fluoro-3,4-dihydroxyphenylalanine (^{18}F-FDOPA), Tc-99m methyl diphosphonate (MDP), Ga-68 somatostatin analogs (SSAs), and I-123/I-131 metaiodobenzylguanidine (MIBG)
- *Anaplastic thyroid cancer*: ^{18}F-FDG.

Differentiated Thyroid Cancer

Assessment of postoperative disease status after initial thyroid surgery in patients with DTC:

- Postoperative serum thyroglobulin (Tg) helps in assessing the persistence of disease or thyroid remnant and predicting possible future disease recurrence. The Tg reaches its nadir by 3–4 weeks postoperatively in most patients.
- Postoperative diagnostic (RAI) 2 mCi I-131 whole-body scan (WBS) ± SPECT/CT may be useful to assess the thyroid remnant mass or residual disease or metastatic focus **(Figs. 2A to C)**.

The indications of postoperative I-131 WBS in clinical decision-making are:
- The WBS is essential when the surgical note does not spell clearly the extent of the thyroid remnant left or neck USG is unclear about the extent of the tissue in and around thyroid bed.
- Also, when the decision to treat is dependent on the WBS results.
- Single-photon emission computed tomography/CT has incremental value and helps in the correct staging of the disease.
- *The activity used*: I-123 (2–3 mCi, oral) or low activity of I-131 (1–2 mCi, oral).
- Scanning after 24–72 hours for I-131[7] and 24 hours for I-123.[8]
- Ideally, therapeutic activity should be administered within 72 hours of the diagnostic WBS to prevent stunning effects.[9-11]

I-131 in the Management of Differentiated Thyroid Cancer

I-131 is offered to DTC patients in three scenarios: (1) for remnant ablation, (2) for adjuvant therapy, and (3) for the treatment of metastases. The last option is noncontroversial; however, the former two options are fraught with controversies.

Radioactive iodine remnant ablation is most controversial. The ATA 2015 guidelines recommend no I-131 remnant ablation in low-risk DTC patients. Remnant ablation is also not advocated in total thyroidectomy patients who has unifocal follicular DTC and even in multifocal micropapillary carcinoma in the absence of other adverse features.[12]

Radioactive iodine adjuvant therapy is considered after total thyroidectomy in intermediate-risk level DTC patients and routinely recommended for triiodothyronine (T3) and thyroxine (T4) high-risk DTC patients.

Activity of ^{131}I used for remnant ablation or adjuvant therapy: Following several randomized controlled trials (RCTs) and multiple meta-analyses that culminated in ATA 2015 guideline recommending for lower activity of I-131 (25–50 mCi) for remnant ablation.[13,14] For adjuvant therapy, administered activities used up to 150 mCi are generally favored.[15]

For the preparation of patients for RAI scanning/treatment—two options are available.
- The first and cheapest option is thyroid hormone withdrawal for 2–4 weeks to raise the TSH level >30 mIU/L. Nowadays, with improved surgical skills, 14–18 days of T4 is sufficient, following total/near-total thyroidectomy, to achieve the desired TSH value.
- The better option, albeit costly option, is recombinant human thyroid-stimulating hormone (rhTSH) (thyrogen) stimulation—an alternative to T4 withdrawal for remnant ablation or adjuvant therapy. However, rhTSH is not yet recommended for I-131 treatment of metastatic DTC.
- Protocol for rhTSH used—two consecutive 0.9 mg of rhTSH intramuscular injections on day 1 and day 2 followed by on day 3 therapy dose of RAI is administered.

Response assessment after initial radioactive iodine therapy: Criteria for the excellent response is defined as no clinical or imaging evidence of tumor by WBS and/or the neck US, 24 hours RAIU <0.2%, and stimulated serum Tg <0.2 ng/mL in the absence of interfering antibodies.

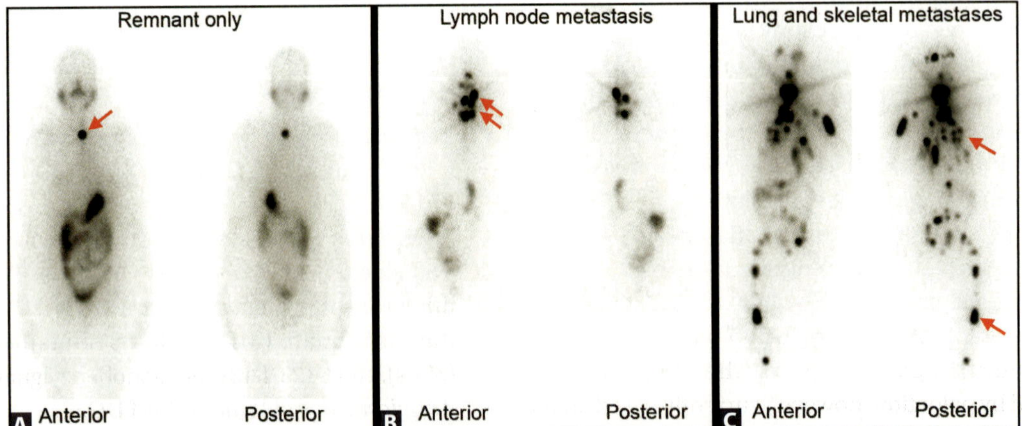

Figs. 2A to C: Pattern of uptake on diagnostic ^{131}I whole-body scan. (A) Focal area of tracer uptake in thyroid bed was suggestive of remnant only (red arrow); (B) The scan shows multiple foci of tracer uptake in neck suggestive of remnant and lymph node metastases (red arrows); (C) Multiple areas of focal tracer uptake in the neck (remnant and nodes), bilateral lungs, and multiple skeletal sites suggestive of metastases (red arrows).

Diagnostic 2 mCi whole-body scan in follow-up: Following remnant ablation or adjuvant therapy, the negative I-131 WBS performed at 6–9 months is considered a successful outcome. This diagnostic WBS is very reassuring to the patient and to the treating physician.

In low-risk and intermediate-risk patients with above criteria, routine diagnostic WBS during follow-up is unnecessary; however, reserved when there is clinical, biochemical, or imaging suspicion of recurrence of the disease.

Management of DTC patients with metastatic disease is a different ball game.
Various options of I-131 administration are described in literature: (1) empiric fixed activity administration; (2) therapy determined by the maximum tolerated dose (MTD), i.e., based on blood dosimetry; and (3) lesional dosimetry.[16]

Radioactive iodine therapy for locoregional metastases:[17]
I-131 WBS detected nodal metastases: RAI may be employed in patients with low volume disease (nonpalpable nodal metastasis). However, for palpable nodes, surgery is generally preferred. If the patient has already undergone extensive neck dissection, radioiodine treatment can be an essential modality if the tumor shows radioiodine avidity. External beam radiation therapy (EBRT) can be used to treat these patients in whom radioiodine is not concentrating on metastases.

Pulmonary metastases: I-131 concentrating diffuse pulmonary metastases should be treated with RAI therapy. Depending on the age of the patient repeated every 9–12 monthly in adults but definitely >12 monthly in children as long as the disease continues to concentrate I-131 in sufficient amount until complete remission is achieved.[18] However, in children, the upper limit of cumulative I-131 activity is recommended to limit within 600 mCi. Macronodular pulmonary metastases are less effective to treat with I-131; treatment may be repeated when the real benefit is demonstrated in the form of a decrease in the size of the lesions, but complete remission is unlikely. Again, the amount of optimal I-131 to be administered is based on above said principles—empiric (100–200 mCi) or based on lesional dosimetry or MTD on limiting pulmonary retention to 80 mCi at 48 hours and 2 Gy to the bone marrow. Pulmonary fibrosis is a rare complication of high cumulative RAI treatment if administered too often and at quick intervals (<6 months). Thus, pulmonary function tests (PFTs) should be performed frequently in this subgroup of patients.

Skeletal metastases:
- The management of skeletal metastases is the most challenging and needs multimodality approach. The objective of I-131 therapy of RAI-avid bone metastases is to improve the quality of life and in a few instances, even better survival outcome seen. Thus, I-131 should be employed, although RAI is rarely curative. I-131 activity is empirically administered (200–250 mCi).

- Symptomatic solitary vertebral metastasis—surgery or EBRT is useful.
- If the patient has multiple skeletal metastases and has metastasis causing spinal cord compression—surgical excision and spinal fixation followed by EBRT are helpful for initial symptomatic relief. Later radioiodine can be used to treat metastases at other sites.

Brain metastases:
- If it is oligometastasis and present in the noneloquent area of brain, surgical resection is possible as it is the best option; otherwise, stereotactic EBRT is used as a palliative measure. These are the mainstay of therapy options for central nervous system (CNS) metastases. RAI may be considered if CNS metastases avidly concentrate I-131.
- Before planning to administer I-131, consider concomitant glucocorticoid therapy to reduce intracranial tension (ICT) to minimize the effects of a potential TSH induced increase in tumor volume/edema and radiation-induced inflammatory response.
- Recombinant human TSH should be used with caution as a sudden increase in tumor volume that might raise the intracranial pressure and results in the compromise of patient safety.

Role of ^{18}F-fluorodeoxyglucose Positron Emission Tomography Scanning in Thyroid Cancer Patients[19,20]

If serum Tg (generally >10 ng/mL) is elevated with negative I-131 imaging, the first investigation is neck ultrasound and if negative, high-resolution computed tomography (HRCT) of the chest should be performed. If both are negative, then ^{18}F-FDG PET scanning should be considered in high-risk DTC patients (TENIS syndrome) **(Figs. 3A and B)**.

[18]F-fluorodeoxyglucose PET scanning is seriously considered in the following conditions:
- Invasive pure Hurthle cell carcinomas
- Poorly DTCs
- Tool for response assessment following systemic or local therapy of metastatic or locally invasive disease.

Radioiodine Refractory Differentiated Thyroid Cancer[21]

Differentiated thyroid cancer that is structurally evident but RAI refractory is defined by anyone of the following criteria: (1) lesion that does not ever concentrate radioiodine from the beginning; (2) lose of the ability to concentrate radioiodine after previously RAI-avid disease; (3) mixed lesions some show radioiodine concentration and others not, or (4) progression despite significant concentration of RAI. The ATA 2015 guideline had one more criterion of RAI-refractory disease, i.e., cumulative dose exceeding 600 mCi despite avid RAI in

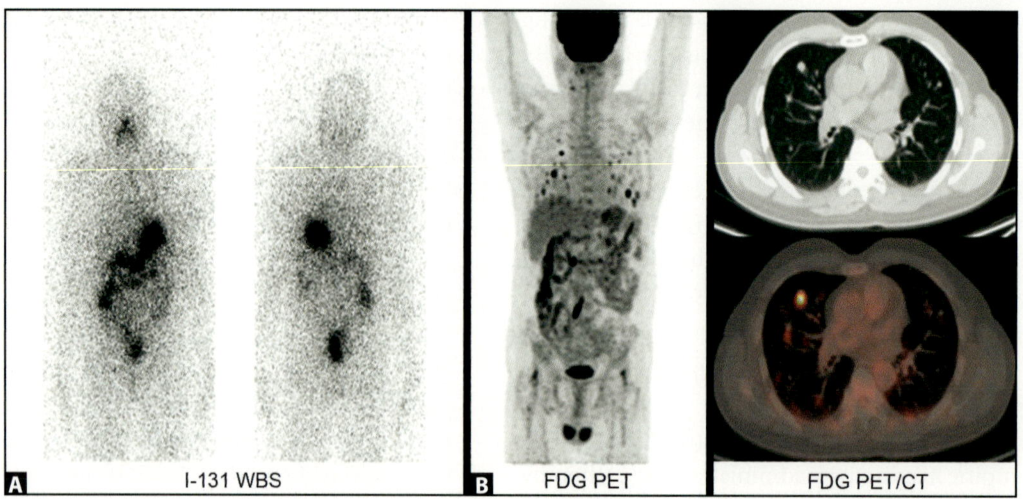

Figs. 3A and B: (A) No abnormal area of focal tracer uptake in the neck or elsewhere in the body in a case of DTC post total thyroidectomy; however, serum thyroglobulin levels were elevated (TENIS syndrome); (B) ^{18}F-FDG PET/CT in the same case, which shows bilateral lung nodules with increased FDG uptake suggesting bilateral lung metastases.
(DTC: differentiated thyroid cancer; ^{18}F-FDG: ^{18}F-fluorodeoxyglucose; PET: positron emission tomography; WBS: whole-body scan)

metastases that are being challenged by Martinique consensus statement.[22]

Management

In patient with RAI-refractory disease, there is no indication for further radioiodine treatment. However, one can argue that patients having mixed lesions, if the vast majority of the lesions are taking RAI, they may be benefitted from a combination of RAI therapy and directed therapy for those few lesions that do not concentrate RAI.

The other option is to monitor such patients on TSH-suppressive therapy with serial radiographic imaging every 3–12 months, particularly those patients, who are stable or minimally progressive and do not have indications for directed therapy.

Role of systemic therapy (tyrosine kinase inhibitors): Tyrosine kinase inhibitors (TKIs) are currently used in RAI-refractory clinically progressive DTCs. The progression-free survival compared to placebo, albeit small, has been demonstrated in four well-conducted RCTs namely (1) vandetanib (VERIFY trial), (2) sorafenib (DECISION trial),[23] (3) lenvatinib (SELECT trial),[24] and (4) axitinib.[25] Apart from the cost, the side effects of these drugs are significant and class-specific. Some of these drugs are the Food and Drug Administration (FDA) and the European Medicines Agency (EMA) approved.

Medullary Thyroid Carcinoma[26]

The patients should be evaluated by imaging procedures if the post total thyroidectomy serum calcitonin level exceeds 150 pg/mL. The imaging could be conventional or molecular or both depending on the availability of the facility for the thorough workup of the patient. This could be neck and chest contrast-enhanced computed tomography (CECT), contrast-enhanced MRI, USG of the liver, and bone scintigraphy.

The molecular imaging in the form of ^{18}F-FDG PET/CT is adequate in the vast majority of cases; however, if available ^{18}F-FDOPA PET/CT can be used to detect persistent or recurrent MTC. Several studies have demonstrated that ^{18}F-FDOPA PET/CT scores better detection of tumor load than ^{18}F-FDG PET/CT. However, later it is universally available and reasonably accurate in identifying patients with progressive disease.

The advantage of ^{68}Ga-DOTANOC PET/CT over above said molecular imaging techniques is for the theranostic applications. The patients with metastatic disease concentrating ^{68}Ga-DOTANOC can be treated with ^{177}Lu-DOTATATE (peptide receptor radionuclide therapy).

The scintigraphy with various planar and even SPECT/CT tracers such as SSAs, MIBG, dimercaptosuccinic acid (DMSA), and gastrin are usually of low sensitivity. MTC is non-RAI avid; thus, there is no role of I-131 in MTC.

Poorly Differentiated Thyroid Cancer

For initial workup of poorly DTC (PDTC), ^{18}F-FDG PET/CT scanning plays an important role for staging and identification of treatable metastatic sites either by EBRT or even by metastasectomy, if possible.

^{18}F-fluorodeoxyglucose PET/CT scanning is a useful tool in the initial staging and follow-up of patients with anaplastic thyroid cancer.

Radioactive iodine imaging or therapy may be used in the initial management of patients with predominantly having DTC with a small undifferentiated component (anaplastic tissue).[27]

◇ PARATHYROID GLAND

Primary hyperparathyroidism (PHPT) is biochemically characterized by an elevated serum parathormone

(PTH) level, serum calcium level, and a decline in serum inorganic phosphates.[28] It is often diagnosed after the unexpected discovery of hypercalcemia in a symptom-free patient. In the symptomatic patient, it may present with osteoporotic fractures, pain, bone lesions, nephrolithiasis, nephrocalcinosis, impaired renal function, abdominal pain, psychiatric symptoms, and cognitive impairments. All those signs and symptoms result in a poor quality of life.[29]

Etiology

About 80% of the patients with PHPT have a single parathyroid adenoma in 80% time, more than one adenoma in 10–11% cases, and all four-gland hyperplasia in <10% of cases. Parathyroid carcinoma, per se producing hyperparathyroidism, is attributed to <1% of cases.[30]

The definitive treatment for PHPT is parathyroidectomy.[31,32] With the advent of the more sensitive preoperative imaging techniques and intraoperative PTH monitoring, limited parathyroid exploration or targeted surgery or minimally invasive parathyroidectomy has achieved wider acceptance rather than four-gland exploration in the past decades.[33] These tools have reduced the duration, extent, and morbidity of surgical exploration.[28]

Parathyroid Scintigraphy (⁹⁹ᵐTc-sestamibi Scintigraphy)

Radiopharmaceutical

⁹⁹ᵐTc-sestamibi

Mechanism of Uptake

⁹⁹ᵐTc-sestamibi, a cationic complex, enters the cytoplasm and stick to mitochondria.[34] Parathyroid adenomas cells, interestingly, have a large number of mitochondria. Therefore, ⁹⁹ᵐTc-sestamibi is likely to be taken up more avidly in adenomas than the surrounding thyroid tissue and with time, the contrast is improved as the slower release would occur from the parathyroid cell compared to the thyroid.[35]

Clinical Indications

Localization of hyperfunctioning parathyroid tissue (adenomas or hyperplasia) in PHPT, the persistent or recurrent disease after initial treatment, and intraoperative localization using a gamma probe, particularly in patients with persistent or recurrent disease.[28]

Protocol/Image Acquisition[28]

Dual-phase ⁹⁹ᵐTc-sestamibi Protocols

During early imaging between 10 and 30 minutes after injection and delayed scanning at 1.5–2.5 hours postinjection time, the high-count images are obtained of the neck and chest. The parathyroid adenoma shall appear as an area of increased uptake on the immediate scan and with time becomes more prominent on the delayed images because of a slower washout from parathyroid than from thyroid (**Figs. 4A and B**). However, some lesions (10–15%) show a faster washout of methoxyisobutylisonitrile (MIBI) by 2–2.5 hours that is as fast as that of the thyroid, thus likely produce a false-negative result.

To prevent false-negative results and characterize the lesion, SPECT/CT plays an important role. SPECT/CT provides the depth information and 3D location regarding the adenoma. It is essential for accurate localization of parathyroid adenomas, particularly for localizing ectopic lesions.[36]

Limitations:

- *False positives*: Certain none parathyroid lesions also concentrate ⁹⁹ᵐTc-sestamibi including thyroid adenomas/carcinomas, reactive cervical lymph nodes, hyperplastic thymus, sarcoidosis, and carcinoid tumor.[37]

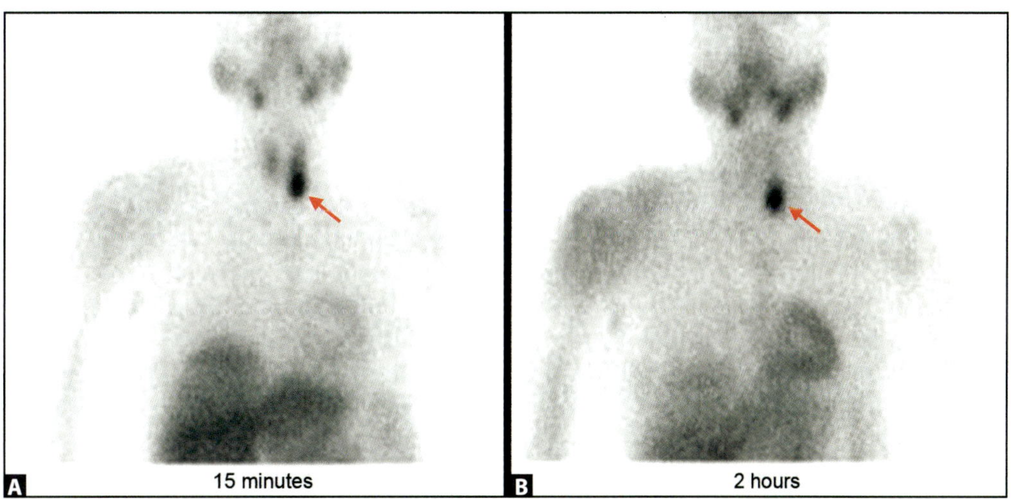

Figs. 4A and B: (A) The early 15-minute and (B) delayed 2 hours images of ⁹⁹ᵐTc-sestamibi scan. (A) Diffuse uptake in the thyroid gland and a focal area of abnormal uptake in relation to left lobe of lower pole region (red arrow); (B) Delayed image shows washout of tracer from thyroid and persistent abnormal uptake in relation to lower pole of left lobe suggesting solitary left parathyroid adenoma (red arrow).

- *False negatives*: Small size (adenomas or hyperplastic glands smaller than 500 mg) and certain adenomas with significant early washout can be missed vide supra.[38]

The localization success rate of single tracer but dual-phase protocol with SPECT/CT is about 64–90%.[39] However, ^{99m}Tc-MIBI scintigraphy has a positive predictive value of 90% in the localization of ectopic parathyroid adenomas.[40] In patients with uremic secondary hyperparathyroidism, the combined USG and sestamibi scintigraphy showed sensitivity about 73% than that of either USG (55%) or MIBI alone (62%) and a specificity of 95% for both procedures. This combination has led to the preoperative diagnosis of ectopic (29%) or supernumerary glands (10%) and concomitant nodular thyroid disease (24%).[41]

Novel Positron Emission Tomography Tracers for Parathyroid Localization

- ^{11}C-methionine, ^{18}F-FDG, and ^{18}F-fluorocholine (^{18}F-FCH) are the PET tracers useful for the detection of parathyroid adenoma.
- Both ^{18}F-FCH and ^{11}C-methionine are sensitive PET tracer for imaging ^{99m}Tc-MIBI SPECT/CT-negative patients with biochemically proven PHPT before reoperation.[42] However, limited availability and cost restrict its use in PHPT patients undergoing the first operation.
- ^{18}F-fluorodeoxyglucose PET/CT is exclusively used in patients with parathyroid carcinoma.[43]
- In the preoperative localization of hyperfunctioning parathyroid tissue, ^{18}F-FCH PET/CT has a sensitivity of about 92% and specificity close to 100%.[44]
- The major advantage of PET tracers is higher resolution associated with PET/CT technology and the shorter imaging time. However, the drawback is like false-positive results from thyroid nodules and inflammatory lymph nodes.[38]

Intraoperative Probe-guided Localization

The intraoperative gamma probe technique with low MIBI doses aids in minimally invasive surgery.[45] Even in patients with negative sestamibi scans, intraoperative use of the gamma probe after preoperative sestamibi injection is useful in localizing parathyroid adenomas.[46,47] The protocol is as follows: Tracer is injected 2 hours before surgery and the probe is used to detect the lesion, first by scanning before skin incision and then after initial exploration. However, this technique is now redundant as intraoperative rapid PTH assay that is widely available in most of the modern hospitals.

◇ ADRENAL GLAND

Functional Imaging of Adrenal Medulla

Pheochromocytoma is the tumor that arises from adrenal medullary chromaffin cells.

Paragangliomas are extra-adrenal tumors; depending on the cell of origin, they are two types: (1) sympathetic PGL and (2) parasympathetic PGL. The former arises from the sympathetic ganglia in the thoracoabdominal and pelvic regions and later from the parasympathetic ganglia in the head and neck regions.

The following inherited syndromes or genetic mutations increase the risk of pheochromocytoma or PGL:
- Multiple endocrine neoplasias—MEN2A and MEN2B
- von Hippel–Lindau (VHL) syndrome
- Neurofibromatosis type 1 (NF1)
- Hereditary paraganglioma syndrome
- Carney–Stratakis dyad [PGL and gastrointestinal stromal tumor (GIST)]
- Carney triad (PGL, GIST, and pulmonary chondroma).

Biochemical Evaluation

Pheochromocytoma produces both epinephrine and norepinephrine.[48] Sympathetic PGLs mainly produce norepinephrine, as norepinephrine to epinephrine conversion depends on phenylethanolamine N-methyltransferase (PNMT). This enzyme requires high concentrations of cortisol levels, which is available in the adrenal gland, hence creating the difference in the biochemical phenotypes of the pheochromocytoma and the PGL.[49] Parasympathetic PGL is largely nonfunctional except in some cases where dopamine and its metabolite 3-methoxytyramine are produced in small quantities.[50]

Rarely, PGLs have been described at unusual sites including orbit, nasal cavity, thyroid, larynx, duodenum, mesentery, urinary bladder, spermatic cord, etc.[51,52]

Malignant pheochromocytoma/paraganglioma (PPGL) is defined as the presence of chromaffin cells in organs/tissues that are typically devoid of chromaffin cells. Common sites of metastases are bones, lungs, and liver. Incidence of metastases in pheochromocytoma is around 10–15% and increased up to 30–40% in extra-adrenal PGL. Risk factors including young age of presentation, succinate dehydrogenase B (SDHB) mutations, large size primary tumor, and dopaminergic phenotype that are associated with malignant forms.[53]

After clinical evaluation, the biochemical workup is essential to characterize whether the tumor is functional or nonfunctional. The next step in the management of these tumors is to locate, characterize the tumor, and determine the extent of disease. Imaging also becomes more critical in situations when these tumors are biochemically silent like head and neck PGL and SDHx mutation-associated PGL. These patients have the germline mutations in up to one-third of patients and it is seen that patients with hereditary tumors often present with the multifocal disease, which should be evaluated by the imaging.

Anatomical imaging modalities provide detailed morphology and local extent.[54] The sensitivity of CT imaging for adrenal lesions is >90%, but for extra-adrenal, recurrent, or metastatic tumors, it is inadequate imaging modality. These imaging modalities tend to miss multifocal PGLs, which are known in hereditary PGL syndromes.[55] Also, these imaging modalities lack specificity with multiple differential diagnoses. Therefore, the need for functional imaging becomes essential as these can scan the whole body in one go and provide useful information with high specificity.

The functional imaging methods are now widely available and have been used extensively in clinical practice.

The older ones for SPECT/CT imaging are ^{123}I/^{131}I-MIBG scintigraphy, ^{111}In-pentetreotide scintigraphy (octreoscan), and ^{99m}Tc-hydrazinonicotinyl-Tyr3-octreotide (^{99m}Tc-HYNIC-TOC) scintigraphy. Most of them are now being replaced by PET tracers, except MIBG scanning.

- *Positron emission tomography/CT tracers*: ^{18}F-FDOPA, ^{18}F-fluorodopamine (^{18}F-FDA), ^{18}F-FDG, and ^{68}Ga-DOTANOC PET/CT (**Figs. 5A and B**).
- All these SPECT and PET tracers have some advantages and disadvantages. The imaging resolution, sensitivity, specificity, ease of tracer synthesis, and availability vary from the tracer to tracer.[56]

- *[123]I/^{131}I-MIBG scintigraphy*: It is a guanethidine analog (structurally similar to norepinephrine), recognized by norepinephrine transporter (NET) and enters the cytoplasm type 1 uptake mechanism. In the cytoplasm, it is stored in the neurosecretory granules via vesicular monoamine transporters 1 and 2.[57] ^{123}I-MIBG scintigraphy is preferable to ^{131}I-MIBG scintigraphy (because better image resolution, less radiation burden, and early imaging 24 hours compared to 48–72 hours for later). The sensitivity of ^{123}I-MIBG is 83–100% and specificity 95–100% for pheochromocytoma, however less sensitivity is 52–75% in extra-adrenal, multiple, or hereditary PGLs.[58]

  • The patient preparation of MIBG scintigraphy is crucial. The thyroid gland needs to be blockade with cold iodine preparation. Several drugs interfere with MIBG uptake, thus need to be stopped for a few days to weeks before tracer injection. The imaging is performed 24–72 hours postinjection of the tracer. I-123 is not widely available and one has to deal with unfavorable dosimetry of ^{131}I imaging. There are factors which limit the wide use of MIBG scintigraphy.

  • *Definite role*: If planning for treatment of known metastatic PGL patients, then the diagnostic ^{123}I/^{131}I-MIBG scan is must before therapy.[54]

- ^{111}In-pentetreotide scintigraphy is popularly known as Octreoscan. Pentetreotide binds to somatostatin receptors (SSTRs) expressed on cell membranes. In parasympathetic head and neck PGLs, Octreoscan has been reported to have better sensitivity about 89–100% compared to ^{131}I/^{123}I-MIBG about 18–50%. However, inferior to ^{123}I-MIBG scintigraphy in abdominal and metastatic PGL.[59,60]

- *[99m]Tc-HYNIC-TOC scintigraphy*: Radiolabeled SSAs have brought new prospects to nuclear oncology for diagnosis and therapy of neuroendocrine tumors. There was a need for technetium-based radiopharmaceutical for NET imaging as ^{111}In-based Octreoscan was prohibitively expensive and not widely available due to patent issues. The first success came in the form of ^{99m}Tc-HYNIC-TOC. This tracer is the low molecular weight with a high affinity for SSTRs. Several characteristics favor this tracer, namely excellent tissue penetration and internalization into the tumor cells after receptor binding.

Advantages of ^{99m}Tc-labeled radiopharmaceuticals are many due to better image quality, short imaging time, cost, and easy availability; however, inferior to ^{68}Ga-DOTANOC PET/CT scan. If there is no PET/CT scanner available, then ^{99m}Tc-HYNIC-TOC could be an alternative for NET imaging using SPECT/CT. Both sensitivity and specificity of ^{99m}Tc-HYNIC-TOC are better than ^{111}In-Octreoscan.[61]

[18]F-6-fluoro-3,4-dihydroxyphenylalanine PET is an amino acid-based PET tracer. It binds to LAT1 (neutral amino acid transporter) with high affinity and is converted into ^{18}F-FDA

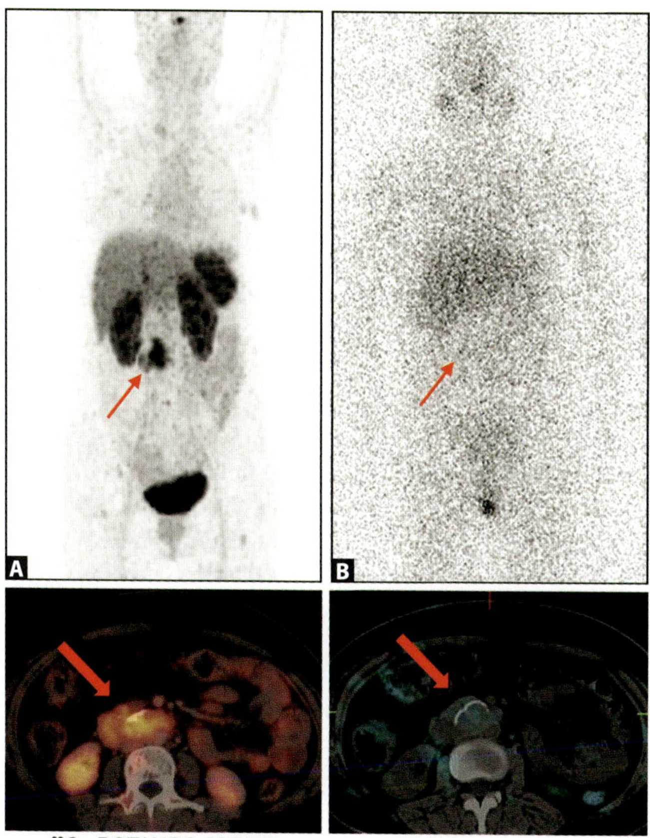

Figs. 5A and B: (A) ^{68}Ga-DOTANOC PET/CT shows somatostatin receptor expression in retroperitoneal soft tissue lesion suggesting paraganglioma (red arrow); (B) ^{131}I-MIBG planar and SPECT/CT images showing no abnormal tracer uptake in the same retroperitoneal lesion (red arrow).
(MIBG: metaiodobenzylguanidine; PET: positron emission tomography; SPECT: single-photon emission computed tomography)

by cytosolic enzyme aromatic L-amino acid decarboxylase (AADC). Then, ^{18}F-FDOPA enters the catecholamine storage vesicles by VMAT1 and 2. Diagnostic ability of ^{18}F-FDOPA PET/CT varies with tumor location and also the genetic status. It is recommended as the functional imaging modality of choice for nonmetastatic head and neck and abdominal PGL with negative germline mutations and also where mutation results are not available.[54] The reported sensitivity and specificity are around 79% and 95%, respectively.

^{68}Ga-DOTATOC or DOTANOC or DOTATATE PET/CT targets somatostatin receptors (SSTR2 and 5). Han et al. in a head-to-head comparison have shown a pooled localization rate of 93% compared to that of ^{18}F-FDOPA PET/CT of 80% in a recent publication.[62]

[18]F-fluorodeoxyglucose PET mechanism: ^{18}F-FDG is taken up by glucose transporter (GLUT) receptors expressed on the cell membrane, then gets phosphorylated to ^{18}F-FDG-6-phosphate by the enzyme hexokinase. This metabolite ^{18}F-FDG-6-P does not undergo further enzymatic conversion and thus, get trapped in cells. Uptake occurs in proportion to the glycolysis rate of cell—a metabolic signature of the cell type. ^{18}F-FDG PET scan is recommended to be used as a functional imaging method in metastatic patients.[54]

Functional Imaging of Adrenal Cortex

Anatomical Imaging

CT scanning is the primary modality of imaging for the adrenal gland. The contrast washout profile helps to characterize various adrenal pathologies. MRI provides high-resolution imaging and can be used for the characterization of the adrenal lesions.

Functional Imaging

Hormonal profiles and anatomic details from CT/MRI are complemented by functional information from adrenal scintigraphy.

Role of functional adrenal cortical imaging:[63]

- Distinguishing unilateral from the bilateral adrenocortical disease
- Cushing's disease (hypercortisolism)
- Different patterns suggest ACTH-dependent or ACTH-independent cause
- Ectopic Cushing's syndrome
- Primary hyperaldosteronism or Conn's syndrome
- Identifying function in adrenal incidentalomas.

Radiopharmaceuticals

Single-photon Emission Computed Tomography Tracers

NP-59 ([131]I-6ß-iodomethyl-19 cholesterol, ^{75}Se-selenomethionyl-19-norcholesterol).

- *Mechanism of uptake*: These molecules are cholesterol analogs and act as a substrate for adrenal steroid hormone synthesis. After uptake, these analogs undergo esterification but are not further metabolized and therefore serve as a marker of tissue cholesterol accumulation.[63]
- *Limitations*: Not commonly used due to limited availability and suboptimal image quality, imaging after 72 hours, and physiologic intestinal uptake results in difficult interpretation.

Positron Emission Tomography Tracers

[11]C or I-123 or ^{18}F metomidate (MTO) and ^{18}F-FDG PET/CT.

[11]C or ^{18}F metomidate:

- *Mechanism of uptake*: MTO enters cells via transporters on the cell surface and binds to 11-beta-hydroxylase, a key enzyme for the synthesis of cortisol and aldosterone.
- This tracer is specific for adrenal cortex.
- It allows for the differentiation of adrenocortical neoplasm from nonadrenocortical tumors; however, differentiation of benign nodule from adrenocortical carcinoma (ACC) is difficult.[64]

[18]F-fluorodeoxyglucose:

- It provides glucose metabolism information
- Useful in imaging ACCs.

◇| CUSHING'S SYNDROME

It is a state of hypercortisolism (inappropriately elevated levels of free plasma glucocorticoids) characterized by typical symptoms and signs of prolonged exposure to excess glucocorticoids.

Adrenocorticotropic Hormone-dependent Causes

Excess of cortisol is due to the stimulation of adrenal glands by ACTH. Commonly source of ACTH is pituitary (Cushing disease), other uncommon reasons are nonpituitary ectopic source—ectopic ACTH syndrome, ectopic corticotropin-releasing hormone (CRH) syndrome. Bronchial carcinoids are the common sources of ectopic ACTH and to some extent, the small cell lung carcinoma, oat cell carcinoma, pancreas, and thymus. Chronic stimulation by ACTH produces macronodular adrenal hyperplasia (autonomous adrenal nodule). Usually, there is bilateral adrenal involvement in the form of hyperplasia with nodule formation.

Adrenocorticotropic Hormone-independent Causes

Excess glucocorticoids are commonly iatrogenic (e.g., pharmacologic doses of exogenous prednisolone, dexamethasone, etc.) or increased cortisol production from adrenal causes (adrenal adenoma and carcinoma). The uncommon causes described in the literature include primary pigmented nodular adrenal hyperplasia, association with Carney syndrome, McCune–Albright syndrome, and ACTH-independent macronodular hyperplasia. Usually, the adrenal involvement in adrenal adenoma and carcinoma is unilateral.

Investigations

Clinical workup of patients suspected to have Cushing's syndrome begins by first to confirm biochemically whether the patient has Cushing's syndrome or not followed by further investigations to find the etiology.

- For the management point of view, ACTH levels are checked first. The next issue is whether one is dealing with ACTH-dependent or ACTH-independent Cushing's syndrome. Depending on biochemical clues, the imaging workup is designed.
- *Imaging options*:
  - Imaging of the adrenal glands—CT (investigation of choice), MRI, and functional imaging
  - Imaging pituitary—MRI of sella (investigation of choice)
  - Imaging for ectopic ACTH/CRH—CT, functional imaging.
- *Patterns of functional adrenal imaging*:[65]
  - *ACTH-dependent Cushing's syndrome*: NP-59 imaging shows symmetric to varying degrees of asymmetric bilateral visualization of the adrenal glands.
  - *Adrenal adenoma*: Unilateral visualization of the gland containing the adenoma with the suppressed contralateral gland.
  - *Adrenal carcinoma*: Nonvisualization of the adrenal glands bilaterally even tumoral cortisol secretion is sufficient to cause hypercortisolism.[66]

- *Ectopic Cushing's syndrome*: ^{111}In-pentetreotide (Ostreoscan), ^{18}F-FDG PET/CT, ^{68}Ga-DOTANOC PET/CT, and ^{18}F-FDOPA PET/CT can be used **(Figs. 6A to E)**.
- In one of the systematic review by Isidori on imaging of ectopic Cushing's syndrome, tumors were localized by CT in 66% (137/207), MRI in 51% (53/103), ^{111}In-pentetreotide in 49% (84/172), ^{18}F-FDG PET in 51% (46/89), ^{18}F-FDOPA PET in 57% (12/21), ^{131}I/^{123}I-MIBG in 30% (4/13), and ^{68}Ga-SSTR PET/CT in 81% (18/22) of cases. Molecular imaging discovered 79% (53/67) of tumors unidentified by conventional radiology.[67]

◇| PRIMARY ALDOSTERONISM

One of the common causes of resistant hypertension is primary aldosteronism. Excess secretion of aldosterone from the adrenal gland results in hypertension and hypokalemia.[68] The cause for excess aldosterone production can be a cortical adenoma or bilateral hyperplasia of the zona glomerulosa.

Biochemical Evaluation

Aldosterone-renin ratio is used to screen high-risk patients suspected to have primary aldosteronism (patient with spontaneous hypokalemia, moderately severe hypokalemia induced by usual doses of diuretics or refractory hypertension).

Imaging

After initial biochemical diagnosis, imaging is used to localize the lesion and find out the possible etiological diagnosis as it significantly impacts the management. Unilateral

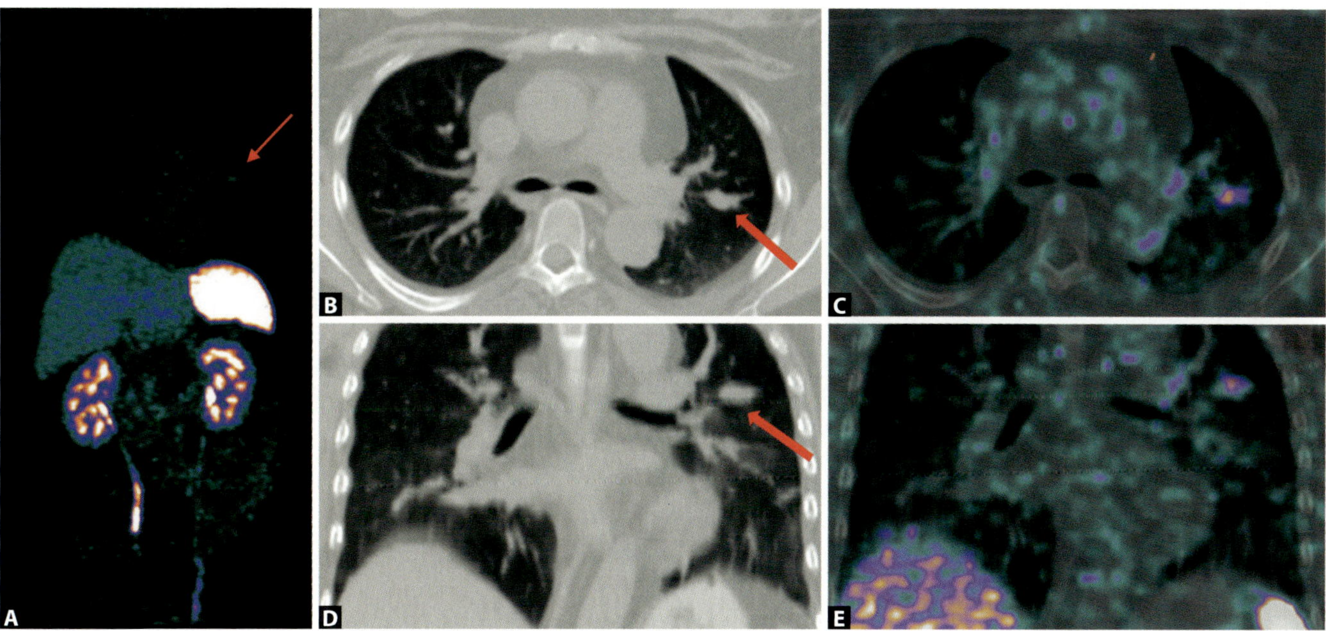

Figs. 6A to E: (A) Maximum intensity projection image (red arrow); (B and C) Axial (red arrow); (D and E) Coronal sections of ^{68}Ga-DOTANOC positron emission tomography (PET)/CT whole-body scan (red arrow) done in case of Cushing's syndrome to rule out the ectopic site of hormone production. The scan shows soft tissue lesion in left lung of upper lobe with somatostatin receptor expression (likely lung carcinoid lesion).

adrenalectomy (for adenoma and unilateral hyperplasia) can result in the normalization of hypokalemia and improving the hypertension control in up to 30–60% of patients; hence, it is essential to localize the lesion.

CT is the preferred initial imaging modality that gives information about laterality of disease (unilateral adenoma, unilateral/bilateral hyperplasia), excludes large adrenal mass which may be ACC and provides information about adrenal vein anatomy to guide adrenal vein sampling. However, there are limitations of structural imaging—limitation in visualizing microadenomas and limitation to differentiate nonfunctioning from functioning aldosterone-producing adenomas.[69] Hence, adrenal vein sampling is used to confirm laterality of the lesion if the surgery is desired, but it is an invasive and expensive procedure; therefore, it should be used in appropriately screened patients.[70]

Functional Imaging

Adrenocortical imaging with (NP-59) along with dexamethasone suppression (1 mg orally every 6 hours for 7 days before NP-59 injection and throughout the imaging period) is to suppress ACTH-dependent component of uptake in the zona fasciculata.[65]

Imaging Patterns

- Unilateral visualization (before the 5th day)—suggestive of aldosteronoma
- Bilateral visualization (before the 5th day)—suggestive of adrenal hyperplasia
- This test is almost abandoned due to poor spatial resolution and better availability of structural and molecular imaging techniques.

11C-metomidate PET/CT has also been used for evaluation for primary aldosteronism, with reported specificity of 87% and sensitivity of 76% for aldosterone-producing adenomas.[71] With a better spatial resolution of PET/CT compared to gamma camera-based images, this modality might be used more often in the future with the full availability of this radiotracer.

◁ ADRENAL INCIDENTALOMA

Any incidentaloma is defined as detection of a lesion in an organ on imaging not performed for the suspected disease of that organ. Adrenal incidentalomas can be seen in up to 4% of patients who undergo imaging for nonadrenal causes like pain in abdomen, low backache, kidney stones, etc.[72]

Clinical Importance

Incidental adrenal lesion can be a primary adrenal or metastatic lesion, functioning or nonfunctioning lesion, and benign or malignant lesion.[72-74] Incidental adrenal lesions (≥1 cm) or even smaller lesions with clinical profile suggestive of hormonal hypersecretion require additional workup to detect

functional nature (hormonal hypersecretion or nonsecretory); to distinguish between benign and malignant lesions, the management of these patients differs. Adrenalectomy is indicated for functional tumors causing significant clinical symptoms and the lesion suspicious for malignancy.

Functional Evaluation

Initial biochemical evaluation includes an overnight dexamethasone suppression test. This test is for cortisol-secreting adenoma. The plasma-free metanephrines or urinary metanephrines are tested to excluding pheochromocytoma. Aldosterone to renin ratio is used to exclude primary aldosteronism in patients with concomitant hypertension and hypokalemia.[75]

Imaging

CT densitometry [Hounsfield unit (HU)], which provides information about the amount of fat within an adrenal lesion, is used for differential diagnosis. On noncontrast computed tomography (NCCT), HU ≤ 10 suggests a lipid-rich adenoma. However, up to 30% of benign adenomas (lipid-poor adenoma) have an attenuation value of >10 HU; thus, it is difficult to diagnose on the basis of CT density benign from malignant lesions.[76]

If the adrenal lesions are indeterminate on initial NCCT and hormonal profile does not indicate significant hormone excess, further evaluation can be considered including CECT (washout pattern of contrast enhancement), MRI (chemical shift imaging), and functional imaging.[75,77]

Functional Imaging Role

Despite the anatomic details from the CT and MRI, functional adrenal imaging using radionuclides (NP-59, 131I/123I-MIBG, 68Ga-DOTANOC, and 18F-FDG) can be utilized in the characterization of incidental adrenal lesions.

NP-59 scintigraphy—to distinguish adrenal adenomas from nonadenomatous lesions (including adrenal metastases, cysts, hemorrhage, lipoma, and myelolipoma).[65]

Patterns: Concordant uptake (focal uptake more on the side of the lesion) is suggestive of adenoma, discordant uptake is indicative of destructive/malignant pathology involving ipsilateral adrenal gland, and normal uptake (symmetrical, nonlateralizing) is suggestive of pseudoadrenal mass (arising from another organ).

123I/131I-MIBG, 68Ga-DOTANOC imaging—can be used to assess for nonhypersecreting pheochromocytoma and evaluation of extra-adrenal pheochromocytoma (PGL), metastatic pheochromocytoma.

18F-fluorodeoxyglucose PET/CT—role as a functional imaging technique in differentiating primary versus metastatic lesion by providing whole-body screening and evaluation and metastatic workup for primary adrenal carcinoma.[78,79]

NEUROENDOCRINE NEOPLASM

Neuroendocrine neoplasms (NENs) are the tumors that arise from the cells of the diffuse neuroendocrine system, which is present in the skin, lung, gastrointestinal tract, hepatobiliary system, urogenital tract, and thyroid.[80] Although commonly involved sites are the gastrointestinal tract including pancreas [gastroenteropancreatic neuroendocrine tumor (GEP-NET)] and lung.[81] Among GEP-NET, the most common site included is the ileum, followed by the rectum and the appendix. Gastric, duodenal, and jejunal NET are less common and the colon is one of the uncommon sites.[82,83] Pancreatic NETs, which are around 10% of all pancreatic neoplasms, constitute approximately 7% of all GEP-NETs.[84]

The hallmark of NETs is the secretion of metabolically active hormones and amines, which can result in specific clinical manifestations. Nonfunctioning NETs are frequent as compared to functioning NETs, hence present late with features of the locally advanced tumor like bowel obstruction, mass effect, or with hepatic metastases.

Pathological Classification

According to the World Health Organization (WHO) (2010) classification, these tumors are classified as:[85]

- *Well-differentiated*:
  - *Gastroenteropancreatic neuroendocrine tumor grade 1 (G1)*: Mitotic count [<2/10 high-power field (HPF)], Ki 67 index (<3%).
  - *Gastroenteropancreatic neuroendocrine tumor grade 2 (G2)*: Mitotic count (2–20/10 HPF), Ki 67 index (3–20%).
- *Poorly differentiated*: Gastroenteropancreatic neuroendocrine tumor grade 3 (neuroendocrine carcinoma) G3: Mitotic count (>20/10 HPF), Ki 67 index (>20%).

In the latest WHO (2017) classification, another category referring to as "NET grade 3 (G3)" has been added.[86] This group represents tumors with high proliferation index but well-differentiated morphology, show different genomic mutations resembling lower grade NET (e.g., MEN1, DAX, ATRX mutations), and have a more indolent clinical course compared to poorly differentiated type tumor which shows mutations involving *p53* and *RB1* genes.

Imaging Techniques

Conventional Imaging

USG, CT, and MRI are used.[87,88]

Functional Imaging

Somatostatin receptor imaging: It is based on the presence of SSTRs on the cell membrane. Well-differentiated NETs have the expression of SSTR.[89]

- Gamma camera-based SSTR imaging—[111]In-pentetreotide
- Positron emission tomography-based SSTR imaging—[68]Ga-DOTATATE/DOTATOC/DOTANOC.

[18]F-fluorodeoxyglucose PET: Assess glucose metabolism in tumor cells. Increased uptake is seen in poorly differentiated neuroendocrine carcinoma (which scarcely expresses SSTRs). It provides prognostic information—increased ^{18}F-FDG uptake is associated with aggressive behavior.[90]

Other radiopharmaceuticals: ^{18}F-FDOPA and ^{18}F-FDA.

Differentiation between well-differentiated neuroendocrine tumors from poorly differentiated neuroendocrine tumors based on functional imaging **(Figs. 7A and B)**:

- ^{68}Ga-DOTANOC PET/CT—SSTRs are highly expressed on the surface of well-differentiated NETs
- ^{18}F-fluorodeoxyglucose PET/CT—increased uptake in G3, neuroendocrine carcinoma (which scarcely expresses SSTRs).

Role of functional imaging in neuroendocrine tumor:[91]

- Initial staging of NETs
- Evaluation of suspected mass which is not readily amenable to endoscopic or percutaneous biopsy.
- Localization of the primary tumor in patients with known metastatic disease, but primary unknown on conventional imaging.
- Evaluation of patients with clinical symptoms and biochemical evidence of NET, but no localization on conventional imaging.
- Restaging
- Selection of patients for peptide receptor radionuclide therapy (PRRT)
- And for response evaluation.

INSULINOMA

Among conventional functional imaging techniques used for GEP-NET, separate mention about insulinoma is required, as we have now functional imaging techniques specific to insulinoma [glucagon-like peptide-1 (GLP-1) receptor imaging] is available.

72-hour Fast Test

Demonstrating inappropriately high serum insulin levels during a prolonged fast. After confirming the biochemical diagnosis, the next step is the localization of the lesion as they can be found anywhere in the pancreas. Preoperative localization usually requires a combination of different noninvasive and invasive imaging methods.[92]

Functional Imaging

- ^{111}In-pentetreotide SPECT/CT (SPECT-based SSTR imaging)
- ^{18}F-FDOPA PET/CT

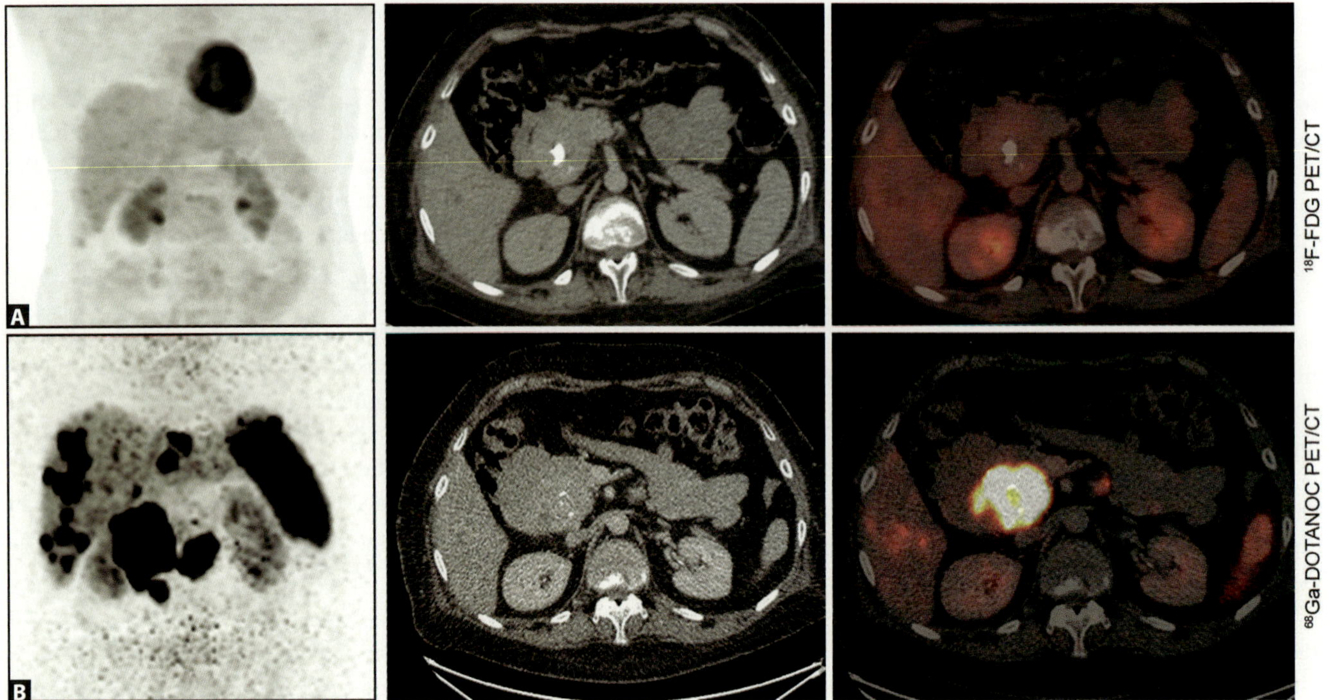

Figs. 7A and B: (A) ¹⁸F-FDG PET/CT; (B) ⁶⁸Ga-DOTANOC PET/CT in a young male presenting with pain in abdomen that shows a large pancreatic mass with multiple liver metastatic lesions which do not show FDG uptake; however, it shows intense DOTANOC uptake (SSTR expression) suggesting well-differentiated NET.
(¹⁸F-FDG: ¹⁸F-fluorodeoxyglucose; NET: neuroendocrine tumor; PET: positron emission tomography; SSTR: somatostatin receptor)

- ⁶⁸Ga-DOTANOC PET/CT (SSTR-PET imaging)
- ¹⁸F-fluorodeoxyglucose PET/CT—role in malignant insulinoma
- Glucagon-like peptide-1 receptor imaging.

Mechanism of Uptake

The GLP-1 receptor has been identified in normal tissues including the pancreas, stomach, brain, and lung. It has been shown that it is highly overexpressed in insulinoma with high incidence (>90%); hence, it can be used as a target for functional imaging.[93] The molecule exendin-4 (a 39 amino acid polypeptide extracted from saliva of the Gila monster) has a structural similarity to mammalian incretin (GLP-1). There is a 53% amino acid sequence homology with incretin.[94] It is a more potent and longer-lasting GLP-1 receptor agonist than GLP-1. It can be radiolabeled with different radionuclides using chelators and used for imaging of GLP-1 receptors.

Single-photon emission computed tomography: ¹¹¹In- and ⁹⁹ᵐTc-labeled exendin-4.

Positron emission tomography: ⁶⁸Ga-DOTA-exendin-4 PET/CT.

Recent studies using ⁶⁸Ga-DOTA-exendin-4 PET/CT have shown good results. The advantage of PET/CT imaging is a shorter imaging time, better tumor-to-background ratio, excellent spatial resolution, and negligible radiation burden. The sensitivity and specificity are acceptable range, varying from 75 to 97%, as reported in the literature.[95,96]

PEPTIDE RECEPTOR RADIONUCLIDE THERAPY

Poorly differentiated NETs are more aggressive tumors compared to well-differentiated ones. Regional and distant metastases are seen in up to 20–40% of cases. Common sites of metastases are lymph nodes and liver; less common sites are lungs, bones, peritoneum, and mesentery.[97]

The theranostics means visualizing the sites of disease (diagnostic imaging) and targeting those sites with bioradio conjugates (radionuclide therapy); thus, functional imaging selects the patients who shall be benefited by PRRT, a crucial role in the management of metastatic NETs.

A host of treatment options are available for metastatic NET. They are classified into surgical options and medical therapies. If possible to do R0 dissection of the primary tumor with oligometastatic tumor surgery, that is the best chance for the patient to have long-term disease-free survival. The currently available medical options are suboptimal. However, a host of options are explored namely long-acting SSAs, interferon-alpha therapy, chemotherapy, molecularly targeted agents including mammalian target of rapamycin (mTOR) inhibitor (everolimus), PRRT, and cytoreductive therapies including transarterial chemoembolization (TACE), radiofrequency ablation (RFA), and selective internal radiation therapy (SIRT) can be used in functionally active tumors to reduce the tumor burden.[97] However, none of them

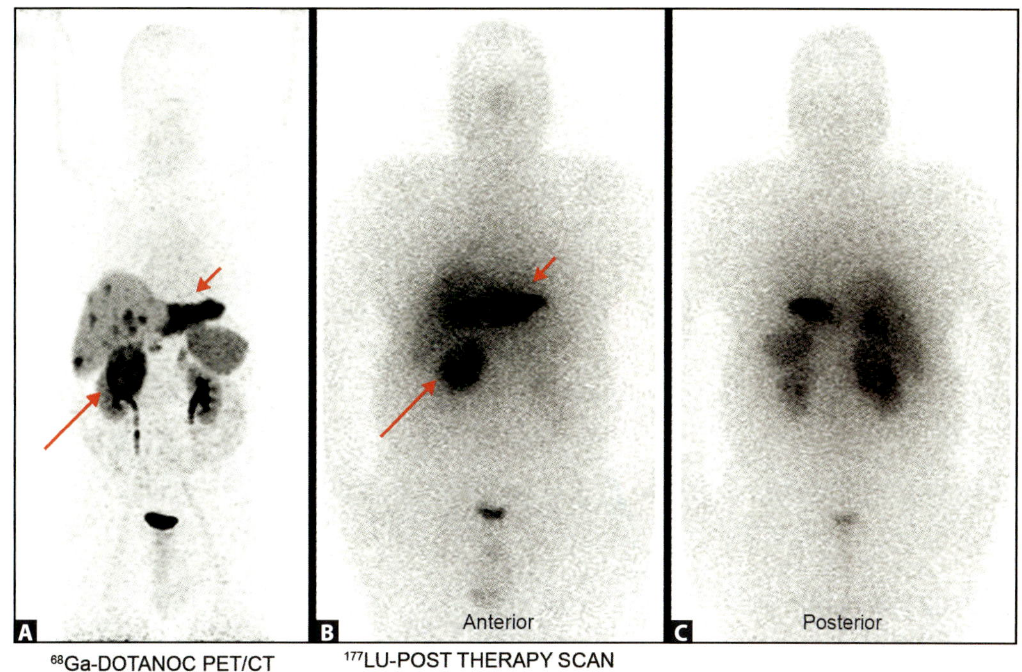

Figs. 8A to C: (A) ⁶⁸Ga-DOTANOC PET/CT maximum intensity projection image shows abnormally increased tracer uptake in large lesion at right renal hilum level (pancreatic NET) with multiple liver metastases (red arrows); (B and C) Post ¹⁷⁷Lu-DOTATATE (PRRT) therapy anterior and posterior planar images show tracer distribution in the region of pancreatic primary and liver metastases (red arrow).
(NET: neuroendocrine tumor; PET: positron emission tomography; PRRT: peptide receptor radionuclide therapy)

is curative; at best, these modalities prolong survival and improve the quality of life.

- Involves the use of SSAs labeled with either an auger/conversion electron emitter (indium ¹¹¹In), beta particle emitting (yttrium ⁹⁰Y, lutetium ¹⁷⁷Lu), or alpha particle-emitting radionuclide (actinium AC-225) **(Figs. 8A to C)**.
- Initially started with ¹¹¹In-octreotide, but now replaced with ¹⁷⁷Lu/⁹⁰Y DOTATATE and recently alpha therapy (²²⁵Ac-DOTATATE) is becoming popular.[98]
- Appropriate candidates for PRRT are the patient with well-differentiated or moderately differentiated NET (WHO grade 1 or 2) with adequate SSTR expression.[99]
- Contraindications—absolute contraindication is pregnancy, severe acute concurrent medical illness, and severe unmanageable psychiatric illness. Relative contraindications include severely compromised renal and hematological dysfunction and breastfeeding, if not yet stopped.
- As SSAs interfere in PRRT, it is mandatory to stop long-acting SSAs for 4 weeks and 24 hours for short-acting SSAs before PRRT infusion is administered.

The kidneys are the critical organ for radiation toxicity because of reabsorption of the radiopeptide and retention of the radiopharmaceutical in proximal convoluted tubules of the kidney. The renal toxicity is prevented by the infusion of positively-charged amino acids (L-lysine and L-arginine) starting before PRRT and continuing after it. The next critical organ is red marrow, particularly in patients with extensive skeletal metastases.

The first international multicentric RCT (NETTER1 trial) using four cycles of ¹⁷⁷Lu-DOTATATE (LUTATHERA) at 8 weeks interval published in 2017 showed a progression-free survival benefit of 28.4 months for PRRT versus 8.4 months for high-dose SSA in midgut NET progressive to standard SSA treatment.[100] Following this landmark research publication, the FDA has approved ¹⁷⁷Lu-DOATATE (LUTATHERA) in the USA for metastatic midgut NETs.

CONGENITAL HYPERINSULINISM/ PERSISTENT HYPERINSULINEMIC HYPOGLYCEMIA OF INFANCY

Congenital hyperinsulinism (CHI) or persistent hyperinsulinemic hypoglycemia of infancy (PHHI) is a rare condition, albeit, a most common cause of prolonged hypoglycemia in neonates. The dysregulation of insulin secretion is a genetic disorder seen both in familial and sporadic forms.[101]

Genetics

Insulin dysregulation results from different mutations including *ABCC8* (most common), *KCNJ11*, *GLUD1*, *GCK1*, *HK1*, *HNF4A*, and *HADH* genes.[102-104]

Genetic information can guide imaging and management. Recessive inactivating mutations in *ABCC8/KCNJ11* are common causes.[105] Paternal uniparental disomy (focal loss of the maternal allele and replacement with the paternal allele) from chromosome 11p15 harboring mutation in *ABCC8/KCNJ11* gene results in hemi- or homozygosity of the abnormal paternal gene that is associated with focal pancreatic disease.[106]

Two different presentations of PHHI are noted either focal or diffuse pancreatic involvement. The patients who fail to respond to medical therapy namely glucose infusion, diazoxide, and octreotide can be taken for surgical intervention. The focal lesion, if present, can be dealt with enucleation or partial pancreatectomy. However, for diffuse pancreatic involvement, near-total pancreatectomy is advocated with associated lifelong morbidity in the form of insulin-dependent diabetes mellitus and exocrine pancreatic insufficiency, a high price to pay.

Evaluation of Focal/Diffuse Variants

The most sophisticated tests are pancreatic venous sampling (PVS) and pancreatic arterial calcium stimulation test, but these methods are technically demanding and invasive.

Structural Imaging

MRI is the best noninvasive test currently used.

Functional Imaging

^{18}F-FDOPA PET/CT.

- This molecular imaging has shown good results either superior or same as compared to previous conventional modalities like PVS and pancreatic arterial stimulation test and the test being noninvasive is preferred more nowadays.[107]
- In a head-to-head comparison study of ^{68}Ga-DOTANOC and ^{18}F-FDOPA, Christiansen et al. have shown the better performance of ^{18}F-FDOPA PET/CT over ^{68}Ga-DOTANOC.[108]

◁ STRUMA OVARII

Struma ovarii is a type of mature ovarian teratoma representing around 2–5% of all ovarian teratomas and 0.5–1% of all ovarian tumors.[109] Ectopic thyroid tissue can be seen in ovarian dermoid cysts; however, it is called struma ovarii when at least 50% or more of the mass is thyroid tissue.[110] The malignant form of struma ovarii is rare occurring in 0.3–5% of these struma ovarii cases.[111] Thyrotoxicosis can be seen in 5–10% of struma ovarii cases.[112]

These patients usually are asymptomatic and often detected incidentally as an ovarian cyst on routine USG checkup. When symptomatic, they typically have nonspecific symptoms including pain in abdomen, palpable lump, menstrual irregularities, and less commonly present with overt signs and symptoms of thyrotoxicosis. Malignant change can be seen in this ectopic thyroid tissue associated with struma ovarii and both papillary and follicular histologies have been reported.[113] Coexistent primary thyroid cancer can be seen along with struma ovarii.[114]

Management

Surgical resection of the primary ovarian mass/cyst is the first step in the management. For benign struma ovarii, cystectomy or unilateral salpingo-oophorectomy is done however, data regarding optimal management and follow-up of malignant struma ovarii is still lacking. Regarding the extent of surgery for the primary ovarian mass, no standard guidelines exist concerning those with malignant struma ovarii. The surgical decision could be total abdominal hysterectomy with bilateral salpingo-oophorectomy with or without omentectomy as done for malignant epithelial ovarian tumors or unilateral salpingo-oophorectomy/oophorectomy or cystectomy for preserving the fertility.[115] However, cystectomy alone in managing these cases is suggested to be suboptimal, though there is no reliable evidence in the literature regarding the prognosis of these patients managed with cystectomy alone.

There is no clear-cut guideline whether RAI should be administered or not. However, adjuvant RAI treatment for malignant struma ovarii has been suggested by few studies, in which they have shown an improved outcome in patients who underwent total thyroidectomy and I-131 ablation after ovarian mass excision compared to the group managed conservatively.[113] To facilitate radioactive I-131 treatment of residual and metastatic disease, removal of the thyroid gland is necessary before RAI therapy can be planned.[116] Total thyroidectomy also allows monitoring with serum Tg levels postoperatively, where increased Tg levels in a patient on suppressive levels of TSH indicate persistent or recurrent disease.[117] The patient can then be followed with serum Tg levels, I-131 WBS, and USG of pelvis.

◁ TUMOR-INDUCED OSTEOMALACIA

Tumor-induced osteomalacia is a rare condition, which presents clinically as bone pain, muscle weakness, and fractures. Biochemically, it is characterized by persistent phosphaturia and hypophosphatemia with inappropriately normal or low levels of 25-hydroxy vitamin D3.[118] It is considered a paraneoplastic condition associated with mesenchymal tumors associated with increased tumor production of fibroblast growth factor-23 (FGF-23).[119]

Role of Imaging

Once the biochemical diagnosis is confirmed, localization of the lesion, which is essential because complete surgical resection of the lesion, results in almost complete resolution of the disease.[120]

Role of Functional Imaging

Functional whole-body imaging provides screening of the whole body for the presence of the active lesion.

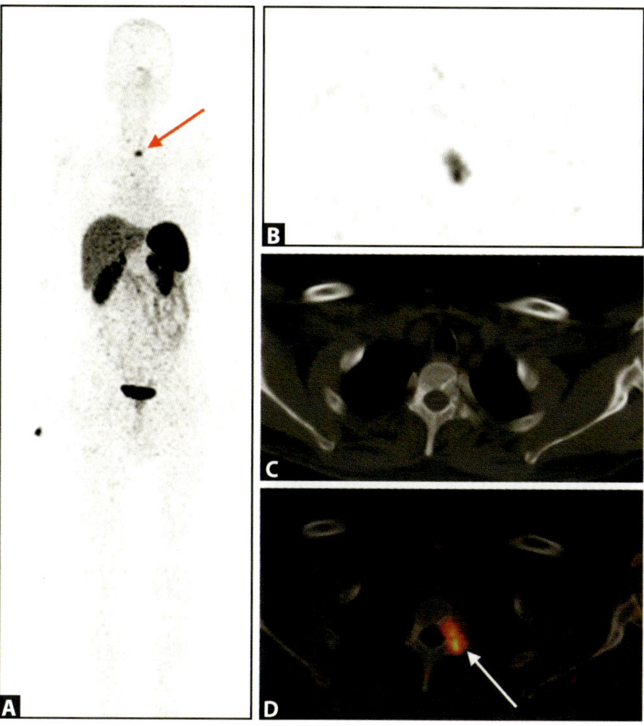

Figs. 9A to D: (A) MIP (red arrow); (B to D) Axial images of ⁶⁸Ga-DOTANOC-PET/CT in a case presenting with multiple bone pains, fractures with persistent phosphaturia and hypophosphatemia suggesting tumor-induced osteomalacia, and shows focal tracer avid lesion in the D2 vertebral body suggesting likely etiology (white arrow).
(MIP: maximum intensity projection; PET: positron emission tomography)

Single-photon emission computed tomography/CT-based tracers:

- ⁹⁹ᵐTc-MDP bone scan—detection of any focal osteoblastic lesion in the skeleton. However, osteoblastic foci may be present at sites of associated fractures (false positive) and the visceral lesion is missed.
- ¹¹¹In-Octreoscan—based on SSTR expression on the lesion.

Positron emission tomography/CT tracers:

- ⁶⁸Ga-DOTANOC PET/CT—based on SSTR expression on the lesion **(Figs. 9A to D)**.
- ¹⁸F-fluorodeoxyglucose PET/CT—based on glucose metabolism.

Somatostatin receptor-based imaging methods have shown excellent results. A study comparing ⁶⁸Ga-DOTATATE PET/CT with Octreoscan and ¹⁸F-FDG PET has demonstrated higher sensitivity and specificity with ⁶⁸Ga-DOTATATE PET/CT; thus, it may be advocated for localization of the phosphaturic tumor.[121] However, in some cases, the tumor may be localized on ¹⁸F-FDG PET/CT, but not on SSA imaging; hence, SSA imaging and ¹⁸F-FDG PET have a complementary role.[122] After localization by functional imaging, the tumor can be better anatomically characterized by CECT or MRI before planning for surgical resection.

Management

Mainstay of therapy is surgical resection if culprit FGF-23 producing mesenchymal tumor could be identified correctly.[118] If surgery is not possible, then image-guided RFA/cryoablation is an option.[123,124] If the offending tumor cannot be localized, medical treatment (which includes phosphorus and active vitamin D supplementation) is done.[122] Octreotide and cinacalcet have been found useful.[125] Recently, one case report showed the potential application of ¹⁷⁷Lu-PRRT in cases of recurrent inoperable phosphaturic mesenchymal tumor of the skull base.[126]

CONCLUSION

Nuclear medicine plays a crucial role in the diagnosis and therapy of many endocrine disorders. To name a few, differentiated thyroid carcinoma with distant metastases, metastatic neuroendocrine tumors whether GEP-NETs or apudomas of neural crest origin are under theranostic domain of nuclear endocrinology. With advent of more specific radiotracers and alpha-based radiopharmaceuticals therapy, nuclear endocrinology is going to play a dominant role in multidisciplinary management of 'difficult to treat' endocrine problems in coming days.

REFERENCES

1. American College of Radiology (ACR). (2019). ACR–SNMMI–SPR Practice Parameter for the Performance of Scintigraphy and Uptake Measurements for Benign and Malignant Thyroid Disease. [online] Available from https://www.acr.org/-/media/ACR/Files/Practice-Parameters/Thy-Scint.pdf. [Last accessed April, 2020].
2. Ballal S, Soundararajan R, Bal C. Re-establishment of normal radioactive iodine uptake reference range in the era of universal salt iodization in the Indian population. Indian J Med Res. 2017;145:358-64.
3. Ross DS, Burch HB, Cooper DS, Greenlee MC, Laurberg P, Maia AL, et al. 2016 American Thyroid Association Guidelines for Diagnosis and Management of Hyperthyroidism and Other Causes of Thyrotoxicosis. Thyroid. 2016;26:1343-421.
4. Damle N, Bal C, Kumar P, Reddy R, Virkar D. The predictive role of 24h RAIU with respect to the outcome of low fixed-dose radioiodine therapy in patients with diffuse toxic goitre. Hormones (Athens). 2012;11:451-7.
5. Read CH, Tansey MJ, Menda Y. A 36-year retrospective analysis of the efficacy and safety of radioactive iodine in treating young Graves' patients. J Clin Endocrinol Metab. 2004;89:4229-33.
6. Boice JD. Radiation and thyroid cancer: what more can be learned? Acta Oncol. 1998;37:321-4.
7. Muratet JP, Daver A, Minier JF, Larra F. Influence of scanning doses of iodine-131 on subsequent first ablative treatment outcome in patients operated on for differentiated thyroid carcinoma. J Nucl Med. 1998;39:1546-50.
8. Silberstein EB. Comparison of outcomes after (123)I versus (131)I pre-ablation imaging before radioiodine ablation in differentiated thyroid carcinoma. J Nucl Med. 2007;48:1043-6.

9. Avram AM, Fig LM, Frey KA, Gross MD, Wong KK. Preablation 131-I scans with SPECT/CT in postoperative thyroid cancer patients: what is the impact on staging? J Clin Endocrinol Metab. 2013;98:1163-71.

10. Chen MK, Yasrebi M, Samii J, Staib LH, Doddamane I, Cheng DW. The utility of I-123 pretherapy scan in I-131 radioiodine therapy for thyroid cancer. Thyroid. 2012;22:304-9.

11. Van Nostrand D, Aiken M, Atkins F, Moreau S, Garcia C, Acio E, et al. The utility of radioiodine scans prior to iodine 131 ablations in patients with well-differentiated thyroid cancer. Thyroid. 2009;19:849-55.

12. Ross DS, Litofsky D, Ain KB, Bigos T, Brierley JD, Cooper DS, et al. Recurrence after treatment of micropapillary thyroid cancer. Thyroid. 2009;19:1043-8.

13. Bal CS, Kumar A, Pant GS. Radioiodine dose for remnant ablation in differentiated thyroid carcinoma: a randomized clinical trial in 509 patients. J Clin Endocrinol Metab. 2004;89:1666-73.

14. Haugen BR, Alexander EK, Bible KC, Doherty GM, Mandel SJ, Nikiforov YE, et al. 2015 American Thyroid Association Management Guidelines for Adult Patients with Thyroid Nodules and Differentiated Thyroid Cancer: The American Thyroid Association Guidelines Task Force on Thyroid Nodules and Differentiated Thyroid Cancer. Thyroid. 2016;26:1-133.

15. Mallick U, Harmer C, Yap B, Wadsley J, Clarke S, Moss L, et al. Ablation with low-dose radioiodine and thyrotropin alfa in thyroid cancer. N Engl J Med. 2012;366:1674-85.

16. Lassmann M, Reiners C, Luster M. Dosimetry and thyroid cancer: the individual dosage of radioiodine. Endocr Relat Cancer. 2010;17:R161-72.

17. Higashi T, Nishii R, Yamada S, Nakamoto Y, Ishizu K, Kawase S, et al. Delayed initial radioactive iodine therapy resulted in poor survival in patients with metastatic differentiated thyroid carcinoma: a retrospective statistical analysis of 198 cases. J Nucl Med. 2011;52:683-9.

18. Chopra S, Garg A, Ballal S, Bal CS. Lung metastases from differentiated thyroid carcinoma: prognostic factors related to remission and disease-free survival. Clin Endocrinol (Oxf). 2015;82:445-52.

19. Leboulleux S, Schroeder PR, Schlumberger M, Ladenson PW. The role of PET in the follow-up of patients treated for differentiated epithelial thyroid cancers. Nat Clin Pract Endocrinol Metab. 2007;3:112-21.

20. Robbins RJ, Wan Q, Grewal RK, Reibke R, Gonen M, Strauss HW, et al. Real-time prognosis for metastatic thyroid carcinoma based on 2-[18F]fluoro-2-deoxy-D-glucose-positron emission tomography scanning. J Clin Endocrinol Metab. 2006;91: 498-505.

21. Brose MS, Smit J, Capdevila J, Elisei R, Nutting C, Pitoia F, et al. Regional approaches to the management of patients with advanced, radioactive iodine-refractory differentiated thyroid carcinoma. Expert Rev Anticancer Ther. 2012;12:1137-47.

22. Tuttle RM, Ahuja S, Avram AM, Bernet VJ, Bourguet P, Daniels GH, et al. Controversies, Consensus, and Collaboration in the Use of 131 I Therapy in Differentiated Thyroid Cancer: A Joint Statement from the American Thyroid Association, the European Association of Nuclear Medicine, the Society of Nuclear Medicine and Molecular Imaging, and the European Thyroid Association. Thyroid. 2019;29:461-70.

23. Brose MS, Nutting CM, Jarzab B, Elisei R, Siena S, Bastholt L, et al. Sorafenib in radioactive iodine-refractory, locally advanced or metastatic differentiated thyroid cancer: a randomised, double-blind, phase 3 trial. Lancet. 2014;384:319-28.

24. Schlumberger M, Tahara M, Wirth LJ, Robinson B, Brose MS, Elisei R, et al. Lenvatinib versus placebo in radioiodine-refractory thyroid cancer. N Engl J Med. 2015;372:621-30.

25. Cohen EE, Rosen LS, Vokes EE, Kies MS, Forastiere AA, Worden FP, et al. Axitinib is an active treatment for all histologic subtypes of advanced thyroid cancer: results from a phase II study. J Clin Oncol. 2008;26:4708-13.

26. Wells SA, Asa SL, Dralle H, Elisei R, Evans DB, Gagel RF, et al. Revised American Thyroid Association guidelines for the management of medullary thyroid carcinoma. Thyroid. 2015;25:567-610.

27. Smallridge RC, Ain KB, Asa SL, Bible KC, Brierley JD, Burman KD, et al. American Thyroid Association guidelines for the management of patients with anaplastic thyroid cancer. Thyroid. 2012;22:1104-39.

28. Greenspan BS, Dillehay G, Intenzo C, Lavely WC, O'Doherty M, Palestro CJ, et al. SNM practice guideline for parathyroid scintigraphy 4.0. J Nucl Med Technol. 2012;40:111-8.

29. Lundgren E, Rastad J, Thrufjell E, Akerstrom G, Ljunghall S. Population-based screening for primary hyperparathyroidism with serum calcium and parathyroid hormone values in menopausal women. Surgery. 1997;121:287-94.

30. Udelsman R. Six hundred fifty-six consecutive explorations for primary hyperparathyroidism. Ann Surg. 2002;235:665-72.

31. Bilezikian JP, Brandi ML, Eastell R, Silverberg SJ, Udelsman R, Marcocci C, et al. Guidelines for the management of asymptomatic primary hyperparathyroidism: summary statement from the Fourth International Workshop. J Clin Endocrinol Metab. 2014;99:3561-9.

32. Russell CF, Edis AJ. Surgery for primary hyperparathyroidism: experience with 500 consecutive cases and evaluation of the role of surgery in the asymptomatic patient. Br J Surg. 1982;69:244-7.

33. Greene AB, Butler RS, McIntyre S, Barbosa GF, Mitchell J, Berber E, et al. National trends in parathyroid surgery from 1998 to 2008: a decade of change. J Am Coll Surg. 2009;209:332-43.

34. Chiu ML, Kronange JF, Piwnica-Worms D. Effect of mitochondrial and plasma membrane potentials on the accumulation of hexakis (2-methoxyisobutylisonitrile) technetium in cultured mouse fibroblasts. J Nucl Med. 1990;31:1646-53.

35. Sandrock D, Menno Mi, Norton JA, Benton CS, Miller DL, Neumann RD. Light- and electron-microscopic analyses of parathyroid tumours explain results of Tl-20l/Tc-99m parathyroid scintigraphy. Eur J Nucl Med. 1989;15:410.

36. Lorberboym M, Minski I, Macadziob S, Nikolov G, Schachter P. Incremental diagnostic value of preoperative 99mTc-MIBI SPECT in patients with a parathyroid adenoma. J Nucl Med. 2003;44:904-8.

37. Demetrius P, William BI, Michel G. Endocrine Surgery, 2nd edition. Boca Raton: CRC Press; 1929.

38. Prabhu M, Damle NA. Fluorocholine PET imaging of parathyroid disease. Indian J Endocrinol Metab. 2018;22:535-41.

39. Insogna KL. Primary hyperparathyroidism. N Engl J Med. 2018;379:1050-9.

40. Roy M, Mazeh H, Chen H, Sippel RS. Incidence and localization of ectopic parathyroid adenomas in previously unexplored patients. World J Surg. 2013;37:102-6.

41. Vulpio C, Bossola M, De Gaetano A, Maresca G, Bruno I, Fadda G, et al. Usefulness of the combination of ultrasonography and 99mTc-sestamibi scintigraphy in the preoperative evaluation of uremic secondary hyperparathyroidism. Head Neck. 2010;32:1226-35.

42. Traub-Weidinger T, Mayerhoefer ME, Koperek O, Mitterhauser M, Duan H, Karanikas G, et al. ^{11}C-methionine PET/CT imaging of 99mTc-MIBI-SPECT/CT-negative patients with primary hyperparathyroidism and previous neck surgery. J Clin Endocrinol Metab. 2014;99:4199-205.

43. Evangelista L, Sorgato N, Torresan F, Boschin IM, Pennelli G, Saladini G, et al. FDG-PET/CT and parathyroid carcinoma: Review of literature and illustrative case series. World J Clin Oncol. 2011;2:348-54.

44. Lezaic L, Rep S, Sever MJ, Kocjan T, Hocevar M, Fettich J. ^{18}F-Fluorocholine PET/CT for localization of hyperfunctioning parathyroid tissue in primary hyperparathyroidism: a pilot study. Eur J Nucl Med Mol Imaging. 2014;41:2083-9.

45. Casara D, Rubello D, Pelizzo MR, Shapiro B. Clinical role of 99mTcO4/MIBI scan, ultrasound and intraoperative gamma probe in the performance of unilateral and minimally invasive surgery in primary hyperparathyroidism. Eur J Nucl Med. 2001;28:1351-9.

46. Buicko JL, Kichler KM, Amundson JR, Scurci S, Kozol R. The sestamibi paradox: Improving intraoperative localization of parathyroid adenomas. Am Surg. 2017;83:832-5.

47. Murphy C, Norman J. The 20% rule: a simple, instantaneous radioactivity measurement defines cure and allows the elimination of frozen sections and hormone assays during parathyroidectomy. Surgery. 1999;126:1023-8.

48. Eisenhofer G, Lenders JW, Goldstein DS, Mannelli M, Csako G, Walther MM, et al. Pheochromocytoma catecholamine phenotypes and prediction of tumour size and location by use of plasma free metanephrines. Clin Chem. 2005;51:735-44.

49. Pamporaki C, Hamplova B, Peitzsch M, Prejbisz A, Beuschlein F, Timmers H, et al. Characteristics of pediatric vs adult pheochromocytomas and paragangliomas. J Clin Endocrinol Metab. 2017;102:1122-32.

50. DeLellis RA, Lloyd RV, Heitz PU, Eng C. Pathology and Genetics of Tumours of Endocrine Organs (IARC WHO Classification of Tumours). France: World Health Organization; 2004.

51. Lee KY, Oh YW, Noh HJ, Lee YJ, Yong HS, Kang EY, et al. Extra-adrenal paragangliomas of the body: imaging features. Am J Roentgenol. 2006;187:492-504.

52. El-Tholoth HS, Al Rasheed S, Alharbi F, Alshammari W, Alzahrani T, Al Zahrani A. Paraganglioma of Urinary Bladder Managed by Laparoscopic Partial Cystectomy in Conjunction with Flexible Cystoscopy: A Case Report. J Endourol Case Rep. 2018;4:15-7.

53. Ayala-Ramirez M, Feng L, Johnson MM, Ejaz S, Habra MA, Rich T, et al. Clinical risk factors for malignancy and overall survival in patients with pheochromocytomas and sympathetic paragangliomas: primary tumour size and primary tumour location as prognostic indicators. J Clin Endocrinol Metab. 2011;96:717-25.

54. Lenders JW, Duh QY, Eisenhofer G, Gimenez-Roqueplo AP, Grebe SK, Murad MH, et al. Pheochromocytoma and paraganglioma: an endocrine society clinical practice guideline. J Clin Endocrinol Metab. 2014;99:1915-42.

55. Jacques AET, Sahdev A, Sandrasagara M, Goldstein R, Berney D, Rockall AG, et al. Adrenal phaeochromocytoma: correlation of MRI appearances with histology and function. Eur Radiol. 2008;18:2885-92.

56. Taïeb D, Hicks RJ, Pacak K. Radiopharmaceuticals in paraganglioma imaging: too many members on board? Eur J Nucl Med Mol Imaging. 2016;43:391-3.

57. Bomanji J, Levison DA, Flatman WD, Horne T, Bouloux PM, Ross G, et al. Uptake of iodine-123 MIBG by pheochromocytomas, paragangliomas, and neuroblastomas: a histopathological comparison. J Nucl Med. 1987;28:973-8.

58. Ilias I, Chen CC, Carrasquillo JA, Whatley M, Ling A, Lazurova I, et al. Comparison of 6-18F-fluorodopamine PET with 123Imetaiodobenzylguanidine and 111In-pentetreotide scintigraphy in localization of nonmetastatic and metastatic pheochromocytoma. J Nucl Med. 2008;49:1613-9.

59. Koopmans KP, Jager PL, Kema IP, Kerstens MN, Albers F, Dullaart RP. 111In-octreotide is superior to 123Imetaiodobenzylguanidine for scintigraphic detection of head and neck paragangliomas. J Nucl Med. 2008;49:1232-7.

60. Tenenbaum F, Lumbroso J, Schlumberger M, Mure A, Plouin PF, Caillou B, et al. Comparison of radiolabeled octreotide and metaiodobenzylguanidine (MIBG) scintigraphy in malignant pheochromocytoma. J Nucl Med. 1995;36:1-6.

61. Krenning EP, de Jong M, Kooij PP, Breeman WA, Bakker WH, de Herder WW, et al. Radiolabelled somatostatin analogue(s) for peptide receptor scintigraphy and radionuclide therapy. Ann Oncol. 1999;10:S23-9.

62. Han S, Suh CH, Woo S, Kim YJ, Lee JJ. Performance of ^{68}Ga-DOTA-Conjugated Somatostatin Receptor Targeting Peptide PET in Detection of Pheochromocytoma and Paraganglioma: A Systematic Review and Metaanalysis. J Nucl Med. 2019;60:369-76.

63. Gross MD, Valk TW, Swanson DP, Thrall JH, Grekin RJ, Beirewaltes WH. The role of pharmacologic manipulation in adrenal cortical scintigraphy. Semin Nucl Med. 1981;11:128-48.

64. Hennings J, Lindhe O, Bergström M, Långström B, Sundin A, Hellman P. [11C]metomidate positron emission tomography of adrenocortical tumors in correlation with histopathological findings. J Clin Endocrinol Metab. 2006;91:1410-4.

65. Avram AM, Fig LM, Gross MD. Adrenal gland scintigraphy. Semin Nucl Med. 2006;36:212-27.

66. Schteingart DE, Seabold JE, Gross MD, Swanson DP. Iodocholesterol adrenal tissue uptake and imaging in adrenal neoplasms. J Clin Endocrinol Metab. 1981;52:1156-61.

67. Isidori AM, Sbardella E, Zatelli MC, Boschetti M, Vitale G, Colao A, et al. Conventional and nuclear medicine imaging in ectopic Cushing's syndrome: a systematic review. J Clin Endocrinol Metab. 2015;100:3231-44.

68. Young WF. Primary aldosteronism: the renaissance of a syndrome. Clin Endocrinol (Oxf). 2007;66:607-18.

69. Young WF, Stanson AW, Thompson GB, Grant CS, Farley DR, van Heerden JA. The role of adrenal venous sampling in primary aldosteronism. Surgery. 2004;136:1227-35.

70. Rossi GP, Sacchetto A, Chiesura-Corona M, De Toni R, Gallina M, Feltrin GP, et al. Identification of the etiology of primary aldosteronism with adrenal vein sampling in patients with equivocal computed tomography and magnetic resonance findings: results in 104 consecutive cases. J Clin Endocrinol Metab. 2001;86:1083-90.

71. Burton TJ, Mackenzie IS, Balan K, Koo B, Bird N, Soloviev DV, et al. Evaluation of the sensitivity and specificity of (11) C-metomidate positron emission tomography (PET)-CT for lateralizing aldosterone secretion by Conn's adenomas. J Clin Endocrinol Metab. 2012;97:100-9.

72. Kloos RT, Gross MD, Francis IR, Korobkin M, Shapiro B. Incidentally discovered adrenal masses. Endocr Rev. 1995;16:460-84.

73. Barzon L, Sonino N, Fallo F, Palu G, Boscaro M. Prevalence and natural history of adrenal incidentalomas. Eur J Endocrinol. 2003;149:273-85.

74. Mantero F, Terzolo M, Arnaldi G, Osella G, Masini AM, Ali A, et al. A survey on adrenal incidentaloma in Italy. Study Group

on Adrenal Tumors of the Italian Society of Endocrinology. J Clin Endocrinol Metab. 2000;85:637-44.

75. Fassnacht M, Arlt W, Bancos I, Dralle H, Newell-Price J, Sahdev A, et al. Management of adrenal incidentalomas: European Society of Endocrinology Clinical Practice Guideline in collaboration with the European Network for the Study of Adrenal Tumors. Eur J Endocrinol. 2016;175:G1-34.

76. Boland GW, Lee MJ, Gazelle GS, Halpern EF, McNicholas MM, Mueller PR. Characterization of adrenal masses using unenhanced CT: an analysis of the CT literature. Am J Roentgenol. 1998;171:201-4.

77. Haider MA, Ghai S, Jhaveri K, Lockwood G. Chemical shift MR imaging of hyperattenuating (>10 HU) adrenal masses: does it still have a role? Radiology. 2004;231:711-6.

78. Yun M, Kim W, Alnafisi N, Lacorte L, Jang S, Alavi A. 18F-FDG PET in characterizing adrenal lesions detected on CT or MRI. J Nucl Med. 2001;42:1795-9.

79. Boland GW, Blake MA, Holalkere NS, Hahn PF. PET/CT for the characterization of adrenal masses in patients with cancer: qualitative versus quantitative accuracy in 150 consecutive patients. Am J Roentgenol. 2009;192:956-62.

80. Schimmack S, Svejda B, Lawrence B, Kidd M, Modlin IM. The diversity and commonalities of gastroenteropancreatic neuroendocrine tumours. Langenbecks Arch Surg. 2011;396:273-98.

81. Yao JC, Hassan M, Phan A, Dagohoy C, Leary C, Mares JE, et al. One hundred years after "carcinoid": epidemiology of and prognostic factors for neuroendocrine tumors in 35,825 cases in the United States. J Clin Oncol. 2008;26:3063-72.

82. Lawrence B, Gustafsson BI, Chan A, Svejda B, Kidd M, Modlin IM. The epidemiology of gastroenteropancreatic neuroendocrine tumors. Endocrinol Metab Clin North Am. 2011;40:1-18.

83. Chang S, Choi D, Lee SJ, Lee WJ, Park MH, Kim SW, et al. Neuroendocrine neoplasms of the gastrointestinal tract: classification, pathologic basis, and imaging features. Radiographics. 2007;27:1667-79.

84. Oberg K. Pancreatic endocrine tumors. Semin Oncol. 2010;37:594-618.

85. Bosman F, Carneiro F, Hruban RH, Theise N. WHO Classification of Tumors of the Digestive System. France: IARC Press; 2010.

86. Lloyd RV, Osamura RY, Kloppel G. WHO Classification of Tumors of Endocrine Organs, 4th edition. France: IARC Press; 2017.

87. Tan EH, Tan CH. Imaging of gastroenteropancreatic neuroendocrine tumors. World J Clin Oncol. 2011;2:28-43.

88. Dumortier J, Ratineau C, Roche C, Lombard-Bohas C, Chayvialle JA, Scoazec JY. Angiogenesis and endocrine tumors. Bull Cancer. 1999;86:148-53.

89. Oberg K. Diagnostic pathways. In: Oberg K (Ed). Handbook of Neuroendocrine Tumors. England: BioScientifica; 2006. pp. 101-21.

90. Bombardieri E, Maccauro M, De Deckere E, Savelli G, Chiti A. Nuclear medicine imaging of neuroendocrine tumors. Ann Oncol. 2001;12:S51-61.

91. Hope TA, Bergsland EK, Bozkurt MF, Graham M, Heaney AP, Herrmann K, et al. Appropriate use criteria for somatostatin receptor PET imaging in neuroendocrine tumors. J Nucl Med. 2018;59:66-74.

92. de Herder WW, Niederle B, Scoazec JY, Pauwels S, Kloppel G, Falconi M, et al. Well-differentiated pancreatic tumor/carcinoma: insulinoma. Neuroendocrinology. 2006;84: 183-8.

93. Reubi JC, Waser B. Concomitant expression of several peptide receptors in neuroendocrine tumors: Molecular basis for in vivo multireceptor tumor targeting. Eur J Nucl Med Mol Imaging. 2003;30:781-93.

94. Meier JJ, Nauck MA. Glucagon-like peptide-1 (GLP-1) in biology and pathology. Diabetes Metab Res Rev. 2005;21:91-117.

95. Pallavi UN, Malasani V, Sen I, Thakral P, Dureja S, Pant V, et al. Molecular Imaging to the Surgeons Rescue: Gallium-68 DOTA-Exendin-4 Positron Emission Tomography-Computed Tomography in Pre-operative Localization of Insulinomas. Indian J Nucl Med. 2019;34(1):14-8.

96. Luo Y, Pan Q, Yao S, Yu M, Wu W, Xue H, et al. Glucagon-Like Peptide-1 Receptor PET/CT with 68Ga-NOTA-Exendin-4 for Detecting Localized Insulinoma: A Prospective Cohort Study. J Nucl Med. 2016;57:715-20.

97. Bodei L, Mueller-Brand J, Baum RP, Pavel ME, Hörsch D, O'Dorisio MS, et al. The joint IAEA, EANM, and SNMMI practical guidance on peptide receptor radionuclide therapy (PRRNT) in neuroendocrine tumours. Eur J Nucl Med Mol Imaging. 2013;40:800-16.

98. Valkema R, De Jong M, Bakker WH, Breeman WA, Kooij PP, Lugtenburg PJ, et al. Phase I study of peptide receptor radionuclide therapy with [In-DTPA]-octreotide: the Rotterdam experience. Semin Nucl Med. 2002;32:110-22.

99. Kwekkeboom DJ, de Herder WW, Kam BL, van Eijck CH, van Essen M, Kooij PP, et al. Treatment with the radiolabeled somatostatin analogue [177Lu-DOTA0, Tyr3] octreotate: toxicity, efficacy, and survival. J Clin Oncol. 2008;26:2124-30.

100. Strosberg J, El-Haddad G, Wolin E, Hendifar A, Yao J, Chasen B, et al. Phase 3 trial of ^{177}Lu-dotatate for midgut neuroendocrine tumors. N Engl J Med. 2017;376:125-35.

101. Fournet JC, Junien C. The genetics of neonatal hyperinsulinism. Horm Res. 2003;59:30.

102. Kane C, Shepherd RM, Squires PE, Johnson PR, James RF, Millia PJ, et al. Loss of functional KATP channels in pancreatic beta-cells causes persistent hyperinsulinemic hypoglycemia of infancy. Nat Med. 1996;2:1344-7.

103. Gills D. (2003). Gene Reviews Monograph on Familial Hyperinsulinism. [online] Available from http://www.ncbi.nlm.nih.gov/books/NBK1375/. [Last accessed April, 2020].

104. Stanley CA, Lieu YK, Hsu BY, Burlina AB, Greenberg CR, Hopwood NJ, et al. Hyperinsulinism and hyperammonemia in infants with regulatory mutations of the glutamate dehydrogenase gene. N Engl J Med. 1998;338:1352-7.

105. Flanagan SE, Kapoor RR, Hussain K. Genetics of congenital hyperinsulinemic hypoglycemia. Semin Pediatr Surg. 2011;20:13-7.

106. Fournet JC, Mayaud C, de Lonlay P, Gross-Morand MS, Verkarre V, Castanet M, et al. Unbalanced expression of 11p15 imprinted genes in focal forms of congenital hyperinsulinism: association with a reduction to homozygosity of a mutation in ABCC8 or KCNJ11. Am J Pathol. 2001;158:2177-84.

107. de Lonlay-Debeney P, Poggi-Travert F, Fournet JC, Sempoux C, Dionisi Vici C, Brunelle F, et al. Clinical features of 52 neonates with hyperinsulinism. N Engl J Med. 1999;340:1169-75.

108. Christiansen CD, Petersen H, Nielsen AL, Detlefsen S, Brusgaard K, Rasmussen L, et al. 18F-DOPA PET/CT and 68Ga-DOTANOC PET/CT scans as diagnostic tools in focal congenital hyperinsulinism: a blinded evaluation. Eur J Nucl Med Mol Imaging. 2018;45:250-61.

109. Yoo SC, Chang KH, Lyu MO, Chang SJ, Ryu HS, Kim HS. Clinical characteristics of struma ovarii. J Gynecol Oncol. 2008;19: 135-8.

110. Outwater EK, Siegelman ES, Hunt JL. Ovarian teratomas: tumor types and imaging characteristics. Radiographics. 2001;21:475-90.

111. Gould SF, Lopez RL, Speers WC. Malignant struma ovarii. A case report and literature review. J Reprod Med. 1983;28:415-9.

112. Ross DS. Syndromes of thyrotoxicosis with low radioactive iodine uptake. Endocrinol North Am. 1998;27:169-85.

113. DeSimone CP, Lele SM, Modesitt SC. Malignant struma ovarii: a case report and analysis of cases reported in the literature with a focus on survival and I131 therapy. Gynecol Oncol. 2003;89:543-8.

114. Goffredo P, Sawka AM, Pura J, Adam MA, Roman SA, Sosa JA. Malignant struma ovarii: a population-level analysis of a large series of 68 patients. Thyroid. 2015;25:211-5.

115. Al Hassan MS, Saafan T, El Ansari W, Al Ansari AA, Zirie MA, Farghaly H, et al. The largest reported papillary thyroid carcinoma arising in struma ovarii and metastasis to the opposite ovary: case report and review of the literature. Thyroid Res. 2018;11:10.

116. Luo J, Xie C, Li Z. Treatment for Malignant Struma Ovarii in the Eyes of Thyroid Surgeons: A Case Report and Study of Chinese Cases Reported in the Literature. Medicine (Baltimore). 2014;93:e147.

117. Rose PG, Arafah B, Abdul-Karim FW. Malignant struma ovarii: recurrence and response to treatment monitored by thyroglobulin levels. Gynecol Oncol. 1998;70:425-7.

118. Chong WH, Molinolo AA, Chen CC, Collins MT. Tumor-induced osteomalacia. Endocr Relat Cancer. 2011;18:53-77.

119. Yamazaki Y, Okazaki R, Shibata M, Hasegawa Y, Satoh K, Tajima T, et al. Increased circulatory level of biologically active full-length FGF-23 in patients with hypophosphatemic rickets/osteomalacia. J Clin Endocrinol Metab. 2002;87:4957-60.

120. Takeuchi Y, Suzuki H, Ogura S, Imai R, Yamazaki Y, Yamashita T, et al. Venous sampling for fibroblast growth factor-23 confirms the preoperative diagnosis of tumor-induced osteomalacia. J Clin Endocrinol Metab. 2004;89:3979-82.

121. El-Maouche D, Sadowski SM, Papadakis GZ, Guthrie L, Cottle-Delisle C, Merkel R, et al. 68Ga-DOTATATE for tumor localization in tumor-induced osteomalacia. J Clin Endocrinol Metab. 2016;101:3575-81.

122. Chong WH, Andreopoulou P, Chen CC, Reynolds J, Guthrie L, Kelly M, et al. Tumor localization and biochemical response to cure in tumor-induced osteomalacia. J Bone Miner Res. 2013;28:1386-98.

123. Hesse E, Rosenthal H, Bastian L. Radiofrequency ablation of a tumor causing oncogenic osteomalacia. N Engl J Med. 2007;357:422-4.

124. Tella SH, Amalou H, Wood BJ, Chang R, Chen CC, Robinson C, et al. Multimodality image-guided cryoablation for inoperable tumor-induced osteomalacia. J Bone Miner Res. 2017;32:2248-56.

125. Geller JL, Khosravi A, Kelly MH, Riminucci M, Adams JS, Collins MT. Cinacalcet in the management of tumor-induced osteomalacia. J Bone Miner Res. 2007;22:931-7.

126. Basu S, Fargose P. 177Lu-DOTATATE PRRT in recurrent skull-base phosphaturic mesenchymal tumor causing osteomalacia: a potential application of PRRT beyond neuroendocrine tumors. J Nucl Med Technol. 2016;44:248-50.

CHAPTER 43

Anesthesia for Endocrine Surgery

Shilpi Misra, Deepak Malviya

INTRODUCTION

Patients with *primary or coexisting endocrine diseases* pose numerous unique challenges during surgical and anesthetic management. *Safe and quality anesthesia practices* mandate a thorough preoperative assessment and preparation of the patient for endocrine surgery.

The most common comorbidity encountered in surgical patients is endocrinopathies. Anesthesia for endocrine surgery is different from that for routine procedures. *The neurotransmitter and hormonal secretion occurring with a deranged endocrinal milieu in the perioperative period can be highly variable and unpredictable.* With recent advances in anesthesia techniques, endocrine anesthesia is now a rapidly evolving specialty.[1]

The underlying endocrinopathies involving pituitary, thyroid, parathyroid, pancreas, adrenal, can have a direct impact on the immediate perioperative management and the surgical outcome.[2-6]

THYROID SURGERY AND ANESTHESIA

Amongst the various endocrine surgical procedure, thyroidectomy is the most common being encountered with the anesthesiologists. The risk of surgical procedure may range from simple solitary nodule excision to potential high risk involved with removal of retrosternal goiter.[7]

Patients may have hypothyroidism or hyperthyroidism with deranged thyroid functions[8] and can have significantly different implications for anesthetic management.

Medical treatment of altered thyroid function (hypothyroidism or hyperthyroidism) may require several weeks to achieve a new steady state. Evaluation and treatment of altered thyroid status is required before taking up the patient for thyroid surgery. Patient's thyroid status guides in predicting sensitivity to drugs commonly administered in the perioperative period, physiological and hemodynamic responses during surgery and anesthesia.

Anesthetic consideration during thyroid surgery involves the following:

- *Difficult airway*: Long-standing thyroid swelling compressing over trachea and retrosternal goiter can pose potential difficult airway management for the anesthesiologist.
- *The positioning of patient and complexity of surgical intervention*: During the surgery after the patient is positioned head-up and extended, the endotracheal tube (ETT) should be checked and secured to avoid tube dislodgement and endobronchial intubation.
- *Potential risk of uncontrolled hemorrhage*: Due to position of thyroid gland in close vicinity to major vessels, intraoperative and postoperative bleeding risks always exist.
- Any associated cardiac derangement and the presence of other comorbidities.

PREANESTHETIC ASSESSMENT

Preoperative optimization for thyroid surgery involves coordinated team effort of endocrinologist, cardiologist, radiologist, surgeon, and anesthesiologist.

HISTORY

Thorough history taking guides for perioperative preparation of the patient and better surgical outcome.

- During preanesthetic evaluation, any symptom related to thyroid derangement (hypo/hyperthyroidism) or any other comorbid medical condition should be assessed.
- Pressure symptoms due to enlarged or long-standing thyroid swelling such as dyspnea, orthopnea, dysphagia, stridor, and voice change should be elicited.
- Factors making patient prone for developing tracheomalacia such as large sized thyroid swelling presenting for long duration should be sought.[9,10]
- Rapidly increasing size of the thyroid swelling suggests the possibility of malignancy or due to hemorrhage that can cause airway management difficulty.
- Multiple endocrine neoplasia (MEN) syndrome should be ruled out in patients presenting with autonomic nervous system dysfunction symptoms.[11]

Primary aim should be to ensure euthyroid state and assessment and preparation for anticipated difficult airway.

EXAMINATION

General Examination

Pulse rate: Resting tachycardia and irregularly irregular rhythm (atrial fibrillation) should be excluded to rule out signs of hyperthyroidism.

The position of trachea should be checked for any deviation from midline and tracheal compression ruled out after listening to stridor.

Examination of Goiter

- The inspection and palpation of the thyroid swelling for size, consistency, mobility, and extent of enlargement should be done.
- Mobile and firm swelling indicates benign while fixed and hard consistency points toward malignancy.
- Large goiter with inability to feel the lower border of the swelling indicates retrosternal extension. The compression effect on the surrounding vital structures because of retrosternal extension of a large thyroid gland may cause superior venocaval obstruction syndrome, pleural and pericardial effusion, and Horner syndrome.[12]

Thyroid surgery is a case of anticipated difficult airway thus thorough *airway examination* should be performed which includes the following:

- Mouth opening by assessing inter incisor gap, loose tooth, artificial denture, protruding incisors, protruding or retrognathic mandible.
- Neck mobility to assess extension and flexion assessment of neck movements (especially atlantoaxial flexion and extension)
- Estimation of hyomental, thyromental and sternomental distance
- Grading of Mallampati score
  Infiltrating malignancy and large swelling with retrosternal extension may make neck movement, and hence intubation, difficult.[13]

Routine Investigations

Hematological

- Complete blood count, thyroid function tests, serum electrolytes (sodium, potassium, and calcium), blood glucose, coagulation profile, and hepatic and renal profile
- Electrocardiogram (ECG) (echocardiography in cases of associated cardiovascular comorbidities)

Indirect Laryngoscopy

Owing to the close proximity of recurrent laryngeal nerve with the thyroid gland, the surgeries have greater risk of nerve injury. IL is thus done to see the normal vocal cord mobility and rule out any pre-existing vocal cord palsy for medicolegal purposes.[14]

Radiological: X-ray chest posteroanterior (PA) view, X-ray neck anteroposterior, and lateral view for assessing any tracheal deviation and compression.

In cases of large-sized thyroid gland with retrosternal extension, *computed tomography (CT) scan or magnetic resonance imaging (MRI)* is performed to delineate the exact location and extension.[15]

Indirect laryngoscopy: To record any pre-existing vocal cord palsy. It is advisable for medicolegal purposes as 3–5% of population invariably has unilateral paralysis of vocal cords.[14]

CONCERNS WITH THYROID DISORDERS

The clinical manifestations of hypothyroidism include reduced cardiac output secondary to decreased stroke volume and heart rate, decreased plasma volume, decreased β-receptor activity, hyponatremia, water retention, depressed ventilatory drive, impaired hepatic metabolism, and gastrointestinal function.

Because of decreased rate of metabolism, the *hypothyroidism state prolongs the recovery from the effects of anesthetic agents.*

Patients with untreated profound hypothyroidism can present as critical emergency, myxoedema coma. Infection, surgical stress, trauma, exposure to cold, drug overdose of narcotic/anesthetic agents can be precipitating factors. Clinical manifestation include hypothermia, hypoventilation, hypotension, bradycardia, and hypoxemia which can progress to congestive heart failure (CHF) and pericardial effusion, if left untreated. Laboratory findings usually found are hypoglycemia, hyponatremia, hyperkalemia, hypercholesterolemia, anemia, decreased PO_2, and raised PCO_2 in arterial blood. The goal of management is to optimize and maintain hemodynamic, respiratory, and metabolic function. Intravenous administration of thyroid hormone therapy, L thyroxine 300–500 µg T4 bolus followed by daily doses of 50 µg/day or 25 µg T3 every 8 hourly for 24–48 hours. Most clinicians prefer L thyroxine because of its predictable onset of action and less adverse cardiac effects. One needs to be cautious while the drug administration as these drugs could precipitate CHF/myocardial ischemia. Intravenous hydration with dextrose saline, temperature regulation, correction of electrolytes and intravenous hydrocortisone is recommended.

Hyperthyroidism, or thyrotoxicosis is characterized by increased circulating levels of unbound thyroid hormones. The clinical manifestation include those of hypermetabolic state. Increased cardiac sensitivity to catecholamines results in hypertension and tachyarrhythmias, high output congestive heart failure. Patients usually present with tremors, hyperreflexia, irritability, nausea, vomiting, diarrhea, hepatic dysfunction, fever and heat intolerance. Hyperthyroid patients are prone for cardiovascular complications such as atrial fibrillation, exaggerated hypertension, and thyroid storm.[16]

Medical treatment for hyperthyroidism is accomplished by administration propylthiouracil (PTU) or methimazole (MMI) to reduce thyroid hormone synthesis. PTU has added advantage of inhibiting peripheral conversion of T4 to T3. High-dose iodine therapy also transiently inhibit new hormone synthesis (Wolff-Chaikoff effect).

Carbimazole, the commonly used drug in hyperthyroidism, poses patient for higher risk of bleeding and postoperative infection because of increased vascularity and reduced white blood cell (WBC) count. Potassium iodide was used previously, but this intervention takes a very long time, usually 4–6 weeks to make patient euthyroid.[17]

Decompensated hyperthyroidism patient can present as thyroid storm with cardinal features of cardiovascular collapse, CHF, arrhythmia, agitation, delirium, seizures/coma, hyperthermia and gastrointestinal disturbances such as diarrhea. Laboratory findings include elevated levels of T_4/T_3 and free T_4, hyperglycemia, leukocytosis with left shift, anemia, hypercalcemia, hypokalemia, and hypercortisolemia.

Thyroid storm is a medical emergency that should be managed to limit the catastrophic systemic effects. The treatment includes rapid alleviation of toxicity by controlled production of thyroid hormone, CHF, general supportive care to treat dehydration with infusion of crystalloid and temperature cooling with acetaminophen, β-adrenergic blockers for rate control, glucocorticoids, and circulatory support.[18]

◇ ANESTHETIC TECHNIQUES

- *General anesthesia in combination with cervical plexus block could safely be used as technique of choice.*
- Regional anesthesia has been used in a selected group of patients and have shown high levels of patient satisfaction.[19]
- Unilateral and bilateral superficial cervical plexus block with local supplementation or deep cervical plexus block have been described for thyroid surgery. Obese patients and patients who cannot communicate verbally are not good candidate for this technique. Deep cervical plexus block carries the associated risk of anesthetizing the phrenic nerve with resulting diaphragm dysfunction.

General Anesthesia

General anesthesia is the preferred anesthetic technique for thyroid surgery. General anesthesia has the advantages of patient comfort, amnesia, and immobility, along with control of the airway. If preoperative assessment anticipates difficult ventilation and intubation, the following preparation should be made.[20]

◇ DIFFICULT AIRWAY MANAGEMENT

Anticipated Difficult Ventilation and Intubation

Long-standing large thyroid swelling is considered as case of difficult ventilation and intubation. The relaxation caused by administration of general anesthesia (anesthetic agents and muscle relaxant) may lead to airway obstruction and inability to ventilate. A difficult airway cart with airway adjuncts such as oropharyngeal, nasopharyngeal airways, laryngeal mask airway (LMA), rigid bronchoscope, and jet ventilation should be kept ready.

Induction could be done in position to have least chance of airway obstruction and convenient for intubation, e.g., semi recumbent/semi supine.

Fiberoptic Intubation

This technique is useful in an anticipated difficult airway scenario such as retrosternal extension of goiter, compression or deviation of trachea, malignancy of thyroid causing fibrosis, and soft tissue involvement or co-existing airway problem (e.g., ankylosing spondylitis) making the laryngoscopic view extremely difficult. As the large thyroid swelling over trachea makes it difficult to perform laryngeal and transtracheal block, inhalational induction with sevoflurane or infusion of dexmedetomidine gives an advantage of least chances of airway obstruction.

Awake fiberoptic intubation should be performed with local/topical anesthesia of airway. Injection glycopyrrolate 0.2 mg IV is given in preoperative area. Nebulization with 4% lignocaine is done and xylometazoline drops put in each nostril. Lignocaine puffs are sprayed on posterior pharynx and tonsillar pillars and fiberoptic bronchoscope is advanced with "spray-as-you-go" technique **(Figs. 1A and B)**. Safe dose of lignocaine (5 mg/kg) should not be exceeded.

Availability of fiberoptic bronchoscope gives an edge over other conventional methods and is a boon to the attending anesthesiologist.

Ventilation through rigid bronchoscope and tracheostomy, which is difficult in cases of midline large swelling over trachea, should be kept as an option in scenarios where none of the above measures help. Intubation with help of bougie may also be used in some cases **(Figs. 2A to C)**.

Airway control often is achieved by intubation with a cuffed ETT. Studies have compared several different devices for intubation. The role of *electromyographic ETT* placement during thyroid surgery in neuromonitoring of recurrent laryngeal nerve has recently been advocated **(Fig. 3)**.[21,22]

Drugs for Intravenous Induction

Preoxygenation with 100% oxygen should always be done prior to induction as it enhances the functional residual volume and avoids rapid desaturation.

Patients are premedicated with injection glycopyrrolate and midazolam, shorter acting opioids such as fentanyl and remifentanil are preferably used. Induction is done with either thiopentone (3–5 mg/kg) or propofol in a dose of 2 mg/kg. In a difficult airway scenario, succinylcholine is preferred relaxant, keeping in mind the contraindications and arrhythmogenic potential. Vecuronium and rocuronium are the muscle relaxant of choice because of cardio stable characteristics. Intubation with armored ETT or Ring, Adair, and Elwyn (RAE) tube (North Pole) reduces the chance of kinking and respiratory obstruction during surgery. After intubation, the air inserted for cuff inflation is noted for absence of leak and

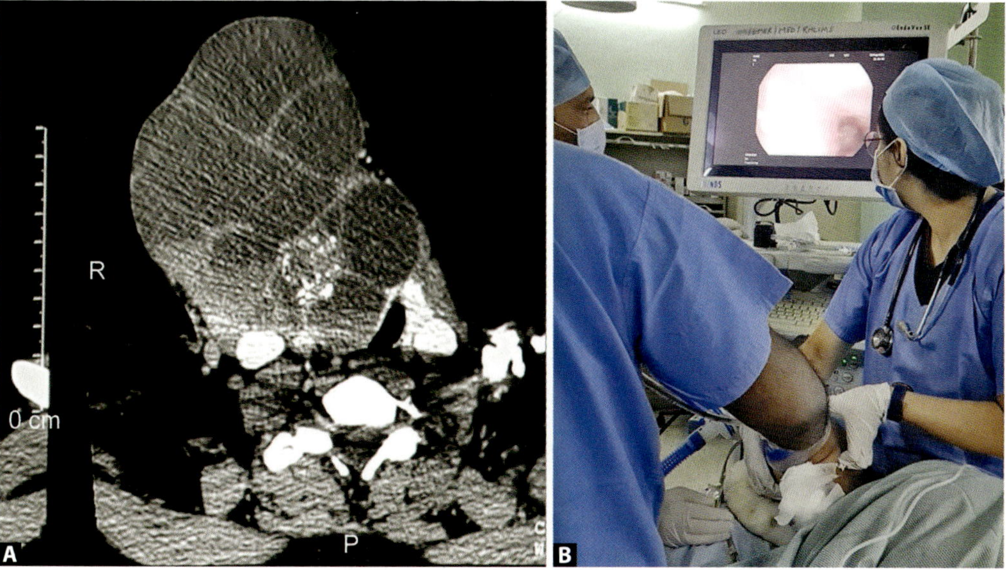

Figs. 1A and B: (A) CT scan with deviated airway; (B) Awake bronchoscopy with "spray-as-you-go" method.

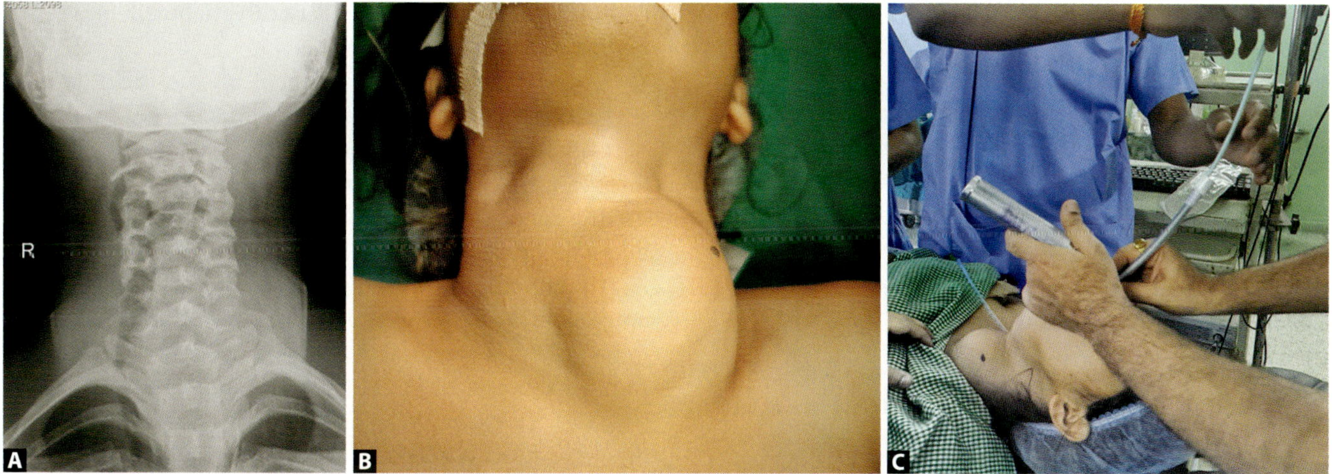

Figs. 2A to C: (A) X-ray neck with deviation of trachea to right; (B) Left STN measuring 8 × 6 × 4; (C) Intubation with help of bougie.

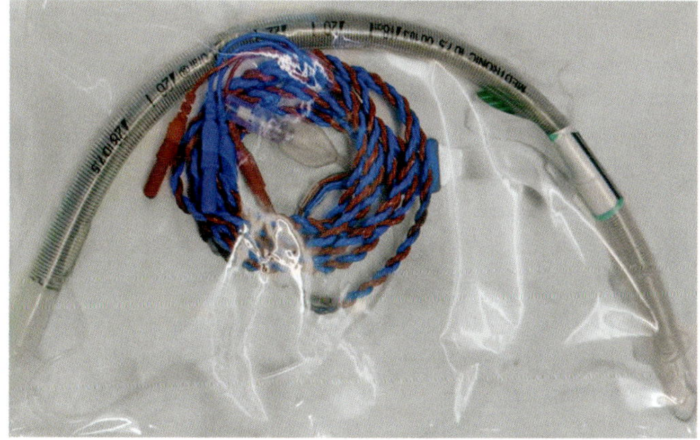

Fig. 3: Neuromonitoring tube.

should be correlated during extubation to rule out chances of tracheomalacia. Maintenance of anesthesia is done with oxygen: Air, inhalational agent, and incremental doses of muscle relaxant.

Positioning

The conventional position of patient during thyroid surgery is slight head up, with the head extended and stabilized using a head ring and sandbag between the scapulae.

Care should be taken during positioning for nerve/soft-tissue compression. Eyes are lubricated and taped and padded well especially those with proptosis and exophthalmos.

Monitoring

Owing to high vascularity and close proximity to airway, the thyroid surgery needs intense hemodynamic monitoring.

Baseline parameters monitored include heart rate, blood pressure, pulse oximetry, end tidal CO_2, and temperature. The muscle relaxant should be supplemented as per neuromuscular monitoring because of high incidence of hyperthyroid patients having associated myasthenia gravis.

Intraoperative administration of steroids, dexamethasone reduces the incidence of postoperative nausea and vomiting (PONV) and airway edema.

Extra vigilance is taken during extubation to reduce chances of stress response leading to accidental hemorrhage. Injection xylocard or dexmedetomidine proves beneficial for smooth extubation. The absence of leak around the deflated cuff should alert anesthesiologist to the possibility of tracheomalacia. Management include prolonged intubation (24-48 hrs postoperatively), although at time tracheostomy is necessary. Other more complicated treatment include Marlex mesh around trachea, tracheopexy or buttressing the trachea with plastic rings. The main disadvantage in carrying out extubation in a deeper plane of anesthesia is the possible failure of elicitation of vocal cord movements.

Some anesthesiologists prefer extubation to be performed with the patient fully awake and breathing spontaneously.

◇ POSTOPERATIVE ANALGESIA

For the prevention of postoperative pain, following strategies are implemented:
- Perioperative administration of paracetamol/nonsteroidal anti-inflammatory drugs/short-acting opioids
- Superficial cervical plexus blockade
- Postoperative infiltration of the wound site with local anesthetics

◇ PARATHYROID SURGERY

The parathyroid hormone (PTH) secreted via parathyroid glands maintain calcium homeostasis by their action mediated through bones and kidneys.[23]

Primary hyperthyroidism is caused by excessive production of PTH by abnormal parathyroid gland leading to elevation of total serum calcium levels. The most common symptoms include urological (nephrolithiasis), gastrointestinal, neuropsychiatric, musculoskeletal, fragility fractures, historically described as "stones, bones, abdominal groans, and psychic moans." Patients may have higher incidence of cardiovascular complications related to hypercalcemia,[24] impaired glucose tolerance, increased fracture risk, and poorer quality of life.[25]

Surgery is indicated in all patients with symptomatic primary hyperparathyroidism and asymptomatic individuals with severe hypercalcemia, markedly reduced creatinine clearance and/or profound osteopenia.

Anesthetic Considerations

Preanesthetic evaluation should include thorough investigations and optimization of clinical manifestation of hypercalcemia such as dehydration, vomiting, cardiovascular, and neuropsychiatric symptoms.[26] The main emphasis during the entire perioperative period is maintenance of normal serum calcium levels and hemodynamic stability. Apart from routine hematological investigation, renal work up is done to rule out nephrolithiasis and planning perioperative renoprotective drugs and fluid management.[27]

Technetium-99m Sestamibi scintigraphy enables to elect the minimally invasive parathyroidectomy approach after precise preoperative localization of parathyroid adenomas.[28]

Anesthesia for Parathyroid Surgery

Anesthesia techniques for parathyroidectomy can be general anesthesia or regional anesthesia. Regional techniques include combinations of deep and superficial cervical plexus blocks.

Cervical plexus block (CPB): The CPB has been used to provide adequate analgesia and anesthesia for the head and neck region and thyroid surgery. Ultrasound guidance has made the CPBs safe and accurate by identification of important landmarks including muscles, cervical vertebrae, large vessels, nerves, and the cervical fascia.

Superficial and deep cervical plexus block can be performed separately or in combination.

Contraindication to block include patient refusal, local infection, and radiation therapy to neck.

The cervical plexus is formed by the anterior division of four upper cervical nerves.

The superficial cervical plexus innervates the skin of the anterolateral neck. The superficial sensory branches are as follows: Lesser occipital (C2, C3), great auricular (C2, C3), transverse cervical (C2, C3), and supraclavicular nerves (C3, C4). The superficial CPB involves a multidirectional or single subcutaneous injection alongside the posterior border of the sternocleidomastoid muscle to block superficial branches of the cervical plexus by landmark or ultrasound technique.

The branches of deep cervical plexus innervate the deeper structure of neck, muscles of anterior neck, and diaphragm.

Deep CPB involves the placement of a needle between the prevertebral fascia and the cervical nerve roots at the C2–C4 level, needle should contact posterior tubercle of transverse process where the spinal nerve at individual levels is located just in front of tubercle. The complication of deep block includes inadvertent injection into the dural cuff or vertebral artery and phrenic nerve palsy. Bilateral deep cervical blocks should be avoided in view of respiratory compromise.

General anesthesia with tracheal intubation and muscle relaxants is still the preferred choice.

The technique and positioning are similar to thyroid surgery with less airway encroachment. Care should be taken during laryngoscopy as lytic lesions because of prolonged hypercalcemia make patients prone for pathological fractures and cervical spine injury. For any anticipated difficult airway, fiberoptic bronchoscope and LMA-assisted intubation should be done.

Positioning

Parathyroidectomy involves bilateral exploration of the neck and removal of the diseased gland or glands. Patient is positioned with neck extended and head up. Eyes should be padded and covered. Extension tubing is attached to intravenous access for drug administration.

Intraoperative monitoring includes noninvasive blood pressure, pulse oximetry, ECG with lead II and V5, temperature, and end-tidal carbon dioxide ($EtCO_2$). Intraoperative frozen section or parathyroid assays if performed can increase the operating times.

Neuromuscular monitoring is recommended for nondepolarizing muscle relaxant administration because of associated muscle weakness. The degree of muscle blockade should be monitored with train of four stimulations before extubation so as to prevent any potential respiratory compromise.

Dyselectrolytemia may cause inadequate reversal due to unpredictable augmentation of nondepolarizing neuromuscular blockade.

◇ HYPERCALCEMIC CRISIS

Severe calcium intoxication with serum calcium levels of 14-16 mg/dL (>3.5 mmol/L) is a rare and potentially life-threatening complication of primary hyperparathyroidism. Although the diagnostic criteria for hypercalcemic crisis are not yet well established, the most generally accepted criteria include an elevated serum intact parathyroid hormone level (iPTH) together with a substantial increase in the serum calcium level higher than 3.5mmol/L, associated with an acute onset of symptoms.

Presentations of hyperparathyroid crisis are heterogeneous, including nausea, vomiting, fatigue, altered sensorium, dehydration, decreased renal function, cardiac arrhythmias, mental alteration, confusion, and coma; if the condition is untreated, it may result in death.[6,7] The treatment of hyperparathyroid crisis begins with aggressive hydration, diuresis, and calcitonin and bisphosphonate administration.

- *Aggressive hydration*: Preferred fluid for infusion is normal saline.
- *Diuresis*: Forced diuresis is done with injection furosemide. Electrolyte imbalance may occur and serum levels of potassium, magnesium, and phosphate must be followed closely.
- Infusion of phosphates and bisphosphonates is treatment of choice for life-threatening hypercalcemia. In cases of calcium intoxication, IV/subcutaneous calcitonin is the agent of choice.
- Corticosteroids act by inhibiting gastrointestinal absorption of calcium in acute phase.

- Cautious use of drugs with very narrow therapeutic index, plicamycin, and mithramycin
- Hemodialysis is used as salvage therapy in patients with renal failure when the above options failed.

Parathyroidectomy is the only curative method for hyperparathyroid crisis. It involves the removal of the overactive gland, thereby lowering the levels of iPTH released into the blood and decreasing serum calcium levels.

Cardiac arrhythmias are common in patients with hyperparathyroid crisis. Hypercalcemia most often shortens ST-segment and consequently reduces QT interval. The presentations of severe cardiac arrhythmia can be highly variable, including tachy-brady syndrome, ventricular tachycardia, ventricular fibrillation, and paroxysmal atrioventricular block. Persistent hypercalcemia can also cause myocardial injury and heart failure.

Preoperative ECG and echocardiography are required to detect the function of cardiac conductivity and contractility.

Difficult airway, fluid depletion, electrolyte disorders, multiple organ dysfunction, hypercoagulability, and cardiac arrhythmias are the primary challenges in anesthetic management.

Postoperative Care

After tumor removal, the anesthesiologist should carefully monitor the circulation. Rapid serum calcium reduction can result in hypotension (loss of vascular tone), heart failure (impaired cardiac contractility), or myocardial infarction. Premature ventricular contractions and ventricular fibrillation can occur during severe hypocalcemia.

The mortality rate associated with hyperparathyroid crisis has gradually declined in recent years due to early diagnoses and improved medical interventions.

Hypocalcemia is the most common complication post-parathyroidectomy. Serum calcium should be routinely checked after surgery.

Hypocalcemia Symptoms

- Perioral tingling and muscular twitching
- *Neurological*: Confusion and seizures
- Tetany[29]

Clinical Assessment

- Chvostek and/or Trousseau sign
- *Cardiorespiratory*: Laryngospasm, prolongation of QT interval, and varied arrhythmias

Treatment

- Oral supplements if the Ca^+ levels are >2 mmol/L
- Intravenous injection of either calcium gluconate/calcium chloride if Ca^+ levels <2 mmol/L. Calcium chloride has three times more elemental calcium in a similar volume of injection.

Management of Postoperative Pain

- *Injection paracetamol/nonsteroidal anti-inflammatory drug (NSAID)*: NSAID to be avoided in patients with renal derangement
- Superficial cervical plexus blocks along with local infiltration.

Pheochromocytoma and Paraganglioma

Pheochromocytomas are neuroendocrine tumors arising in the adrenal medulla. These tumors may be benign or malignant. *The secretion of vasoactive substances, including the catecholamines (dopamine, norepinephrine, and epinephrine), leads to clinical manifestation of the tumor.* A neuroendocrine chromaffin tumor arising outside of the adrenal medulla is referred to as *paraganglioma*. Most pheochromocytomas are intra-adrenal (90%). Rarely, extra adrenal pheochromocytoma can be found in the paraganglia cells of the sympathetic nervous system, and the organ of Zuckerkandl.[30]

"Rule of 10" was previously associated with these tumors quoting as 10% of the tumors are bilateral, 10% are extra-adrenal, and 10% of the tumors are malignant. Pheochromocytoma may coexist with other syndromes such as MEN syndromes (MEN 2A and 2B), von Recklinghausen disease, and von Hippel Landau syndrome.[31,32]

There is higher prevalence of this tumor in females as compared to males in a ratio of 60:40.[33]

Pathophysiology of Catecholamine-secreting Pheochromocytoma

Symptoms of pheochromocytoma are mainly due to the excessive secretions of the catecholamines and to a smaller extent to some other hormones and peptides including somatostatin, calcitonin, and other adrenocorticotropic hormones (ACTHs), etc.[34]

Clinical Manifestations

- Paroxysmal tachycardia, hypertension (paroxysmal in 65% and sustained in 35% approximately), headache, palpitations, episodic sweating, and feeling of doom
- *Cardiovascular*: Arrhythmias, dilated cardiomyopathy, and peripheral vasoconstriction leading to cardiac failure
- *Neurological*: Anxiety, psychosis, and nervousness
- *Catastrophic*: Acute pulmonary edema, cardiac failure, severe metabolic acidosis, or fulminant toxemia during pregnancy[35]
- Clinical manifestation may differ with size of tumor, small tumors (<25 g) have typically brief paroxysms of catecholamine-induced symptoms, because released catecholamines are quickly taken up by postganglionic adrenergic neuron. Patients with larger tumors (>50 g), which are often malignant, may have sustained hypertension between paroxysmal attacks.[36]

Diagnosis through Investigation

- Free catecholamines/plasma catecholamines in a 24-hour period urine collection by high performance liquid chromatography confirm diagnosis.[37]
- *Imaging*: CT-scan or MRI for localization of tumor[38]

Anesthetic Considerations

Patients with pheochromocytoma are prone to intraoperative cardiovascular sequelae, hypertension, tachycardia, dysrhythmias, cardiac ischemia or myocardial dysfunction,[39] hemodynamic instability owing to intravascular volume depletion, metabolic acidosis, and hyperglycemia.

Patients may present in shock, caused by either the secreted products of the tumor or some complication of the disease, such as myocardial infarction, cardiac failure, or dissected/ruptured aorta.

Thus, acute manifestations of an unsuspected pheochromocytoma must be considered in the differential diagnosis of many intraoperative clinical scenarios.

Preoperative Optimization

The goal of preoperative medication is to normalize blood pressure and heart rate, optimize glucose, electrolyte, assessment of other end organ function (cardiomyopathy), and to rule out any other associated syndrome. Sustained adrenergic stimulation leads to diminution of red cell mass and plasma volume making the patients prone for hypovolemia. Patients may present with poor glycemic control due to anti-insulin effects of catecholamines.

A number of regimens have been reported to reduce blood pressure during surgical resection of pheochromocytoma.

ANTIHYPERTENSIVE DRUGS FOR PHEOCHROMOCYTOMAS

- α-*adrenergic blockade* is physiologically complex because activation of α_2-adrenergic receptors, which are presynaptic, reduces catecholamine secretion, whereas activation of α_1-adrenergic receptors, which are postsynaptic, causes vasoconstriction.[40]
  - Phenoxybenzamine, a nonselective, noncompetitive, α-adrenergic blocker that covalently binds to α-adrenergic receptors, has been a mainstay of therapy. It reduces the vasoconstrictive effects of the catecholamines and maintains intravascular blood volume. Phenoxybenzamine dosage is started with 10–20 mg twice daily initially and titrated gradually to control and stabilize blood with maximum dose of 250 mg/day. The usual duration to alleviate symptom is 10–14 days although the catecholamine-induced cardiomyopathy may take several weeks of adrenergic blockade.
  - Prazosin is a competitive α-adrenergic blocking agent. Potential advantage of prazosin, a more selective α_1

blocker than phenoxybenzamine, is that after tumor resection α-adrenergic receptors can return quickly to normal function, thereby restoring physiological regulation of vascular tone and blood pressure. A disadvantage of competitive α-adrenergic blockade is the possibility that massive concentrations of catecholamines released by the tumor can overwhelm the competitive receptor antagonist, resulting in clinical manifestations including hypertension. Covalent, noncompetitive deactivation of α-adrenergic receptors as with phenoxybenzamine can withstand a surge in circulating catechol levels.[41] However, following resection of the tumor and removal of excess circulating catecholamines, permanent deactivation of α-adrenergic receptors by phenoxybenzamine may result in hypotension refractory to α-adrenergic agonists for days until new receptors are synthesized.

The choice of α-adrenergic blockade is an individual and institutional practice for optimal preoperative pharmacological control of pheochromocytoma.

- β-*adrenergic blockade* is commonly used to control tachycardia. β-adrenergic *blocking drugs must never be administered before initiation of α-blockade.* If done so, the unopposed α-adrenergic activation in the vasculature would result in dangerous elevation of blood pressure.
- *Calcium channel blockers* such as diltiazem and nifedipine have been used for preoperative control of tachyarrhythmias and hypertension. They act by blocking catecholamine-mediated influx of calcium into vascular smooth muscles thus preventing coronary artery spasm or myocarditis. They are usually administered to supplement adrenoceptor blockers in patients with poor blood pressure control.[42]
- *False neurotransmitters* such as α-methyl-p-tyrosine act as enzyme tyrosine hydroxylase inhibitors, thus blocking the synthesis of catecholamines. These are particularly given to patients with inoperable malignant tumor and who are resistant to α-1 blockade.[43]
- *Magnesium sulfate* has established a perioperative role during pheochromocytoma resection. It inhibits catecholamine release from adrenal medulla,[44] acts as α-adrenergic antagonist,[45] produces direct arteriolar dilation, and has antiarrhythmics properties.

◇ PREANESTHETIC ASSESSMENT

Pre-anesthesia checkup (PAC) should include thorough history taking and clinical examination to evaluate cardiac manifestation and end-organ damage.[46]

The preoperative optimization of tachyarrhythmias, hypertension, glycemic control, volume status, electrolyte levels, and counselling is essential for successful outcome postoperatively.[47]

Planning for perioperative management involves co-operation between an anesthesiologist, a surgeon, a cardiologist, and an endocrinologist.

Preoperative Investigations

Investigations

- *Hematological*: Complete blood count, serum electrolytes (sodium, potassium and calcium), blood glucose, coagulation profile, hepatic and renal profile
- ECG and echocardiography
- *Radiological*: Chest X-ray PA view
- Pulmonary function test

Perioperative Anesthetic Management

Anesthetic management of pheochromocytoma is quite challenging to concerned anesthesiologist owing to catecholamine-induced hemodynamic and cardiac manifestation perioperatively.

Laparoscopy is the preferred surgical approach for abdominal pheochromocytoma resection. However, open surgery may be required depending on the exact location of the lesion (e.g., neck paraganglioma) or anatomic variation of an abdominal tumor.

Invasive hemodynamic monitoring and central venous monitoring should be done to assess volume status and cardiac performance, and the utility of a central route for delivering vasoactive or inotropic drugs. Intraoperative transesophageal echocardiography (TEE) is recommended if there is concern for cardiomyopathy.

Anesthetic goal is to manage hemodynamic instability due to catecholamine surge during surgical manipulation of tumor.

General anesthesia with epidural analgesia is the anesthetic technique of choice. The regional anesthesia provides suppression of the stress response along with the analgesia.[48] Adrenergic crisis due to catecholamine surge can be observed during:

- Laryngoscopy and intubation
- Positioning of patient
- Stress response during surgical incision and manipulation of the tumor[49]

The main objective during these phases is maintenance of hemodynamic stability and normovolemia.

Preoperative medication with benzodiazepines such as midazolam is calm anxious patients, thus reducing the level of sympathetic output. Induction agent of choice are injection propofol, etomidate, or barbiturates in combination with synthetic opioids. Titrated doses of short-acting opioids such as fentanyl or sufentanil are given. Morphine is avoided as the histamine release can stimulate catecholamine release.[49]

Endotracheal intubation is facilitated with rocuronium, *cis*-atracurium and vecuronium, which are devoid of histamine-releasing effects and are cardio stable. Histamine-releasing muscle relaxant tubocurarine, atracurium, and mivacurium are avoided. Rocuronium should be considered in cases of rapid sequence induction.[50]

Maintenance of anesthesia is done with Oxygen: Air, incremental doses of nondepolarizing muscle relaxant, and inhalational agent. Isoflurane and sevoflurane are the preferable agents, as they are cardioprotective as compared to halothane and enflurane with potentially arrhythmogenic potential to catecholamine. Desflurane, although quickly titratable, can stimulate the sympathetic nervous system which could be deleterious in these patients.[51]

To blunt the sympathetic stress response during intubation and laryngoscopy, intravenous boluses of esmolol, lidocaine, or additional opioids can be considered.[5]

◇ MONITORING

- The baseline hemodynamic parameters, temperature, urine output
- Invasive monitoring with arterial and central venous line for titrating doses of various antihypertensive and fluid replacement intraoperatively
- Electrolyte and glucose monitoring

Exaggerated hemodynamic responses may result during laryngoscopy. Insufflation of the abdomen with CO_2 for laparoscopy and direct manipulation of the tumor may stimulate the release of catecholamines from tumors. Once the major draining vein of the tumor is ligated, plasma catecholamine levels usually decline precipitously. Hypotension often ensues. Volume repletion, infusions of α-adrenergic agonists such as phenylephrine, and cessation of vasodilators can be used to support hemodynamics. Phenoxybenzamine produces sustained deactivation of α-adrenergic receptors, which limits the response to phenylephrine. Vasopressin may circumvent this problem. Hypoglycemia should be specifically anticipated and treated as needed.

Analgesia through epidural catheter is supplemented with local anesthetics alone or in combination with opioids.

Most common drugs used to manage hypertensive episodes intraoperatively are nitroprusside, phentolamine, trimethaphan, nitroglycerine, or nicardipine. Intravenous magnesium infusions have also been used successfully.[34] The bolus dosage and infusion have been discussed earlier **(Table 1)**.

Depending on the hemodynamic status and signs of reversal, the extubation can be done on table or later in the intensive care unit (ICU). Reversal agent is a combination of neostigmine (onset of cholinergic effects) and glycopyrrolate (coincide with antimuscarinic effects), producing minimal tachycardia.

Table 1: Drugs used during intraoperative management of pheochromocytoma/paraganglioma.

Drugs	Dose	Indication
α-adrenergic blockers:		
• Phenoxybenzamine	• 20–30 mg/day initially, then can be increased to 60–250 mg/day days (1 mg/kg daily in three divided doses) until blood pressure is controlled	• Preoperative preparation may be achieved in 10–14 days
• Phentolamine	• 2.5–5 mg IV at 1 mg/minute, repeated every 5 minutes until blood pressure is controlled	• Used for prevention of hypertensive crisis
	• Continuous infusion, 100 mg/500 mL D_5W, infusion rate adjusted to targeted blood pressure	• Treatment of acute hypertensive crisis
Beta-adrenergic blockers:		Used preoperatively only after complete α-adrenergic blockade is achieved to effect
• Atenonol	Dose titrated to effect	
• Metoprolol,		
• Propronanolol,		
• Esmolol		
• Labetalol		
Arteriovenodilator:		Used intraoperatively for treatment of acute hypertensive episodes or tachycardia
• Sodium nitroprusside	• 0.5–10 µg kg^{-1} minute^{-1} IV/infusion rate adjusted to targeted blood pressure	• Treatment of acute hypertensive episodes
• Nitroglycerine	• 0.5–10 µg kg^{-1} minute^{-1} IV, infusion rate adjusted to targeted blood pressure	• Treatment of acute hypertensive episodes
• Doxazosin	• 2–16 mg/day, orally	• Preoperative preparation
Calcium-channel blockers:		
• Diltiazem	• 60–120 mg/day	• Preoperative preparation
	• 30–90 mg/day	
• Nifedipine	• 20–60 mg/day, three divided doses/orally	• Preoperative preparation and intraoperative hemodynamic control
• Nicardipine	• 0.5–10.0 µg kg^{-1} minute^{-1} IV infusion rate adjusted to targeted blood pressure, or IV bolus 1–2 mg	
Magnesium sulfate	• Bolus 2–4 g	• Preoperative control of hypertensive crisis
	• Infusion 1–2 g/hour IV	• Control of intraoperative hemodynamics
False transmitters α-methyl para tyrosine	Start at 250 mg orally, 4 times per day; increase to maximum of 4 g/day	Preoperative depletion of catecholamine stores

(IV: intravenous)

Postoperative Management

Vigilant monitoring is required in the ICU/high-dependency unit (HDU) for high chances of hypertensive, hypotensive, or hypoglycemic episodes postoperatively.[52]

- *Persistent hypotension causes*:
  - Decline in plasma catecholamine levels following tumor resection
  - Residual effects of adrenergic-blocking drugs
  - Intra-abdominal bleed (rare)[53]
- *Postoperative hypertension causes*:
  - Postoperative pain
  - It may take several days to week to normalize urinary excretion of catecholamines and metabolites thus causing raised blood pressure.
  - Residual tumor[54]
- *Hypoglycemia*: Dramatic rise in insulin levels after surgical resection
- Electrolyte derangements

Above parameters should be monitored strictly in the postanesthesia care unit (PACU).

With the better understanding of pathophysiology, advanced monitoring, effective and safer cardiac medication, the outcome of pheochromocytoma surgery has significantly improved.

Anesthesia for Adrenal Cortical Surgery

The outer portion of the adrenal gland lying on the superior aspect of kidney is adrenal cortex. This endocrine gland secretes three classes of steroid:

1. *Glucocorticoids (cortisol)*: Excessive production causes *Cushing syndrome*
2. *Mineralocorticoids*: Hypersecretion of aldosterone leads to *Conn syndrome*
3. Androgens (sex hormones)

◇ CONN SYNDROME/PRIMARY HYPERALDOSTERONISM

Conn syndrome/primary hyperaldosteronism is caused by hypersecretion of the major adrenal mineralocorticoid aldosterone by hyperplastic adrenal glands, mineralocorticoid-secreting adenomas, or, rarely, cancers.[55] The principle effect of mineralocorticoid is maintenance of electrolyte and fluid balance by stimulating sodium reabsorption at the expense of potassium and hydrogen ions; thus resulting in extracellular fluid expansion. Renin–angiotensin system, hyponatremia, hyperkalemia, or pituitary-induced ACTH release affect aldosterone secretion.

Angiotensin-II produced via renin–angiotensin system facilitates the conversion of cholesterol to pregnenolone and the conversion of corticosterone to aldosterone.

Secondary hyperaldosteronism usually presents in severe cardiac failure, nephritic syndrome, and advanced liver disease is due to renin–aldosterone axis activation induced by increased levels of renin.

Clinical Manifestation in Conn

Hypertension (5–13% of secondary hypertension and <1% of essential one),[56] hypokalemic alkalosis, hypomagnesemia, skeletal muscle weakness, and fatigue.[57]

Cardiac manifestations:

- Arrhythmias due to electrolyte imbalance
- Rare incidence of CHF because of fluid retention secondary to hypernatremia[58]

Investigations to Confirm Diagnosis

Blood Investigations

- *Electrolyte levels*: Plasma potassium and sodium
- Biochemical test for renin and aldosterone level
  - *Conn syndrome*: Decreased renin with high aldosterone, high aldosterone to renin ratio
  - *Secondary hyperaldosteronism*: Raised renin level

Radiological

- Magnetic resonance imaging, angiogram-CT, and ultrasonography of adrenal gland
- Adrenal scintigraphy with ^{131}I-labeled or ^{75}Se-labelled precursors of aldosterone differentiates between an adenoma and hyperplasia.[59]

Management

- Medical management with spironolactone[60] (aldosterone antagonist) for hyperplasia
- Surgical removal for adrenal adenoma with laparoscopic or open approach

Anesthetic Considerations

The primary concerns such as hemodynamic instability and electrolyte imbalance should be dealt with during perioperative period.

Preoperative goals include:

- Optimization of cardiovascular status and hypertension
- Correction of electrolyte and metabolic derangement
- Intravascular fluid management

Hypokalemia is known to have baroreceptor suppressive effect[61] and combined with metabolic alkalosis prolongs nondepolarizing neuromuscular blocking agent's action.

Perioperative Management

- Unilateral or bilateral adrenalectomy may be performed to treat Conn syndrome depending on the pathology. If bilateral adrenal resection or manipulation is planned, a stress dose of cortisol should be considered preoperatively and continued for 24 hours.
- Surgery planned unilateral or bilateral adrenalectomy via laparoscopically or open laparotomy. Laparoscopic approach remains gold standard.[62,63]

- Monitoring includes pulse oximetry, noninvasive blood pressure, temperature, end-tidal carbon dioxide, electrocardiography, and urine output.
- Invasive monitoring with arterial and central venous cannulation guides for volume replacement and managing hemodynamic instability.
- During induction, etomidate must be avoided because of interference with cortisol synthesis. Neuromuscular blockade monitoring with a twitch monitor is done to supplement muscle relaxant.
- Vigilant hemodynamic monitoring is required as the manipulation of adrenal gland during dissection and resection may lead to catecholamine surge leading to intraoperative hypertension.[64]
- To avoid adrenal suppression-induced cardiovascular and electrolyte disturbances, stress dose of cortisol should be considered perioperatively in cases of bilateral adrenal resection or patients with chronic steroid administration.[65]
- After completion of surgery, assessment of adequate reversal of neuromuscular blocking agent (a sustained head lift for 5 seconds or a strong handgrip), and good ventilatory effort should be observed before extubation.
- Postoperative management includes pain-free stay and electrolyte and vital monitoring, since potassium deficiency may be observed as long as a week after surgery.[66]

Glucocorticoid Action

1. *Catabolic*: Metabolism of carbohydrates, fats, and proteins and promotes gluconeogenesis.
2. Essential for maintaining cardiovascular response to catecholamines. It possesses weak mineralocorticoid activity.
3. Immunosuppression and delayed wound healing

Regulation of glucocorticoid activity involves a negative feedback mechanism through hypothalamopituitary axis.

◇| CUSHING SYNDROME

Overproduction of cortisol by the adrenal cortex or exogenous glucocorticoid therapy leads to the complexity of clinical manifestation which includes hypertension, hyperglycemia, increased intravascular fluid volume, hypokalemia, obesity, fragile bones and myopathies, metabolic alkalosis, and psychological changes.

Cushing disease associated with pituitary adenoma may present with neurological symptoms visual disturbances, headache, and elevated intracranial pressure.

The inappropriate secretion may be due to a primary pituitary ACTH-producing tumor (70%), ectopic production of ACTH (15%), or secondary to an adrenal tumor (15%).[67]

The other tumors having associated Cushing syndrome are pheochromocytoma, sarcoidosis, pancreatic acinar cell carcinoma, malignant gastrinoma, bronchial carcinoid lung tumor, pancreatic neuroendocrine tumor, and mesenteric neuroendocrine carcinoma.[68,69]

Laboratory Diagnosis

Screening

- Increased blood cortisol and excessive plasma ACTH level
- *24-hour urinary free cortisol*: Elevated urinary 17-hydroxycorticosteroids[70]
- *Dexamethasone suppression test* can determine the origin of glucocorticoid hypersecretion. It leads to suppression of serum cortisol in Cushing of pituitary origin because of negative feedback control but not of adrenal Cushing or ectopic ACTH secretion.[71]

Radiological imaging is done after the screening through biochemical tests. Angiogram-CT, MRI, or ultrasonography of adrenal gland help in confirming the diagnosis.[72] Technetium-99-labeled octreotide scintigraphy examinations can detect ectopic glucocorticoid secreting tissues.[73]

Anesthetic Considerations

- *Difficult airway*: Owing to the presence of central obesity with facial fat thickening, these patients may present as anticipated difficult airway for the anesthesiologist. Difficult airway cart and fiberoptic bronchoscope must be kept ready before induction.
- *Pulmonary*: Severe obesity leads to decreased chest wall compliance, functional residual capacity (FRC), and increased oxygen consumption. The patients are prone for rapid desaturation in the presence of *reduced pulmonary reserve*.
- Obstructive sleep apnea is common in these patients making them prone to develop pulmonary hypertension.
- *Cardiovascular*: Hypertension and left ventricular hypertrophy
- Hyperglycemia and increased risk of thromboembolic events
- Osteoporotic changes need care during intubation and positioning for surgery.
- Hypokalemia and fluid retention require preoperative optimization.[51]

Thorough preanesthetic check-up for clinical manifestations and preoperative optimization of hypertension, hyperglycemia, hypokalemia, and coagulopathy is warranted. Oral hypoglycemic agents are substituted with insulin before surgery for better glycemic control.[74]

Prevention of perioperative venous and pulmonary thromboembolism advocates low molecular weight heparin (LMWH), lower-extremity compression devices,[75] and early postoperative mobilization.

Perioperative Management

Surgical approach for adrenalectomy can be open or laparoscopic. Laparoscopic adrenalectomy remains gold standard.

Anesthesia plan takes into consideration possible difficult airway management, rapid sequence induction, standard and/or invasive monitoring.

Anesthetic technique of choice is general anesthesia with epidural analgesia. Epidurally delivered analgesia minimizes the respiratory depressant effect caused by systemically administered opioids.

Epidural insertion in Cushing disease is difficult owing to obesity and osteoporotic changes. Thus it should be done before induction in sitting position and catheter tested for satisfactory function.[76] Lower doses of drugs are required through epidural because of decreased volume of the epidural space secondary to higher intra-abdominal pressures and engorged vessels.

Large bore intravenous catheter and central vein cannulation are accessed for facilitation of fluids and drugs in titrated manner. Perioperative monitoring includes baseline pulse oximetry, noninvasive blood pressure, temperature, end-tidal carbon dioxide, electrocardiography, and urine output.

Invasive monitoring includes invasive blood pressure and central venous monitoring.[77]

Premedication include drugs for aspiration prophylaxis, H2-receptor blockers/metoclopramide as these patients have increased risk for gastric aspiration. In view of anticipated difficult airways and hypoxia, deep sedation is avoided.

Preoxygenation is must as the decreased FRC in Cushing predisposes them for rapid hypoxemia.[78] Rapid sequence induction with cricoid pressure is preferred because of anticipated difficult airway and increased chances of pulmonary aspiration.

Intravenous induction is done with drugs dosed according to ideal weight, propofol or barbiturates are preferred agents of choice with short-acting opioids.[79] Neuromuscular blocking agents should be titrated according to monitoring owing to myopathy and resulting muscle weakness.

Maintenance of anesthesia is done with oxygen: Air, volatile inhalational anesthetic, incremental doses of muscle relaxant, and epidural supplementation of local anesthetic. Desflurane or sevoflurane with relatively low lipid solubility are preferred inhalational agent. Nitrous oxide should be avoided in patients with pulmonary hypertension.

Care should be taken during positioning and taping of the patient, in view of fragile bones and skin changes. The intravascular fluid status, serum glucose, and electrolytes are monitored perioperatively and managed accordingly. The patients are prone for hypoventilation, atelectasis, and hypoxia as a consequence of reduced FRC.

Neuromuscular blockade should be reversed with neostigmine and glycopyrrolate combination and after assessing complete neuromuscular reversal, the patient should be extubated fully awake and following commands. During the stay in PACU, the upright sitting position and analgesia through the epidural catheter decreases the chance of pulmonary complications by facilitating breathing efforts and reducing chances of atelectasis and hypoventilation.

Hydrocortisone replacement therapy may be necessary and should be started at the time of resection of the tumor.[51] Chronic suppression of the contralateral adrenal gland or resection of both glands can lead to acute hypocortisolism.

Postoperative Management

- *Pain management*: Epidural Analgesia with/intravenous paracetamol
- *Early mobilization*: Reduced chances of thromboembolism
- Hypertension and hyperglycemia control

Steroid replacement therapy becomes necessary, especially after bilateral adrenalectomy.

PERIOPERATIVE STEROID COVER IN CUSHING SYNDROME

Patients at risk for adrenal suppression and perioperative adrenal insufficiency should be assessed and the patient's risk for adrenal crisis must be weighed against the risks of unnecessary steroid supplementation. ACTH stimulation test is done for assessing the integrity of the hypothalamic-pituitary-adrenal axis (HPAA) **(Table 2)**.

Table 2: Steroid supplementation.

Anticipated surgical stress	Preoperative	Intraoperative	Postoperative
Minor	25 mg or usual steroid dose	None, unless complications	Resume usual replacement postoperative day 1 (POD 1)
Moderate	50–75 mg or usual steroid dose, whichever is higher	50 mg IV	20 mg IV q8h on POD 1, then resume preoperative replacement dose on POD 2
Major	100–150 mg or usual steroid dose, whichever is higher, within 2 hours of start of procedure	50 mg IV q8h after initial dose	50 mg IV q8h, or 150 mg continuously over 24 hours for 2–3 day, then reduce dose by 50% per day until preoperative regimen is reached

(IV: intravenous)

Patients at risk include:

- Patients demonstrated to have secondary adrenal insufficiency.
- Patients with chronic steroid therapy/treated with a glucocorticoid for >3 weeks in doses equivalent to at least 20 mg/day of prednisone/clinical features of Cushing syndrome
- Bilateral adrenalectomy

Patients with normal response to administration of cosyntropin/who have been treated with any dose of glucocorticoid for <3 weeks do not require perioperative supplementation.

In case of unavailability of testing, the stress-dose steroids based on the patient's perioperative condition (*e.g.*, degree of hemodynamic stability) and surgical risk.

Perioperative Steroid Dose[80,81]

Refer **Table 2**.

For Postoperative

- *Minor*: Resume usual replacement postoperative day 1 (POD 1)
- *Moderate*: 20 mg IV q8h on POD 1, then resume preoperative replacement dose on POD 2
- *Major*: 50 mg IV q8h, or 150 mg continuously over 24 hours for 2–3 days, then reduce dose by 50% per day until preoperative regimen is reached.

◇| REFERENCES

1. Bajwa SS, Kalra S. Endocrine anesthesia: a rapidly evolving anesthesia specialty. Saudi J Anaesth. 2014;8(1):1-3.
2. Bajwa SS, Sehgal V. Anesthesia and thyroid surgery: The never ending challenges. Indian J Endocrinol Metab. 2013;17: 228-34.
3. Bajwa SS, Sehgal V. Anesthetic management of primary hyperparathyroidism: a role rarely noticed and appreciated so far. Indian J Endocr Metab. 2013;17:235-9.
4. Yong SL, Coulthard P, Wrzosek A. Supplemental perioperative steroids for surgical patients with adrenal insufficiency. Cochrane Database Syst Rev. 2012;12:CD005367.
5. Bajwa SS, Bajwa SK. Implications and considerations during pheochromocytoma resection: a challenge to the anesthesiologist. Indian J Endocrinol Metab. 2011;15: S337-44.
6. Bajwa SS, Bajwa SK. Anesthesia and intensive care implications for pituitary surgery: recent trends and advancements. Indian J Endocrinol Metab. 2011;15:S224-32.
7. Dionigi G, Dionigi R, Bartalena L, Tanda ML, Piantanida E, Castano P, et al. Current indications for thyroidectomy. Minerva Chir. 2007;62:359-72.
8. Farling PA. Thyroid disease. Br J Anesth. 2000;85:15-28.
9. Kandaswamy C, Balasubramanian V. Review of adult tracheomalacia and its relationship with chronic obstructive pulmonary disease. Curr Opin Pulm Med. 2009;15:113-9.
10. Balasubramanian S, Kannan R, Balakrishnan K. Post-operative tracheomalacia after surgery on the thyroid and the aerodigestive tract. Internet J Surg 2009;19:2.
11. Rapini RP, Bolognia JL, Jorizzo JL. Dermatology, volume 2 set. St. Louis: Mosby; 2007. p. 858.
12. White ML, Doherty GM, Gauger PG. Evidence-based surgical management of substernal goiter. World J Surg. 2008;32:1285-300.
13. Bouaggad A, Nejmi SE, Bouderka MA, Abbassi O. Prediction of difficult tracheal intubation in thyroid surgery. Anesth Analg. 2004;99:603-6.
14. Chin SC, Edelstein S, Chen CY, Som PM. Using CT to localize side and level of vocal cord paralysis. Am J Roentgenol. 2003;180:1165-70.
15. Marshall P. Oxford Handbook of Anaesthesia. Oxford: Oxford University Press; 2002. p. 301.
16. Rosato L, Avenia N, Bernante P, De Palma M, Gulino G, Nasi PG, et al. Complications of thyroid surgery: Analysis of a multicentric study on 14,934 patients operated on in Italy over 5 years. World J Surg. 2004;28:271-6.
17. Meier DA, Brill DR, Becker DV. Procedure guideline for therapy of thyroid disease with 131 iodine. J Nucl Med. 2002;43: 856-61.
18. Danzi S, Klein I. Thyroid hormone and the cardiovascular system. Med Clin North Am. 2012;96(2):257-68.
19. Hisham AN, Aina EN. A reappraisal of thyroid surgery under local anaesthesia—back to the future? ANZ J Surg. 2002;724: 287-9.
20. Malhotra S, Sodhi V. Anaesthesia for thyroid and parathyroid surgery. Contin Educ Anaesth Crit Care Pain. 2007;7(2):55-8.
21. Dixit H, Kamat L, Potdar M, Modi T. Role of electromyography endotracheal tube in preventing recurrent laryngeal nerve injury during thyroid surgery: a case report. Airway trauma during difficult intubation... from the frying pan into the fire? Indian J Anaesth. 2017;61(5):435-7.
22. Tsai CJ, Tseng KY, Wang FY, Lu IC, Wang HM, Wu CW, et al. Electromyographic endotracheal tube placement during thyroid surgery in neuromonitoring of recurrent laryngeal nerve. Kaohsiung J Med Sci. 2011;27(3):96-101.
23. Mihai R, Farndon JR. Parathyroid disease and calcium metabolism. Br J Anaesth. 2000;85(1):29-43.
24. Lundgren E, Lind L, Palmér M, Jakobsson S, Ljunghall S, Rastad J. Increased cardiovascular mortality and normalised serum calcium in patients with mild hypercalcaemia followed up for 25 year. Surgery. 2001;130:978-85.
25. Sheldon D, Lee FT, Neil NJ, Ryan JA. Surgical treatment of hyperparathyroidism improves health related quality of life. Arch Surg. 2002;137:1022-8.
26. Fraser WD. Hyperparathyroidism. Lancet. 2009;374:145-58.
27. Bajwa SS, Sharma V. Peri-operative renal protection: the strategies revisited. Indian J Urol. 2012;28:248-55.
28. Dijkstra B, Healy C, Kelly LM, McDermott EW, Hill AD, O'Higgins NO. Parathyroid localization: current practice. JR Coll Surg Ed. 2002;47:599-607.
29. Dickerson RN. Treatment of hypocalcemia in critical illness-part 2. Nutrition. 2007;23:436-7.
30. Manger WM, Gifford JW Jr. Pheochromocytoma: A clinical overview. In: Swales JD (Ed). Textbook of Hypertension. Oxford: Blackwell Scientific; 1994. pp. 941-58.

31. Khairi MR, Dexter RN, Burzynski NJ, Johnston CC. Mucosal neuroma, pheochromocytoma and medullary thyroid carcinoma: Multiple endocrine neoplasia type 3. Medicine. 1975;54:89-112

32. Bouloux PM. Multiple endocrine neoplasia. Surgery. 1987;1:1180-5.

33. Manger WM, Gifford RW. Pheochromocytoma. New York: Springer-Verlag; 1977.

34. Prys-Roberts C. Pheochromocytoma: recent progress in its management. Br J Anaesth. 2000;85(1):44-87.

35. Fahmy N, Assad M, Bathijad P, Whittier FC. Postoperative acute pulmonary edema: a rare presentation of pheochromocytoma. Clin Nephrol. 1997;48:122-4.

36. Breivik H. Perianaesthetic management of patients with endocrine disease. Acta Anaesthesiol Scand. 1996;40(8 Pt 2): 1004-15.

37. Jones DH, Reid JL, Hamilton CA, Allison DJ, Welbourn RB, Dollery CT. The biochemical diagnosis, localization and follow up of pheochromocytoma: The role of plasma and urinary catecholamine measurements. QJ Med. 1980;49: 341-61.

38. Hodin R, Lubitz C, Phitayakorn R, Stephen A. Diagnosis and management of pheochromocytoma. Curr Probl Surg. 2014;51(4):151-87.

39. Kinney MA, Narr BJ, Warner MA. Perioperative management of pheochromocytoma. J Cardiothorac Vasc Anesth. 2002;16: 359-69.

40. Langer SZ. Presynaptic regulation of the release of catecholamines. Pharmacol Rev. 1981;32:337-62.

41. Roizen MF, Hunt TK, Beaupre PN, Kremer P, Firmin R, Chang CN, et al. The effect of alpha adrenergic blockade on cardiac performance and tissue oxygen delivery during excision of pheochromocytoma. Surgery. 1983;94:941-5.

42. Proye C, Thevenin D, Cecat P, Petillot P, Carnaille B, Verin P, et al. Exclusive use of calcium channel blockers in preoperative and intraoperative control of pheochromocytomas: Hemodynamics and free catecholamine assays in ten consecutive patients. Surgery. 1989;106:1149-54.

43. Engelman K, Jequier E, Udenfriend S, Sjoerdsma A. Metabolism of alpha-methyltyrosine in man: Relationship to its potency as an inhibitor of catecholamine biosynthesis. J Clin Invest. 1968;47:568-76.

44. James MF, Beer RE, Esser JD. Intravenous magnesium sulfate inhibits catecholamine release associated with tracheal intubation. Anesth Analg. 1989;68:772-6.

45. James MF, Cork RC, Harlen GM, White JF. Interactions of adrenaline and magnesium on the cardiovascular system of the baboon. Magnesium. 1988;7:37-43.

46. Van Vliet PD, Buchel HB, Titus JL. Focal myocarditis associated with pheochromocytoma. N Engl J Med. 1966;74: 1102-8.

47. Desmonts JM, le Houelleur J, Remond P, Duvaldestin P. Anaesthetic management of patients with pheochromocytoma: a review of 102 cases. Br J Anaesth. 1977;49:991-8.

48. Roizen MF, Horrigan RW, Koike M, Eger IE 2nd, Mulroy MF, Frazer B, et al. A prospective randomized trial of four anesthetic techniques for resection of pheochromocytoma. Anesthesiology. 1982;57:A43.

49. Bogdonoff DL. Pheochromocytoma: Specialist cases that all must be prepared to treat? J Cardiothor Vasc Anesth. 2002;16:267-9.

50. Stoelting RK, Dierdorf SF. Endocrine disease adrenal gland dysfunction. In: Stoelting RK, Diedorf SF (Eds). Anesthesia and co-existing disease, 4th edition. Philadelphia: Churchill Livingstone; 2002. pp. 425-34.

51. Roizen MF. Anesthetic complications of concurrent diseases. In: Miller RD (Ed). Anesthesia, 5th edition. Philadelphia: Churchill Livingstone; 2000. pp. 903-1015.

52. Singh G, Kam P. An overview of anaesthetic issues in Pheochromocytoma. Ann Acad Med Singapore. 1998;27:843-8.

53. Hull CJ. Pheochromocytoma: diagnosis, pre-operative preparation, and anaesthetic management. Br J Anaesth. 1986;58:1453-68.

54. Desmonts JM, Marty J. Anaesthetic management of patients with pheochromocytoma. Br J Anaesth. 1984;56:781-9.

55. Wheeler MH, Harris DA. Diagnosis and management of primary aldosteronism. World J Surg. 2003;27(6):627-31.

56. Calhoun DA. Aldosteronism and hypertension. Clin J Am Soc Nephrol. 2006;1(5):1039-45.

57. Weigel RJ, Oberhelman HA, Steven K. Endocrine surgery: adrenalectomy. In: Jaffe RA, Samuels SI (Eds). Anesthesiologist's Manual of Surgical Procedures, 2nd edition. Philadelphia: Lippincott Williams and Wilkins; 1999. pp. 481-4.

58. Zannad F. Aldosterone and heart failure. Eur Heart J. 1995;16: 98-102.

59. Heald A. Adrenocortical hormones. Anaesth Intensive Care Med. 2002;;3;327-9.

60. French G, Low J, Thompson J. Endocrine and metabolic disease. In: Allman KG, Wilson IH (Eds). Oxford Handbook of Anaesthesia. Oxford: Oxford University Press; 2001. pp. 72-107.

61. Winship SM, Winstanley JHR, Hunter JM. Anaesthesia for Conn's syndrome. Anaesthesia. 1999;54:564-74.

62. Lertakyamanee N, Somprakit P, Buranakijaroen P, Lertakyamanee J, Nimmanwudipong T, Sriussadaporn S. Anesthesia and laparoscopic adrenalectomy for primary aldosteronism. J Med Assoc Thai. 2001;84(6):798-803.

63. Edwin B, Raeder I, Trondsen E, Kaaresen R, Buanes T. Outpatient laparoscopic adrenalectomy in patients with Conn's syndrome. Surg Endosc. 2001;15(6):589-91.

64. Domi R, Sula H. Pheochromocytoma, the challenge to anesthesiologist. J Endocrinol Metab. 2011;1(3):97-100.

65. Shaikh S, Verna H, Yadav N, Jauhari M, Bullangowda J. Application of steroid in clinical practice: a review. ISRN Anesthesiology. 2012;2012:985495.

66. Celen O, O'Brien MJ, Melby JC, Beazley RM. Factors influencing outcome of surgery for primary aldosteronism. Arch Surg. 1996;131:646-50.

67. Bayraktar F, Kebapcilar L, Kocdor MA, Asa SL, Yesil S, Canda S, Demir T, et al. Cushing's syndrome due to ectopic CRH secretion by adrenal pheochromocytoma accompanied by renal infarction. Exp Clin Endocrinol Diabetes. 2006;114(8): 444-7.

68. Kumar M, Kumar V, Talukdar B, Mohta A, Khurana N. Cushing syndrome in an infant due to cortisol secreting adrenal pheochromocytoma: a rare association. J Pediatr Endocrinol Metab. 2010;23(6):621-5.

69. Park SY, Rhee Y, Youn JC, Park YN, Lee S, Kim DM, et al. Ectopic Cushing's syndrome due to concurrent corticotropin-releasing hormone (CRH) and adrenocorticotropic hormone (ACTH) secreted by malignant gastrinoma. Exp Clin Endocrinol Diabetes. 2007;115(1):13-6.

70. Newell-Price J, Bertagna X, Grossman AB, Nieman LK. Cushing's syndrome. Lancet. 2006;367(9522):1605-17.

71. Vaughan ED, Jr. Diseases of the adrenal gland. Med Clin North Am. 2004;88(2):443-66.

72. Arnaldi G, Angeli A, Atkinson AB, Bertagna X, Cavagnini F, Chrousos GP, et al. Diagnosis and complications of Cushing's syndrome: a consensus statement. J Clin Endocrinol Metab. 2003;88(12):5593-602.

73. Esfahani AF, Chavoshi M, Noorani MH, Saghari M, Eftekhari M, Beiki D, et al. Successful application of technetium-99m-labeled octreotide acetate scintigraphy in the detection of ectopic adrenocorticotropin-producing bronchial carcinoid lung tumor: a case report. J Med Case Rep. 2010;4:323.

74. Pomposelli JJ, Baxter JK, 3rd, Babineau TJ, Pomfret EA, Driscoll DF, Forse RA, Bistrian BR. Early postoperative glucose control predicts nosocomial infection rate in diabetic patients. JPEN J Parenter Enteral Nutr. 1998;22(2):77-81.

75. Geerts WH, Bergqvist D, Pineo GF, Heit JA, Samama CM, Lassen MR, et al. Prevention of venous thromboembolism: American College of Chest Physicians Evidence-Based Clinical Practice Guidelines (8th Edition). Chest. 2008;133(6 Suppl): 381S-453S.

76. Vierra MA, Howard KH. Operations for morbid obesity. In: Jaffe RA, Samuels SI (Eds) Anesthesiologist's Manual of Surgical Procedures, 2nd edition. Philadelphia: Lippincott, Williams and Wilkins; 1999. pp. 352-6.

77. Domi R. Cushing' surgery: Role of the anesthesiologist. Indian J Endocr Metab. 2011;15:322-8.

78. Berthoud MC, Peacock JE, Reilly CS. Effectiveness of preoxygenation in morbidly obese patients. Br J Anaesth. 1991;67:464-6.

79. Juvin P, Vadam C, Malek L, Dupont H, Marmuse JP, Desmonts JM. Postoperative recovery after desflurane, propofol, or isoflurane anesthesia among morbidly obese patients: a prospective, randomized study. Anesth Analg. 2000;91:714-9.

CHAPTER 44

Role of Radiotherapy in Endocrine Tumors

Punita Lal, Shagun Misra, Sidharth Pant, Shaleen Kumar

◇ THYROID CARCINOMA

According to GLOBOCAN, thyroid cancer is the most commonly diagnosed endocrine cancer with an estimated incidence of 5.6 lakhs in 2018 and ranking it ninth most common cancer overall.[1] There is a male preponderance with an M:F ratio of 3:1. Mortality with thyroid cancer is low comprising 0.4% of all cancer deaths.[1] Differentiated thyroid carcinoma (DTC) and anaplastic thyroid cancer (ATC) are the most common subtypes arising from follicular epithelial cells. The C or parafollicular cells are the calcitonin cells derived from the neural crest which is the cell of origin for medullary thyroid carcinoma (MTC). Rare tumors such as lymphoma and sarcoma usually arise from the immune cells and stromal cells of the thyroid gland.[2]

Differentiated Thyroid Carcinoma

Differentiated thyroid carcinoma comprises broadly papillary thyroid carcinoma (PTC) and follicular thyroid carcinoma (FTC). PTC comprises 90% of DTC and is bilateral in one-third cases with indolent behavior and excellent prognosis; however, there are unfavorable variants in PTC such as anaplastic transformation, tall cell papillary variants, and columnar variants which usually have a higher potential for recurrence with relatively poor prognosis. PTC is characterized by extrathyroidal invasion into adjacent soft tissue in up to 15% of patients and 30% have clinically evident lymph node (LN) enlargement. Distant metastasis usually occurs in <10% of patients in these cases.[3] FTC, on the other hand, comprises 5–10% of all thyroid malignancies and is usually more aggressive than PTC. These tumors typically do not show extrathyroid invasion or lymphadenopathy. They are usually characterized by either tumor invasion through tumor capsule or invasion into an underlying blood vessel. Distant metastasis may be found in nearly one-fifth of patients at presentation.[4] Hurthle cell carcinoma is a relatively rare variant of follicular thyroid cancer, accounting for 3–5% of all DTCs, according to the American Cancer Society.[4] Tall cell papillary variants and insular thyroid carcinomas (rare thyroglobulin-producing neoplasm) are considered more aggressive than well-differentiated carcinomas of papillary or follicular cell origin and are considered an intermediate group of tumors.[3,4]

Differentiated thyroid carcinoma generally has an excellent prognosis while oncologic outcomes worsen as the stage progresses.[5] The prognostic factors identified to predict the risk of death and postoperative outcomes are the patient's age, local invasion, tumor size, completeness of resection, and metastasis at presentation. The Mayo Clinic developed the MACIS (*M*etastasis, patient *A*ge, *C*ompleteness of resection, local *I*nvasion and tumor *S*ize) nomogram, which, based on all these factors, predicts the 20-year survival and also has management implications. With a score of <6 (low risk), the survival is 99% at 20 years while for a score of ≥8 (high risk), the survival falls to 24%.[6] At the Mayo Clinic, postoperative radioactive iodine (RAI) therapy is offered for high-risk groups or patients with a diagnosis of FTC or occasionally Hurthle cell carcinoma (less likely to take up RAI). The primary management for DTC is surgery, which includes hemithyroidectomy or total thyroidectomy with or without neck dissection. Neck dissection has two components—central compartment neck dissection and lateral neck dissection. As per the American Thyroid Association (ATA), patients who present with clinically palpable central nodes should undergo total thyroidectomy with therapeutic central compartment (level VI) neck dissection. For early stage (T1 or T2), clinically node-negative patients, thyroidectomy alone is advised. Therapeutic lateral neck compartmental LN dissection along with primary thyroidectomy is recommended in patients with biopsy-proven lateral cervical LNs. Patients are further stratified based on the ATA risk stratification.[7] In low-risk patients, DTC is confined to the thyroid gland without capsular invasion and are clinically node-negative or have <5 pathological nodes with micrometastases (<0.2 cm in the largest dimension) and intermediate-risk patients have aggressive histology with a microscopic invasion of disease into extrathyroidal soft tissues. Other features include clinically N1 or pathologically involved LNs (<3 cm in largest dimension). High risk is defined when there is a macroscopic perithyroidal extension of disease and complete resection with negative margins is not possible. Also, there is evidence of distant metastasis or pathologically N1 disease ≥3 cm in the greatest dimension. Intermediate- and high-risk patients are offered RAI. Following RAI, long-term use of levothyroxine (LT4) is considered optimal for patients with structural residual carcinoma or high risk for recurrence to maintain thyroid-stimulating hormone (TSH) levels < 0.1 mU/L.[7] The rationale behind the use of LT4 is to suppress the TSH and, therefore, inhibit the activation of cells from the thyroid follicular epithelium.

The role of external beam radiotherapy (EBRT) in the adjuvant setting for differentiated thyroid cancers is controversial due to the lack of any level I evidence supporting its benefit after radical surgery and RAI therapy. However, pooled analysis of retrospective studies comprising locally advanced-stage disease patients has shown superior 5-year locoregional relapse-free survival with radiation therapy (RT) versus no RT with a risk ratio of 1.39 [95% confidence interval (CI): 1.23–1.58, $p < 0.001$].[5] The risk of locoregional recurrences is usually high, around 20% (range: 2.5–58.1%), when adjuvant EBRT is omitted[8] in these patients. Locally advanced stage (T4) tumors that have a high likelihood of gross/microscopic residual disease due to the presence of other high-risk features such as age >45 years, extrathyroid extension, and tumors with low capacity to concentrate RAI should undergo adjuvant EBRT as recommended by the American Head and Neck Society[9] and ATA.[7] In the absence of these high-risk features, adjuvant EBRT is not routinely recommended, especially if complete resection has been done. Nodal metastasis alone is not an indication of adjuvant EBRT as adjuvant RAI provides acceptable locoregional control.[9] In terms of overall survival (OS), based on the meta-analysis and systematic reviews, adjuvant RT does not confer any OS benefit;[5,8] however pooled retrospective analysis showed improvement in cause specific survival (CSS) in elderly patients with T4 disease with no evidence of gross residual disease (81 vs. 64%, $p = 0.04$).[10] In fact, the CSS showed significant improvement even in those with gross residual disease (74.1 vs. 49.7%, $p = 0.01$).[11]

Keeping the level of evidence available toward EBRT efficacy in DTC and, the associated acute and late toxicities that accompany radiotherapy, the decision of treatment is challenging, and therefore a "case-by-case" decision-making approach has been adopted. Delivering radiotherapy to a patient with thyroid cancer is fraught with technical challenges, due to the anatomy of this region. It is associated with significant acute and late toxicities. The acute toxicities include mucositis (>Grade 3 seen in about 20% cases), dermatitis (>Grade 3 seen in 12% cases), dysphagia (>Grade 3 seen in 17% cases), and hoarseness of voice.[12] Late sequelae often seen are neck fibrosis, chronic laryngeal edema (3%), and esophageal or tracheal stenosis (2%).[13,14]

The role of chemotherapy in DTC is more limited. It has been tested in advanced or metastatic diseases which are incurable to surgery or do not have RAI uptake. Advanced-stage DTC is usually treated with systemic chemotherapy as they cannot concentrate iodine, and therefore RAI is not recommended. Doxorubicin has shown to have moderate activity in DTC and is, therefore, approved palliative treatment for advanced thyroid cancer. The reported overall response rates with doxorubicin are 20–30%.[15] The Eastern Cooperative Oncology Group (ECOG) has published a randomized study with advanced DTC comparing single-agent doxorubicin (60 mg/m² intravenously every 3 weeks) with the combination of doxorubicin plus cisplatin (40 mg/m²) 3 weekly.[16] The maximum cumulative dose of doxorubicin allowed was 550 mg/m². Of the 84 eligible advanced DTC patients, the investigators reported an overall response rate of 17% (7/41 patients) in the doxorubicin arm, which was significantly lower than the combination arm—26% [11/43 cases, its (CR)]. To sum up the role of cytotoxic chemotherapy, it is generally recommended in patients with metastatic DTC who have progressed on RAI therapy.[7]

Undifferentiated Thyroid Carcinoma (Anaplastic Carcinoma)

Anaplastic thyroid cancer accounts for <5% of thyroid cancer diagnosed; however, it is a highly aggressive tumor with an estimated median survival of fewer than 5 months.[17,18] Elderly patients with advanced-stage, larger tumor size, and elevated white blood cell count are known adverse prognostic factors in these tumors.[19,20] The goal of treatment is usually palliative as patients mostly present with bulky metastatic LNs and distant metastasis. ATC is considered a stage IV disease and should be treated as a systemic disease even in the absence of metastasis.[17] Patients with the locoregional disease should undergo gross tumor resection with minimal morbidity followed by adjuvant chemoradiotherapy for the best outcomes.[17,21] The role of surgery is based on resectability, extent of local invasion, and structures involved. The goal of surgery is to attempt complete surgical excision as debulking does not improve outcomes and, therefore, carry a poor prognosis. Definitive radiotherapy with or without chemotherapy should be offered in such situations. Delayed surgery may be considered at a later date if the patient's condition permits.[21] Commonly used concurrent chemotherapy agents are paclitaxel (30–60 mg/m²), doxorubicin, or cisplatin (40 mg/m²). Doxorubicin has proven to be the most efficacious chemotherapy, with a response rate of 22%, usually given (20 mg/m² weekly) and is continued as adjuvant (50 mg/m² 3-weekly) up to a cumulative dose of 550 mg/m². The major issue of concern with doxorubicin, especially when given concurrently with radiation, is "radiation recall" phenomenon.[17] In patients with unresectable disease and poor performance status, palliative EBRT is beneficial in alleviating local symptoms and preventing/delaying asphyxia-related situations.[21] The Collaborative Anaplastic Thyroid Cancer Health Intervention Trials (CATCHIT) Group did a phase-II study in 96 ATC patients with the residual or disseminated disease despite surgery or local radiation therapy and reported a response rate of 53% in 19 evaluable patients with grade 2 or less toxicity.[22] Recently, there has been increasing evidence for paclitaxel being a more efficacious radiosensitizing agent in comparison to traditionally used chemotherapeutic agents. Paclitaxel in induction setting was assessed in 13 patients with ATC stage IVB (n = 9) and IVC (n = 4) and observed a response rate of 33 and 25%, respectively. They reported an improved OS in patients with stage IVB disease (p = 0.02) when compared to those with no chemotherapy; however, no advantage was seen in stage IVC patients. There is evidence of a positive dose–response relationship in ATC leading to OS benefit with EBRT doses between 60 and 75 Gy.[18] There is no therapeutic role of RAI as ATC does not concentrate iodine.

Medullary Thyroid Carcinoma

Medullary thyroid carcinoma arises for parafollicular cells of the thyroid gland and accounts for <5% of all thyroid cancers. The presentation is mostly sporadic (80%); however, some cases (20%) are associated with familial syndromes (multiple endocrine neoplasia; MEN IIa, IIb, and pure familial MTC). Familial MEN syndrome is inherited in an autosomal-dominant fashion because of a germline point mutation in the *RET* gene on chromosome 10q11.2. MEN2A is associated with MTC in virtually all patients along with pheochromocytoma, hyperparathyroidism, Cushing's syndrome, and cutaneous lichen amyloidosis. In MEN2B, MTC usually develops in infancy and is associated with typical facies, ophthalmologic abnormalities (thickened and everted eyelids, mild ptosis), skeletal malformations (marfanoid body habitus, narrow long facies, pes cavus, pectus excavatum, high-arched palate, scoliosis, and slipped capital femoral epiphyses), and a generalized ganglioneuromatosis throughout the aerodigestive tract. Primary management includes total thyroidectomy with central neck dissection in all cases. Compartment-oriented lateral neck dissection is indicated when clinically involved. There is no role for adjuvant I-131 therapy as they do not concentrate iodine to a degree that is curative. MTC is a slowly progressive disease with a relatively good 10-year survival (Stage I—100%, Stage II—93%, Stage III—71%, Stage IV—21%).[23] High incidence of locoregional relapse (LRR) is reported in patients with residual disease, perithyroidal extension, or LN metastases, and those at risk of airway obstruction and, therefore, adjuvant EBRT should be offered in such situations as it reduces the risk of LRR by 38%.[23,24] A systemic review looking into the role of EBRT in MTC did not find any significant effect on OS.[23]

External Beam Radiotherapy

The decision to give EBRT, treatment volumes, and dose prescription is individualized for each patient according to his risks for LRR. Prescription dose and radiotherapy planning do not vary, based on histology and stage of the disease. Randomized data considering the treatment-related factors is lacking due to the relative rarity of the disease. A typical EBRT planning has the following features: (1) Reproducible and comfortable patient's treatment position, using an immobilization device and obtaining a volumetric CT scan dataset of the patient in treatment position; (2) Defining target volume(s) and organs at risk using the volumetric planning image dataset; (3) Dose prescription for the various target volume(s) based on the extent of disease and defining dose–volume constraints for organs at risk (OARs); (4) Radiotherapy treatment planning using either forward planning technique [three-dimensional conformal radiotherapy (3D-CRT)] or inverse planning (intensity-modulated radiotherapy—IMRT); (5) Plan evaluation and modifications until accepted by treating physician and transfer of patient's plan to treatment machine; (6) Plan implementation on the treatment machine includes verification of the patient's treatment position and treatment delivery using appropriate quality assurance (QA) procedures throughout the treatment.

Radiotherapy planning techniques for DTC usually range from two-dimensional (2-D) planning using conventional X-ray images and defining RT portals based on the anatomical bony landmark to 3D-CRT forward planning wherein we determine beam orientation and design beam apertures and compute a 3D dose distribution according to the prescribed dose, and finally, IMRT inverse planning in which a computer optimization program uses the pre-fed optimization parameters such as dose–volume constraints for OARs and coverage parameters for the target to initiate treatment planning system optimization process, to generate beam fluences. After multiple iterations, a desired 3D dose distribution is achieved to meet the prespecified dose–volume objectives.

Simulation

Patients with thyroid malignancy usually undergo CT scan simulation in a supine position with arms at their side and the neck extended from the vertex of the skull through the entire chest **(Fig.1)**. For immobilization, a standard thermoplastic head and neck cast with a standardized neck rest is used for reproducibility and to reduce movement of the neck and shoulder to a minimum. Radiopaque fiducial markers are placed on the immobilization device based on patient anatomy and close to the region of interest for aiding in tumor localization. CT scan external lasers are aligned with the external fiducial markers placed on the immobilization cast for generating an external reference point and to check for any patient rotatory (roll) or transverse movement (lateral or longitudinal). The external reference points are marked on the cast with the help of the laser, after the CT is acquired, for future reference during treatment delivery. Slices 3–5 mm thick are obtained from the base of the skull to the carina to assess LNs of the neck and upper mediastinum. For gross residual disease, a bolus is placed to cover the clinically palpable area during simulation. The iodinated intravenous contrast (iohexol) is recommended for better visualization of residual disease or involved LN and vascular anatomy. IV contrast is only given after ensuring that the serum creatinine levels of the patient are within normal range or estimated glomerular filtration rate (eGFR) > 60 mL/min/1.73 m^2.

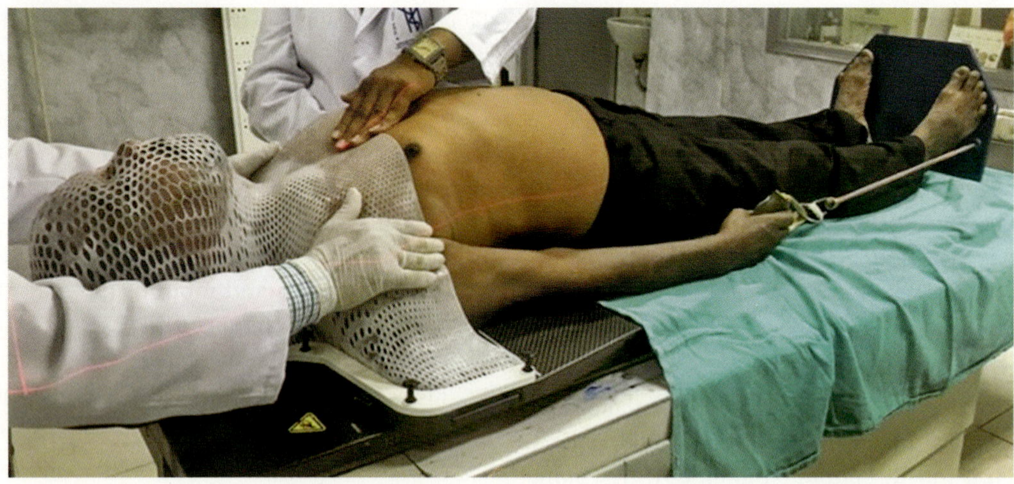

Fig. 1: Patient undergoing simulation for radiotherapy planning. Immobilization cast is being made for stabilizing the head, neck, and shoulder region. A shoulder retractor has been used to pull the shoulders down and out of the radiation field, as much as possible.

Defining Target Volume

In the 2D era, thyroid cancer was typically treated with simple, heavily anteriorly weighted anterior–posterior:posterior–anterior (AP:PA) fields. Alternatively, lateral or oblique fields were used, but this required using a customized bolus to deal with the issue of treating the level of the shoulder. The typical AP/PA field border would extend superiorly at the level of the mastoid process shielding the mandible, inferiorly just below the carina, and laterally extending to cover medial two thirds of the clavicle. At a spinal cord tolerance of 45 Gy, the fields were shrinked to encompass gross disease or involved nodes with perinodal extension.

Target volumes are defined based on the recommendations from International Commission on Radiation Units (ICRU). Gross tumor volume (GTV) represents any visible residual primary disease or grossly involved LN on CT scan while clinical target volume (CTV) usually includes the area with the presumed highest risk of microscopic disease beyond 0.5–1.0 cm of GTV (high-risk CTV) or postoperative thyroid bed in case of complete resection, areas of positive margin, extrathyroidal extension, or involved resected LN regions. Unresected clinically negative regional cervical LN (levels II–V), central compartment (level VI), and upper mediastinal (level VII LNs) which are at moderate risk of recurrence comprise the low-risk CTV. Since the thyroid gland is a midline structure, crossover lymphatics mandates treating neck nodes on both sides **(Figs. 2A to C)**. A planning target volume (PTV) isotropic margin of 3–5 mm is given around the CTV to account for day-to-day movements in a patient's setup. OAR is segmented on the CT scan and includes spinal cord, parotid gland, brainstem, trachea, esophagus, mandible, oral cavity, cochleae, pharyngeal constrictors, brachial plexus, and lungs. Due to complex anatomy and proximity to OARs, IMRT is the preferred technique[7,21,24] for thyroid cancers to selectively protect critical organs and blood vessels and simultaneously give a maximal dose to the target area **(Figs. 3A and B)**.

The dose schedule varies depending on the intent of radiation treatment as follows:

- *Adjuvant radiotherapy dose and fractionation* **(Figs. 4A and B)**:
  - *For high-risk PTV (high-risk CTV + 3–5 mm)*: 60–66 Gy in 1.8–2 Gy per fraction
  - *For low-risk PTV (low-risk CTV + 3–5 mm)*: 54–56 Gy in 1.8–2 Gy per fraction
  - *Definitive EBRT after incomplete resection (R2) or unresectable disease*:
    - *Gross disease (GTV)*: 66–70 Gy in 1.8–2 Gy per fraction
    - *High-risk CTV*: 60–66 Gy in 1.8–2 Gy per fraction
    - *Low-risk CTV*: 45–54 Gy in 1.6–1.8 Gy per fraction
- *Palliative EBRT dose and fractionation*:
  - *For bony or soft-tissue metastasis*: 8 Gy/single fraction; 30 Gy/10 fractions; 20 Gy/5 fractions.
  - *For central nervous system (CNS) (brain) metastasis*: 30 Gy in 10 fractions
  - Dose constraints for OAR[25]
  - *Parotid*: Mean dose ≤25 Gy for both glands or mean dose <20 Gy for single gland
  - *Mandible*: Volume receiving 50 Gy (V50) should be <31–32%.
  - *Glottic/supraglottic larynx*: Mean dose ≤44 Gy
  - *Spinal cord*: Maximum point dose (D_{max}) should be <50 Gy.
  - *Esophagus*: Volume receiving 35 Gy (V35) <50% or V30 <40%.

Conclusion

There is compelling evidence to support that adjuvant RT in high-risk DTC after curative surgery and RAI-improved locoregional control. Prospective studies are required to fully define the role of RT in DTC. Anaplastic thyroid carcinoma is a rare aggressive tumor with high rates of metastasis with surgery

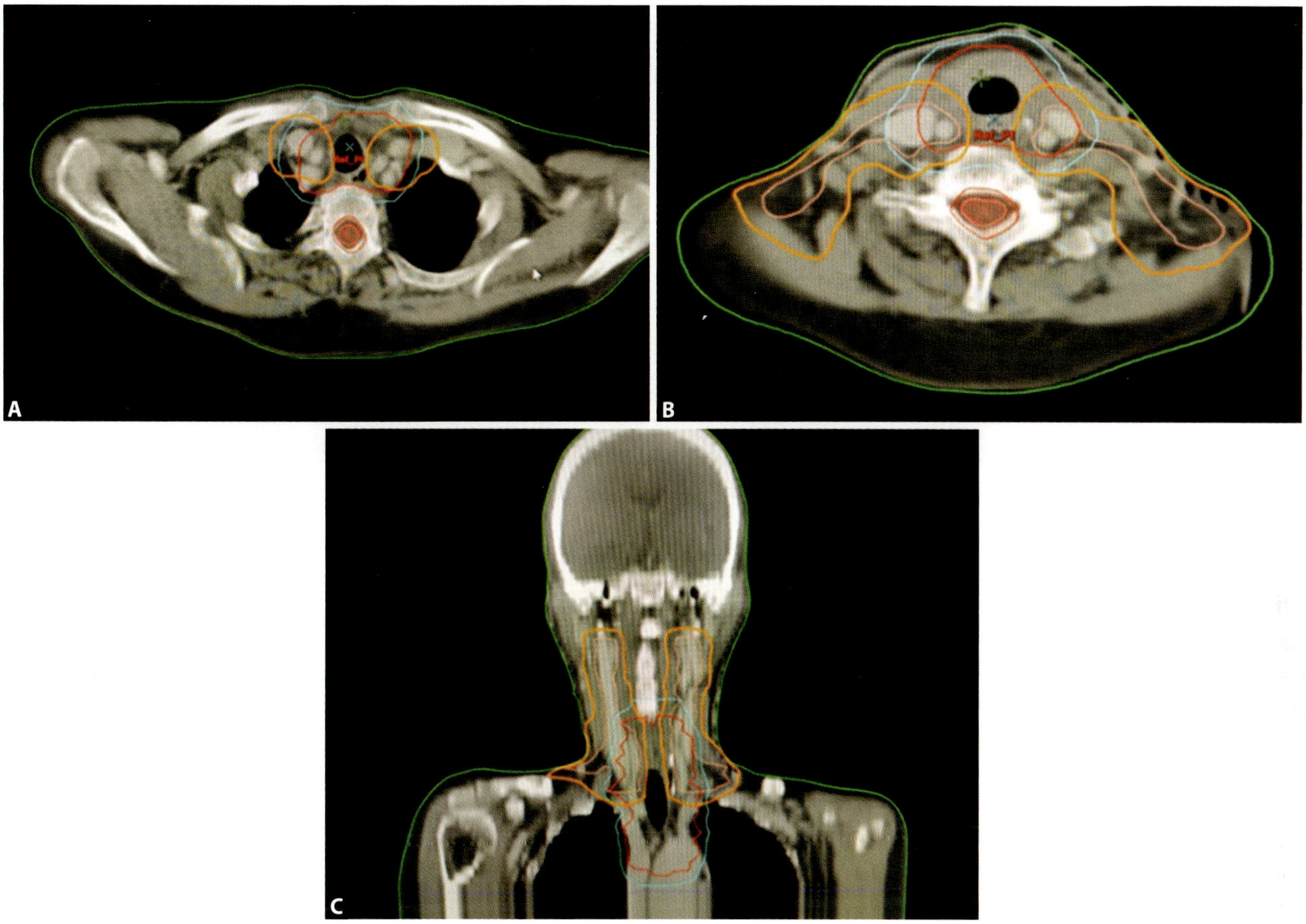

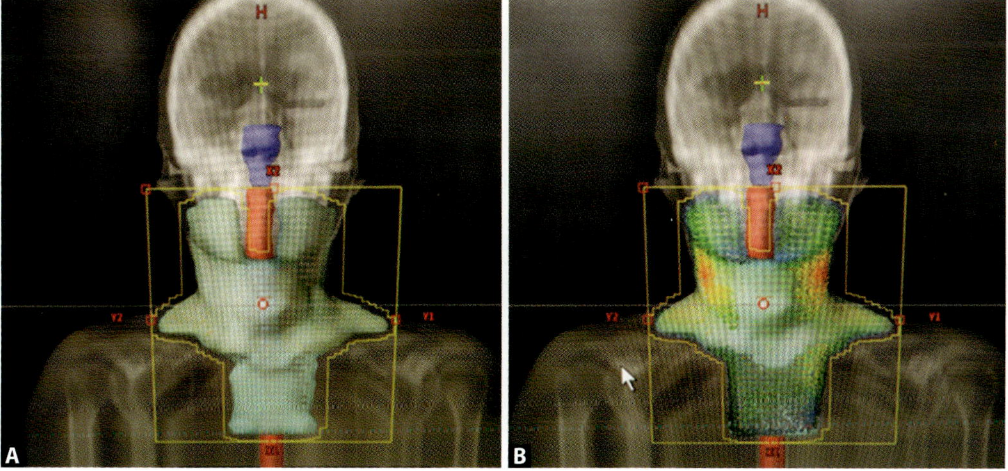

Figs. 2A to C: Axial and coronal sections of contrast-enhanced CT scan done for radiotherapy planning (RTP) scan showing high-risk and low-risk clinical target volume (CTV) and planning target volume (PTV).

Figs. 3A and B: Digitally reconstructed radiograph (DRR) image showing anteroposterior (AP) field arrangements with 95% dose distribution.

as the only curative option. OS is poor and, therefore, more effective systemic and local therapies are urgently needed. The role of radiotherapy remains palliative in these tumors.

◇ ADRENOCORTICAL TUMORS

Adrenocortical tumor (ACC) is a rare disease and is highly malignant with a poor prognosis. The 5-year survival rate ranges from 16 to 47%[26,27] with a median survival for stage III/IV disease between 8 and 28 months.[28] The overall rate of recurrence is 84%.[28-30] Adjuvant treatment with systemic therapy following radical surgery reduces the risk of relapse to 50%.[30] All patients with ACC should undergo adrenalectomy. Resectability and biology of the disease (proliferative index based on mitosis count or Ki67 expression) are the most important factors predicting the outcome in ACC.

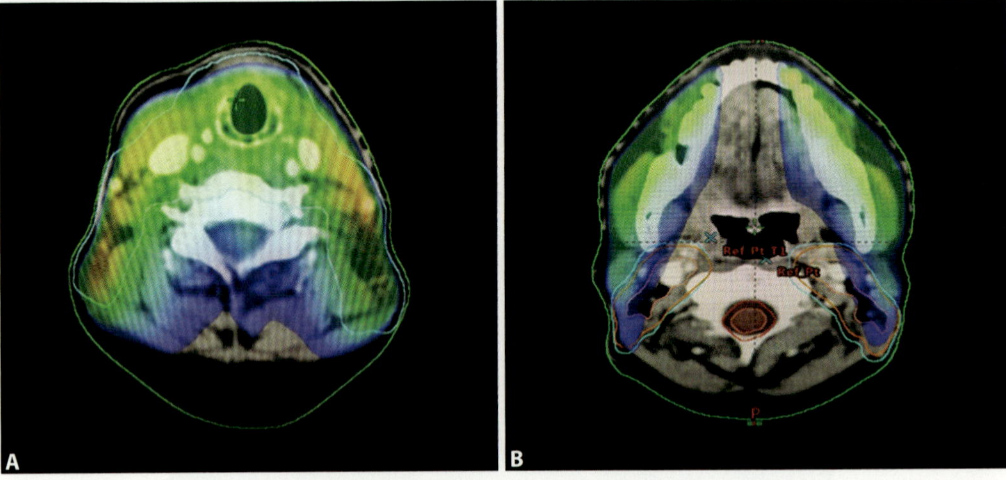

Figs. 4A and B: 95% dose distribution.

Based on the expert panel consensus in the second annual International Adrenal Cancer Symposium 2008[31] held in Michigan, patients with potential residual disease (R1 or Rx resection) and/or Ki67 > 10% were considered as a high-risk group and should be treated with adjuvant mitotane therapy. Stage I/II and some patients in stage III with RO resection, tumor size < 8 cm, and Ki-67 ≤ 10% were considered as low-/intermediate-risk group. In such patients, administration of adjuvant mitotane therapy is at the discretion of the treating physician; however, observational follow-up is also justified.[32] Local relapse of 37% has been reported even after complete surgical excision with negative margins.[33] No randomized prospective data are defining the role of adjuvant EBRT due to the rarity of the disease and lack of use of radiotherapy as an adjuvant. Currently, indications of EBRT are based on various retrospective series which are subject to selection bias. However, there is evidence that omission of adjuvant EBRT is associated with 4.7 times the risk of local failure.[28] Therefore, based on the German ACC registry results,[32] EBRT as an adjuvant is recommended in patients with microscopic/macroscopic disease or situations where the margin status is unknown and presence of lymphovascular or tumor capsule invasion with a high Ki-67 index > 20%.[28,34-36]

Mitotane is an adrenocorticolytic drug that has been used in the treatment of ACC since the 1970s. It is a chemical congener of the insecticide dichlorodiphenyltrichloroethane (DDT) with specific activity on the adrenal cortex. Mitotane is the recommended adjuvant chemotherapy for ACC and also salvage chemotherapy in recurrent settings. For patients who are unresectable or medically inoperable, mitotane has been used as the primary therapy as well with a good response rate. In patients with measurable disease, overall response rates of 14–36% have been reported;[37] however, the recurrence rate is still very high after mitotane therapy with 50% of patients recurring within 5 years.[30] Mitotane in the adjuvant setting is given at a dose of 1.5 g/day which is gradually increased within 4–6 days to 6 g/day. During right-sided radiotherapy, dose beyond >3 g/day is not recommended. Treatment is continued for 2–4 years and dosage should be adjusted according to patient tolerability. Common side effects observed are gastrointestinal side effects—nausea, vomiting, diarrhea, anorexia; adrenal insufficiency; primary hypogonadism in men; and hypercholesterolemia and hypertriglyceridemia.

External Beam Radiotherapy

Initial radiotherapy portals (phase I) should encompass tumor bed including—posteriorly, diaphragm and parts of the thoracic wall in case of infiltration; laterally, to encompass preoperative tumor volume with adequate margins; cranially, up to the diaphragm crus/apex; and inferiorly, till the kidney hilum. Regional lymphatic (para-aortic LNs, bilateral) to be included regional lymph nodes such as para-aortic LN should be included in cases of node positive disease, large tumor size and/or tumor infiltrating the adrenal capsule).[34,38] In phase II, treatment volume is reduced excluding the uninvolved regional lymphatics and only treating the tumor bed as described above. Concurrent cytotoxic chemotherapy is not recommended as there is no data to suggest otherwise.[38]

Radiotherapy Dose Fractionation[38]

- *Adjuvant EBRT after R0 or R1 resection **(Figs. 5 and 6)**:* 54 Gy @1.8 Gy per fraction in 30 fractions
  - *Phase I: 45 Gy/25#; Phase II: 9 Gy/5#*
- *Adjuvant EBRT after (R2) or unresectable disease:* 59.4 Gy @1.8 Gy per fraction in 33 fractions
  - *Phase I: 45 Gy/25#; Phase II: 14 Gy/8#*
- *Palliative EBRT:* For soft-tissue recurrence or large unresectable mass: 20 Gy/5#
  - *For bone metastasis: 8 Gy/1#; 20 Gy/5#; 30 Gy/10#*

Dose constraints for OARs: Spinal cord: D_{max} <50 Gy **(Fig. 7)**
- Small bowel: V15 <120 cc
- *Bowel bag (entire potential space with the peritoneal cavity): V45 <195 cc*
- *Stomach*: Whole organ should receive < 45 Gy.
- *Liver*: Mean dose <30–32 Gy

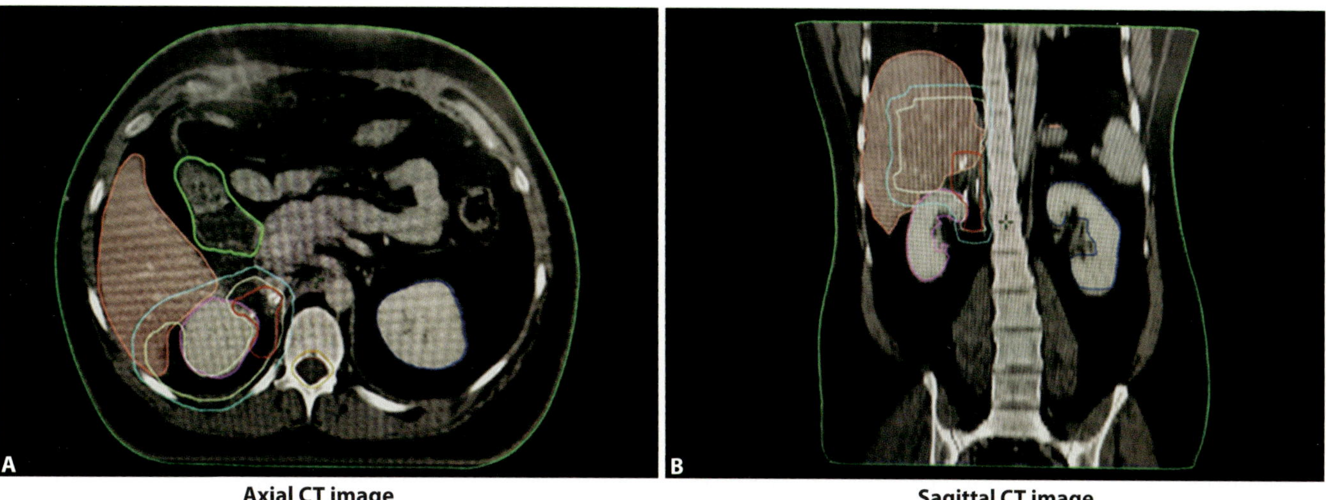

Figs. 5A and B: *Target volumes:* Clinical target volume and planning target volume. *Organs at risk:* Kidney (right and left), duodenum, spinal cord, and liver.

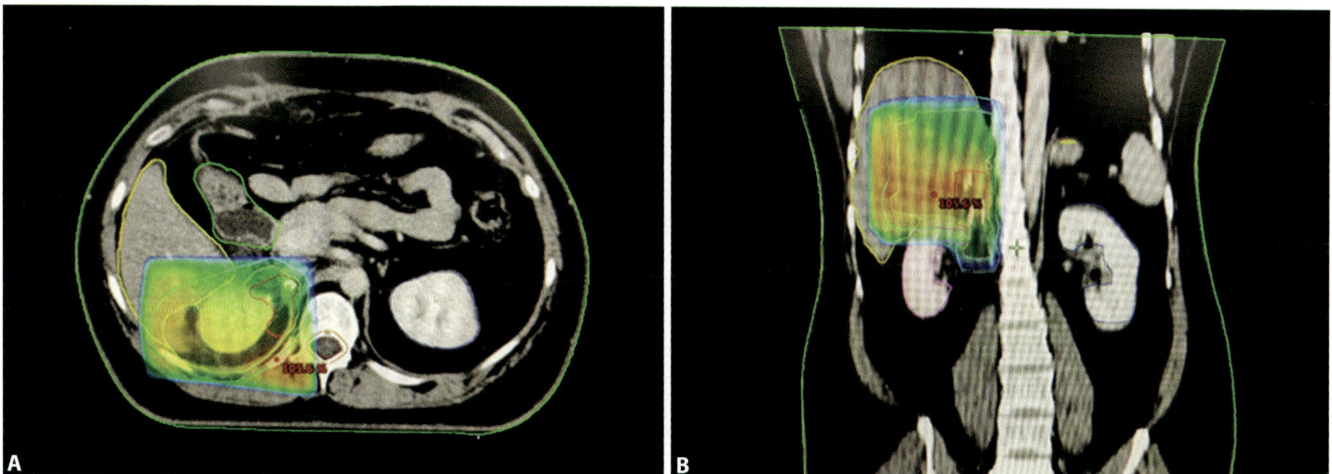

Figs. 6A and B: 95% dose distribution.

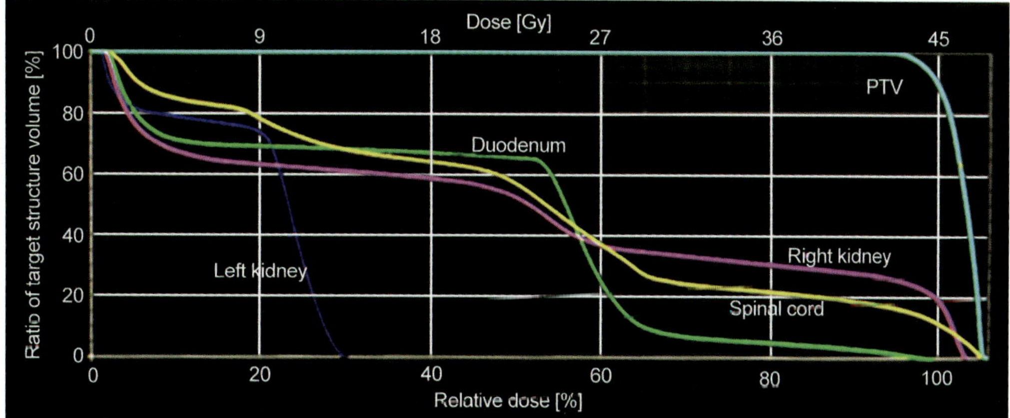

Fig. 7: Dose-volume histogram displaying dose received with respect to volume of organs at risk (OAR) and target (PTV: planning target volume)

Conclusion

Adrenocortical tumor is a rare tumor and most patients are amenable for surgery. Evidence for adjuvant radiotherapy is predominantly based on retrospective data; however, it has significant therapeutic potential in terms of reducing local recurrence even though it is still debatable whether this translates into improved OS, and therefore prospective studies are required to provide robust evidence for radiotherapy.

◇| PANCREATIC ISLET CELLS TUMOR

The pancreatic islets are small islands of cells that produce hormones representing the endocrine functions of the pancreas. The hormones produced in these cells are insulin, glucagon, somatostatin, pancreatic polypeptide, and ghrelin, which are produced by five different types of cells, namely alpha, beta, delta, gamma, and epsilon. The incidence of pancreatic islet cell carcinoma is 1 per 100,000 patient population making it an extremely rare tumor.[39] These are slow-growing tumors and generally produce symptoms as a result of mass effect in the pancreatic area or local extension into adjacent organs. The liver is the most common site for distant metastasis.[40] Surgery is the mainstay of treatment. In one of the largest series of 98 patients reported in the literature, <10% of patients received adjuvant radiotherapy of whom survival-related outcomes were not reported.[41] They found that broadly these tumors are divided into two groups (functional and nonfunctional tumors) and that the most important prognostic factors were the patient's age and extent of tumor. In another case series reporting outcomes in three patients with unresectable islet cell tumors of the pancreas receiving definitive RT in one and palliative RT in two patients, the authors concluded that RT is a viable and effective treatment option for palliation of symptoms in advanced disease.[42] All patients eventually died not before surviving for 9 months/39 months and 6 years after receiving RT. Conventional doses of 4,650 cGy were used in one patient while in the other two patients, 1,250 cGy palliative doses were given.[42]

Parathyroid Cancer

Parathyroid carcinoma is one of the rarest of all endocrine malignancies. The estimated prevalence is 0.005% of all solid malignancies.[43] The majority of cases often coexists with primary hyperparathyroidism (PHPT). The incidence of parathyroid cancer ranges from 0.5 to 5% of cases of PHPT.[44,45] Parathyroid carcinoma is commonly diagnosed when patients undergo surgery for PHPT and the removed tumor shows malignant features on pathological examination. Radical surgical resection is the only effective treatment modality and consists of en bloc resection of the primary lesion, determining the prognosis of these patients.[46] Clinically, suspicious ipsilateral regional LNs should also be removed. Local recurrence after curative treatment is high with a rate of 33–82% at 5 years.[45,47]

Parathyroid carcinomas are usually radiotherapy resistant suggesting a limited role of radiotherapy although one case series claimed to achieve locoregional control in four postoperative patients with negative margins when given adjuvant EBRT.[48] However, conflicting results have been reported in literature where four out of five patients (80%) receiving adjuvant EBRT experienced local recurrence;[46] thus further exploration is needed to justify the role of EBRT in the adjuvant setting. In patients with unresectable disease, palliative EBRT can be offered to alleviate symptoms. There is no standard dose-fractionation schedule recommended for PTH carcinoma. In the Mayo Clinic experience, the patient received 66–70 Gy in 2 Gy per fraction completing in 33–35 fractions using 6- or 10-MV photon beams.[48]

◇| REFERENCES

1. Ferlay J, Colombet M, Soerjomataram I, Mathers C, Parkin DM, Piñeros M, et al. Estimating the global cancer incidence and mortality in 2018: GLOBOCAN sources and methods. Int J Cancer. 2019;144(8):1941-53.
2. Jemal A, Siegel R, Ward E, Hao Y, Xu J, Thun MJ. Cancer statistics, 2009. CA Cancer J Clin. 2009;59(4):225-49.
3. Hay ID. Papillary thyroid carcinoma. Endocrinol Metab Clin North Am. 1990;19(3):545-76.
4. Grebe SK, Hay ID. Follicular thyroid cancer. Endocrinol Metab Clin North Am. 1995;24(4):761-801.
5. Jacomina LE, Jacinto JKM, Co LBA, Yu KKL, Agas RAF, Co JL, et al. The role of postoperative external beam radiotherapy for differentiated thyroid carcinoma: a systematic review and meta-analysis. Head Neck. 2020;42(8):2181-93.
6. Hay ID, Thompson GB, Grant CS, Bergstralh EJ, Dvorak CE, Gorman CA, et al. Papillary thyroid carcinoma managed at the Mayo Clinic during six decades (1940–1999): temporal trends in initial therapy and long-term outcome in 2444 consecutively treated patients. World J Surg. 2002;26(8):879-85.
7. Haugen BR, Alexander EK, Bible KC, Doherty GM, Mandel SJ, Nikiforov YE, et al. 2015 American Thyroid Association Management Guidelines for Adult Patients with Thyroid Nodules and Differentiated Thyroid Cancer: The American Thyroid Association Guidelines Task Force on Thyroid Nodules and Differentiated Thyroid Cancer. Thyroid. 2016;26(1):1-133.
8. Fussey JM, Crunkhorn R, Tedla M, Weickert MO, Mehanna H. External beam radiotherapy in differentiated thyroid carcinoma: a systematic review. Head Neck. 2016;38(Suppl 1):E2297-305.
9. Kiess AP, Agrawal N, Brierley JD, Duvvuri U, Ferris RL, Genden E, et al. External-beam radiotherapy for differentiated thyroid cancer locoregional control: a statement of the American Head and Neck Society. Head Neck. 2016;38(4):493-8.
10. Brierley J, Tsang R, Panzarella T, Bana N. Prognostic factors and the effect of treatment with radioactive iodine and external beam radiation on patients with differentiated thyroid cancer seen at a single institution over 40 years. Clin Endocrinol (Oxf). 2005;63(4):418-27.
11. Chow SM, Yau S, Kwan CK, Poon PCM, Law SCK. Local and regional control in patients with papillary thyroid carcinoma: specific indications of external radiotherapy and radioactive iodine according to T and N categories in AJCC 6th edition. Endocr Relat Cancer. 2006;13(4):1159-72.
12. Romesser PB, Sherman EJ, Shaha AR, Lian M, Wong RJ, Sabra M, et al. External beam radiotherapy with or without concurrent chemotherapy in advanced or recurrent non-anaplastic non-medullary thyroid cancer. J Surg Oncol. 2014;110(4):375-82.
13. Schwartz DL, Lobo MJ, Ang KK, Morrison WH, Rosenthal DI, Ahamad A, et al. Postoperative external beam radiotherapy for differentiated thyroid cancer: outcomes and morbidity with conformal treatment. Int J Radiat Oncol Biol Phys. 2009;74(4):1083-91.

14. Terezakis SA, Lee KS, Ghossein RA, Rivera M, Tuttle RM, Wolden SL, et al. Role of external beam radiotherapy in patients with advanced or recurrent nonanaplastic thyroid cancer: Memorial Sloan-Kettering Cancer Center experience. Int J Radiat Oncol Biol Phys. 2009;73(3):795-801.

15. Gottlieb JA, Hill CS. Chemotherapy of thyroid cancer with adriamycin. Experience with 30 patients. N Engl J Med. 1974;290(4):193-7.

16. Shimaoka K, Schoenfeld DA, DeWys WD, Creech RH, DeConti R. A randomized trial of doxorubicin versus doxorubicin plus cisplatin in patients with advanced thyroid carcinoma. Cancer. 1985;56(9):2155-60.

17. Nagaiah G, Hossain A, Mooney CJ, Parmentier J, Remick SC. Anaplastic thyroid cancer: a review of epidemiology, pathogenesis, and treatment. J Oncol. 2011;2011:542358.

18. Pezzi TA, Mohamed ASR, Sheu T, Blanchard P, Sandulache VC, Lai SY, et al. Radiation therapy dose is associated with improved survival for unresected anaplastic thyroid carcinoma: Outcomes from the National Cancer Data Base. Cancer. 2017;123(9):1653-61.

19. Sugitani I, Miyauchi A, Sugino K, Okamoto T, Yoshida A, Suzuki S. Prognostic factors and treatment outcomes for anaplastic thyroid carcinoma: ATC Research Consortium of Japan cohort study of 677 patients. World J Surg. 2012;36(6):1247-54.

20. Kebebew E, Greenspan FS, Clark OH, Woeber KA, McMillan A. Anaplastic thyroid carcinoma. Treatment outcome and prognostic factors. Cancer. 2005;103(7):1330-5.

21. Smallridge RC, Ain KB, Asa SL, Bible KC, Brierley JD, Burman KD, et al. American Thyroid Association Guidelines for Management of Patients with Anaplastic Thyroid Cancer. Thyroid. 2012;22(11):1104-39.

22. Ain KB, Egorin MJ, DeSimone PA. Treatment of anaplastic thyroid carcinoma with paclitaxel: phase 2 trial using 96 hour infusion. Collaborative Anaplastic Thyroid Cancer Health Intervention Trials (CATCHIT) Group. Thyroid. 2000;10(7):587-94.

23. Rowell NP. The role of external beam radiotherapy in the management of medullary carcinoma of the thyroid: a systematic review. Radiother Oncol. 2019;136:113-20.

24. Wells SA, Asa SL, Dralle H, Elisei R, Evans DB, Gagel RF, et al. Revised American Thyroid Association guidelines for the management of medullary thyroid carcinoma. Thyroid. 2015;25(6):567-610.

25. Patrik Brodin N, Tomé WA. Revisiting the dose constraints for head and neck OARs in the current era of IMRT. Oral Oncol. 2018;86:8-18.

26. Koschker AC, Fassnacht M, Hahner S, Weismann D, Allolio B. Adrenocortical carcinoma: improving patient care by establishing new structures. Exp Clin Endocrinol Diabetes. 2006;114(2):45-51.

27. Abiven G, Coste J, Groussin L, Anract P, Tissier F, Legmann P, et al. Clinical and biological features in the prognosis of adrenocortical cancer: poor outcome of cortisol-secreting tumors in a series of 202 consecutive patients. J Clin Endocrinol Metab. 2006;91(7):2650-5.

28. Sabolch A, Feng M, Griffith K, Hammer G, Doherty G, Ben-Josef E. Adjuvant and definitive radiotherapy for adrenocortical carcinoma. Int J Radiat Oncol Biol Phys. 2011;80(5):1477-84.

29. Stojadinovic A, Ghossein RA, Hoos A, Nissan A, Marshall D, Dudas M, et al. Adrenocortical carcinoma: clinical, morphologic, and molecular characterization. J Clin Oncol. 2002;20(4):941-50.

30. Terzolo M, Angeli A, Fassnacht M, Daffara F, Tauchmanova L, Conton PA, et al. Adjuvant mitotane treatment for adrenocortical carcinoma. N Engl J Med. 2007;356(23):2372-80.

31. Berruti A, Fassnacht M, Baudin E, Hammer G, Haak H, Leboulleux S, et al. Adjuvant therapy in patients with adrenocortical carcinoma: a position of an international panel. J Clin Oncol. 2010;28(23):e401-402; author reply e403.

32. Fassnacht M, Johanssen S, Fenske W, Weismann D, Agha A, Beuschlein F, et al. Improved survival in patients with stage II adrenocortical carcinoma followed up prospectively by specialized centers. J Clin Endocrinol Metab. 2010;95(11):4925-32.

33. Bellantone R, Ferrante A, Boscherini M, Lombardi CP, Crucitti P, Crucitti F, et al. Role of reoperation in recurrence of adrenal cortical carcinoma: results from 188 cases collected in the Italian National Registry for Adrenal Cortical Carcinoma. Surgery. 1997;122(6):1212-8.

34. Fassnacht M, Hahner S, Polat B, Koschker AC, Kenn W, Flentje M, et al. Efficacy of adjuvant radiotherapy of the tumor bed on local recurrence of adrenocortical carcinoma. J Clin Endocrinol Metab. 2006;91(11):4501-4.

35. Fassnacht M, Allolio B. What is the best approach to an apparently nonmetastatic adrenocortical carcinoma? Clin Endocrinol (Oxf). 2010;73(5):561-5.

36. Ho J, Turkbey B, Edgerly M, Alimchandani M, Quezado M, Camphausen K, et al. Role of radiotherapy in adrenocortical carcinoma. Cancer J. 2013;19(4):288-94.

37. Pommier RF, Brennan MF. An eleven-year experience with adrenocortical carcinoma. Surgery. 1992;112(6):963-70; discussion 970-1.

38. Polat B, Fassnacht M, Pfreundner L, Guckenberger M, Bratengeier K, Johanssen S, et al. Radiotherapy in adrenocortical carcinoma. Cancer. 2009;115(13):2816-23.

39. Moldow RE, Connelly RR. Epidemiology of pancreatic cancer in Connecticut. Gastroenterology. 1968;55(6):677-86.

40. Broder LE, Carter SK. Pancreatic islet cell carcinoma. I. Clinical features of 52 patients. Ann Intern Med. 1973;79(1):101-7.

41. Venkatesh S, Ordonez NG, Ajani J, Schultz PN, Hickey RC, Johnston DA, et al. Islet cell carcinoma of the pancreas. A study of 98 patients. Cancer. 1990;65(2):354-7.

42. Torrisi JR, Treat J, Zeman R, Dritschilo A. Radiotherapy in the management of pancreatic islet cell tumors. Cancer. 1987;60(6):1226-31.

43. Lee PK, Jarosek SL, Virnig BA, Evasovich M, Tuttle TM. Trends in the incidence and treatment of parathyroid cancer in the United States. Cancer. 2007;109(9):1736-41.

44. Iihara M, Okamoto T, Suzuki R, Kawamata A, Nishikawa T, Kobayashi M, et al. Functional parathyroid carcinoma: Long-term treatment outcome and risk factor analysis. Surgery. 2007;142(6):936-43; discussion 943.e1.

45. Kleinpeter KP, Lovato JF, Clark PB, Wooldridge T, Norman ES, Bergman S, et al. Is parathyroid carcinoma indeed a lethal disease? Ann Surg Oncol. 2005;12(3):260-6.

46. Schaapveld M, Jorna FH, Aben KKH, Haak HR, Plukker JTM, Links TP. Incidence and prognosis of parathyroid gland carcinoma: a population-based study in The Netherlands estimating the preoperative diagnosis. Am J Surg. 2011;202(5):590-7.

47. Kebebew E. Parathyroid carcinoma. Curr Treat Options Oncol. 2001;2(4):347-54.

48. Munson ND, Foote RL, Northcutt RC, Tiegs RD, Fitzpatrick LA, Grant CS, et al. Parathyroid carcinoma: is there a role for adjuvant radiation therapy? Cancer. 2003;98(11):2378-84.

CHAPTER 45

Thymectomy for Myasthenia Gravis

Surendra Kumar Agarwal

INTRODUCTION

Myasthenia gravis (MG) is a disease involving the neuromuscular system and is autoimmune in nature. Thymus, as a seat of T-cell mediated immunity, is thought to be responsible for its pathogenesis and thymectomy (surgical excision of thymus gland) is a widely used procedure in the treatment of MG. This chapter will summarize the basic embryology, anatomy, histology, and physiology of thymus, followed by pathophysiology of MG, investigations, and various modalities of treatment and role of thymectomy in MG, types of thymectomy, and results of thymectomy in MG, both with and without presence of thymoma.

THYMUS GLAND

The Greek word *thumos*, meaning the soul, is the word from which the name of the thymus gland is derived, as it was believed to be the seat of soul in the body.[1] In the second century AD, Galen described the evolution of the thymus with growth of the individual with growing of the gland till 2–3 years of age, reaching maximum weight by puberty and followed by shrinkage thereafter.[2,3] He also termed it an *organ of mystery*. Later, in 1777, William Heusan confirmed Galen's findings of evolution of thymus.[4]

ANATOMY

The thymus gland is a bilobed, roughly "H"-shaped structure, situated in the anterosuperior mediastinum (**Figs. 1 and 2**), anterior to the pericardium and left innominate vein. The upper parts of the lobes extend into the base of neck on either side and may be attached to the thyroid gland by the thyrothymic ligaments, while the lower parts of the lobe on each side lie over the pericardium up to the level of 4th–5th costal cartilages. The two lobes are joined in the middle by strands of connective tissues. The anatomical relations of thymus include the sternum, upper four costal cartilages and neck muscles anteriorly, pericardium, aortic arch and branches and left innominate vein posteriorly, and mediastinal pleura, lungs, and phrenic nerves laterally. There is a wide variety in shape, size, and extent of gland among the individuals and during various parts of the life cycle of the individual. In addition, accessory thymus tissue (both micro- and macroscopic) may be found outside the thymic capsule

anywhere from neck to the diaphragm and in the anterior mediastinal fat. The arterial supply comes from the branches of both the internal mammary arteries and sometimes from inferior thyroid and pericardiophrenic arteries. Venous drainage is through small veins accompanying these arterial branches in addition to a main venous trunk which is centrally located and runs on the posterior surface of the thymus, joining veins from the posterior surface of the thymus

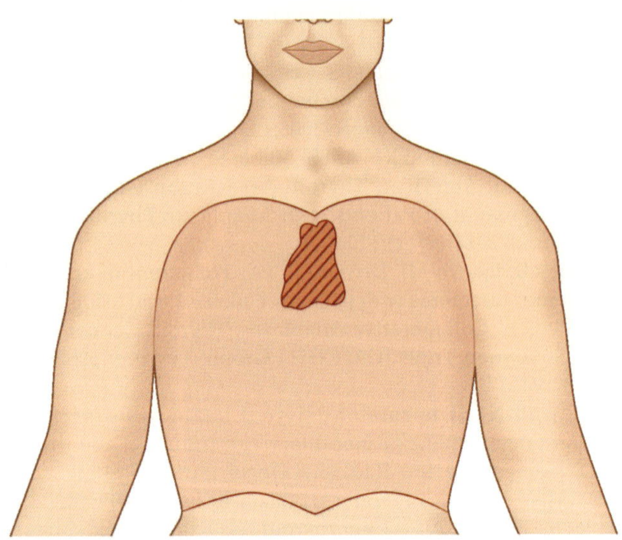

Fig. 1: Thymus gland.

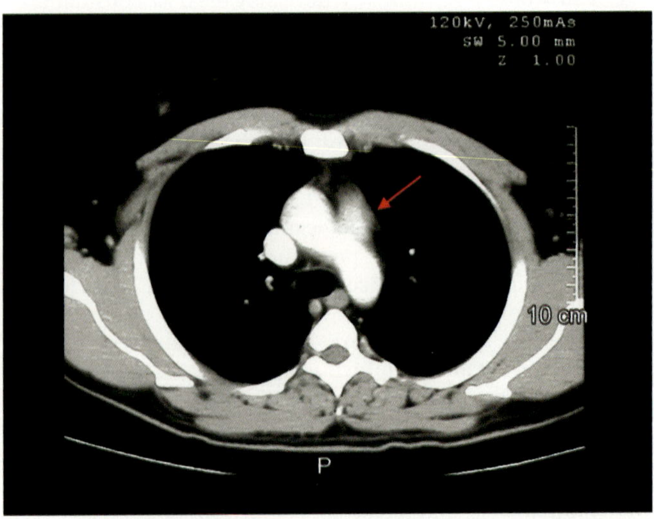

Fig. 2: CECT chest showing a small thymoma (arrow).

at various levels and drains in the left innominate vein. Lymphatic drainage is to the anterior mediastinal, hilar, and internal mammary lymph nodes. No lymphatic vessels enter the thymus. The gland is supplied by both sympathetic and parasympathetic nerves.[5,6]

Embryology

The development of the thymus starts in 6th week of gestation and it arises from 3rd and possibly 4th pharyngeal pouches as an outpouching containing all three germinal layers.[7,8] From 8th to 9th week of gestation, thymus migrates caudally, resulting in joining (not fusion) of both lobes and its final position in mediastinum **(Fig. 3)**. Initially, it is made of purely epithelial cells. By 10th week of gestation, lymphoid cells migrate from fetal liver and bone marrow. This results in lobulations and then differentiation into cortex and medulla which is completed by 14–16 weeks of gestation. Parathyroid glands also develop from the 3rd and 4th pharyngeal pouches and their development and caudal migration are intimately associated with the development of the thymus gland.

The thymus is largest (vis-a-vis the body weight) at birth and is most active till puberty. After puberty, it starts involution and by the age of 40 years, it becomes small and most of the tissue becomes fatty tissue. The mechanism of this involution is not fully understood, but there seems to be a role of sex hormones and cytokines.

Histology

The thymus is covered with a fibrous capsule that sends septa to the interior parenchyma of the gland and thus makes the thymus a lobular structure. Each lobule is approximately 0.5–2 mm in size. Each lobule consists of a cortex and a medulla, with medulla extending into the adjoining lobules.[6] As far as cellular composition is concerned, the cortex primarily contains lymphocytes, mostly T-lymphocytes (thymocytes), along with some epithelial and mesenchymal cells. The medulla mainly contains epithelial cells and few

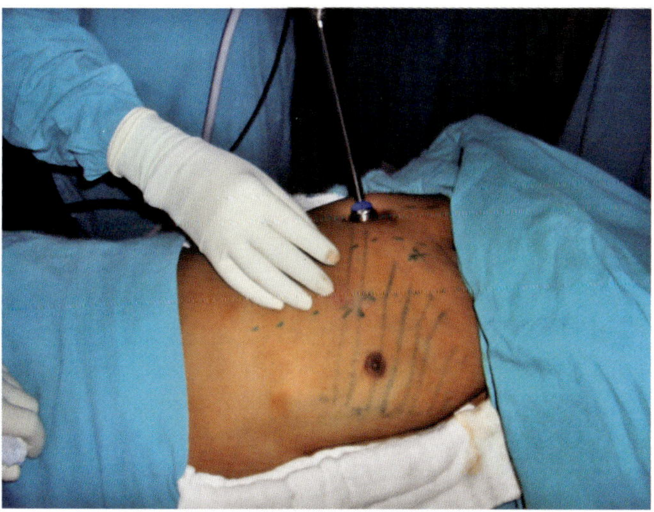

Fig. 3: Markings for port placement in VATS approach.

lymphocytes with characteristic Hassall corpuscles (oval to round, keratinized structures containing epithelial cells). Other cells such as macrophages and myoid cells are also present in the thymus gland.[2] Apart from reticular fibers, a network of epithelial reticular cells (epitheliocytes) forms a three-dimensional network of meshes, both in cortex and in medulla, in which lie the thymocytes. There are six types of thymic epitheliocytes with type 1 located in subcapsular and perivascular portions, types 2–4 located in cortex, and types 5 and 6 located in medulla. They are different in shape, size, and function.[9]

PHYSIOLOGY/FUNCTION

The thymus was in search of a function for centuries and was also termed as the organ of mystery. It was only in 1960s that studies started unraveling the role of thymus in development of the immune system.

Thymus is a primary lymphoid organ, intimately associated with the development of immune response to the pathogens including tumor cells while maintaining self-tolerance to prevent autoimmunity by processing and maturation of T-lymphocytes. Although most of the T-cell maturation is completed before birth, the thymus continues to release naïve T-cells all through life, although at a reduced rate, especially after involution which occurs mostly after 40 years of age.[9]

Development of T-cell mediated immunity is a complex process and requires interplay of thymic epithelial cells with lymphocytes and there is a role of various growth factors and cytokines in this process. Briefly, bone marrow-derived immature T-lymphocytes [prothymocytes (PTC)] enter the thymus through circulation at the corticomedullary junction and initially pass to the subcapsular portion of the cortex and then move to medulla while undergoing a four-stage process of development.[10] This process results in smaller cell size, expression of various receptors (for antigens and cytokines), and rearrangement of *T-cell receptor (TCR)* gene for T-cell receptor expression on cell surface along with T-cell competence generation.

Initially, PTCs are double negative, i.e., negative for CD4 as well as CD8 coreceptors which then become double positive expressing both the coreceptors. These cells start expressing various TCR receptors that can identify and bind with millions of different antigens including self-antigens. The thymic epithelial cells present major histocompatibility complex (MHC) class I molecules and MHC class II molecules to double positive cells in the cortex that results in development of CD4–/CD8+ (cytotoxic) T-cells and CD4+/CD8– (helper) T-cells, respectively. Simultaneously, there are both positive and negative selections that result in only those T-cells surviving and being released in circulation that recognize the antigens in context of MHC I/II antigens present on host cells while simultaneously deleting cells with receptors to self-antigen to avoid development of autoimmunity. Negative selection primarily occurs in medulla. Only about 5% of the PTCs entering the thymus survive and ultimately enter the circulation as naïve T-cells capable of recognizing only foreign antigens and mounting an adequate immune response against millions of antigens with the help of various other cells including B-lymphocytes. The process of positive and negative selection involves apoptosis. There are some other T-cells (regulatory T-cells and natural killer cells) that also get released in the circulation from the thymus and help in immune response of the body toward pathogens.[11]

◇| MYASTHENIA GRAVIS

Myasthenia gravis is an autoimmune disorder, affecting neuromuscular junction and resulting in impaired transmission of neurologic impulse. The primary pathology is destruction/impaired function of acetylcholine receptor (AChR) on which acetylcholine released from vesicles of nerve ending acts for transmission of impulse. This results in fatigable weakness of various muscles of the body. This is variable during the course of disease as well as day.

The estimated prevalence of MG is 0.5–12.5 per 100,000 persons.[12] The disease can occur at any age and has a female preponderance, especially after puberty and before menopause.

Pathophysiology

Pathogenesis of MG involves development of autoantibodies against AChR, which is primarily concentrated on the postsynaptic surface on neuromuscular junction in about 80% patients. Antibodies against muscle-specific kinase (MuSK) and low-density lipoprotein receptor protein 4 (LPR4) are found in approximately 5–20% patients while rest have no antibodies on currently available assays. These autoantibodies either destroy AChR through binding with it and activation of complement cascade, or endocytosis and degradation of AChR–antibody complex. The antibodies can also hamper activation of AChR. AChR autoantibodies producing B-lymphocytes are found in thymus and are produced with the help of CD4+ T-helper lymphocytes.

Reduction in AChR, along with repeated stimulation, results in inadequate activation of postsynaptic membrane potential. The muscle fiber fails to contract, leading to weakness. The fatigability results from the fact that with repeated stimulation, less and less acetylcholine is released from presynaptic nerve vesicles which becomes inadequate for activation of a lesser number of available AChR on the postsynaptic membrane.

Clinically, the patient presents with reduced muscle strength with repeated activity which is variable due to various factors such as disease severity, infections, and drugs. Ocular and palpebral muscles are the most commonly involved muscles with resultant ptosis and diplopia. The onset of symptoms may be acute or chronic. The symptoms may be unilateral or bilateral. Generalized muscle weakness, more of the proximal muscles of upper limbs, is also present in about 80% MG patients. Symptoms usually worsen over the course of the day with maximum in the evening with repeated use of affected muscles. Bulbar presentation may be in form of dysphagia, dysarthria, and respiratory muscle weakness. Dysphagia, dysarthria, neck muscle weakness, loss of facial expression, and respiratory muscle weakness may be present in varying degrees at various time points in the same patient. A life-threatening presentation is respiratory muscle weakness requiring intubation and artificial ventilation is termed myasthenic crisis.

Diagnosis

Diagnosis is based on clinical examination (and specific clinical tests), serum antibody testing (against AChR, MuSK, and LPR4 antigens) by radioimmunoassay, electromyography (with repeated stimulation), and single muscle-fiber electromyography.[13] Classical response to intravenous edrophonium, which is an anticholinesterase, is almost a diagnostic test for MG but should be conducted with caution to avoid complications. Ice pack and rest test are also useful clinical tests for diagnosis of MG.[12]

Classification of MG is based on various factors **(Table 1)**: Muscle groups involved (ocular or generalized), age at onset (early—before 40–50 years or late—after 40–50 years of age), according to autoantibody present (AChR/MuSK/LPR4/antibody negative), and whether thymoma is present or absent.[13]

Osserman classification of MG is based on muscles involved and progression of disease **(Table 2)** and classifies it in five stages: (1) Class I—only ocular muscle involvement; (2) Class IIa—generalized muscle involvement; (3) Class IIb—bulbar manifestation; (4) Class III—rapid progression of

Table 1: Clinical basis of classification of myasthenia gravis.

Basis of classification	Classification
Involved muscle groups	Ocular/generalized
Age at onset	Early (before 40–50 years)/late (after 40–50 years) of age
Autoantibody present	AChR/MuSK/LPR4/antibody negative
Thymoma	Present/absent

(AChR: acetylcholine receptor; LPR4: low-density lipoprotein receptor protein 4; MuSK: muscle-specific kinase)

Table 2: Osserman classification of myasthenia gravis.

Class	Description
I	Only ocular muscle involvement
IIa	Generalized muscle involvement
IIb	Bulbar manifestations (dysphagia, dysarthria, etc.)
III	Rapid progression of generalized bulbar disease and respiratory muscle weakness
IV	Class I or II patients, presenting with progressive symptoms within 2 years, i.e., rapid progression of disease

generalized bulbar disease and respiratory muscle weakness; and (5) class IV—those with class I or II, presenting with progressive symptoms within 2 years, i.e., rapid progression of disease.[13]

A more detailed classification has been given by the Myasthenia Gravis Foundation of America (MGFA) along with a scoring system for disease severity.[14] This classification and scoring system is useful for standardization of results of treatment, especially when comparing various modes of therapy during research.

Treatment

Treatment of MG involves a medical and surgical approach. Medical treatment primarily includes symptomatic treatment (with anticholinesterases such as pyridostigmine) and immunosuppression (with steroids, azathioprine, mycophenolate mofetil, cyclosporine, complement inhibiting antibodies, etc.). Intravenous immunoglobulin (IVIG) and plasmapheresis, though sometimes used for long-term therapy, are primarily used for either acute exacerbation of MG or during preoperative preparation of a patient prior to thymectomy.[12,13]

Surgery for Myasthenia Gravis

Surgical treatment primarily involves thymectomy which may be done through various approaches described below. Although the first thymectomy for MG was performed by Sauerbruch[15] in 1912, it was revived and popularized by Blalock[15] in 1939. Thymectomy has now been established as a treatment that, if used for correct indication, results in remission/improvement along with decreased requirement of medical treatment.

Rationale of thymectomy for MG: It is based on the fact that thymic abnormalities (hyperplasia in 60–70% and thymoma in 10–20% cases with MG) are present in most patients with MG and presence of anti-AChR autoantibodies.

Although it has been used extensively for treatment of MG, there have been debates about its utility as compared to medical treatment. Various studies including randomized controlled studies and meta-analyses have now confirmed that in properly selected cases, thymectomy is better as compared to medical treatment alone.

Indications: Despite a 100-year history of thymectomy for treatment of myasthenia gravis, no clear-cut indications have been defined and are still being debated. A summary of indications of thymectomy for MG are given here:

- *MG with presence of thymoma*: As thymectomy is indicated in all patients with thymoma, with or without MG, it remains class 1 indication for thymectomy in MG. Complete resection of thymoma and total thymectomy are a must for remission/improvement in MG symptoms as well as to prevent recurrence of thymoma.[16] In case

of thymoma being unresectable, methods to make it resectable in the form of radiotherapy and chemotherapy may be employed to make it resectable.[17] A detailed discussion of management of thymoma is beyond the scope of this chapter.

- *Nonthymomatous MG*: In patients with MG without thymoma (which comprise most of the patients with MG), thymectomy has been proved to be superior to medical management alone, especially those with AChR antibody positivity. Patients with MuSK antibody positive MG do not respond as well to thymectomy and so the role of thymectomy in these patients is controversial. In the patients with seronegative MG (i.e., in those where no antibody is detected), surgery might be beneficial, especially if generalized symptoms are present.

In terms of symptoms, thymectomy is equally beneficial whether the symptoms are mild, moderate, or severe. Some reports indicate that the results may be better in patients with mild symptoms.[18] But the role of surgery in patients with only ocular MG (Osserman class I) is still debatable. Recent years have seen more patients with ocular MG alone being offered thymectomy through minimally access route.

The surgery is usually offered in the first 3 years of development of MG as there are indications that the remission rates are better in patients operated early in the course of the disease but there is no confirmatory literature.[13]

Although there are no studies confirming any age limit for thymectomy, most surgeons do not offer it to elderly patient, especially those over 60 years of age. The rationale behind is the fact that the thymus is usually involuted in elderly and also the fact that the risks of surgery, especially trans-sternal, are more in this age group. Similarly, thymectomy in prepubertal patients with MG is reserved for patients with generalized symptoms and anti-AChR positivity who either have inadequate response to medical therapy or in whom immunosuppression is to be avoided.

Preoperative Preparation

The patients should be evaluated and managed for thymectomy by a team of surgeon, neurologist, and anesthetist. Preoperative evaluation should include contrast-enhanced CT scan or MR scan of the chest for proper delineation of thymus anatomy. This is invaluable in staging and planning of surgery for thymoma. Positron emission tomography–computed tomography (PET-CT) is required in patients suspected to have thymoma. Patients should be operated upon when they are optimally controlled with symptomatic treatment and lowest possible dose of steroids/immunosuppressants. This reduces the risk of postoperative complications. Role of pulmonary function testing and optimization with the help of a pulmonologist, if needed, cannot be overemphasized. Some patients with severe symptoms/crisis may require plasmapheresis or IVIG to tide over the crisis and to prepare the patient for surgery. This also helps with the postoperative recovery of these patients. The anticholinesterases should be continued till the day of surgery (last dose on the morning of surgery) and must be restarted as soon as the patients is able to take orally.

Anesthesia

Surgery is usually performed under general anesthesia with endotracheal intubation. Single lung ventilation is required for video-assisted thoracoscopic or robotic thymectomies. Recently, some surgeons are performing thymectomy with laryngeal mask or even awake surgery with high thoracic spinal block.

Muscle relaxants and depolarizing neuromuscular blocking agents are avoided. Anticholinesterases and steroids are given intraoperatively as per the protocol or requirement of the patient.

Monitoring during surgery includes ECG, noninvasive blood pressure, oxygen saturation by pulse oximetry, airway pressure and tidal capnometry, and other measures of respiration and anesthesia. Neuromonitoring with nerve stimulator may also be employed, if available.

Surgical Techniques

There are many techniques for doing thymectomy, especially in patients without thymoma and those with thymic hyperplasia or early stage thymoma indicating that there is no one technique, which is really superior. All the techniques result in equivalent response as for as MG is concerned but each has its proponents. The basic tenet is a total thymectomy along with extended dissection to remove any ectopic thymic tissue, if present.

The MGFA has developed a system to classify various techniques. As the techniques are evolving, this classification also needs to evolve with time. A modified version is given in **Table 3**.[14]

Briefly, the approaches may be described as follows:
- *Trans-sternal approach*: This is the most commonly employed approach and is invaluable for patients with stage II or more advanced thymoma. It has also been

described as the "gold standard" of thymectomy. General anesthesia with endotracheal intubation is utilized for surgery. Median sternotomy is performed with the help of a sternal saw and thymectomy is done while directly visualizing the thymus. The whole of thymus, along with thymoma, if present, is removed including both the cervical extensions, all the fatty tissue surrounding the thymus gland and the tissue in aortopulmonary window, and other areas surrounding the thymus. The extent of this extended dissection is variable, with some surgeons advocating extended dissection for achieving long-lasting and complete relief from MG symptoms. Care is taken to avoid injury to innominate vein, pericardium, phrenic, recurrent laryngeal and vagus nerves, and thoracic duct. One should avoid opening the pleura. Chest is closed in layers after putting one or more chest drains as per requirement.
- *Transcervical thymectomy*: This is one of the most commonly performed approaches, alone or in combination with various approaches. Isolated transcervical thymectomy is said to be associated with lesser morbidity as compared to transsternal approach while providing equivalent results for relief from MG. Surgery is performed under general anesthesia. A single-lung ventilation may be employed, especially if videoscopic techniques are employed. Basically, it involves a curvilinear incision of approximately 5 cm about 1 cm above the suprasternal notch. After developing plane below platysma muscle, extending from inferior aspect of thyroid cartilage to sternal notch vertically and anterior aspect of sternocleidomastoid muscles laterally. Strap muscles are split in the midline vertically and retracted laterally. The superior poles of thymus are visualized by cautery dissection at the upper end of manubrium to remove ligamentous attachments. The superior poles of thymus are dissected in the neck, up to the inferior thyroid veins, and their attachment to the thymus is ligated and divided. The dissection is then extended behind the manubrium and both the lobes of thymus glands are removed with the help of blunt and sharp dissection anteriorly behind the sternum, posteriorly above the pericardium, and laterally up to phrenic nerves on both sides. Cautery or ultrasonic energy device, along with liberal use of clips, is used for complete hemostasis. Special attention is given toward veins that lie on the posterior aspect of the gland, may be more than one in number, and usually drain into an innominate vein. The surgery is helped by use of special retractors such as Cooper's retractor or a special hook to lift up the manubrium. One may also use a videoscope to help in proper visualization of the thymus in anterior mediastinum. In some situations, one may extend the incision vertically on the upper part of sternum and do a partial upper sternotomy, extending on one side a "J" or both sides as "T" at the 3rd intercostal space to help

Table 3: The Myasthenia Gravis Foundation of America classification of various types of thymectomy (modified).

Classification	Description
T1	Transcervical thymectomy (may be basic, extended, extended with partial upper sternal split and extended with videoscope help)
T2	VATS thymectomy (may be classic unilateral right or left VATS, bilateral VATS with extended cervical, bilateral VATS alone and robotic)
T3	Trans-sternal (standard or extended)
T4	Trans-sternal thymectomy with transcervical extension
T5	Infrasternal thymectomy (videoscopic subxiphoid, combined subxiphoid, and transcervical, robotic)

(VATS: video-assisted thoracic surgery)

with the dissection and complete removal of the thymus. The sternum, if cut, is closed with two steel wires and one drain is put in the anterior mediastinum and taken out from the neck. The rest of the incision is closed in layers in usual fashion.

- *Combined transcervical and trans-sternal thymectomy*: Also called maximal thymectomy or extended cervicomediastinal thymectomy, it has been advocated by some surgeons as the ideal operation. This combined both sternotomy and a cervical incision to achieve wide exposure in both the mediastinum and the neck. This helps in en bloc removal of all the thymus along with suspected ectopic thymus in cervicomediastinal fat tissue. The main utility of this procedure is in patients with thymoma and thymic carcinoma. This is supposed to result in removal of almost 100% of the thymic tissue and is supposed to provide better outcome.

- *Video-assisted thymectomy*: Video-assisted thoracic surgery thymectomy or VATS thymectomy is a procedure that has gained popularity in the last two decades and has been helpful in extending the indications of thymectomy in patients with MG (including elderly and patients with lesser grade of symptoms) due to lesser morbidity and hospital stay along with early return to work associated with this procedure. Although it is most commonly done from the right side, it can be done from the left side as well. Some surgeons perform bilateral VATS thymectomy to achieve extended thymectomy, especially dissection in the aortopulmonary window. An extension of this procedure is called video-assisted transthoracic extended thymectomy (VATET) and involves bilateral VATS and a cervical incision to help with bilateral dissection of mediastinal fat along with thymus and completer removal of superior lobes of the thymus along with fatty tissue from the neck. VATET is supposed to be conceptually more complete thymectomy as it allows complete visualization of both sides of mediastinum and includes the neck dissection in addition.

Steps involve semi-supine decubitus position with chosen hemithorax elevated by about 30° and three ports (5 or 10 mm as required)—one in sixth intercostal space in the midaxillary line for 30° videoscope, second in third intercostal space at midaxillary line and third in sixth intercostal space, anterior-to-anterior axillary line. The latter two ports are put under direct vision through videoscope and are used for instruments. Lung is deflated with sponge stick. Adhesions are divided if present. CO_2 insufflation is done at 8–12 mm Hg. Proper visualization and blunt and sharp dissection are employed and thymus is removed as described above. The aortopulmonary window must be cleared and superior poles are removed by traction and dissection from below. Hemostasis is achieved by ultrasonic device. Hemoclips are used liberally, especially for thymic veins. The resected specimen is put in a specimen bag and removed. Chest tube is placed through the third port

and incisions are closed in usual fashion after removing the ports.

A modification of the VATS procedure involves uniportal thymectomy and is done through a 3–4 cm long incision in anterior to midaxillary line in fifth intercostal space. A tissue retractor and dedicated instruments are required for this procedure and it involves greater skill and experience of the surgeon as well as better co-ordination between surgeon and assisting staff.

Contraindications, though none absolute, to VATS thymectomy include morbid obesity, coagulopathy, thick bilateral pleural adhesions, and patient being unable to tolerate single-lung ventilation due to concomitant pulmonary disease.

Complications include bleeding that may require conversion, nerve injury, and chylothorax.

- *Robotic-assisted thoracoscopic surgery (RATS) thymectomy*: Robotic thymectomy employs use of da Vinci (Intitutive Surgical, Inc., CA, USA) robotic system and is an extension of VATS thymectomy. The advantages include superior 3D visualization, better, high-definition optics, ×12 magnification, and more agile arms that allow precise dissection. It also allows filtration of tremors and avoids fatigue. Magnification also helps in identification of nerves and vessels to avoid injury and easier control, respectively. Again, it can be done from right, left, or both sides. Many surgeons prefer the left-side approach as the left lobe of the thymus is larger and aortopulmonary window is easier to dissect from left side. Trocar placement is slightly different from that for VATS (fourth intercostal space in the anterior axillary line, third intercostal space in the anterior axillary line, and sixth intercostal space slightly anterior to anterior axillary line). Central port holds the camera while cranial port has the robotic arm connected to the dissector and caudal port has the robotic arm with bipolar forceps. The dissection starts near phrenic nerve in the middle of pericardium and then proceeds cranially, clearing aortopulmonary window, and reaching till the left brachiocephalic vein. Then the dissection is carried to the right side till the right lung is visible. Both the superior poles are grasped sequentially and brought down using traction and blunt dissection. Then thymic vein/s are identified and tackled with hemoclips or ultrasonic energy device. Then the dissection is proceeded to free all of the thymus both from the back of sternum and from pericardium. As much as possible, fatty tissue in anterior mediastinum is also removed along with the thymus.

Increased cost and increase in operating time due to need for docking and undocking of the robot are the main disadvantages of this procedure. Also, in case of major bleeding, conversion is time consuming (due to undocking) and difficult.

- *Subxiphoid thymectomy*: This technique has been introduced in the last decade by Kiddo et al. and is not a commonly utilized approach. This technique uses a subxiphoid incision to enter the anterior mediastinum and allows visualization of bilateral mediastinal spaces. A videoscope is utilized for better visualization that may be placed through the same incision or through ports in thorax (unilateral or bilateral) as for VATS. Sometimes, cervical incision is also added to achieve extended thymectomy to remove all the possible ectopic thymic tissue along with the thymus. Cooper's retractor for lifting the manubrium and a hook to lift lower sternum are also employed to increase the space for dissection and better visualization. Robotic assistance may also be employed with this approach.

- *Thoracotomy*: Although a common approach used for excision of large thymoma extending into the pleural cavity, this approach is not utilized for MG patients without thymoma or those with small thymomas or thymic hyperplasia. Left or right thoracotomy may be utilized as per the preoperative radiological findings regarding extent of tumor.

Complications

As the patients with MG may have respiratory muscle weakness, it is essential to do as much preoperative preparation as possible to avoid postoperative respiratory complications. In the current year, the mortality is <1%. Most patients can be extubated in the operation theater or in the postoperative unit immediately or within 24 hours after surgery (as soon as possible). Apart from bleeding, nerve injuries mentioned above, infections, and chylothorax, all of which are uncommon with modern surgical techniques and in hands of experienced surgeons, a dreaded complication is myasthenic crisis that may occur in as much as 6% patients and requires proper management including ventilatory care, anticholinesterases, and plasmapheresis or IVIG for treatment. Risk factors for development of crisis include preoperative presence of bulbar symptoms, preoperative respiratory weakness with vital capacity <2 L, AChR antibody levels of >100 nmol/L, and excessive bleeding during surgery.

Postoperative Management

As described above, early extubation and mobilization of the patient are the main goals in the postoperative period. Close observation and monitoring are needed to look for any signs of respiratory muscle weakness and vital capacity may be measured 3–4 times a day for this. Respiratory physiotherapy and, if required, bronchoscopy should be utilized. Anticholinesterases are started as early as possible, through a nasogastric tube if needed. Plasmapheresis and IVIG should be readily available and utilized if the respiratory condition of the patient worsens. Drains are removed after a day or after based on the drainage pattern. Most patients can be moved to ward after 24 hours and discharged in 3–5 days

after surgery. Minimally invasive techniques have reduced the recovery time and many patients can start normal work as early as 1 week after surgery.

Results of Thymectomy

Although thymectomy has been used for treatment of MG for over 70 years, the exact role of thymectomy is still not defined. Similarly, exact role of thymic abnormalities and other factors is still being elucidated.

There has been a controversy in the role of thymectomy for MG, especially in the absence of thymoma. This is due to many reasons. It is known that even incomplete thymectomy and, in few patients, medical therapy alone may result in complete remission of the disease. It is possible that if the mass of immunogenic thymus tissue is below a critical level, achieved either through thymectomy or immunosuppression, MG remission may occur. But there is no currently available method to prove this hypothesis nor is there any way to find out ectopic thymic tissue by the currently available imaging techniques. Although many cohort and case control studies supported the role of thymectomy, it was not until 2016 that a randomized clinical trial conclusively proved the role of thymectomy for MG. In a Cochrane review published in 2013, no studies could be included (empty review) and the conclusion was that there is insufficient evidence in support of thymectomy for MG in absence of thymoma. The same was the opinion of the American Academy of Neurology in the "International Consensus Guidance for Management of Myasthenia Gravis" which was published in 2016. It recommended that "In nonthymomatous MG, thymectomy is performed as an option to potentially avoid or minimize the dose or duration of immunotherapy or if patient fails to respond to an initial trial of immunotherapy or has intolerable side effects from that therapy."[19]

The trial by myasthenia gravis treatment (MGTx) group enrolled 126 patients from 36 centers between 2006 and 2012. The patients were randomized to either surgical arm (thymectomy plus prednisone) or nonsurgical group (prednisone alone). The inclusion criteria included age 18–65 years, MG duration <5 years, MGFA clinical classes II–IV, and increased levels of anti-AChR antibodies. The primary outcome was defined as time-weighted quantitative average MG score and average dose of prednisone required over a follow-up of 3 years. The surgical group showed a significant difference on both the outcome parameters (6.15 vs. 8.99 and 44 vs. 60 mg, respectively; p <0.001 for both). In addition, use of azathioprine (17 vs. 48%; p < 0.001) and hospital admissions for exacerbations (9 vs. 37%; p < 0.001) were also lower in the surgery group. It is to be noted that the surgery was performed via a transsternal approach and included extended thymectomy, so the results cannot be applied to minimally invasive methods of thymectomy where extended resection of thymus is not often possible. The same has been advocated by the latest guidelines of the American Academy of Neurology where transsternal extended thymectomy is now recommended for treatment of MG but there is a caution over use of minimally invasive techniques for thymectomy.

The latest review and meta-analysis[19] found that the chance of remission with thymectomy was greater than medical treatment alone [odds ratio (OR) of the difference 2.34, 95% confidence interval (CI): 1.79–3.05]. Rates of remission range from 14 to 42% in the surgical groups versus 0 to 32% in the medical group in various studies. Similarly, the combined rates of remission plus clinical and/or pharmacological improvement were higher in the surgical group (OR: 4.10, 95% CI: 2.25–7.44). At present, it is not possible to differentiate between various surgical methods, age groups, gender, etc., in terms of results. The proponents of minimally invasive techniques suggest that these techniques are associated with lesser pain, scars, and early recovery and return to work and have reported good results in individual study. A randomized clinical trial has been proposed to address the role of various techniques of thymectomy for treatment of MG. Till then, it may be concluded that thymectomy is superior to medical treatment alone for MG. Although transsternal extended thymectomy should be the gold standard, other techniques may be associated with good results and lesser morbidity in hands of expert surgeons who may be able to achieve near total excision of thymus and ectopic thymic tissue.

CONCLUSION

- Myasthenia gravis is a disease of neuromuscular junction, autoimmune in nature, and is associated with varying degrees of muscle weakness.
- Thymus has a role in immune-pathogenesis of the disease, but the exact mechanism is still not known.
- Thymectomy should be performed in all patients with thymomatous MG.
- Role of surgery in nonthymomatous MG is established with recent clinical trials including randomized clinical trial.
- Trans-sternal extended thymectomy is the gold standard as of now.
- Minimally invasive techniques of thymectomy may also offer equally good response for MG and are superior to transsternal approach in terms of cosmesis, pain, and return to work.
- One should strive for extended thymectomy, regardless of the approach, for better and lasting relief.

REFERENCES

1. Zdrojewicz Z, Pachura E, Pachura P. The thymus: a forgotten, but very important organ. Adv Clin Exp Med. 2016;25: 369-75.
2. Nishino M, Ashiku SK, Kocher ON, Thurer RL, Boiselle PM, Hatabu H. The thymus: a comprehensive review. Radiographics. 2006;26:335-48.
3. May MT. Galen on the usefulness of the parts of the body. Ithaca, NY: Cornell University Press; 1968. p. 30.
4. Hewson W. Experimental enquiries III. In: Cadell T (Ed). Experimental enquiries into the properties of the blood. London: J Johnson; 1777. pp. 1-223.
5. Safieddine N, Keshavjee S. Anatomy of the thyroid gland. Thorac Surg Clin. 2011;21:191-5.
6. Shields TW. 'The thymus'. In: Shields TW, LoCicero J, Reed CE, Feins RH (Eds). General Thoracic Surgery, Volume 2, 7th edition. Philadelphia, PA: Lippincott Williams and Wilkins; 2009. pp. 2059-67.
7. Lele SM, Lele MS, Anderson VM. The thymus in infancy and childhood: embryologic, anatomic, and pathologic considerations. Chest Surg Clin N Am. 2001;11:233-53.
8. Gordon J, Manlery NR. Mechanisms of thymus organogenesis and morphogenesis. Development. 2011;138:3865-78.
9. Palumbo C. Embryology and anatomy of the thymus gland. In: Lavini C, Moran CA, Morandi U, Schoenhuber R (Eds). Thymus Gland Pathology. Milano: Springer,; 2008. pp. 13-8.
10. Thapa P, Farber DL. The role of the thymus in the immune response. Thorac Surg Clin. 2019;29:123-31.
11. Pearse G. Normal structure, function and histology of the thymus. Toxicol Pathol. 2006;34:504-14.
12. Mukkharesh L, Kaminski HJ. A neurologist's perspective to understanding of myasthenia gravis. Clinical perspectives of etiologic factors, diagnosis and preoperative treatment. Thorac Surg Clin. 2019;29:143-50.
13. Aydin Y, Ulas AB, Mutlu V, Colak A, Eroglu A. Thymectomy in myasthenia gravis. Eurasian J Med. 2017;49:48-52.
14. Jaretzki A III, Barohn RJ, Ernstoff RM, Kaminski HJ, Keesey JC, Penn AS, et al. Task force of the medical scientific advisory board of the myasthenia gravis foundation of America. Ann Thorac Surg. 2000;70:327-34.
15. Blalock A. Thymectomy in the treatment of myasthenia gravis: report of 20 cases. J Thorac Surg. 1944;13:316-39.
16. Kondo K, Monden Y. Thymoma and myasthenia gravis: a clinical study of 1,089 patients from Japan. Ann Thorac Surg. 2005;79:219-24.
17. Scorsetti M, Leo F, Trama A, D'Angelillo R, Serpico D, Maacerelli M, et al. Thymoma and thymic carcinomas. Crit Rev Oncol Hematol. 2016;99:332-50.
18. Mao Z, Hu X, Lu Z, Hackett ML. Prognostic factors of remission in myasthenia gravis after thymectomy. Eur J Cardiothorac Surg. 2015;48:18-24.
19. Cataneo AJM, Felisberto G Jr, Cataneo DC. Thymectomy in nonthymomatous myasthenia gravis—systematic review and meta-analysis. Orphanet J Rare Dis. 2018;13:99.

Index

Page numbers followed by *b* refer to box, *f* refer to figure, *fc* refer to flowchart, and *t* refer to table.